Comprehensive ENT

Series Editor

Cemal Cingi, Department of Otorhinolaryngology, Medical Faculty,
Eskişehir Osmangazi University, Eskisehir, Türkiye

As technology progresses, there are continuous advances in every medical subspeciality, and otorhinolaryngology/ENT is a particularly outstanding example of this. ENT lends itself well to the development of innovative and sophisticated solutions, including those affecting the vital area of airway management. Rhinoplasty and related cosmetic procedures are now a well-established part of ENT practice, and make major contributions to patient well-being, quality of life and social function. The series also covers the key principles involved in the use of social media for advertising and sharing cosmetic outcomes, from minor procedures to full-scale surgical operations. The series gathers ENT and related sub-specialty experts from across the globe and translates their knowledge into easily accessible, well-structured summaries of the current state of knowledge, with accompanying illustrations, diagrams and summary tables. Each volume is under the leadership of editors who are thoroughly familiar with the area covered and understands exactly which information is of most relevance and interest to those entering the field for the first time or seeking to update their existing knowledge. The series both outlines precisely the current state of the art in each area of ENT practice and shows where the future of the feld may lie. The fundamental scientifc basis of various disorders is covered, including molecular and cellular aspects, as well as diagnostic practice and the appropriate use of investigations. Historical aspects will be covered where they cast light on the general direction of the specialty. The latest developments in clinical management, disease prevention and public health aspects are described. The series shows how these multiple scientifc and clinical aspects can be best understood in supporting an individual, personalized approach to patient care that fts the patient-centered ethos of twenty-frst century ENT healthcare.

Hasan Yüksel • Ozge Yilmaz
Nuray Bayar Muluk • Charles M. Myer
Editors

Pediatric Airway Diseases

Springer

Editors
Hasan Yüksel
Department of Pediatric Pulmonology
and Department of Pediatric Allergy
and Immunology
Celal Bayar University,
School of Medicine
Manisa, Türkiye

Nuray Bayar Muluk
Department of Otorhinolaryngology
Kırıkkale University
Kırıkkale, Türkiye

Ozge Yilmaz
Department of Pediatric Allergy
and Immunology
Celal Bayar University,
School of Medicine
Manisa, Türkiye

Charles M. Myer
Academic Health Center
University of Cincinnati
Cincinnati, OH, USA

ISSN 2731-6742 ISSN 2731-6750 (electronic)
Comprehensive ENT
ISBN 978-3-031-74855-4 ISBN 978-3-031-74853-0 (eBook)
https://doi.org/10.1007/978-3-031-74853-0

This Springer imprint is published by the registered company Springer Nature Switzerland AG
The registered company address is: Gewerbestrasse 11, 6330 Cham, Switzerland

Contents

Part II Diagnostic Testing

Part III Symptoms and Signs Related with Upper and Lower Respiratory Tract Diseases

Part I

General Concepts of Upper Respiratory Tract for Pediatric Pulmonology

Embryological Origins of the Upper and Lower Respiratory Tract

1

Şeyda Demir Yüksel, Georgina Siordia, and H. Alper Bağrıyanık

1.1 Introduction to Upper Respiratory System

The development of the upper respiratory tract begins very early during the embryonic period and involves the embryonic leaves from the pharyngeal arches and the intermediate lamina from the primitive intestine. The organization and differentiation of laryngotracheal primordia are induced by the migration of neural crest-derived cells under the control of many genes. The laryngotracheal structures are present from the end of the embryonic period, but their maturation continues throughout the fetal period [1].

Ş. D. Yüksel
Department of Histology and Embryology, Faculty of Medicine, Dokuz Eylul University, Balcova, Izmir, Türkiye

Department of Histology and Embryology, Health Sciences Institute, Dokuz Eylul University, Balcova, Izmir, Türkiye

G. Siordia
Department of Pathology, UMAE Hospital de Pediatría, CMN-SXXI, IMSS, Ciudad de México (CdMx), Mexico

H. A. Bağrıyanık (✉)
Department of Histology and Embryology, Faculty of Medicine, Dokuz Eylul University, Balcova, Izmir, Türkiye

Department of Histology and Embryology, Health Sciences Institute, Dokuz Eylul University, Balcova, Izmir, Türkiye

Stem Cell and Organoid Technologies Lab, Izmir Biomedicine and Genome Center (iBG-izmir), Balcova, Izmir, Türkiye
e-mail: alper.bagriyanik@deu.edu.tr

H. Yüksel et al. (eds.), *Pediatric Airway Diseases*, Comprehensive ENT,
https://doi.org/10.1007/978-3-031-74853-0_1

1.1.1 Oral Cavity

The primordium of the mouth (stomodeum) is identified from the third week, rostrally by a bilaminar oropharyngeal or oronasal membrane, composed of ectoderm in its external layer and endoderm in the internal layer, separating the amniotic cavity from the anterior primitive intestine and the primitive pharynx. This membrane will disappear between 26 and 30 days after embryogenesis. At this moment, the floor is already well delimited by the mandible, the lateral walls by the maxillary processes and the caudal region by the frontonasal process [2].

1.1.2 Nasal Cavity

They form from the nasal placodes, which are thickenings of the surface ectoderm that form during the fifth week of development. The nasal placodes invaginate giving rise to the nasal foveas, which expand dorsally cranial to the stomodeum, until they converge to form a single cavity that will later be divided. The nasal passages continue to deepen until, during the sixth week, they are separated from the oral cavity by a temporary membrane called the oronasal membrane [3].

When the oronasal membrane disappears, communication between the nasal passages and the oral cavity is established through two openings called nasal choanae, which open on both sides of the midline in the most dorsal region of the roof of the oral cavity [3].

The mesenchyme surrounding the epithelium of the nasal cavity is a derivative of neural crest cells; In subsequent stages, this mesenchyme forms a cartilage capsule (nasal capsule) that will give rise to the nasal septum in the midline and the lateral nasal wall [4]. Shortly after the degeneration of the oronasal membrane, a plug of epithelial cells forms in the external region of the primitive nasal cavity, so this communication with the outside is temporarily occluded. At the end of the fourth month, this plug disappears [5].

1.1.3 Palate

During the initial stages, there is communication between the nasal cavity and the oral cavity until the formation of the palate, which is usually in the rostral region since the posterior part maintains extensive communication with the pharynx. The separation of both cavities begins during the sixth week with the fusion of the nasal prominences and the maxillary prominences.

The primary palate will also give rise to the anterior triangular third of the incisive foramen and will include the four maxillary incisors.

At the end of the eighth week, the two secondary palatine processes will end up fusing with the primary palate to form the definitive palate. During this same time, the nasal septum grows to separate the left and right nasal passages, and its lower portion will merge with the definitive palate [6].

1.1.4 Primitive Pharynx

It corresponds to the most cranial region of the primitive intestine that originates from the oropharyngeal membrane to the respiratory diverticulum. The neural crest cells migrate to this site during the fourth week and are arranged around the endoderm, which, when they proliferate, give rise to the pharyngeal arches. Toward the fourth week, you can see the four pairs of pharyngeal arches formed by the nucleus of the mesenchyme surrounded by the superficial ectoderm and covered inside by the endoderm of the pharyngeal intestine, the latter invaginates between the pharyngeal arches to give rise to the pouches, pharyngeal, which participates in the formation of the glands of the neck. The invagination of the ectoderm will give rise to the grooves or clefts and the muscles will originate from the presomitic mesoderm and the precordial plate that migrate toward the pharyngeal arches [2].

1.1.5 Upper Airway Anomalies

Upper respiratory tract anomalies represent a broad group of pathological entities whose early diagnosis and timely treatment greatly reduce fetal and neonatal mortality. Although there are currently imaging studies that are routinely performed on pregnant women, there is still work to be done to significantly reduce morbidity and mortality in the perinatal period.

1.1.6 Cleft Lip/Palate

Orofacial clefts are the most common orofacial malformations in humans and include cleft lip, cleft lip with or without cleft palate, and cleft palate only. Cleft palate only is a birth defect that occurs when only the secondary palate is involved and can affect the hard palate and/or the soft palate, sometimes limited to one cleft uvula, due to a failure in the fusion of facial processes during crucial periods in the embryonic development. It represents one-third of all oral clefts and affects about 1–25 per 10,000 newborns worldwide [7, 8].

The etiology of the cleft palate only is multifactorial and involves both genetic and environmental risk factors [9]. Multiple recognized syndromes associated with cleft lip and palate have been identified [10] and they can be alone or in combination with other malformations, mainly cardiac [11].

1.1.7 Choanal Atresia

A rare anomaly, defined as anatomical narrowing of the posterior openings of the nasal cavity, associated with hypoplasia of the nasopharynx, an anomaly that usually occurs in cases of craniofacial and mandibulofacial dysostosis [12].

It can occur unilaterally or bilaterally and be associated with other obstructive anomalies of the upper airway. Its clinical presentation can vary from acute airway obstruction to chronic recurrent sinusitis. The exact cause of this congenital anomaly has not yet been described, however, some probable causes have been accepted, such as the lack of obliteration of the oropharyngeal membrane, the abnormal presence of the mesoderm in the posterior region of the forming nasal cavity, or the aberrant migration of neural crest cells [13].

This anomaly may be seen associated with other defects remembered by the mnemonic CHARGE (coloboma, heart disease, atresia choanae, retarded growth and retarded development and/or CNS anomalies, genital hypoplasia, and ear anomalies) [6].

1.1.8 Laryngomalacia

It is another of the most frequent anomalies of the upper airway and represents the main cause of respiratory stridor in newborns. It occurs during inspiration and worsens during feeding, crying, supine position, and when the infant is agitated [14].

Although the cause of the illness is not entirely understood, short aryepiglottic folds, a lengthy, curved epiglottis, and extra arytenoid mucosa prolapsing into the glottis are also present with anatomical anomalies usually linked to it [14].

There are multiple classifications 1165 [15] although the most practical current classification of this pathology corresponds to the one proposed by Holinger and Konior [16], which takes into account the direction in which the collapse of the supraglottic region occurs: Type A, which occurs toward the posterolateral region, in which there is a collapse of the arytenoid and aryepiglottic folds; Type B, in which there is a complete collapse of the supraglottic structures; Type C, in which a collapse of the anterior region occurs, in this case, the epiglottis is the one that collapses during the inspiration process [16].

1.1.9 Laryngeal Atresia

Laryngeal atresia, categorized as a variant of congenital high airway obstruction syndrome (CHAOS), represents a rare and frequently life-threatening medical condition. Laryngeal atresia arises due to the failure of laryngeal recanalization during the embryological period. The mortality rate of laryngeal atresia is high. Over the last decade, advancements in the early detection of the condition during the antenatal period, coupled with the implementation of diverse antenatal and peripartum management strategies, have contributed significantly to enhancing its outcomes [17].

1.1.10 Laryngeal Webs

Laryngeal web is an uncommon congenital condition leading to airway stenosis. The symptoms exhibited by individuals with a laryngeal web vary widely, ranging from asymptomatic cases to severe respiratory dysfunction that poses a potentially life-threatening situation, often necessitating emergency tracheostomy shortly after birth, depending on the extent of atresia severity [18].

The origin of the congenital laryngeal web stems from the abnormal development of the larynx by the tenth week of gestation, often associated with syndromes such as 22q11.2 deletion syndrome. 22q11.2 deletion syndrome is present in 30% of individuals diagnosed with the congenital laryngeal web [19].

1.1.11 Congenital Subglottic Stenosis

Congenital subglottic stenosis (SGS) refers to the constriction of the subglottic space beneath the vocal cords. This condition arises due to a deformity in the cricoid cartilage and the inability of the laryngeal lumen to undergo proper rechanneling during embryogenesis [20].

Congenital subglottic stenosis (SGS) is the primary laryngeal anomaly that often leads to the need for tracheostomy in children under one. Detecting subglottic stenosis prenatally is not a standard practice. In cases where severe difficulty in breathing emerges at birth, immediate intubation is essential, followed by a prompt tracheotomy to ensure proper ventilation and oxygenation for the newborn [21]. However, for individuals with mild to moderate congenital subglottic stenosis (SGS), the condition tends to ameliorate with age. Tracheostomy is needed for fewer than 50% of such patients.

1.1.12 Laryngeal Cleft

Laryngeal cleft is a congenital anomaly where a gap in the posterior laryngotracheal wall enables the passage of food and liquid from the esophageal lumen to the airway, resulting in aspiration. The incidence of laryngeal cleft anomaly is rare, estimated to be between 1 in 10,000 to 1 in 20,000.

The severity of the anomaly can vary from mild to severe, depending on how large the gap is between the esophagus and the airway.

Patients with small clefts do not need surgery. If there is aspiration and difficulty breathing, the cleft is closed with sutures [22, 23].

1.1.13 Tracheoesophageal Fistula

Tracheoesophageal fistula (TEF) is a foregut malformation that causes an abnormal connection between the trachea, bronchus, and esophagus. It is a rare, life-threatening congenital anomaly. TEF treatment is usually performed through surgical intervention in the first days following birth. Nevertheless, it is crucial not to overlook the substantial rates of recurrence and mortality linked with the surgical procedure, with recurrent TEF reported in 3–20% of infants following the repair of TEF. The etiology of TEF is largely unknown but is thought to be multifactorial. However, it has been reported that 10% of TEF patients have chromosomal anomalies, most commonly trisomy [23, 24].

1.1.14 Tracheal Bronchus

Tracheal bronchus (TB) is a rare congenital anomaly. Children diagnosed with a tracheal bronchus commonly exhibit symptoms such as recurring pneumonia and atelectasis. Surgical interventions in pediatrics are the preferred approach for patients dealing with tracheal bronchus, tracheal stenosis, recurrent pneumonia, and atelectasis. No treatment is necessary for individuals without tracheal stenosis or those experiencing minimal or no symptoms (Shi-Min [25]).

1.2 Introduction to Lower Respiratory System

The respiratory system consists of the lungs and their conducting airways. Facilitating the exchange of gases between blood and air, it provides oxygen to the organism while enabling the removal of carbon dioxide. The development of the respiratory system is intricate, involving coordinated epithelial morphogenesis and mesenchymal development. The lower respiratory tract is early in development in mammals, yet critical steps in alveolar maturation occur after birth. The components of the lower respiratory tract encompass the larynx, trachea, bronchi, and lungs.

The development of the human lung is initiated with the emergence of the tracheal bud from the primitive foregut endoderm during the fourth week of intrauterine life and continues until early childhood. Survival at birth hinges on adequate lung development and maturation during the intrauterine period. Aberrations in bronchopulmonary development lead to congenital lung malformations, and inadequate development is believed to contribute to bronchopulmonary dysplasia [26–28].

1.2.1 General Overview of Lower Respiratory System Development

The lung endoderm becomes specialized within the ventral endoderm of the primitive foregut, approximately during weeks 4–5 of gestation in humans [29]. This specification occurs through the expression of the transcription factor NKX2.1. The respiratory bud, positive for NKX2.1, starts to elongate in the ventral direction, giving rise to the future tracheal tube [30]. Simultaneously, early growth and differentiation are facilitated by growth factors such as FGF10, produced from the pulmonary mesenchyme [31]. Immediately following the formation of the tracheal tube, the hedgehog (shh) signaling pathway, present within the endoderm, is activated to promote the development of extensively branched airways [32]. There are several molecular signaling pathways that regulate cellular differentiation within these airways. SOX2 is necessary for epithelial differentiation in the airways, and the loss of expression has been observed to lead to the loss of secretory and ciliated cells [33]. The activation of the Notch signaling pathway, in turn, leads to an increase in mucus-secreting cells [34]. FOXJ1, on the other hand, has been shown to be necessary for the differentiation of multi-ciliated epithelium in the airways [35]. The branching of developing lobular and segmental bronchi from the trachea concludes with the formation of distal alveoli.

1.2.2 Mesenchyme Development

Upon its formation, the respiratory bud becomes encircled by lateral plate mesoderm. Subsequently, this lateral plate mesoderm will give rise to various mesenchymal lineages within the lungs and trachea. The signaling factors secreted by this mesenchyme, such as FGFs, WNTs, BMPs, and TGFβ, enable branching morphogenesis, epithelial and endothelial differentiation, as well as postnatal alveogenesis to occur [36]. In addition, throughout all stages of endodermal development, lung mesoderm (mesenchyme) interacts with lung endoderm [37] giving rise to mesenchymal-derived cells within the lung, including smooth muscle cells, vascular smooth muscle cells, interstitial fibroblasts, and pericytes [38, 39].

1.2.3 Larynx and Trachea Development

The larynx originates from the fourth and sixth pharyngeal arches. Around the fourth week, the laryngotracheal diverticulum, formed in the caudal part of the foregut, serves as the initial respiratory primordium, progressively giving rise to the formation of the larynx, trachea, and lungs. Initially, it emerges as a laryngotracheal groove beneath the primitive foregut, and subsequently elongates and develops into the laryngotracheal diverticulum. The mesenchyme surrounding the region where the larynx will form later contributes to the formation of the laryngeal cartilages: thyroid, cricoid, arytenoid, and epiglottis The epithelium of the larynx, on the other hand, derives from the endoderm. Initially elongated, the laryngeal orifice transforms into a "T" shape later on [40]. The epithelial cells lining the canal begin to rapidly proliferate, and this swift proliferation leads to a temporary closure of the laryngeal lumen. By the tenth week, re-canalization recreates the channel. During re-canalization, the laryngeal ventricle forms a pair of lateral depressions, which are surrounded by tissue that will eventually give rise to the vocal and vestibular folds [27].

The trachea, as described earlier, arises from the separation of the laryngotracheal diverticulum from the foregut. This separation involves the initial formation of tracheoesophageal ridges, which later grow and fuse with each other, creating the tracheoesophageal septum. This septum divides the cranial portion of the foregut into ventral and dorsal segments. From the ventral portion, the trachea and subsequently the bronchi leading to the lungs develop, while the dorsal portion gives rise to the esophagus (Fig. 1.1) [41].

1.2.4 Lung Development

The aim of bronchopulmonary development is to establish an efficient gas exchange organ with a broad surface area where blood and air remain in close contact with the outside environment. Lung development has traditionally been categorized into five histological stages. These are the embryonic, pseudoglandular, canalicular, saccular, and alveolar stages (Fig. 1.2).

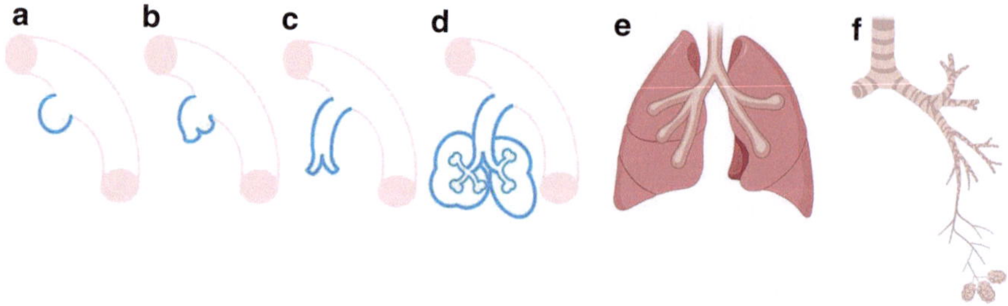

Fig. 1.1 Respiratory system development. (**a**) The initial emergence of the respiratory draft from the ventral aspect of the primitive gut as the laryngotracheal groove. (**b**) Subsequently, the separation of the primitive trachea from the primitive gut through tracheoesophageal folds. (**c**) The separation of the embryonic larynx and the two main branches of the trachea from the primitive gut. (**d**) The formation of primitive lobar bronchi by branching from the primary bronchi. (**e**) The branching of segmental bronchi. (**f**) The development of bronchioles and alveoli

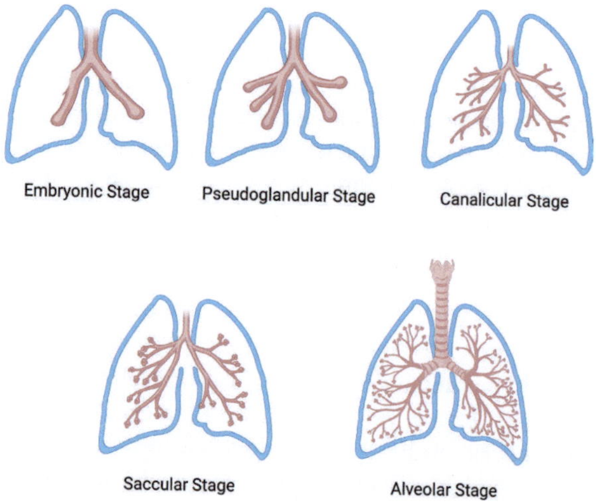

Fig. 1.2 Lung development stages. (Figure was created with BioRender.com)

1.2.4.1 Embryonic Stage

Following the formation of the primitive gut, the lung bud emerges as an epithelial outgrowth on the ventral aspect of the future esophagus. During organogenesis in weeks 4–7, this primitive lung bud undergoes branching to give rise to two lung buds located on either side of the future esophagus. The epithelium of the lung derives from the endoderm and the mesodermal germ layer of the connective tissue. By the seventh week, the initial branching of the primary lobar and segmental bronchi becomes more distinct, signifying the segmental branching of the airways. Experimental studies have demonstrated that this branching is directed by the mesenchyme [41].

1.2.4.2 Pseudoglandular Stage

By the end of the seventh week, each lung resembles a small tubulo-acinar gland, thus this stage is termed "Pseudoglandular." Between weeks 7 and 17 of gestation, lung buds undergo branching, leading to the formation of pre-acinar airways. In this stage, the epithelium of the primitive airways begins to proliferate and differentiate from proximal to distal regions [42]. In this stage, the tubes forming the airways are lined with high columnar epithelium. Neuroendocrine, ciliated, and goblet cells begin to emerge, while mesenchymal cells initiate the formation of cartilage and smooth muscle cells. Cuboidal cells in the distal region start to differentiate by accumulating glycogen. Glycogen serves as a source of energy for cell differentiation and later becomes a crucial component of surfactant, which will cover the respiratory pathways. The distal cuboidal cells represent immature type 2 alveolar epithelial cells. After this stage, the entire conducting airway tree, comprising 20 generations, has developed, and vascularization has occurred.

1.2.4.3 Canalicular Stage

The main events observed during the period spanning weeks 16–25 of gestation include the initiation of the air–blood barrier formation and surfactant secretion. Bronchioles emerge in this stage, and the lumens of bronchi and bronchioles expand, accompanied by increased vascularization [27]. By the 20th week, cuboidal epithelium differentiates into type 1 and type 2 cells. Type 1 epithelial cells cover the majority of the alveolar surface, including the air–blood barrier. Type 2 epithelial cells store surfactant with their intracellular storage organelles called lamellar bodies [43]. Therefore, they are crucial for lung function. As a consequence of the expansion of distal air sacs, cuboidal epithelium begins to flatten, giving rise to regions with a thin air–blood barrier. Subsequently, the flattened epithelial cells come into contact with the capillaries. During this period, pulmonary vascular development encompasses increased capillary proliferation and characterization around airspaces in peripheral mesenchyme. Despite the contact of capillaries with the epithelium, it is not until the 23rd week that capillaries approach and reach their closest proximity to the alveolar epithelium [44]. The capillaries beneath the epithelial cells flatten and differentiate into type 1 epithelial cells.

1.2.4.4 Saccular Stage

It is the stage spanning weeks 24–38 of gestation during which the vital functions required for the fetus to survive are established. In this phase, primary terminal air sacs are formed, and surfactant secretion from type 2 cells occurs. At the onset of the saccular stage, the airways terminate in thin-walled terminal sacs. Subsequently, these sacs give rise to alveolar ducts and alveolar sacs. Production of surfactant begins around the 26th week of gestation and continues gradually throughout the lung parenchyma [45]. The secretion of surfactant into the lumen of the airways occurs around the 30th week of gestation.

By covering the alveolar surface, surfactant reduces the surface tension at the air–liquid interface, thereby facilitating lung expansion in the postnatal period. During the canalicular and saccular stages, blood vessels grow both longitudinally and transversely. Additionally, during the saccular stage, fetal cortisol concentration increases, which is critical for postnatal lung respiration. Cortisol contributes to surfactant synthesis, tissue remodeling, and differentiation of alveolar epithelial cells [46].

1.2.4.5 Alveolar Stage

During this stage, the newly formed sacs continue to develop through a process called alveolarization, which starts at birth and continues until the third year of postnatal life. This process commences around the 36th week of gestation and extends up to 3 years after birth. These air sacs are divided by septa, leading to the formation of alveoli. The septa comprise myofibroblasts, lipofibroblasts, endothelial cells, and pericytes [26].

In addition to the division of alveolar ducts into terminal alveoli, this stage also involves pulmonary angiogenesis to maximize the lung surface area for gas exchange. While the formation of airways is completed by birth, the shaping of the parenchyma occurs during the postnatal period.

It is now widely accepted that over 85% of alveoli are formed after birth. This means that the mammalian lung is not fully mature at birth. Therefore, this stage is referred to as the alveolar stage. The primary mechanism responsible for this is the connective tissue that divides the alveolar sacs, known as septa. Initially thick, these septa gradually become thinner over time [47].

1.2.5 Congenital Respiratory System Defects

The diagnosis and treatment of congenital lung malformations have shown significant advancements in the last decade. Progress in imaging technologies has enabled earlier and more accurate diagnoses, consequently facilitating timely interventions in utero or, when necessary, after birth. These developments have raised survival rates from 60% to 95% [48].

1.2.5.1 Tracheal Agenesis

Tracheal agenesis is extremely rare, occurring in 1 in 50,000 to 1 in 100,000 live births, and it often leads to fatal outcomes. The cervical trachea is typically absent, and the bronchus or carina is connected to the esophagus. It is classified into three types [49]. Type 1 represents 20% of cases, with upper tracheal agenesis. The bronchi are normal, and there is a tracheoesophageal fistula. Type II, which is the most commonly observed type, accounting for 60% of cases, involves complete tracheal agenesis. The bronchi are normal, and a fistula exists between the carina and the esophagus. In Type III, the bronchi arise separately from the esophagus.

The presence of the tracheoesophageal or bronchoesophageal fistula is crucial for the life-saving treatment of critically ill newborns with tracheal agenesis, as it allows for esophageal intubation and mechanical ventilation [50].

1.2.5.2 Congenital Tracheal Stenosis

Congenital tracheal stenosis (CTS) is a rare condition with an estimated incidence of 1 in 64,500 births. CTS involves a true embryological abnormality of the tracheal skeleton, characterized by the presence of complete tracheal rings instead of half rings along the stenotic segment and the determination of a fixed narrow tracheal lumen. Surgical intervention is often required for its management [51].

1.2.5.3 Lung Agenesis

Agenesis of one or both lungs is the absence of development of one or both lungs, a condition that is highly rare. It emerges due to the failure of respiratory buds to develop. Unilateral lung agenesis is more common than bilateral lung agenesis [52]. Unilateral lung agenesis does not necessarily impair the individual's ability to sustain life.

1.2.5.4 Lung Hypoplasia

Congenital diaphragmatic hernia (CDH) is a rare birth defect characterized by incomplete development of the diaphragm, resulting in the herniation of abdominal organs into the chest cavity. It leads to cardiorespiratory developmental anomalies. One of these anomalies, impaired lung development (pulmonary hypoplasia), is characterized by compromised branching morphogenesis, immature pulmonary epithelium and mesenchyme, and a significant reduction in alveolar units, all of which contribute to impaired gas exchange. In high-income countries, the mortality rate among CDH patients has remained around 20–30% since the 1990s; however, in low- and middle-income countries, the mortality rate can exceed 90%. CDH treatment disproportionately consumes healthcare resources compared to other conditions affecting full-term infants that require complex, multidisciplinary neonatal intensive care [53].

References

1. Fayoux P, Devisme L, Maltezeanu A, Thierry B. Embriología de las vías aéreas superiores. EMC Otorrinolaringol. 2023;52:1–10. https://doi.org/10.1016/S1632-3475(23)47949-0.
2. Moore KL, Persaud TVN, Torchia MG. The developing human: clinically oriented embryology. Elsevier; 2018.
3. Jankowski R, Márquez S. Embryology of the nose: the evo-devo concept. World J Otorhinolaryngol. 2016;6:33. https://doi.org/10.5319/wjo.v6.i2.33.
4. Mammoto T, Mammoto A, Torisawa Y, et al. Mechanochemical Control of Mesenchymal Condensation and Embryonic Tooth Organ Formation. Dev Cell. 2011;21:758–69. https://doi.org/10.1016/j.devcel.2011.07.006.
5. Som PM, Naidich TP. Illustrated review of the embryology and development of the facial region, part 1: early face and lateral nasal cavities. Am J Neuroradiol. 2013;34:2233–40. https://doi.org/10.3174/ajnr.A3415.
6. Ansari A, Bordoni B. Embryology, face. 2023.
7. Mossey PA, Little J, Steegers-Theunissen R, et al. Genetic interactions in nonsyndromic orofacial clefts in Europe—EUROCRAN study. Cleft Palate Craniofac J. 2017;54:623–30. https://doi.org/10.1597/16-037.
8. Vyas T, Gupta P, Kumar S, et al. Cleft of lip and palate: a review. J Family Med Prim Care. 2020;9:2621. https://doi.org/10.4103/jfmpc.jfmpc_472_20.
9. Martinelli M, Palmieri A, Carinci F, Scapoli L. Non-syndromic cleft palate: an overview on human genetic and environmental risk factors. Front Cell Dev Biol. 2020;8. https://doi.org/10.3389/fcell.2020.592271.
10. Oner DA, Tastan H. Cleft lip and palate: epidemiology and etiology. Otorhinolaryngol Head Neck Surg. 2020;5:10.15761/OHNS.1000246.

11. Azadgoli B, Munabi NCO, Fahradyan A, et al. Congenital heart disease in patients with cleft lip/palate and its impact on cleft management. Cleft Palate Craniofac J. 2020;57:957–66. https://doi.org/10.1177/1055665620924915.
12. Rajan R, Tunkel DE. Choanal atresia and other neonatal nasal anomalies. Clin Perinatol. 2018;45:751–67. https://doi.org/10.1016/j.clp.2018.07.011.
13. Hengerer AS, Brickman TM, Jeyakumar A. Choanal atresia: embryologic analysis and evolution of treatment, a 30-year experience. Laryngoscope. 2008;118:862–6. https://doi.org/10.1097/MLG.0b013e3181639b91.
14. Jain D, Jain S. Management of stridor in severe laryngomalacia: a review article. Cureus. 2022;14:e29585. https://doi.org/10.7759/cureus.29585.
15. Walner DL, Neumann DB. The classification of laryngomalacia. Ann Otolaryngol Rhinol. 2017;4:1165.
16. Holinger LD, Konior RJ. Surgical management of severe laryngomalacia. Laryngoscope. 1989;99:136–42. https://doi.org/10.1288/00005537-198902000-00004.
17. Teoh KW, Merchant K, Tan JSK, et al. Laryngeal atresia, an unexpected encounter of 'cannot ventilate, cannot oxygenate' at birth. Otolaryngol Case Rep. 2023;28:100533. https://doi.org/10.1016/j.xocr.2023.100533.
18. Abe Y, Hirade T, Koike D, et al. Laryngeal web with 22q11.2 deletion syndrome. Int J Pediatr Adolesc Med. 2022;9:182–4. https://doi.org/10.1016/j.ijpam.2022.02.001.
19. Lawlor CM, Dombrowski ND, Nuss RC, et al. Laryngeal web in the pediatric population: evaluation and management. Otolaryngol Head Neck Surg. 2020;162:234–40. https://doi.org/10.1177/0194599819893985.
20. Varela P, Schweiger C. Congenital airway anomalies. Semin Pediatr Surg. 2021;30:151055. https://doi.org/10.1016/j.sempedsurg.2021.151055.
21. Rovó L, Erdélyi E, Tóbiás Z, et al. Slide laryngotracheoplasty for congenital subglottic stenosis in newborns and infants. Laryngoscope. 2020;130:E199. https://doi.org/10.1002/lary.28192.
22. Martha VV, Vontela S, Calder AN, et al. Laryngeal cleft: a literature review. Am J Otolaryngol. 2021;42:103072. https://doi.org/10.1016/j.amjoto.2021.103072.
23. Strychowsky JE, Rahbar R. Laryngotracheoesophageal clefts. Semin Pediatr Surg. 2016;25:128–31. https://doi.org/10.1053/j.sempedsurg.2016.02.005.
24. Brosens E, Felix JF, Boerema-de Munck A, et al. Histological, immunohistochemical and transcriptomic characterization of human tracheoesophageal fistulas. PLoS One. 2020;15:e0242167. https://doi.org/10.1371/journal.pone.0242167.
25. Yuan S-M. Tracheal bronchus in children. J Coll Physicians Surg Pak. 2023;33:684–90. https://doi.org/10.29271/jcpsp.2023.06.684.
26. Gkatzis K, Taghizadeh S, Huh D, et al. Use of three-dimensional organoids and lung-on-a-chip methods to study lung development, regeneration and disease. Eur Respir J. 2018;52:1800876. https://doi.org/10.1183/13993003.00876-2018.
27. Moore KL, Persaud TVN, Torchia MG. The developing human: clinically oriented embryology. 8th ed. Elsevier; 2007.
28. Wert SE. Normal and abnormal structural development of the lung. In: Fetal and neonatal physiology. Elsevier; 2017. p. 627–641.e3.
29. Goss AM, Tian Y, Tsukiyama T, et al. Wnt2/2b and β-catenin signaling are necessary and sufficient to specify lung progenitors in the foregut. Dev Cell. 2009;17:290–8. https://doi.org/10.1016/j.devcel.2009.06.005.
30. Harris-Johnson KS, Domyan ET, Vezina CM, Sun X. β-Catenin promotes respiratory progenitor identity in mouse foregut. Proc Natl Acad Sci. 2009;106:16287–92. https://doi.org/10.1073/pnas.0902274106.
31. Weaver M, Dunn NR, Hogan BLM. Bmp4 and Fgf10 play opposing roles during lung bud morphogenesis. Development. 2000;127:2695–704. https://doi.org/10.1242/dev.127.12.2695.
32. Menshykau D, Blanc P, Unal E, et al. An interplay of geometry and signaling enables robust lung branching morphogenesis. Development. 2014;141:4526–36. https://doi.org/10.1242/dev.116202.

33. Tompkins DH, Besnard V, Lange AW, et al. Sox2 is required for maintenance and differentiation of bronchiolar Clara, ciliated, and goblet cells. PLoS One. 2009;4:e8248. https://doi.org/10.1371/journal.pone.0008248.
34. Guseh JS, Bores SA, Stanger BZ, et al. Notch signaling promotes airway mucous metaplasia and inhibits alveolar development. Development. 2009;136:1751–9. https://doi.org/10.1242/dev.029249.
35. Chen J, Knowles HJ, Hebert JL, Hackett BP. Mutation of the mouse hepatocyte nuclear factor/forkhead homologue 4 gene results in an absence of cilia and random left-right asymmetry. J Clin Invest. 1998;102:1077–82. https://doi.org/10.1172/JCI4786.
36. Goss AM, Tian Y, Cheng L, et al. Wnt2 signaling is necessary and sufficient to activate the airway smooth muscle program in the lung by regulating myocardin/Mrtf-B and Fgf10 expression. Dev Biol. 2011;356:541–52. https://doi.org/10.1016/j.ydbio.2011.06.011.
37. Yang L, Zhou F, Zheng D, et al. FGF/FGFR signaling: from lung development to respiratory diseases. Cytokine Growth Factor Rev. 2021;62:94–104. https://doi.org/10.1016/j.cytogfr.2021.09.002.
38. El Agha E, Al Alam D, Carraro G, et al. Characterization of a novel fibroblast growth factor 10 (Fgf10) knock-in mouse line to target mesenchymal progenitors during embryonic development. PLoS One. 2012;7:e38452. https://doi.org/10.1371/journal.pone.0038452.
39. Moiseenko A, Kheirollahi V, Chao C-M, et al. Origin and characterization of alpha smooth muscle actin-positive cells during murine lung development. Stem Cells. 2017;35:1566–78. https://doi.org/10.1002/stem.2615.
40. van den Broek P, Brinkman WFB. Congenital laryngeal defects. Int J Pediatr Otorhinolaryngol. 1979;1:71–8. https://doi.org/10.1016/0165-5876(79)90030-2.
41. Mullassery D, Smith NP. Lung development. Semin Pediatr Surg. 2015;24:152–5. https://doi.org/10.1053/j.sempedsurg.2015.01.011.
42. Metzger RJ, Klein OD, Martin GR, Krasnow MA. The branching programme of mouse lung development. Nature. 2008;453:745–50. https://doi.org/10.1038/nature07005.
43. Otto-Verberne CJM, Have-Opbroek AAW, Balkema JJ, Franken C. Detection of the type II cell or its precursor before week 20 of human gestation, using antibodies against surfactant-associated proteins. Anat Embryol (Berl). 1988;178:29–39. https://doi.org/10.1007/BF00305011.
44. deMello DE, Sawyer D, Galvin N, Reid LM. Early fetal development of lung vasculature. Am J Respir Cell Mol Biol. 1997;16:568–81. https://doi.org/10.1165/ajrcmb.16.5.9160839.
45. Burri P. Fetal and postnatal development of the lung. Annu Rev Physiol. 1984;46:617–28. https://doi.org/10.1146/annurev.physiol.46.1.617.
46. Jobe AH, Ikegami M. Lung development and function in preterm infants in the surfactant treatment era. Annu Rev Physiol. 2000;62:825–46. https://doi.org/10.1146/annurev.physiol.62.1.825.
47. Carlson BM. Human embryology and developmental biology. 5th ed. Elsevier; 2014.
48. Zobel M, Gologorsky R, Lee H, Vu L. Congenital lung lesions. Semin Pediatr Surg. 2019;28:150821. https://doi.org/10.1053/j.sempedsurg.2019.07.004.
49. Floyd J, Campbell DC Jr, Dominy DE. Agenesis of the trachea. Am Rev Respir Dis. 1962;86:557–60.
50. Tazuke Y, Okuyama H, Uehara S, et al. Long-term outcomes of four patients with tracheal agenesis who underwent airway and esophageal reconstruction. J Pediatr Surg. 2015;50:2009–11. https://doi.org/10.1016/j.jpedsurg.2015.08.014.
51. Varela P, Torre M, Schweiger C, Nakamura H. Congenital tracheal malformations. Pediatr Surg Int. 2018;34:701–13. https://doi.org/10.1007/s00383-018-4291-8.
52. Xie L, Zhao J, Shen J. Clinical diagnostic approach to congenital agenesis of right lung with dextrocardia: a case report with review of literature. Clin Respir J. 2016;10:805–8. https://doi.org/10.1111/crj.12282.
53. Zani A, Chung WK, Deprest J, et al. Congenital diaphragmatic hernia. Nat Rev Dis Primers. 2022;8:37. https://doi.org/10.1038/s41572-022-00362-w.

Histological Characteristics of the Upper Respiratory Tract: Continuum with Lower Respiratory Tract

2

Elgin Turkoz Uluer, Muhammed Yusuf Pekmezci, Ralph Epaud, and Mahmud Kemal Ozbilgin

2.1 Introduction

The respiratory system is responsible for the process of respiration, from the initial inhalation in the nasal passages to the final exchange of oxygen and carbon dioxide in the alveoli of the lungs. Its core function includes transporting, purifying, and enabling the exchange of these gases, crucial for supporting cellular metabolism. The circulatory system collaborates closely to distribute oxygen to body cells and remove carbon dioxide.

In addition to its primary role, the respiratory system contributes to vocalization and the sense of smell. It has an endocrine function, produces hormones, and aids in immune responses. The system comprises three key components: air conduction passages, the respiratory area, and motor structures, supported by mucosal linings and structural elements.

As air travels toward the alveoli, it undergoes heating, humidification, and purification facilitated by specialized respiratory mucosa. This mucosa, consisting of various cell types, traps and removes particles, preventing them from reaching the alveoli. The system's multifaceted functions, including vocalization, make it essential for sustaining life and overall well-being.

E. T. Uluer (✉) · M. Y. Pekmezci · M. K. Ozbilgin
Department of Histology and Embryology, Faculty of Medicine, Manisa Celal Bayar University, Manisa, Turkey

R. Epaud
Service de Pédiatrie Générale, Centre Hospitalier Intercommunal de Créteil, Créteil, France

Univ Paris Est Creteil, INSERM, IMRB, Créteil, France

Centre des Maladies Respiratoires Rare, Respirare®, Créteil, France
e-mail: ralph.epaud@chicreteil.fr

H. Yüksel et al. (eds.), *Pediatric Airway Diseases*, Comprehensive ENT,
https://doi.org/10.1007/978-3-031-74853-0_2

2.2 Nasal Cavity

The nose is partitioned into two nasal cavities, distinguished as right and left, by a central area comprising cartilage and bone. The anterior portion of each cavity is enlarged and establishes a connection with the external environment via the anterior naris or nostrils. The posterior part of the nasal cavity is adjacent to the nasopharynx, the superior section of the pharynx, through the posterior naris. The front wall of the anterior naris is constructed of fibrous connective tissue and cartilage. Except for the anterior naris, each nasal cavity is enclosed by a solid barrier formed of bone and hyaline cartilage. In the lateral bony walls, three conchae (superior, medial, and inferior) are present. Each nasal cavity is further divided into three sections: the vestibule, located directly behind the anterior naris, as well as the respiratory and olfactory regions.

2.2.1 Vestibule

The external surface of the nose is covered by the skin with a stratified squamous epithelium. This skin, distinguished by the presence of large sebaceous glands, extends into the front section of the vestibule. Within this area, both sebaceous and sweat glands exist, along with thick hairs known as vibrissae. These hairs function to eliminate large particles from the inhaled air. The secretions from the sebaceous glands in the vestibule aid in trapping these particles. Collagen fibers connect the dermis of the vestibule to the perichondrium of the hyaline cartilage. Deeper within the vestibule, the epithelium transitions into respiratory epithelium, and sebaceous glands are not observed in this region.

2.2.2 Respiratory Mucosa

The nasal cavity is covered by the respiratory mucosa, which is a type of pseudostratified ciliated columnar epithelium. Within the underlying layer called lamina propria, there are mucous glands and serous crescents situated beneath the basal lamina. This lamina propria extends into the surrounding periosteum or perichondrium, which encases the bone or cartilage tissues adjacent to it. In the middle portion of the nasal cavities, the surface is relatively smooth, but there are folds on lateral walls called turbinates or conchae. These turbinates serve to enlarge the surface area and are covered by the respiratory epithelium. The presence of these turbinates induces air turbulence, leading to improved warming of the air and increased interaction of particles with the mucous membrane. Among these turbinates, the largest one is the inferior turbinate, which possesses a thicker mucous membrane. Extensive networks of interconnected veins are located within the lamina propria of the lower and middle turbinates. These venous plexuses contribute to air warming, and the autonomic nervous system is responsible for regulating and controlling this process.

2.2.3 Olfactory Mucosa

The olfactory mucosa is a small region situated in the upper part of the nasal cavities and contiguous lateral and medial nasal walls. This mucosa is coated with pseudostratified columnar epithelium; however, it lacks goblet cells within the epithelial layer, and a clearly discernible prominent basal lamina cannot be identified. The yellow-brown pigment found in the olfactory mucosa stands out under a microscope due to its coloration. Within the olfactory epithelium, there exist four distinct cell types: supporting cells, basal cells, olfactory receptor cells, and brush cells.

2.2.3.1 Cells of Olfactory Mucosa

Supporting Cells

Supporting cells are the most numerous cells within the olfactory epithelium. It features a narrow base and a wide, prismatic-shaped apical region, measuring around 50–60 μm in length. The nucleus, which is oval and rich in heterochromatin, is positioned in the upper apical third of the cell. This distinct placement aids in easily distinguishing these cells from others. Numerous microvilli are present on the apical surface. The apical cytoplasm contains yellow pigment granules and a substantial number of mitochondria, contributing to the distinctive coloration of the olfactory epithelium. Abundant tonofibrils, a significant presence of rough endoplasmic reticulum (rERs), and a lesser amount of smooth endoplasmic reticulum (sERs) are observed in the cytoplasm.

These cells are linked to neighboring olfactory cells through adherence-type junction complexes, although gap and tight junction complexes are not evident. The role of support cells parallels that of glial cells within the central nervous system. They enwrap mature olfactory cells, ensuring electrical isolation. Additionally, they form connections with each other through tight junction complexes, establishing a barrier in the apical region. This network of support cells provides both mechanical and metabolic support to olfactory nerve cells. Also, these cells synthesize and secrete "odorant binding proteins," which are small and water-soluble proteins.

Basal Cell

Basal cells are stem cells and progenitors of the other mature cell types. The cells are small, rounded cells and form an irregular single row along the basal membrane, without extending toward the lumen. Their cytoplasm contains an abundance of filamentous structures, while the nucleus, stained with a darker shade, assumes an oval shape, and is located in the lower region of the olfactory cell nuclei. Basal cells encompass the initial segment of olfactory nerve axons. Their cytoplasm contains relatively few organelles [1].

Olfactory Receptor Cell (Bipolar Neuron)

It is typically situated in the lower two-thirds of the epithelial layer, positioned between supporting cells. The protrusion on the outer (apical) side is short, resembling a dendrite, while the inner (basal) extension is lengthy, like an axon, defining the bipolar nature of this neuron. Neurofibrils can be discerned in the cytoplasm due to their silver appearance. The circular nucleus resides beneath the supporting cells. This neuron spans from the base membrane to the cavity, enveloped by supporting cells. The dendrites that extend into the nasal cavity measure 0.5 μm in thickness and 200 μm in length.

The olfactory cells have a single dendrite that projects toward the cavity and exhibits small bulges referred to as olfactory vesicles. These vesicles each sprout about 6–10 cilia that project in various directions, collectively forming a mesh-like structure on the upper surface. These cilia are anchored to basal bodies within the olfactory vesicle and extend radially in parallel to the mucosal surface. Airborne odor molecules dissolve in the mucus layer upon entering the respiratory tract. By binding to the odor-binding proteins, these molecules transport to the olfactory receptors on the plasma membrane of the cilia and then trigger an action potential. This electrical signal then travels through the incredibly thin (0.2 μm) basal extensions (axons) of the olfactory cells.

Upon leaving the epithelium, these axonal extensions pass through the lamina propria and approximately 20 of them come together to create the visible "olfactory fila." Although these nerve fibers lack a myelin sheath. Schwann cells envelop them after departing from the epithelial layer. This unique property of Schwann cells guides the formation of new synapses during cell regeneration, as described by Nomura et al. [2].

The olfactory fila traverse the lamina cribrosa of the ethmoid bone and establish connections with sensory neurons in the olfactory bulb. The lifecycle of olfactory cells lasts around 1 month, and these neurons are among the few types in the human body capable of proliferation.

Brush Cell (Microvillar Cell)

The primary distinguishing characteristic of these cells is the existence of prominent microvilli on their upper surfaces. The lower surface of these cells extends toward the basal lamina. These cells are present in limited numbers in the olfactory epithelium.

There are two distinct types of these cells. Type I brush cells function similar to absorptive cells seen in the digestive and respiratory epithelium and their nuclei are aligned with the nuclei of the supporting cells. They are in smaller numbers compared to Type II cells. Some have even proposed that type II cells constitute a new, fifth cell type within the olfactory mucosa. Type II cell nuclei are situated above the nuclei of supporting cells and lack brush-like border characteristics.

Research has demonstrated their robust activity of Na^+, K^+-ATPase on the lower surface, indicating their role in cellular transport. It is posited that type II cells potentially play a role in generating and upholding the distinct structure of the mucus layer that coats the olfactory mucosa, as outlined by Asan and Drenckhahn [3].

2.2.3.2 The Lamina Propria

The lamina propria of the olfactory epithelium is firmly attached to the periosteum and comprises loose connective tissue that has abundant capillaries, veins, and lymphatic vessels. Within the lamina propria, unmyelinated fibers of the olfactory nerve coexist with myelinated nerve fibers. Lymphatic vessels within this region are connected to the subarachnoid space in the brain through capillaries that course within the olfactory fila. Consequently, infections originating in the nasal mucosa can potentially spread to the meninges.

2.2.3.3 Olfactory Glands (Bowman's Glands)

Olfactory glands are branched tubuloalveolar glands situated in the lamina propria and are composed of serous acini. The secretory ducts of these glands are lined with cubic cells and traverse through the epithelium to reach the surface. This configuration enables the excretory duct cells to be visible in the olfactory epithelium, as discussed by Nomura et al. Similar to sustentacular cells, the gland cells contain lipofuscin granules. Excretory ducts exhibit similarity to acinar cells in the basal portion of the epithelium, appearing as slender cells surrounded by connective tissue in the upper portion of the epithelium. Bowman's glands constantly produce secretions that clean the apical surfaces of olfactory cells and facilitate the reception of new stimuli. These secretions from the glands also contain immunoglobulin A (IgA) and lysozyme, both of which are produced by plasma cells situated in the connective tissue enveloping the gland [4, 5].

2.3 Paranasal Sinuses

Paranasal sinuses are air-filled cavities located within the ethmoid, sphenoid, maxillary, and frontal bones. These spaces are interconnected with the nasal cavity. The mucous membrane that covers these sinuses is tightly attached to the periosteum. The mucosal surface of the sinuses is lined with a respiratory epithelium. However, this epithelium is thinner and contains many Goblet cells. The underlying lamina propria is composed of loose connective tissue abundant in blood vessels, and it contains a limited number of small seromucous glands. The mucus produced through ciliary activity is expelled into the nasal passages. The epithelium that lines the paranasal sinuses, nose, and nasopharynx is coated with a layer of mucus. This mucus layer is in constant motion toward the oropharynx due to the coordinated movement of kinocilia.

2.4 Pharynx

The pharynx is composed of three distinct segments. The upper section, which connects to the nasal cavity, is referred to as the nasopharynx; the middle portion, which opens into the mouth, is known as the oropharynx; and the lower part that connects to the larynx is termed the laryngopharynx. The lining epithelium of the pharynx is primarily the respiratory epithelium, but there exists a small region of stratified squamous epithelium (oral mucosa) on the posterior wall where it contacts the soft palate. The lamina propria, a loose connective tissue layer, is rich in elastic fibers and contains numerous lymphocytes, as well as mucous and serous glands. Lymphocytes tend to congregate around the openings of the Eustachian tubes into the nasopharynx, forming the tonsilla tubalis. Similarly, on the posterior wall, they cluster to create the pharyngeal tonsil. Waldeyer's lymphatic ring is formed by the collective presence of the tonsilla lingualis and tonsilla palatina, situated behind the tongue, along with other tonsils. The lamina propria connects to the lateral walls of the pharynx through the submucosal layer and is directly linked to the muscle tissue on the posterior wall. While the diameter of the nasopharynx might change, its passageway remains capable of both opening and fully closing.

2.5 Larynx

The larynx is an elongated, slender tubular structure measuring 4–5 cm in length, characterized by its irregular morphology. It serves as a vital conduit connecting the pharynx to the trachea. Beyond its role in phonation, the larynx also fulfils the crucial function of averting the passage of liquid and solid substances into the trachea during the process of swallowing. The laryngeal framework comprises cartilaginous tissue, with both singular and paired cartilages constituting its architectural components. The solitary cartilages encompass the thyroid, cricoid, and epiglottis, while the twofold cartilages encompass the corniculate, cuneiform, and arytenoid cartilages. Ligaments interconnect these cartilages, with intrinsic and extrinsic muscular components orchestrating the intricate movements of the cartilaginous framework. Intrinsic muscles govern the tension of the vocal cords, while extrinsic muscles orchestrate the laryngeal movements required for swallowing.

Among the individual laryngeal cartilages, the thyroid and cricoid cartilages are responsible for shaping the laryngeal structure. The epiglottis, located loosely on the anterior surface of the larynx, functions in closing the laryngeal orifice during the act of swallowing. The laryngeal lumen encompasses two pairs of folds. The upper pair, termed the vestibular fold (also known as the false vocal cord or false plica vocalis), remains immobile. Comprising loose connective tissue, seromucous glands, lymphoid tissue, and adipocytes, the vestibular fold resides in the superior aspect of the false fold. The true vocal fold (also referred to as the true chord or true plica vocalis) resides within the lower section of the false fold. This dynamic region plays a central role in sound production, with its movements directed by the vocal muscle, a type of skeletal muscle. A ventricle, characterized by a deep slit-shaped recess, is positioned between these folds. The vocal cords' free edges, composed of elastic connective tissue, comprise the vocal ligament. Intricately controlled by the intrinsic laryngeal muscles, the tension of the vocal cords governs the vibration of air traversing the aperture between the cords (rima glottis) (Fig. 2.1).

The laryngeal surface is enveloped by a lining of respiratory epithelium. The orchestrated ciliary motion inherent to this respiratory epithelial layer facilitates the propulsion of the overlaying mucus toward the oral cavity. Additionally, distinct regions of the epiglottis facing the pharynx, the initial section of the laryngeal

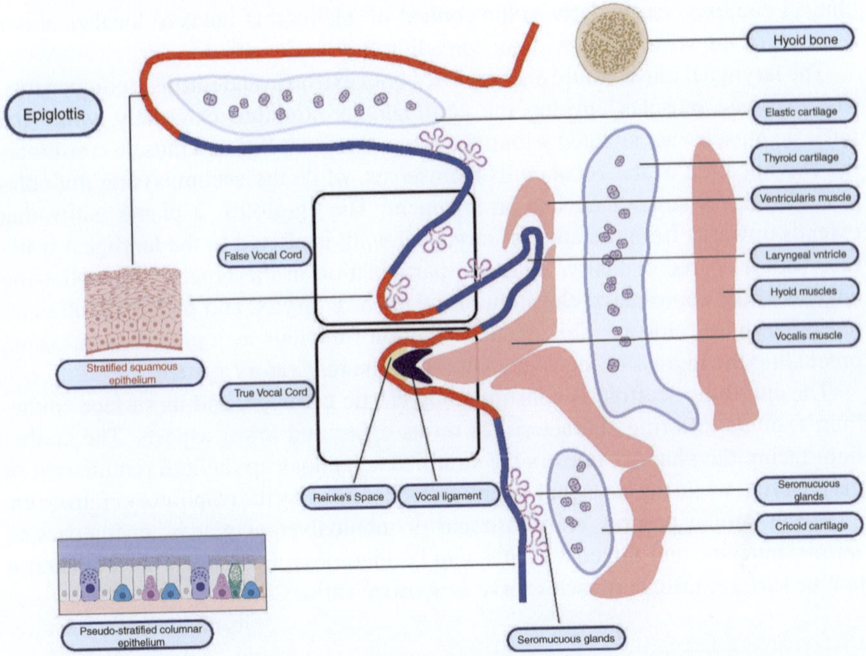

Fig. 2.1 Diagram of a human larynx. The larynx, connecting the pharynx and trachea, comprises singular and paired cartilages, controlled by muscles for voice and swallowing. Notably, the laryngeal surface features respiratory epithelium, but distinct areas, such as the epiglottis and the initial part of the laryngeal surface and the epithelial layer covering the true vocal folds, exhibit stratified squamous epithelium. The lamina propria contains elastic fibers and various gland types. Extrinsic and intrinsic muscles surround and regulate the laryngeal structure, while the epiglottis aids in swallowing protection. The epiglottis consists of elastic cartilage with varying surface epithelium. In the lamina propria are glands including serous and mucous glands. (This figure was created with biorender.com)

surface, and the epithelial layer encompassing the true vocal folds exhibit a configuration characterized by the stratified squamous epithelium.

The lamina propria represents a matrix of loose connective tissue, interspersed with a substantial quantity of mast cells and lymphocytes distributed throughout the connective framework. This lamina propria is notably abundant in elastic fibers, a constituent notably forming the vocal ligaments composed of elastic fibers.

Numerous serous and mucous glands are distributed within the lamina propria, with mucous glands predominating in this milieu. Notably, the presence of seromucous glands and lymphatic vessels does not align with the level of the vocal cords. Noteworthy also is the relatively inconspicuous manifestation of the submucosal layer in the laryngeal configuration, characterized by a seamless transition from the surrounding lamina propria. A notable clinical consideration is the absence of submucosal tissue behind the epiglottis and above the vocal ligaments, contributing to their firm attachment to the underlying structures. This feature becomes pivotal in clinical contexts, particularly in the context of edema that tends to localize above the level of the vocal cords without spreading further downward.

The laryngeal musculature encompasses both extrinsic and intrinsic components. The extrinsic muscles envelop the cartilaginous structure externally, while the intrinsic muscles are situated within the internal region. Striated muscle constitutes the classification of the vocal cords themselves, while the encompassing musculature assumes a smooth muscle arrangement. The epiglottis, a planar entity that extends upwards from the anterior laryngeal wall, is affixed to the laryngeal structure with a degree of laxity. Its active participation in the process of swallowing engenders the coordinated elevation of the trachea, larynx, and pharynx, culminating in laryngeal closure. This dynamic motion functions as a protective measure, precluding the ingress of ingested matter into the respiratory system.

The epiglottic scaffold is constituted by elastic cartilage, and its surface epithelium exhibits differing characteristics on its upper and lower aspects. The epithelium facing the pharynx mirrors the stratified squamous epithelium reminiscent of the pharynx, while the laryngeal-facing surface is lined by the respiratory epithelium.

In the lamina propria, an assortment of tubuloalveolar glands, encompassing serous, mucous, and mixed variants, can be identified. Positioned on the anterior tongue surface, taste corpuscles serve as sensory entities [4, 5].

2.6 Trachea

The human trachea is about 2.5 cm in diameter and 11–12 cm in length. Extending from the cricoid cartilage at the base of the larynx to the fourth thoracic vertebra, the trachea bifurcates into the right and left primary bronchi. Hyaline cartilage, forming a C-shaped structure, maintains tracheal lumen patency, while the connected smooth muscle bundle controls lumen width, enabling efficient expulsion of foreign bodies or mucus during rapid air passage, such as during coughing.

Histologically, the trachea comprises four layers: the innermost tunica mucosa, covered with respiratory epithelium and an elastic fiber-rich lamina propria; the relatively dense connective tissue of the tunica submucosa; a C-shaped layer of hyaline cartilage beneath the submucosa; and the outermost tunica adventitia. The epithelium is characterized by typical respiratory epithelium, including pseudostratified columnar epithelium with ciliated and goblet cells, accompanied by a substantial basal lamina (Fig. 2.2). On an ultrastructural level, electron microscopy distinguishes five distinct cell types.

2.6.1 Cells of Trachea Epithelium

2.6.1.1 Ciliated Columnar Cells

Ciliated columnar cells, the most numerous cells (30%) of the tracheal epithelium, these elongated cells exhibit basal nuclei positioning. The apical surface of these cells has numerous cilia, intricately connected to basal bodies within the apical

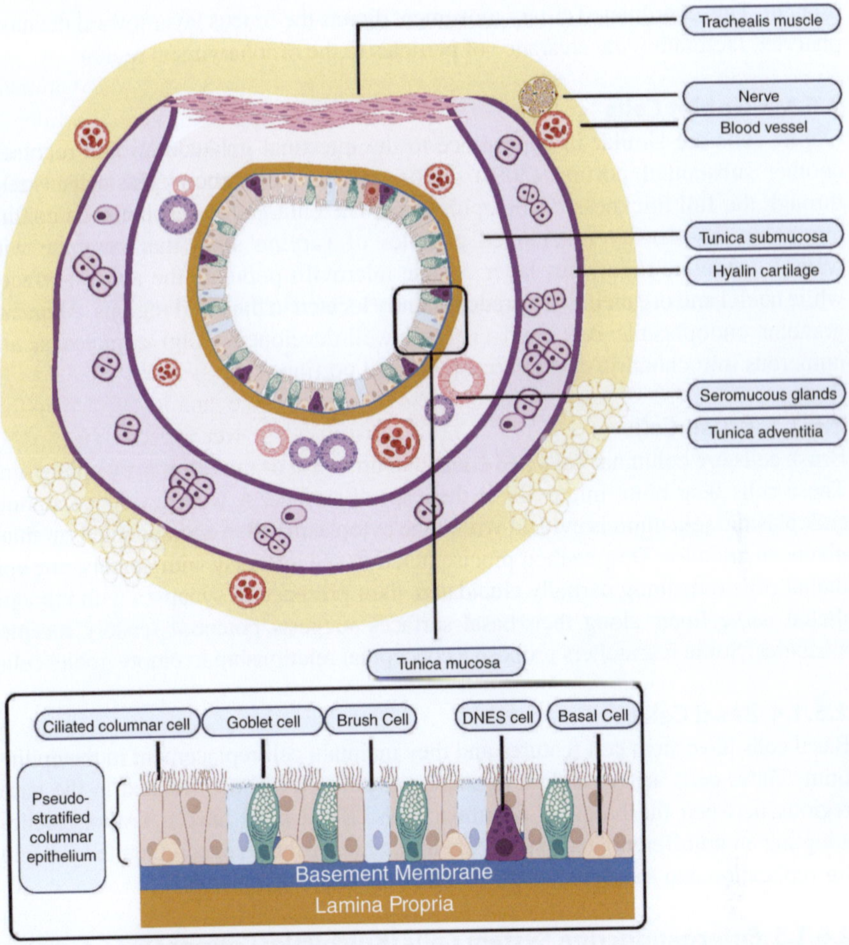

Fig. 2.2 Diagram of a human trachea. This illustration showcases the human trachea, an essential part of the respiratory system, featuring a cross-section to highlight its anatomy and histological composition. The trachea, measuring about 2.5 cm in diameter, begins at the cricoid cartilage and extends to the fourth thoracic vertebra before dividing into the primary bronchi. Layers such as tunica mucosa with specialized respiratory epithelium, tunica submucosa with dense connective tissue, C-shaped hyaline cartilage, and the outer tunica adventitia are illustrated, emphasizing their roles in maintaining the tracheal structure and functionality. Additionally, the presence of smooth muscle bundles controlling lumen width and cellular components like ciliated and goblet cells is depicted, enhancing understanding at a microscopic level. (This figure was created with biorender.com)

cytoplasm. The Golgi complex is small and located near the upper nucleus, accompanied by an abundance of mitochondria. These motile cilia have a continual, rhythmic beating motion of 1000–1500 cycles/min, propelling the mucus layer at a rate of 5–20 mm/min in narrower airways and 0.5–1 mm/min in the trachea and principal bronchi. This coordinated ciliary movement directs the mucus layer toward the nasopharynx, facilitating the clearance of particles to the oropharyngeal region.

2.6.1.2 Goblet Cells

Goblet cells are similar in appearance to the intestinal goblet cells and represent another substantial portion (30%) of the cellular population. The cells extend through the full thickness of the epithelium. The enlarged apical domains contain numerous low-density mucinogen granules of varying sizes that combine with water to generate the mucus layer. Sparse microvilli populate the apical surfaces, while nuclei and organelles are predominantly located in the basal regions. Abundant granular endoplasmic reticulum cisterns, well-developed Golgi complexes, and numerous mitochondria characterize this basal portion.

2.6.1.3 Brush Cells

Brush cells are columnar cells and constitute up to 3% of the respiratory epithelium. These cells bear blunt microvilli at their apical surface. A well-developed smooth endoplasmic reticulum is evident within the cytoplasm, often accompanied by small glycogen granules. Despite their precise function and interplay with neighboring epithelial cells remaining partially elucidated, their presence of synapses with intraepithelial nerve fibers along their basal surfaces suggests potential sensory receptor attributes. Some researchers propose a conceptual relationship to empty goblet cells.

2.6.1.4 Basal Cells

Basal cells have stem cell features and they maintain cell replacement in the epithelium. These cells are pyramidal in shape and their nuclei are situated in the basal regions between the bases of columnar cells. Basal cells have a few organelles, adopting an undifferentiated aspect. Their notable attributes encompass the capacity for replication and transformation into other cellular constituents.

2.6.1.5 Enteroendocrine System Cells (Kulchitsky Cells or DNES Cells)

Enteroendocrine cells occur singly in the trachea and exhibit numerous membrane-bounded, dense-core granules. These granules, averaging 100–300 nm in diameter, primarily occupy basal cell locations. Within this category, a subset displays the staining profile like catecholamine-storing cells. Furthermore, certain types bear a resemblance to cells releasing enteropeptides (serotonin, calcitonin, and gastrin-releasing peptide) in the epithelial context. Both subsets are conjectured to exert regulatory influences over mucous and serous gland secretory functions within the lamina propria.

2.6.2 Lamina Propria

Beneath the tracheal epithelium lies the basement membrane, measuring 25–40 μm in thickness, exhibiting a uniform and luminous aspect under light microscopy. Collagen fibers present organized alignment. Chronic irritation from smoking induces increased thickness.

The lamina propria appears as a typical loose connective tissue. Serous and mucous glands are situated within this matrix, discharging their secretions into the tracheal lumen. Connective tissue harbors lymphocytes and neutrophils, often forming lymphoid nodules in localized aggregations. Cellular, plasma cells, mast cells, eosinophils, and fibroblasts are additionally noted, collectively constituting the bronchial lymphatic tissue (BALT). A discernible elastic membrane, visible with specialized tissue dyes, separates the deep lamina propria from the submucosa.

2.6.3 Submucosa and Adventitia

The submucosal layer, characterized by loose connective tissue, hosts scattered serous crescents alongside numerous mucous glands. These glands release glycoproteins via ducts lined with cuboidal epithelium. Abundant vascular structures, encompassing blood and lymphatic vessels, are discernible. The submucosa is contiguous with cartilage perichondrium.

Arranged in a horseshoe or “C” configuration, the tracheal cartilage, numbering between 16 and 20, resides beneath the submucosa. This hyaline cartilage array is stacked in a rearward orientation, interspersed with fibroelastic membranes. Age-related fibrous tissue augmentation occurs in these membranes. Thick bundles of smooth muscle interpose between the posterior cartilage ends, supported by collagen-elastic fibers. This architecture facilitates tracheal diameter modulation during respiration.

Continuity with adjacent connective tissues (esophagus and neck) is maintained by the adventitia, forming the outermost layer of loose connective tissue. The inferior thyroid artery predominantly supplies blood to the trachea. Parasympathetic fibers originate from the recurrent branch of the vagus nerve, while sympathetic fibers arise from the truncus sympathicus [4, 5].

2.7 Lungs

2.7.1 Pleura

The pleura is a serous membrane that lines the inner surface of the thoracic cavity. It consists of two layers: the parietal pleura, which covers the chest wall, and the visceral pleura, which envelops the lung’s outer surface. These two layers converge at the hilus region, forming a closed sac. Both the parietal and visceral pleura are composed of a single layer of mesothelial cells covering an underlying connective tissue rich in elastic fibers. This connective tissue is continuous with the lung parenchyma’s elastic fibers. The blood vessels supplying the visceral pleura originate from the pulmonary and bronchial arteries, while nerves come from the vagus and bronchial sympathetic nerves. Conversely, the parietal pleura receives its blood supply from the intercostal arteries and nerves. Between the visceral and parietal pleura lies a potential space containing approximately 30–50 cm^3 of serous fluid. This fluid is secreted by the mesothelial cells and serves to lubricate the pleura.

2.7.2 Bronchi

The bronchi divide into two main parts: extrapulmonary bronchi, which remain outside the lungs, and intrapulmonary bronchi, which extend within the lung. The trachea bifurcates into the right and left primary bronchi at the fourth thoracic vertebra, known as extrapulmonary bronchi. These primary bronchi enter the lungs through the hilum region (intrapulmonary bronchi) and branch into secondary and tertiary bronchi. Beyond the bronchi, the respiratory tree progresses into bronchioles, culminating in the terminal bronchiole. The respiratory bronchiole follows, representing the first site of gas exchange in this part. Approximately 20 branching divisions occur from the trachea to the respiratory bronchioles. Subsequent divisions lead to the formation of alveolar ducts and alveolar sacs. Alveoli constitute the primary structural and functional unit of the lung.

Throughout the course of the respiratory tree toward the alveoli, notable histological changes occur. The diameter decreases, glands and goblet cells decrease in number, epithelial length shortens, while smooth muscle and elastic tissue increase. The primary bronchi resemble the trachea structurally but are smaller in diameter and have thinner walls. They enter the lungs alongside pulmonary arteries, veins, and lymphatic vessels. The right bronchus is wider and more vertically oriented than the left.

Secondary (lobar) bronchi form when primary bronchi enter the lung and divide, resulting in three on the right and two on the left. Consequently, the right lung has three lobes and the left lung has two. Tertiary (segmental) bronchi emerge from secondary bronchi branching, leading to bronchopulmonary segments. These segments are separated by connective tissue and are significant for lung surgical procedures. There are approximately ten bronchopulmonary segments in each lung.

Segmental branches further divide into subsegmental branches, eventually forming segments into lobules. The branching pattern in the bronchial tree is dichotomous, resulting in 9–12 branch divisions. In intrapulmonary bronchi, the histological structure is similar to primary bronchi but characterized by shorter epithelium, fewer goblet cells, and irregularly shaped cartilage that entirely encircles the bronchi to maintain their open position (Fig. 2.3). Two layers of smooth muscle fibers are present between the fibroelastic fibers of the lamina propria and the cartilage tissue. The submucosa consists of dense connective tissue with numerous serous and mucous glands. Lymphocytes are abundant in the lamina propria among the epithelial cells, and lymph nodes are primarily found at the bifurcation regions of the bronchial tree.

2.7.3 Bronchioles

Bronchioles, the terminal branches of bronchi, enter lung lobules and further divide into 5–7 terminal bronchioles with a 1 mm diameter. Large bronchioles have a single-layer columnar epithelium with goblet cells, while small bronchioles have a cuboidal epithelium with Club cells. Cartilage and glands are absent.

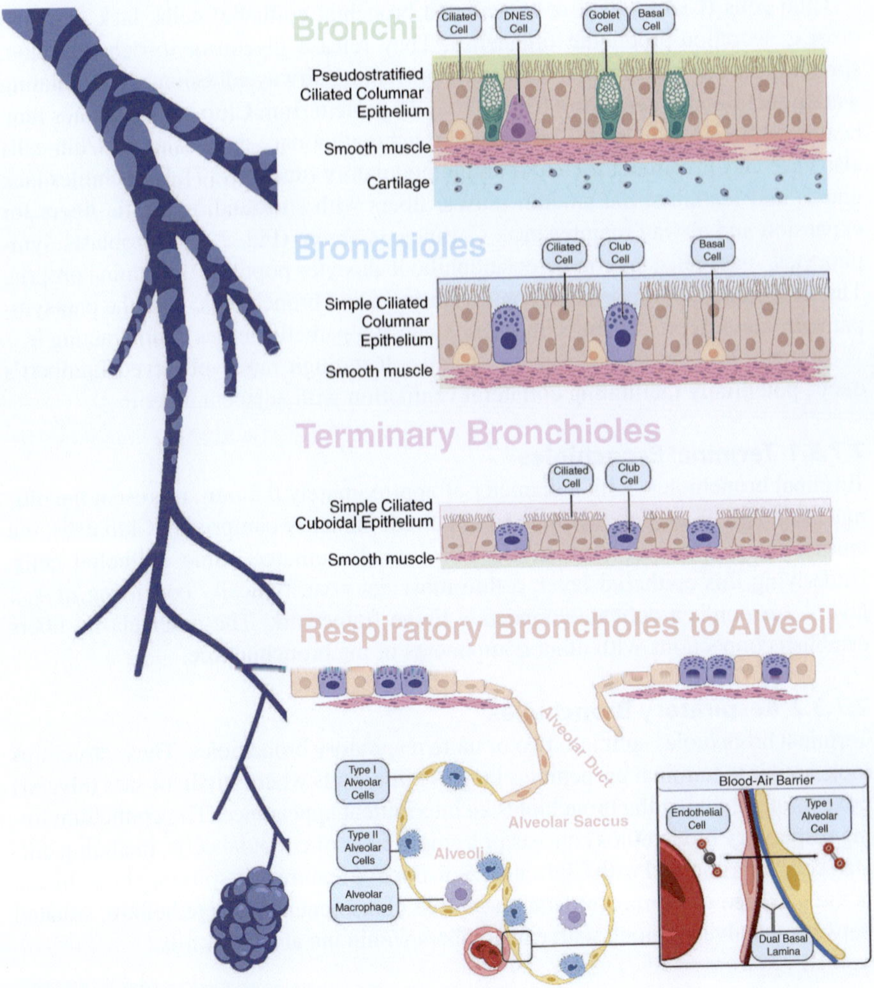

Fig. 2.3 Diagram of a human bronchiole tree. Respiratory epithelium in bronchi is composed of pseudostratified columnar cells rich in ciliated and goblet cells. The hyaline cartilage forms the structural support, maintaining bronchial lumen patency. The lamina propria beneath comprises elastic fiber-rich tissue. The bronchioles are absent of cartilage but have spiral smooth muscle in the lamina propria and varying epithelial cell types: single-layered columnar or cuboidal cells, including goblet cells and Club cells. Terminal bronchioles have delicate connective tissue rich in elastic fibers within the lamina propria, and predominantly cuboidal epithelial cells like Club cells. The respiratory bronchioles to alveoli image highlights the transition, showcasing the thin-walled structures, smooth muscle, and the critical role of Type I alveolar cells for gas exchange. It further includes the alveolar canals and saccules, which are tiny air-filled sacs that facilitate gas exchange. The lamina propria in alveoli is rich in collagen and elastic fibers. (This figure was created with biorender.com)

Club cells (Clara cells), or nonciliated bronchial epithelial cells, lack cilia and possess secretion-producing organelles. They release glycoprotein-rich secretion, similar in function to alveolar surfactant, preventing airway adhesion and facilitating watery secretion by removing Cl^- ions. CC16 protein from Club cells indicates lung health, while KL-6 indicates advanced bronchopulmonary dysplasia [6]. Club cells also have anti-inflammatory and immunomodulatory functions [7]. Bronchioles lack glands and feature spiral smooth muscle fibers with surrounding elastic fibers for expansion and airway maintenance. Cartilage is absent (Fig. 2.3). Fibroblasts, lymphocytes, mast cells, and rarely eosinophilic leukocytes populate the lamina propria. The autonomic nervous system controls bronchi and bronchioles, with the parasympathetic vagus nerve causing constriction and sympathetic nerves counteracting it.

Bronchioles can connect directly to alveoli through rarely observed Lambert's ducts, potentially facilitating collateral ventilation with adjacent alveoli.

2.7.3.1 Terminal Bronchioles

Terminal bronchioles, with a diameter of approximately 0.5 mm, represent the ultimate segment of the conducting airways. Predominantly comprising Club cells, the epithelium of terminal bronchioles also includes ciliated cubic epithelial cells. Underlying this epithelial layer, a thin muscular coat, typically consisting of 1–2 layers, surrounds a delicate connective tissue framework. The outer elastic fibers establish connections with other components of the bronchial tree.

2.7.3.2 Respiratory Bronchioles

Terminal bronchioles split into two or more respiratory bronchioles. These structures look similar to terminal bronchioles but have thin walls where small air sacs (alveoli) poke through, giving the bronchioles an intermittent appearance. The epithelium lining respiratory bronchioles consists of a single layer of cuboidal cells, including ciliated cells intermingled with Club cells. A distinctive feature of respiratory bronchioles is the presence of prominent smooth muscle fibers beneath the epithelium, situated between the alveoli, along with elastic fibers within the alveolar walls.

2.7.4 Ductus Alveolaris

Respiratory bronchioles transform into ductus alveolaris, with 2–11 branches. These ducts are lined with alveoli. In narrower regions away from the alveoli, they contain ciliated epithelial cells and elastic-rich connective tissue. Single alveolar sacs or atria connect to the ductus alveolaris, forming a complex network of elastic and reticular fibers at their openings, allowing for alveolar expansion during inhalation and contraction during exhalation.

2.7.5 Alveoli

The alveoli, constituting the terminal segment of the respiratory tree, serve as the anatomical and functional keystones within the pulmonary system. Their remarkably thin walls facilitate the crucial exchange of carbon dioxide (CO_2) and oxygen (O_2). Although each individual alveolus boasts a modest volume of approximately 200 μm^3, their collective abundance, numbering between 150 and 250 million per lung, results in an extensive gas exchange interface, totaling roughly 75 m^2. This perfusion of alveoli significantly contributes to the lung's characteristic spongy architecture.

For the essential task of gas exchange between the inhaled air and the bloodstream, the alveolar walls possess a specialized configuration. A rich network of capillaries envelops the alveoli, affording a substantial surface area, albeit somewhat smaller at approximately 60 m^2. The intervening tissue that separates the capillaries from the alveoli bears the designation "interalveolar septum." Within these regions, the alveolar epithelium and capillary endothelium are in close proximity, facilitating the intricate process of gas exchange.

Blood arriving from the pulmonary artery, laden with carbon dioxide, undergoes oxygenation within the alveoli, catalyzing the exchange of oxygen for carbon dioxide. The oxygenated blood subsequently returns to the heart via the pulmonary veins and circulates throughout the entire body. The structural integrity of the septum is reinforced by Type III collagen fibers, which provide crucial support.

In regions contiguous to the alveoli, the interstitial tissue, primarily composed of connective tissue, is notably diminished. Additionally, certain regions feature pores ranging from 8 to 60 μm in diameter, referred to as Kohn's intervals. These intervals, while generally not implicated in normal ventilation, facilitate airflow in instances of atelectasis (lung collapse) and obstructions [8].

When scrutinizing the alveolar structure, two primary cell types, namely Type I and Type II cells, predominate (Fig. 2.3).

2.7.5.1 Type I Alveolar Cell (Squamous Alveolar Cell, Small Alveolar Cell)

Type I alveolar cells, making up 40% of alveolar cells, form a continuous, squamous monolayer covering a substantial 95% of the alveolar surface. Their unique ultrastructure includes a centrally located nucleus, minimal cytoplasmic thickness, and abundant pinocytotic vesicles. Tight junctions and desmosomes connect these cells, which are intimately associated with a network of capillaries in the interalveolar septum.

2.7.5.2 Type II Alveolar Cell (Septal Cell, Large Alveolar Cell)

Type II alveolar cells, occupying approximately 60% of the alveolar cell population, cover 5% of the alveolar surface. These cuboidal cells are typically found in clusters of two or three at the alveolar corners. Type II cells exhibit a vesicular cytoplasm when observed under a light microscope and are often referred to as "granular pneumocytes." These vesicles are multilamellar bodies containing concentric or parallel lamellae inside, surrounded by a unit membrane with a diameter of 1–2 μm at the ultrastructural level. Histochemical investigations have revealed these structures to be rich in phospholipids, glycosaminoglycans, and proteins. This surfactant is vital, reducing surface tension, enhancing lung compliance, stabilizing alveoli, and providing immunity against pathogens, particularly in allergic responses [9]. The surfactant, comprising 90% lipids and 10% protein, coats the inner surfaces of alveoli as a film. When the alveolar epithelium is damaged, type II alveolar cells proliferate and differentiate into the damaged cell [4, 5].

References

1. Carlson BM. Human embryology and developmental biology. 5th ed. Philadelphia: Elsevier Saunders; 2014.
2. Nomura T, Takahashi S, Ushiki T. Cytoarchitecture of the normal rat olfactory epithelium: light and scanning electron microscopic studies. Arch Histol Cytol. 2004;67:159–70.
3. Asan E, Drenckhahn D. Immunocytochemical characterization of two types of microvillar cells in rodent olfactory epithelium. Histochem Cell Biol. 2005;123:157–68.
4. Kierszenbaum A, Tres L. Histology and cell biology: an introduction to pathology. Elsevier; 2011. p. 720. ISBN: 978-0-323-07842-9.
5. Pawlina W, Ross MH. Histology: a text and atlas: with correlated cell and molecular biology. 7th ed. Lippincott Williams & Wilkins; 2018.
6. Rokicki W, Rokicki M, Wojtacha J, Dzeljijli A. The role and importance of club cells (Clara cells) in the pathogenesis of some respiratory diseases. Kardiochirurgia i Torakochirurgia Polska. 2016;13:26–30.
7. Karnati S, Graulich T, Oruqaj G, Pfreimer S, Seimetz M, Stamme C, Mariani TJ, Weissmann N, Mühlfeld C, Baumgart-Vogt E. Postnatal development of the bronchiolar club cells of distal airways in the mouse lung: stereological and molecular biological studies. Cell Tissue Res. 2016;364:543–57.
8. Bastacky J, Goerke J. Pores of Kohn are filled in normal lungs: low-temperature scanning electron microscopy. J Appl Physiol. 1992;73:88–95.
9. Zuo YY, Veldhuizen RAW, Neumann AW, Petersen NO, Possmayer F. Current perspectives in pulmonary surfactant—inhibition, enhancement and evaluation. Biochim Biophys Acta Biomembr. 2008;1778:1947–77.

3 Structural and Physiological Basis of the Upper Respiratory Tract

Oğuzhan Oğuz, Nuray Bayar Muluk, and Felicia Manole

3.1 Nasal Anatomy and Physiology

3.1.1 Anatomy of the Nose

The external nose consists of paired nasal bones and upper and lower lateral cartilages. Internally, the nasal septum divides the nasal cavity into a right and left side. The lateral nasal wall consists of inferior and middle turbinates and occasionally a superior or supreme turbinate bone. The opening of the sinuses also is found under the middle turbinates on the lateral nasal wall. The lacrimal system drains into the nasal cavity below the anterior inferior aspect of the inferior turbinates [1].

As in the rest of the upper respiratory tract, nasal membranes are composed of ciliated pseudostratified glandular columnar epithelium. Cilia beat in unison to propel mucus from the nasal cavity and paranasal sinuses toward the nasopharynx where it can be swallowed. Mucociliary transport relies on mucus production and ciliary function. Normally, the nose and paranasal sinuses produce approximately 1 quart of mucus in 24 h. The amount of mucus produced can more than double when the nose and/or sinuses are inflamed. Mucus contains IgA, immunoglobulin E, and muramidase. A study by Uzeloto et al. indicated that mucociliary clearance is negatively impacted by active and passive smoking [2].

O. Oğuz
Department of Audiology, Health Services Vocational School, Istanbul Nişantaşı University, Istanbul, Turkey

Dr. Oğuzhan Oğuz Wellnose Clinic, Istanbul, Turkey

N. Bayar Muluk (✉)
Department of Otorhinolaryngology, Faculty of Medicine, Kırıkkale University, Kırıkkale, Turkey

F. Manole
Department of ENT, Faculty of Medicine, University of Oradea, Oradea, Romania

H. Yüksel et al. (eds.), *Pediatric Airway Diseases*, Comprehensive ENT,
https://doi.org/10.1007/978-3-031-74853-0_3

Blood and autonomic nerve supply control secretions and the level of congestion of nasal membranes. General innervation to the nose is from the autonomic nervous system; the parasympathetic nerves supply the resting tone and control secretions. Contributions of nerve supply are from the facial nerve originating at the inferior salivatory nucleus and following along the distribution of the facial nerve through the sphenopalatine ganglion. Blood supply to the nose comes from branches of the internal and external carotid artery systems. Terminal branches of the internal maxillary artery supply most mucosal surfaces of the nasal cavity. Contributions from the ophthalmic artery of the internal carotid artery system supply the posterior aspect of the nasal cavity [1].

Olfactory nerve endings originate in the olfactory bulb under the frontal lobe and pass directly through the cribriform plate as second-order neurons entering the nasal cavity. Olfactory nerves are found on the superior portion of the septum, superior turbinates, and cribriform region [1].

3.1.1.1 Skin and Soft Tissues

Like the underlying bony-cartilaginous framework of the nose, the overlying skin may also be divided into vertical thirds. The skin of the upper third is fairly thick but tapers into a thinner, mid-dorsal region. The inferior third regains the thickness of the upper third owing to the more sebaceous nature of the skin in the nasal tip. The dorsal skin is usually the thinnest of the three sections of the nose. The difference in skin thickness must be appreciated during dorsal reduction [3].

The nasal muscles are encountered deep into the skin and consist of four principal groups: the elevators, the depressors, the compressor, and the dilators. The elevators include the procerus and levator labii superioris alaeque nasi. The depressors are made up of the alar nasalis and depressor septi nasi. The compressor of the nose is the transverse nasalis, whereas the dilators are the dilator naris anterior and posterior. The muscles are interconnected by an aponeurosis termed the nasal superficial musculoaponeurotic system (SMAS) [4].

The internal nasal lining consists of squamous epithelium in the vestibule. This transitions to pseudostratified ciliated columnar respiratory epithelium with abundant seromucinous glands within the nose [4].

3.1.1.2 Blood Supply and Lymphatics

The nose, like the rest of the face, has an abundant blood supply. The arterial supply to the nose may be principally divided into (1) branches from the internal carotid, namely, the branches of the anterior and posterior ethmoid arteries from the ophthalmic artery, and (2) branches from the external carotid, namely, the sphenopalatine, greater palatine, superior labial, and angular arteries [4].

The external nose is supplied by the facial artery, which becomes the angular artery coursing over the superomedial aspect of the nose. The sellar and dorsal regions of the nose are supplied by branches of the internal maxillary artery (namely, the infraorbital) and ophthalmic arteries (which are from the internal carotid system) [4].

Internally, the lateral nasal wall is supplied by the sphenopalatine artery posteroinferiorly and by the anterior and posterior ethmoid arteries superiorly. The nasal septum also derives its blood supply from the sphenopalatine and the anterior and posterior ethmoid arteries with the added contribution of the superior labial artery (anteriorly) and the greater palatine artery (posteriorly). The Kiesselbach plexus, or the Little area, represents a region in the anteroinferior third of the nasal septum, where all three of the chief blood supplies to the internal nose converge [4].

Veins in the nose essentially follow the arterial pattern. They are significant for their direct communication with the cavernous sinus and for their lack of valves; these features potentiate the intracranial spread of infection. Even with the abundant blood supply of the nose, smoking does compromise postoperative healing [4].

Lymphatics arise from the superficial mucosa and drain posteriorly to the retropharyngeal nodes and anteriorly to the upper deep cervical nodes and/or submandibular glands [4].

3.1.1.3 Nerves

The sensation of the nose is derived from the first two branches of the trigeminal nerve. The following outline effectively delineates the respective sensory distribution of the nose and face of the trigeminal nerve [4].

Ophthalmic Division

The ophthalmic division includes the following [4]:

- Lacrimal: Skin of lateral orbital area except lacrimal gland
- Frontal: Skin of forehead and scalp, including the supraorbital (eyelid skin, forehead, and scalp) and supratrochlear (medial eyelid and medial forehead) skin
- Nasociliary: Skin of the nose and mucous membrane of anterior nasal cavity.

On a more detailed level, the nasociliary portion of the ophthalmic division includes the following [4]:

- Anterior ethmoid: Anterior half of nasal cavity: (1) internal: ethmoid and frontal sinuses and (2) external: nasal skin from rhinion to tip
- Posterior ethmoid: Superior half of the nasal cavity, namely, the sphenoid and ethmoids
- Intratrochlear: Medial eyelids, palpebral conjunctiva, nasion, and bony dorsum

Maxillary Division

The maxillary division includes the following [3]:

- Maxillary
- Infraorbital: External nares
- Zygomatic
- Superior posterior dental
- Superior anterior dental: Mediates sneeze reflex

- Sphenopalatine: Divides into lateral and septal branches and conveys sensation from posterior and central regions of the nasal cavity

Parasympathetic Nerve Supply

The parasympathetic supply is derived from the greater superficial petrosal (GSP) branch of cranial nerve VII. The GSP joins the deep petrosal nerve (sympathetic supply), which comes from the carotid plexus to form the vidian nerve in the vidian canal. The vidian nerve travels through the pterygopalatine ganglion (with only the parasympathetic nerves forming synapses here) to the lacrimal gland and glands of the nose and palate via the maxillary division of the trigeminal nerve [4].

3.1.1.4 Bony Anatomy

Superiorly, the paired nasal bones are attached to the frontal bone (see the images below). Superolaterally, they are connected to the lacrimal bones, and inferolaterally, they are attached to the ascending processes of the maxilla. Posterosuperiorly, the bony nasal septum is composed of the perpendicular plate of the ethmoid, shown in the second image below. Posteroinferiorly lies the vomer, which in part forms the choanal opening into the nasopharynx. The floor consists of the premaxilla and the palatine bones [4].

The lateral nasal walls contain three pairs each of small, thin, shell-like bones: the superior, middle, and inferior conchae, which form the bony framework of the turbinates. Lateral to these curved structures lies the medial wall of the maxillary sinus.

Inferior to the turbinates lies a space called a meatus, with names that correspond to the above turbinate, e.g., superior turbinate and superior meatus. The roof of the nose internally is formed by the cribriform plate of the ethmoid. Posteroinferior to this structure, sloping down at an angle, is the bony face of the sphenoid sinus [4].

3.1.1.5 Cartilaginous Pyramid

The cartilaginous septum extends from the nasal bones in the midline above to the bony septum in the midline posteriorly, then down along the bony floor. It assumes a quadrangular shape. Its upper half is flanked by two triangular-to-trapezoidal cartilages, called the upper lateral cartilages, which are fused to the dorsal septum in the midline and attached to the bony margin of the pyriform aperture laterally by loose ligaments. The inferior ends of the upper lateral cartilages are free. The internal area or angle formed by the septum and upper lateral cartilage constitutes the internal valve. Adjacent sesamoid cartilages may be found lateral to the upper lateral cartilages in the fibroareolar connective tissue. These are found variably [4].

Beneath the upper lateral cartilages lie the lower lateral cartilages, shown below. The paired lower lateral cartilages swing out from medial attachments to the caudal septum in the midline, called the medial crura, to an intermediate crus area. They finally flare out superolaterally as the lateral crura. These cartilages are frequently mobile, in contradistinction to the upper lateral cartilages [4].

3.1.1.6 Structure

External Nasal Anatomy

The first image below depicts the external nasal anatomy. Nasal subunits include the dorsum, sidewalls, hemilobules, alae, soft triangles, and columella [5]. Ethnic influences can result in different appearances of the nose [6] as follows: Caucasian, leptorrhine; African American, platyrrhine; Hispanic, paraleptorrhine; and Asian, subplatyrrhine. The external valve is a variable area dependent on the size, shape, and strength of the lower lateral cartilage [4].

Internal Nasal Anatomy

The septum is a midline bony and cartilaginous structure that divides the nose into two similar halves. Regarding the lateral nasal wall and paranasal sinuses, the superior, middle, and inferior concha form the corresponding superior, middle, and inferior meatus on the lateral nasal wall. The superior meatus is the drainage area for the posterior ethmoid cells and the sphenoid sinus. The middle meatus provides drainage of the anterior ethmoid and the maxillary and frontal sinuses. The inferior meatus provides drainage of the nasolacrimal duct [5].

The internal nasal valve involves the area bounded by upper lateral cartilage, septum, nasal floor, and anterior head of the inferior turbinate. This makes up the narrowest portion of the nasal airway in the leptorrhine nose. Generally, an angle wider than 15° is needed in this area. The width of the nasal valve can be increased with spreader grafts and flaring sutures [4].

3.1.2 Nasal Physiology

3.1.2.1 Nasal Airflow

Air flows superiorly into the nares, determined by its position and the anterior nasal valve. The airstream then turns posteriorly approximately 90° and flows into the nasopharynx. The airstream then turns inferiorly 90° through the pharynx and larynx and flows into the trachea toward the lungs. The anterior nasal valve is located 1.5–2 cm posterior to the anterior nares and is the narrowest portion of the upper airway. The narrow portion of the upper airway allows close contact between the airstream and mucosal surfaces. Humidification occurs by evaporation of moisture from the mucosal blanket. Air is humidified to 75–80%. Warming of inspired air to 36 °C results from contact between air and the rich blood supply of the nasal membranes, especially the inferior turbinate mucosa [1].

Adults condition more than 14,000 L of air/day, requiring more than 680 g of water, approximately 20% of our daily water intake [3].

The sniff is also an important part of nasal airflow; it provides a way to force air into the superior nasal vault and into better contact with the olfactory mucosa. Information on nasal airflow also can be found in the Medscape Reference article Nasal Aerodynamics [1].

With regard to the human nasal cycle, Williams and Eccles proposed a model for the central control of airflow patterns, in which in-phase and reciprocal airflow changes are explained through the incorporation of a hypothalamic center and two brainstem half centers [7, 8].

3.1.2.2 Abnormal Nasal Physiology

Environmental allergies are the most common causes of inflammation of nasal membranes, followed by inhaled irritants (e.g., cigarette smoke, perfumes, various chemicals, and other noxious odorants) [1].

Nonallergic, or vasomotor, rhinitis results from dysfunction of the autonomic nervous system or blood flow changes from iatrogenic or drug-related causes [3]. Increases in blood flow or parasympathetic tone or decreases in the sympathetic tone increase congestion and drainage of the nasal cavity. Conversely, reduction of blood flow, suppression of the parasympathetic system, and stimulation of the sympathetic system decrease nasal congestion and discharge. Supplemental female hormones or hormonal changes caused by pregnancy or menstruation may affect nasal systems. Any medications taken for hypertension or cardiac dysfunction may affect nasal physiology [1].

Nasal physiology also is affected by anatomic deformities that may have a varying effect on congestion, drainage, and olfaction. Septal deviation and enlarged turbinates can affect airflow into the nasal cavity, transforming it from a laminar pattern to a more turbulent pattern (see the images below). Turbulent airflow causes further irritation to nasal membranes, with a resultant increase in nasal drainage and congestion [1].

3.2 Larynx Anatomy and Physiology

3.2.1 Larynx Anatomy

3.2.1.1 Cartilages of the Larynx

Cricoid Cartilage

The cricoid cartilage is a ring of hyaline cartilage located at the inferior aspect of the larynx and is the only complete ring of cartilage around the trachea. It has the shape of a "signet ring," with a broad portion posterior to the airway (lamina of cricoid cartilage) and a narrower portion circling anteriorly (arch of cricoid cartilage). The posterior surface of the lamina contains two oval depressions, which serve as attachment sites for the posterior cricoarytenoid muscles, separated by a vertical midline ridge that serves as an attachment to the esophagus [9].

At the junction of the lamina with the arch, small, round articular facets exist on the outer posterolateral surface of each side of the ring that articulate with the inferior horn of the thyroid cartilage. The lower border of the cricoid cartilage is connected to the first tracheal ring by the cricotracheal ligament. The upper border of the cricoid cartilage gives attachment to the cricothyroid ligament on the anterior midline, the cricothyroid muscles on the lateral aspects, and the bases of a pair of arytenoid cartilages on both sides of the posterior aspect [9].

Thyroid Cartilage

The thyroid cartilage is the largest of the laryngeal cartilages. It is formed by a right and a left lamina that are separated posteriorly and joined together at an acute angle in the anterior midline, forming the laryngeal prominence, commonly known as Adam's apple. The laryngeal prominence is more apparent in men because the angle between the two laminae is more acute in men (90°) than in women (120°) [9].

The superior thyroid notch is a V-shaped notch immediately above the laryngeal prominence, while the inferior thyroid notch is less distinct and located in the midline along the base of the cartilage (see the image below). The two laminae are quadrilateral in shape and form the lateral surfaces of the thyroid cartilage that extend obliquely to cover each side of the trachea [9].

The posterior aspect of each lamina is elongated to form a superior horn and an inferior horn. The medial surfaces of the inferior horns articulate with the outer posterolateral surface of the cricoid cartilage. The inferior border of the thyroid cartilage is attached to the cricoid cartilage by the cricothyroid membrane in the midline and the cricothyroid muscles on either side. The superior horn along with the entire superior edge of the thyroid cartilage is attached to the hyoid bone by the thyrohyoid membrane [9].

Epiglottis

The epiglottis is a leaf-shaped cartilage that moves down to form a lid over the glottis and protects the larynx from aspiration of foods or liquids being swallowed. It is attached by its stem to the midline of the inner aspect of the thyroid cartilage, about halfway between the angle of the laryngeal prominence and the inferior notch [9].

It is attached via the thyroepiglottic ligament and projects posterosuperiorly to cover the superior opening of the larynx. The midline of the superior surface of the epiglottis is also attached to the body of the hyoid bone via the hyoepiglottic ligament. The mucous membrane covering the upper anterior part of the epiglottis reflects off the sides of the epiglottis, giving rise to the glosso-epiglottic folds. The aryepiglottic folds are mucosal folds on the posterior surface of the epiglottis. The depressions on either side of the median fold, between the root of the tongue and the epiglottis, are called the valleculae epiglottica [9].

Arytenoid Cartilages

The arytenoid cartilages form the part of the larynx to which the vocal ligaments and vocal folds attach. They are pyramidal in shape and have three surfaces, a base, and an apex. They are located superior to the cricoid cartilage in the posterior part of the larynx, with the base of the arytenoid cartilages articulating on either side with the posterior aspect of the upper border of the cricoid lamina. The anterior angle of the base of the arytenoid cartilage is elongated to form a vocal process for attachment of the vocal ligament, while the lateral angle is elongated to form a muscular process for attachment of the posterior and lateral cricoarytenoid muscles [9].

The posterior surface of the arytenoid cartilage gives attachment to the arytenoid muscle. The anterolateral surface has two depressions for attachment to the false vocal cord (vestibular ligament) and the vocalis muscle. The medial surface has a mucosal lining that forms the lateral aspect of the respiratory part of the glottis. The apex of the arytenoid cartilage is pointed and articulates with the corniculate cartilage [9].

Corniculate Cartilages

The corniculate cartilages are two small, conical cartilages that articulate with the apices of the arytenoid cartilages, serving to extend them posteriorly and medially. They are located in the posterior parts of the aryepiglottic folds of mucous membrane [9].

Cuneiform Cartilages

The cuneiform cartilages are two small, club-shaped cartilages that lie anterior to the corniculate cartilages in the aryepiglottic folds. They form small, whitish elevations on the surface of the mucous membrane just anterior to the arytenoid cartilages [9].

3.2.1.2 Ligaments of the Larynx

Extrinsic Ligaments

The thyrohyoid membrane is a broad fibroelastic ligament that spans between the superior border of the thyroid cartilage and the hyoid bone above. It contains an aperture on the lateral surfaces of each side for the superior laryngeal arteries, nerves, and lymphatics [9].

The hyoepiglottic ligament extends from the midline of the superior surface of the epiglottis to the body of the hyoid bone, located anterosuperiorly. The cricotracheal ligament connects the lower border of the cricoid cartilage to the upper border of the first tracheal cartilage ring [9].

Intrinsic Ligaments

The conus elasticus, a submucosal membrane, extends superiorly from the anterior arch of the cricoid cartilage and attaches to the thyroid cartilage anteriorly and the vocal processes of the arytenoid cartilages posteriorly. The free superior margin of the conus elasticus is thickened to form the vocal ligament, which forms the vocal folds (true vocal cords) once covered by mucosa [9].

The quadrangular membrane, another submucosal sheet, extends between the lateral aspects of the epiglottis and the anterolateral surface of the arytenoid cartilages on each side. The free lower inferior margin of this membrane is thickened to form the vestibular ligament, which forms the vestibular folds (false vocal cords) once covered by mucosa [9].

3.2.1.3 Cavities of the Larynx

Laryngeal Cavity

The laryngeal central cavity is tubular in shape and lined with mucosa. The superior aspect of the cavity (laryngeal inlet) opens into the pharynx, inferior and posterior to the tongue. The inferior aspect of the cavity is continuous with the lumen of the trachea [9].

The laryngeal cavity may be divided into three major regions: the vestibule, the middle, and the infraglottic space. The vestibule is the upper portion of the cavity, in between the laryngeal inlet and the vestibular folds. The middle portion of the cavity, or the voice box, is formed by the vestibular folds above and the vocal folds below. The infraglottic space is the lower portion of the cavity, in between the vocal folds and the inferior opening of the larynx into the trachea [9].

Laryngeal Ventricles and Saccules

On either side of the middle laryngeal cavity, between the vestibular and vocal folds, the mucosa bulges laterally to form troughs known as the laryngeal ventricles. The laryngeal saccules are tubular extensions of each ventricle anterosuperiorly between the vestibular fold and the thyroid cartilage. It is thought that the walls of these saccules contain many mucous glands that lubricate the vocal folds [9].

Rima Vestibuli and Rima Glottidis

The rima vestibuli is the triangular-shaped opening between the two adjacent vestibular folds. The apex lies anterior and the base is formed by the posterior wall of the laryngeal cavity. The rima glottidis is a narrower, triangular-shaped opening that lies beneath the rima vestibuli, formed by the two adjacent vocal folds [9].

Piriform Recesses

The piriform recesses (piriform sinuses) are present on either side of the anterolateral wall of the laryngopharynx. They are bounded medially by the aryepiglottic folds and laterally by the thyroid cartilage and thyrohyoid membrane. They are a common place for food to become trapped [9].

3.2.1.4 Muscles of the Larynx

Cricothyroid Muscles

The cricothyroid muscles are attached to the anterolateral surfaces of the arch of the cricoid cartilage and expand superiorly and posteriorly to attach to the inferior border of the thyroid cartilage. They are the only laryngeal muscles supplied by the external branch of the superior laryngeal nerve, a branch of the vagus nerve (cranial nerve [CN] X) below the base of the skull [9].

These muscles function to elevate the anterior arch of the cricoid cartilage and depress the posterior portion of the thyroid cartilage lamina. This produces tension and elongation of the vocal cords, resulting in higher-pitch phonation [9].

Posterior Cricoarytenoid Muscles

The posterior cricoarytenoid muscles extend from the oval depressions on the posterior surface of the cricoid lamina on each side and extend upward to the muscular process of the arytenoid cartilage on the same side. These muscles function to rotate the arytenoid cartilages laterally, thereby abducting the vocal cords. Their action opposes that of the lateral cricoarytenoid muscles. The posterior cricoarytenoid muscles receive innervation from the recurrent laryngeal branch of the vagus nerve (CN X) [9].

Lateral Cricoarytenoid Muscles

The lateral cricoarytenoid muscle on each side extends from the upper border of the arch of the cricoid cartilage to the muscular process of the arytenoid cartilage on the same side. These muscles function to rotate the arytenoid cartilages medially, thereby adducting the vocal cords. The lateral cricoarytenoid muscles receive innervation from the recurrent laryngeal branch of the vagus nerve (CN X) [9].

Transverse Arytenoid Muscle

The transverse arytenoid muscle is a single muscle that extends between the posterior surfaces of each arytenoid cartilage. Its main function is the adduction of the vocal cords, and it is innervated by both recurrent laryngeal branches of the vagus nerves (CN X) [9].

Thyroarytenoid Muscles

The thyroarytenoid muscles run from a vertical line on the interior surface of the thyroid cartilage angle and adjacent to the external surface of the cricothyroid ligament to the anterolateral surface of the arytenoid cartilage. Each muscle consists of two parts: the vocalis and thyroepiglottic part [9].

The vocalis part lies deep and inferior, parallel with the vocal ligament to which it is attached at the posterior end. The thyroepiglottic part is occasionally described as a separate muscle; it lies superior and continues into the aryepiglottic fold, where some fibers extend to the margin of the epiglottis. These muscles function to draw the arytenoid cartilages forward, thereby relaxing and shortening the vocal cords, while also rotating the arytenoid cartilages inward, thus adducting the vocal folds and narrowing the rima glottis. The thyroarytenoid muscles receive innervation from the recurrent laryngeal branch of the vagus nerve (CN X) [9].

3.2.1.5 Nerves of the Larynx

Superior Laryngeal Nerve

The superior laryngeal nerves arise from the inferior ganglia of the vagus nerve and receive a branch from the superior cervical sympathetic ganglion on each side of the upper neck. They descend adjacent to the pharynx on either side, behind the internal carotid artery, and divide into internal and external branches [9].

The external branch (external laryngeal nerve) descends beneath the sternothyroid muscle and supplies the cricothyroid muscle. Injury to this nerve during thyroidectomy or cricothyrotomy causes hoarseness of the voice and an inability to produce high-pitched sounds [9].

The internal branch (internal laryngeal nerve) pierces the thyrohyoid membrane and supplies sensory innervation to the laryngeal cavity down to the level of the vocal folds. It is responsible for the cough reflex [9].

Recurrent Laryngeal Branch of the Vagus Nerve (CN X)

The recurrent laryngeal branches of the vagus nerves ascend into the larynx within the groove between the esophagus and the trachea. The left recurrent laryngeal nerve originates in the thorax, looping under the aortic arch before ascending, while the right recurrent laryngeal nerve originates in the neck [9].

These nerves are responsible for supplying sensory innervation to the laryngeal cavity below the level of the vocal folds, as well as motor innervation to all laryngeal muscles except the cricothyroid. Since the nerves run immediately posterior to the thyroid gland, they are at risk of injury during thyroidectomies. Unilateral nerve damage presents with voice changes, including hoarseness. Bilateral nerve damage may result in aphonia (inability to speak) and breathing difficulties [9].

3.2.1.6 Vessels of the Larynx

Arteries

The superior and inferior laryngeal arteries supply the majority of blood to the larynx. The superior laryngeal artery originates from the superior thyroid branch of the external carotid artery and enters the larynx with the internal branch of the superior laryngeal nerve through the lateral aperture of the thyrohyoid membrane. The inferior laryngeal artery originates from the inferior thyroid branch of the thyrocervical trunk, which is a branch of the subclavian artery. It ascends into the larynx within the groove between the esophagus and the trachea, along with the recurrent laryngeal branch of the vagus nerve (CN X) [9].

Veins

The superior and inferior laryngeal veins drain the larynx and share the same course as the arteries. The superior laryngeal veins drain into the superior thyroid veins, which empty into the internal jugular veins. The inferior laryngeal veins drain into the inferior thyroid veins, which both empty into the left brachiocephalic vein [9].

Lymphatics

The lymphatic vessels that drain above the vocal folds travel along the superior laryngeal artery and drain to the deep cervical lymph nodes at the bifurcation of the common carotid artery. The lymphatic vessels that drain below the vocal folds travel along the inferior thyroid artery and drain to the upper tracheal lymph nodes [9].

3.2.1.7 Functional Anatomy of the Larynx

Swallowing

During swallowing, the rima glottidis, rima vestibuli, and vestibule are closed. The backward motion of the tongue forces the epiglottis over the opening of the glottis to cover the laryngeal inlet and prevent aspiration of swallowed material into the lungs. The larynx also moves upward and forward, which helps to open the esophagus for the passage of the swallowed material [9].

Respiration

During respiration, the rima glottidis, rima vestibuli, and vestibule are open. The vocal folds may be further abducted during forced inspiration, by the action of the posterior cricoarytenoid muscles, thus widening the rima glottidis and increasing the diameter of the laryngeal airway [9].

Phonation

During phonation, the vocal cords and arytenoid cartilages are adducted. When air is forced through the closed rima glottidis, the vocal cords vibrate against one another to produce sounds [9].

3.2.2 Function and Physiology of the Larynx

The upper airway in adult humans traverses the digestive tract in the region of the pharynx, complicating its sphincteric protection of the lower airway. By sharing a common passageway with the upper digestive system, the larynx is also compromised in its respiratory performance by resultant ventilatory turbulence and, therefore, resistance. Thus, the anatomic configuration in adult humans that benefits phonatory purposes of the larynx simultaneously serves to compromise its sphincteric and respiratory functions. This functional dilemma is resolved at the laryngopharyngeal level by two important organic modifications: structural adaptation and delicate coordination among the three basic laryngeal functions as determined by precisely organized brainstem reflexes [10].

From a structural point of view, the protective function of the adult human larynx is admittedly precarious by virtue of its low position in the neck. Other mammalian species are provided with a relatively high-riding larynx, affording it a close approximation with structures of the posterior nasal cavities. The intranarial position of the larynx, securing a continuous airway from the nose to the bronchi, therefore, decreases the risk of pulmonary contamination by swallowed matter. This structural modification is most obvious among certain cetaceans and herbivores but appears to a lesser degree among carnivores that use an elongated epiglottis to affect nasolaryngeal connection during deglutition. In this regard, Negus considers the epiglottis to serve secondarily in an olfactory capacity, ensuring that inspired air enters exclusively through the nose. By a series of anatomic demonstrations in macrosmatic animals, this contention appears very convincing and is supported by later histologic work identifying epiglottic chemoreceptors similar in structure to taste buds of the oral cavity, implying epiglottic participation in chemosensory perception as well [11].

In adult humans, the characteristic flat, shield-like configuration of the epiglottis serves to direct swallowed food laterally into the pyriform fossae, away from the midline laryngeal aperture. Furthermore, in adult humans, the elevation of the larynx toward the nasal cavity during the height of deglutition exaggerates this protective function. Implicit in this maneuver is the role of the aryepiglottic folds, which consist of mucous membrane, connective tissue, and muscle, extending from the epiglottic framework to the arytenoid bodies posteriorly. These lateral folds act as ramparts to the larynx, allowing food to pass on either side of the epiglottis along the gutter produced between each fold and the lateral pharyngeal wall. In this capacity, the cartilages of Santorini and Wrisberg, also called corniculate and cuneiform cartilages, respectively, are contained in the aryepiglottic folds to provide added support and stiffness to these ramparts of the laryngeal aperture. Therefore, from a structural perspective alone, it would appear that the primary role of the supraglottic larynx in adult humans lies in its protection of the lower airway [10].

In the human larynx the ability to perform as an effective valve depends on the unique shelf-like configuration of its superior and inferior folds bilaterally represented. The ventricular folds or false cords, which are located superiorly, act as exit valves, preventing the escape of air from the lower respiratory tract. When positioned by muscular contraction, they seal even more tightly as tracheal pressure is increased from below. This feature of adducted false cords occurs independently of muscle tone, a phenomenon attributable to their unique shape, which is characterized by the down-turned direction of their free margins. Such a configuration is made possible by the lateral ventricles and is exaggerated by the superior extension of the laryngeal saccules [10].

On the other hand, the true cords behaved as a one-way valve in the opposite direction, obstructing the ingress of air. When approximated in the cadaver, the true cords offered little resistance to pressure from below but resisted a pressure head from above exceeding 140 mmHg. Their ability to resist pressure from above was not influenced by closure of the false cords [10].

The false cords, therefore, prevent the egress of air from the lungs, and the true cords with their up-turned margins are capable of impeding its ingress [10]. Therefore, it is not surprising that expectorative functions of the larynx remain unimpaired in bilateral laryngeal paralysis. In this regard, passive closure of the false cords alone appears essential to effective cough production. The valvular component of the true cords, on the other hand, is implicated in the clinical difficulty experienced in overcoming laryngeal spasms by abrupt pressure peaks of positive pressure ventilation that only further serve to protectively seal the true cords. Therefore, from a structural perspective, the false cords provide an expectorative function, whereas the true cords assume a protective role in respiration [10].

Further structural modifications in humans are relevant. The short arytenoid vocal processes in humans effectively increase the relative length of the membranous true cords. Although obviously benefiting the phonatory characteristic of the larynx by maximizing its vibratory surface, these short vocal processes compromise its respiratory capacity. In this regard, Negus calculates the optimum arytenoid length to be 7/10 the length of the true cords, allowing a maximum cross-sectional area at the glottis produced by the pivotal motion of the arytenoid bodies. Such an optimum ratio of arytenoid to vocal cord length is found in the gazelle, with humans possessing a 4:10 ratio instead [10].

3.2.2.1 Reflex Glottic Closure

Reflex glottis closure is facilitated by (1) expiratory phase, (2) decreased arterial partial pressure of carbon dioxide (pCO_2), (3) increased arterial partial pressure of oxygen (pO_2), (4) negative intrathoracic pressure, and (5) hyperthermia. On the other hand, reflex glottic closure is inhibited by (1) inspiratory phase, (2) increased arterial pCO_2, (3) decreased arterial pO_2, (4) positive intrathoracic pressure, and (5) hypothermia [10].

In early inspiration, the mean threshold stimulus measured 0.37 V, 0.1 ms, whereas in late inspiration, the mean threshold measured 0.36 V, 0.1 ms. In early expiration, the mean threshold measured 0.28 V, 0.1 ms, whereas in late expiration, the mean threshold measured 0.29 V, 0.1 ms. In the spontaneously breathing subject, therefore, the threshold of reflex glottic closure seemed to increase on inspiration and decrease on expiration. In other words, reflex glottic closure occurred more readily in expiration than inspiration [10].

Effect of Carbon Dioxide

The threshold of the glottic closure reflex was determined with respect to precisely controlled variations in arterial pCO_2. The mean and range of three separate determinations were obtained in hypocapnia, normocapnia, and hypercapnia. For example, hypocapnia was produced by hyperventilating on room air, normocapnia by administering room air during spontaneous respiration, and hypercapnia by administering 10% CO_2 during spontaneous breathing. Arterial blood gas determinations were confirmed in each test situation, such that arterial O_2 tension (95 mmHg) remained constant throughout this test period [10].

In the spontaneously breathing subject, iSLN stimuli were precisely phase-locked to early inspiration and early expiration to avoid variations caused by the respiratory phase. During early inspiration, the mean threshold of the glottic closure reflex measured 0.21 V at pCO_2 of 25 mmHg, 0.37 V at pCO_2 of 40 mmHg, and 0.56 V at pCO_2 of 60 mmHg. During early expiration, the threshold of the glottic closure reflex measured 0.21 V at pCO_2 of 25 mmHg, 0.28 V at pCO_2 of 40 mmHg, and 0.40 V at pCO_2 of 60 mmHg [10].

3.2.2.2 Neurophysiology of Respiratory Function

Pertinent to respiratory laryngeal function is the role of the cricothyroid muscle, known to be a vocal cord adductor and isotonic tensor. We have demonstrated that this muscle contracts phasically with inspiration [12]. Although its inspiratory adductor role would appear counterproductive to inspiration by narrowing the glottic aperture, its role in cord lengthening actually enhances the cross-sectional diameter of the glottis by increasing its anteroposterior dimension by 30%. Therefore, it would appear that both posterior cricoarytenoid and cricothyroid muscles are driven by the medullary respiratory center, the level of their activity regulated in eupneic breathing by afferent impulses originating in the chest. Although posterior cricoarytenoid contraction increases the horizontal diameter of the glottic chink, its anteroposterior diameter is increased by phasic inspiratory contraction of the cricothyroid muscle [10].

In addition to its inspiratory function, cricothyroid expiratory activity is an equally important consideration. In eupneic states, expiratory flow and duration are principal determinants of respiratory frequency. As others have demonstrated in both animal and human investigations, variations in respiratory rate result primarily from changing the duration of the expiratory phase rather than the inspiratory phase of the respiratory cycle [13, 14].

On a mechanical ventilator we observed the following interesting phenomenon. Cricothyroid activity is evoked by positive intratracheal pressure, its contraction synchronized with the phase of the ventilator. When the respiratory rate is mechanically increased from 20 to 40/min, cricothyroid activity appears to track synchronously with this rate change [10].

3.2.2.3 Neurophysiology of Phonation

The phonatory function of the larynx is probably the least well understood of its three basic functions. Because of advances in the investigative technique, many established hypotheses based on animal models have been challenged, owing in large measure to the advent of more sophisticated technology based on human study [15–17]. High-speed cinematography, improved endoscopic techniques with the use of the laryngeal stroboscope, and direct human EMG measurements made possible by hooked wire electrodes are largely responsible for these newer additions [10].

It is generally agreed that speech results from the production of a fundamental tone at the larynx and is modified by resonating chambers of the upper aerodigestive tract. Intelligible speech, therefore, represents the combined effect of the larynx, tongue, palate, and related structures of the oral vestibule. The production of the fundamental tone is due to the vibration of the vocal folds against each other, generated by the passage of air between them. Vocal cord vibrations may be a passive phenomenon representing the basis of the aerodynamic theory of sound generation. Such a theory finds support in the observation that the completely paralyzed larynx is capable of producing sound, as is the cadaver larynx when subglottic pressure is forcefully increased. Obviously, phonation ceases when a tracheotomy is performed for diversionary purposes [10].

The aerodynamic theory of sound production therefore replaces the neurochronaxic theory. The central generation of recurrent laryngeal nerve impulses produced cord vibrations by active contraction of the thyroarytenoid muscles. Each vibration, therefore, represented the result of beat-by-beat impulses through the recurrent laryngeal nerve. This theory, no longer accepted, is of historical interest only [10].

Although sound production may be considered a passive function, the regulation of its acoustic quality is not a passive phenomenon. Rather, vocal cord shaping and positioning are under active neural regulation [18].

The cricothyroid (CT) muscle increases the fundamental frequency (F0) by tensing the vocal fold. The vocal fold is stretched, elongated, thinned, and slightly adducted to the paramedian position as the vocal fold is lowered within the larynx. These changes reduce the cross-sectional area of the vocal fold, reducing vibratory mass and increasing F0. Vocalis muscle (Voc), on the other hand, generates the opposite effect as it loosens and thickens the vocal fold. In addition, as it increases glottal resistance, it contributes to vocal intensity as subglottal pressure is increased. Vocal control, therefore, is achieved by the coordinated efforts of respiratory, laryngeal, and articulatory muscles capable of producing great variations of tonal qualities characterizing the human voice [10].

References

1. Archer SM. Nasal physiology. In: Meyers AD, editor. Medscape. Updated 16 Nov 2021. https://emedicine.medscape.com/article/874771-overview#a2. Accessed 21 Jun 2023.
2. Uzeloto JS, Ramos D, Silva BSA, et al. Mucociliary clearance of different respiratory conditions: a clinical study. Int Arch Otorhinolaryngol. 2021;25(1):e35–40.
3. Naclerio RM, Pinto J, Assanasen P, Baroody FM. Observations on the ability of the nose to warm and humidify inspired air. Rhinology. 2007;45(2):102–11.
4. Chang EW. Nasal anatomy. In: Meyers AD, editor. Medscape. Updated 23 Jul 2015. https://emedicine.medscape.com/article/835134-overview#a2. Accessed 21 Jun 2023.
5. Jafek BW. Anatomy and physiology of the nose. In: Jafek BW, Stark AK, editors. ENT secrets. Philadelphia, PA: Hanley & Belfus; 1996. p. 77–83.
6. Heidari Z, Mahmoudzadeh-Sagheb H, Khammar T, Khammar M. Anthropometric measurements of the external nose in 18-25-year-old Sistani and Baluch aborigine women in the southeast of Iran. Folia Morphol (Warsz). 2009;68(2):88–92.
7. Williams M, Eccles R. A model for the central control of airflow patterns within the human nasal cycle. J Laryngol Otol. 2016;130(1):82–8.
8. Kahana-Zweig R, Geva-Sagiv M, Weissbrod A, Secundo L, Soroker N, Sobel N. Measuring and characterizing the human nasal cycle. PLoS One. 2016;11(10):e0162918.
9. Vashishta R. Larynx anatomy. In: Gest TR, editor. Medscape. Updated 7 Dec 2017. https://emedicine.medscape.com/article/1949369-overview#a2. Accessed 21 Jun 2023.
10. Sasaki CT. Anatomy and development and physiology of the larynx. Part 1 Oral cavity, pharynx and esophagus. GI Motility online. 2006. https://doi.org/10.1038/gimo7. https://www.nature.com/gimo/contents/pt1/full/gimo7.html. Accessed 21 Jun 2023.
11. Lalonde ER, Eglitis JA. Number and distribution of taste buds on the epiglottis, pharynx, larynx, soft palate, and uvula in human newborn. Anat Rec. 1961;140:91.
12. Suzuki M, Kirchner JA, Murakami Y. The cricothyroid as a respiratory muscle. Ann Otol Rhinol Laryngol. 1970;79:1.
13. Bendixon HH, Smith GM, Mead J. Pattern of ventilation in young adults. J Appl Physiol. 1964;19:195.
14. Remmers JE, Bartlett D Jr. Reflex control of expiratory airflow and duration. J Appl Physiol. 1977;42:80.
15. Stevens K, Hirano H. Vocal fold physiology. Tokyo: Tokyo University Press; 1981.
16. Bless DM, Abbs JH. Vocal fold physiology contemporary research and clinical issues. San Diego: College Hill Press; 1983.
17. Baer T, Sasaki CT, Harris K. Laryngeal function in phonation and respiration. Boston: Little, Brown; 1987.
18. Hirano M. Laryngeal muscles in singing. In: Hirano M, Kirchner JA, Bless D, editors. Neurolaryngology: recent advances. Boston: Little, Brown; 1987.

Congenital Anomalies of the Upper Respiratory Tract

4

Emine Körkuyu Yardımcı, Cemal Cingi, Emmanuel P. Prokopakis, and Nuray Bayar Muluk

4.1 Introduction

Infants and young children often experience morphological and functional obstruction due to congenital anomalies of the upper airway, which includes the nasal oropharynx and extends to the subglottis. As a result, they may have trouble breathing. This section will examine the most frequent upper airway congenital anomalies according to their primary anatomic location [1]. In children younger than 2½ years old, anomalies of the larynx account for 85% of cases of stridor. It is vital to distinguish between self-limiting and terminal conditions while working with these patients [2].

E. K. Yardımcı
Department of Otolaryngology, Head and Neck Surgery, Adana Çukurova Public Hospital, Adana, Turkey

C. Cingi
Department of Otorhinolaryngology, Medical Faculty, Eskisehir Osmangazi University, Eskisehir, Turkey
e-mail: cemal@ogu.edu.tr

E. P. Prokopakis
Department of Otorhinolaryngology, University of Crete, School of Medicine, Crete, Greece

N. Bayar Muluk (✉)
Department of Otorhinolaryngology, Faculty of Medicine, Kırıkkale University, Kırıkkale, Turkey

H. Yüksel et al. (eds.), *Pediatric Airway Diseases*, Comprehensive ENT, https://doi.org/10.1007/978-3-031-74853-0_4

4.2 Congenital Anomalies of the Nose and Nasopharynx

Newborns must breathe through their noses, so any blockage there could be dangerous. Some possible causes include choanal atresia, a narrowed pyriform aperture, and even malignant tumors, including glioma, encephalocele, dermoid, and teratoma.

4.2.1 Choanal Atresia

In congenital choanal atresia, bone or soft tissue at birth blocks the nasal cavity's posterior choanae. The congenital nasal airway defect known as choanal atresia (CA) is associated with various symptoms, from complete airway obstruction to chronic sinusitis. Roederer first recognized this medical condition in 1755 [3]; later, in 1829, Oto et al. provided additional information about the deformity of the palatine bones. Only one in every 5000–7000 babies is diagnosed with choanal atresia [4]. In 1910, researchers found that bony atresia accounted for 90% of deformity cases, while membrane atresia accounted for 10%. One research of 63 patients found that 29% had pure bone atresia, 71% had mixed membranous and bone atresia, and no pure membranous atresia was detected [5] based on CT scans and histologic investigation (Fig. 4.1).

The clinical appearance of CA can range from acute airway obstruction to chronic recurrent sinusitis, with the latter being more common in patients with CHARGE syndrome and craniofacial deformities.

This problem should be diagnosed soon after delivery. A 6 or 8 Fr suction catheter is inserted via the nostrils, methylene blue dye is tested, cotton swabs are used, and a laryngeal mirror is used for the initial clinical evaluation. Understanding the cause of nasal blockage by measuring the amount of resistance experienced is possible. A deviation of the nasal septum or inferior turbinate is likely to cause an obstruction 1–2 cm from the ala rim in neonates, while an obstruction 3–3.5 cm

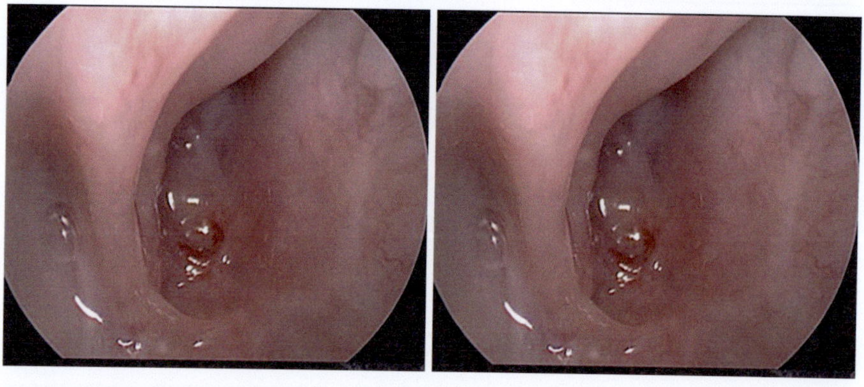

Fig. 4.1 Endoscopic view of the atretic plate of the choanal atresia

from the alar rim indicates the level posterior choanae [6]. After the infant has been appropriately prepared, including nasal decongestion and mucus suctioning, the diagnosis of choanal atresia can be confirmed via examination with a flexible nasal endoscope. A CT scan is recommended for diagnosing choanal atresia because it can more clearly define the anatomy of the atretic area, such as the thickness of the atretic plate and the existence and thickness of a bony plate. CT helps distinguish choanal atresia from other causes of nasal obstruction and elucidates the condition's nature and severity. Pyriform aperture stenosis, nasolacrimal duct cysts, enlarged turbinates, septal dislocation and deviation, antrochoanal polyp, and nasal neoplasm [7] are all potential causes.

Choanal atresia is treated with a surgical procedure. The goals are to restore choanal patency while minimizing invasiveness, preventing recurrences, and interfering with the patient's natural craniofacial growth. Surgery for unilateral choanal atresia can be delayed until school age when the area's anatomy is more similar to that of adults and is, therefore, less urgent. However, it must be observed for signs of a breathing disorder. The saline nasal spray is another option for maintaining a clear nasal passage. When available, a McGovern nipple, an intraoral nipple with a large opening created by cutting off its end and securing it in the mouth with ties around the infant's occiput, is used to maintain an adequate oral airway until the atresia plate can be perforated and the infant can breathe normally. The proposed surgical routes are transpalatal, transeptal, sublabial, transanal, and transnasal. Before the emergence of the endoscopic endonasal method in recent decades, the transpalatal procedure was the norm. Since the endoscopic endonasal technique for the repair of choanal atresia is effective with fewer surgical complications than traditional procedures [6, 7], many surgeons are increasingly turning to it. Comparison and meaningful interpretation of various studies are difficult, if not impossible, due to differences in surgical techniques, duration of stenting, or use of adjunct therapy (e.g., mitomycin), and the lack of standardized outcome measures (i.e., a definition for choanal patency and surgical failure) [6].

4.2.2 Pyriform Aperture Stenosis

Rare and potentially fatal neonatal nasal obstruction [8] is caused by congenital nasal pyriform stenosis (CNPS). The pyriform aperture is the frontmost and smallest of the nasal airway openings made of bone. Laterally, it is bounded by the maxillary nasal process; inferiorly, by the horizontal process of the maxilla and the anterior nasal spine; and superiorly, by the nasal bones themselves (position 9). CT scans can accurately diagnose pyriform aperture stenosis by acquiring thin (1.5–3.0 mm), continuous axial sections in a plane parallel to the anterior hard palate. Showing the narrowing on consecutive sections is crucial because oblique imaging can produce a false impression of narrowing [9]. In infants aged 0–6 months, the pyriform sinus should measure between 8.8 and 17.2 mm (median width = 13.5 mm). If a term child has a pyriform aperture width of less than 3 mm on one side or the combined width of both pyriform apertures is less than 8 mm, then the diagnosis is CNPS [10].

After a diagnosis of CNPS has been made, initial care often consists of conservative measures such as topical nasal decongestants, humidification, the insertion of an oral airway, and lavage feeding. When this does not work, surgery via a sublabial technique to enlarge the bone inlet is considered [11].

4.2.3 Cleft Lip Nasal Deformity

A cleft lip and/or palate is one of the most common congenital nose defects [2]. Patients with cleft lips, including those with incomplete clefts, almost always have a degree of nasal malformation. Cleft lip and nasal deformities are frequent, although the degree to which they manifest depends on the severity of the lip deformity. The degree of nasal malformation on either side of the face in those with bilateral clefts is proportional. Defects in the alar cartilage on the cleft side, the septum, the columella, the nasal tip, and the entire nasal pyramid all contribute to nasal deformity. Significant contributions to nasal asymmetry come from the malposition of maxillary segments, maxilla hypoplasia, and maxilla clefting. Structural and functional abnormalities also influence nasal deformity in the orbicularis oris muscle [2, 12, 13].

Cleft lip and nasal deformity treatment options include primary and revision rhinoplasty. When repairing a cleft lip for the first time, many surgeons re-drape the skin and soft tissue envelope over the lower lateral cartilage. A more medial anchoring of the skin-soft tissue envelope on the lower lateral cartilage may help restore the nostril's rounded look. This amendment further defines the tip subunit. Later, during a second treatment, the alar base is repositioned using a chondrocutaneous sliding flap procedure, which is frequently paired with installing a columellar strut or shield graft to project the columella, which has been abnormally shortened. There are typically several steps involved in this secondary process. Stage 1, which occurs between ages 4 and 6, focuses mainly on esthetic enhancement. Stage 2, typically completed between the ages of 8 and 12, follows the completion of orthodontic treatment and aims to provide an ideal skeletal structure. It is best to wait until skeletal maturity for a more permanent rhinoplasty. Therefore, it is done between the ages of 16 and 18. There have been cases of both open and closed rhinoplasty [2, 12].

4.2.4 Nasolacrimal Duct Cysts

Twenty percent of neonates are born with a deficiency in nasolacrimal drainage, but dacryocystocele, the most severe variant, is exceptionally uncommon. It occurs in approximately 2% of all births. Ninety percent of dacryocystoceles occur on one side only [2].

Differentiating tumors and locating intracranial communication are aided by CT and MRI imaging. CT is simple and fast, and the diagnostic features include cystic dilatation of the lacrimal sac, NLD dilatation, and the appearance of a homogeneous, well-defined, thin-walled, fluid-attenuating mass in the intranasal cavity [14]. Even though MRI can characterize the lesion's substance without exposing the patient to radiation, CT is the preferred imaging method.

Most cases of asymptomatic dacryocystocele are cured spontaneously by age one [15], making conservative management with lacrimal sac massage an option. When symptoms of dacryocystitis manifest, including pain, fever, purulent discharge, and congested eyes, it is necessary to administer broad-spectrum antibiotics. Cellulitis of the orbit and face can be a complication of untreated dacryocystitis [15]. Excessive swelling of the lacrimal sac can cause persistent canthal asymmetry and anisometropic amblyopia by narrowing the lid fissure or causing corneal astigmatism. Patients with large exterior or intranasal cysts who develop apnea or stridor may require surgical procedures such as lacrimal probing by an ophthalmologist and intranasal endoscopic cyst marsupialization by an otorhinolaryngologist [16].

4.2.5 Encephaloceles

A meningocele or meningoencephalocele is an abnormal protrusion of the meninges (the membranes surrounding and protecting the brain) outside the cranium. Encephalocele occurs in about 1 in 35,000 births worldwide but is nearly six times more common in Southeast Asia, where it is reported in 1 in 6000 births. Its etiology is unknown, but a herniation may cause it because of improper closure of the fonticulus frontalis. The sporadic occurrence of encephaloceles in families with a history of central nervous system (CNS) developmental defects [2, 17] suggests a genetic component to the disease's etiology. Due to the importance of embryological development, an encephalocele should be investigated in the differential diagnosis of any nasal, maxillofacial, or frontal tumor in a newborn. With a median age of presentation between 15.5 and 21 months, it is pretty unusual for an encephalocele to be diagnosed in a patient who is significantly older than average [18].

Nasal endoscopy is crucial to the diagnostic process since it provides insight into the nasal mass's origin, location, and size. MRI is helpful for defining soft tissue connections to the CNS, while a CT scan is excellent for assessing the bone structure of the skull base. Contrast enhancement and sagittal reconstruction are also helpful imaging aides for encephaloceles [2, 19].

Traditional neurosurgical treatment for encephaloceles has been a transcranial approach, which carries the risk of complications like loss of smell, post-operative intracerebral hemorrhage, cerebral edema, epilepsy, and frontal lobe dysfunction, which can lead to memory and attention problems [19, 20]. With the development of endoscopic sinus surgery, doctors can now treat basal encephaloceles with a less-invasive intranasal technique [20].

4.2.6 Dermoids of the Nasal Cavity

Nasal dermoid and sinus cysts (NDSCs) are uncommon congenital abnormalities. They are the most prevalent congenital nasal midline lesions [2, 21]. Midline nasal dermoid cysts and fistulas occur in 1 in 20,000 to 1 in 40,000 people [22] annually. In children, NDSCs account for 61% of median lesions [23], 11% of dermoid cysts in the head and neck, and 1% of dermoid cysts overall. Some NDSCs also have a second fistula in the inner canthus, and the fistula orifice is usually found on the nose's median line. However, it can also be found on the face's median line, between the eyebrow and the nasal columella. In severe cases, patients may experience complications such as meningitis, cellulitis, osteomyelitis, cerebrospinal fluid leakage, frontal abscess, dead bone formation, and inward growth of the lesions that can reach the nasal bone ossification center. The fistula presents as a needle-like orifice with a white cheese-like substance or fine hair discharged after extrusion. The cyst presents as an elastic round mass at the median line of the nose.

Symptoms and indicators, along with imaging tests like CT and MRI, are used to make a diagnosis. Most cases of NDSCs require surgical intervention. Optimal access for the removal of the cyst, fistula, and sick bone tissue; restoration of the skull base to cease cerebrospinal fluid leaking; promotion of nasal reconstruction; and post-operative cosmesis [24] are all prerequisites for surgical removal of the dermoid and cyst.

4.3 Craniofacial Anomalies

4.3.1 Pierre Robin Syndrome

In infants born with Pierre Robin Syndrome, the lower jaw is underdeveloped (micrognathia), the tongue is positioned posteriorly (glossoptosis), and the roof of the mouth is open (cleft palate) [25, 26]. Premature breathing and feeding difficulties are possible outcomes of this combination [26]. The Pierre Robin sequence can occur in isolation or as part of a syndrome with accompanying symptoms. The condition arises by itself in roughly 20–40% of cases [26]. Pierre Robin syndrome has mysterious origins [25]. Most solitary occurrences of the Pierre Robin sequence may be traced back to changes (mutations) in the DNA close to the SOX9 gene [26]. Surgery to aid breathing and dietary changes to prevent choking are examples of individualized approaches that may be part of the treatment plan [25].

4.3.2 Treacher-Collins Syndrome

The facial bones and other tissues cannot develop normally due to Treacher-Collins syndrome (TCS). Symptoms range from hardly perceptible to quite severe. Most patients with this disorder have small jaws and chins (a condition known as micrognathia) and undeveloped cheekbones. Other characteristics include but are not limited to ocular problems, hearing loss, and cleft palate [2, 27]. Mutations in TCOF1, POLR1C, or POLR1D have been linked to TCS [28]. The TCOF1 and POLR1D genes cause autosomal dominant inheritance [13, 27]. About 60% of autosomal dominant cases, however, are not inherited from a parent and are caused by a novel mutation in the gene [27]. Autosomal recessive inheritance is the norm when the POLR1C gene is at fault [28]. Sometimes, doctors cannot pinpoint where the problem originated in the family tree.

4.3.3 Crouzon Syndrome

In patients with Crouzon syndrome, the skull bones fuse too soon (a condition known as craniosynostosis). The head and face may not develop normally as a result of this obstruction to skull growth. Crouzon syndrome is characterized by features such as a tiny, "beak-shaped" nose, an undeveloped upper jaw, and wide-set, protruding eyes [29, 30]. Cleft lip and palate, hearing loss, and rotten teeth are frequent characteristics. Even within a single family, affected members can differ in how severely they experience symptoms. The majority of people with intellectual disability have average intelligence [29, 31]. Crouzon syndrome is an autosomal dominant disorder caused by mutations in the FGFR2 gene. Surgery is an option for patients seeking to avoid difficulties, enhance function, and promote positive psychological and social growth [29].

4.3.4 Down Syndrome

Children with Down syndrome (DS) often experience difficulties in the areas of the ear, nose, and throat (ENT). This includes chronic rhinitis, sinusitis, chronic ear infections, and middle ear effusions that lead to hearing loss, airway obstruction, and sleep apnea. Many of these ENT issues also call for surgical treatments, and unique anesthetic concerns must be considered when treating children with Down syndrome [2, 13]. Subglottic stenosis, post-operative airway blockage, and cervical spine issues all fall under this category. The treatment outcomes for these ENT symptoms of DS have improved as the care of children with DS has become more consistent and proactive. The prevalence of hearing loss, chronic rhinitis, and sleep apnea/sleep-disordered breathing in people with DS has decreased, thanks to aggressive medicinal and surgical interventions [32].

4.3.5 Apert Syndrome

One reason for craniofacial condition or deformity is Apert syndrome, sometimes called acrocephalosyndactyly. This infrequent congenital disorder is characterized by premature fusion of the cranial sutures (craniosynostosis) and deformity of the skull, hands, face, and feet [2]. It is an autosomal dominantly inherited congenital disability with a prevalence of 1 in 50,000 to 1 in 80,000 live births. These missense substitutions in fibroblast growth factor receptor 2 (FGFR2), which cause Apert syndrome, are located between the protein's second and third extracellular immunoglobulin domains and map to the chromosomal band 10q26. The father's aging has been linked to the appearance of Apert syndrome in offspring. Early, definitive diagnosis is crucial to differentiate Apert syndrome from other craniosynostosis, such as Carpenter syndrome, Crouzon disease, Pfeiffer syndrome, and Saether-Chotzen syndrome. The most effective treatment for Apert syndrome requires a team of specialists, including but not limited to neonatologists, neurosurgeons, craniofacial surgeons, plastic surgeons, otolaryngologists, orthodontists, orthopedic surgeons, ophthalmologists, radiologists, geneticists, clinical psychologists, and speech and language pathologists. Apert syndrome has a favorable adult prognosis if diagnosed and treated early [33, 34].

4.4 Congenital Anomalies of the Oropharynx and Larynx

4.4.1 Thyroglossal Duct Cyst

With a prevalence of 7%, thyroglossal duct cysts are the most common congenital cervical anomaly. They can appear anywhere the thyroid travels, from the bottom of the tongue to the lower neck. The hyoid bone is typically involved, and the cysts manifest as nodules in the center of the neck [35]. A thyroglossal duct cyst develops when the thyroglossal duct, which runs from the foramen cecum in the tongue to the thyroid in the neck, does not entirely close during embryonic development. In the third week of gestation, the thyroid forms as a median extension of the primitive pharynx. The foramen cecum, where the tongue's front two-thirds meet its back one-third, is where the thyroid primordium forms. From there, the thyroid travels down toward the front of the neck, where it comes into proximity to the hyoid bone as it forms. By the seventh week of pregnancy [2], it has settled into its permanent location in the inferior pre-tracheal neck.

The thyroglossal duct connects the thyroid gland to the foramen cecum and is the remaining narrow tubular structure at the base of the thyroid. In roughly half of humans, the distal section of the duct develops into the pyramidal lobe of the thyroid gland. The thyroglossal duct is typically involuted when pregnancy reaches the ninth week. Secretion from the epithelial lining of the duct can cause inflammation and thyroglossal duct cyst development if even a tiny part of the duct remains after removal [36]. About 7% of people have thyroglossal duct cysts. The hyoid bone is frequently involved with these cysts. They are between 15% and 20% above the hyoid, 25–65% below the hyoid, and 20–25% above the infrahyoid [36, 37].

When starting with imaging, ultrasound is the gold standard. Ultrasound is accessible, affordable, and painless. It is beneficial for treating youngsters because it does not involve ionizing radiation or anesthesia. Although computed tomography (CT) and magnetic resonance imaging (MRI) can be used to assess thyroglossal duct cysts and normal thyroid tissue, ultrasound is typically adequate for this purpose [38] (Fig. 4.2).

Due to the low risk of malignancy associated with thyroglossal duct cysts, surgical excision is recommended to prevent reinfection. High recurrence rates (45–55%) are seen after simple excision of thyroglossal duct cysts. Recurrence rates are significantly lower after the Sistrunk surgery, making it the gold standard in surgical care. More tissue from the base of the tongue and the middle third of the hyoid bone must be removed during surgery for this procedure [39].

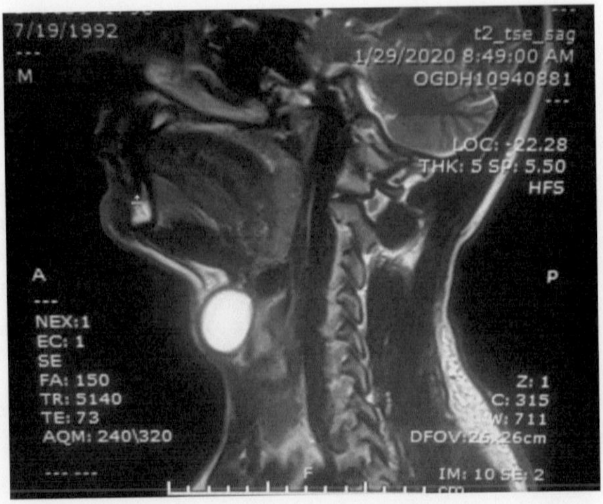

Fig. 4.2 Pre-operative MRI showing thyroglossal cyst

4.4.2 Laryngomalacia

Most cases of neonatal stridor can be traced back to laryngomalacia, and symptoms typically present themselves in the first few days of life [13]. Feeding, weeping, and lying supine all worsen the already modest stridor. Symptoms worsen in half of all instances within the first 6 months of life, but almost all cases of laryngomalacia improve by the time a child turns one [13, 40]. One in five newborns diagnosed with laryngomalacia will develop a life-threatening condition requiring emergency surgery due to severe airway blockage and feeding difficulties. Apnea, cyanosis, severe retractions, and failure to thrive are all signs that a youngster needs surgery. Cor pulmonale is diagnosed in the most severe of cases [13, 40, 41].

Flexible transnasal fiberoptic laryngoscopy is used to confirm the diagnosis [2, 40]. Short aryepiglottic folds and prolapse of the cuneiform cartilages are defining features. The epiglottis may be firmly coiled (-shaped) in some people. The supraglottic structures typically collapse on inspiration due to the Bernoulli effect [2, 40]. Even in healthy newborns, an omega-shaped epiglottis can cause breathing difficulties, most commonly seen in those with laryngomalacia [2]. Infants with laryngomalacia may also experience airway complications due to a second synchronous lesion. Children with more severe laryngomalacia are more likely to develop secondary lesions, with reported rates ranging from 8% to 58% [2].

In the 10% of children who need surgical intervention, this can often be scheduled within a few weeks of presentation as an elective procedure. It is wise to treat gastroesophageal reflux disease (GER) before surgery [40]. Supraglottoplasty (aryepiglottoplasty) has replaced previous methods of treatment [2, 40]. It is an endoscopic treatment that is quick and successful in treating the laryngeal pathology of infants [40]. The short aryepiglottic fold is divided to do a supra-glottoplasty [2, 42]. Alternately, the tissue underlying the arytenoids, the aryepiglottic folds, or the posterior section of the epiglottis [43] may be excised if the supraglottis is prolapsing. Preventing post-operative stenosis requires protecting the inter arytenoid mucosa [2, 43]. Laryngeal edema may compromise the airway after supraglottoplasty, making overnight supervision in the ICU necessary. Extubation is typically done within the first 24 h after surgery. Some youngsters still have problems breathing after surgery. Fiberoptic laryngoscopy at the bedside can distinguish between laryngeal edema and chronic laryngomalacia. The swelling of the larynx can be reduced by treating reflux. Sometimes the larynx looks fine after surgery, but the baby still has trouble breathing. Tracheotomy is sometimes necessary in cases of laryngomalacia with an underlying neurologic component [2, 40]. Supraglottic stenosis, the most worrisome complication, may develop in up to 4% of cases [2, 44], but it is still uncommon.

4.4.3 Vocal Fold Paralysis

One of the most common causes of infant stridor is vocal fold paralysis. The stridor has a musical sound, either inspiratory or biphasic. Bilateral vocal fold paralysis (VFP) is more often congenital than unilateral VFP. Causes of VFP in infants range from birth trauma to thoracic disease or surgery to the hydrocephalus and Chiari malformation of the brainstem to idiopathic causes [2, 45]. A tracheotomy should be performed on a baby with stridor and retractions because of bilateral paralysis.

Diagnosis is made for laryngomalacia, with an awake flexible transnasal fiberoptic laryngoscopy [40] (Fig. 4.3). Idiopathic bilateral VFP should include a brain MRI to rule out an Arnold-Chiari malformation or other intracranial cause of brainstem compression [46]. A small, dynamic glottis and collapsing supraglottic tissues in infants can make the diagnosis of VFP challenging [2].

The second most prevalent cause of congenital stridor is paralysis of the vocal cords at birth [47]. Individuals with unilateral VFP may have trouble feeding, aspirating their food, or crying weakly. Paralysis can resolve on its own in up to half of children by age 1. Therefore, decannulation surgeries are typically postponed until after this time frame [40]. Decannulating airway surgery aims to keep the patient's voice and prevent further aspiration. A variety of surgical procedures, including laser cordotomy, endoscopic or open partial or whole adenoidectomy, endoscopically guided or open vocal process lateralization, and posterior cricoid cartilage grafting, are available for patients with vocal cord paralysis [13, 48]. There is no one best solution available. Maintaining a tracheotomy in a child is often recommended prior to decannulation to guarantee a secure airway. Unlike idiopathic cord paralysis, acquired bilateral vocal cord paralysis can be difficult to cure, and decannulation may require more than one therapy. Patients undergoing these procedures may benefit from continuous positive airway pressure (CPAP) or a high-flow nasal cannula to treat stridor after extubation. Before a kid may return to a regular diet after surgery, the risk of aspiration should be evaluated using a video swallow study. Certain textures, and fragile fluids, may increase the risk of aspiration in the first few weeks after surgery [40].

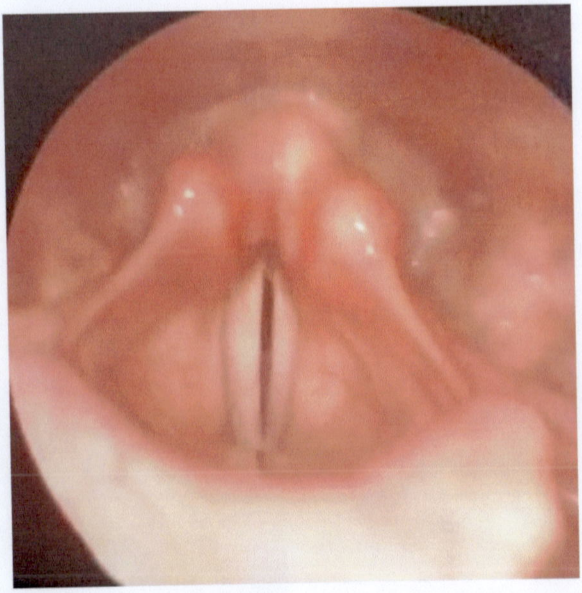

Fig. 4.3 Endoscopic view of the bilateral vocal fold paralysis

4.4.4 Webs of the Larynx

A laryngeal web indicates that the glottic airway was not successfully recanalized during the first few weeks of development. The majority of glottic webs (95%) are located in the front of the glottis; nonetheless, glottic webs are highly uncommon, accounting for only 5% of congenital laryngeal anomalies [40] (Fig. 4.4). They result from delayed or halted recanalization of the primitive larynx, generally occurring between the eighth and tenth weeks of embryonic development. Congenital subglottic stenosis, trachea-esophageal fistulas, and specific syndromes [49] are other congenital deformities that can occur in tandem. The relatively high connection frequency with 22q11 microdeletion makes genetic inquiry and counseling essential [49], even though a gene has not been identified as the cause of this deformity. All patients with congenital anterior glottic webs should be referred for genetic investigation due to the high prevalence of chromosome 22q11.2 deletion syndrome among those affected by this condition (over 50%). Numerous phenotypes, such as DiGeorge's syndrome, velocardiofacial syndrome, conotruncal anomaly face syndrome, and sporadic or familial cardiac problems, are caused by the same microscopic and submicroscopic deletions. Genetic testing and a complete cardiovascular examination should be performed on all patients diagnosed with the laryngeal web [22]. Abnormal cries or respiratory discomfort are the most common symptoms reported by parents of newborns. In the first few hours or days of life, if a baby with an anterior glottic web presents with significant airway compromise, the web is severed, and airway management is necessary immediately. Although newborns are extraordinarily tolerant of airway impairment, the clinician should know that even infants with a moderate to severe glottic web may initially present with only minor

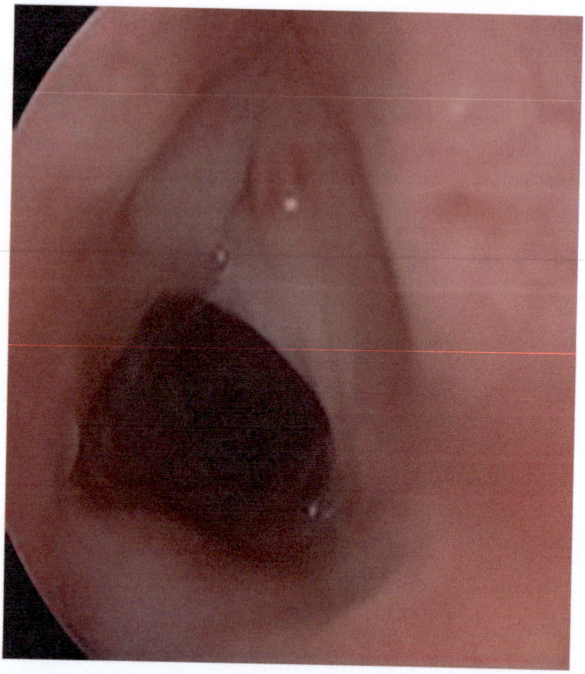

Fig. 4.4 Endoscopic view of the anterior laryngeal web

airway symptoms. During a newborn's first several months, these symptoms often worsen. Biphasic stridor and retractions are very noticeable in newborns with moderate to severe webs, especially when these infants are disturbed or feeding [40, 50].

In most cases, an open approach is necessary to successfully treat an anterior laryngeal web so that the subglottic constriction can be addressed. It is not generally recommended to do definitive surgery on a child younger than 6–12 months of age due to the perioperative dangers and technical difficulties of operating on a small airway [51]. When an infant is born with a thick glottic web, the first step is to decide if the repair should be done in the neonatal or pediatric periods. Due to the technical advantages of operating on a more prominent larynx, late repair is preferred in children with a mild or moderate web and no clinical airway compromise. By the time a child reaches age 4, it may be possible to restore the damage and improve the sound of their voice in time for school. Early correction may be performed in children with more severe glottic impairment. An alternative is to perform a tracheotomy and schedule surgery later. About 40% of patients with thick webs need this method [40]. Endoscopic therapy with laser division may be effective in unusual circumstances where the web is small [22].

4.4.5 Subglottic Stenosis

When the laryngeal lumen is less than 4.0 mm in a full-term baby or 3.5 mm in a premature neonate with no history of intubation or surgical trauma, the diagnosis of congenital subglottic stenosis (CSS) is made [52, 53] (Fig. 4.5). Congenital stenosis

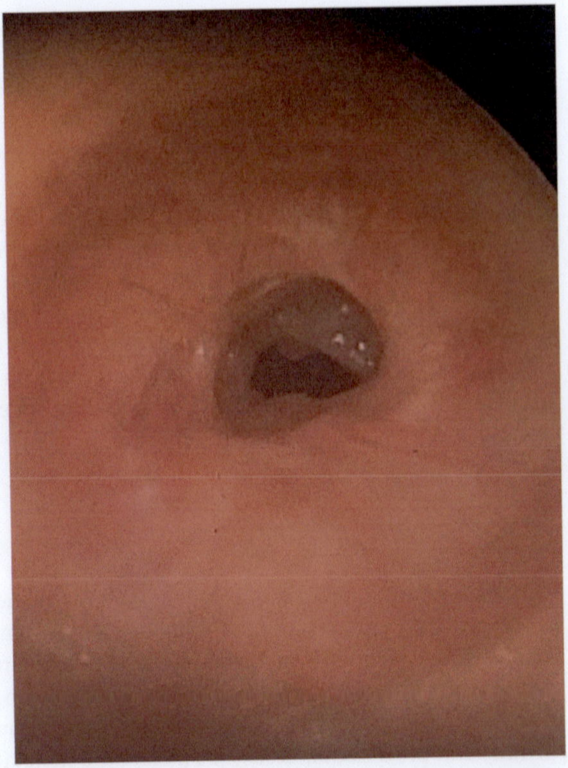

Fig. 4.5 Endoscopic view of the subglottic stenosis

or atresia of the larynx is the result of inadequate fetal airway recanalization during embryogenesis (about the tenth week of gestation). CSS is not seen as a singular condition but as part of a more extensive congenital syndrome. The syndromes 22q11.2 deletion (DiGeorge syndrome), Fraser syndrome, VACTERL/VATER association, and CHARGE syndrome all involve CSS [53, 54]. Cotton proposed the current system for grading laryngeal stenosis in 1984, and Myer modified it in 1989. Endoscopy determines the degree of blockage and its anatomical location [54]. Airway stenosis is categorized as grade I if it is between 50% and 70% narrow, grade II if it is between 71% and 99% (with visible lumen), and grade IV if it is completely blocked [53].

The size and length of stenosis in a nonintubated airway may be discerned through radiologic examination. Imaging techniques such as chest X-ray, fluoroscopy, and films of the soft tissues of the neck taken during inspiration and expiration can all be helpful. High-kilovolt airway film, however, is the most crucial study to date. The characteristic steepling seen in patients with CSS and the possibility of tracheal stenosis may be seen on these films. The latter is more common in patients with complete tracheal rings and can make rigid endoscopy dangerous for the patient. Endoscopic examination is necessary for a proper evaluation of CSS. Dynamic vocal fold function can be studied with the help of flexible fiberoptic endoscopy. Hopkins rigid endoscopes provide the most thorough analysis. It is essential to thoroughly examine the endolarynx, including a careful grading of the CSS [40, 55].

The standard treatment for a newborn with subglottic stenosis is to perform a tracheostomy and evaluate the infant's airway every 3 months to determine if reconstructive surgery is necessary. Under general anesthesia, a cricoid split can be performed anteriorly or posteriorly to widen the cricoid lumen. Laryngotracheal reconstruction is the gold standard treatment for subglottic stenosis that has developed over time. In laryngotracheal reconstruction, the larynx is exposed from the hyoid above to the tracheostomy below by a second incision made above the tracheostomy at the cricoid level. The larynx is incised precisely down the middle, and the lumen is entered above the superior thyroid notch. A graft of costal cartilage widens the cricoid ring. The graft is kept from collapsing with the use of a silastic stent. It is crucial to precisely oppose the anterior commissure during incision closure [56].

4.4.6 Subglottic Hemangioma

Premature infants often develop subglottic infantile hemangiomas, a benign vascular abnormality. The occurrence of cutaneous hemangiomas in more than half of patients with a subglottic hemangioma suggests the presence of a synchronous subglottic lesion [40]. The likelihood of developing a subglottic hemangioma is higher in patients whose hemangioma is located in the beard distribution (i.e., the chin, jawline, and preauricular areas) [57]. Infantile hemangiomas occur in females at a rate of 2:1 compared to males [2]. Pathologically, these tumors are characterized by uniform, significantly positive staining for erythrocyte-type glucose transporter protein isoform 1 (GLUT-1) and endothelial proliferation. Biphasic stridor with retractions are symptoms, and they are most noticeable when the youngster is angry or eating. There may also be a barking cough, like that of croup. Apnea, cyanosis, and "dying spells" can happen with severe airway obstruction.

Transnasal flexible laryngoscopy with the patient awake is preferable for the initial assessment. It may make it possible to see the damaged subglottis, and more importantly, it should eliminate other potential causes of neonatal stridor, such as laryngomalacia and paralysis of the vocal folds. A laryngoscopy and bronchoscopy performed in the operating room under general anesthesia are necessary for a child with increasing stridor and a standard glottic and supraglottic evaluation. A radiographic examination of the neck and an MRI scan (T2-weighted gadolinium contrast) can help diagnose the narrowing of the subglottis [2, 40].

Most people need some treatment, and doctors often use multiple approaches. Subglottic hemangiomas are traditionally treated with systemic steroids, which often cause at least partial hemangioma regression in most children [2]. Subglottic hemangiomas can cause airway obstruction, and typical surgical treatment involves performing a tracheotomy and hoping for spontaneous involution. Reports of success using a CO_2 laser to decannulate a tracheostomy have been mixed.

4.4.7 Laryngeal Cysts

Rare causes of respiratory obstruction in children include saccular cysts and laryngoceles [2]. It is located superiorly between the vestibular fold and the inner side of the thyroid cartilage, and the laryngeal saccule is a tiny diverticulum containing many mucous glands at the anterior end of the laryngeal ventricle [58]. Mucus-filled congenital saccular cysts extend laterally into the false vocal and aryepiglottic fold. In the initial few days of birth, babies with these cysts often have trouble breathing, their cries are muted, and they have trouble swallowing [59]. Internal, external, or combined dilatation and herniation of the saccule characterize a laryngocel. Sometimes there are air-fluid levels within laryngoceles, giving the appearance of spherical lumps in the neck or supraglottic region [2]. Saccular cysts generate persistent symptoms due to mucoid fluid within the cyst, whereas laryngoceles cause occasional upper airway blockage and hoarseness due to episodic filling with air.

The results of needle aspiration, marsupialization, or endoscopic excision for managing saccular cysts have historically been unsatisfactory, often necessitating repeated surgeries and tracheotomy installation. The author prefers an anterior cervical approach, with the superior border of the thyroid alar cartilage being found and the thyrohyoid membrane being incised along its superior border. This method allows the cyst to be reached and carefully dissected free before removal. Thyroid cartilage may be removed to facilitate cyst removal and reattachment [40, 59].

4.4.8 Laryngeal Cleft

Clefts of the larynx, esophagus, or windpipe are extremely unusual congenital disabilities. Failure of the laryngotracheal groove to fuse during development causes laryngeal clefts [2]. Associated defects affecting the patient's airway or other organ systems are common. Tracheomalacia (present in >80% of patients) and tracheoesophageal fistula (TEF) formation (present in 20% of patients) are two of the most common airway abnormalities seen in these patients. GER and anogenital abnormalities have been linked to a lack of airway development. Opitz-Frias syndrome, which includes hypertelorism, anogenital abnormalities, and posterior laryngeal clefting, is the most prevalent syndrome involving this congenital disability [4]. Benjamin and Inglis [2, 60] suggested a helpful anatomic classification and divide posterior laryngeal clefts into the following four subtypes [2, 60]:

- Type 1: supraglottic inter arytenoid cleft present to, but not below, the level of the true vocal folds. This cleft could also be considered a deep inter arytenoid notch.
- Type 2: Partial cricoid cleft that extends into, but not through, the posterior cricoid cartilage.
- Type 3: Total cricoid cleft with or without extension of the cleft into the cervical trachea.
- Type 4: Cleft extending to the thoracic trachea [2, 60].

Coughing (particularly during eating), difficulty feeding, and respiratory discomfort (depending on the depth of the split) are some of the earliest signs of a laryngeal cleft. Cyanosis (especially in those with other underlying health problems or abnormalities), aspiration, recurrent lung infections, stridor, wheezing, failure to thrive, and cyanosis are some of the other symptoms that may be present. Clefts of types III and IV are linked to more severe respiratory symptoms, including frequent episodes of pneumonia and increased mucus production. In most cases, types III and IV symptoms appear within the first week of life [2, 60].

Rigid bronchoscopy and esophagoscopy are the gold standard for diagnosis. In contrast, other methods such as flexible nasopharyngoscopy, fiberoptic endoscopic evaluation of swallowing, video fluoroscopy-barium swallow, and flexible bronchoscopy are helpful. The cleft is frequently missed or misinterpreted during initial evaluation with flexible or rigid bronchoscopy due to redundant mucosa in the posterior glottis [40].

Several surgical methods have been explored in recent decades for treating laryngeal cleft. In 1967, Evans [61] stated that Jahrsdoerfer and colleagues described the anterior method, which entails exposing the cleft via thyrotomy, cricoidotomy, and trachea-fissure to the first and second rings to provide direct access to the posterior cleft and permit microsurgical closure. Due to the potential for laryngeal instability and long-term laryngeal development problems, some publications have recommended avoiding the anterior approach [61, 62]. Avoiding the laryngofissure has also been described for the lateral pharyngotomy approach [61]. According to other researchers [63], the risk of laryngeal instability with the anterior approach can be reduced with careful closure under magnification, correct stenting with a nasotracheal tube, and appropriate post-operative care in the intensive care unit. A lateral pharyngotomy with a right thoracotomy approach or an anterior approach with a median sternotomy has been employed for a more extensive cleft involving the thoracic trachea [64].

4.5 Conclusion

Assessing a newborn with respiratory distress requires expert knowledge of upper airway embryological development and congenital abnormalities. Most infants experiencing respiratory distress (58%) were in the 1–6 months age range. Laryngomalacia, subglottic stenosis, laryngeal web, and vocal fold paralysis were not strongly associated with age, sex, family history, or other congenital disabilities. Diagnosis is typically made through endoscopy. The severity of an illness determines how it is treated.

References

1. Daniel SJ. The upper airway: congenital malformations. Pediatr Respir Rev. 2006;7(Suppl 1):S260–3.
2. Truong MT, Messner AH. Evaluation and management of the pediatric airway. In: Cummings pediatric otolaryngology. Elsevier; 2015. p. 309–22.
3. Flake CG, Ferguson CF. Congenital choanal atresia in infants and children. Ann Otol Rhinol Laryngol. 1964;73:458–73. https://doi.org/10.1177/000348946407300216.

4. Ramsden JD, Campisi P, Forte V. Choanal atresia and choanal stenosis. Otolaryngol Clin N Am. 2009;42(2):339–52.
5. Brown OE, Pownell P, Manning SC. Choanal atresia: a new anatomic classification and clinical management applications. Laryngoscope. 1996;106(1 Pt 1):97–101. https://doi.org/10.1097/00005537-199601000-00019.
6. Kwong KM. Current updates on choanal atresia. Front Pediatr. 2015;3:52.
7. Andaloro C, La Mantia I. Choanal atresia. StatPearls. Last update 27 Sept 2020.
8. Brown OE, Myer CM, Manning SC. Congenital nasal pyriform aperture stenosis. Laryngoscope. 1989;99:86–91.
9. Ey EH, Han BK, Towbin RB, Jaun WK. Bony inlet stenosis is a cause of nasal airway obstruction. Radiology. 1988;168:477–9.
10. Belden CJ, Mancuso AA, Schmalfuss IM. CT features of congenital nasal piriform aperture stenosis: initial experience. Radiology. 1999;213:495–501.
11. Devambez M, Delattre A, Fayoux P. Congenital nasal pyriform aperture stenosis: diagnosis and management. Cleft Palate Craniofac J. 2009;46:262–7.
12. Mulliken JB. Bilateral complete cleft lip and nasal deformity: an anthropometric analysis of staged to synchronous repair. Plast Reconstr Surg. 1995;96:9.
13. Rutter MJ. Evaluation and management of upper airway disorders in children. Semin Pediatr Surg. 2006;15:116–23.
14. Rand PK, Ball WS Jr, Kulwin DR. Congenital nasolacrimal mucoceles: CT evaluation. Radiology. 1989;173:691–4. https://doi.org/10.1148/radiology.173.3.2813773.
15. Shashy RG, Durairaj VD, Holmes JM, Hohberger GG, Thompson DM, Kasperbauer JL. Congenital dacryocystocele associated with intranasal cysts: diagnosis and management. Laryngoscope. 2003;113:37–40. https://doi.org/10.1097/00005537-200301000-00007.
16. Yin T, van der Meer G. Neonatal airway obstruction in bilateral congenital dacryocystocoele: case report and review of the literature. Int J Pediatr Otorhinolaryngol. 2017;92:161–4. https://doi.org/10.1016/j.ijporl.2016.11.027.
17. Kallen K. Maternal smoking, body mass index, and neural tube defects. Am J Epidemiol. 1998;147:1103–11.
18. Rahbar R, Resto VA, Robson CD, Perez-Atayde AR, Goumnerova LC, McGill TJ, et al. Nasal glioma and encephalocele: diagnosis, and management. Laryngoscope. 2003;113:2069–77.
19. Phillips CD. Neuroradiologic imaging in craniofacial surgery. In: Lin KY, Ogle RC, Jane JA, editors. Craniofacial surgery: science and surgical technique. Philadelphia: Saunders; 2002. p. 153–60.
20. Marshall AH, Jones NS, Robertson IJA. Endoscopic management of basal encephaloceles. J Laryngol Otol. 2001;115:545–7.
21. Hughes GB, Sharpino G, Hunt W, et al. Management of the congenital midline nasal mass—a review. Head Neck Surg. 1980;2:222–33.
22. Messner AH, Richardson MA, editors. Cummings otolaryngology-head and neck surgery.
23. Littlewood AH. Congenital nasal dermoid cysts and fistulas. Plast Reconstr Surg Transplant Bull. 1961;27:471–88.
24. Ni K, Li X, Zhao L, Jiali W, Liu X, Shi H. Diagnosis and treatment of congenital nasal dermoid and sinus cysts in 11 infants. Medicine (Baltimore). 2020;99(21):e19435. Published online 2020 May 22. https://doi.org/10.1097/MD.0000000000019435.
25. Pierre Robin syndrome. MedlinePlus. 29 Oct 2013. http://www.nlm.nih.gov/medlineplus/ency/article/001607.htm.
26. Isolated Pierre Robin sequence. Genetics Home Reference (GHR). Aug 2013. https://ghr.nlm.nih.gov/condition/isolated-pierre-robin-sequence.
27. Treacher Collins syndrome. Genetics Home Reference. Jun 2012. http://ghr.nlm.nih.gov/condition/treacher-collins-syndrome. Accessed 27 Oct 2014.
28. Vazquez M-P. Treacher Collins syndrome. Orphanet. Jan 2014. http://www.orpha.net/consor/cgi-bin/OC_Exp.php?lng=en&Expert=861. Accessed 27 Oct 2014.
29. Crouzon syndrome. Genetics Home Reference. Feb 2008. http://ghr.nlm.nih.gov/condition/crouzon-syndrome. Accessed 7 Nov 2015.

30. Arnaud E, Collett C, Di Rocco F. Crouzon disease. Orphanet. Nov 2013. http://www.orpha.net/consor/cgi-bin/OC_Exp.php?lng=en&Expert=207.
31. O'Neill MJF. Crouzon syndrome. OMIM. 18 Mar 2016. http://www.omim.org/entry/123500.
32. Shott SR. Down syndrome: common otolaryngologic manifestations. Am J Med Genet. 2006;142C:131. https://doi.org/10.1002/ajmg.c.30095.
33. Gazi SR, Manu PS, Vijayalakshmi S. Apert's syndrome—a rare craniofacial anomaly. Southeast Asian J Case Rep Rev. 2014;3:645–67.
34. Satyanand T, Sachin K, Mohit S. Etiology, symptoms and treatment of Apert syndrome, a congenital disorder: an overview. Int J Pharm Bio Sci. 2010;1:1–7.
35. Garcia E, Osterbauer B, Parham D, Koempel J. The incidence of microscopic thyroglossal duct tissue superior to the hyoid bone. Laryngoscope. 2019;129(5):1215–7.
36. Ma J, Ming C, Lou F, Wang ML, Lin K, Zeng WJ, Li ZC, Liu XF, Zhang TS. Misdiagnosic analysis and treatment of pyriform sinus fistula in children. Zhonghua Er Bi Yan Hou Tou Jing Wai Ke Za Zhi. 2018;53(5):381–4.
37. Ross J, Manteghi A, Rethy K, Ding J, Chennupati SK. Thyroglossal duct cyst surgery: a ten-year single institution experience. Int J Pediatr Otorhinolaryngol. 2017;101:132–6.
38. Povey HG, Selvachandran H, Peters RT, Jones MO. Management of suspected thyroglossal duct cysts. J Pediatr Surg. 2018;53(2):281–2.
39. Pucher B, Jonczyk-Potoczna K, Kaluzna-Mlynarczyk A, Kurzawa P, Szydlowski J. The central neck dissection or the modified Sistrunk procedure in the treatment of the thyroglossal duct cysts in children: our experience. Biomed Res Int. 2018;2018:8016957.
40. Rutter MJ. Congenital laryngeal anomalies. Braz J Otorhinolaryngol. 2014;80(6):533–9.
41. Richter GT, Wooten CT, Rutter MJ, Thompson DM. Impact of supraglottoplasty on aspiration in severe laryngomalacia. Ann Otol Rhinol Laryngol. 2009;118:259–66.
42. Loke D, Ghosh S, Panarese A, et al. Endoscopic division of the aryepiglottic folds in severe laryngomalacia. Int J Pediatr Otorhinolaryngol. 2001;60:59–63.
43. Senders CW, Navarete EG. Laser supraglottoyplasty for laryngomalacia; are specific anatomical defects more influential than associated anomalies on the outcome? Int J Pediatr Otorhinolaryngol. 2001;57:235–44.
44. Gandhi S, Oswal V, Thekedar P, et al. Role of transoral CO2 laser surgery for severe pediatric laryngomalacia. Eur Arch Otorrinolaringol. 2011;268:1479–83.
45. Miyamoto RC, Parikh SR, Gellad W, Licameli GR. Bilateral congenital vocal cord paralysis: a 16-year institutional review. Otolaryngol Head Neck Surg. 2005;133:241–5.
46. Choi SS, Tran LP, Zalzal GH. Airway abnormalities in patients with Arnold-Chiari malformation. Otolaryngol Head Neck Surg. 1999;121:720–4.
47. Ada M, Isildak H, Saritzali G. Congenital vocal cord paralysis. J Craniofac Surg. 2010;21(1):273.
48. Hartnick CJ, Brigger MT, Willging JP, Cotton RT, Myer CM 3rd. Surgery for pediatric vocal cord paralysis: a retrospective review. Ann Otol Rhinol Laryngol. 2003;112:1–6.
49. Trey LA, Lambercy K, Monnier P, Sandu K. Management of severe congenital webs-12 year review. Int J Pediatr Otorhinolaryngol. 2016;86:82–6.
50. Cohen SR. Congenital glottic webs in children. A retrospective review of 51 patients. Ann Otol Rhinol Laryngol Suppl. 1985;121:2–16.
51. Avelino MAG, Pazinatto DB, Rodrigues SO, Maunsell R. Congenital laryngeal webs: from diagnosis to surgical outcomes. Braz J Otrhinolaryngol. 2022;88:497.
52. Hartnick CJ, Cotton RT. Congenital laryngeal anomalies. Laryngeal atresia, stenosis, webs, and clefts. Otolaryngol Clin N Am. 2000;33(6):1293–308.
53. Tesmera P, Wróblewska-Seniuka K, Mazelaa J, Szydłowskib J. Congenital laryngeal stenosis and concomitant birth defects in a term newborn: a case report. Biomed Hub. 2020;5:1.
54. Blanchard M, Leboulanger N, Thierry B, Blancal JP, Glynn F, Denoyelle F, et al. Management specificities of congenital laryngeal stenosis: external and endoscopic approaches. Laryngoscope. 2014;124(4):1013–8.
55. Myer CM 3rd, O'Connor DM, Cotton RT. The proposed grading system for subglottic stenosis is based on endotracheal tube sizes. Ann Otol Rhinol Laryngol. 1994;103:319–23.

56. Morrissey MS, Bailey CM. Diagnosis and management of subglottic stenosis after neonatal ventilation. Arch Dis Child. 1990;65(10):1103–4.
57. Orlow SJ, Isakoff MS, Blei F. Increased risk of symptomatic hemangiomas of the airway in association with cutaneous hemangiomas in a beard distribution. J Pediatr. 1997;131:643–6.
58. Janfaza P, Montgomery WW, Randolph GW. Anterior regions of the neck. In: Janfaza P, Nadol JB, Galla R, Fabian RL, Montgomery WW, editors. Surgical anatomy of the head and neck. Philadelphia, PA: Lippincott Williams & Wilkins; 2001. p. 629–74.
59. Cotton RT, Prescott CAJ. Congenital anomalies of the larynx. In: Cotton RT, Myer III CM, editors. Practical pediatric otolaryngology. Philadelphia, PA: Lippincott-Raven Publishers; 1999. p. 497–513.
60. Benjamin B, Inglis A. Minor congenital laryngeal clefts: diagnosis and classification. Ann Otol Rhinol Laryngol. 1989;98:417–20.
61. Evans JG. Management of the cleft larynx and tracheoesophageal clefts. Ann Otol Rhinol Laryngol. 1985;94:627–30.
62. Donahoe PK, Gee PE. Complete laryngotracheoesophageal cleft: management and repair. J Pediatr Surg. 1984;19:143–8.
63. Froehlich P, Truy E, Stamm D, Morgan A, Floret D, Chappuis JP. Cleft larynx: management and one-stage surgical repair by anterior translaryngotracheal approach in two children. Int J Pediatr Otorhinolaryngol. 1993;27:73–8.
64. Cotton RT, Schreiber JT. Management of laryngotracheoesophageal cleft. Ann Otol Rhinol Laryngol. 1981;90:401–5.

Immunological Defense Mechanisms of the Respiratory System

5

Neslihan Edeer Karaca, Ayse Aygun, and Tsvetelina Velikova

The respiratory tract continuously faces inhaled air containing microbial organisms, airborne pollutants, particles, noxious gases, and allergens. The pulmonary immune system must also cope with potentially harmful threats and react rapidly to protect the host [1–3]. Different physical, secretory, and cellular factors are involved in the immune response in the lung parenchyma and airways, constituting the two functional areas of the respiratory system.

The airway epithelium and submucosa serve as the respiratory primary defense system as both a mechanical and immunological barrier [4]. Pulmonary host defense has evolved innate and specific immune mechanisms. The airway epithelium mainly comprises ciliated columnar cells and secretory (goblet) cells that provoke mucociliary elimination of inhaled antigens. Apart from providing a physical barrier, the epithelium is immunologically active by secreting diverse antimicrobial peptides, releasing chemokines, cytokines, and growth factors, modulating adaptive immunity, and remodeling with tissue repair. In the mucosa, there are macrophages, dendritic cells (DCs), plasma cells, innate lymphoid cells (ILC), natural killer (NK) cells, and T lymphocytes [1–3]. Epithelial T lymphocytes in the mucosa are mainly $CD8^+$ T cells; in the lamina propria, $CD4^+$ T cells are abundant [1, 3, 5]. There are also areas of lymphoid tissue (LT) in the airway mucosa, namely, nasal mucosa-associated LT (NALT) and bronchus-associated LT (BALT) [6]. This tissue is not encapsulated and is in direct contact with epithelial mucosa. In the lung parenchyma, there are alveolar macrophages and small proportions of T and B lymphocytes and dendritic cells. Innate and adaptive immunity have significant protective and therapeutic roles against infections and inflammation in the respiratory tract (Fig. 5.1).

N. E. Karaca (✉) · A. Aygun
Department of Pediatric Immunology, Ege University Faculty of Medicine, Izmir, Türkiye

T. Velikova
Sofia University, Faculty of Medicine, "St. Kliment Ohridski", Sofia, Bulgaria

H. Yüksel et al. (eds.), *Pediatric Airway Diseases*, Comprehensive ENT,
https://doi.org/10.1007/978-3-031-74853-0_5

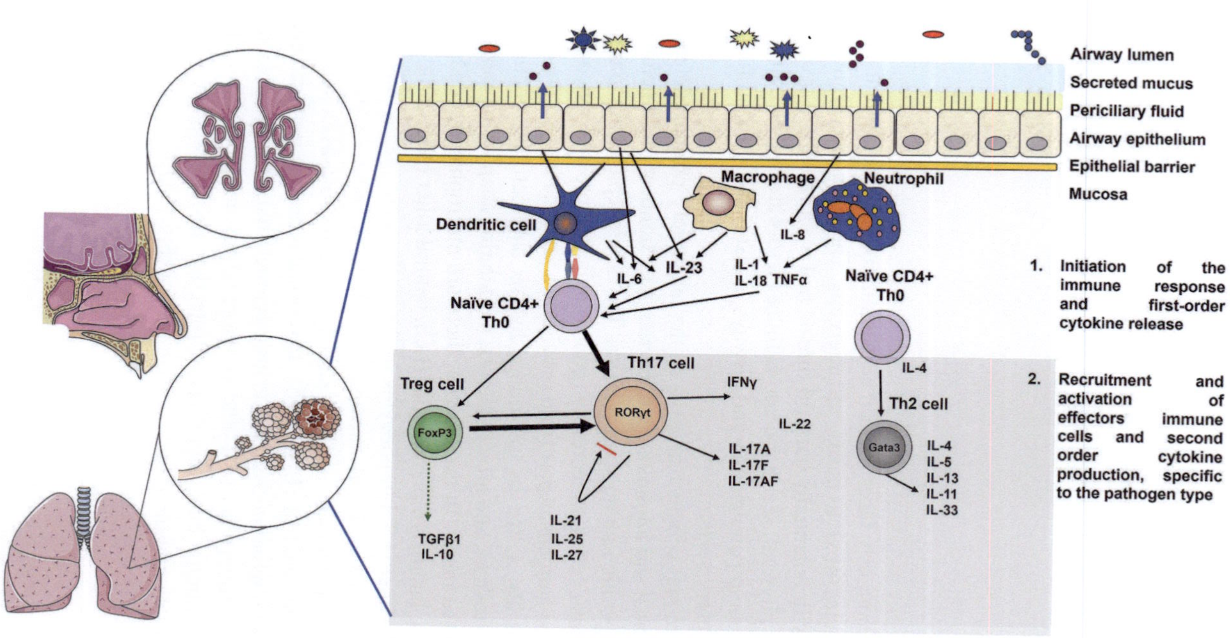

Fig. 5.1 Immune response in the respiratory tract. Mucosa in the upper and lower airways is constantly exposed to environmental and infectious agents, such as LPS, flagellin, pilin, and other bacterial antigens, as well as various allergens (dust, etc.). Epithelial cells are central in defending respiratory mucosal membrane by both secreting type I and II interferons, lactoferrin, defensins, nitric oxide, etc. into the airway lumen, and communicating with the immune cells in the mucosa by releasing chemokines (such as MP-1, IL-8, MCP-1, and RANTES) and cytokines (IL-6, IL-1b, TNF-α, etc.) to activate immune cells into the mucosa. Epithelial cells along with macrophages, dendritic cells, mast cells, and neutrophils are the first line of defense, involved in direct pathogen clearance (via IFN-γ production, phagocytosis, etc.) and via direct attraction, recruitment, and activation of effector cells (innate lymphoid cells, tissue-resident T cells, NK, and NKT cells). This two-tiered immune response eventually leads to pathogen clearance and tissue repair. Furthermore, because of the proinflammatory signals, naïve T cells along with FoxP3+ T regulatory cells predominantly differentiate into Th17 cells, which are engaged in the clearance of pathogens. (Parts of the figure were drawn by using pictures from Servier Medical Art. Servier Medical Art by Servier, licensed under a Creative Commons Attribution 3.0 Unported License. https://creativecommons.org/licenses/by/3.0/)

5.1 Innate Immunity

The initial phase of lung defense involves the innate immune system, including defensive structures throughout the airway lumen and lung parenchyma, antimicrobial agents, alveolar macrophages, DCs, neutrophils, NK cells, and ILCs [1–3].

1. The *airway epithelium* is at the interface of the human body between the external inhaled environment and the internal tissues. It forms a complex physicochemical and mechanical barrier supplemented by mucociliary clearance to provide the first line of defense against inhaled pathogens. The airway mucus covering the respiratory tract's luminal surface entraps inhaled pathogens, including infectious agents, and eliminates them by the coordinated beating of the cilia. Epithelial cells maintain epithelial integrity by attaching to their neighbors by tight junctions, adherens junctions, gap junctions, and desmosomes [7]. These structures form an impermeable and effective mechanical barrier to most pathogens and permit the maintenance of an ionic gradient for the directional exchange of many nutrients, water, and gases [7, 8]. The upper airway epithelial cells efficiently prevent microparticles >10 μm and a large percentage of particles >5 μm from reaching the lower airways via direct prevention of their passage through the nasopharyngeal mucosa [8, 9]. The particles entrapped are either exhaled with cough or ingested with mucus into the gastrointestinal tract. If pathogens crack structural defenses, the innate immune system mediators of the upper respiratory tract, including salivary lysozyme, peroxidase, and lactoferrin, function with antimicrobial activity. Lower respiratory system airways are also lined with epithelial cells and beating cilia. Approximately 90% of particles >2–3 μm trapped within the mucus are transported through the mucociliary escalator from the bronchioles to the trachea and exhaled with the help of a cough [7].
2. The *airway mucus* is a viscoelastic gel secreted continuously by intraepithelial goblet cells and by mucous cells of submucosal glands toward the surface of the epithelium. The airway lining fluid is composed of different proteins, such as *mucins and antimicrobial substances* (lysozyme, lactoferrin, and defensins), cytokines, antiproteases, and antioxidant proteins [10–12]. The airway damage can be induced from microbes as well as from several factors that are produced during inflammatory reactions and phagocytosis. *Lysozyme* destroys the walls of the microbes and fungus. It also has the protective role of inhibiting the destructive effects of oxidative factors produced during inflammation [13].

   Defensins are cationic peptides secreted by neutrophils (α-defensin) and epithelial cells (β-defensins) [10]. These peptides exhibit antimicrobial activity against various types of bacteria, mycobacteria, fungi, and some enveloped viruses by promoting chemokine production and subsequent migration of host inflammatory cells, inducing phagocytosis, complement activation, and $CD4^+$ T-cell proliferation [10, 13]. *Lactoferin* can bind with iron and prevent the utilization of elemental iron by pathogenic bacteria [14, 15].

   Collectins, or collagen-like lectins, are another family of small proteins with important anti-pathogen properties [16]. Their role is to inhibit the invasion of epithelial cells by several respiratory viruses and facilitate the phagocytosis and subsequent clearance of target microorganisms. These molecules exhibit a wide range of specificities. They interact with pathogens through their lectin domains and regulate the functions of T lymphocytes, macrophages, dendritic cells, and neutrophils. Important collectins are the mannose-binding lectin (MBL) and surfactant proteins A and D [16–18]. Collectins cannot destroy microbes directly; they are responsible for enhancing macrophage phagocytosis.

3. The respiratory tract *microbiome*, a collection of microorganisms (bacteria, viruses, fungi, and archaea) residing in the respiratory mucosa, maintains a symbiotic relationship with the host. It acts as a barrier against the invasion of pathogens and plays an essential role in maintaining the balance between immune tolerance and inflammation [19].
4. Mast cells and plasma cells, which secrete IgA, are among the primary cells present in the lamina propria. The *secretory IgA* barrier facilitates the beneficial local microbiome's permanence and helps to eliminate noxious agents, such as pathogens and pollutant particles, by inhibiting their adherence to the epithelium [15].
5. *Complement*, a complex protein system, is a critical component of the innate immune response. The complement system plays a crucial role in the defense against invading pathogens through bacterial lysis, stimulation of phagocytosis, the recruitment of immune cells to infected tissue, and the promotion of the inflammatory response. Although complement is well characterized in the serum, complement activity is also present in the lung [20]. Alveolar macrophages and pulmonary alveolar type II epithelial cells synthesize and secrete complement proteins C2, C3, C4, C5, and Factor B, whereas bronchiolar epithelial cells can generate C3 [21]. Once complement is activated by the hydrocarbons on the outer membrane of the microorganisms or the collectins, the cascade leads to cell death by the final formation of the lytic membrane attack complex (C5–C9), which forms pores on the target cell membrane.
6. If the microorganism overcomes the mucociliary escalator and defensive proteins, it reaches its target, the *respiratory epithelial cells*. As mentioned before, these cells act as an effective mechanical barrier to the microorganism entry and dissemination into the submucosa. Respiratory epithelial cells produce antimicrobial and immunomodulatory molecules such as interferons, lactoferrin, and defensins. These cells express receptors within the basolateral epithelial membrane, serving as an entry site for several viruses. Under steady-state conditions, the epithelial cells of both the bronchi and the alveoli have essential roles in maintaining tolerance by producing the anti-inflammatory cytokines interleukin (IL)-10 and TGF-β [19]. In case of exposure to exogenous microorganisms or tissue damage of any sort, the airway epithelium senses antigens via pattern recognition receptors (PRR) such as Toll-like receptors (TLR), RIG-I-like receptors (RLR), Nod-like receptors (NLR), and C-type lectin receptors [22–24]. When PRRs recognize the molecular structures common to pathogens, called pathogen-associated molecular patterns (PAMPs), they activate intracellular down-stream signaling pathways that ultimately result in the translocation of

NF-kB from the cytoplasm to the nucleus and the transcription of chemokines and proinflammatory cytokines (IL)-8, monocyte chemotactic protein-1, lymphocyte chemoattractant factor (IL-16), IL-6, IL-8, and interferon (IFN)-β. Subsequently, adhesion molecules increase to attract neutrophils and macrophages to the inflammatory site.

7. Professional antigen-presenting cells (APC), such as *DCs and alveolar macrophages* in the lungs, are vital in directing adaptive immune responses to inflammation, which infectious pathogens invade or tolerate after most environmental exposures and commensals [25]. They detect PAMPs through PRRs and release chemoattractant and inflammatory cytokines, including tumor necrosis factor-alpha (TNF-α), IL-1β, IL-12, and IL-6, into the alveolar space. IL-12 augments NK cell activity microenvironmentally, and large amounts of IFN-γ secreted by NK cells enhance the antimicrobial function of the alveolar macrophages [26]. The microorganisms captured by APCs are subsequently transported to the draining hilar and mediastinal lymph nodes to commence an adaptive immune response. Dendritic cells and alveolar macrophages present epitopes of ingested pathogens through endocytosis or phagocytosis on major histocompatibility complex class I (MHC-I) or MHC-II protein complex to naïve $CD8^+$ or $CD4^+$ T cells, respectively. The second set of signals delivered via costimulatory molecules expressed on the cell surface of activated APCs activates T cells, initiating an adaptive immune response.
8. *ILCs* are innate immune cells belonging to the lymphoid lineage but lacking adaptive antigen-specific receptors [27]. Depending on their ability to synthesize and release cytokines and their transcription factor profile, ILCs are divided into three major helper-like subsets, ILC1, ILC2, and ILC3, which are considered the innate counterparts of T helper 1 (Th1), Th2, and Th17 cells, respectively. ILC1 cells, which include NK cells, secrete IFN-γ and TNF-α, and express the T-box transcription factor T-bet or eomesodermin (Eomes). ILC2 cells produce IL-4, IL-5, IL-9, and IL-13 in response to IL-25, IL-33, and thymic stromal lymphopoietin and express high levels of the Th2 signature transcription factor GATA-3. ILC3 cells release IL-17, IL-22, and GM-CSF at mucosal sites, functioning as early orchestrators of lung tissue remodeling and fibrogenesis. Although representing a small portion of the pulmonary immune cells, ILCs play a significant role in early protective antimicrobial responses and facilitate the acquisition of adaptive immunity. They also play pathogenic roles in inflammation, allergy, autoimmunity, and tissue fibrosis [28].
9. *Neutrophils* are recruited rapidly to the site of inflammation following stimulation by chemotactic factors such as chemokines (CXCL1–8, CXCL-12, CCL2, and CCL17), lipid mediators (eicosanoids/leukotrienes), C5a, and interleukins (i.e., IL-8) released from the damaged lung tissues [29]. They localize mainly in the bronchoalveolar space, engaging in short-term host–pathogen interactions. Activated neutrophils eliminate microorganisms by phagocytosis, oxidative burst, degranulation, and by means of NETosis (neutrophil extracellular traps formation) [1, 29].

5.2 Adaptive Immunity

Adaptive immunity involves a tightly regulated interplay between antigen-presenting cells and the effectors, T and B lymphocytes, which facilitate pathogen-specific immunologic effector pathways, immunologic memory generation, and regulation of host immune homeostasis. Cell-mediated immunity is controlled by T cells, and humoral immunity is controlled by antibody-producing B cells. Highly mobile lymphocytes traffic to secondary lymphoid organs after developing in the primary lymphoid organs (thymus and bone marrow) and serve to capture circulating antigens from lymph. T cells are primed in the lymphoid areas, often influenced by innate immune system signals provided by APCs migrating to the secondary lymphoid organs. Naive lymphocytes undergo a stepwise process of activation, proliferation, clonal expansion, and differentiation to become effector cells that can migrate to the lung and mediate antimicrobial immune responses [30].

The activation of T helper cells by APC causes them to differentiate into different subtypes with specific functions mediated by cytokine secretion and cell-to-cell contact. T helper 1 cells secrete cytokines such as IFN-γ, IL-6, and IL-12 and play a crucial role in cellular response formation [15]. Th2 cells help humoral responses by providing a second signal to B cells, mostly through IL-4 secretion and CD40/CD40L interaction. During the first encounter with an antigen (pathogen), long-lived memory T and B cells are established. In subsequent encounters with the same pathogen, the memory cells are quickly activated to yield a more rapid and robust protective response. The activated B cells secrete antibodies circulating in the body and coat the microbes, targeting them for efficient phagocytosis. T follicular helper cells (Tfh) control the critical interactions in the germinal centers essential for the maturation of memory B cells and long-lived high-affinity antibody-producing plasma cells [31]. Another subset of $CD4^+$ T cells differentiates into a pool of memory T helper cells. Activated $CD8^+$ cytotoxic T lymphocytes (CTL) cause apoptosis of the infected host cells. Some CTLs differentiate into memory cytotoxic T cells, which have the role of fast restoration of the CTL response with secondary antigen contacts. A similar destruction mechanism occurs when NK cells interact with the virally infected cell [31]. They contain granules with IFN-γ and TNF-α in their cytoplasm. NK cells form pores in the membranes of target cells by perforin. Granzymes pass through the pores, and together with cytokines, they initiate apoptosis, resulting in the death of infected cells.

After the control of infection, clones from the antigen induces the infection to circulate, creating lymphocytes that are specific to the circulating antigen. Initially, these lymphocytes are observed in small populations; however, they can act fast upon the recolonization of the known antigen, giving the immune system the time to produce more specific lymphocytes.

Lymphocytes can be found either singly or in clusters in the airway lamina propria and the submucosa [3, 15]. Effector and memory $CD4^+$ and $CD8^+$ T cells and B cells are present in the airway mucosa (in the intraepithelial and within the underlying lamina propria). They may play a role in the constitution of BALT, which has a significant role in local immunological homeostasis in the respiratory tract. Most intraepithelial T cells express CD8+, whereas CD4+ T cells are more frequently found in the lamina propria. B cells contribute to local antigen presentation in the lymph nodes that drain the lungs. Some B cells differentiate into plasma cells. Plasma cells located in the lamina propia mainly produce IgA but also IgM to clear inhaled pathogens [32, 33]. IgG subclasses are also present in the alveoli and airway secretions.

The lungs are a major site of entry of innocuous inhaled antigens and presumably by commensal microorganisms into the body. The absolute requirement of the pulmonary immune system is to limit the infectious and inflammatory consequences of inhaled agents while maintaining tolerance to harmless aeroallergens. The immune response in the lung must be tightly regulated such that pathogens are cleared. Furthermore, immunopathology due to chronic or excessive inflammation is avoided. Critical antimicrobial monitoring and downregulation of the activated immune response are vital to protect the lung from inflammatory damage. The immune homeostasis and tolerance in the lung are maintained by a complex network of cells and molecules interacting with lung stromal cells, such as regulatory T cells (Tregs), resident interstitial lung macrophages, plasmacytoid dendritic cells, γδT cells, cytokines IL-10, and TGF-β [33–35]. The coordinated and close interplay between resident (airway epithelial cells) and infiltrating immune cells is important to establish the protective respiratory innate and adaptive immune responses.

References

1. Nicod LP. Lung defenses: an overview. Eur Respir Rev. 2005;14:45.
2. Wilmott RW, Khurana-Hershey G, Stark JM. Current concepts on pulmonary host defense mechanisms in children. Curr Opin Pediatr. 2000;12(3):187–93.
3. Chaudhuri N, Sabroe I. Basic science of the innate immune system and the lung. Paediatr Respir Rev. 2008;9(4):236–42.
4. Denney L, Ho LP. The role of respiratory epithelium in host defense against influenza virus infection. Biomed J. 2018;41(4):218–33.
5. Naderi W, Schreiner D, King CG. T-cell-B-cell collaboration in the lung. Curr Opin Immunol. 2023;81:102284.
6. Heier I, Malmström K, Sajantila A, Lohi J, Mäkelä M, Jahnsen FL. Characterisation of bronchus-associated lymphoid tissue and antigen-presenting cells in central airway mucosa of children. Thorax. 2011;66(2):151–6.
7. Bustamante-Marin XM, Ostrowski LE. Cilia and mucociliary clearance. Cold Spring Harb Perspect Biol. 2017;9(4):a028241.
8. Tsai KS, Grayson MH. Pulmonary defense mechanisms against pneumonia and sepsis. Curr Opin Pulm Med. 2008;14(3):260–5.
9. Fokkens WJ, Scheeren RA. Upper airway defence mechanisms. Paediatr Respir Rev. 2000;1(4):336–41.
10. Zhang P, Summer WR, Bagby GJ, Nelson S. Innate immunity and pulmonary host defense. Immunol Rev. 2000;173:39–51.
11. Ridley C, Thornton DJ. Mucins: the frontline defence of the lung. Biochem Soc Trans. 2018;46(5):1099–106.
12. Devine DA. Antimicrobial peptides in defence of the oral and respiratory tracts. Mol Immunol. 2003;40(7):431–43.
13. Laube DM, Yim S, Ryan LK, Kisich KO, Diamond G. Antimicrobial peptides in the airway. Curr Top Microbiol Immunol. 2006;306:153–82.

14. Campione E, Cosio T, Rosa L, Lanna C, Di Girolamo S, Gaziano R, Valenti P, Bianchi L. Lactoferrin as protective natural barrier of respiratory and intestinal mucosa against coronavirus infection and inflammation. Int J Mol Sci. 2020;21(14):4903.
15. Iwasaki A, Foxman EF, Molony RD. Early local immune defences in the respiratory tract. Nat Rev Immunol. 2017;17(1):7–20.
16. Sano H, Kuroki Y. The lung collectins, SP-A and SP-D, modulate pulmonary innate immunity. Mol Immunol. 2005;42(3):279–87.
17. Kishore U, Greenhough TJ, Waters P, Shrive AK, Ghai R, Kamran MF, Bernal AL, Reid KB, Madan T, Chakraborty T. Surfactant proteins SP-A and SP-D: structure, function and receptors. Mol Immunol. 2006;43(9):1293–315.
18. Nayak A, Dodagatta-Marri E, Tsolaki AG, Kishore U. An insight into the diverse roles of surfactant proteins, SP-A and SP-D in innate and adaptive immunity. Front Immunol. 2012;3:131.
19. Rogers GB. The lung microbiome. Emerg Top Life Sci. 2017;1(4):313–24.
20. Varsano S, Kaminsky M, Kaiser M, Rashkovsky L. Generation of complement C3 and expression of cell membrane complement inhibitory proteins by human bronchial epithelium cell line. Thorax. 2000;55(5):364–9.
21. Strunk RC, Eidlen DM, Mason RJ. Pulmonary alveolar type II epithelial cells synthesize and secrete proteins of the classical and alternative complement pathways. J Clin Invest. 1988;81(5):1419–26.
22. Bauer RN, Diaz-Sanchez D, Jaspers I. Effects of air pollutants on innate immunity: the role of Toll-like receptors and nucleotide-binding oligomerization domain-like receptors. J Allergy Clin Immunol. 2012;129(1):14–26.
23. Le J, Kulatheepan Y, Jeyaseelan S. Role of toll-like receptors and nod-like receptors in acute lung infection. Front Immunol. 2023;14:1249098.
24. Takeda K, Kaisho T, Akira S. Toll-like receptors. Annu Rev Immunol. 2003;21:335–76.
25. Byrne AJ, Mathie SA, Gregory LG, Lloyd CM. Pulmonary macrophages: key players in the innate defence of the airways. Thorax. 2015;70(12):1189–96.
26. Lai HC, Chang CJ, Lin CS, Wu TR, Hsu YJ, Wu TS, Lu JJ, Martel J, Ojcius DM, Ku CL, Young JD, Lu CC. NK cell-derived IFN-γ protects against nontuberculous mycobacterial lung infection. J Immunol (Baltimore, MD: 1950). 2018;201(5):1478–90.
27. Mjösberg J, Spits H. Human innate lymphoid cells. J Allergy Clin Immunol. 2016;138(5):1265–76.
28. Mikami Y, Takada Y, Hagihara Y, Kanai T. Innate lymphoid cells in organ fibrosis. Cytokine Growth Factor Rev. 2018;42:27–36.
29. Effah CY, Drokow EK, Agboyibor C, Ding L, He S, Liu S, Akorli SY, Nuamah E, Sun T, Zhou X, Liu H, Xu Z, Feng F, Wu Y, Zhang X. Neutrophil-dependent immunity during pulmonary infections and inflammations. Front Immunol. 2021;12:689866.
30. Hasenberg M, Stegemann-Koniszewski S, Gunzer M. Cellular immune reactions in the lung. Immunol Rev. 2013;251(1):189–214.
31. Pilette C, Ouadrhiri Y, Godding V, Vaerman JP, Sibille Y. Lung mucosal immunity: immunoglobulin-A revisited. Eur Respir J. 2001;18(3):571–88.
32. Lee CM, Oh JE. Resident memory B cells in barrier tissues. Front Immunol. 2022;13:953088.
33. Allard B, Panariti A, Martin JG. Alveolar macrophages in the resolution of inflammation, tissue repair, and tolerance to infection. Front Immunol. 2018;9:1777.
34. Xu J, Xiao N, Zhou D, Xie L. Disease tolerance: a protective mechanism of lung infections. Front Cell Infect Microbiol. 2023;13:1037850.
35. Kawasaki T, Ikegawa M, Kawai T. Antigen presentation in the lung. Front Immunol. 2022;13:860915.

Innate and Adaptive Immunity of the Respiratory System

6

Esra Hazar, Mehmet Ali Karaselek, and Sevgi Keles

6.1 Introduction

The respiratory tract (RT) is a complex system that provides gas exchange and oxygenation of the blood, while at the same time forming a physical and immunological barrier between the external environment and tissues. Hereby, the respiratory tracts are constantly exposed to inhaled agents including allergens, pollutants, commensal or pathogenic microorganisms, and respiratory pathogens [1]. The RT compromises the upper (URT) and lower respiratory tracts (LRT), and drains the localized lymphoid tissue including cervical and mediastinal lymph nodes to start a localized immune response against antigens. The tract is covered with a barrier that is composed of a mucus layer, cilia, and airway epithelial cells. The first line of defense starts in URT or LRT by interaction between environmental agents and this barrier in the respiratory tract. This barrier is supported by a complex network of immune systems which is composed of innate and adaptive immune systems. These systems recognize and react to a wide variety of stimuli. They also eliminate unwanted pathogens to keep the tract free from infections. This system also regulates maximizing pathogen clearance while minimizing excessive inflammation and tissue injury. Maintaining balance in the respiratory tract during injury or infection is crucial to host survival [2]. The distribution of these protective mechanisms contributes to the pathogenesis of many pulmonary diseases. Many diseases, such as asthma, allergies, and acute or chronic lung diseases, result from dysregulated responses in the airways. In addition, numerous infectious agents, including viral, bacterial,

E. Hazar
Pediatric Allergy and Immunology Unit, Faculty of Medicine, Alanya Alaaddin Keykubat University, Antalya, Turkey

M. A. Karaselek · S. Keles (✉)
Pediatric Allergy and Immunology Unit, Faculty of Medicine, Necmettin Erbakan University, Konya, Turkey

H. Yüksel et al. (eds.), *Pediatric Airway Diseases*, Comprehensive ENT, https://doi.org/10.1007/978-3-031-74853-0_6

fungal, and protozoan, target airway cells for replication, then cause direct damage to barrier sites by triggering inflammation-related tissue damage.

The respiratory immune system is composed of innate and adaptive immune systems. Less-virulent pathogens are generally obliterated by the primary defense like mucociliary clearance and alveolar macrophage, which is a part of innate immunity in the tract. Contrary, virulent microorganisms and most of the inhaled antigens/pathogens need to be eliminated by the inflammatory process initiated by the innate immune system. In the early phase of infection with a respiratory pathogen, there is a balance between pathogen clearance and immune response which is closely controlled by the epithelial immune cell axis. Dysregulation in this response can cause serious tissue damage. In the late stages of infection, a balance must be established between inflammation and tissue repair to recover proper lung function. On the other hand, dysregulated airway response to pathogens by innate and adaptive immune systems results in hyperinflammatory syndromes, site destruction in the respiratory tract leading to a sequela such as lung fibrosis. As a consequence, innate and adaptive pulmonary immune responses are strictly regulated to maintain this homeostasis following injury and infection [1]. Hence, knowing the role of adaptive and innate immune responses in the respiratory tract is important to understanding the pathophysiology and improving the management of respiratory diseases. Here, we have summarized various aspects of immune hemostasis which is regulated by innate and adaptive immune responses in the respiratory tract.

6.2 Innate Immunity

The innate immune system is the first line of defense against inhaled materials, and nonspecifically identifies the microorganisms by recognition of their common microbial motifs. Thus, it provides a nonspecific response against antigens. Innate immunity is contributed by epithelial cells, dendritic cells, macrophages, neutrophils, innate lymphoid cells, and monocytes, which respond rapidly to inhaled materials. Activation of these innate immunity cells induces the production of anti-microbial peptides, chemokines, and cytokines [2]. The intercellular communication between the airway and the immune cells is facilitated by complement factors, lipid mediators, chemo-attractants, and chemokines. The biological function of chemokines is relayed by different cytokines, including several interleukins and thymic stromal lymphopoietin (TSLP). These substances, secreted by local airway cells, generate customized immunological responses [2, 3]. Important components of theinnate immunity system in the respiratory tract are summarized in the following part of the chapter and in Fig. 6.1 [1].

6.2.1 Mucosal Immunity in the Respiratory System

The epithelium is the primary defense line against airborne harmful microorganisms. It captures particles in the air and removes them from the airways. The primary function of this epithelia is to be a physical boundary between the airways and

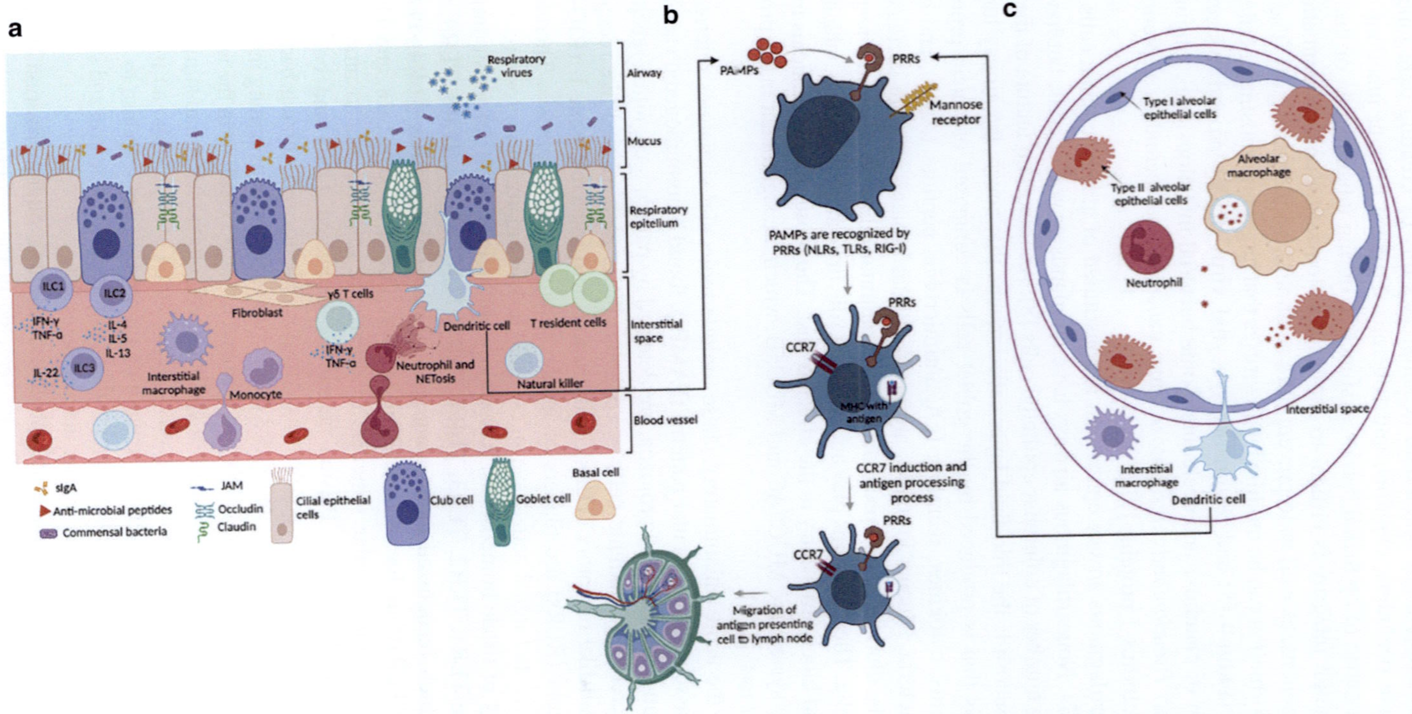

Fig. 6.1 Components and cells of innate immunity in the respiratory tract showing at the mucosal barrier (**a**), activation of antigen-presenting cells by antigens (**b**), and additional cells in the lower respiratory system (**c**)

vascular structures. The epithelium accomplishes this by creating tight junctions that include occludins, claudins, and adherens. Damage to tight junctions is an important cause of epithelial barrier dysfunction during inflammation of the lung. The epithelial integrity is critical to avoid the colonization and dissemination of microorganisms, as well as to prevent fluid accumulation in the lung [4]. The tight junction formation can be modified with viruses that target the epithelium. Influenza disrupts claudin-4 [5] and respiratory syncytial virus (RSV) [6] and reduces the expression of claudin-1 and occludins. Some bacterial infections, e.g., lung infection due to *Pseudomonas aeruginosa,* may cause edema secondary depletion of zonula occludins-1 proteins [7].

The cartilaginous airway epithelium is constituted of glands, ciliated cells, and goblet cells. Noncartilaginous airways have no glands or goblet cells, but have an increasing number of columnar epithelial cells [8]. An important feature of the pulmonary mucosa is the thin fluid layer called mucus that covers the airway lumen. The mucus that is produced by the goblet cells is composed of mucin proteins, complements, cytokines, secretory IgA, antimicrobial peptides (AMP), and commensal bacteria. Mucins in mucus are extra-cellular proteins that are secreted by goblet cells, club cells, and pseudostratified columnar ciliated cells of the respiratory epithelia. These proteins play an important role in viral transmission, which can capture and block virus entry in the affected host. The most prevalent mucins in the respiratory system are MUC5AC and MUC5B, which are significant in the protective barrier task [1, 9].

During the acute inflammatory phase, unique molecular signatures referred as pathogen-associated molecular patterns (PAMPs), found in immunogenic vaccines, bacteria, fungi, viruses, and protozoa, are detected by pattern recognition receptors (PRRs) secreted by immune cells of epithelia. PRRs such as Nod-like receptors (NLRs), Toll-like receptors (TLRs), and retinoic acid inducible gene I- (RIG-I-)-like receptors (RLRs) are players of innate immunity and apoptosis. Therefore, PR-intermediated signal paths have an essential task in inflammatory responses and the stability of tissue homeostasis. Respiratory epithelia and cells of innate immunity secrete TLR1, TLR2, TLR3, TLR4, TLR5, TLR6, TLR7, TLR8, TLR9, and TLR10, which recognized distinct antigens. While TLR1, TLR2, TLR4, TLR5, TLR6, and TLR10 are located at the cell surface, TLR3, TLR7, TLR8, and TLR9 are locatede in intracellular vesicules (endoplasmic reticulum, endosome, lysosome, and endolysosome). Plasma membrane-associated TLRs and endosome membrane-associated TLRs are primarily responsible for recognizing bacteria in the lung, while TLR3, TLR7, and TLR8 detect virus nucleic acids in lung infections [10]. Studies have shown that dsRNA recognized by TLR3 (such as in the influenza virus) was the most potent activator of epithelial cells in the lung, and stimulates a potent cytokine and chemokine response. TLR2 and TLR5 promote an increased response of the airway epithelium, leading to a more efficient response to bacteria and allergens. TLR4 is capable of recognizing Gram-negative bacteria and stimulating upregulation of TLR3 in alveolar macrophages [4].

Another subtype of PRRs is the nucleotide-binding oligomerization domain (NOD)-like receptors (NLRs). NLRs are secreted in the cytoplasm and nucleus.

There are more than 20 receptors in the NLR family. There are four kinds of effector domains with specific functional features that allow the NLR to be divided into five different subfamilies: NLRA, NLRB, NLRC, NLRP, and NLRX. The human NLRC is a subfamily of NLR composed of five members (NLRC1–5). NLRC1 and NLRC2, also called NOD1 and NOD2, are the two major components of the NLRC subfamily [10].

NOD1 is widely expressed in respiratory epithelia, endothelia, smooth muscles, and leukocytes. However, NOD2 expression is limited in myeloid cells, which include dendritic cells, macrophages, and human bronchial epithelial cells. Following ligand recognition, NLRC members induce the activation of distinct signaling paths through CARD–CARD interactions with several types of proteins. While NOD1 and NOD2 both recognize different ligands via leucine-rich repeat (LRR) domains, they act through the same protein called receptor-interacting serine/threonine-protein kinase 2 (RIPK2). RIPK2-mediated activation gives rise to the regulation of several pathways involved in different cellular responses, including inflammatory responses through nuclear factor kappa-light-chain-enhancer of activated B cells (NF-κB) and mitogen-activated protein kinase (MAPK) activation. NOD1 or NOD2 codependent induction of these paths can interfere with other PRRs, e.g., TLRs [11].

NLRP is the biggest NLR sub-family counting 14 members. At a minimum, five of the NLRP elements, including NLRP1, NLRP3, NLRP6, NLRP7, and NLRP12, can activate the generation of inflammasome, and modulate the release of IL1β and IL18 in response to different damage-associated molecular pattern (DAMP) or microbe-associated molecular pattern (MAMP). NLRP1 inflammasome is the first identified intracellular molecule capable of activating pro-caspase 1. NLRP3 is the well-characterized member of the NLRP sub-family, and the most studied inflammasome. The initial signal by DAMP or MAMP inflammatory stimulus induces NF-κB-mediated NLRP3 expression. Following the first signal, the NLRP3 stimulation is driven by a secondary signal, which is induced by a broad range of stimuli, in particular bacterially sourced molecules such as LPS, endogenous DAMP such as ATP, viral RNA, hyphae of fungi, or exposed to other environmentally irritating substances. NLRP1 is expressed in the digestive and respiratory epithelial immune cells and brain. NLRP3 is expressed in various immune cells (macrophages, dendritic cells, neutrophils, and T and B lymphocytes). In addition, NLRP3 is found in respiratory and intestinal epithelium [10, 11].

Antimicrobial peptides (AMPs) are widely expressed in the lung, serving as the initial defensive line for protection against infection. Defensins (alpha and beta), surfactant proteins, RegIIIγ, and LL-37 are some AMPs in the respiratory system. Defensins are primarily expressed in neutrophils and epithelial cells. Alpha defensins have a potent anti-viral impact by targeting viral particles and disrupting their capability to invade cells. Beta-defensins also act as chemokines, indirectly enhancing immunity to infections. LL-37 secreted by myeloid and epithelial cells is a member of the cathelicidin family. It has antimicrobial properties by inhibiting LPS and disrupting the bacterial membrane. It also promotes the expression of IL-8 and activation of the epithelial growth factor receptor (EGFR) in epithelial cells [4].

One other significant anti-microbial peptide is regenerating islet-derived 3 γ (RegIIIγ), which is particularly targeting Gram-positive bacteria. It is vital for the elimination of methicillin-resistant *Staphylococcus aureus* (MRSA) associated pneumonia. STAT3 regulates the expression of RegIIIγ, which is highly expressed in the lung epithelium during MRSA infection [12].

Surfactant proteins A (SP-A) and D (SP-D) are known to be members of the collectin AMP family. The binding of collectins to pathogens leads to opsonization and subsequent phagocytosis. SP-D has a potent anti-infective activity against influenza and is proposed as a promising treatment to boost mucosal immunity during influenza epidemics [13]. SP-C has been demonstrated to have immunomodulatory effects in lung repair through JAK/STAT activation after acute respiratory distress syndrome (ARDS) [14].

The complement system is composed of plasma proteins that serve as immune system effectors by inducing phagocytosis, increasing active inflammatory mediators, and targeting the pathogen's membrane [4]. Overactivation of complement may lead to damaged tissues. For example, H5N1 avian influenza has been reported to cause acute lung injury and ARDS by leading the hyperactivation of complement. In this model, the inhibition of complement activation helps to reduce injury in the lung [15].

6.2.1.1 Cells of Innate Immunity

The major cells of the innate immune system are epithelial cells, neutrophils, dendritic cells, macrophages, monocytes, and innate lymphoid cells. Alveolar epithelial cells (AECs) are one of the important cells of innate immunity in the lung. Both AEC I and AEC II coordinate different immune pathways to provide homeostasis in the lung. AEC I covers almost 99% of the lung surface area. Besides acting as a physical barrier, both AEC I and AEC II have a crucial role in the lung's immune response. However, AEC II is more immunologically active. These cells produce several immune factors such as cytokines and chemokines that are responsible for immune cell activation and differentiation. They act as antigen-presenting cells for specific T cells [2].

Macrophages are the other important cells of the innate immunity to response to infections. They express numerous surfaces, vesicular and cytosolic PRR to detect signals, and start appropriate immune responses. Following its activation, these cells phagocytize, directly kill infectious agents, then recruit other innate immune cells by releasing numerous cytokines and chemokines. After stimulation, in circulation, monocytes are differentiated into dendritic cells (DCs) or macrophages, and initiate innate immune response in the lung. On the other hand, tissue-resident macrophages are present in the lung. These macrophages are the initial responders and have significant tasks in homeostasis, immunomodulation, and tissue repair. Macrophages in the lungs are classified into two groups: alveolar macrophages (AMs) and interstitial macrophages (IMs). AMs are supposed to have a central role in a clearance of pathogens, while IMs act as a major immunomodulator of adaptive immunity because of their elevated expression of MHCII [4]. Both macrophages produce robust responses to a wide range of stimuli. AMs promote viral clearance during RSV and influenza infection. But AMs may not always be useful. In human metapneumovirus infection, AMs mediate an early entrance into the lung, and facilitate replication as well as the secretion of inflammatory factors, promoting lung pathology [16]. Furthermore, AMs are potential reservoirs of HIV-1, which disrupt the phagocytosis function of AMs, making patients prone to respiratory infections. As innate immune cells, AM is also responsible for maintaining a suppressed environment through the production of TGF-B that drives Treg development [17].

Dendritic cells (specialized antigen-presenting cells) present in the respiratory tract offer inhaled pathogens as the processed peptides to antigen-specific T cells before they migrate to the lymph nodes. DCs represent the intermediary between innate and adaptive immunity systems. They serve an important role in virus infections such as H1N1 or RSV by inducing the secretion of type I interferon and activating the adaptive immune mechanisms.

Neutrophils are involved in the early response of innate immunity. They are the predominant leukocytes in the circulation. They have both direct and indirect antimicrobial efficacies in innate immunity. They kill infectious agents directly using phagocytosis, by forming neutrophil extracellular traps (NETs), or by the activation of other innate immune cells like macrophages. Neutrophils are the early and more plentiful immune cells entering the respiratory system in acute inflammation. Neutrophils are involved in the removal of pathogens and cellular material from the airways mediated by phagocytosis, degranulation, and the release of NETs [1]. The formation of NETs, called NETosis, is a form of programmed death of neutrophils distinct from apoptotis and necrosis. NETosis, when deregulated, has been shown to exacerbate inflammation leading to microvascular thrombosis, and contributes to viral acute respiratory distress syndrome (ARDS) [18]. In human A/H1N1 and A/H7N9 influenza infection, NETs have been shown to increase the alveolar permeability and lead to disease aggravation. Elevated biomarkers of NETs have been associated with both severe influenza and, more recently, COVID-19 [19, 20].

Innate lymphoid cells (ILCs) are self-regenerating, tissue-resident innate cells present in the airways. ILCs share many features with traditional CD4 and CD8 T cells. Different from lymphocytes, ILCs do not have expression of antigen-specific cell receptors (TCRs), and are responsive to cytokine production. ILCs are classified into three groups (ILC1s, ILC2s, ILC3s) that are roughly similar to Th1, Th2, and Th17/22 cells. ILC1 cells are essential for immune surveillance, and respond against airborne pathogens in an early manner, primarily through the production of IFN-γ and TNFα. ILC2s mimic Th2 lymphocytes, and express type 2 cytokines including IL-4, IL-5, and IL-13 in response to IL-25, IL-33, and thymic stromal lymphopoietin (TSLP). ILC2s are significant cells in allergic reactions, asthma, and clearance of helminths from the lung. ILC3s are mimic to Th17/Th22 lymphocytes. They are the largest group of ILCs found in the human lung, but the literature emphasizing the task of the ILC3s is quite few. ILC3s mainly produce IL-22 in the lung, and they are essential for tissue regeneration after viral infection. IL-17 expression of ILC3s may play a role in defending against extra-cellular bacteria and fungi. These cells have transcriptional plasticity and may adopt niche-specific functional roles according to environmental cytokines [1, 4].

$\gamma\delta$ T cells are a subset of T lymphocytes that possess innate immune cell characteristics and are thought to serve the connection between innate and adaptive immune systems. Early in development, they translocate to mucosal surfaces, and they are assessed as tissue-resident T cells. $\gamma\delta$ T cells are central to the elimination of numerous infections. During *Pneumocystis carinii* infection, $\gamma\delta$ T cells stimulate host immunity through interactions with CD8+ T cells and local IFN-γ production. In tuberculosis infection, they release IFN-γ and trigger macrophages to generate nitric oxide. In other bacterial infections, $\gamma\delta$T cells are essential for TNF-α and IFN-γ generation and bacterial clearance, establishing those cells as a significant element of the innate immune system [4].

6.3 Adaptive Immunity

The innate immune response is the first defense mechanism against pathogens that cause infection. In addition to the innate immune system, cells of the adaptive immune system also play a role in the elimination of pathogens in the respiratory system. The adaptive immune response comes into play later than the innate immune response but could not have a protective effect without the support of the local innate immune system and stromal cells [21]. Whereas innate immune responses are triggered within minutes following the detection of PAMPs, the adaptive immune response is highly antigen-specific and develops over several days to several weeks [1].

The respiratory adaptive immune system consists of cellular and humoral immunity with soluble mediators such as cytokines, adaptive immune system's cells migrate into tissue when activated by infection or tissue damage [22, 23]. This system involves T cells, including CD8+ T cells, which are mainly in charge of directly killing infected cells, and CD4+ T cells (or Th1), which mediate additional stimulation of adaptive cytolytic immunity or B-cell-mediated responses (Th2), and B cells, which are involved in the production of antibodies to neutralize pathogens or stimulate additional functional responses in innate cells [1, 22].

6.3.1 Cells of Cellular Immunity: T Cells and Their Subsets

T cells, which are important cells of the adaptive immune system, interact with other immune system cells and perform many tasks such as the production of immunomodulatory cytokines and killing antigen-specific infected cells. Thus plays an important role in the control of infections in the respiratory system. T cells working in the respiratory system can generally be divided into two groups: T cells that respond to acute infection and memory T cells (TMC) that form after infection and maintain the immune response for a long time [1].

Cytotoxic CD8+ T cells (CTLs), which produce an acute response against the infectious agent, are cells that secrete anti-inflammatory cytokines such as IL-10, and they recognize the class I MHC bound peptide presented by antigen-presenting cells (APCs) such as dendritic cells [24]. These cells kill the infected cells through the secretion of cytolytic enzymes. Although CTLs play a critical role in the response to the infectious agent, dysregulated responses in these cells can cause severe lung damage [23, 25, 26].

Other T cells in the adaptive immune system are CD4+ helper T cells, which differentiate into various subsets including Th1, Th2, Th17, follicular T (Tfh), and regulatory T (Treg) under the influence of cytokines in the microenvironment [1]. In addition to activating macrophages, Th1 cells are involved in the response to intracellular lung infection through IFN-γ and IL-2 cytokines. Th2 cells, which secrete IL-4, IL-5, and IL-13 cytokines, are involved in allergic inflammation and in the response to parasitic infections [27]. Th17 cells not only produce cytokines involved in the innate immune response in the lungs but also support the integrity of the epithelium by stimulating the proliferation of epithelial cells. IL-17A and IL-22 cytokines, which are produced by CD4+ T cells, are very important in homeostasis and tissue repair. As a part of mucosal immunity, they are associated with innate immune defense [4].

CD4+ FoxP3+ Tregs, which are formed in the later stages of pulmonary inflammation, are cells that are important in maintaining airway tolerance through IL-10 and TGF-β production. In addition to immune tolerance, Treg cells stimulate tissue repair, induce differentiation of type I and type II pneumocytes, and inhibit fibrocyte aggregation and proliferation [28]. T follicular helper (Tfh) cells are cells that help develop B-cell-mediated humoral responses to infection.

In the late phase of acute infections/inflammation, both CD4+ and CD8+ memory T cells (TMC) develop in the respiratory system. TMCs are present in the upper and lower respiratory tracts and play an important role in the prevention of viral infections. TMCs are cells that respond rapidly to infections and quickly perform their effector functions when they encounter an infectious agent. In addition, TMCs not only eliminate the infectious agent but also maintain tissue integrity through the cytokines and chemokines they secrete [29]. These T cells are long-lived, and express CD69+ CD103+ following re-infection or vaccination, then called T resident helper (T_{RH}) cells. TRH (T_{RH}) cells are not circulating cells, and remain stable in the mucosal site throughout their lifetime. These cells, recently identified following influenza infection in mice, are functionally similar to Tfh and TCM cells [30]. These cells are both phenotypically and functionally distinct from effector memory T (TEM) cells and reside in the respiratory mucosa throughout life to function by increasing the expression of integrins and selectins as needed [1, 31].

6.3.2 Cells of Humoral Immunity: B Cells and B Cell Subsets

Similar to T cells, B cells migrate to the lymph node after encountering antigens and settle in the T/B cell region of the lymph node. In this region, some of the B cells differentiate into short-lived plasma cells, while others move toward the germinal center where maturation occurs. In the germinal center, B cells expand clonally and differentiate into long-lived plasma cells and/or memory B cells (BMCs) with the help of Tfh cells [32].

In the early stages of infection, short-lived plasma cells form, and cause the release of low-affinity IgG and IgA at the site of infection. On the other hand, in the later stages of infection, plasma cells secreting high-affinity immunoglobulin are formed. IgA is more commonly found in the respiratory mucosa, and both IgA and IgG have been shown to be effective against infections in the respiratory tract [33]. Due to mechanisms by which a tissue-specific cell is directed to a specific tissue or organ, antigen-specific IgA+ B cells differentiate into monomeric IgA (mIgA)-producing plasma cells before differentiating into polymeric IgA (pIgA)-producing plasma cells to migrate toward the effector site [24]. pIgA forms a complex with the polymeric Ig receptor (pIgR) expressed by epithelial cells. This results in the formation of secretory IgA [34]. The synthesis of IgA antibodies and the production of tissue-resident memory T cells (TMC) are important features of adaptive immune responses. Secreted mucosal IgA prevents antigens and pathogens from invading the mucosa by various mechanisms [35]. During the recovery phase after acute pulmonary inflammation, B cells can differentiate into memory cells or like T cells, can reside in the airways as tissue-resident memory B (BRM) [34, 36]. In the light of current information, BRM cells, together with other cells of the respiratory tract, are thought to be important mediators of protective humoral responses against pulmonary infections and airway immune surveillance.

As a result, the respiratory system is a highly complex system for human health, interacting with the external environment and playing a critical role as the first-line defense against lung injury caused by inhaled pathogens and toxins. There is enormous complexity among cellular and humoral immune responses in the airways following infection and vaccination. Innate immune cells in the lung respond to non-antigen-specific signals from their environment, enabling them to mobilize quickly in the presence of a threat. Adaptive immunity, which develops following the innate immune response, is highly antigen-specific and it is important in long-lasting immunity.

Conflict of Interest None.
There is no conflict of interest of any authors.

References

1. Mettelman RC, Allen EK, Thomas PG. Mucosal immune responses to infection and vaccination in the respiratory tract. Immunity. 2022;55(5):749–80.
2. Gopallawa I, Dehinwal R, Bhatia V, et al. A four-part guide to lung immunology: invasion, inflammation, immunity, and intervention. Front Immunol. 2023;14:1119564. https://doi.org/10.3389/fimmu.2023.1119564.
3. Parker D, Prince A. Innate immunity in the respiratory epithelium. Am J Respir Cell Mol Biol. 2011;45(2):189–201. https://doi.org/10.1165/rcmb.2011-0011RT.
4. Galeas-Pena M, McLaughlin N, Pociask D. The role of the innate immune system on pulmonary infections. Biol Chem. 2019;400(4):443–56. https://doi.org/10.1515/hsz-2018-0304.
5. Short KR, Kasper J, van der Aa S, et al. Influenza virus damages the alveolar barrier by disrupting epithelial cell tight junctions. Eur Respir J. 2016;47(3):954–66. https://doi.org/10.1183/13993003.01282-2015.

6. Kast JI, McFarlane AJ, Głobińska A, et al. Respiratory syncytial virus infection influences tight junction integrity. Clin Exp Immunol. 2017;190(3):351–9. https://doi.org/10.1111/cei.13042.
7. Higgins G, Fustero Torre C, Tyrrell J, et al. Lipoxin A4 prevents tight junction disruption and delays the colonization of cystic fibrosis bronchial epithelial cells by Pseudomonas aeruginosa. Am J Physiol Lung Cell Mol Physiol. 2016;310(11):L1053–61. https://doi.org/10.1152/ajplung.00368.2015.
8. Wittekindt OH. Tight junctions in pulmonary epithelia during lung inflammation. Pflugers Arch. 2017;469(1):135–47. https://doi.org/10.1007/s00424-016-1917-3.
9. Kim KC. Role of epithelial mucins during airway infection. Pulm Pharmacol Ther. 2012;25(6):415–9. https://doi.org/10.1016/j.pupt.2011.12.003.
10. Zhang H, He F, Li P, et al. The role of innate immunity in pulmonary infections. Biomed Res Int. 2021;2021:6646071. https://doi.org/10.1155/2021/6646071.
11. Alvarez-Simon D, Ait Yahia S, de Nadai P, et al. NOD-like receptors in asthma. Front Immunol. 2022;13:928886. https://doi.org/10.3389/fimmu.2022.928886.
12. Choi SM, McAleer JP, Zheng M, et al. Innate Stat3-mediated induction of the antimicrobial protein Reg3γ is required for host defense against MRSA pneumonia. J Exp Med. 2013;210:551–61.
13. Hillaire MLB, van Eijk M, Vogelzang-van Trierum SE, et al. Recombinant porcine surfactant proteinD inhibits influenza A virus replication ex vivo. Virus Res. 2014;181:22–6. https://doi.org/10.1016/j.virusres.2013.12.032.
14. Jin H, Ciechanowicz AK, Kaplan AR, et al. Surfactant protein C dampens inflammation by decreasing JAK/STAT activation during lung repair. Am J Physiol Cell Mol Physiol. 2018;314:L882–92. https://doi.org/10.1152/ajplung.00418.2017.
15. Sun S, Zhao G, Liu C, Wu X, et al. Inhibition of complement activation alleviates acute lung injury induced by highly pathogenic avian influenza H5N1 virus infection. Am J Respir Cell Mol Biol. 2013;49:221–30. https://doi.org/10.1165/rcmb.2012-0428OC.
16. Kolli D, Gupta MR, Sbrana E, et al. Alveolar macrophages contribute to the pathogenesis of human metapneumovirus infection while protecting against respiratory syncytial virus infection. Am J Respir Cell Mol Biol. 2014;51(4):502–15. https://doi.org/10.1165/rcmb.2013-0414OC.
17. Cribbs SK, Lennox J, Caliendo AM, et al. Healthy HIV-1-infected individuals on highly active antiretroviral therapy harbor HIV-1 in their alveolar macrophages. AIDS Res Hum Retroviruses. 2015;31(1):64–70. https://doi.org/10.1089/AID.2014.0133.
18. Yang H, Biermann MH, Brauner JM, et al. New insights into neutrophil extracellular traps: mechanisms of formation and role in inflammation. Front Immunol. 2016;7:302. https://doi.org/10.3389/fimmu.2016.00302.
19. Zhu L, Liu L, Zhang Y, et al. High level of neutrophil extracellular traps correlates with poor prognosis of severe influenza A infection. J Infect Dis. 2018;217(3):428–37. https://doi.org/10.1093/infdis/jix475.
20. Zuo Y, Yalavarthi S, Shi H, et al. Neutrophil extracellular traps in COVID-19. JCI Insight. 2020;5(11):e138999. https://doi.org/10.1172/jci.insight.138999.
21. Iwanaga N, Devarajan P, Shenoy AT. Editorial: Adaptive immunity to respiratory pathogens. Front Immunol. 2023;14:1174178. https://doi.org/10.3389/fimmu.2023.1174178.
22. He X, Chen X, Wang H, et al. Recent advances in respiratory immunization: a focus on COVID-19 vaccines. J Control Release. 2023;355:655–74. https://doi.org/10.1016/j.jconrel.2023.02.011.
23. Stambas J, Lu C, Tripp RA. Innate and adaptive immune responses in respiratory virus infection: implications for the clinic. Expert Rev Respir Med. 2020;14(11):1141–7. https://doi.org/10.1080/17476348.2020.1807945.
24. Sato S, Kiyono H. The mucosal immune system of the respiratory tract. Curr Opin Virol. 2012;2(3):225–32. https://doi.org/10.1016/j.coviro.2012.03.009.
25. Schmidt ME, Varga SM. The CD8 T cell response to respiratory virus infections. Front Immunol. 2018;9:678. https://doi.org/10.3389/fimmu.2018.00678.

26. Guo K, Yombo DJK, Xu J, et al. The chemokine receptor CXCR3 promotes CD8+ T cell-dependent lung pathology during influenza pathogenesis. Preprint at bioRxiv. 2022; https://doi.org/10.1101/2022.02.14.480379.
27. Schattgen SA, Thomas PG. TRH cells, helpers making an impact in their local community. Sci Immunol. 2021;6(55):eabf2886. https://doi.org/10.1126/sciimmunol.abf2886.
28. D'Alessio FR, Tsushima K, Aggarwal NR, et al. CD4+CD25+Foxp3+ Tregs resolve experimental lung injury in mice and are present in humans with acute lung injury. J Clin Invest. 2009;119(10):2898–913. https://doi.org/10.1172/JCI36498.
29. Rakhra K, Abraham W, Wang C, et al. Exploiting albumin as a mucosal vaccine chaperone for robust generation of lung-resident memory T cells. Sci Immunol. 2021;6(57):eabd8003. https://doi.org/10.1126/sciimmunol.abd8003.
30. Swarnalekha N, Schreiner D, Litzler LC, et al. T resident helper cells promote humoral responses in the lung. Sci Immunol. 2021;6(55):eabb6808. https://doi.org/10.1126/sciimmunol.abb6808.
31. Purwar R, Campbell J, Murphy G, et al. Resident memory T cells (T(RM)) are abundant in human lung: diversity, function, and antigen specificity. PLoS One. 2011;6(1):e16245. https://doi.org/10.1371/journal.pone.0016245.
32. Pereira JP, Kelly LM, Cyster JG. Finding the right niche: B-cell migration in the early phases of T-dependent antibody responses. Int Immunol. 2010;22(6):413–9. https://doi.org/10.1093/intimm/dxq047.
33. Barker KA, Etesami NS, Shenoy AT, et al. Lung-resident memory B cells protect against bacterial pneumonia. J Clin Invest. 2021;131(11):e141810. https://doi.org/10.1172/JCI141810.
34. Johansen FE, Braathen R, Brandtzaeg P. Role of J chain in secretory immunoglobulin formation. Scand J Immunol. 2000;52(3):240–8. https://doi.org/10.1046/j.1365-3083.2000.00790.
35. Strugnell RA, Wijburg OL. The role of secretory antibodies in infection immunity. Nat Rev Microbiol. 2010;8(9):656–67. https://doi.org/10.1038/nrmicro2384.
36. Onodera T, Takahashi Y, Yokoi Y, et al. Memory B cells in the lung participate in protective humoral immune responses to pulmonary influenza virus reinfection. Proc Natl Acad Sci U S A. 2012;109(7):2485–90. https://doi.org/10.1073/pnas.1115369109.

Immune Responses to Respiratory Infections

7

Ezgi Topyildiz, Francesco Cinetto, and Guzide Aksu

7.1 Introduction

The respiratory system is a complex system representing both a physical and immunological barrier between the external environment and the blood and tissues. It provides gas exchange and oxygenation of the blood and is a crucial component of the body's defenses against various pathogens that can cause infections. In response to harmful microorganisms entering the respiratory tract, such as viruses, bacteria, fungi, and protozoa, a complex and multifaceted response occurs. Respiratory cells and innate immune cells initiate the clearing and resolution of infection, followed by the intervention of adaptive immune cells. A range of cellular and molecular mechanisms are involved in this immune response, which is responsible for identifying, neutralizing, and eliminating invading pathogens [1]. Recurrent and severe respiratory tract infections, particularly if caused by atypical pathogens, are indeed listed among the key warning signs that should raise the suspicion of an Inborn Error of Immunity (IEI), both in pediatric and adult patients [2].

Acute respiratory tract infections (ARTIs) are the leading cause of symptomatic illness worldwide and are frequently caused by viruses, although bacteria and fungi can also cause ARTIs [3]. Both innate and adaptive defense systems are involved in antimicrobial immunity [4].

E. Topyildiz
Department of Pediatric Allergy and Immunology, Acıbadem Healthcare Group, Ataşehir Hospital, Istanbul, Turkey

F. Cinetto
Rare Diseases Referral Center, Internal Medicine 1, Department of Medicine (DIMED), AULSS2 Marca Trevigiana, Ca' Foncello Hospital, University of Padova, Podova, Italy

G. Aksu (✉)
Department of Pediatric Immunology, Ege University Faculty of Medicine, Izmir, Turkey

H. Yüksel et al. (eds.), *Pediatric Airway Diseases*, Comprehensive ENT, https://doi.org/10.1007/978-3-031-74853-0_7

Respiratory epithelial cells form the first physical barrier to infection and express Toll-like receptors (TLRs) and other pattern recognition receptors (PRRs), such as retinoic acid-inducible gene I (RIG I), which recognize viral components and can produce antiviral IFNs in response [4–7]. Mucus provides a physical barrier to prevent microorganisms from being captured and removed by mucociliary clearance. Additionally, mucins serve as scaffolds for antimicrobial proteins. The innate defense system includes neutrophils, eosinophils, basophils, monocytes, macrophages, dendritic cells (DCs), natural killer (NK), and natural killer T (NKT) cells.

Innate immune system cells use PRRs to identify viral replication in infected host cells, which triggers the early response to viral airway infections. Pattern recognition receptors recognize components of the bacterial cell wall (lipopolysaccharides and peptidoglycans), structures of potential pathogens, and intracellular components of pathogens, including DNA and RNA.

Toll-like receptors are among the most widely studied and well-known PRRs. In particular, TLR7 and TLR8 are effective against viruses with single-stranded RNA, such as influenza virus, SARS-CoV-2, rhinovirus, and respiratory syncytial virus (RSV). In human cells, they detect single-stranded RNA, which is absent during normal metabolic processes. When TLR7 and TLR8 recognize pathogenic structures, they initiate the production of antiviral type I and type III interferons (IFNs), resulting in a direct inhibitory effect on viral replication. In addition, these interferons (α, β, and λ) promote the activation of nearby cells' antiviral defenses [4, 8].

The bacteria that can cross the mucus layer reach the epithelial surface, where they are rapidly detected by numerous PRRs like those in viruses. Lipoteichoic acids of pneumococci and *S. aureus* are recognized by TLR-2, whereas the lipoproteins and lipopolysaccharides of *H. influenzae* can be recognized by TLR-2 and TLR-4, respectively [9]. In the context of pneumococci immunity, lack of molecules downstream of the IL-1 receptor (IRAK-4, MyD88, etc.) or the absence of a functional spleen is also associated with increased rates of invasive disease. As with most of these diseases, the period of greatest susceptibility to invasive pneumococcal disease is early childhood [10]. Circulating monocytes respond to virus-induced inflammatory signals and contribute to antiviral immunity by infiltrating infected tissues [11]. They can, however, also cause damage to the host tissues by causing local inflammation. Their activation results in the production of IFN-I, which is a signal that further activates NK cells, other monocytes, and CD8+ T cells [11]. In accordance with this, mice lacking C–C chemokine receptor type 2 (CCR2) have displayed impaired monocyte recruitment, leading to a decrease in the priming of CD8+ T cells directed against the influenza virus and a delay in the clearance of the virus [11–13].

Dendritic cells (DCs) have a crucial role in antiviral immunity by acting as a link between the innate and adaptive immune systems. There are three distinct types of DCs involved in this interaction: conventional type 1 DCs (cDC1), conventional type 2 DCs (cDC2), and plasmacytoid DCs (pDCs) [11]. Dendritic cells lining the upper respiratory tract mature into antigen-presenting cells when activated. The activation of DCs increases levels of class I and class II key tissue compatibility complex molecules and induces a wide variety of costimulatory and adhesion molecules and inflammatory cytokines essential for T-cell responses. Unlike cDCs, which perform their functions primarily through T cells, pDCs produce high levels of type I IFNs. These IFNs play an essential role in antiviral immunity, although their importance in respiratory viral infections may vary [11]. For instance, although pDCs are the main source of IFN-I in RSV infection, they are also needed to produce IFN-I and generate antiviral immunity following influenza infection [11, 14–17]. Moreover, the importance of type I IFNs has been recently highlighted in response to SARS-COV-2 infections; indeed, inborn errors of, and auto-antibodies against type I IFNs underlie life-threatening COVID-19 pneumonia [18].

Natural killer cells are members of the innate lymphoid cells (ILCs) family. Their function includes the production of effector cytokines and the destruction of infected cells, which are essential for the antiviral response [11].

The depletion and dysfunction of NK cells, which are crucial to the clearance of viral infections, increase the risk of respiratory viral infections. Type 1 ILCs, which contribute to limiting viral infections, are innate counterparts of IFN-γ-producing T helper 1 (Th1) cells [11, 19, 20]. In addition, certain components of the innate immune system target respiratory pathogens [4]. For example, NKT cells have receptors that can recognize lipids when they are presented on major tissue compatibility complex (MHC)-like molecules such as CD1c on innate immune cells. iNKT cells may inhibit the immunosuppressive activity of myeloid suppressor cells during influenza A infection and shorten the duration of the infection [4, 21–23].

Unlike viruses, bacteria are attacked by immune proteins known as complement proteins when they enter the circulation. Complement proteins are involved in killing bacteria through three pathways: the classical complement pathway, the alternative complement pathway, and the lectin pathway. The first step of the classical complement pathway requires antibodies to bind to the surface of the target bacteria. The antibodies are then targeted by a specific complement protein complex. Once bound, it initiates the disassembly and remodeling of complement complexes that produce opsonins that tag bacteria for destruction. At the end of this pathway, the membrane attack complex (MAC) is formed. MAC can localize to Gram-negative bacteria cell membranes, but not to Gram-positive bacteria cell membranes. This process produces pores that facilitate the entry of membrane-damaging molecules such as lysozyme into bacteria, making them susceptible to osmotic lysis. The alternative complement pathway does not require antibodies. In this pathway, complement proteins of a complex known as C3 bind directly to bacteria and activate downstream components of the complement cascade. This results in the formation of MAC, which causes lysis of the bacteria. During the lectin pathway, mannan-binding lectin (MBL) attaches to proteins containing mannose residues found in some bacterial species [24]. The importance of complement in defense against respiratory infections is recapitulated by the clinical features of patients with primary complement deficiencies [25].

Even though innate immune responses are responsible for the initial control of microbial spread, adaptive immunity must be active to ensure the complete clearance of the pathogen. Adaptive immunity encompasses both humoral responses mediated by B cells and cellular immunological responses mediated by T cells.

After intimate contact with innate immune cells, humoral and cellular immunity work together to stimulate adaptive responses. In contrast to innate immunity, which responds quickly to respiratory infections without having any antigen specificity, adaptive immune responses take time to develop antigen specificity while also forming long-term memory [26].

Pathogenic peptide fragments are collected by macrophages, monocytes, and DCs, which are then presented to T cells that recognize MHC molecules or the human leukocyte antigen (HLA)—the MHC peptide complex [4]. In this way, T cells are activated and antigen-specific B cells are instructed. As soon as the naive B cells are activated, they produce antibodies or migrate to the infection site with T cells to destroy the infected cells (Fig. 7.1). When naive CD4+ T lymphocytes are activated, they differentiate into specific types of helper T lymphocytes (e.g., Th1, Th2, or Th17) and expand clonally according to the cytokine environment during activation [27]. For example, in influenza infection, CD4+ T cells generally promote the differentiation and activation of antibody-producing B cells while also

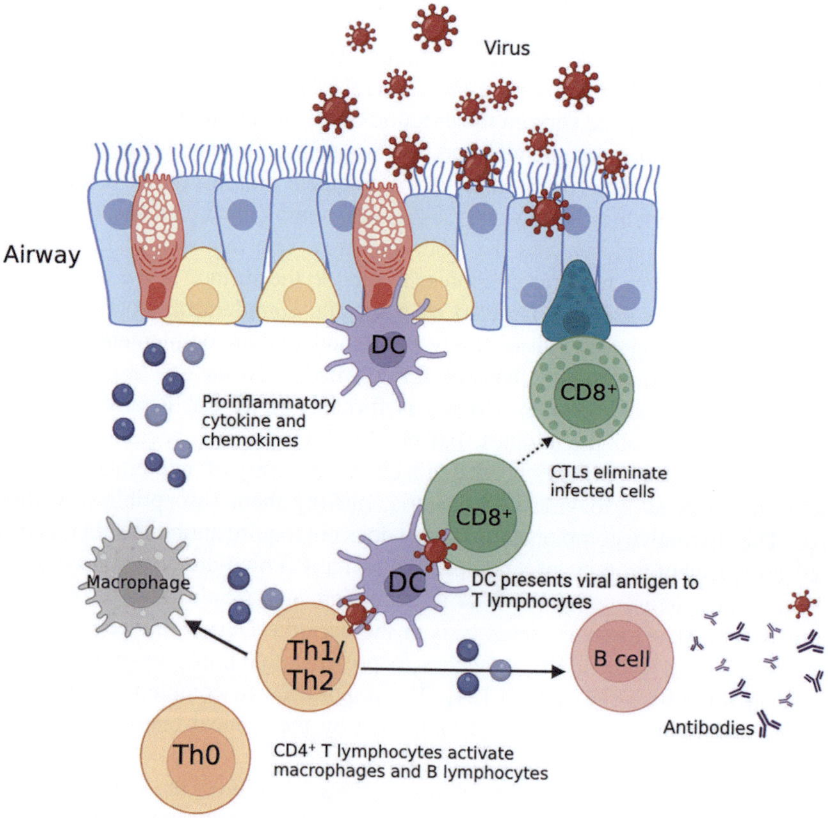

Fig. 7.1 Mechanism of immune response

promoting the stimulation of CD8+ T-cell responses. Some CD4+ T cells exhibit cytolytic activity mediated by perforin after influenza infection [11]. The CD8+ T cells recognize and eliminate virus-infected cells through mechanisms mediated by perforins and granzymes or apoptosis. Furthermore, virus-specific CD8+ T cells are capable of generating both anti-inflammatory interleukin (IL)-10 and pro-inflammatory mediators such as tumor necrosis factor (TNF) and IFN-γ, thereby maintaining the balance with effective antiviral responses [11, 28]. It is observed that, following the clearance of the virus, these two pro-inflammatory mediators are reduced. For IL-10 to be produced in lung tissues, IL-27 (released by mononuclear cells and neutrophils) and IL-2 (produced by T CD4+ lymphocytes) are required [27]. As well as CD4+ and CD8+ T lymphocytes and regulatory T cells (Tregs) are involved in immune response modulation. A large number of regulatory interleukins are produced by these cells, such as IL-10 and transforming growth factor-β1 (TGF-β1) and inhibitory molecules such as CTLA-4 (cytotoxic T-lymphocyte-associated protein) [27]. Following clearance, part of the effector T cells converts into circulating and tissue-resident memory T cells, providing long-term immunity against re-infection, while others undergo apoptosis during the contraction phase [29].

Bacterial infections sometimes occur as superinfection following viral infections. In this situation, macrophages usually represent the first line of defense. These macrophages are also responsible for recruiting and activating other immune cells and controlling the spread of bacterial infections. Inflammatory response to extracellular bacteria, such as *S. pneumoniae*, is primarily driven by neutrophil infiltration and secondarily by a late adaptive immunity regulated by Th1 and Th17 cells. Additionally, the production of specific antibodies against the microorganisms is provided by B lymphocytes [27]. Of note, IgM, IgG, and IgA are fundamental in the response against bacteria, and particularly capsulated bacteria, as shown by the recurrence of *S. pneumoniae* and *H. influenzae* infections in patients with primary antibody deficiencies (PAD), often leading to airway remodeling and bronchiectasis [30]. Notably, the evaluation of the antibody response to vaccination is part of the diagnostic process of common variable immunodeficiency. In these patients with a suspicion of PAD, the assessment of the response to pneumococcal polysaccharide vaccines is used as a gold standard to assess T-independent antibody responses [31]. In particular, between IgG subclasses, IgG2 plays a prominent role as an anti-polysaccharide antibody. Also, specific antibody deficiencies are reported, in which a specific inability to mount an antibody response against purified *Streptococcus pneumoniae* capsular polysaccharide antigens is detected. This may occur despite normal total IgG, IgA, and IgM levels and preserved antibody responses to protein antigens [32].

Fungi are ubiquitous indoor and outdoor microorganisms that will likely increase in prevalence and antigenicity with global climate change. Fungi contain cell wall molecules such as β-glucan and chitin and secrete biologically active proteases and glycosidases. Innate immune cells, such as airway epithelial cells and dendritic cells, are equipped with cell surface molecules that respond to these fungal products, leading to the production of cytokines and proinflammatory mediators. As a result, protection against fungal infection is enhanced by generating the adaptive arm of antifungal immunity, including Th1, Th2, and Th17-type CD4+ T cells [33].

In conclusion, immune responses to respiratory infections are complex processes involving both innate and adaptive components. The immune system's ability to recognize, neutralize, and eliminate pathogens is a remarkable defense mechanism that helps maintain respiratory health. The clinical picture of patients affected by IEI clearly recapitulates the importance of the different branches of the immune system in the response against respiratory pathogens and helps in understanding the mechanisms [34]. The knowledge of these responses is crucial to the development of effective therapies and preventive strategies for a wide variety of respiratory infections.

References

1. Baroody FM, Naclerio RM. Immunology of the upper airway and pathophysiology and treatment of allergic rhinitis. In: Flint PW, Haughey BH, Lund VJ, et al., editors. Cummings otolaryngology: head and neck surgery, vol. 1. 5th ed. St. Louis, MO: Mobsy; 2010. p. 597–623.
2. Jeffrey Modell Foundation. Primary immunodeficiency resource centre. http://www.info4pi.org/library/educational-materials/10-warning-signs. Accessed 7 Mar 2017.
3. GBD 2015 LRI Collaborators. Estimates of the global, regional, and national morbidity, mortality, and aetiologies of lower respiratory tract infections in 195 countries: a systematic analysis for the Global Burden of Disease Study 2015. Lancet Infect Dis. 2017;17(11):1133–61. https://doi.org/10.1016/S1473-3099(17)30396-1.
4. Govers C, Calder PC, Savelkoul HFJ, Albers R, van Neerven RJJ. Ingestion, immunity, and infection: nutrition and viral respiratory tract infections. Front Immunol. 2022;13:841532. Published 2022 Feb 28. https://doi.org/10.3389/fimmu.2022.841532.
5. Fahy JV, Dickey BF. Airway mucus function and dysfunction. N Engl J Med. 2010;363(23):2233–47. https://doi.org/10.1056/NEJMra0910061.
6. Ioannidis I, Ye F, McNally B, Willette M, Flaño E. Toll-like receptor expression and induction of type I and type III interferons in primary airway epithelial cells. J Virol. 2013;87(6):3261–70. https://doi.org/10.1128/JVI.01956-12.
7. Tengroth L, Millrud CR, Kvarnhammar AM, Kumlien Georén S, Latif L, Cardell LO. Functional effects of Toll-like receptor (TLR)3, 7, 9, RIG-I and MDA-5 stimulation in nasal epithelial cells. PLoS One. 2014;9(6):e98239. Published 2014 Jun 2. https://doi.org/10.1371/journal.pone.0098239.
8. Kotenko SV, Durbin JE. Contribution of type III interferons to antiviral immunity: location, location, location. J Biol Chem. 2017;292(18):7295–303. https://doi.org/10.1074/jbc.R117.777102.
9. Zola TA, Lysenko ES, Weiser JN. Mucosal clearance of capsule-expressing bacteria requires both TLR and nucleotide-binding oligomerization domain 1 signaling. J Immunol. 2008;181(11):7909–16. https://doi.org/10.4049/jimmunol.181.11.7909.
10. Picard C, Puel A, Bustamante J, Ku CL, Casanova JL. Primary immunodeficiencies associated with pneumococcal disease. Curr Opin Allergy Clin Immunol. 2003;3(6):451–9. https://doi.org/10.1097/00130832-200312000-00006.
11. Wei X, Narasimhan H, Zhu B, Sun J. Host recovery from respiratory viral infection. Annu Rev Immunol. 2023;41:277–300. https://doi.org/10.1146/annurev-immunol-101921-040450.
12. Lee AJ, Chen B, Chew MV, et al. Inflammatory monocytes require type I interferon receptor signaling to activate NK cells via IL-18 during a mucosal viral infection. J Exp Med. 2017;214(4):1153–67. https://doi.org/10.1084/jem.20160880.
13. Aldridge JR Jr, Moseley CE, Boltz DA, et al. TNF/iNOS-producing dendritic cells are the necessary evil of lethal influenza virus infection. Proc Natl Acad Sci USA. 2009;106(13):5306–11. https://doi.org/10.1073/pnas.0900655106.

14. Hikono H, Kohlmeier JE, Ely KH, et al. T-cell memory and recall responses to respiratory virus infections. Immunol Rev. 2006;211:119–32. https://doi.org/10.1111/j.0105-2896.2006.00385.x.
15. Eisenbarth SC. Dendritic cell subsets in T cell programming: location dictates function. Nat Rev Immunol. 2019;19(2):89–103. https://doi.org/10.1038/s41577-018-0088-1.
16. Smit JJ, Rudd BD, Lukacs NW. Plasmacytoid dendritic cells inhibit pulmonary immunopathology and promote clearance of respiratory syncytial virus. J Exp Med. 2006;203(5):1153–9. https://doi.org/10.1084/jem.20052359.
17. GeurtsvanKessel CH, Willart MA, van Rijt LS, et al. Clearance of influenza virus from the lung depends on migratory langerin+CD11b− but not plasmacytoid dendritic cells. J Exp Med. 2008;205(7):1621–34. https://doi.org/10.1084/jem.20071365.
18. Bastard P, Zhang Q, Zhang SY, Jouanguy E, Casanova JL. Type I interferons and SARS-CoV-2: from cells to organisms. Curr Opin Immunol. 2022;74:172–82. https://doi.org/10.1016/j.coi.2022.01.003.
19. Bi J. NK cell dysfunction in patients with COVID-19. Cell Mol Immunol. 2022;19(2):127–9. https://doi.org/10.1038/s41423-021-00825-2.
20. Lujan RA, Vrba SM, Hickman HD. Antiviral activities of group I innate lymphoid cells. J Mol Biol. 2022;434(6):167266. https://doi.org/10.1016/j.jmb.2021.167266.
21. Juno JA, Keynan Y, Fowke KR. Invariant NKT cells: regulation and function during viral infection. PLoS Pathog. 2012;8(8):e1002838. https://doi.org/10.1371/journal.ppat.1002838.
22. Diana J, Lehuen A. NKT cells: friend or foe during viral infections? Eur J Immunol. 2009;39(12):3283–91. https://doi.org/10.1002/eji.200939800.
23. Ho LP, Denney L, Luhn K, Teoh D, Clelland C, McMichael AJ. Activation of invariant NKT cells enhances the innate immune response and improves the disease course in influenza A virus infection. Eur J Immunol. 2008;38(7):1913–22. https://doi.org/10.1002/eji.200738017.
24. Gil E, Noursadeghi M, Brown JS. *Streptococcus pneumoniae* interactions with the complement system. Front Cell Infect Microbiol. 2022;12:929483. Published 2022 Jul 28. https://doi.org/10.3389/fcimb.2022.929483.
25. Skattum L, van Deuren M, van der Poll T, Truedsson L. Complement deficiency states and associated infections. Mol Immunol. 2011;48(14):1643–55. https://doi.org/10.1016/j.molimm.2011.05.001.
26. Stambas J, Lu C, Tripp RA. Innate and adaptive immune responses in respiratory virus infection: implications for the clinic. Expert Rev Respir Med. 2020;14(11):1141–7. https://doi.org/10.1080/17476348.2020.1807945.
27. Borzutzky Schachter A, Morales Matamala P. Immunological defense mechanisms of the respiratory system. In: Bertrand P, Sánchez I, editors. Pediatric respiratory diseases. Cham: Springer; 2020. https://doi.org/10.1007/978-3-030-26961-6_6.
28. Hua L, Yao S, Pham D, et al. Cytokine-dependent induction of CD4+ T cells with cytotoxic potential during influenza virus infection. J Virol. 2013;87(21):11884–93. https://doi.org/10.1128/JVI.01461-13.
29. Sun J, Madan R, Karp CL, Braciale TJ. Effector T cells control lung inflammation during acute influenza virus infection by producing IL-10. Nat Med. 2009;15(3):277–84. https://doi.org/10.1038/nm.1929.
30. Durandy A, Kracker S, Fischer A. Primary antibody deficiencies. Nat Rev Immunol. 2013;13(7):519–33. https://doi.org/10.1038/nri3466.
31. Bonilla FA. Vaccines in patients with primary immune deficiency. Immunol Allergy Clin N Am. 2020;40(3):421–35. https://doi.org/10.1016/j.iac.2020.03.004.
32. Sorensen RU, Edgar D. Specific antibody deficiencies in clinical practice. J Allergy Clin Immunol Pract. 2019;7(3):801–8. https://doi.org/10.1016/j.jaip.2019.01.024.
33. Bartemes KR, Kita H. Innate and adaptive immune responses to fungi in the airway. J Allergy Clin Immunol. 2018;142(2):353–63. https://doi.org/10.1016/j.jaci.2018.06.015.
34. Conti F, Marzollo A, Moratti M, Lodi L, Ricci S. Inborn errors of immunity underlying a susceptibility to pyogenic infections: from innate immune system deficiency to complex phenotypes. Clin Microbiol Infect. 2022;28(11):1422–8. https://doi.org/10.1016/j.cmi.2022.05.022.

Respiratory Microbiome 8

Ülkü Rabia Korkmaz, Omer Faruk Cetiner, Asha Rani, Ravi Ranjan, and Ayşe Bilge Öztürk

8.1 Introduction

The human body hosts a complex community of microorganisms called "microbiota," the number of which is 10 times more than the total human cell count [1]. Microbial species belonging to this heterogeneous community exhibit different dynamics according to time and place [2]. They are affected by the environment and are in active communication both with the host and among themselves [2].

Human microbiota, which has become increasingly popular in the last 20 years, has now begun to be defined as our "**last organ**" [1]. As only less than 1% of the bacteria can be cultured in the laboratory [3], therefore, bacterial laboratory culture is no longer the gold standard for understanding the role of microbiota in greater detail. Today, genetic molecular analysis of polymorphic bacterial 16SrRNA gene sequencing is considered the main method to characterize microbiota [2, 3]. Since

Ü. R. Korkmaz
Institute of Asthma and Allergy Prevention, Helmholtz Zenter Munich, Neuherberg, Germany
e-mail: ulku-rabia.korkmaz@helmholtz-munich.de

O. F. Cetiner
Istanbul Faculty of Medicine, Istanbul University, Istanbul, Turkey

A. Rani
Department of Food Science, University of Massachusetts Amherst, Amherst, MA, USA
e-mail: arani@umass.edu

R. Ranjan
Genomics Resource Laboratory, Institute for Applied Life Sciences, University of Massachusetts Amherst, Amherst, MA, USA
e-mail: ranjan@umass.edu

A. B. Öztürk (✉)
Department of Allergy and Immunology, Medeniyet University Faculty of Medicine, Istanbul, Turkey

H. Yüksel et al. (eds.), *Pediatric Airway Diseases*, Comprehensive ENT,
https://doi.org/10.1007/978-3-031-74853-0_8

the beginning of the 2000s, gene sequencing technology with high data output has been widely used, and its routine use in the fields of proteomics, metabolomics, and epigenomics has led to the historical microbiology term "microbiota" [2]. This rapid technological development has also led to promising options in the prevention of diseases and personalized medicine [3].

The entire gene summation of all microbes (bacteria, bacteriophage, fungi, protozoa, and viruses) belonging to the microbiota of a specific environment is termed the "microbiome" [3]. The "Human Microbiome Project-HMP" is one of the most comprehensive international projects which has led to over 200 scientific studies in the literature. The HMP project was planned as an open data portal in 2007 [4] and this project defined the normal microbiomes of the nasal, oral, skin, gastrointestinal tract, and urogenital regions of healthy people.

When "The Human Microbiome Project-HMP" was planned, human airways were not sampled because the lungs were thought to be sterile, but the role of airway microbiota in disease and health is now well established [5]. Since its discovery, the role of the respiratory microbiome in the pathogenesis of various lung diseases has been investigated. A growing body of scientific data from observational clinical studies and laboratory studies supports the role of microbiota in the pathogenesis of airway disease and healthy lungs [5]. Our microbiota may play a key modulatory role in immune, metabolic, and cellular functions, activating disease-related inflammatory signals, increasing airway disease susceptibility and disease severity, as well as directing different phenotypes [3, 6].

Airways are directly exposed to allergens, microbes, and other irritants, and inhaled air contains 10^4–10^6 bacterial cells/m^3 [7]. Lung microbiota occurs by the balance of microbial immigration, microbial elimination, and the relative reproduction rates of its members [3]. Temperature, pH, oxygen tension, nutrient availability, local microbial competition, host epithelial cell interactions, activation of inflammatory cells, and concentration of inflammatory cells all have an effect on the microbiota [3]. The healthy lung has a diverse microbiota and the most prevalent phyla in the airways are Bacteroidetes and Firmicutes. Streptococcaceae (Firmicutes), Veillonellaceae (Firmicutes), Prevotellaceae (Bacteroidetes), Fusobacteriaceae (Fusobacteria), Neisseriaceae (Betaproteobacteria), Porphyromonadaceae (Bacteroidetes), and Lachnospiraceae (Firmicutes) are the most prevalent bacteria found in healthy lung airways [3].

Although it is well known that the intestinal microbiota has a critical importance for human physiology, the "lung microbiota" of healthy individuals has been a less studied subject. Lung microbiota has long been accepted as sterile, and routine sampling encounters various difficulties. Despite its low density and reduced bacterial load, lung microbiota plays a primary role in maintaining a balance between the immune system and epithelial responses [3]. Local and distant effects of the bacterial load of the lung have a decisive effect on many respiratory diseases, including asthma [3, 6, 8].

Although the results of childhood asthma studies have been highly variable because of the different methods used to assess bacterial populations, however, there are extensive data available on childhood asthma and microbiota. This chapter aims to summarize the current literature on airway microbiota, with a focus on childhood asthma studies, to provide a comprehensive approach to the respiratory microbiome and its relationship with airway disease. Accumulating evidence indicates that the airway microbiome may provide valuable predictive insights for the diagnosis of asthma, a basis for identifying risk factors and potential targets for treatment options [6]. In this review, we provide the most essential concepts and recent developments related to the airway microbiome in the context of pediatric asthma. This review also highlights the noteworthy studies that have contributed significantly to advancing our understanding of airway microbiomes.

8.2 Childhood Asthma and Respiratory Microbiome

8.2.1 Childhood Asthma

Childhood asthma, the most prevalent disease of childhood, is identifiable by its phenotype characterized by initial recurrent wheezing, followed by the occurrence of airway obstruction and narrowing within the initial 6 years of life [9, 10]. Approximately 3–5% of individuals develop persistent wheeze symptoms from childhood into adulthood [11]. The subsequent existence of numerous proinflammatory cells, such as mast cells, eosinophils, T-lymphocytes, macrophages, or neutrophils, leads to bronchial constriction, mucosal edema, and increased mucus production [12]. Although in older children and adults the prevalence of asthma is associated with serum IgE level, asthma development is independent of the IgE level at birth [13]. While there has been significant advancement in comprehending the pathogenic mechanisms (risk and protective factors, phenotypes, triggers, etc.) and distinctions between children and adults in asthma, our understanding of effective prevention strategies remains incomplete.

Microbial colonization starts in utero, and it is influenced by many factors, including maternal microbiome, infection, the season of birth, mode of birth, pet exposure, breastfeeding, farming, the existence of older siblings, and use of antibiotics in early life [14–17]. A delicate balance is maintained by microbes, which could be beneficial or harmful. During early life, chronic microbial (viral, bacterial, and fungal) infection or colonization by microbial agents in the lower airway could result in impaired mucociliary clearance that stimulates an increase in mucus production and ultimately contributes to the development of asthma [18, 19].

Newborns born in summer exhibited higher bacterial richness and specific profiles, with an increased abundance of Gram-negative α-proteobacteria and Gram-positive Bacilli in their nasopharynx at 1 month, contrasting with those born in other seasons, suggesting that birth season influences the early colonization of specific pathogens in the upper airways [20]. Another study highlighted peak colonization periods for *M. catarrhalis* in fall/winter and for *H. influenzae* in winter/spring, reflecting regular cycles of colonization and clearance in healthy children. The observed rise in *M. catarrhalis* and *H. influenzae* detection during winter is likely attributed to an uptick in viral respiratory infections, such as influenza, creating more opportunities for secondary infections by bacterial pathogens [21].

Interestingly, infants who have experienced respiratory illnesses accompanied by wheezing in their first year tend to exhibit lower lung function levels even before the onset of any lower respiratory diseases than infants without wheezing-related illness [22, 23]. This suggests that respiratory infections are associated with childhood asthma and may also impact the development and severity of asthma [24]. However, the crucial factor in shaping host immune responses lies in the nature, type, and timing of exposure to microbes [25, 26]. While viral infections appear to play a significant role in initiating wheezing and respiratory distress in early life, exposure to specific bacterial species may have a protective effect [23].

On the other hand, epidemiological studies have indicated that living in a microbial-rich environment in early life protects against developing asthma, particularly in children exposed to farming [27–31]. Recent data on farming indicate that DNA from mattress dust consists of *Clostridium* and *Facklamia* species which were positively associated with farming [32]. Whether the inhalation of metabolites of environmental bacteria contributes to this strong inverse association of asthma with bacterial diversity is not clearly understood [32]. Another outstanding study from Depner et al. revealed that the presence of asthma was positively correlated with a particular operational taxonomic unit from the genus *Moraxella* in children without exposure to farming. However, in children from farming environments, *Moraxella* colonization showed no association with asthma [32]. von Mutius et al. identified 84 farming and nonfarming families in rural regions of Southern Germany and Switzerland. This study suggested that the degree of environmental exposure to endotoxins and other bacterial wall components plays a significant role as a protective determinant in preventing the onset of atopic diseases during childhood [33]. Furthermore, the meta-analyses show that the protective "farm effect" is stronger than what individuals brought up in inner cities can experience by exposure to pets, daycare, and siblings.

8.2.2 Asthma Exacerbation

Asthma exacerbations represent a significant factor contributing to morbidity and, in severe cases, mortality of children affected by asthma [34]. Various factors can contribute to asthma exacerbation, including infections, underuse of asthma control medications, or exposure to allergens or pollutants. Although asthma exacerbations may occur at any time during the year, seasonal factors play a crucial role in childhood asthma. This is particularly prevalent during autumn and spring in temperate climates when viral respiratory tract infections are most widespread [34]. Viral infections play a pivotal role, contributing significantly to as many as 90% of exacerbations [35]. On the other hand, summer exacerbations were associated with compromised pulmonary function, sensitivity to *Alternaria* spp., elevated blood eosinophil counts, increased doses of inhaled corticosteroids (ICS), and a history of exacerbation in the preceding season [35].

8.3 Bacteriome

In 2010, the first distinctive microbiome analysis from bronchoscopy was obtained using 16S rRNA gene marker sequencing technology in eight healthy individuals [36]. Interestingly, the identified bacteria in the lower airways were found to be distinct from those in the upper respiratory tract [36]. The bacteria associated with lower chronic respiratory conditions might be colonized commensally in the upper and lower respiratory tracts of healthy individuals [37]. While it is not well defined whether the upper or lower microbiome is more relevant for asthma occurrence, the bacterial burden in the upper airway is greater than the lower airway. The inflammatory condition in the local airway impacts the lower airway health using postnasal drip or aspiration, resulting in the downward translocation of pathogens [38, 39]. Colonization of the respiratory tract with bacterial pathogens triggers cell recruitment and inflammation in the airways via enhancing inflammatory response to allergens [40].

A study conducted in the Copenhagen Childhood Birth Cohort, involving 321 neonates monitored over their first 5 years of life, aimed to explore the potential relationship between bacterial colonization of the hypopharynx in asymptomatic neonates and the development of asthma [19]. The findings indicated that colonization with *Streptococcus pneumoniae*, *Haemophilus influenzae*, and *Moraxella catarrhalis* in the airway or a combination were at greater risk for recurrent wheeze and exacerbation, as well as asthma development via an increase in blood eosinophil and serum IgE levels [19, 41]. Subsequent follow-up studies indicated that these bacteria are associated with asthma exacerbations [42]. Similarly, a prospective cohort study of 234 children with acute respiratory infections revealed that colonization with *Streptococcus* in the nasopharynx (NP) during the critical first year of life is linked to childhood asthma development [42]. Additionally, the Finish Birth Cohort Study (STEPS) made significant progress in understanding the nasal airway microbiome by identifying five different microbiota profiles in 923 infants at the age of 2, including *Moraxella*-dominant, *Streptococcus*-dominant, *Dolosigranulum*-dominant, *Staphylococcus*-dominant, and Corynebacteriaceae-dominant profiles [43, 44]. Among these microbiotas, *Moraxella* species were associated with a greater risk of respiratory diseases later in childhood [44].

A Childhood Asthma birth cohort study involving infants in the first 2 years of life indicated that the nasopharyngeal *Staphylococcus*-dominant microbiome in the first 6 months of life was associated with an increased risk of recurrent wheezing by age 3 years and asthma that persisted throughout childhood [45]. Moreover, this path was linked with early allergen sensitization. Furthermore, in cases of wheezing, the identification of the prevalence of *Moraxella* was correlated with the persistence of asthma into later childhood [45]. Upon subsequent follow-up of the same cohort, the frequency of both upper and lower respiratory tract infections was linked to asthma development by the age of 7 [46].

Another study focusing on nasal microbiome highlighted the association of pediatric asthma with Proteobacteria and *Moraxella* [47]. A study involving nasal blow samples from 214 children highlighted that airway microbiota colonization is differentially associated with the risk of loss of asthma control and severe exacerbation [48]. Specifically, airway microbiota dominated by the *Corynebacterium* and *Dolosigranulum* cluster was associated with a lower risk of asthma compared to microbiota dominated by more pathogenic bacteria such as *Staphylococcus*, *Streptococcus*, and *Moraxella* [45]. Likewise, a study highlighted that *Moraxella catarrhalis*, an opportunistic human respiratory pathogen, has been identified as a dominant species of nasal airway microbiotas of children (age range 6–17 years) who experience a greater frequency of exacerbation [49]. Furthermore, in vitro findings demonstrate that strains from *Moraxella catarrhalis* may cause epithelial damage and elevate the expression of IL-8 and IL-33 [44]. Microbial taxonomic analysis from Chile revealed that the nasal mucosa was dominated by a high abundance of *Moraxella*, *Dolosigranulum*, *Haemophilus*, *Corynebacterium*, *Streptococcus*, and *Staphylococcus*, whereas the oral mucosa was characterized by a high abundance of *Streptococcus*, *Haemophilus*, *Gemella*, *Veillonella*, *Neisseria*, and *Porphyromonas* in asthmatic children [50]. Kim et al. demonstrated in a cross-sectional case–control study an elevated proportion of Firmicutes in upper airway samples among individuals with asthma compared to control as well as children with asthma remission [51]. In addition, atypical bacteria such as *Mycoplasma pneumoniae* and *Chlamydophila pneumoniae*, recognized as common respiratory pathogens, have been linked to asthma, wheezing, and asthma exacerbations in children [52–54].

Unlike the upper respiratory microbiota, there are only a few studies that have reported the potential association between the lower airway microbiota and asthma [36, 55–57]. Hilty et al. collected samples of lower airways from children with and without asthma [36]. Microbiome analysis indicated that children with asthma are richer in Firmicutes phyla and *Haemophilus* genus [36]. The use of a mouse model of *Haemophilus* infection demonstrated that corticosteroid treatment, the main treatment to reduce airway inflammation in people with asthma, promotes *Haemophilus influenzae* persistence, which suggests that this bacterium may respond directly to corticosteroid via influencing biofilm formation [58]. In line, Ovaalbumin (OVA)-induced *Haemophilus influenzae*-infected mouse shows that a combination of infection and allergic airway disease promotes bacterial persistence, leading to the development of steroid-resistant neutrophilic asthma [59] via immune modulation [60]. Moreover, bronchoalveolar lavage (BAL) pellets from children who underwent bronchoscopy over 20 months with severe asthma showed significantly enriched abundance of *Bacteroides*, *Faecalibacterium*, *Roseburia*, *Ruminococcus*, *Parabacteroides*, *Romboutsia*, *Alistipes*, *Eubacterium*, and other five bacteria in comparison to control, whereas *Proteus* and *Capnocytophaga* showed higher abundance in samples from individuals without severe asthma compared to those with the condition [57].

While association with bacteria and its potential risk for asthma development is already multifarious, an additional layer of complexity might be added by potential interaction between viruses and bacteria to shape host microbiome relationships by altering mucosal surfaces. Following virus infection, cells may decrease the antibacterial peptides and induce bacterial colonization and replication both directly and indirectly via the upregulation of adherence receptors [61]. The nested cohort of 118 with confirmed respiratory syncytial virus (RSV), which is one of the most common causes of upper and lower acute respiratory infections (ARIs), indicated that higher nasopharyngeal detection and abundance of *Lactobacillus* during infancy were consistently associated with a reduced risk of subsequent wheezing illnesses at age 2 [62].

Evidence has shown that the microbiome is associated with asthma pathogenesis, but how microbiota and their metabolites shape immune pathways to drive asthma is still not fully understood. Depending on bacterial species, immune modulation alters. While Proteobacteria species provoke T helper (Th) 17 inflammation, which is associated with noneosinophilic asthma, some *Acinetobacter* species are associated with Th2/eosinophilic asthma [63]. Bronchoalveolar lavage from children aged from 4 to 32 months with wheezing has demonstrated that an increase in the alveolar macrophages and neutrophil, but not of eosinophil and mast cells, suggests an association between bacterial colonization and initiating event of allergic asthma [64].

8.4 Virome

Viral infections have been repeatedly and consistently associated with wheezing [65–67]. Various evidence indicates that viral infections exacerbate asthma [68–70]. Among the plethora of respiratory viruses, in particular, rhinovirus (RV) stands out as the predominant single trigger for exacerbations, accounting for as much as 76% of wheezing episodes in children [67, 71–73]. In addition, early-life rhinovirus wheezing illnesses and aeroallergen sensitization are the most potent risk factors for asthma at school age [74]. Rhinoviruses (RVs) can induce a range of illnesses, spanning from asymptomatic infections to severe conditions affecting the lower respiratory tract [75]. RV also regulates airway hyperresponsiveness, a key characteristic feature of asthma [76]. The Copenhagen prospective study on asthma childhood (COPSAC) has identified RV as a pathogen inducing severe respiratory disease potential [42, 77]. Data have highlighted that RV-induced bronchiolitis was more strongly associated with the risk of developing wheeze and childhood asthma [73]. Notably, RV as a cause of first-time wheezing in children using corticosteroid treatment could be effective. Clinical trials indicate that children who got a short dose of oral corticosteroids not only wheezed less in the following year [78, 79] but also had a 30% lower risk of developing asthma over the next 4–7 years [79, 80].

Children prone to developing asthma may have a tendency to create an inflammatory environment favoring Th2 responses, along with a connection to specific risk genes like CDHR3 [71]. Factors like weakened interferon responses, a compromised airway barrier, environmental exposures (like an imbalanced airway microbiome), and nutritional deficiencies (low vitamin D and fish oil) increase the risk of infections from viruses, including RV [71]. Whether viral illnesses actually cause asthma is still a topic of active debate.

Another prevalent respiratory virus, respiratory syncytial virus (RSV), is among the most significant risk factors for the onset of wheezing in infants and young children. In 1959, Witting and Glasser outlined the epidemiological link between childhood viral bronchiolitis and the later development of repeated wheezing and/or asthma [81]. Since then, numerous studies have indicated the relationship between asthma and RSV [82–84]. The follow-up at age 18 years, involving 46 of 47 subjects with RSV and 92 of 93 controls, revealed that severe early RSV bronchiolitis is linked to a higher prevalence of persistent allergic asthma into early adulthood, with small airway dysfunction (LCI) associated with current asthma and airway inflammation [85]. Early-life severe RSV infection has been linked to the onset of childhood wheezing illnesses during infancy and the development of childhood asthma [86]. However, to definitively determine causality, the effect of interventions that prevent, delay, or reduce the severity of the initial RSV infection on childhood asthma needs to be investigated.

The mechanisms linking these viruses to asthma development are distinct, with RV generally a risk for later atopic asthma, while RSV is more likely to be associated with later nonatopic asthma [71]. Another notable difference is that in children hospitalized for lower respiratory tract illness, while RSV is frequently detected until about 12 months of age, RV becomes more common in older children [87]. Makrinioti et al. performed the first meta-analysis that directly compares between-virus differences in the magnitude of virus-recurrent wheeze and virus-childhood asthma outcomes [88]. The preschool wheeze and childhood asthma development association comparison between RSV- and RV-induced bronchiolitis analysis shows that the RV-induced bronchiolitis group was more strongly associated with the risk of developing wheeze and childhood asthma [88].

Other commonly identified viruses include human bocavirus (hBOV) and human metapneumovirus (HMPV), with detection rates reaching 10–25%, followed by the parainfluenza virus, adenovirus, coronavirus, and influenza virus, each generally accounting for less than 10% [71].

Nasal biopsy analysis from 49 children infected with HMPV showed that infection is a leading cause of respiratory tract infection in the first years of life [89, 90]. Moreover, an association was observed between infection with HMPV and the diagnosis of an asthma exacerbation [90]. However, the connection between HMPV infection and asthma was intriguing. Conflicting reports exist on a potential link between this infection and asthma [91]. Nevertheless, the existence of a correlation between the presence of a virus and symptoms of respiratory tract disease does not necessarily imply a causal relationship.

In addition, scientists highlighted the possible relationship of hBOV wheezy infection with nonspecific markers of atopy in Polish children [92]. Another report highlighted that 11.6% of hospitalized children with exacerbations of asthma were infected with Bocavirus [93].

Epidemiologic studies indicated that H1N1 induces severe complications in the lower respiratory tract, including bronchitis pneumonia, and atelectasis even in atopic children without any history of either an asthma attack or asthma treatment [94].

8.5 Mycobiome

Research conducted by Charlson et al. (2012) identified fungal communities in BAL and oropharyngeal wash (OW) samples obtained from six healthy individuals. The fungal communities observed in the OW samples of these healthy volunteers were predominantly composed of fungal species already recognized in the oral cavity, with *Candida* and *Aspergillus* being notable examples [95]. Fungi identified in BAL specimens from these subjects exhibited fewer fungal quantities compared to samples from OW [95]. Numerous sequence reads were linked to the genera *Davidiellaceae*, *Aspergillus*, *Penicillium*, and *Polyporales*, implying that fungal inhabitants are present at a diminished density in the alveolar regions of the lungs in contrast to the upper respiratory tract [96]. Continuous exposure to fungal allergens may contribute to fungal colonization which potentially promotes a major shift in bacterial microbiome and exacerbates the challenges in managing asthma symptoms clinically [97]. Fungi are a well-recognized source of indoor and outdoor allergens for individuals with atopic disease. The predominant associations involve three distinct fungal groups: Ascomycota, Basidiomycota, and Deuteromycota [67].

Fluctuations in seasons can lead to heightened spore production from fungi, contributing to worsened asthma symptoms and increased pediatric morbidity [98]. A study revealed a correlation between seasons and changes in the composition of fungal microbiota in samples from children with respiratory illnesses [49]. An increase in respiratory symptoms during the spring was linked to an increase in *Malassezia*, whereas those occurring in the fall were associated with an enrichment of allergenic fungi, *Candida* and *Cladosporium* [49].

Numerous studies have explored the correlation between exposure to fungi, sensitization, and the exacerbation of asthma in childhood. In particular, filamentous fungal species belonging to the *Aspergillus*, *Alternaria*, *Cladosporium*, *Penicillium*, and *Didymella* genera (in the phylum Ascomycota) generate spores that can serve as allergens, potentially triggering bronchial asthma in individuals with atopic tendencies [99–101]. Among them, *Alternaria* is one of the most well-studied airborne fungi in terms of allergic potency [102]. Although *Alternaria* spp. typically exist in lower atmospheric concentrations compared to other airborne allergenic spores, they exhibit the highest sensitization rate among atopic patients, estimated to range from 13% to 17% [103]. Analysis of BAL pellets from children who underwent bronchoscopy indicated that *Rhodosporidium*, *Pneumocystis*, *Leucosporidium*, and *Rhodotorula* were substantially increased in severe asthmatic individuals compared with nonasthmatic. In contrast, *Davidiella*, *Cryptococcus*, and *Sterigmatomyces* were more prevalent in the nonasthmatic individual [57]. Tham et al. have shown that the risk of child and adolescent asthma hospitalization is linked to exposures to various outdoor fungal spore types, including *Alternaria*, *Leptosphaeria*, *Cladosporium*, *Sporormiella*, *Coprinus*, and *Drechslera* [104]. This association is particularly notable in individuals sensitized to *Cladosporium* [104]. Although informative and providing a detailed account of microbial characteristics in these asthmatic groups, these studies do not establish a causal relationship between the identified airway mycobiome signatures and the development of asthma. In a study involving 280 children from Boston, exposure to *Alternaria* in classrooms was linked to prolonged asthma symptoms in children already sensitized to *Alternaria*. This association was observed in comparison to sensitized children exposed to lower levels of *Alternaria* in classrooms over 2 weeks [105]. Another study by Welsh et al. (2016) examined sputum cultures from children with acute exacerbation or stable asthma and discovered elevated concentrations of *Aspergillus fumigatus* in the sputum of children experiencing exacerbation, indicating a potential role of this fungal species in asthma manifestations [106].

Aspergillus, a genus of mold that includes various species of fungi, is associated with hypersensitivity respiratory disorders, conditions include *Aspergillus*-induced asthma, allergic bronchopulmonary aspergillosis (ABPA), allergic *Aspergillus* sinusitis (AAS), and hypersensitivity pneumonitis [107]. In 1953, the most extensively documented case of asthma linked to fungal was ABPA, initially identified as a distinct entity that develops following sensitization to mostly *A. fumigatus* allergen [63]. The prevalence of ABPA is on the rise, it is impacting 1–3% of all asthmatics globally [108]. In individuals with asthma, fungal spores are entangled within the thick and adhesive secretions that typically characterize the airways [107]. This continuous exposure can exacerbate asthma, potentially leading to a more severe manifestation of the condition [108].

While fungal spores are prevalent in substantial quantities outdoors, they are also commonly found in indoor environments, primarily resulting from mold growth facilitated by ventilation systems that assist in their dispersion [68, 69]. A more recent issue has arisen with the recognition that numerous households contain significant quantities of fungi. In multiple studies conducted across Europe, Canada, and the United States, findings revealed the presence of mold in homes ranging from 15% to 36% [70–74]. A study conducted on 640 infants from Cincinnati elevated that the presence of major mold caused the likelihood of recurrent wheezing by nearly two-fold in infants, five-fold in infants sensitized to food or aeroallergens, and six-fold in aeroallergen-sensitized [75]. A prospective birth cohort study suggested a direct relationship between the amount of indoor fungal exposure and the incidence of respiratory tract infection in the first year of life [76].

Evidence from the experimental mouse model indicates that prevalent fungal colonizers in the gut can influence the immune system, potentially making the host more susceptible to allergic airway inflammation. Changes in the mycobiome induced by antibiotic treatment and the intestinal increase of *Candida albicans* [109, 110], *Candida parapsilosis* [111], or *Wallemia mellicola* [112] have been associated with heightened severity of allergic airway inflammation in mice. In addition, the expansion of filamentous fungi (*Aspergillus amstelodami*, *Epicoccum nigrum*, and *Wallemia sebi*) subsequent to antifungal treatment exacerbated allergic airway responses in animal research [113, 114]. Furthermore, a study analyzing fecal samples from infants who later developed the atopic/wheeze phenotype revealed a higher proportion of total sequenced fungal reads, a significant increase in fungal 18S recovered DNA, and an overrepresentation of *Pichia kudriavzevii* at 3 months of age [115]. These findings suggest a correlation between early gut fungal overgrowth and the subsequent development of asthma, uncovering fungal alterations associated with heightened susceptibility to asthma by school age.

These investigations highlighted the significant role of fungi in exacerbating asthma, affecting both children and adults. The origins of this impact are often traced back to immune sensitization during infancy or childhood. However, not every encounter with fungi leads to asthma-inducing sensitizations. Like bacteria, some fungal exposures may be protective, highlighting the complex interplay between specific fungal species' immunogenicity and host immune susceptibilities. Although not all fungal exposures negatively affect immune development, certain genera, such as *Alternaria* and *Aspergillus*, consistently correlate with sensitization in asthmatics and increased asthma severity. Improvements are still needed in fungal taxonomic databases, as well as in bioinformatics algorithms capable of effectively accommodating the greater variability in read length and the increased frequency of genetic insertions and deletions within the regions commonly utilized in most mycobiome sequencing approaches.

The microbiome represents a new frontier in respiratory medicine, and further research is needed to elucidate the potential mechanisms underlying the pathophysiological processes of airway disease other than asthma in pediatric and adult populations. Not only bacteria but also fungi and viruses are collectively linked to clinical outcomes, including periods of exacerbation, severity of disease, and response to treatment. In the future, the development of personalized microbiota-based therapies may help alleviate clinical symptoms and decelerate the progression of airway disease using the integration of data regarding microbiota with technological advances such as next-generation sequencing and omics.

References

1. Berg G, Rybakova D, Fischer D, et al. Microbiome definition re-visited: old concepts and new challenges. Microbiome. 2020;8(1):103.
2. Morgan XC, Huttenhower C. Chapter 12: Human microbiome analysis. PLoS Comput Biol. 2012;8:e1002808.
3. Öztürk AB, Ranjan R, Rani A, Yazıcı D, Bavbek S. Microbiota—the unseen players in adult asthmatic airways. Turk Thorac. 2021;22(1):75–82.
4. Human Microbiome Project Consortium. Structure, function and diversity of the healthy human microbiome. Nature. 2012;486(7402):207–14.
5. Mathieu E, Escribano-Vazquez U, Descamps D, Cherbuy C, Langella P, Riffault S, Remot A, Thomas M. Paradigms of lung microbiota functions in health and disease, particularly, in asthma. Front Physiol. 2018;21(9):1168.
6. Ozturk AB, Turturice BA, Perkins DL, Finn PW. The potential for emerging microbiome-mediated therapeutics in asthma. Curr Allergy Asthma Rep. 2017;17(9):62.
7. Hasleton PS. The internal surface area of the adult human lung. J Anat. 1972;112(Pt 3):391–400.
8. Oğuzülgen K, Öztürk AB, Bacceoğlu A, et al. Inhaler steroid use changes oral and airway bacterial and fungal microbiome profile in asthma patients. Int Arch Allergy Immunol. 2024;185(1):10–9.
9. Kocevar VS, Bisgaard H, Jönsson L, et al. Variations in pediatric asthma hospitalization rates and costs between and within Nordic countries. Chest. 2004;125(5):1680–4.

10. Adams PF, Hendershot GE, Marano MA. Current estimates from the National Health Interview Survey, 1996. Vital Health Stat 10. 1999(200):1–203.
11. Strachan DP, Butland BK, Anderson HR. Incidence and prognosis of asthma and wheezing illness from early childhood to age 33 in a national British cohort. BMJ. 1996;312(7040):1195–9.
12. Jackson DJ, Gangnon RE, Evans MD, et al. Wheezing rhinovirus illnesses in early life predict asthma development in high-risk children. Am J Respir Crit Care Med. 2008;178(7):667–72.
13. Halonen M, Stern D, Taussig LM, et al. The predictive relationship between serum IgE levels at birth and subsequent incidences of lower respiratory illnesses and eczema in infants. Am Rev Respir Dis. 1992;146(4):866–70.
14. Fuchs O, Bahmer T, Rabe KF, et al. Asthma transition from childhood into adulthood. Lancet Respir Med. 2017;5(3):224–34.
15. Thavagnanam S, Fleming J, Bromley A, Shields MD, Cardwell CR. A meta-analysis of the association between caesarean section and childhood asthma. Clin Exp Allergy. 2008;38(4):629–33.
16. Xue M, Dehaas E, Chaudhary N, O'Byrne P, Satia I, Kurmi OP. Breastfeeding and risk of childhood asthma: a systematic review and meta-analysis. ERJ Open Res. 2021;7(4):00504.
17. Hansen R, Gerasimidis K, Turner S. Asthma causation and the gastrointestinal microbiome and metabolome: might there be a signal, or is it just noise? J Allergy Clin Immunol. 2019;144(2):401–3.
18. Martin RJ, et al. A link between chronic asthma and chronic infection. J Allergy Clin Immunol. 2001;107(4):595–601.
19. Bisgaard H, Hermansen MN, Buchvald F, et al. Childhood asthma after bacterial colonization of the airway in neonates. N Engl J Med. 2007;357(15):1487–95.
20. Schoos AM, Kragh M, Ahrens P, et al. Season of birth impacts the neonatal nasopharyngeal microbiota. Children (Basel). 2020;7(5):45.
21. DeMuri GP, Gern JE, Eickhoff JC, et al. Dynamics of bacterial colonization with Streptococcus pneumoniae, Haemophilus influenzae, and Moraxella catarrhalis during symptomatic and asymptomatic viral upper respiratory tract infection. Clin Infect Dis. 2017;66(7):1045–53.
22. Al-Shamrani A, Bagais K, Alenazi A, Alqwaiee M, Al-Harbi AS. Wheezing in children: approaches to diagnosis and management. Int J Pediatr Adolesc Med. 2019;6(2):68–73.
23. Lloyd CM, Saglani S. Early-life respiratory infections and developmental immunity determine lifelong lung health. Nat Immunol. 2023;24(8):1234–43.
24. Guilbert TW, Denlinger LC. Role of infection in the development and exacerbation of asthma. Expert Rev Respir Med. 2010;4(1):71–83.
25. Olszak T, An D, Zeissig S, Vera MP, et al. Microbial exposure during early life has persistent effects on natural killer T cell function. Science. 2012;336(6080):489–93.
26. Cereta AD, Oliveira VR, Costa IP, et al. Early life microbial exposure and immunity training effects on asthma development and progression. Front Med (Lausanne). 2021;8:662262.
27. Pechlivanis S, von Mutius E. Effect of farming on asthma. Acta Med Acad. 2020;49(2):144–55.
28. Ober C, Sperling AI, von Mutius E, Vercelli D. Immune development and environment: lessons from Amish and Hutterite children. Curr Opin Immunol. 2017;48:51–60.
29. Kirjavainen PV, Karvonen AM, Adams RI, et al. Farm-like indoor microbiota in non-farm homes protects children from asthma development. Nat Med. 2019;25(7):1089–95.
30. von Mutius E. The microbial environment and its influence on asthma prevention in early life. J Allergy Clin Immunol. 2016;137(3):680–9.
31. Eder W, Ege MJ, von Mutius E. The asthma epidemic. N Engl J Med. 2006;355(21):2226–35.
32. Birzele LT, Depner M, Ege MJ, et al. Environmental and mucosal microbiota and their role in childhood asthma. Allergy. 2017;72(1):109–19.
33. von Mutius E, Braun-Fahrländer C, Schierl R, et al. Exposure to endotoxin or other bacterial components might protect against the development of atopy. Clin Exp Allergy. 2000;30(9):1230–4.
34. Moorman JE, Akinbami LJ, Bailey CM, et al. National surveillance of asthma: United States, 2001-2010. Vital Health Stat 3. 2012(35):1–58.

35. Cohen HA, Blau H, Hoshen M, Batat E, Balicer RD. Seasonality of asthma: a retrospective population study. Pediatrics. 2014;133(4):e923–32.
36. Hilty M, Burke C, Pedro H, et al. Disordered microbial communities in asthmatic airways. PLoS One. 2010;5(1):e8578.
37. Dick S, Turner S. The airway microbiome and childhood asthma—what is the link? Acta Med Acad. 2020;49(2):156–63.
38. Budden KF, Shukla SD, Rehman SF, et al. Functional effects of the microbiota in chronic respiratory disease. Lancet Respir Med. 2019;7(10):907–20.
39. Kozik AJ, Holguin F, Segal LN, et al. Microbiome, metabolism, and immunoregulation of asthma: an American Thoracic Society and National Institute of Allergy and Infectious Diseases Workshop Report. Am J Respir Cell Mol Biol. 2022;67(2):155–63.
40. Lee YG, Jeong JJ, Nyenhuis S, et al. Recruited alveolar macrophages, in response to airway epithelial-derived monocyte chemoattractant protein 1/CCl2, regulate airway inflammation and remodeling in allergic asthma. Am J Respir Cell Mol Biol. 2015;52(6):772–84.
41. Bisgaard H, Hermansen MN, Bønnelykke K, et al. Association of bacteria and viruses with wheezy episodes in young children: prospective birth cohort study. BMJ. 2010;341:c4978.
42. Kraft M. The role of bacterial infections in asthma. Clin Chest Med. 2000;21(2):301–13.
43. Teo SM, Mok D, Pham K, et al. The infant nasopharyngeal microbiome impacts severity of lower respiratory infection and risk of asthma development. Cell Host Microbe. 2015;17(5):704–15.
44. Toivonen L, Hasegawa K, Waris M, et al. Early nasal microbiota and acute respiratory infections during the first years of life. Thorax. 2019;74(6):592–9.
45. Tang HHF, Lang A, Teo SM, et al. Developmental patterns in the nasopharyngeal microbiome during infancy are associated with asthma risk. J Allergy Clin Immunol. 2021;147(5):1683–91.
46. Toivonen L, Forsström V, Waris M, Peltola V. Acute respiratory infections in early childhood and risk of asthma at age 7 years. J Allergy Clin Immunol. 2019;143(1):407–410.e6.
47. Pérez-Losada M, Authelet KJ, Hoptay CE, Kwak C, Crandall KA, Freishtat RJ. Pediatric asthma comprises different phenotypic clusters with unique nasal microbiotas. Microbiome. 2018;6(1):179.
48. Zhou Y, Jackson D, Bacharier LB, et al. The upper-airway microbiota and loss of asthma control among asthmatic children. Nat Commun. 2019;10(1):5714.
49. McCauley K, Durack J, Valladares R, et al. Distinct nasal airway bacterial microbiotas differentially relate to exacerbation in pediatric patients with asthma. J Allergy Clin Immunol. 2019;144(5):1187–97.
50. Ramos-Tapia I, Reynaldos-Grandón KL, Pérez-Losada M, Castro-Nallar E. Characterization of the upper respiratory tract microbiota in Chilean asthmatic children reveals compositional, functional, and structural differences. Front Allergy. 2023;4:1223306.
51. Kim BS, Lee E, Lee MJ, et al. Different functional genes of upper airway microbiome associated with natural course of childhood asthma. Allergy. 2018;73(3):644–52.
52. Wark PA, Johnston SL, Simpson JL, Hensley MJ, Gibson PG. Chlamydia pneumoniae immunoglobulin A reactivation and airway inflammation in acute asthma. Eur Respir J. 2002;20(4):834–40.
53. Cunningham AF, Johnston SL, Julious SA, Lampe FC, Ward ME. Chronic Chlamydia pneumoniae infection and asthma exacerbations in children. Eur Respir J. 1998;11(2):345–9.
54. Johnston SL, Blasi F, Black PN, Martin RJ, Farrell DJ, Nieman RB, TELICAST Investigators. The effect of telithromycin in acute exacerbations of asthma. N Engl J Med. 2006;354(15):1589–600.
55. Durack J, Boushey HA, Lynch SV. Airway microbiota and the implications of dysbiosis in asthma. Curr Allergy Asthma Rep. 2016;16(8):52.
56. First NJ, Parrish KM, Martínez-Pérez A, et al. Bordetella spp. block eosinophil recruitment to suppress the generation of early mucosal protection. Cell Rep. 2023;42(11):113294.
57. Goldman DL, Chen Z, Shankar V, Tyberg M, Vicencio A, Burk R. Lower airway microbiota and mycobiota in children with severe asthma. J Allergy Clin Immunol. 2018;141(2):808–811.e7.

58. Earl CS, Keong TW, An SQ, et al. Haemophilus influenzae responds to glucocorticoids used in asthma therapy by modulation of biofilm formation and antibiotic resistance. EMBO Mol Med. 2015;7(8):1018–33.
59. Essilfie AT, Simpson JL, Dunkley ML, et al. Combined Haemophilus influenzae respiratory infection and allergic airways disease drives chronic infection and features of neutrophilic asthma. Thorax. 2012;67(7):588–99.
60. Brown MA, Jabeen M, Bharj G, Hinks TSC. Non-typeable Haemophilus influenzae airways infection: the next treatable trait in asthma? Eur Respir Rev. 2022;31(165):220008.
61. Bosch AA, Biesbroek G, Trzcinski K, Sanders EA, Bogaert D. Viral and bacterial interactions in the upper respiratory tract. PLoS Pathog. 2013;9(1):e1003057.
62. Rosas-Salazar C, Shilts MH, Tovchigrechko A, et al. Nasopharyngeal Lactobacillus is associated with a reduced risk of childhood wheezing illnesses following acute respiratory syncytial virus infection in infancy. J Allergy Clin Immunol. 2018;142(5):1447–1456.e9.
63. Simpson JL, Daly J, Baines KJ, et al. Airway dysbiosis: Haemophilus influenzae and Tropheryma in poorly controlled asthma. Eur Respir J. 2016;47(3):792–800.
64. Le Bourgeois M, Goncalves M, Le Clainche L, Benoist MR, Fournet JC, Scheinmann P, de Blic J. Bronchoalveolar cells in children < 3 years old with severe recurrent wheezing. Chest. 2002;122(3):791–7.
65. Kusel MM, de Klerk NH, Holt PG, Kebadze T, Johnston SL, Sly PD. Role of respiratory viruses in acute upper and lower respiratory tract illness in the first year of life: a birth cohort study. Pediatr Infect Dis J. 2006;25(8):680–6.
66. Lemanske RF Jr, Jackson DJ, Gangnon RE, et al. Rhinovirus illnesses during infancy predict subsequent childhood wheezing. J Allergy Clin Immunol. 2005;116(3):571–7.
67. Johnston SL, Pattemore PK, Sanderson G, et al. Community study of role of viral infections in exacerbations of asthma in 9-11 year old children. BMJ. 1995;310(6989):1225–9.
68. Gern JE, Busse WW. Relationship of viral infections to wheezing illnesses and asthma. Nat Rev Immunol. 2002;2(2):132–8.
69. Kuruvilla ME, Lee FE, Lee GB. Understanding asthma phenotypes, endotypes, and mechanisms of disease. Clin Rev Allergy Immunol. 2019;56(2):219–33.
70. Zhao L, Luo JL, Ali MK, Spiekerkoetter E, Nicolls MR. The human respiratory microbiome: current understandings and future directions. Am J Respir Cell Mol Biol. 2023;68(3):245–55.
71. Jartti T, Bønnelykke K, Elenius V, Feleszko W. Role of viruses in asthma. Semin Immunopathol. 2020;42(1):61–74.
72. Turunen R, Koistinen A, Vuorinen T, Arku B, Söderlund-Venermo M, Ruuskanen O, Jartti T. The first wheezing episode: respiratory virus etiology, atopic characteristics, and illness severity. Pediatr Allergy Immunol. 2014;25(8):796–803.
73. Heymann PW, Carper HT, Murphy DD, et al. Viral infections in relation to age, atopy, and season of admission among children hospitalized for wheezing. J Allergy Clin Immunol. 2004;114(2):239–47.
74. Rubner FJ, Jackson DJ, Evans MD, et al. Early life rhinovirus wheezing, allergic sensitization, and asthma risk at adolescence. J Allergy Clin Immunol. 2017;139(2):501–7.
75. Esquivel A, Busse WW, Calatroni A, et al. Effects of omalizumab on rhinovirus infections, illnesses, and exacerbations of asthma. Am J Respir Crit Care Med. 2017;196(8):985–92.
76. Lo D, Kennedy JL, Kurten RC, Panettieri RA Jr, Koziol-White CJ. Modulation of airway hyperresponsiveness by rhinovirus exposure. Respir Res. 2018;19(1):208.
77. Bisgaard H. The Copenhagen Prospective Study on Asthma in Childhood (COPSAC): design, rationale, and baseline data from a longitudinal birth cohort study. Ann Allergy Asthma Immunol. 2004;93(4):381–9.
78. Jartti T, Gern JE. Role of viral infections in the development and exacerbation of asthma in children. J Allergy Clin Immunol. 2017;140(4):895–906.
79. Lehtinen P, Ruohola A, Vanto T, Vuorinen T, Ruuskanen O, Jartti T. Prednisolone reduces recurrent wheezing after a first wheezing episode associated with rhinovirus infection or eczema. J Allergy Clin Immunol. 2007;119(3):570–5.

80. Lukkarinen M, Lukkarinen H, Lehtinen P, Vuorinen T, Ruuskanen O, Jartti T. Prednisolone reduces recurrent wheezing after first rhinovirus wheeze: a 7-year follow-up. Pediatr Allergy Immunol. 2013;24(3):237–43.
81. Wittig HJ, Glaser J. The relationship between bronchiolitis and childhood asthma; a follow-up study of 100 cases of bronchiolitis. J Allergy. 1959;30(1):19–23.
82. Sigurs N, Bjarnason R, Sigurbergsson F, Kjellman B. Respiratory syncytial virus bronchiolitis in infancy is an important risk factor for asthma and allergy at age 7. Am J Respir Crit Care Med. 2000;161(5):1501–7.
83. Stein RT, Sherrill D, Morgan WJ, et al. Respiratory syncytial virus in early life and risk of wheeze and allergy by age 13 years. Lancet. 1999;354(9178):541–5.
84. Sigurs N, Gustafsson PM, Bjarnason R, et al. Severe respiratory syncytial virus bronchiolitis in infancy and asthma and allergy at age 13. Am J Respir Crit Care Med. 2005;171(2):137–41.
85. Sigurs N, Aljassim F, Kjellman B, et al. Asthma and allergy patterns over 18 years after severe RSV bronchiolitis in the first year of life. Thorax. 2010;65(12):1045–52.
86. Rosas-Salazar C, Chirkova T, Gebretsadik T, et al. Respiratory syncytial virus infection during infancy and asthma during childhood in the USA (INSPIRE): a population-based, prospective birth cohort study. Lancet. 2023;401(10389):1669–80.
87. Feldman AS, He Y, Moore ML, Hershenson MB, Hartert TV. Toward primary prevention of asthma. Reviewing the evidence for early-life respiratory viral infections as modifiable risk factors to prevent childhood asthma. Am J Respir Crit Care Med. 2015;191(1):34–44.
88. Makrinioti H, Hasegawa K, Lakoumentas J, et al. The role of respiratory syncytial virus- and rhinovirus-induced bronchiolitis in recurrent wheeze and asthma—a systematic review and meta-analysis. Pediatr Allergy Immunol. 2022;33(3):e13741.
89. Eddens T, Parks OB, Williams JV. Neonatal immune responses to respiratory viruses. Front Immunol. 2022;13:863149.
90. Williams JV, Harris PA, Tollefson SJ, et al. Human metapneumovirus and lower respiratory tract disease in otherwise healthy infants and children. N Engl J Med. 2004;350(5):443–50.
91. Rawlinson WD, Waliuzzaman Z, Carter IW, Belessis YC, Gilbert KM, Morton JR. Asthma exacerbations in children associated with rhinovirus but not human metapneumovirus infection. J Infect Dis. 2003;187(8):1314–8.
92. Sobkowiak P, Mikoś M, Bręborowicz A, Szczepankiewicz A. Human bocavirus and metapneumovirus in acute wheezing in children-is there a link with atopy? Clin Respir J. 2020;14(12):1201–7.
93. Mandelcwajg A, Moulin F, Menager C, Rozenberg F, Lebon P, Gendrel D. Underestimation of influenza viral infection in childhood asthma exacerbations. J Pediatr. 2010;157(3):505–6.
94. Hasegawa S, Hirano R, Hashimoto K, Haneda Y, Shirabe K, Ichiyama T. Characteristics of atopic children with pandemic H1N1 influenza viral infection: pandemic H1N1 influenza reveals 'occult' asthma of childhood. Pediatr Allergy Immunol. 2011;22(1 Pt 2):e119–23.
95. Ghannoum MA, Jurevic RJ, Mukherjee PK, et al. Characterization of the oral fungal microbiome (mycobiome) in healthy individuals. PLoS Pathog. 2010;6(1):e1000713.
96. Charlson ES, Diamond JM, Bittinger K, et al. Lung-enriched organisms and aberrant bacterial and fungal respiratory microbiota after lung transplant. Am J Respir Crit Care Med. 2012;186(6):536–45.
97. van Tilburg Bernardes E, Pettersen VK, Gutierrez MW, et al. Intestinal fungi are causally implicated in microbiome assembly and immune development in mice. Nat Commun. 2020;11(1):2577.
98. Trivedi M, Denton E. Asthma in children and adults-what are the differences and what can they tell us about asthma? Front Pediatr. 2019;7:256.
99. O'Hollaren MT, Yunginger JW, Offord KP, et al. Exposure to an aeroallergen as a possible precipitating factor in respiratory arrest in young patients with asthma. N Engl J Med. 1991;324(6):359–63.
100. Goldman DL, Huffnagle GB. Potential contribution of fungal infection and colonization to the development of allergy. Med Mycol. 2009;47(5):445–56.

101. Hughes KM, Price D, Torriero AAJ, Symonds MRE, Suphioglu C. Impact of fungal spores on asthma prevalence and hospitalization. Int J Mol Sci. 2022;23(8):4313.
102. Myszkowska D, Bogawski P, Piotrowicz K, et al. Co-exposure to highly allergenic airborne pollen and fungal spores in Europe. Sci Total Environ. 2023;905:167285.
103. Arbes SJ Jr, Gergen PJ, Elliott L, et al. Prevalences of positive skin test responses to 10 common allergens in the US population: results from the third National Health and Nutrition Examination Survey. J Allergy Clin Immunol. 2005;116(2):377–83.
104. Tham R, Vicendese D, Dharmage SC, et al. Associations between outdoor fungal spores and childhood and adolescent asthma hospitalizations. J Allergy Clin Immunol. 2017;139(4):1140–1147.e4.
105. Baxi SN, Sheehan WJ, Sordillo JE, et al. Association between fungal spore exposure in inner-city schools and asthma morbidity. Ann Allergy Asthma Immunol. 2019;122(6):610–615.e1.
106. Welsh K, Pashley CH, Satchwell J, et al. Colonisation with filamentous fungi and acute asthma exacerbations in children. Eur Respir J. 2016;48(Suppl 60):PA3354.
107. Shah A. Aspergillus-associated hypersensitivity respiratory disorders. Indian J Chest Dis Allied Sci. 2008;50(1):117–28.
108. Agarwal R, Chakrabarti A, Shah A, et al. Allergic bronchopulmonary aspergillosis: review of literature and proposal of new diagnostic and classification criteria. Clin Exp Allergy. 2013;43(8):850–73.
109. Noverr MC, Noggle RM, Toews GB, Huffnagle GB. Role of antibiotics and fungal microbiota in driving pulmonary allergic responses. Infect Immun. 2004;72(9):4996–5003.
110. Noverr MC, Falkowski NR, McDonald RA, McKenzie AN, Huffnagle GB. Development of allergic airway disease in mice following antibiotic therapy and fungal microbiota increase: role of host genetics, antigen, and interleukin-13. Infect Immun. 2005;73(1):30–8.
111. Kim YG, Udayanga KG, Totsuka N, Weinberg JB, Núñez G, Shibuya A. Gut dysbiosis promotes M2 macrophage polarization and allergic airway inflammation via fungi-induced PGE_2. Cell Host Microbe. 2014;15(1):95–102.
112. Skalski JH, Limon JJ, Sharma P, et al. Expansion of commensal fungus Wallemia mellicola in the gastrointestinal mycobiota enhances the severity of allergic airway disease in mice. PLoS Pathog. 2018;14(9):e1007260.
113. Wheeler ML, Limon JJ, Bar AS, et al. Immunological consequences of intestinal fungal dysbiosis. Cell Host Microbe. 2016;19(6):865–73.
114. Li X, Leonardi I, Semon A, et al. Response to fungal dysbiosis by gut-resident CX3CR1(+) mononuclear phagocytes aggravates allergic airway disease. Cell Host Microbe. 2018;24(6):847–856.e4.
115. Arrieta MC, Arévalo A, Stiemsma L, et al. Associations between infant fungal and bacterial dysbiosis and childhood atopic wheeze in a nonindustrialized setting. J Allergy Clin Immunol. 2018;142(2):424–434.e10.

Communication with Sick Children

9

Burak Çakir, Alberto Adalid, and Öznur Bilaç

9.1 Introduction

Childhood is referred to as the first 18-year period of life, and this period can be examined in subgroups. The first month of life is considered the newborn period, while the ages of 0–2 are referred to as the infancy period. Subsequently, the period can be divided into early childhood and preschool age. The school age is followed by the adolescent (teenage) period, and an individual who has reached the age of 18 is considered an adult.

9.2 Essential Features of Communication with Children in Childhood

The behavioral and cognitive development of children generally follows a specific sequential order. However, the pace of development can vary from child to child, being either slow or rapid [1]. Life, growth and development are interconnected, therefore communication should encompass all three aspects [2]. The manner of communication should be age-appropriate for the child, which is a fundamental principle. Another fundamental principle is recognizing the presence of the family in the relationship established with the child [3].

B. Çakir
Uşak University Training and Research Hospital, Uşak, Turkey

A. Adalid
Private Psychoanalyst and Psychotherapist, Mexico City, Mexico

Mexican Association of Group Psychoanalytic Psychotherapy (AMPAG), Mexico City, Mexico

Ö. Bilaç (✉)
Manisa Celal Bayar University Hospital, Manisa, Turkey

H. Yüksel et al. (eds.), *Pediatric Airway Diseases*, Comprehensive ENT,
https://doi.org/10.1007/978-3-031-74853-0_9

Communication should be "child and young people-centered communication" rather than "adult-centered communication." Child and young people-centered communication does not simply involve inserting child characters or speaking in child-specific jargon. It means developing communication strategies that activate appropriate ways of seeing, hearing, imagining, and creating for each age group. The essence lies in creating communication strategies that engage the abilities of observation, listening, imagination, and creativity specific to each developmental stage, in order to be able to perceive and interpret the child and young people in terms of intentional mental states: their needs, desires, feelings, beliefs, goals, purpose, and reasons [4].

In establishing and maintaining a relationship between doctors and pediatric patients within the boundaries of respect, various techniques are recommended for different age groups. However, it is important to view these techniques as tools that can address needs rather than treating them as one-size-fits-all solutions to every problem.

Certainly, effective communication with pediatric patients involves specific techniques across all age groups. When referring to or addressing a child, using their name is essential. When doctors encounter a child patient, it is important to introduce themselves, state their role, and provide information about the purpose and content of the meeting. This approach encourages collaboration between the medical professional, the child, and the family. Without this, families might withhold certain information, assuming that some topics are of no concern to the physician. Having a space in the examination room where the child can engage in play is beneficial. However, there should not be excessively noisy or distracting items that hinder the consultation and examination. When conversing with children, it is crucial to avoid accusatory, stigmatizing, authoritative, judgmental, critical, or condescending behavior. Communication barriers, such as providing excessive and unsolicited information, conveying excessive reassurance, stubbornly defending a particular perspective, using clichéd expressions, and asking closed-ended, short questions that hinder the expression of the child's emotions, should also be avoided. Praising children should be done frequently, expressed genuinely, and encouraged to be heard by others. Conversely, if criticism is necessary, it should be done in private, communicated clearly, combined with justified praise, and avoided when the child is upset. Waiting for the child to calm down is advised [5].

9.3 Characteristics of Communication with an Infant

In the presence of an infant, the behavior of healthcare professionals should be adjusted in a way that considers the child an intentional mental agent. For this reason, when entering the examination room, the physician should enter slowly without frightening the child, because that ecosystem is a foreign one for him. During the examination, the information provided by the caregiver should be listened to attentively, and respectful behavior should be displayed. As parents or caregivers spend more extended periods of time with the child, they can detect any problems related to the child's health earlier. Babies, during this period, rely heavily on body language, so their body movements should be observed closely. Approaching the baby rapidly should be avoided, and a certain distance should be maintained. When speaking to parents, a smiling expression and a gentle tone of voice should be used. When interacting with the baby, maintaining eye contact and sitting at the same level are crucial. The healthcare professional should always keep in mind to be open and flexible, and be able to adapt to any further interference proposed in this model [6].

As discomfort might arise when transitioning to the examination table, if possible, physical examinations are better conducted with the baby in the mother's arms for the sake of comfort.

9.4 Communication Characteristics with Pediatric Patients

When children are brought in for examination by their parents, involving the child in the conversations and listening to their complaints is of utmost importance. While listening to their complaints, it is beneficial to understand how these complaints make them feel in terms of their emotional states, as this helps the child express themselves, build self-confidence, and feel understood. If an apprehensive child is encountered who prefers to remain silent, it is not appropriate to conduct the consultation solely with the parent as if the child is not present in the examination room. If there is an object in the examination room that captures the child's attention, initiating communication with the child through that object initially can enhance rapport and increase the child's willingness to engage [6].

Children in this age group might be active and energetic. In such cases, redirecting the child's focus to their movements is important, as parents' attention might be divided when recounting complaints, potentially leading to an incomplete medical history. Similarly, the physician's perception of the child's behavior might become negative, hindering the establishment of trust-based communication. Maintaining eye contact with the child during the examination, playing with toys intermittently, and most importantly, leaving the potentially unsettling examination component until the end are advisable. Concluding the examination by rewarding the child can be a highly effective practice [7].

Listening plays a pivotal role in establishing healthy communication with children. It is one of the fundamental ways of gaining information, understanding, and learning. When communicating with children, it is crucial to listen carefully to what they are trying to convey before saying anything to them. When a child perceives that they are being listened to, they will find it easier to express their emotions and thoughts to the person in front of them [8]. In communication, paying attention to both verbal and nonverbal messages of the other person is important. Alongside the responses provided during listening, the listener's body posture and physical presence in a listening stance also carry significance. As one immerses oneself in the act of listening, body posture, eye contact, facial expressions, head movements, physical proximity, and touch become influential factors that directly shape the communication process [9]. Therefore, while being attentive listeners, individuals should be mindful of their own nonverbal cues, as these nonverbal elements contribute greatly to the overall communication dynamic.

- *Body posture*: A relaxed body posture signifies readiness and openness to listen. The listener's relaxed and natural demeanor can make the person being listened to feel more comfortable and attended to. Maintaining eye contact with the person's face during communication will have a significant impact on both the listener and the speaker. When communicating with a child who has come to the hospital, it is crucial for healthcare professionals to align themselves with the child's height or raise the child to their own eye level. Having the adult and child at the same distance allows the removal of barriers, equalizing the positions of the child and the adult. Being at the same level as the child who is speaking with the healthcare professional enables the child to establish eye contact, notice the facial expressions of the speaking adult, observe their gestures, and consequently focus on the conversation. This alignment will help the child better comprehend what is being said to them.
- *Eye contact*: Establishing eye contact during communication is essential for the child to better understand the adult and to grasp what the child is trying to convey. Maintaining eye contact with a child who has come to the hospital while communicating can make the child feel listened to by the person they are communicating with, consequently leading them to feel respected. If the adult avoids making eye contact with the child, it could create a sense of insecurity in the child.
- *Facial expression*: A smiling face, a warm and friendly approach, and a genuinely kind facial expression can significantly impact communication. Children, especially in unfamiliar environments like hospitals, are greatly influenced by individuals who are approachable and wear a warm expression. Communication with such individuals, who make them feel more comfortable and secure, might be easier for children.
- *Head movements*: Nodding one's head during listening is an expression of showing interest in the speaker and what is being said. This action conveys the message "I understand you" to the person being spoken to, allowing them to receive the message that they are being understood. When healthcare professionals communicate with children and use head movements to express approval while listening, it can encourage the child to continue speaking.
- *Physical proximity*: When a child who has come to the hospital shares their concerns, being physically close to them and engaging in a face-to-face conversation can make them feel much more connected to the healthcare professional. This sense of closeness can foster trust in the person they are speaking to, enabling them to express themselves more comfortably and easily.
- *Touch*: Physical contact and touch in communication reflect intimacy, emotions, and closeness. It can also lead to sudden changes in emotional state. During communication with a child, gestures like touching their shoulder or gently stroking their head can make them more willing to engage in conversation. Touching signifies acknowledging an individual's physical presence and expressing value. However, it is important to remember to avoid any forms of touch that might make the child uncomfortable.

- *Passive listening*: In passive listening, nonverbal active listening behaviors are exhibited, such as silence and attentive nonverbal gestures (nodding, leaning forward, etc.), which demonstrate openness and attentiveness to the messages from the other party. In passive listening, "silence" is a powerful element that allows the person to have the opportunity to speak. It evokes a sense of acceptance in the speaker, providing them with an opportunity to express themselves. When communicating with children, remaining silent can encourage them to continue speaking. Children, especially when they have a problem, may find it difficult to express themselves and may require moments of silence. In some cases, the listener may need to provide certain reactions to indicate that they are actively listening, such as nodding, leaning forward, smiling, or using affirmations like "yes" or "uh-huh." Some individuals also need encouragement to speak. To support their conversation, using phrases like "I understand," "Is that right?" "Tell me more," or "Do you want to continue?" can create an opening for them to share further. Children who experience fear and anxiety during medical examinations or treatments in a hospital setting might have difficulty expressing themselves. As healthcare professionals, remaining silent while listening and providing the aforementioned reactions can facilitate communication.
- *Active listening*: Active listening is a form of listening where the listener indicates that they understand or can understand the speaker by providing feedback, paraphrasing, or repeating what the speaker has said. Active listening is an extremely important aspect of communication and involves showing that the listener is engaged and paying attention. By actively participating in the conversation, the listener can demonstrate their comprehension and create a more effective communication exchange.
- We can exemplify active listening based on a dialogue between mother and child.

  M: "Do you remember that today you have an appointment with the dentist?. You're getting braces on your teeth. Are you ready? We need to leave."
  C: "Mom, my stomach hurts. I don't want to go…"
  M: "I see, where does it hurts?, that can be an uncomfortable feeling."
  C: "Yes, I don't like how it feels."
  M: "Do you think it might have something to do with going to the dentist?"
  C: "Maybe. Will they give me a shot?"
  M: "You're wondering if they'll give you a shot when they put on the braces."
  C: "Yes."
  M: "Not knowing what will happen can make you feel confused."
  C: "I don't want to feel pain. Actually, I'm afraid of it hurting."
  M: "I understand you, I think that can be a frightening experience. When we arrive you can ask the dentist what will happen and all the doubts you have about the braces. Do you think that's a good idea?"

As seen in the example above, the mother can put herself under his child's skin to understand his emotional and mental states, such as confusion, discomfort, and fear about going to the dentist. Taking into consideration the developmental levels of children while being curious about how the world looks from their perspective and how our own perspective may influence how we see someone else's behavior is crucial. This way the child can have a safe haven, since the mother relates to the child's mental states and intentions, as well as letting the child know her own affects and behaviors toward him or her [10].

In conclusion, communication stands at the core of human life and is essential for the continuation of relationships. When establishing effective and healthy communication with children, it is crucial to allow them the opportunity to be themselves as much as possible. Children who can communicate freely, openly, and healthily with the people around them will be able to lead their lives in a happy and successful manner according to their developmental potential. All adults who approach children considering their emotions and motivations, while seeing their reactions and behaviors, regardless of the context, will be able to establish effective and healthy communication with them.

There are certain key strategies to keep in mind:

- How does the child or young person know that I want to listen to him/her?
- Help the child or young person and the family to get a shared understanding of why he or she is there, its goals, and what the problem is.
- Be sure that the child or young person understands the choices available to him or her and their pros and cons.
- Explore his/her views and preferences.
- Help them all to reach a shared agreement on key problems, plans, and what is going to happen next.

References

1. Dwyer Hall, Holly. "Mentalization-based treatment for children: a time-limited approach: by Nick Midgley, Karin Ensink, Karin Lindqvist, Norka Malberg, & Nicole Muller, Washington, DC, American Psychological Association, 2017, 268.
2. Midgley, Nick; Ensink, Karin; Lindqvist, Karin; Malberg, Norka; Muller, Nicole. Mentalization-Based Treatment for Children. American Psychological Association, 2011.
3. Barclay S. Recognizing and managing conflict between patients, parents and health professionals. Pediatr Child Health. 2016;26(7):314–8.
4. Midgley, Nick, and Ioanna Vrouva, eds. Minding the child: Mentalization-based interventions with children, young people and their families. Routledge, 2013.
5. Allen, Jon G. Mentalizing in the development and treatment of attachment trauma. Routledge, 2018.
6. Ritter RH Jr, Reis MD, Rascoe TG. Interviewing techniques. In: Textbook of family medicine e-book. Elsevier; 2011. p. 166.
7. Lorin MI. General principles of communicating with pediatric patients and family members. In: Communicating with pediatric patients and their families: the Texas Children's Hospital guide for physicians, nurses and other healthcare professionals; 2015. p. 11–25.
8. Sacks D, Westwood M. An approach to interviewing adolescents. Paediatr Child Health. 2003;8(9):554–6.
9. Bernzweig J, Takayama JI, Phibbs C, Lewis C, Pantell RH. Gender differences in physician-patient communication. Evidence from pediatric visits. Arch Pediatr Adolesc Med. 1997;151:586–91.
10. Kolucki B, Lemish D. Communicating with children. UNICEF; 2011. ISBN: 978-0-578-09512-7.

Communication with Sick Child's Parents 10

Can Cemal Cingi

10.1 Introduction

Children, like adults, frequently inquire about the nature of their sickness, treatment, and eventual death. Answers to queries should be forthcoming, truthful, and age-appropriate. Adolescent and child patients benefit from age-appropriate explanations of their condition, symptom management, and end-of-life planning. Adolescents are more likely to feel comfortable talking to doctors if they are actively involved in their care planning [1, 2].

Children's communication needs to consider their age, stage of development, and any neurological abnormalities they may have. The child should be the focus of all communication, while parents may also be involved in discussions about care depending on the child's age. When addressing the child's care, including all appropriate family members is essential [3].

One method to use when communicating with kids is [1]

- Please communicate with the youngster at their developmental level [4].
- Draw, read, and play with age-appropriate toys and games for your child [5].
- Communicate openly and earn trust by providing straightforward answers to queries.
- Spend quality time together and talk about things other than their health.
- Be willing to listen to and rehash conversations regarding care; give kids a break from their parents and other caregivers [6].

C. C. Cingi (✉)
Communication Design and Management Department, Faculty of Communication Sciences, Anadolu University, Eskisehir, Turkey

H. Yüksel et al. (eds.), *Pediatric Airway Diseases*, Comprehensive ENT,
https://doi.org/10.1007/978-3-031-74853-0_10

10.2 Communication with Family

Parents of children with terminal illnesses say that challenges in talking to doctors and nurses about the child's impending death rank high on their list of sources of stress [7]. Including family members in the care planning process is essential to having open discussions about treatment options. It can be challenging to gauge the child's and their parents' comprehension while discussing the child's life-limiting disease in the same conversation [1, 8].

When communicating with families in the aftermath of a child's death, it's essential to keep a few things in mind:

- Be straightforward, concise, and empathic when conveying the child's health information. Plan the conversations, considering timing and surroundings
- Assess prior knowledge and what needs to be shared
- Allow for silence and acknowledge emotions
- Plan for future meetings
- Assess prior knowledge and what needs to be discussed
- Be clear, concise, and empathetic when delivering information about the child's condition [9]

10.3 Communication Tips for Parents of Pediatric Patients

Let Them Warm Up to You
When coming in for their initial visit, many young patients experience anxiety. You want them to feel at ease, so allow them time to get to know you and the setting.

This is a perfect use case for your waiting area! Having something fun for kids to do while they wait is a significant benefit. But once they're inside the examination room, their nerves could start to act up again.

Engage these patients in conversation about anything but their illness. This facilitates communication and sets the stage for a future working partnership. Please provide them with off-topic inquiries during your visit.

This may concern their academics, extracurriculars, or weekend plans. You might also inquire about their entertainment preferences, such as their preferred film or book.

Asking inquiries along these lines will encourage conversation on familiar ground. It's an excellent opportunity to connect with them more individually. The patient's confidence in you and comfort with the visit will increase. In addition, this will demonstrate to the parents that you are concerned for their child [10].

10.3.1 Create a Relaxing Setting

It's not a direct method of communication, but it can make things go more smoothly. Exam rooms, especially for toddlers, are stressful due to the strong odors and intense lighting. If they are anxious to begin with, something else will be needed.

However, if you improve their surroundings, they will be more at ease. Decorating waiting areas and appointment rooms with lighthearted themes might help patients feel more at ease.

Small, sanitized toys or plush animals that kids can hold throughout the exam may also help children relax.

Talking to patients is the most remarkable approach to gauging their level of relaxation. Please inquire as to whether or not there is anything you can do for the patient to improve their level of ease. As a result, people may feel more comfortable opening up to you.

It's a helpful tool for figuring out how to make the facility safer for future patients. When people are at ease, they are more receptive to communicating with you [10].

10.3.2 Talk to Them Where They're At

There is a wide range of linguistic competence among age groups. Babies and toddlers don't talk like school-aged kids. Teenagers are still considered pediatric patients, although their communication styles differ significantly from younger children's.

Guests of all ages will have a better time if you tailor your message to their demographic. Acting goofy in front of the youngest pediatric patients can help them feel more at ease.

Having something in common with a youngster their age makes them feel more at ease around you.

Adopt an adult tone when conversing with adolescent students. They demand that grown-ups treat them equally, not like children. Teenagers are more likely to listen to advice when it is delivered with respect and as though they are adults.

However, any disparities in development must be taken into account. Tailoring your approach to each child patient is essential, as some may be mature beyond their years.

Patients who are developmentally delayed may also have difficulty maintaining a conversation at a typical adult level. Therefore, it is crucial to tailor your communication to the patient's age and stage of development [10].

10.3.3 The Appointment Process, Explained

Young patients may feel uneasy because of the unknown. A step-by-step explanation of the procedure can help calm their nerves about what's to come.

Preparing children for even the most basic of situations will assist. Make sure they know the stethoscope will likely be cool to the touch before you use it on them. During the uncomfortable sections of the appointment, you can try talking to the patient to divert them.

You can even let them assist you through the scheduled time. Kids learn best via doing. Allow them to participate in some aspects of the appointment even if they cannot replace a doctor. This will help them feel safer and more confident. They will have a good time, a bonus [9].

10.3.4 Don't Misuse the Terms

Always try to utilize simple, straightforward language. This material is more for the parents of very young patients. Many people aren't familiar with medical terminology, so using more straightforward language when communicating with their parents is crucial.

If you explain it to older children properly, they may be able to understand. You'll need to utilize more straightforward language or find a way to connect it to a concept they already know and comprehend [10].

The use of appropriate body language is an integral part of effective communication. If you can, sit down with your pediatric patients so you're both on the same level.

Their concerns and fears won't be eased if you stand over them. If you need help getting to the kids' level, have them sit on their parents' laps instead.

When speaking to the patient, make direct eye contact with them. Your focus should be on the patient, not on the parents. Parents must remain involved in the discussion. However, kids need to realize that their care is tailored to them.

Only communicating while wearing the mask won't help, either. Drop it whenever you can, engage in conversation, and flash a grin. These subtle cues convey a lot. You don't want to provide a bad image that would make your young patients nervous by reading your face. Despite the gravity of the issue, strive to have a positive outlook [10].

10.3.5 Parental Involvement

Although the juvenile patient is your primary concern, you should also talk to their parents. Because children look to their parents for leadership, this is critical.

The presence of a person the youngster knows and trusts in the talk will likely put them at ease [10].

10.3.6 Consult the Parent on Anything

We discussed how various children are at different stages of growth before. The easiest way to speak with the youngster in this situation is first to talk with the parent to find out where the kid is. Their parents will have the most insight into their children's communication styles.

Parents can break the ice with their reserved or reticent children. If you ask a patient's parents what's bothering them, you can better understand how to put them at ease.

When youngsters have questions they can't figure out, they might turn to their parents for guidance. To ask a child about their health history is to put them on the spot and likely increase their anxiety levels. Children may not know their parents' medical history, allergies, or vaccinations, but their parents would [10].

10.3.7 Treat Your Parents with Respect

Most parents would do whatever to ensure their kids are safe and healthy. They can be as challenging to deal with as the patient themselves when they are as anxious as their children. They could jump to conclusions and become annoyed or uneasy. The patient may become distressed as a result.

Have a private dialogue with the parents outside of the patient's presence. You should remain calm and patient even if the parent is worried or upset.

They're more likely upset about the circumstance than angry with you. Help them comprehend by responding to their inquiries and providing explanations where necessary. Give them resources that can help them learn as well [10].

10.4 Coordinating Care When Your Child Is Ill

The fact that their kid will become sick occasionally is a given for all parents. It's common for youngsters to contract a cold from a classmate and then spread it to their family at home. Many parents have experienced this, as it is practically inevitable at certain seasons of the year.

A sick child can throw a wrench into a co-parenting couple's plans and cause tension in the household. Read these valuable guidelines for co-parenting a sick child [11] before your child contracts their subsequent illness.

10.4.1 Discuss Your Child-Care Arrangements with Each Other

Your child may need to stay home from school if their illness is severe. They may also be too exhausted to be transported between the homes of their parents [11].

In such cases, your parenting plan or visiting arrangements must be worked out between you and your co-parent. Your parenting plan may have provisions for this, so you should look there. Keep up with the routine if your youngster is healthy enough to travel between houses or for a visit [11].

If your child is genuinely ill, you should decide as a family. If your child needs to relax and recover, staying in their current location may be preferable. The stress will make their disease worse and last longer. Communicating clearly and keeping good records of parenting decisions that depart from the norm is essential.

It is usually up to the parent the child is staying with to make arrangements for the child to miss school. If you cannot take care of your child full-time, talk to your partner about sharing that responsibility. This may already be covered if you have a right of first refusal clause in your parenting agreement [11].

10.4.2 Inform Your Co-parent of the Specifics

When handing off parental duties to your co-parent, ensure everyone understands their responsibilities. Put all drugs and their dosages and administration times down on paper. Before entrusting someone else with your child, ensure they know how things have been going so far [11].

When you've finished communicating the necessary information, your co-parent can take over. Have faith in their ability to nurse your child back to health and commit to doing what is in the child's best interest. Although it may be challenging to relinquish control, you must do so in this situation [11].

10.4.3 Exhibit Cohesion

Maintain a cheerful environment for your ill youngster. Treat your co-parent with respect before your child, and consider increasing your co-parent's visitation rights. They could make more frequent phone or text checks. If your kid is genuinely sick, consider inviting them to spend time with them [11].

A child can benefit from seeing their parents work together as co-parents at any time, but the effect is magnified when one is ill. Feel free to set aside your differences and focus on getting your sick child well again if that youngster is yours. Put aside your differences and work together as a team for the sake of your child [11].

It's not easy to deal with a sick kid, but you must do it effectively when it happens. Before your child is sick, discuss how you'll improve them quickly and implement your plans [11].

10.5 Talking to One's Siblings and Pals

Children with life-limiting illnesses may have a different concept of death and dying than children of the same age. This comprehension results from their participation in discussions about their sickness and its management, as well as their exposure to the deaths of other children [8].

Siblings and close friends of a child with a terminal disease need to have discussions about death and dying that are appropriate for their age. Parents and caregivers often have their losses to contend with. The palliative care team members may need to help them to have these conversations [1, 12].

Siblings can gain from:

- being included in family conversations
- being given information about their sibling's condition

- being given time to discuss concerns with medical professionals
- making connections with support groups or other children dealing with similar circumstances
- receiving individualized attention and care
- being encouraged to express negative emotions like sadness and anger
- having these feelings and emotions normalized [13, 14]

They are reassured about their own health and permitted to visit their sick sibling.

10.6 Conclusion

When talking to kids, keeping their developmental level in mind is essential [15, 16]. Age-appropriate strategies for communicating with kids are outlined in the below [17–22].

Stability can be fostered for children of all ages by upholding consistent routines and expectations. Having "regular" family time that isn't constantly focused on the child's condition is also beneficial. To keep things as normal as possible for their sick kid, parents often need guidance in recognizing how these reminders impact their child's life [20–22].

References

1. PCC4U. Topic 3 | Activity 5: Communication with children and their families. https://pcc4u.org.au/learning/topics/topic3/t3_section2/t3_activity5/. Accessed 4 Oct 2023.
2. Wiener L, Zadeh S, Battles H, Baird K, Ballard E, Osherow J, Pao M. Allowing adolescents and young adults to plan their end-of-life care. Pediatrics. 2012;130(5):897–905.
3. CareSearch. Communicating with health professionals. 2011. www.caresearch.com.au/caresearch/tabid/1107/Default.aspx. Accessed 6 Dec 2012.
4. Zwaanswijk M, Tates K, van Dulmen S, Hoogerbrugge PM, Kamps WA, Beishuizen A, Bensing JM. Communicating with child patients in pediatric oncology consultations: a vignette study on child patients', parents', and survivors' communication preferences. Psychooncology. 2011;20(3):269–77.
5. Rollins JA. Tell me about it: drawing as a communication tool for children with cancer. J Pediatr Oncol Nurs. 2005;22(4):203–21.
6. Turner J, Clavarino A, Yates P, Hargraves M, Connors V, Hausmann S. Development of a resource for parents with advanced cancer: what do parents want? Palliat Support Care. 2007;5(2):135–45.
7. Sandler I. Parental grief and palliative care require attention. Pediatr Adolesc Med. 2004;158(6):590–1.
8. Bluebond-Langner M, Belasco J, DeMesquita Wanda M. "I want to live, until I don't want to live anymore": involving children with life-threatening and life-shortening illnesses in decision making about care and treatment. Nurs Clin North Am. 2010;45(3):329.
9. Klick JC, Hauer J. Pediatric palliative care. Curr Probl Pediatr Adolesc Health Care. 2010;40(6):120–51.
10. Clark M. Common sense pediatric patient and parent communication tips. https://etactics.com/blog/pediatric-patient-parent-communication-tips. Accessed 4 Oct 2023.

11. 4 Tips for co-parenting when your child is sick. OurFamilyWizard Blog. https://www.ourfamilywizard.com/blog/4-tips-co-parenting-when-your-child-sick. Accessed 4 Oct 2023.
12. Carlile M. Understanding grief and bereavement in the palliative care setting. In: O'Connor M, Lee S, Aranda S, editors. Palliative care nursing: a guide to practice. Ascot Vale, VIC: Ausmed Publications; 2012. p. 271–89.
13. Abrams M. The well sibling: challenges and possibilities. Am J Psychother. 2009;63(4):305–17.
14. Brown E, Warr B, Smallman A. Supporting the child and the family in paediatric palliative care. London: Jessica Kingsley Publishers; 2007.
15. Sisk BA, et al. Prognostic disclosures to children: a historical perspective. Pediatrics. 2016;138(3):e20161278. https://doi.org/10.1542/peds.2016-1278.
16. Muriel AC, et al. Measuring psychosocial distress and parenting concerns among adults with cancer: the Parenting Concerns Questionnaire. Cancer. 2012;118(22):5671–8.
17. Moore C, Pengelly M, Rauch P. Communicating with children when a parent is dying. In: Kissane D, Bultz B, Butow P, editors. Handbook of communication in oncology and palliative care. Oxford: OUP; 2010.
18. Cancer Council Australia. Need support? Talking to kids about cancer 2015. Mar 2018. https://www.cancercouncil.com.au/cancer-information/for-family-and-friends/talking-to-kids-about-cancer/support-and-information/.
19. Kopchak Sheehan D, et al. Telling adolescents a parent is dying. J Palliat Med. 2014;17(5):512–20.
20. CareSearch. Talking with children. 2018. https://bit.ly/2TRotYi.
21. Meier DE. The human connection of palliative care: ten steps for what to say and do. 2018. https://youtu.be/7kQ3PUyhmPQ.
22. Rauch P, Arnold R. What do I tell the children? Fast facts and concepts. 2018. https://www.mypcnow.org/blank-uftnj.

Part II

Diagnostic Testing

11 Radiologic Evaluation of Upper Respiratory System

Gonca Koc, Aloisia Paloma Hernandez Morales, and Huseyin Hudaver Alper

11.1 Introduction

The upper airway is defined as the airway passage located between the nostrils and the trachea. It consists of the nasal passage, pharynx (naso- and oropharynx), and larynx. Diseases of upper airway and its obstructive pathologies are more common in children due to certain anatomical and physiological characteristics specific to the respiratory system: The children have enlarged adenoid tissue and narrower nasopharynx compared to adults. Conus elasticus lining the region between the vocal cords and the cricoid is vulnerable to edema related to its loose connective tissue. Children also have weaker respiratory muscles to compensate the respiratory distress [1]. Laryngeal rest during current expiration, a variable resistance mechanism, allows maintaining a stable and adequate residual functional capacity through a compliant rib cage and lung. The variety of the symptoms and the fact that they are not specific to the disease, clinicians (pediatricians, otolaryngologists) may need to implement radiological imaging to establish a diagnosis. The basic radiological imaging method in the upper airway diseases is radiography of associated anatomic region, subsequently computed tomography (CT) can also be obtained. Although magnetic resonance imaging (MRI) is not acquired in the emergency setting due to

G. Koc (✉)
Department of Radiology, King Hamad University Hospital, Royal Medical Services, Muharraq, Bahrain
e-mail: gonca.koc@khuh.org.bh

A. P. H. Morales
Department of Radiology, Instituto Nacional de Enfermedades Respiratorias, Ismael Cosío Villegas, México City, Mexico

H. H. Alper
Division of Pediatric Radiology, Department of Radiology and Medical Imaging, Ege University School of Medicine, Izmir, Turkey

H. Yüksel et al. (eds.), *Pediatric Airway Diseases*, Comprehensive ENT,
https://doi.org/10.1007/978-3-031-74853-0_11

its prolonged examination time, has significant contribution to the diagnosis of tumoral lesions of the airway and sleep apnea. In this section, pediatric upper airway diseases will be discussed according to the anatomical regions. First, the diseases specific to the anatomical regions, subsequently the common diseases that may affect all regions will be discussed with a specific emphasize on their radiological findings.

11.2 Nasal Cavity

The nasal cavity forms the initial part of the airway as anteriorly connected to the external environment with the nasal vestibule. Posteriorly, it has continuity with the nasopharynx via choanae. The borders of the nasal cavity are; cranially cribriform plate of the ethmoid bone, caudally the hard and soft palate, laterally the turbinates, and medial walls of the maxillary sinuses. Due to the direct connection between the nasal cavity and paranasal sinuses, their diseases are closely related. During the childhood, the most common disease is the inflammatory-infectious diseases. The physical examination is the basic diagnostic method of the diseases of paranasal cavity. The radiological imaging, particularly CT and MRI, should be reserved for the chronic, complicated inflammatory, and neoplastic diseases.

11.2.1 Choanal Atresia

The definition of choanal atresia is the lack of development of the posterior part of the nasal cavity (choana) and therefore the interruption of the connection between the nasal cavity and the nasopharynx. The incidence is 1 per 5000–7000 live births [2]. It can be encountered as uni- or bilateral forms. The bilateral forms occur less frequently. Since the neonates present with respiratory distress immediately following the birth due to compulsory nasal breathing during the neonatal period, surgery is an emergency [3]. Children with unilateral choanal atresia show the symptoms of unilateral nasal discharge and congestion at later stages. CT scan obtained following the failure to advance the nasogastric tube is the first choice imaging method for confirmation of choanal atresia and surgical planning. There are two forms of choanal atresia: In the bony atresia, the lateral walls of the nasal cavity bend medially and the enlarged vomer come together to cover the choana. In membranous atresia, bony structures are generally normal. The posterior nasal cavity and nasopharynx connection is interfered with a thin membrane. In the CT examination of the nasopharynx accumulation of a small amount of water-soluble contrast material dripped through the nostrils at the level of atretic choana might be helpful in making the diagnosis of choanal atresia (Fig. 11.1).

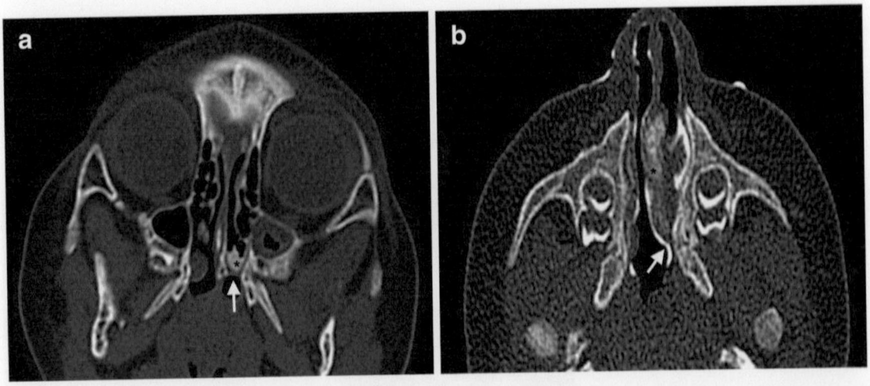

Fig. 11.1 CT images of membranous and bony atresia of the choana. (**a**) One-month-old boy with left-sided membranous type choanal atresia. Thin membrane separating choana and nasopharynx is seen (white arrow). The water-soluble contrast medium is accumulated within the atretic pouch of the choana (black asterisk). (**b**) Three-month-old boy with left-sided bony type choanal atresia. Vomer is thickened (black asterisk) and bent laterally to obstruct the choana (white arrow)

11.2.2 Rhinosinusitis

Rhinitis is defined as the inflammation of the nasal mucosa. However, since it is almost always accompanied with the inflammation of the paranasal sinuses, the use of the term rhinosinusitis would be more accurate. Rhinosinusitis can be classified as acute (less than 1 month) or chronic (more than 3 months); and as viral or bacterial. In children, most cases occur as viral rhinosinusitis. The American Academy of Pediatrics defines acute bacterial sinusitis as a persistent illness with nasal discharge of any quality and/or daytime cough lasting for >10 days without improvement, a worsening clinical course, a severe onset of symptoms with concurrent fever (temperature ≥ 39 °C), and purulent nasal discharge for at least 3 consecutive days [4]. Since the radiological imaging does not change the treatment approach, it is not recommended for the diagnosis of uncomplicated acute rhinosinusitis [5]. Radiography is not beneficial for the diagnosis and follow-up of acute/chronic rhinosinusitis of pediatric patients due to difficulty in positioning and evaluating particularly the ethmoid sinuses. Furthermore, paranasal sinus opacification on CT and MRI can be encountered even in healthy children without a clinical sign of rhinosinusitis. Therefore, radiological imaging has a limited role in the diagnosis (6). As recommended by the American College of Radiology, the imaging modality of choice should be paranasal sinus CT without intravenous (IV) contrast administration for surgical planning if functional sinus surgery is planned for chronic or recurrent rhinosinusitis, and as paranasal and brain CT/MRI with IV contrast if rhinosinusitis/invasive fungal sinusitis with intracranial or orbital complication is suspected [6].

Complications of the rhinosinusitis occur in the form of spread of the infection to the orbit, intracranial region, or bone. Orbital complications are the most common and develop with the dispersal of ethmoid or frontal sinus

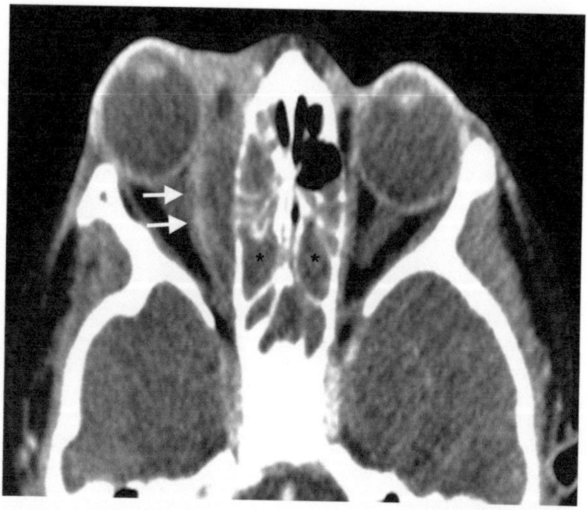

Fig. 11.2 Subperiosteal abscess. CT orbits with intravenous contrast administration of a 12-year-old boy reveals right-sided subperiosteal abscess (white arrows) and bilateral ethmoid sinusitis (black asterisk)

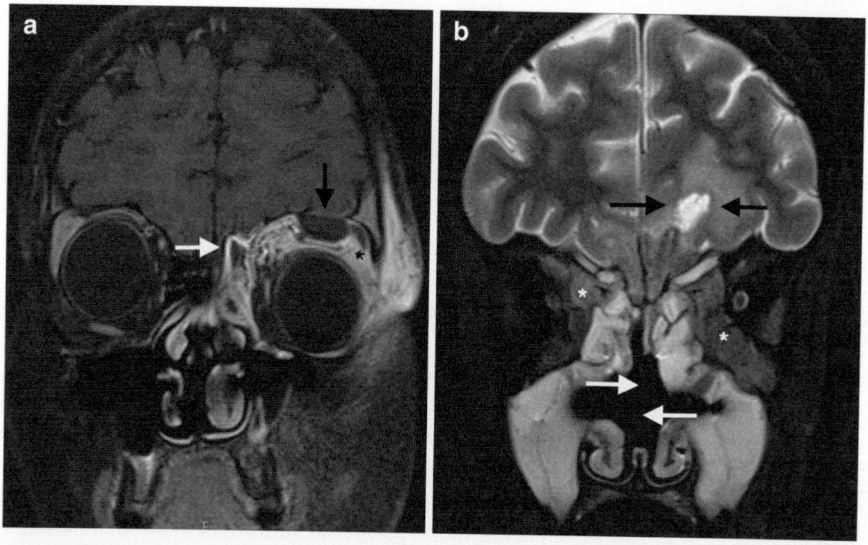

Fig. 11.3 Orbital and intracranial abscess as the complication of rhinosinusitis. (**a**) Postcontrast T1-weighted coronal MR image of 10-year-old girl with left-sided ethmoid sinusitis (white arrow), intraorbital abscess (black arrow), and orbital cellulitis (black asterisk). (**b**) T2-weighted coronal MR image of a 15-year-old boy previously diagnosed with leukemia and fungal sinusitis. Pansinusitis, defect of nasal septum (white arrows) associated with fungal infection, intracranial abscess (black arrow), and intraorbital extension of the infection (white asterisks) are seen

infections. Orbital complications are as follow, preseptal cellulitis, orbital cellulitis, orbital abscess, subperiosteal abscess, and cavernous sinus thrombosis (Figs. 11.2 and 11.3). In orbital complications, a favorable response to medical treatment compared to particularly intracranial complications is expected [7].

Pottt's Puffy tumor is the subperiosteal abscess of the frontal bone caused by the extension of rhinosinutis. Intracranial spread is the most serious complication and appears as inflammation of any structure within the brain or intracranial abscess.

11.2.3 Sinonasal Polyposis and Antrochoanal Polyp

Nasal polyp is a benign and inflammatory growth of the nasal mucosa and its extension into the nasal cavity and/or paranasal sinuses. It is often associated with chronic and allergic rhinosinusitis and less common during the childhood. Nasal polyposis might be a sign of cystic fibrosis, immune deficiency, or ciliary dyskinesia in children [8].

A single polyp is albeit rarely encountered in anywhere in the nasal cavity. When it originates from the maxillary sinus antrum and extends posteriorly to the choana is called as antrochoanal polyp. The major symptom caused by anthrochoanal polyp is chronic nasal obstruction.

The radiological findings associated with nasal polyps are expansion of the sinus ostia and remodeling of the bony walls of the nasal cavity and sinuses without causing any destruction. On MRI, they are hyperintense on T2 and hypointense on T1-weighted images, and might peripherally enhance following IV gadolinium injection. If sinonasal surgery is planned, a paranasal sinus CT or MRI examination, preferably without IV contrast, can be obtained for preoperative planning (Fig. 11.4).

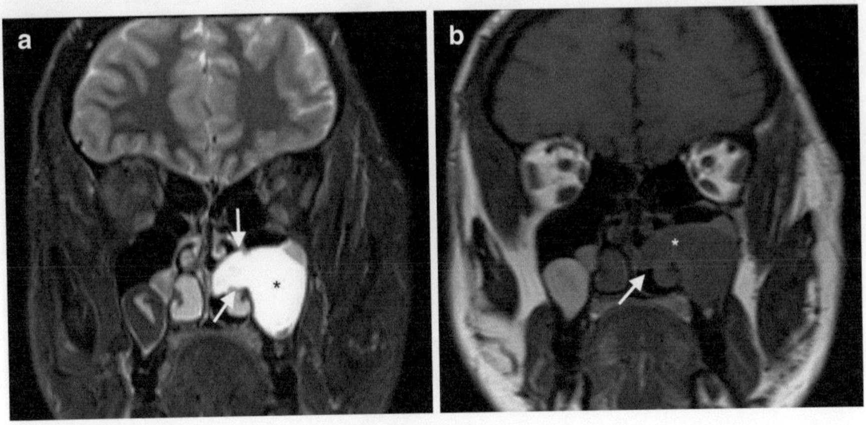

Fig. 11.4 MR images of antrochoanal polyp. (**a**) T2-weighted MR image reveals left-sided antrochoanal polyp filling left maxillary sinus (asterisk) and extending to the nasal cavity via accessory maxillary sinus ostium (white arrow). It is hyperintense on T2-weighted image. (**b**) T1-weighted MR image, note enlarged maxillary sinus accessory ostium (asterisk) and extension of antrachoanal polyp into the nasal cavity (white arrow)

11.2.4 Juvenile Nasopharyngeal Angiofibroma

Albeit rare, nasopharyngeal angiofibroma is the most common benign tumor of the nasal cavity [9]. It is a locally aggressive and highly vascular tumor frequently encountered in adolescent boys. Patients usually present with nasal congestion and bleeding. The common thought of its origin is sphenopalatine foramen. Extension of the tumor in all directions, primarily by filling the pterygopalatine fossa, and intracranial extension may also be encountered. Due to its increased blood supply, biopsy may cause excessive bleeding. Therefore, radiological diagnosis is extremely important. The most important radiological findings of the tumor on CT and MRI are typical location of pterygopalatine fossa and intense contrast enhancement following IV contrast medium administration (Fig. 11.5). CT is useful in revealing bony erosion. On MRI, dot like signal void areas are indicative of increased vascularity of the tumor.

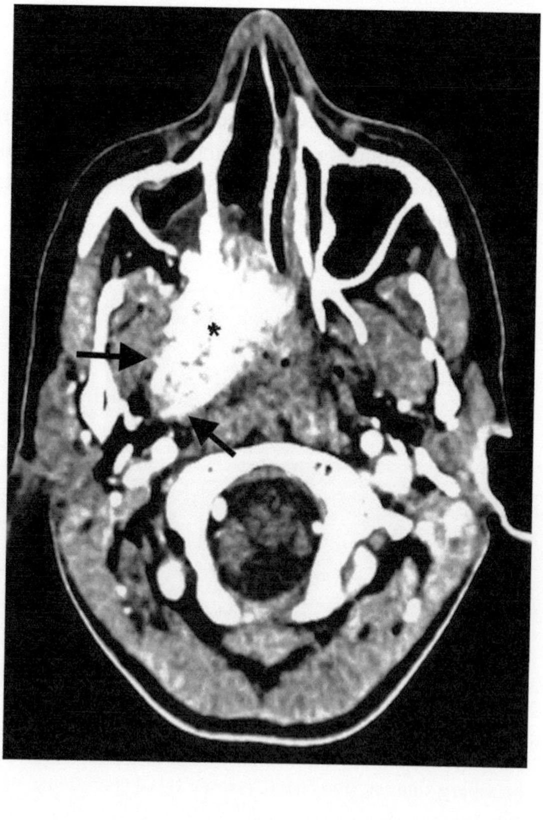

Fig. 11.5 Contrast-enhanced CT image of 14-year-old boy reveals vividly enhancing right-sided nasopharyngeal angiofibroma (asterisk). It is filling pterigopalatine fossa and extending to the posterior of right nasal cavity, parapharyngeal, and masticator spaces (black arrows)

11.3 Pharynx

Pharynx is divided into three parts: nasopharynx, oropharynx, and hypopharynx.

11.4 Nasopharynx

Nasopharynx is continuous with the nasal cavity and forms the uppermost part of the pharynx. Its borders are the skull base above and the soft palate below.

11.4.1 Adenoid Hypertrophy

The posterior and superior walls of the nasopharynx are rich in lymphoid tissue. Hypertrophy of nasopharyngeal lymphoid tissue in children, particularly between the ages of 3–6, is called as adenoid hypertrophy or nasopharyngeal lymphoid hypertrophy and probably due to recurrent infections and allergic conditions [10, 11]. Adenoid hypertrophy may cause chronic adenoiditis; chronic sinusitis, snoring, sleep apnea due to obstruction of nasopharynx; otitis media, serous otitis media related with the obstruction of the eustachian tube, and either medical or surgical treatment might be required [12]. The presence of adenoid hypertrophy and the degree of airway obstruction can be evaluated by flexible fiberoptic nasal endoscopy or lateral neck radiograph. Different results have been reported in the literature by comparing these two methods [13, 14]. Airway patency can be evaluated by measuring the adenoid/nasopharynx ratio (thickness of the adenoid in the craniocaudal direction/distance between basiocciput and hard palate) on lateral radiograph (Fig. 11.6). However, with lateral neck radiography the radiation exposure is the main concern. If the radiography is not obtained with optimum positioning and timing (with the neck in slight extension and at the end of inspiration) may lead to misinterpretation of the exact obstruction of the nasopharynx. Although it is presumed that hypertrophied adenoid regresses after the age of 6–7, can be encountered incidentally in imaging at later ages. Adenoid hypertrophy has typical CT and MRI appearance that helps differentiate from nasopharynx cancer: It grows symmetrically with a smooth surface and the Rosenmüller fossa is not obliterated. Following IV contrast administration, hypo- and hyperintense lines from front to back, especially on MR images, are in favor of adenoid hypertrophy (Fig. 11.7).

11.4.2 Nasopharyngeal Carcinoma

Nasopharyngeal carcinoma is encountered less frequently in children compared to adults and constitutes less than 1% of childhood cancers [15]. It usually occurs during the adolescence. Since the clinical findings are nonspecific and mostly related with the obstruction of the nasopharynx and eustachian tube, locally advanced tumors are most likely to be encountered at the time of diagnosis. It is seen as a mass

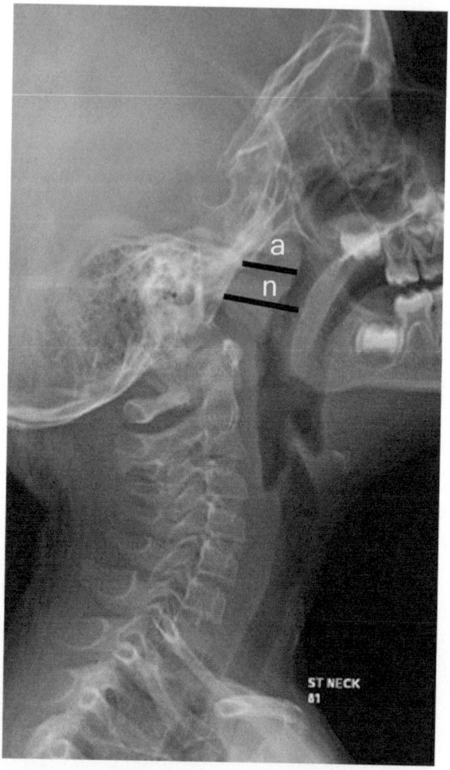

Fig. 11.6 Lateral neck radiograph of 6-year-old boy with adenoid hypertrophy. Measurement of adenoid/nasopharynx ratio is shown. *a* adenoid; *n* nasopharynx

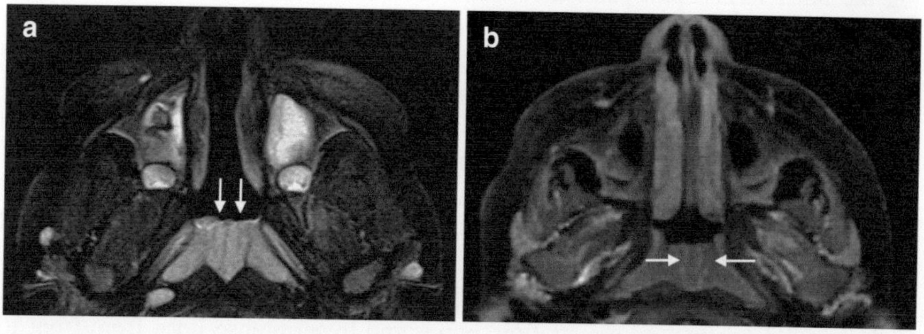

Fig. 11.7 Adenoid hypertrophy of a 14-year-old girl. (**a**) T2-weighted MR image shows homogenous adenoid hypertrophy with smooth surface (white arrows). (**b**) On T1-weighted contrast-enhanced MR image, note the hypo- and hyperintense vertical lines suggesting adenoid hypertrophy rather than carcinoma (white arrows)

in the posterior wall of the nasopharynx, which often grows asymmetrically and obliterates the Rosenmüller fossa. In contrast-enhanced examinations, the typical linear pattern observed in adenoid hypertrophy disappears, the lesion enhances heterogeneously. The involvement of the parapharyngeal, prevertebral, and masticatory spaces; skull base indicates locally advanced disease. MRI with IV contrast is the

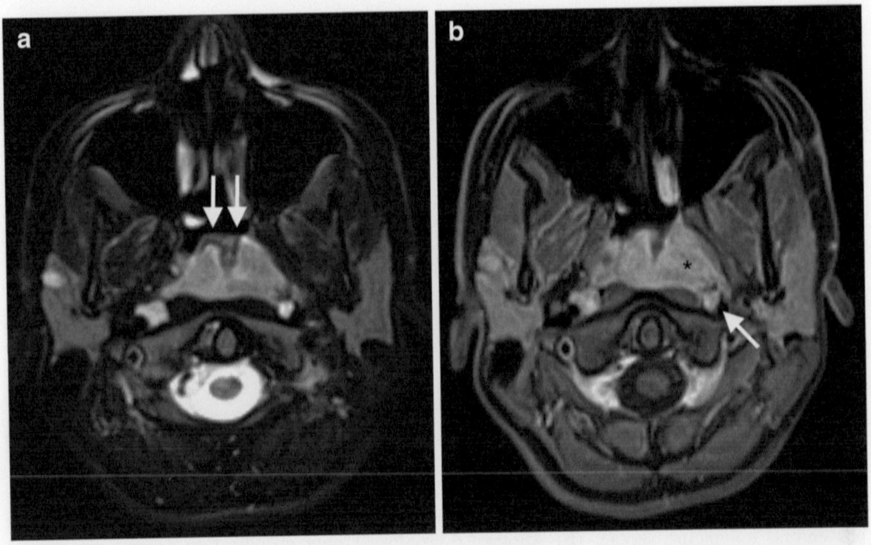

Fig. 11.8 MR images of 13-year-old boy with nasopharynx carcinoma. (**a**) T2-weighted axial image. Note the irregular surface of nasopharyngeal mass (white arrows). (**b**) T1-weighted post-contrast image is revealing asymmetric nasopharyngeal mass more prominent on the left (asterisk). Lateral retropharyngeal lymph node is also seen (white arrow)

choice of imaging to reveal the extent of the disease and has mostly been replaced CT. MRI is also superior to CT in demonstrating the lateral retropharyngeal lymph nodes, which are the primary nodal spread site of the disease [16] (Fig. 11.8).

11.5 Oropharynx

Oropharynx is the middle part of the pharynx that is continuous with the oral cavity. The borders; superiorly and anteriorly soft palate, inferiorly upper border of the epiglottis, posteriorly the posterior wall of the pharynx. It contains the root of the tongue and palatine tonsils.

11.5.1 Thyroglossal Duct Cyst

The development of the thyroid gland begins with the proliferation of endodermal cells at the base of the tongue in the third week of gestation. It then descends from the root of the tongue through the thyroglossal canal, anterior to hyoid bone and larynx, to its normal location in the neck. Thyroglossal duct cyst develops due to incomplete obliteration of the thyroglossal duct and is the most common congenital cystic neck lesion of children. Approximately 65% of the cases has infrahyoid localization and tongue root localization is extremely rare (1–2%) [17]. It typically has midline or paramedian location.

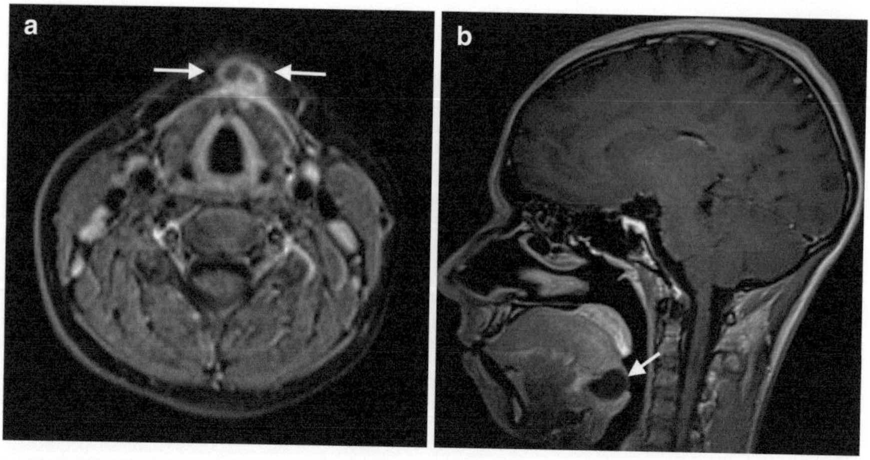

Fig. 11.9 Thyroglossal duct cysts with various locations. (**a**) T1-weighted postcontrast image shows a thick-walled cystic lesion with median location at the level hyoid bone (white arrows). It has central enhancing septae. (**b**) Another thyroglossal duct cyst of root tongue on sagittal T1-weighted MR image (white arrow)

Patients with thyroglossal duct cyst present with painless soft tissue swelling of the neck. When infected redness of the skin and pain may also be added to the clinical scenario. Diagnosis is mostly based on clinical findings. Ultrasonography (US) helps establish cystic nature of the lesion. In the oropharynx, imaging with MRI or CT is required for the delineation of the lesion. CT reveals a homogeneous, hypodense, thin-walled cystic lesion with no significant contrast enhancement if it is not infected. While high signal intensity on T2-weighted MR images is expected, its signal on T1-weighted images varies depending on proteinaceous or hemorrhagic content. The thick wall and internal septae would suggest infection or hemorrhage (Fig. 11.9).

11.5.2 Hypertrophied Palatine Tonsils and Peritonsiller Abscess

Palatine tonsils are lymphoid tissue clusters located on both lateral walls of the oropharynx, showing continuity with the soft palate at the top and front, the root of the tongue at the bottom and front, and the posterior wall of the pharynx in the back. Tonsillitis is mostly viral and 30% bacterial caused by group A beta hemolytic streptococcus. The diagnosis is solely based on clinical findings. In conjunction with inflammation of the nasopharyngeal adenoid tissue, it may cause airway obstruction. If any complication is suspected imaging methods are considered.

Peritonsillar abscess is the most common infection of the neck region and occurs when tonsillitis turns into cellulitis and then into abscess [18]. Radiological imaging has an important role in the diagnosis and management of the treatment. CT neck with IV contrast administration is the choice of imaging modality (Fig. 11.10).

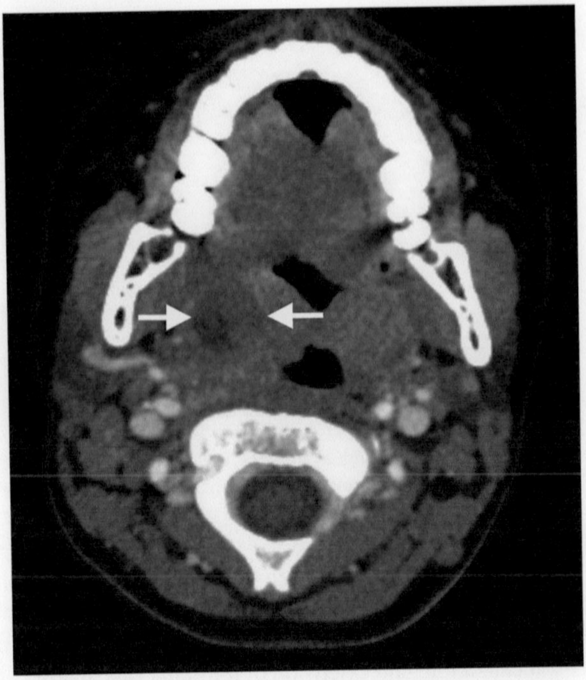

Fig. 11.10 Contrast-enhanced CT image of 12-year-old girl with peritonsillar abscess. Right-sided hypodense, rounded peritonsillar abscess is seen (white arrows)

11.6 Hypopharynx

Hypopharynx forms the most distal part of the pharynx and is continuous with the oropharynx above, the cervical esophagus below. It starts at the level of hyoid bone above and ends just below the cricoid cartilage consisting of three parts: Pyriform sinuses, posterior pharyngeal wall, and postcricoid region [19].

11.6.1 Retropharyngeal Abscess

The retropharyngeal region is a potential space located posterior to the pharynx. It extends from the skull base to the mediastinum below, is surrounded by the prevertebral muscles posteriorly and the carotid sheath on the sides. It contains lymph nodes and fatty tissue [20]. The retropharyngeal abscess is frequently encountered in early childhood, up to 4–5 years of age, as this is the age group that upper respiratory tract infections are more common. The abscess is thought to occur as a result of lymph adenitis of this region. Rarely, trauma caused by the foreign body aspiration may be the reason for the abscess. Early diagnosis and treatment are profoundly important since delay may lead to respiratory tract obstruction, mediastinal extension and cause sclerosing mediastinitis.

Lateral nasopharyngeal radiography should be obtained during the inspiration with the neck in slight extension. Normally the thickness of the soft tissue anterior to the second cervical vertebra does not exceed the thickness of ½ vertebral body. When this

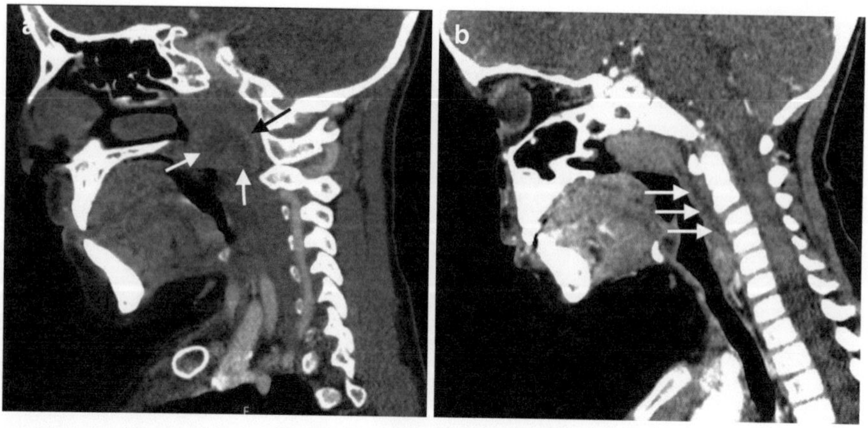

Fig. 11.11 Retropharyngeal abscess vs. fluid. (**a**) Sagittal reformatted contrast-enhanced CT image of 8-year-old boy revealing retropharyngeal abscess (white arrows) with enhancing capsule (black arrow). (**b**) Retropharyngeal fluid of 5-year-old boy (white arrows)

is the case, it might be the sign of infection of the retropharyngeal region. The radiograph should also be examined carefully for the presence of a foreign body. Intravenous contrast-enhanced CT of the neck is the gold standard imaging method in the diagnosis, localization, and extension of retropharyngeal abscess. A hypodense, peripherally enhancing fluid collection is defined as retropharyngeal abscess (Fig. 11.11). Treatment includes abscess drainage and antibiotics. Since the treatment is usually conservative, other infections of retropharyngeal region as retropharyngeal edema, cellulitis, and phlegmon that reveal nonloculated fluid collection without any capsular enhancement should be differentiated from retropharyngeal abscess.

11.6.2 Lymphatic Malformation

As the most common vascular malformation of the neck, the majority of lymphatic malformations are located in the cervical region [21]. The diagnosis might be established antenatally; however, patients may also present with various symptoms related with intralesional bleeding and infection in the postnatal period. They develop due to drainage obstruction of the lymphatic channels to venous system. If the size of the lesion large enough might cause airway compression.

The first-line imaging method is US. The lesion consists of single or multiple cysts with various sizes and contains septa. The echogenicity of the cyst content alters depending on whether it is complicated by bleeding or infection. MRI with IV contrast is the modality of choice due to its higher soft tissue resolution to show extent of the lymphangioma. The signal intensity of the cysts varies depending on whether the content is hemorrhagic or proteinaceous. Lack of solid component and contrast enhancement solely in the septa and cyst walls distinguishes lymphangioma from teratoma (Fig. 11.12).

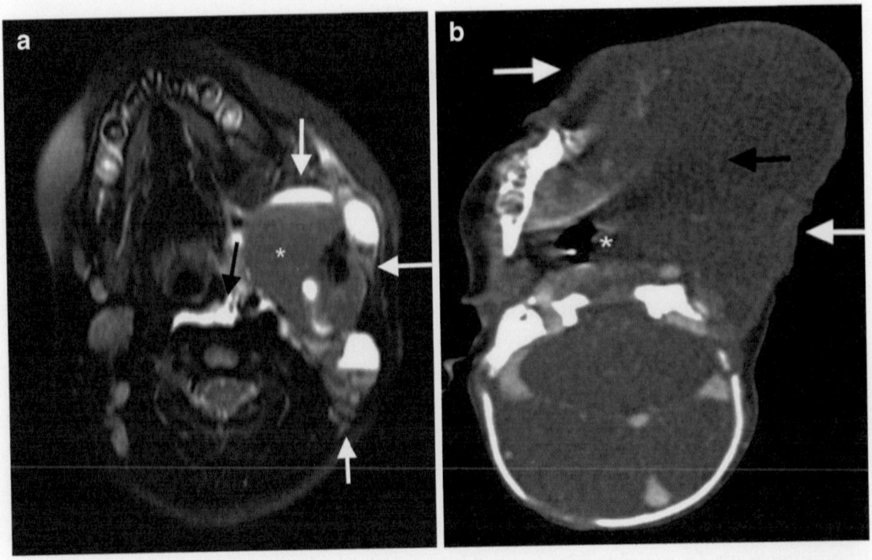

Fig. 11.12 Lymphatic malformation of the neck. (**a**) Two-year-old girl presented with soft tissue swelling of the neck. T2-weighted axial MR image shows left-sided multiloculated cystic lesion of the neck (white arrows). It has hypointense component suggesting hemorrhage (white asterisk) and retropharyngeal extension (black arrow). (**b**) Contrast-enhanced CT neck of newborn with antenatal diagnosis of lymphatic malformation and respiratory distress. Left-sided cystic mass of the neck (white arrows), with enhancing septae (black arrow) and airway compression (white asterisk)

11.6.3 Hemangioma and Venous Malformations

Hemangiomas and vascular malformations of the head and neck region constitute of 60% of vascular lesions of childhood and may affect airway when they seat deep and reach big sizes [22]. Infantile hemangiomas present after few weeks following birth while vascular malformations are usually encountered at birth.

Hemangioma is a benign vascular tumor and characterized as solid mass lesion. When it is located at airway usually diagnosed with bronchoscopy during the first 1.5–2 years of life at rapidly growing phase due to obstructive respiratory symptoms. When bronchoscopic findings are vague or for the delineation of the extension of the lesion radiological imaging is conducted. On CT vivid enhancement of the lesion following contrast administration is suggestive of the diagnosis of hemangioma. MRI would be more advantageous due to its higher soft tissue resolution and lack of radiation exposure. Significant increased signal on T2-weighted images and vivid and early enhancement on postcontrast images are the features indicative of hemangioma.

Venous anomalies usually present at birth and grow proportionally as the child grows up. They are blue, soft, compressible lesions and may enlarge during valsalva maneuver. Superficial lesions may be diagnosed with US and Doppler US with radiological findings of vascular channels with slow flow. When the lesions have deeper extensions MRI may help show the extent of the lesion.

If the lesions are causing airway compromise, treatment options for hemangioma are propranolol, steroids, laser ablation, surgical excision of the lesion. Venous malformations are decreased in size with Sirolimus and embolization and following surgical resection might be conducted.

11.6.4 Lymphoma

In children, lymphoma is the most common malignant tumor of the head and neck region. It often arises with lymph node involvement. While extranodal involvement is observed at a rate of approximately 30% in non-Hodgkin lymphoma, it is extremely rare in Hodgkin's disease [23]. Involvement of the sinonasal region and Waldeyer's ring may be associated with airway-related symptoms and be observed as polypoid masses with smooth surfaces in the submucosal region. Advanced imaging of masses can be performed with contrast-enhanced CT or MRI (Fig. 11.13). CT is superior in revealing bone destruction, while MRI is superior in showing soft tissue extension and intracranial spread. The masses have soft tissue density on CT. On MRI, the lesions are hypointense on T1-weighted image and hypo- or hyperintense on T2-weighted image. It may show diffusion restriction and contrast enhancement with varying degrees.

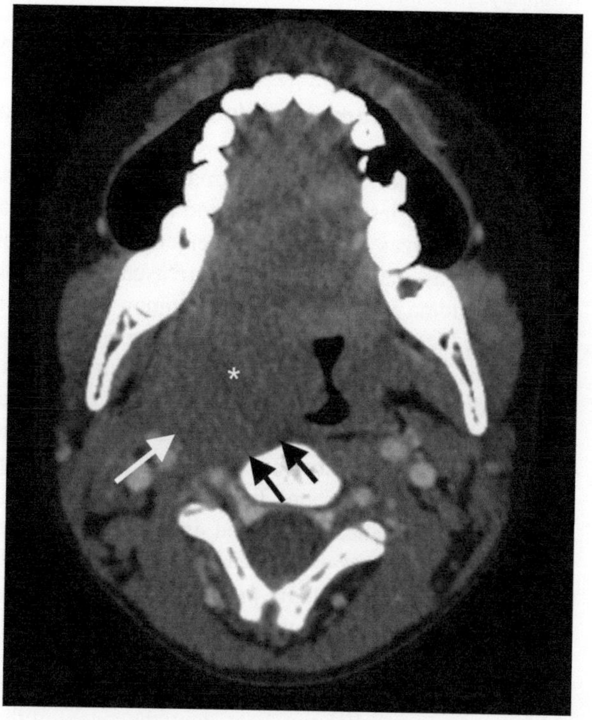

Fig. 11.13 Eight-year-old girl with right-sided tonsil mass. Axial CT image is revealing mass of right tonsil obliterating prevertebral (black arrows) and right parapharyngeal spaces (white arrow). The patient was diagnosed as Burkitt lymphoma

11.6.5 Rhabdomyosarcoma

Rhabdomyosarcoma (RMS) is the most common malignant tumor of head and neck following lymphoma in children [24]. The average age at diagnosis is under 5–6 years old, and 72–81% of cases are diagnosed before the age of 10 [25]. Rhabdomyosarcomas located in the sinonasal cavity and parapharyngeal space are defined as parameningeal RMS and have the worst prognosis due to their close relation to cranium and advanced local disease at the time of diagnosis. Findings of skull base invasion, intracranial extension, and cranial nerve invasion are encountered in approximately 1/3 of the cases [25]. Patients may often present with persistent, nonspecific or sometimes airway-related symptoms (such as nasal congestion). In the presence of a rapidly growing head and neck mass in the childhood age group, RMS should be at the forefront of the differential diagnosis list.

Although radiological findings are nonspecific, imaging plays a key role to define the local extension, staging, and evaluation of treatment response. US can be utilized to identify superficial lesions and to reveal their solid nature. However, the lesions usually have deep location. MRI is the first-line imaging method due to its capability of showing the location and local spread of the lesions due to its high spatial and contrast resolution. The lesion is hypo-isointense relative to the muscle on T1-weighted images and hyperintense on T2-weighted images, might be heterogeneous due to bleeding or necrosis. Significant enhancement with IV contrast material and diffusion restriction are other features of RMS (Fig. 11.14). CT should be reserved for the investigation of lung metastases to minimize radiation exposure.

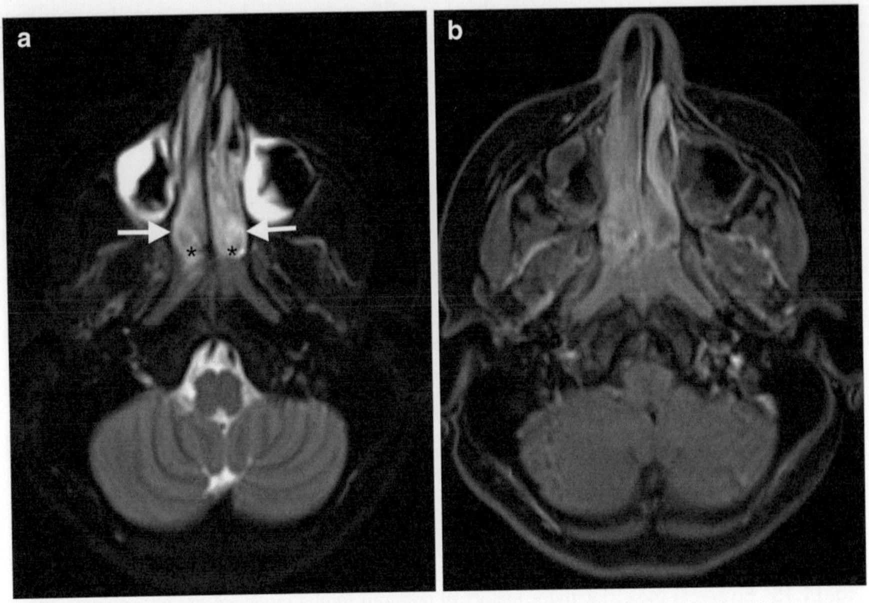

Fig. 11.14 Ten-year-old boy with rhabdomyosarcoma. (**a**) Axial T2-weighted MR image showing T2 hyperintense and slightly heterogeneous mass filling both nasal cavity more prominently on the right (arrows) and chonoae (asterisk). (**b**) On postgad axial T1-weighted image the mass is enhancing vividly with some heterogeneity

11.7 Larynx

The larynx locates between the hypopharynx and the trachea. It basically has a cartilage structure and is divided into three parts by the vocal cords: supraglottic, glottic, and infraglottic.

11.7.1 Subglottic Stenosis

The subglottic region is defined as the region between the inferior of the vocal cords and the inferior border of cricoid cartilage. Stenosis may be congenital or acquired. Necrosis due to pressure created by the cuff during the prolonged intubation is the most common cause of subglottic stenosis. Congenital and idiopathic forms are encountered less frequently, and congenital subglottic stenosis may be accompanied by pathologies such as tracheoesophageal fistula and vascular ring anomalies.

Bronchoscopy is the basic imaging method in the diagnosis. However, 3 plane CT and MRI images can be implemented in the diagnosis and surgical planning. Virtual endoscopy and VRT images of CT may further help understand the degree and length of the stenosis (Fig. 11.15). Contrast-enhanced CT images also rule out the possibility of vascular compression.

11.7.2 Laryngotracheal Papillomatozis

The causative agent of laryngotracheal papillomatosis is human papilloma virus. Children develop the disease by ingesting the virus from a contaminated birth canal during birth. It is the most common laryngeal neoplasia of the childhood [26]. The

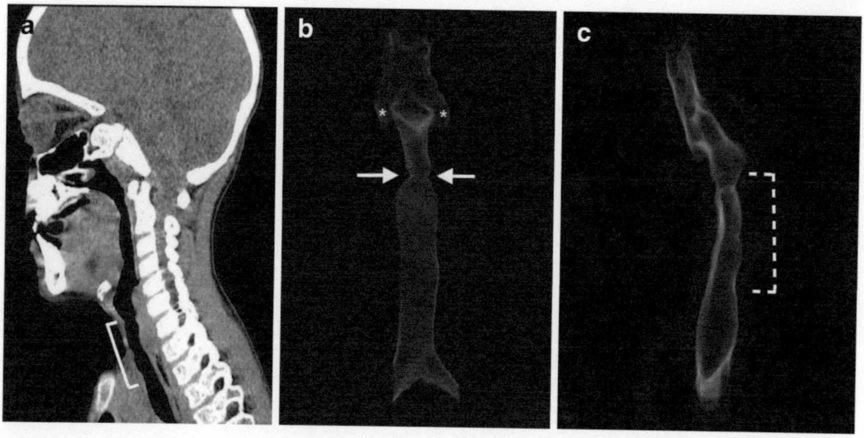

Fig. 11.15 Five-year-old girl with the history of previous intubation is presenting with inspiratory stridor. (**a**) Sagittal CT image reveals long segment subglottic stenosis of the trachea. (**b**, **c**) Volume-rendered 3D CT images on coronal and sagittal plain help better visualization of the stenosis. Arrows on coronal image show the narrowest segment (asterisk pyriform sinuses)

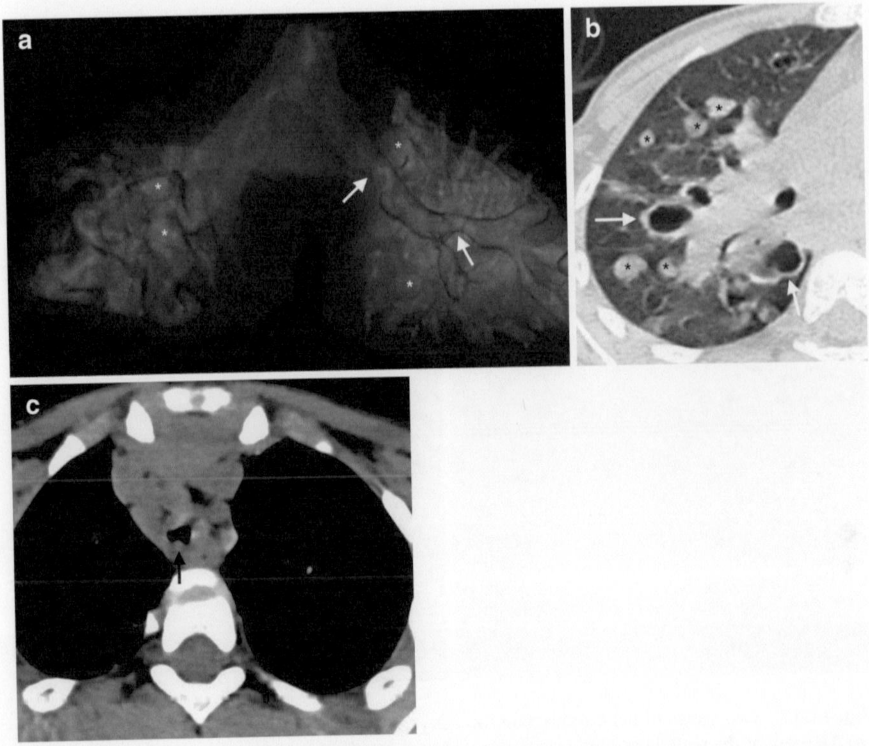

Fig. 11.16 Five-year-old girl with laryngotracheal papillomatosis. (**a**) On 3D CT volume-rendered image, multiple filling defects of left main and lower lobe bronchi created by papillomatosis (arrows). Cystic lung nodules of both lungs are also seen (asterisks). (**b**) Axial CT image of right lung reveals cysts (arrows) and nodules (asterisks) of the lung. (**c**) On axial CT image, circumferential tracheal stenosis, by papillomatosis (black arrow)

papillomas may spontaneously regress, but in 1% the disease spreads to the lungs and cause respiratory symptoms [27]. The symptoms usually present prior to age of 5 [27]. Multiple surgical procedures and tracheostomy may be needed to ensure the airway patency. In decreasing recurrency frequency of the papillomas, some non-surgical treatments including interferon alfa, cidofovir, indol-3-carbinol, celecoxib, heat shock of protein have been investigated and seem to be promising [28].

CT is the basic imaging method to reveal polypoid lesions of the airway. A large number of polyps of various sizes originating from the larynx, trachea, and bronchi are encountered. When the disease spreads to the lungs, nodules and cavitations are seen, with lower lobes distribution. Over time, cavities tend to coalesce (Fig. 11.16).

11.7.3 Croup

Croup or laryngotracheobronchitis is defined as infection of upper airway caused by viral agents in early childhood. The causative agent is often rhinosincytial virus or parainfluenza, and children aged 6 months to 3 years are mostly affected [29]. Cases

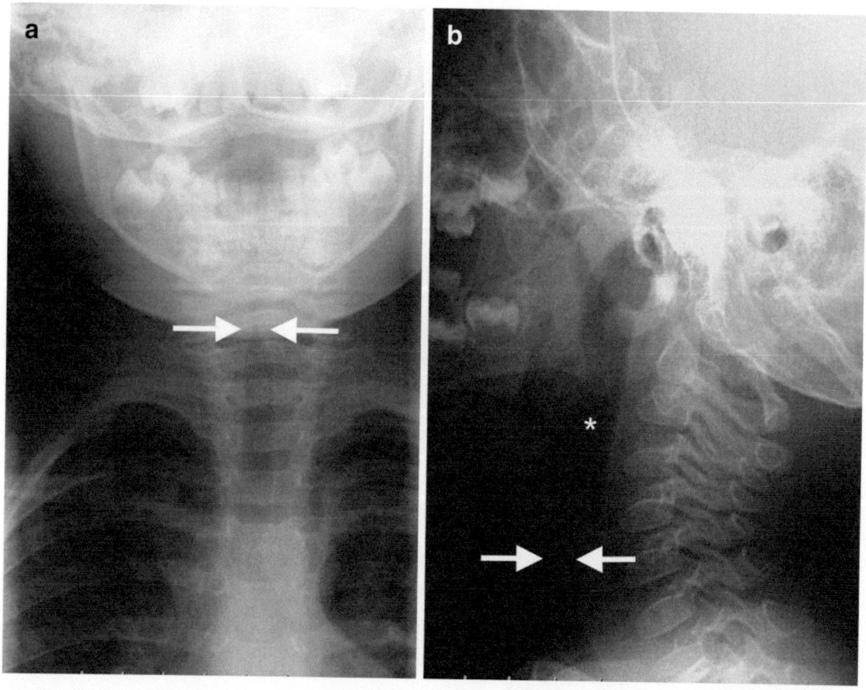

Fig. 11.17 Two views of neck radiograph of a 2-year-old boy presented with inspiratory stridor. (**a**) AP view of the neck is showing significant narrowing of subgottic trachea (arrows) compatible with Steeple sign. (**b**) On lateral view dilatation of the hypopharynx (asterisk) and narrowed subglottic trachea (arrows) are again noted

present with inspiratory stridor and dog-barking cough. The diagnosis is made clinically. When lateral and AP radiographs of the neck are obtained for the differential diagnosis of foreign body aspiration, retropharyngeal abscess, and epiglottitis, which may cause similar symptoms, narrowing of the subglottic airway called as Steeple sign is observed. Subglottic stenosis and dilatation of the hypopharynx (occurs to overcome airway resistance) are typical findings of the disease observed on radiographs (Fig. 11.17).

11.7.4 Epiglottitis

Epiglottitis is a rapid inflammatory process of epiglottis usually caused by bacterial agents. Haemophilus influenzae type B, prior to introduction of the vaccination, was the foremost etiologic agent of the epiglottitis. Due to widespread immunization of Hemophilus influenza type B, the incidence of the disease amongst children has been decreased [30]. Patients rapidly present with the symptoms of fever, difficulty in swallowing and breathing, anxiety. The diagnosis is usually established clinically and with direct visualization of the epiglottitis via laryngoscopy. Lateral neck radiography acquired in erect position in order to secure airway may help make the diagnosis with the findings of thickened epiglottitis (thumb sign) and aryepiglottic folds, increased prevertebral soft tissue thickness, and dilated hypopharyngeal air column.

CT and MRI of the neck are not preferable due to airway compromise in supine position. The treatment of epiglotitits is including intravenous antibiotherapy, steroid, supportive therapy as intravenous fluid and oxygen.

11.7.5 Foreign Body Aspiration

Aspiration of foreign body into the airways is of particular concern in infants and preschool young children and fourth leading cause of death [31]. Organic material, particularly food with rounded shape including peanuts, fruit, and candies are most often aspirated. When the aspirated material is involving upper airway the main symptoms are usually sudden onset coughing and respiratory distress. If the patient is clinically stable the radiological evaluation may start with lateral neck and two views chest radiography. Radiopaque foreign bodies can be vizualized with the radiographs. In case the aspirated material is not demonstrated with physical examination or radiographs prior to endoscopic procedures and for delineation of postraumatic complications CT of neck and/or chest might be acquired with low dose protocols (Fig. 11.18). The removal of foreign body from upper airway is conducted via laryngoscopy.

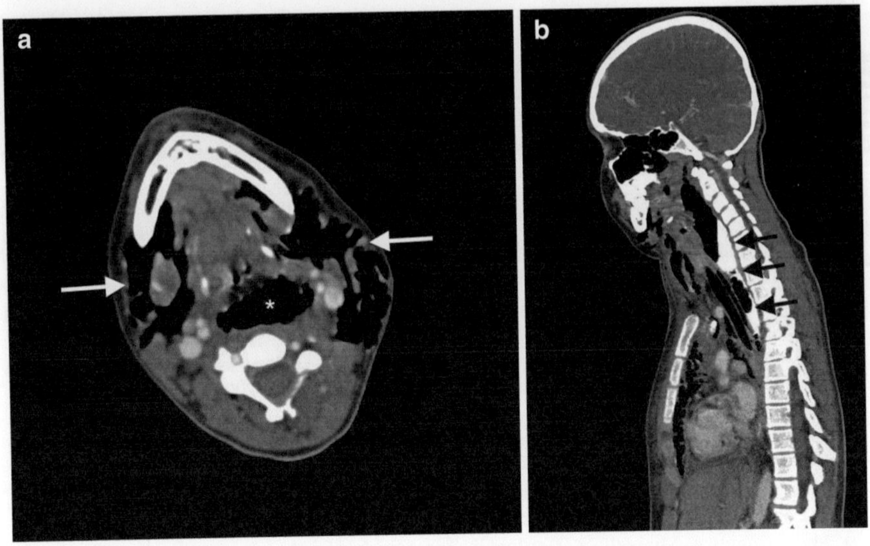

Fig. 11.18 Fourteen-year-old girl, with posttraumatic retropharyngeal collection, its mediastinal extension, and subcutaneous emphysema caused by aspirated foreign body. (**a**) Axial CT image of the neck reveals air-filled retropharyngeal collection (asterisk) and soft tissue emphysema of bilateral cervical chain (white arrows). (**b**) Sagittal contrast-enhanced CT image of the neck and chest show retropharyngeal collection extending down to the mediastinum filled with air and water-soluble contrast medium (black arrows)

References

1. Adewele L. Anatomy and assessment of pediatric airway. Pediatr Anaesth. 2009;19(suppl 1):1–8.
2. Kwong KM. Current updates on choanal atresia. Front Pediatr. 2015;3:52.
3. Newman JR, Harmon P, Shirley WP, Hill JS, Woolley AL, Wiatrak BJ. Operative management of choanal atresia: a 15-year experience. JAMA Otolaryngol Head Neck Surg. 2013;139:71–5.
4. Wald ER, Applegate KE, Bordley C, Darrow DH, Glode MP, Marcy SM, et al. Clinical practice guideline for the diagnosis and management of acute bacterial sinusitis in children aged 1 to 18 years. Pediatrics. 2013;132:e262–80.
5. American College of Radiology. ACR appropriateness Criteria® radiation dose assessment introduction. https://www.acr.org/-/media/ACR/Files/Appropriateness-Criteria/RadiationDoseAssessmentIntro.pdf. Accessed 30 Sept 2021.
6. Glasier CM, Mallory GB Jr, Steele RW. Significance of opacification of the maxillary and ethmoid sinuses in infants. J Pediatr. 1989;114:45–50.
7. Al-Madani MV, Khatatbeh AE, Rawashdeh RZ, Al-Khtoum NF, Shawagfeh NR. The prevalence of orbital complications among children and adults with acute rhinosinusitis. Braz J Otorhinolaryngol. 2013;79(6):716–9.
8. Heath J, Hartzell L, Putt C, Kennedy JL. Chronic rhinosinusitis in children: pathophysiology, evaluation, and medical management. Curr Allergy Asthma Rep. 2018;18:37.
9. Danhnert W. Radiology review manual. 4th edn. Ear, nose and throat disorders. Philadelphia: Lippincott Williams and Wilkins; Juvenile angiofibroma. p. 325.
10. Drago L, Esposito S, De Vecchi E, Marchisio P, Blasi F, Baggi E, et al. Detection of respiratory viruses and atypical bacteria in children's tonsils and adenoids. J Clin Microbiol. 2008;46:369–70.
11. Cho K-S, Kim SH, Hong S-L, et al. Local atopy in childhood adenotonsillar hypertrophy. Am J Rhinol Allergy. 2018;32:160–6.
12. Arambula A, Brown JR, Neff L. Anatomy and physiology of the palatine tonsils, adenoids, and lingual tonsils. World J Otorhinolaryngol Head Neck Surg. 2021;7:155–60.
13. Mlynarek A, Tewfik M, Hagr A, et al. Lateral neck radiography versus direct video rhinoscopy in assessing adenoid size. J Otolaryngol. 2004;33:360–5.
14. Caylakli F, Hizal E, Yilmazer C. Correlation between adenoid-nasopharynx ratio and endoscopic examination of adenoid hypertrophy: a blind, prospective clinical study. Int J Pediatric Otorhinolaryngol. 2009;73:1532–5.
15. Ries LAG, Smith MA, Gurney JG, Linet M, Tamra T, Young JL, Bunin GR, editors. Cancer incidence and survival among children and adolescents: United States SEER program 1975–1995. National Cancer Institute, National Institutes of Health: Bethesda; 1999.
16. Tang L, Li L, Mao Y, Chen Y, Sun Y, Liao X, et al. Retropharyngeal lymph node metastasis in nasopharyngeal carcinoma detected by magnetic resonance imaging prognostic value and staging categories. Cancer. 2008;113:347–54.
17. Nakayama S, Kimachi K, Nakayama K, Ikebe T, Ozeki S. Thyroglossal duct cyst occurring in the floor of the mouth: report of 2 cases. J Oral Maxillofac Surg. 2009;67:2690–3.
18. Ruben RJ. Randomized controlled studies and the treatment of middle-ear effusions and tonsillar pharyngitis: how random are the studies and what are their limitations? Otolaryngol Head Neck Surg. 2008;139(3):333–9.
19. Mukherji SK. The pharynx. In: Som PM, Curtin HD, editors. Head and neck imaging. 4th ed. St Louıs, MO: Mosby; 2003. p. 1465–520.
20. Mnatsakanian A, Minutello K, Bordoni B. Anatomy, head and neck, retropharyngeal space. In: StatPearls. Treasure Island, FL: StatPearls Publishing; 2022.
21. Synder EJ, Sarma A, Borst AJ, Tekes A. Lympathic anomalies in children: update on imaging diagnosis, genetics, and treatment. AJR. 2022;218:1089–101.
22. Gorostidi F, Glasson N, Salati V, Sandu K. Pediatric vascular anomalies with airway compromise. J Oral Pathol Med. 2022;6; 51(10):88–96.

23. Urquhart A, Berg R. Hodgkin's and non Hodgkin's lymphoma of the head and neck. Laryngoscope. 2001;111:1565–9.
24. Sengupta S, Pal R. Clinicopathological correlates of pediatric head and neck cancer. J Cancer Res Ther. 2009;5:181–5.
25. Raney RB, Meza J, Anderson JR, Fryer CJ, Donaldson SS, Breneman JC, et al. Treatment of children and adolescents with localized parameningeal sarcoma: experience of the intergroup rhabdomyosarcoma study group protocols IRS-II through-IV, 1978–1997. Med Pediatr Oncol. 2002;38:22–32.
26. Aggünlü L, Erbas G. Recurrent respiratory papillomatosis with lung involvement. Diagn Interv Radiol. 2009;15(2):93–5.
27. Carifi M, Napolitano D, Morandi M, Dall'olio D. Recurrent respiratory papillomatosis current and future perspectives. Ther Clin Risk Manag. 2015;11:731–8.
28. Kumar N, Preciado D. Airway papillomatosis: new treatments for an old challenge. Front Pediatr. 2019;7:383.
29. Peltola V, Heikkinen T, Ruuskanen O. Clinical courses of croup caused by influenza and para-influenza viruses. Pediatr Infect Dis J. 2002;21(1):76–8.
30. Butler DF, Myers AL. Changing epidemiology of Haemophilus influenzae in children. Infect Dis Clin N Am. 2018;32(1):119–28.
31. Tsang JE, Sun J, Ooi GC, Tsang KW. Endobronchial foreign body presenting as exacerbation of asthma. Case Rep Emerg Med. 2017;2017:6863083.

Radiologic Evaluation of Lower Respiratory System

12

Sevinç Taşar and Recep Savaş

12.1 The Differences in the Lower Respiratory Tract in Children and Adults Are as Follows [1]

- In infants, contrary to adults, infections such as bronchiolitis can lead to significant respiratory distress.
- The larynx, trachea, and bronchi have thinner walls compared to lumen diameter. Consequently, the lumen can collapse easily during inspiration.
- Children have shorter tracheas compared to adults, making it easier for tubes to enter the bronchi during endotracheal intubation.
- Newborns have a barrel-shaped thorax, which gradually transforms into a cylindrical shape as they age.
- In newborns and early childhood, the diaphragm muscle is more effective in ventilation due to the weakness of intercostal muscles and the prevalence of cartilage over bone in the thorax. This leads to a focus on abdominal breathing.
- Intra-abdominal organs and mediastinal structures affect breathing.
- Proximal and distal airways grow proportionally up to the first 5 months. However, after 1 year, growth is more prominent in the distal airways. Consequently, up to the age of 5, resistance in the distal airways is higher than in adults.
- Bronchospasm is rare in children, especially in the first 6 months, due to insufficient bronchial musculature.
- In children, bronchial walls can easily adhere to eachother due to insufficient cartilage support. This leads to positive pleural pressure during expiration in

S. Taşar
Pediatric Radiology, University of Health Sciences Ümraniye Training and Research Hospital, İstanbul, Türkiye

R. Savaş (✉)
Department of Radiology, Faculty of Medicine, Ege University, Izmir, Turkey

H. Yüksel et al. (eds.), *Pediatric Airway Diseases*, Comprehensive ENT,
https://doi.org/10.1007/978-3-031-74853-0_12

obstructive pulmonary diseases, potentially causing the collapse of the respiratory tract.

- The number of alveoli rapidly increases until the age of eight to ten. After this age, while the formation of new alveoli significantly decreases, structural development in the existing alveoli becomes more prominent. As collateral airways (Lambert and Kohn pores) do not develop before the age of 8 years, telectasis and pleural-based round pneumonia are more likely to be observed (Fig. 12.1).
- In children, lung compliance is lower than in adults, making the lungs more susceptible to collapse. Surfactant reduces surface tension and enhances lung compliance. Respiratory distress syndrome, which is secondary to surfactant deficiency, may develop in premature infants (Fig. 12.2).

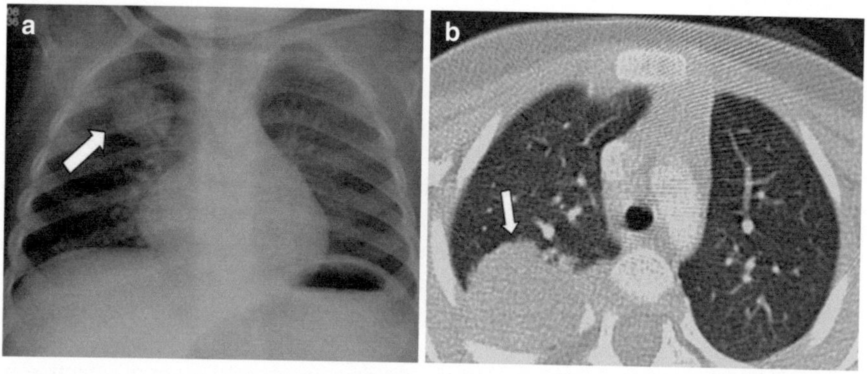

Fig. 12.1 On the PA chest X-ray (**a**), a nodular opacity is evident in the upper zone of the right lung. Simultaneously, in the CT examination (**b**) of the patient, a consolidated area, consistent with pleural-based round pneumonia, is observed in the upper lobe posterior in the axial section

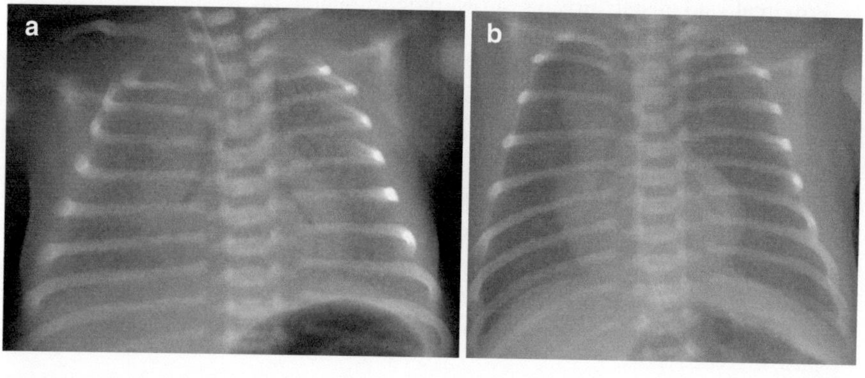

Fig. 12.2 On the first day of birth, a 29-week-old newborn presented with diffuse, hazy, granular pulmonary airspace opacification on CXR (**a**). After 5 days of surfactant treatment, chest X-ray findings returned to normal (**b**)

12.2 Imaging Methods Used in Respiratory System Diseases

- Plain Radiography
- Fluoroscopy
- Ultrasonography (US)—Color Doppler US
- Computed tomography (CT)
  - High-resolution computed tomography (HRCT)
  - Spiral tomography
  - CT angiography
- Magnetic resonance imaging (MRI) and MR angiography
- Angiography
- PET

12.2.1 Plain Radiography

Chest radiography offers several advantages, including easy acquisition, availability, and cost-effectiveness. Despite significant advancements in radiological imaging methods today, chest radiography remains the most commonly and initially preferred imaging method for diagnosing, monitoring, and assessing treatment response in pediatric respiratory system diseases (Fig. 12.3). It allows for the evaluation of the lungs, heart, airways, major vascular structures, and bone structures such as vertebrae, ribs, and the clavicle.

Chest radiography is obtained during full inspiration in cooperative older pediatric patients and during quiet inspiration in uncooperative infants and young children. For infants and young children (under 5 years), a standard chest X-ray is taken in the anterior-posterior position, while in older patients, it is taken in the posterior-anterior position. In neonates, X-rays can be obtained within incubators using modern mobile X-ray equipment. Certain areas, such as the anterior-upper mediastinum, retrocardiac, and sub-diaphragmatic lung regions, may not be well evaluated due to being in superposition and may require lateral radiographs for assessment.

Lateral X-rays are taken close to the pathology side to enhance the visibility of lesions. If the side is not specified, a left lateral chest X-ray is taken to minimize cardiac magnification. In lateral X-rays, density decreases from top to bottom, making it useful for detecting small infiltrates in hidden areas, such as the retrocardiac region, which can be challenging to detect on anterior-posterior X-rays. While lateral radiographs were previously used to detect pleural fluid, ultrasonography is now the preferred imaging method for this purpose due to its portability. It is essential to minimize unnecessary radiation exposure to nonthoracic structures like the lower neck, proximal upper extremity, and upper abdomen by using proper collimation and shielding [2].

When interpreting X-rays, it is crucial to ensure that both hemithoraxes of the patient are equally pressed against the detector, as unequal compression can lead to misleading radiolucent appearances. The symmetry of the X-ray can be assessed practically by examining the ribs. On the side of rotation, the ribs appear shorter

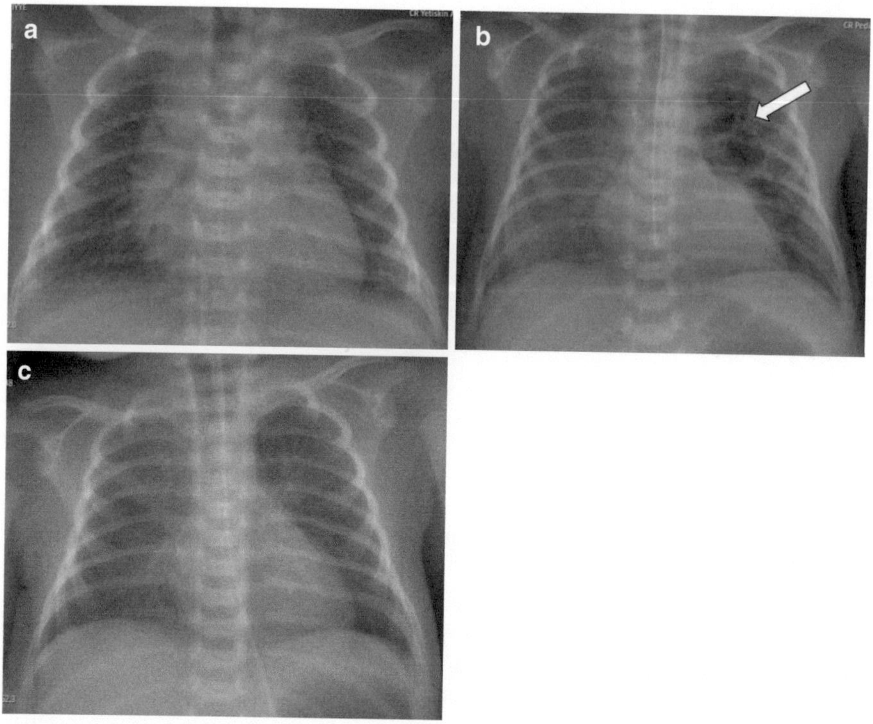

Fig. 12.3 In the case of a newborn with a gestational age of 28 weeks, on the first day of life, a chest X-ray (CXR) reveals diffuse hazy granular pulmonary airspace opacification (**a**). The patient received mechanical ventilation and surfactant treatment within the first 5 days of life, and a focal radiolucent area consistent with pulmonary interstitial emphysema is observed in the left lung. It is challenging to distinguish this condition from congenital pulmonary airway malformation (CPAM) based on this image alone (**b**). By the 17th day of treatment, the lungs appear normal (**c**)

anteriorly and longer posteriorly. Obtaining inspiratory radiography in young children can be challenging. In a good inspiratory radiograph, the diaphragmatic border should align with the fifth and sixth anterior ribs or the tenth and 11th posterior ribs on the posterior-anterior view. In infants, unlike in adults, the thorax expands in all directions, diaphragmatic movement is minimal, and distinguishing between inspiration and expiration is difficult.

12.2.1.1 The Thymus

The thymus gland is visible on chest radiographs from birth to 3 years of age, with its largest volume occurring, particularly during the first 2 years [3]. Its contours appear convex until the first 4 years of age, after which they become concave. In a normal thymus gland, there should be no compression of adjacent anatomical structures. At the junction of the thymus gland with the heart, you may observe the "cardiothymic notch," and its more prominent form is referred to as the "sail sign" (Fig. 12.4a). Additionally, the "wave sign" can be seen due to the pressure exerted by the ribs (Fig. 12.4b).

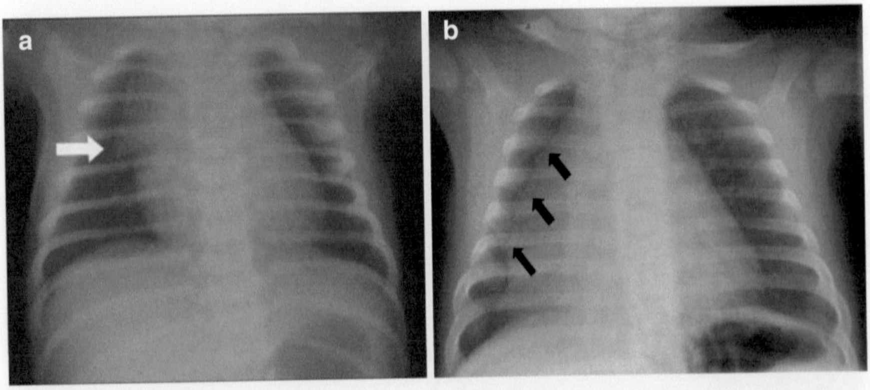

Fig. 12.4 The extension of the thymus toward the minor fissure is referred to as the "sail sign" (**a**). Its indentation into the intercostal spaces is known as the "wave sign" (**b**)

Prominent thymus tissue can create the appearance of a mediastinal mass. This can be differentiated using ultrasonography, where the normal thymus exhibits echogenicity similar to that of the liver (Fig. 12.5).

Thymus tissue is very soft. Even in marked hyperplasia, it does not compress the surrounding tissues. It can change shape with breathing and position. It contracts and elongates on inspiration and shortens and expands on expiration. It does not change the location of the tracheobronchial tree.

Thymus size can be reduced by stress (fever, infection, congenital heart and lung disease, malnutrition, and chemotherapy). When the stress factor disappears, rebound hypertrophy can be observed. Those with abnormal findings on a direct X-ray are first evaluated by ultrasound (US) and then by MRI if necessary. On MRI, the normal thymus has a homogeneous signal and an intermediate signal on T2-weighted images, similar to the spleen and lymph nodes.

Tracheal Buckling

Anterior and rightward displacement of the trachea due to ligamentous laxity is physiologic and is called tracheal buckling in young infants (Fig. 12.6). This becomes more evident in expiration. Normal deviation to the left is observed only when the aortic arch is located to the right of the trachea.

Hilum

The hilar regions are not prominent in the neonatal period. Hilar density gradually increases with age. Unlike adults, hilar growth in children is usually secondary to an acute infection, not a tumor. In infancy, it can also be seen secondary to congenital anomalies such as bronchogenic cysts. It may be difficult to distinguish the vein from nodal enlargement. In nodal enlargement, the outer contour of the hilum becomes convex.

Diaphragm

Normally, the left hemidiaphragm is lower than the right due to the impact of the heart. There should be no more than a 2 cm height difference between the two

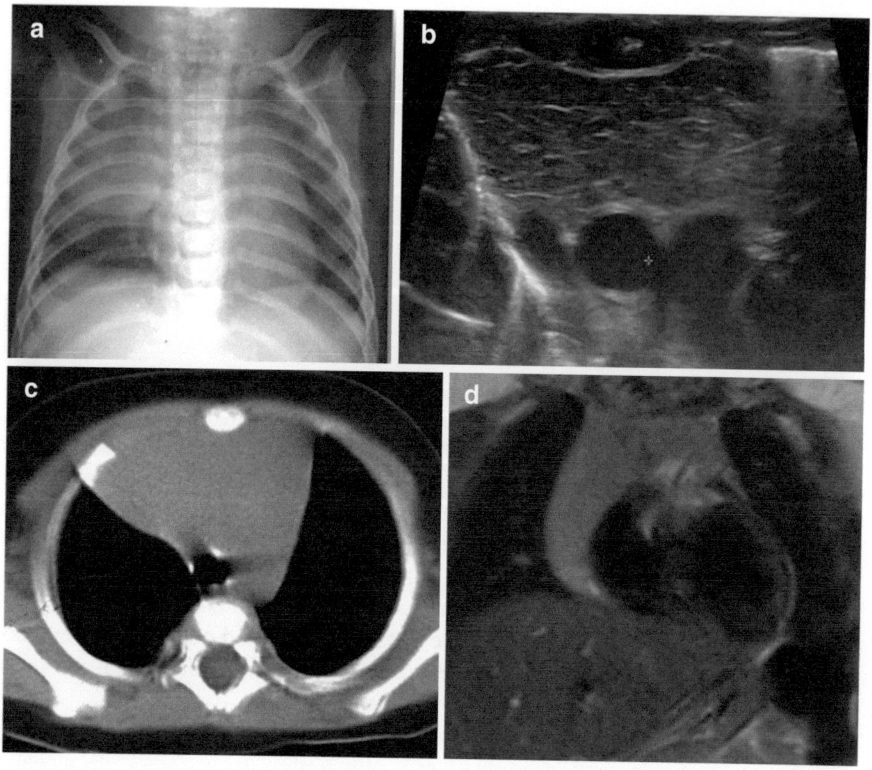

Fig. 12.5 The appearance of normal thymus tissue on chest X-ray, ultrasonography, CT, and MRI in a 2-year-old patient. Ultrasonographically, scattered hyperechoic foci resembling a starry sky are observed in a homogeneous background

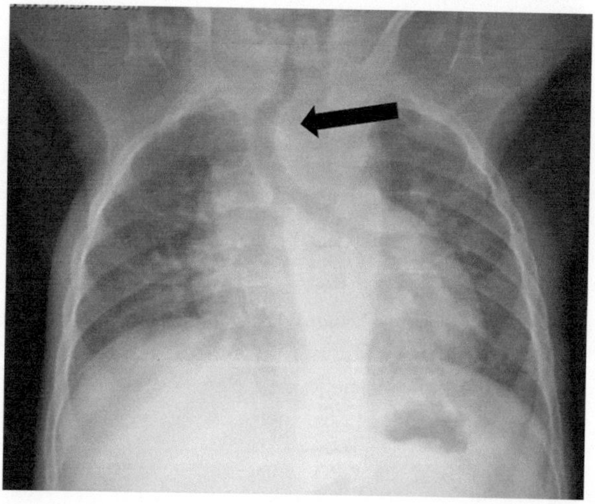

Fig. 12.6 Normal rightward displacement of the trachea; tracheal buckling

diaphragms. In case of increased aeration, the diaphragms are bilaterally flattened, the distance between the ribs is widened, and the anterior-posterior diameter is increased on the lateral radiograph. Increased aeration in children is more common in viral infections. It may be a sign of excessive ventilator pressure in an intubated child. If there is asymmetric lobar overinflation, advanced examination methods are used to detect possible underlying bronchial compression (e.g., mediastinal bronchogenic cyst), an anomaly (congenital lobar emphysema), or a mass causing partial obstruction in the bronchus (endobronchial granuloma) (Fig. 12.7).

Sometimes the diaphragm of the dense hemithorax is observed high in cases such as pulmonary aplasia. In these cases, the mediastinum is displaced toward the

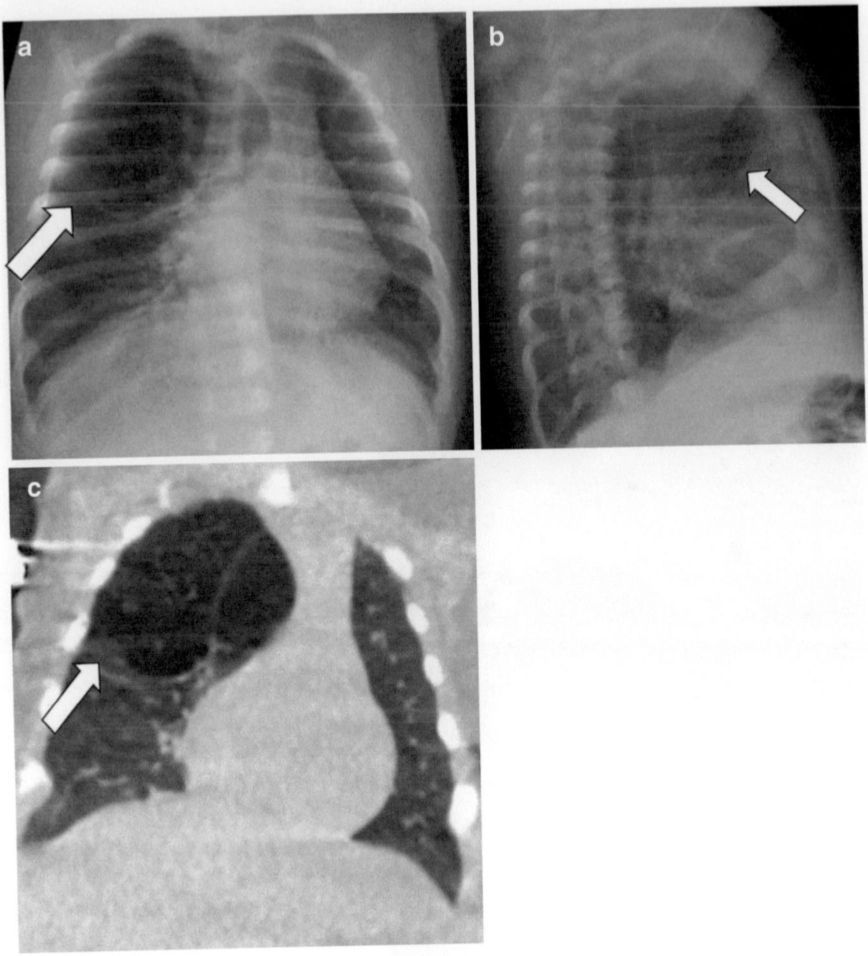

Fig. 12.7 In a newborn diagnosed with congenital lobar emphysema, focal lucency in the upper zone of the right lung on the chest X-ray (**a**), flattening in the diaphragm on the lateral radiograph (**b**), and a hypodense area in the upper lobe due to air trapping on the CT examination (**c**) are observed

dense hemithorax because of volume loss. Other causes of asymmetrical lung volumes include diaphragmatic paresis/paralysis and a large abdominal mass. The diaphragm may also be elevated, apparently secondary to a collection of subpulmonic fluid. Diaphragm contours in the neonatal period should be evaluated for possible congenital diaphragmatic hernia (Fig. 12.8).

Mediastinal Borders

The normal structure of the mediastinum should always be reviewed. On the left side, you should look for the thymus, aortic arch, pulmonary conus, hilus, and left

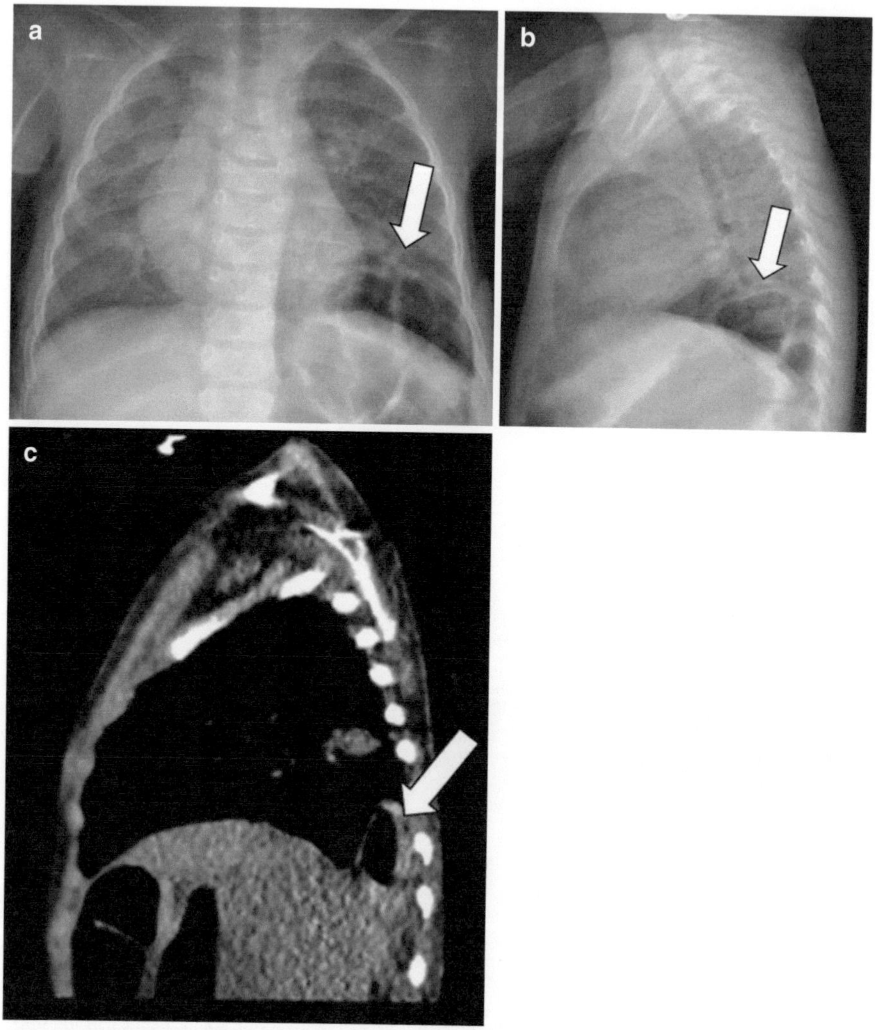

Fig. 12.8 In the bilateral chest radiograph, there is an appearance secondary to intestinal and herniation in the left hemithorax posterior (**a**, **b**). With CT, herniation of the intestinal loops into the hemithorax from the defective area in the diaphragm was demonstrated (**c**)

heart border; on the right side, you should consider the thymus, azygos vein, hilus, and right heart border. The thymus may be misleading in young children, but it should be checked that the posterior paraspinal section can be easily observed since the thymus is located anteriorly. Disturbances in the paraspinal lines or increased opacity at the apex suggest posterior mediastinal masses (meningocele, neuroenteric cyst, duplication cyst, neurogenic tumor, and infection). Erosions in adjacent bone tissues are caused by infection or suggest malignancy. Any abnormal appearance of the thymus suggests an anterior mediastinal mass lesion (thymic hyperplasia, germ cell tumor, T-cell lymphoma, and thymoma). The other mass lesion in the mediastinum usually originates from the middle mediastinum. In young children, this mass is usually a congenital abnormality such as a bronchogenic cyst or duplication cyst. An older child may have enlarged lymph nodes secondary to infective and neoplastic processes.

Lung Opacities

The contours of the mediastinum are used to locate the localization of opacities in the lungs. The differential attenuation of two adjacent structures defines the silhouette sign. For example, the loss of the upper mediastinal outline indicates upper lobe opacification, the loss of the heart borders is the result of right middle lobe or lingular opacification, and the loss of diaphragmatic definition is caused by lower lobe pathology.

Atelectasis and consolidations cause the lung to appear opaque. Volume loss in atelectasis and volume increase in consolidations with air bronchograms are distinctive. In volume loss, mediastinal shift toward the ipsilateral hemithorax, elevation of the diaphragm, and convergence of the ribs are observed. The hilum may be displaced toward the atelectasis, and noncollapsed lung may show compensatory overinflation. In acute atelectasis, a displaced endotracheal tube, foreign body aspiration, or mucus occlusion are causes that should not be considered first. In chronic atelectasis, extrinsic airway obstruction (bronchogenic cyst, mediastinal lymphadenopathy, neoplasia), or chronic infection (e.g., tuberculosis) are more likely causes. Consolidation is the replacement of air in terminal airspaces. It is the uptake of fluid, mucus, or cellular material. Clinical history, accompanying lymphadenopathy, or the presence of pleural effusion is important for differential diagnosis. Bilateral pulmonary edema presents as perihilar patchy consolidation with pleural fluid.

Ground-glass change describes increased attenuation of the lung with preserved bronchial and vascular signs. It is a nonspecific finding with a wide etiology, including infection, and interstitial and alveolar diseases.

CT/MRI is needed to elucidate the underlying cause of focal and multifocal lung opacities other than pneumonia. The cause of a solitary parenchymal lesion may be congenital malformations such as sequestration, congenital pulmonary adenomatoid malformation, and vascular anomaly. Also, a lung abscess may have no apparent gas-fluid level and can be observed as a round mass.

In multifocal lesions, infective (tuberculosis, fungal, septic embolism), inflammatory (LCH) processes, common interstitial lung diseases, and metastasis form the priority diagnosis list.

In children, lower respiratory tract infections remain a major cause of morbidity and mortality. Various pathogens such as viruses, bacteria, bacteria-like organisms, mycobacteria, fungi, and parasites, either alone or in combination, may affect the peripheral airways (bronchiolitis) or the alveoli (pneumonia).

Pneumonia can cause morbidity in children, with the potential development of various acute and chronic complications. Medical imaging is used to confirm or exclude the presence of pneumonia. However, it is also useful in the detection of underlying anomalies in recurrent infections and the evaluation of complications (Fig. 12.9).

Cystic Lung Diseases

Cystic sequelae lesions can be observed in necrotizing pneumonia, infective processes with cavitation (Staphylococcus aureus, tuberculosis, fungus), and abscesses. A lung abscess usually includes both liquid and gas. With the CXR, the gas-liquid

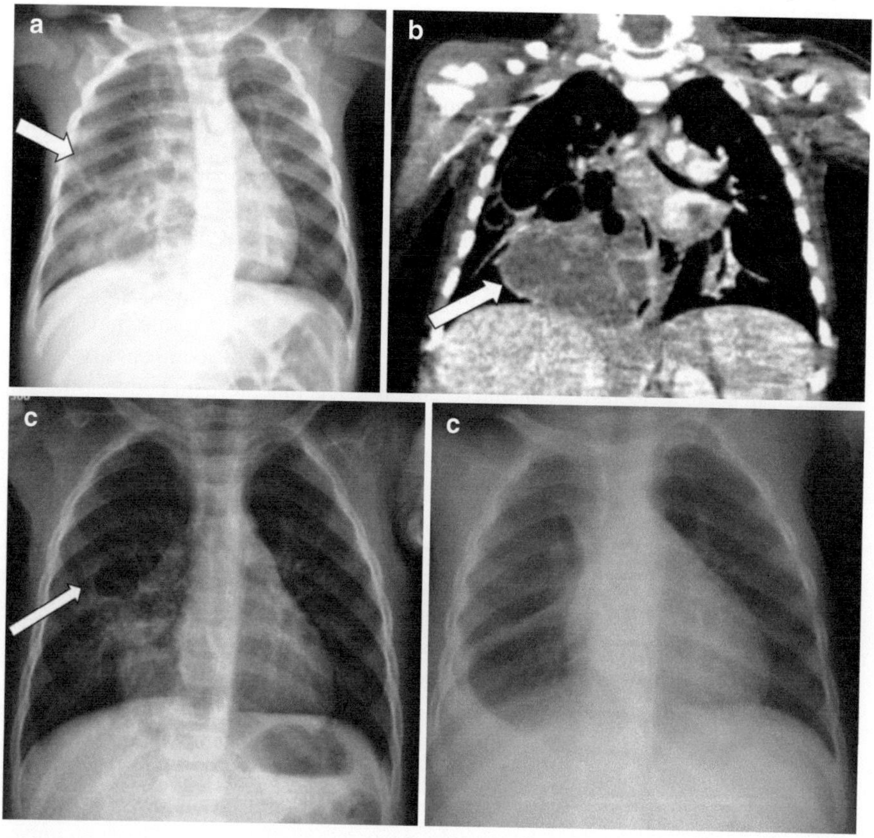

Fig. 12.9 There is an increase in opacity in the middle-lower zone of the right lung on the chest X-ray (**a**). Contrast-enhanced thorax CT examination reveals dense cystic lesions (**b**). After medical treatment, there was still a cystic mass in the right lung (**c**). The patient was operated on, and the pathological diagnosis was CPAM. Control chest X-ray shows postoperative changes after surgery (**d**)

level can be overlooked, sometimes appearing as nodular opacity. Multifocal, multicystic parenchymal lesions may be congenital cystic adenomatoid malformation, Langerhans cell histiocytosis nodules at the cavitating stage, granulomatosis with polyangiitis, or necrotizing vasculitis.

Pulmonary İnterstitial Emphysema (PIE)

PIE is a complication that can occur when high ventilator pressures are used. Rarely, it can be seen spontaneously in babies who have never been ventilated. It is the escape of air into the intestinal tract as a result of alveolar leakage. It is in the form of lace-like linear lucency extending from the pulmonary hilum toward the periphery. If complicated, pneumothorax or pneumomediastinum also develops.

Unilateral Hyperlucent Lung

(a) **Chest Wall Abnormality:** Poland syndrome is a congenital unilateral aplasia of the pectoralis muscles. The characteristic radiographic findings include unilateral hyperlucency of the lung related to the lack of soft tissues in the chest wall.

(b) **Pneumothorax**

Pneumothorax is the presence of air between the leaves of the pleura. It often develops spontaneously or after chest trauma in pediatric patients. It is caused by the transthoracic pressure difference in newborns. Pneumothorax can be fatal if not diagnosed and treated promptly. The main feature of pneumothorax on a chest radiograph is the white visceral pleural line. In most cases, a nonvascular hyperlucent pneumothorax area is also observed adjacent to the visceral pleura. CT is generally used in complicated cases. A progressive pneumothorax may present as a life-threatening tension pneumothorax that causes the mediastinal contralateral shift, increased intercostal distance, and the appearance of a flattened hemidiaphragm.

(c) **Lung Parenchymal Abnormality**

- *Bronchial atresia* is a congenital anomaly that results from the focal obliteration of a proximal segmental or subsegmental bronchus. The development of the distal airways is normal. However, preserved ventilation via collateral pathways leads to air trapping and hyperinflation. The atretic bronchus becomes filled with secretions and forms a bronchocele. The radiographic appearance of bronchial atresia is a round or oval branching opacity representing the bronchocele with an associated area of hyperlucency in the adjacent lung parenchyma (Fig. 12.10).
- *Congenital lobar emphysema* is characterized by progressive hyperinflation of a lobe. The most likely cause is thought to be air trapping with a check valve mechanism as a result of ineffective expiration secondary to malaise or stenosis in the bronchial cartilage.
- *Congenital pulmonary airway malformations* are multicystic masses of segmental lung tissue with disorganized hamartomatous and adenomatoid proliferation that communicate with the bronchial tree. The diagnosis is usually made on antenatal ultrasound in the neonatal period [4]. If large, they may cause pulmonary hypoplasia, with resultant respiratory distress syndrome.

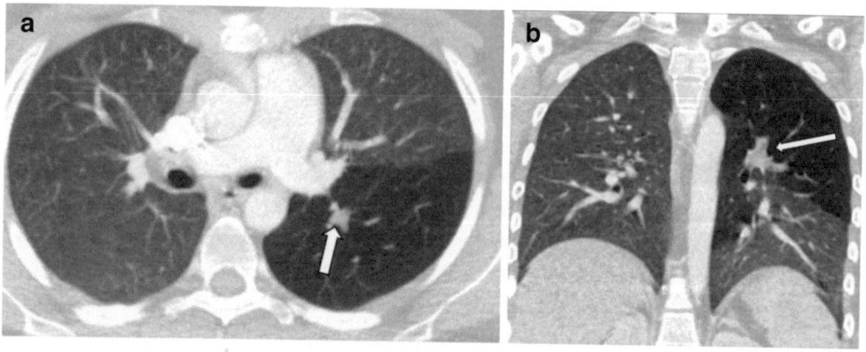

Fig. 12.10 The CT scans show a bronchocele appearance, which indicates a mucus-filled atresic bronchus with an air trapping area around it, located in the posterior of the upper lobe of the left lung, as observed in the parenchymal window on both axial (**a**) and coronal (**b**) sections

  - *Swyer-James Syndrome* usually develops during childhood as a sequela of postinfectious bronchiolitis obliterans. It is generally characterized by unilateral small lung with hyperlucency and air trapping and diminished vascularity. It can be unilateral or bilateral, also be lobar and segmental, and subsegmental involvement with a pathy distribution [5].

(d) **Pulmonary Vasculature Abnormality**

In conditions such as pulmonary agenesis and proximal interruption of the pulmonary artery, herniation secondary to compensatory hyperinflation in the contralateral lung and a unilateral hyperlucent lung occur.

In pulmonary artery sling, an aberrant course of the left pulmonary artery may cause impingement of the right main bronchus that can lead to right-lung air trapping and hyperinflation.

In Scimitar syndrome, also known as venolobar syndrome or hypogenetic lung syndrome, a hyperlucent appearance occurs in the contralateral lung secondary to right lung hypoplasia.

(e) **Central Airway Abnormality**

  - **Foreign Body Aspiration**
  - Foreign body aspiration is the most common cause of intraluminal airway abnormalities in children aged 6 months to 3 years. Most of the aspirated foreign bodies are nonradiopaque foodstuffs. The typical clinical picture is acute cough and wheezing. Foreign body aspiration should also be suspected in a child without a history of asthma presenting with recurrent lobar pneumonia. The radiographic appearance depends on the size, location, duration, and nature of the aspirated material. Radiopaque foreign bodies can be easily identified on radiographs. Obstructive lobar or segmental hyperinflation or atelectasis may be observed in the aspiration of a nonradiopaque foreign body. Inspiration-expiratory radiographs are evaluated with fluoroscopy to better evaluate air trapping. In case of clinical suspicion, bronchoscopy and CT can be performed if necessary. Foreign body can be directly identified

with CT, as well as secondary changes such as retained secretions, hyper-aeration, atelectasis, and consolidation.

- The right main bronchus is shorter and wider than the left, making a narrow angle with the trachea; therefore, foreign bodies are more likely to escape into the right main bronchus in children.
- Endobronchial Tumors

Endobronchial tumors are rare in the pediatric population but should be considered in the differential diagnosis when no other abnormality is present. This list includes carcinoid tumor, papilloma, adenoid cystic carcinoma, mucoepidermoid carcinoma, myofibroblastic tumor, and metastasis.

12.2.2 Fluoroscopy

Fluoroscopy can be used to evaluate dynamic large airway and lung abnormalities, such as airway obstruction, air trapping, and diaphragmatic paralysis. Use of fluoroscopic techniques and equipment should be optimized to minimize radiation exposure.

Fluoroscopy, a dynamic method, is used to evaluate diaphragm movements and mediastinal displacement in patients with air trapping, especially in cases of foreign body aspirations. Paradoxical movement is investigated with fluoroscopy in diaphragmatic paralysis or eventration. Nowadays, diaphragmatic movements are often evaluated with ultrasound (US), especially in pediatric patients.

12.2.3 Ultrasound

Evaluation of the lungs with ultrasound is typically performed with the patient in the supine or upright position. The lateral decubitus view or the supraclavicular and suprasternal notch view may be beneficial in some selected patients. Ultrasound is a valuable and common imaging modality used in the evaluation of the thorax in pediatric patients. It is easy to apply, cost-effective, noninvasive, and does not expose patients to radiation. It has many advantages, such as being portable and providing real-time imaging.

Lung and Mediastinum: US can be used to characterize lesions that present as peripheral opacities on chest X-rays (atelectasis, consolidation, lung necrosis, lung abscess, congenital lung lesions, and masses). Vascular structures in cases of pulmonary sequestration or blood flow in cases involving a neoplasm can also be evaluated with Color Doppler US (Fig. 12.11).

Pleura: It indicates whether the opaque appearance on the chest X-ray is due to pleural fluid or parenchymal lesion. Additionally, ultrasound can visualize the internal debris, septations, and pleural thickening often associated with parapneumonic collections (Fig. 12.12).

It is used to determine whether the pleural effusion is loculated or free by positioning the patient and as a guide imaging method in interventional procedures such

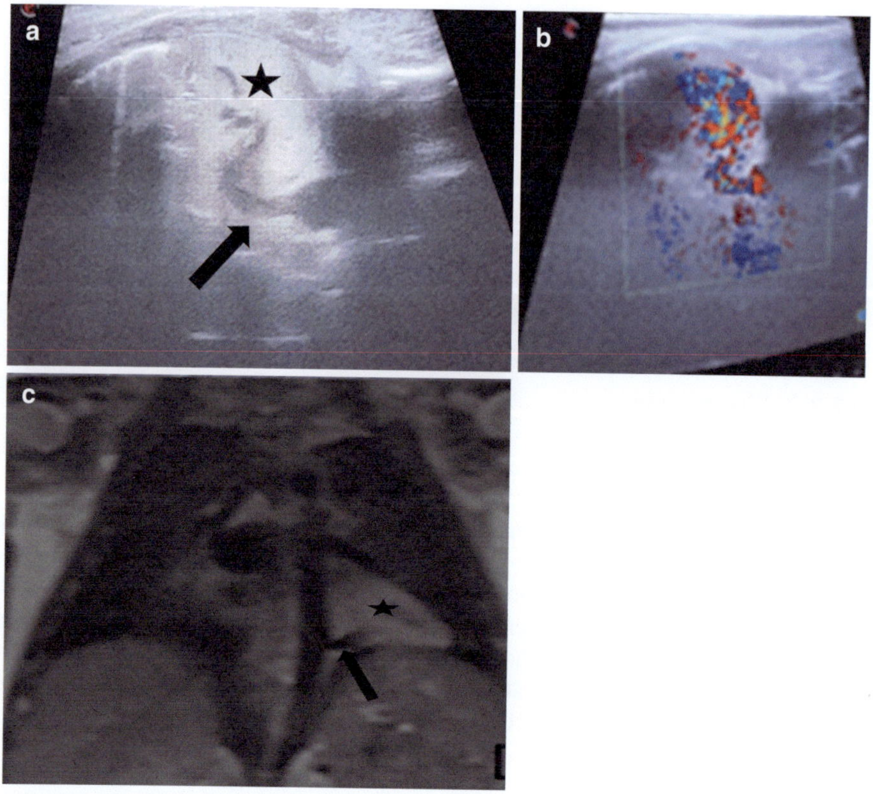

Fig. 12.11 In the US and Doppler US, examination performed while the patient is in the prone position, sequestered lung tissue (star), whose systemic artery (arrow) is selected, is observed in the posterobasal region of the left lung lower lobe (**a**, **b**). The presence of sequestered tissue (star) and the feeding artery (arrow) was confirmed in the noncontrast coronal plan MRI performed with mild sedation (**c**)

as thoracentesis. It may be more sensitive than radiography in the evaluation of pneumothorax in supine patients [6]. CT is insufficient to differentiate between pleural effusion and empyema. Effusion content and septa can be evaluated better with ultrasonography. For this reason, it is necessary to evaluate with ultrasound after a plain X-ray.

In the neonatal intensive care unit (NICU), lung ultrasound (LUS) can be used to diagnose the etiology of neonatal respiratory distress. These diseases include HMD (hyaline membrane disease), transient neonatal tachypnea, neonatal pneumonia, pneumothorax, neonatal pulmonary atelectasis, and congenital anomalies (Fig. 12.13).

In Pneumothorax, the first diagnostic method is plain radiography. However, an anteriorly located pneumothorax may be difficult to detect in neonates or infants, especially in the supine position. In the NICU, we can also use the US to detect pneumothorax.

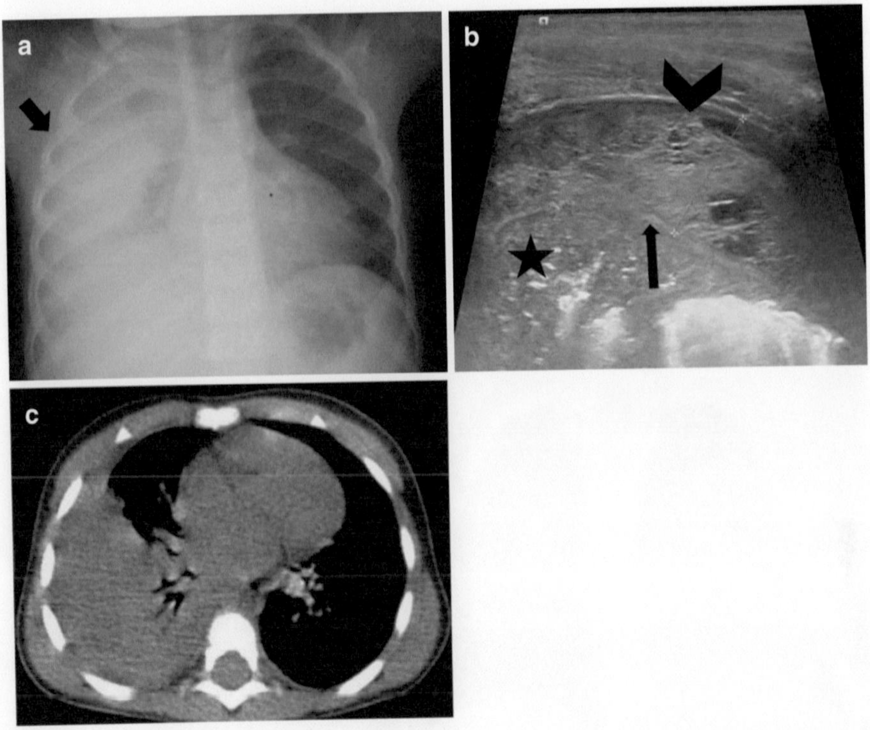

Fig. 12.12 Almost all of the right hemithorax is opaque in the chest X-ray, and the diaphragm line and heart contour cannot be distinguished (**a**). In the US examination, dense pleural fluid (arrowhead) compatible with empyema is observed adjacent to the consolidated lung tissue (star) and visceral pleura (arrow) (**b**). In this complicated pneumonia patient, the empyema border cannot be distinguished from the consolidated tissue in the noncontrast CT examination (**c**)

The change or disappearance of artifacts observed in normal lungs gives us clues about some parenchymal diseases. Among these, "A lines" denote pleural reverberation artifacts, and "B lines" denote vertical short sheen. Normally, there are 2–3 B lines at most in each intercostal space. An increase in the B lines represents increased alveolar or interstitial fluid retention. We suspect pneumothorax if the B lines converge and cast a shadow as a single beam, and we do not see the sliding movement of the lung on the dynamic US (Fig. 12.14).

12.2.4 Computed Tomography

CT is currently the most sensitive way of imaging the lungs due to its high spatial resolution. With the widespread use of multidetector row CT scanners (MDCT), there has been a significant increase in the number of CT exams. As a result of rapid technological developments in radiology, the duration of the examination has considerably shortened. Completing the exam within seconds is particularly important in pediatric patients who may not be able to follow breath-hold commands.

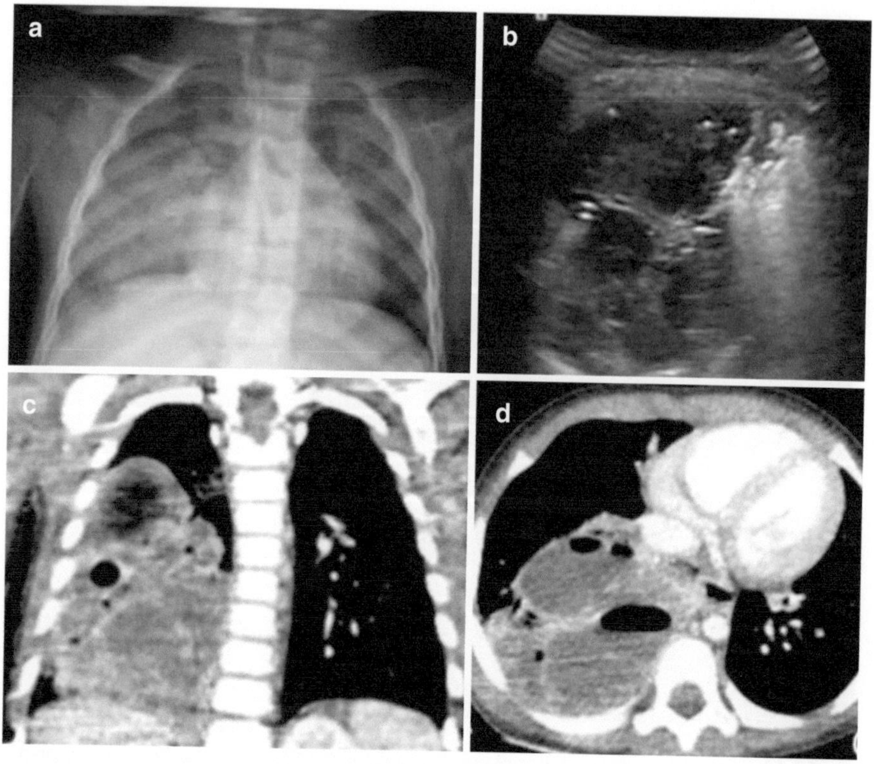

Fig. 12.13 In a mature newborn, there is an opaque appearance in a wide area in the right hemithorax on chest X-ray (**a**), and this area was found to belong to a mass consisting of multiple cysts larger than 2 cm in diameter on US examination (**b**). In the next stage, findings correlated with the contrast-enhanced CT examination (**c**, **d**). The pathology result of the operated patient was CPAM (congenital pulmonary airway malformation)

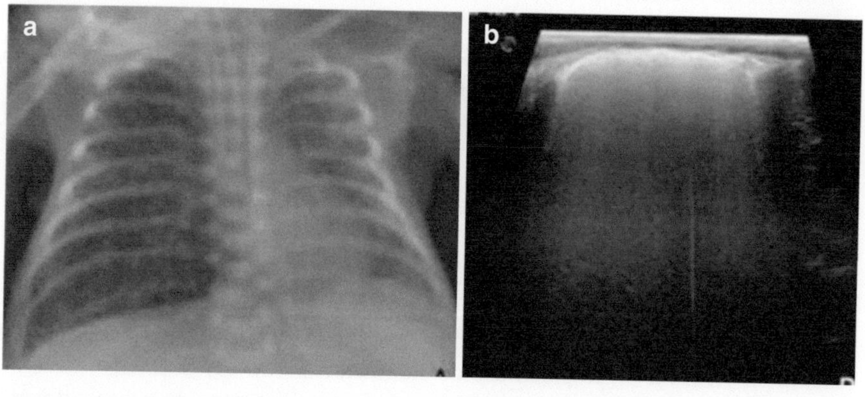

Fig. 12.14 A newborn with a history of mechanical ventilation has pulmonary interstitial emphysema, especially in the right lung, and a pneumothorax that cannot be clearly distinguished on plain radiographs (**a**). On US examination, comet tail artifacts originating from the pleura consistent with pneumothorax disappeared. We also see that the sliding of the lung has disappeared in the dynamic examination. Since it is a real-time dynamic method, it is also used to evaluate diaphragmatic movements in phrenic nerve injuries (**b**)

The increase in radiation exposure from CT, especially in children, is an important problem. An effective anteroposterior chest X-ray dose is 0.05 milliSievert (mSv), while the thorax conventional CT dose is 7.0 mSv (10 mm interval), HRCT dose is 0.7 mSv, and thin section low-dose CT is 0.2 mSv [7]. In the respiratory system, the most common radiological method is CT in cases that cannot be diagnosed by chest radiography and US. Good interpretation of chest radiography findings can prevent many unnecessary CT examinations. The higher radiosensitivity and longer life expectancy of children, combined with the increased use of CT, make it necessary to reduce the CT radiation dose while maintaining diagnostic image quality. There are chest CT protocols that use variable tube voltages and tube currents, often determined by body size [8]. Lowering the kV (kilovolt) from 120 to 100 reduces the dose by 30–70%. When the dose is reduced, there is an increase in image noise [9]. Automatic exposure control (AEC) is a method of dose reduction and common application in MDCT. The lowest dose for which diagnostic data is provided and noise can be tolerated is achieved with automatic exposure systems [10]. Electrocardiogram-triggered sequential scanning may be used in CT to achieve fewer motion artifacts and a lower radiation dose [11].

CT scan can be performed with or without contrast material, depending on the clinical problem. In routine the use of precontrast and postcontrast (dual-phase) chest CT should be avoided in pediatric patients as much as possible to minimize radiation exposure.

CT is valuable in evaluating not only lungs, but also vascular abnormalities (Fig. 12.15), mediastinal, hilar, and chest wall abnormalities also can be assessed. However, the soft tissue contrast resolution of CT is not as good as MRI.

Postprocessed and reconstructed CT images such as multiplanar reformatted (MPR) and volüme rendering techniques considerably increase the diagnostic accuracy of pediatric chest CT [12].

Modern MDCT scanners, with an increasing number of detector rows, have further enhanced performance, with faster scan times (improved temporal resolution) and a wider scan range. When this is combined with the use of smaller detector elements, it enables reduced partial volume artifacts. Thoracic CT in a spiral mode in children, without the need for breath-holding and with minimal respiratory, cardiac, and patient motion artifacts, reduces reliance on sedation and general anesthesia. Using postprocessing software to restructure the overlapping thin sections due to isotropic imaging, they are presented as two-dimensional or three-dimensional displays with a resolution close to the original.

Thoracic CT is frequently used to evaluate metastasis when scanning or when a solitary pulmonary nodule is suspected, and in symptomatic patients with a normal chest X-ray. It is also the most useful method in the characterization of diffuse lung diseases.

Maximum intensity projection (MIP), a multiplanar reconstruction method is used to extract contrast-enhanced anatomic structures than adjacent structures, as in CT angiography. These thicker slabs are useful in detecting and localizing micronodular (Fig. 12.16) or microtubular patterns [13].

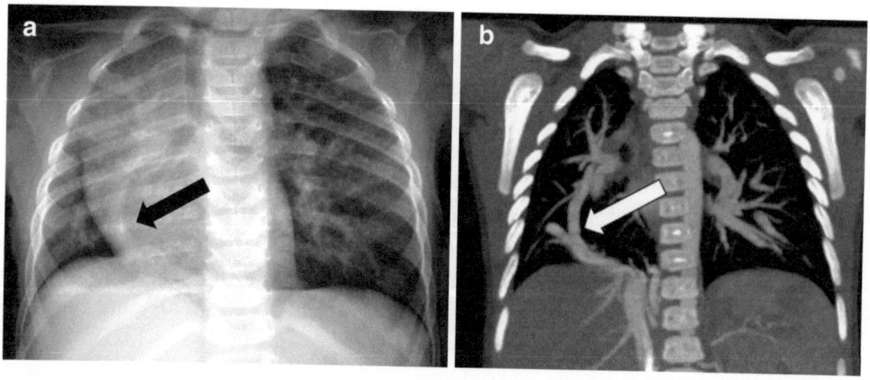

Fig. 12.15 It is observed that a convex-shaped linear density in the hypoplasic right lung lower zone on the PA chest X-ray (**a**), belongs to an abnormal pulmonary venous return anomaly in coronal MIP CT images consistent with scimitar syndrome (arrows: Turkish sword) (**b**)

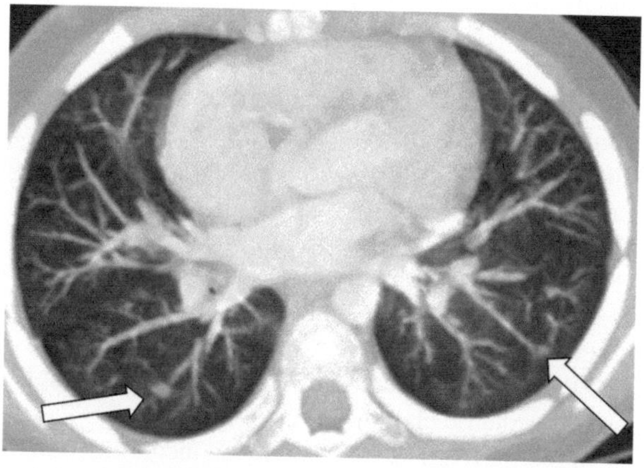

Fig. 12.16 A 10-year-old girl with nodules that were difficult or impossible to select in the CT examination taken to determine the etiology of fever could be detected more easily with MIP images

With volumetric imaging, the bronchial tree and cardiovascular system are better evaluated (Fig. 12.17). MDCT is now widely used as a replacement for conventional angiography in the evaluation of cardiovascular diseases (Fig. 12.18). MDCT is now widely used as a replacement for traditional angiography because it does not require invasive intervention and sedation. The total radiation dose in MDCT is significantly lower than in conventional angiography. Although MDCT plays an important role in the diagnosis of pulmonary embolism, arteriovenous malformation, aneurysm, and dissection, conventional angiography has the advantage of allowing therapeutic intervention.

Static Airway CT is mainly performed to assess fixed airway narrowing or stenosis. It is acquired in infants and young children while they breathe freely, and in older children, they hold their breath at the end of inspiration with the fast scan speed of multidetector CT. Dynamic Airway CT is performed in a paired inspiratory and expiratory phase to evaluate a large airway disorder, most commonly tracheobronchomalacia. The resultant effective dose from this paired study is typically in the range of 3.5–7.5 mSv [14].

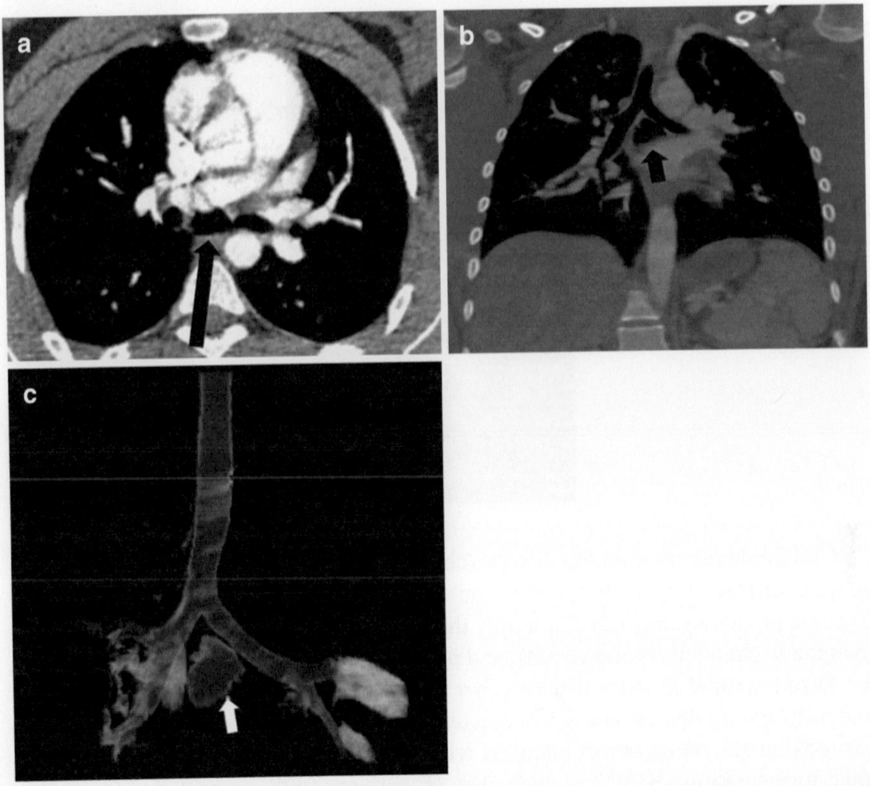

Fig. 12.17 A 15-year-old female patient with stridor. In the axial and coronal plane contrast CT examination, there is a lobulated contoured air-filled diverticular formation associated with the left main bronchus (**a**, **b**). In 3D images obtained from thin-section CT images, the relationship between the diverticula and the left main bronchus can be more clearly identified (**c**)

Minimum intensity projection (MinIP) can be used to show the central airway and air trapping in the lungs. Sometimes, expiratory CT is required to confirm air trapping. For this, patient cooperation or anesthesia is mandatory. In uncooperative infants and young children, lateral decubitus CT may be used as an alternative [15].

The HRCT technique is taken with a section thickness of 1 mm and a gap of 10 mm. It is mostly preferred in bronchiectasis, bronchiolitis obliterans, and interstitial lung diseases. The HRCT technique should not be used for metastasis screening because there are areas of the lung that are not examined. The classic HRCT technique still may be used in pediatric patients because of the overall decreased radiation exposure compared with volumetric data acquisition.

The HRCT technique is taken with a section thickness of 1 mm and a gap of 10 mm. It is mostly preferred in bronchiectasis, bronchiolitis obliterans, and interstitial lung diseases. The HRCT technique should not be used for metastasis screening because there are areas of the lung that are not examined. The classic HRCT technique may still be used in pediatric patients because of the overall decreased radiation exposure compared to volumetric data acquisition.

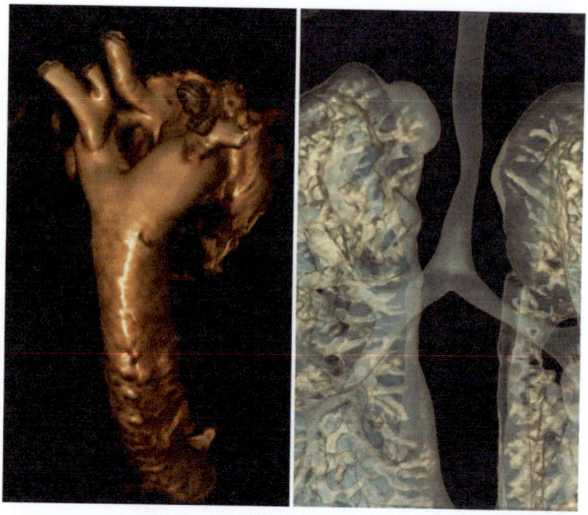

Fig. 12.18 3D reconstructive images obtained from MDCT, double aortic arch (**a**), and compression of the trachea (**b**)

Childhood interstitial lung disease (chILD) encompasses a heterogeneous group of rare diffuse lung diseases that can develop due to acute or chronic causes. Disease processes may affect not only the interstitium but also the alveoli, airways, lymphatic channels, blood vessels, and pleural spaces. Plain radiography is the first preferred method in these diseases, but it may be normal in some cases. Some of the diffuse lung diseases have a characteristic pattern that allows a specific diagnosis to be made, while others manifest with a nonspecific appearance requiring further investigation. HRCT is indicated in patients with suspected diffuse lung disease to demonstrate the pattern and distribution of these opacities radiologically (Fig. 12.19).

12.2.5 Magnetic Resonance Imaging (MRI)

There are some limitations in chest MRI due to the low signal-to-noise ratio of the lung, lengthy examination time, and cardiac-respiratory motion artifacts. In most pediatric patients, it requires sedation. There are some technical methods to improve MRI, like parallel imaging and multichannel body-array coils to reduce examination time. Moreover, electrocardiogram triggering, respiratory triggering, and navigator gating may be used to suppress motion artifacts. The lack of ionizing radiation and the superior soft tissue imaging are advantages of MRI (Fig. 12.20). MRI is also useful in the evaluation of spinal canal extension, especially in neurogenic tumors located in the posterior mediastinum (Fig. 12.21). Additionally, the cellularity of thoracic masses may be evaluated with diffusion-weighted imaging. Central airways and cardiovascular structures can be assessed with black-blood MRI without using a contrast agent [16]. Also, the allergy risk of contrast material used in MRI is lower than the risk of allergy to the contrast agent in CT. In addition, tracheobronchomalacia can be diagnosed with real-time dynamic airway MRI.

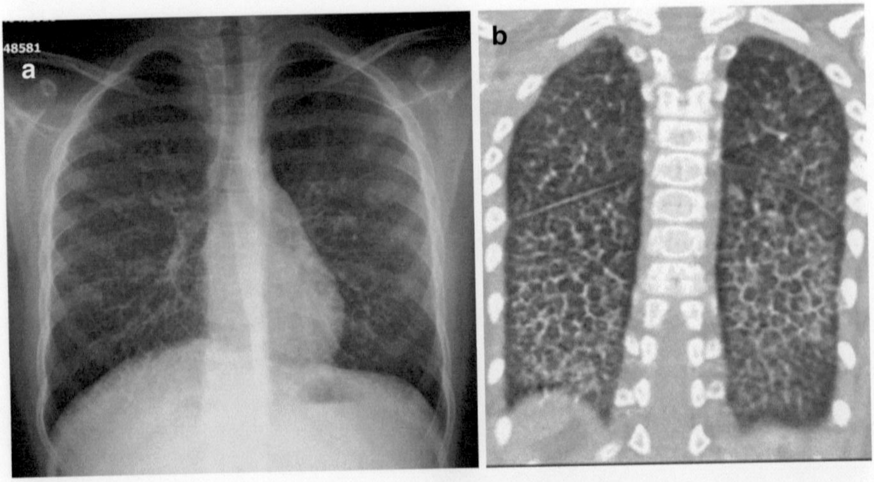

Fig. 12.19 A 14-year-old boy with diffuse reticulonodular and ground glass opacities observed in both lungs. In the coronal section CT examination, there are diffuse interlobular septal thickenings, more prominent in the lower lobes

CT or MRI can be used in the evaluation of lymphoma, leukemia-related infiltration, thymus-located cysts and tumors (Fig. 12.22).

Although diagnostic accuracy is still largely unknown, three-dimensional volumetric MRI images can contribute to diagnosis in most modern scanners.

12.2.6 Angiography

Computed tomography, magnetic resonance angiography, and digital subtraction angiography (DSA) are the radiological modalities used to demonstrate the pulmonary vascular tree. In recent years, noninvasive imaging methods have been increasingly utilized. With the widespread use of MRI and CT, the indications for conventional angiography for diagnostic purposes have significantly decreased. Angiography in pediatric patients is mostly used for therapeutic purposes, such as vascular tumor embolization, arteriovenous fistula embolization before surgery, or vascular stenosis requiring angioplasty (Fig. 12.23).

12.2.7 Positron Emission Tomography (PET)

In pediatric patients, PET is useful for evaluating intrathoracic tumors, including Hodgkin and non-Hodgkin lymphoma, rhabdomyosarcoma, osteosarcoma, Ewing sarcoma, and neuroblastoma. PET offers an advantage over anatomic imaging by detecting metabolically active viable tissue. Therefore, PET is employed in oncologic imaging for both initial diagnosis and monitoring metabolic responses to treatment.

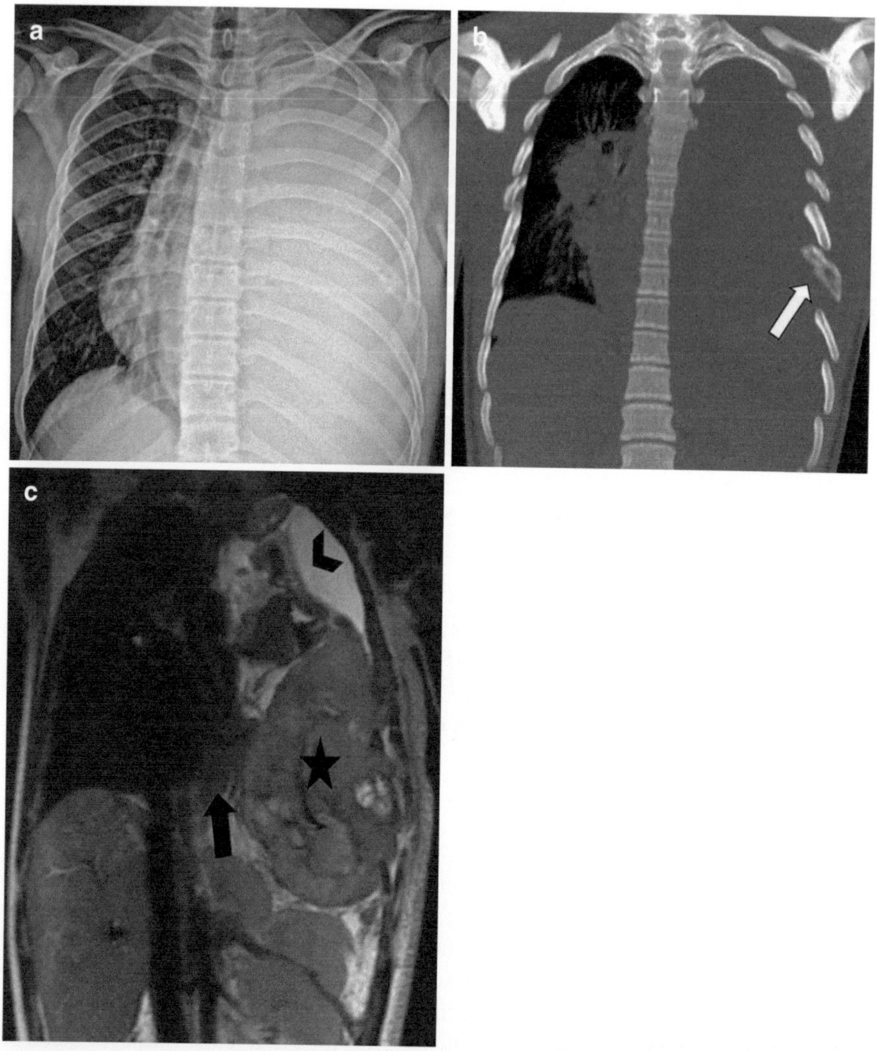

Fig. 12.20 There is a mass lesion that fills the left hemithorax and causes a rightward shift in the mediastinal structures. The diaphragmatic border cannot be selected. The relationship of the mass with the bone was shown in the PA chest X-ray (**a**) and coronal CT (**b**) examination. There is lytic expansile destruction in the left rib (white arrow). In coronal MRI, dense fluid in the vicinity of the mass in the left hemithorax (arrowhead) and collapse in the lung are selected (black arrow) (**c**). Pathology was Ewing sarcoma

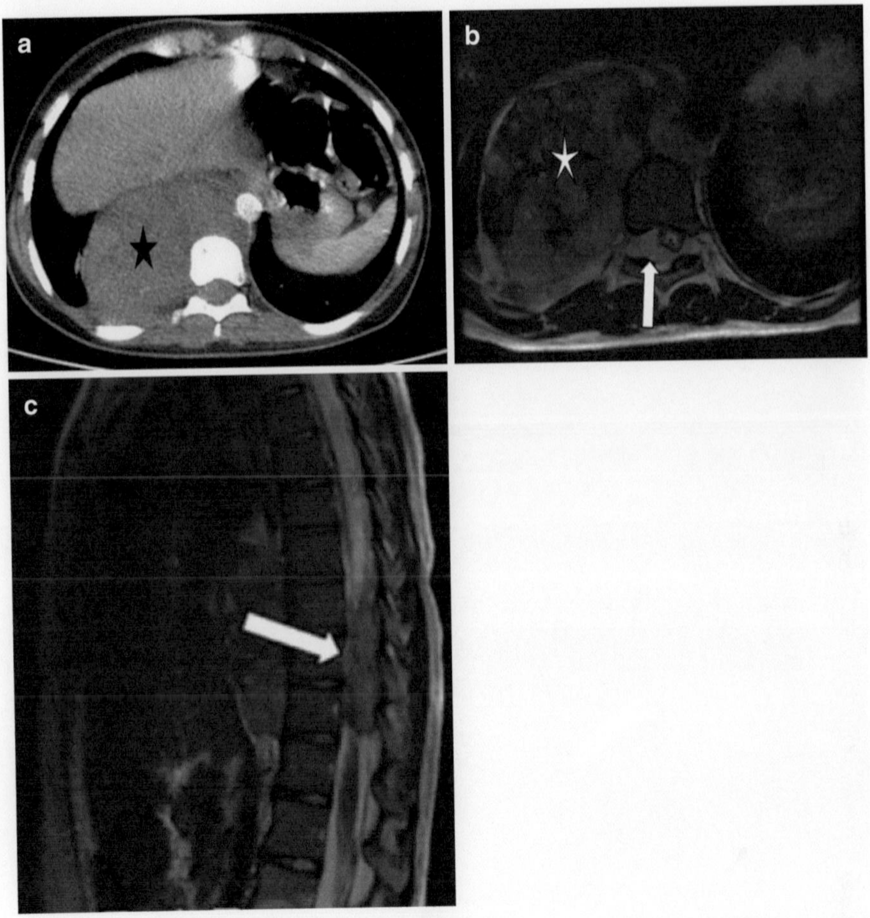

Fig. 12.21 The patient diagnosed with neuroblastoma has a paravebral mass in the posterior mediastinum (**a**) in the axial CT image. Spinal canal extension and cord compression are observed in axial and sagittal MRI (**b, c**)

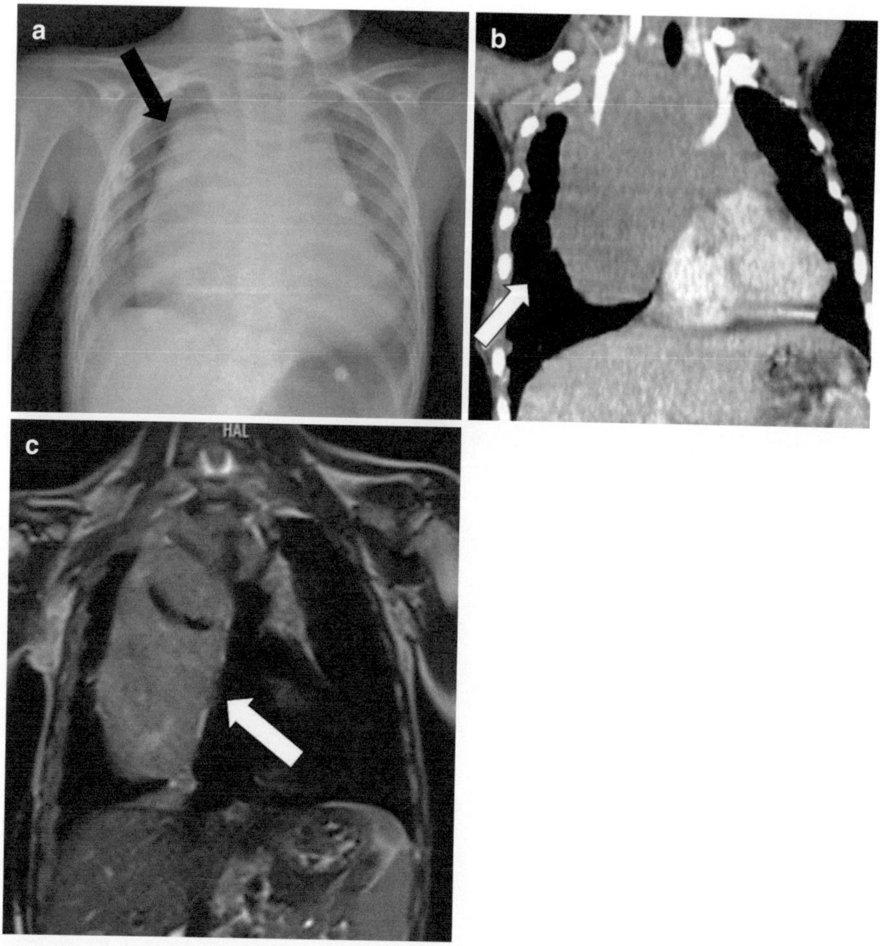

Fig. 12.22 Chest X-ray, CT, and MRI revealed a giant mass lesion surrounding the vascular structures in the anterior mediastinum. On MRI, an involvement compatible with pleural metastasis is also observed on the right

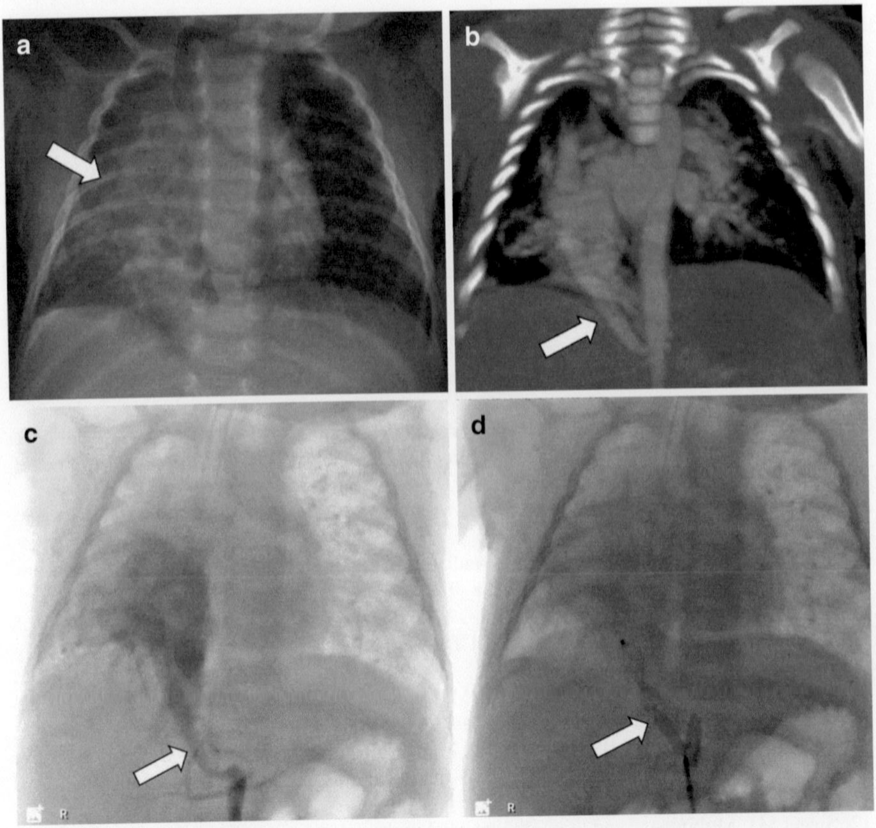

Fig. 12.23 Six-month-old girl. In the newborn period, opacity was detected in the right hemithorax and she received pneumonia treatment (**a**). However, because the clinical and radiological findings persisted despite the treatment, a contrast-enhanced thorax CT examination was performed (**b**). In CT and angiography examinations, sequestered lung tissue and its systemic vascularization were identified (**c**, **d**). Angiography was performed to occlude the aberrant vessel

12.3 Conclusion

Using imaging methods such as Ultrasound (US), Computed Tomography (CT), and Magnetic Resonance Imaging (MRI) following a chest X-ray with a well-defined algorithm is crucial for the benefit of both the patient and the physician. Effective communication between clinicians and radiologists is essential to select the most appropriate imaging modality for the specific disease or symptom. This should consider factors such as minimizing ionizing radiation exposure, accessibility, and cost-effectiveness. The choice of imaging modality should always be made with the patient's best interests and health in mind.

References

1. Costanzo LS. Costanzo physiology. Google Kitaplar. https://books.google.com.tr/books?id=lkdFEAAAQBAJ&printsec=frontcover&hl=tr&source=gbs_ge_summary_r&cad=0#v=onepage&q&f=false.
2. Soboleski D, Theriault C, Acker A, Dagnone V, Manson D. Unnecessary irradiation to non-thoracic structures during pediatric chest radiography. Pediatr Radiol. 2006;36(1):22–5. https://doi.org/10.1007/s00247-005-0016-y.
3. Ayşe E, Aslan T, Kiper N. ÇOCUK GÖĞÜS HASTALIKLARINDA TANI YÖNTEMLERİ.
4. Chest radiology: the essentials. Google Kitaplar. https://books.google.com.tr/books?id=RZBT7KGMEb4C&printsec=frontcover&hl=tr&source=gbs_ge_summary_r&cad=0#v=onepage&q&f=false.
5. Moore ADA, Godwin JD, Dietrich PA, Verschakelen JA, Henderson WR. Swyer-James syndrome: CT findings in eight patients. Am J Roentgenol. 1992;158(6):1211–5. www.ajronline.org.
6. Rambhia SH, D'Agostino CA, Noor A, Villani R, Naidich JJ, Pellerito JS. Thoracic ultrasound: technique, applications, and interpretation. In: Current problems in diagnostic radiology, vol. 46. Mosby Inc.; 2017. p. 305–16.
7. Mayo JR, Aldrich J, Müller NL. Radiation exposure at chest CT: a statement of the fleischner society. Radiology. 2003;228(1):15–21.
8. Kim JE, Newman B. Evaluation of a radiation dose reduction strategy for pediatric chest CT. Am J Roentgenol. 2010;194(5):1188–93.
9. Siegel MJ, Schmidt B, Bradley D, Suess C, Hildebolt C. Radiation dose and image quality in pediatric CT: effect of technical factors and phantom size and shape. Radiology. 2004;233(2):515–22.
10. Lee CH, Goo JM, Lee HJ, Ye SJ, Park CM, Chun EJ, et al. Radiation dose modulation techniques in the multidetector CT era: from basics to practice. Radiographics. 2008;28(5):1451–9.
11. Pauls S, Aschoff AJ, Wahl J, Brambs HJ, Fleiter TR. Multi-detector row CT: is prospective electrocardiographic triggering improving the detection of small pulmonary tumors? Acad Radiol. 2005;12(5):614–9.
12. Siegel MJ. Multiplanar and three-dimensional multi-detector row CT of thoracic vessels and Airways in the Pediatric Population. Radiology. 2003;229(3):641–50.
13. Remy J, Remy-Jardin M, Artaud D, Fribourg M. Multiplanar and three-dimensional reconstruction techniques in CT: impact on chest diseases. Eur Radiol. 1998;8(3):335–51.
14. Lee EY, Boiselle PM. Tracheobronchomalacia in infants and children: multidetector CT evaluation. Radiology. 2009;252(1):7–22.
15. Choi SJ, Choi BK, Kim H, Lee S, Choi S, Park S, et al. Lateral decubitus HRCT: a simple technique to replace expiratory CT in children with air trapping. Pediatr Radiol. 2002;32(3):179–82.
16. Yedururi S, Paul Guillerman R, Chung T, Braverman RM, Dishop MK, Giannoni CM, et al. Multimodality imaging of tracheobronchial disorders in children. Radiographics. 2008;28(3):1–75.

13 Fundamentals of Upper Respiratory Tract Endoscopy

Semih Ak, Nuray Bayar Muluk, and Sheng-Po Hao

13.1 Introduction

The upper aerodigestive tract must be evaluated endoscopically for a correct diagnosis. Laryngoscopes, bronchoscopes, and esophagoscopes, both rigid and flexible, are among the tools at your disposal. The surgeon now has access to a wide range of procedures for collecting data for an accurate diagnosis and, in some situations, for implementing a therapeutic intervention, many of which can be done in an outpatient setting. A precise diagnosis, tumor staging, and the exclusion of concomitant lesions are all possible by surgical endoscopy. The gold standard is to examine thoroughly and biopsy a lesion while the patient is under general anesthesia. A sufficient biopsy specimen must be acquired regardless of the endoscopic approach employed for a histologic diagnosis.

The purpose of an endoscopic examination of the equine upper airway is to detect any anatomical or functional abnormalities in the nasal passages, nasal septum, turbinates, maxillary aperture, pharynx, guttural pouches (sometimes called auditory tube diverticulum), larynx, or palate. Endoscopic examination of the nasal and pharyngeal airways [1] requires a thorough understanding of normal nasopharyngeal anatomy.

S. Ak
Mehmet Akif İnan Training and Research Hospital, Şanlıurfa, Turkey

N. Bayar Muluk (✉)
Department of Otorhinolaryngology, Faculty of Medicine, Kırıkkale University, Kırıkkale, Turkey

S.-P. Hao
Department of Otorhinolaryngology, Shin Kong Wu Ho-Su Memorial Hospital, and Fu Jen Catholic University, Taipei, Taiwan

H. Yüksel et al. (eds.), *Pediatric Airway Diseases*, Comprehensive ENT,
https://doi.org/10.1007/978-3-031-74853-0_13

13.2 Nasal Diagnostic Procedures

A head and neck surgeon can view the nasal vault through a nasal speculum using light sources that offer illumination and coaxial vision. Paying close attention to mucosal color, edema, and discharge, as well as the effect of vasoconstriction, is done both before and after nasal decongestion. The nasal septum, turbinates, and vault can be partially seen using this method [2], but only under certain conditions.

Nose endoscopy is a procedure in which the nose and sinus passages are examined under direct, high-quality visual observation. As an objective diagnostic technique, otolaryngologists routinely use it to assess nasal mucosa, sinonasal architecture, and nasal disease. A rigid endoscope or a flexible fiberoptic endoscope can be used to perform a nasal endoscopy. Flexible and inflexible endoscopies are generally well tolerated [3] when performed by trained professionals.

Rigid nasal endoscopes have different lens angles (0, 60, and 90°), making it possible to see hidden features during conventional anterior rhinoscopy. To see deeper structures or those off-axis from the nasal aperture [2], rigid nasal endoscopy is an excellent tool for your disposal.

The rigid endoscope allows the endoscopist to see more clearly, take tissue samples, prevent epistaxis, and even do minor surgeries [4, 5]. The nasal cavity and sinuses can be viewed in detail with the help of a rigid endoscope, which ranges in diameter from 2.7 to 4 mm and has angled tips (often between 0 and 70°) [3].

The advantages of nasal endoscopy for diagnostic purposes include enhanced lighting, increased magnification, and pinpoint navigation to diseased regions. As a result, doctors have a better chance of making a correct diagnosis. In one research, nearly 40% of patients with routine exams on anterior rhinoscopy had nasal pathology revealed by rigid nasal endoscopy [6]. Patients with sinonasal symptoms often benefit from endoscopic evaluation before and after surgery and during medicinal treatment [3].

13.2.1 Indications

Patients presenting to an otolaryngologist's clinic should be evaluated with nasal endoscopy because of its apparent involvement in diagnosing sinonasal illness.

- Intra-nasal examination: If you have an endoscopy, you can thoroughly check the patients' nasal passages and sinuses [3]
- The evaluation of the patient's response to medical treatment (e.g., resolution of polyps, purulent secretions, or mucosal edema and inflammation after treatment with topical nasal steroids, antibiotics, oral steroids, and antihistamines)
- Evaluate the patient's response to unilateral disease (e.g., resolution of polyps, purulent secretions, mucosal edema, and inflammation after treatment with…
- Evaluation and biopsy of nasal masses or lesions
- Examination of the Nasopharynx for Lymphoid Hyperplasia, Eustachian Tube Dysfunction, and Nasal Obstruction

- Diagnosis and Management of Epistaxis
- Diagnosis and Management of Cerebrospinal Fluid (CSF) Leak
- Diagnosis and Management of Hyposmia or Anosmia
- Evaluation of Cerebrospinal Fluid (CSF) Leak
- Foreign body evaluation and management in the nose.

13.2.2 Contraindications

There are no guaranteed risks associated with nasal endoscopy. However, some patient groups should avoid it. It is essential to take extra precautions while performing nasal endoscopy on individuals using anticoagulants or having a history of bleeding disorders. A vasovagal episode [3] can also occur in a nervous patient or a patient with cardiovascular illness.

13.2.3 Anatomical Features

The septum is a bony and cartilaginous partition running along the middle of the nose, creating two equal chambers on either side. The superior, middle, and inferior conchas produce the superior, middle, and inferior meatus on the lateral nasal wall, leading to the paranasal sinuses. The superior meatus is the drainage area for the posterior ethmoid cells and the sphenoid sinus. The maxillary and frontal sinuses, as well as the anterior ethmoid, drain through the middle meatus. The nasolacrimal duct is exhausted through the inferior meatus [3].

The upper lateral cartilage, septum, nasal floor, and anterior head of the inferior turbinate form the boundaries of the internal nasal valve. This is the most constricted part of the nasal passage in a leptorrhine [3].

13.2.4 Technical Considerations

Objective methods for diagnosing chronic rhinosinusitis (CRS) include nasal endoscopy and imaging [7]. Endoscopy provides a variety of preoperative and postoperative applications in the care of patients with sinonasal symptoms [3].

The presence of polyps, discharge, edema, scarring, or adhesions and crusting are all factors that are taken into account by the Lund-Kennedy endoscopic grading system to determine the severity of nasal and paranasal sinus pathology [8]. Bilateral endoscopic staging is performed before diagnosis, surgery, and at suggested follow-up intervals of 3, 6, 12, 24, and 36 months.

Between 0 and 20, the Lund-Kennedy scale measures how likely someone is to take action. Absence (zero points), presence (one point), and presence (three points) of polyps in the middle meatus are recorded. There are three levels of discharge severity: nil (0), minimal (1), and severe (2). Edema, scarring, and crusting are each evaluated as absence (0), mild (1), or severe (2). Interrater agreement studies assessing the reliability of the Lund-Kennedy endoscopic scoring system reveal that, in many cases, two independent observers agree on the examination findings. Adding nasal endoscopy to treating patients with CRS has led to more precise diagnoses [9]. Endoscopic findings enhance the specificity, positive predictive value, and negative predictive value of assessment for CRS when used with established symptom criteria [7, 10] [11]. This development shows that the use of diagnostic endoscopy may assist in lessening the requirement for computed tomography (CT) and reduce expenditures and radiation exposure [3].

The authors of a best-practice article published by a triological society on nasal endoscopy's involvement in the diagnosis of CRS determined that the test alone has low sensitivity but has repeatedly proven reasonable specificity in identifying CRS, making it a helpful confirmatory test. High diagnosis accuracy of nasal endoscopy was also identified in patients meeting both symptom criteria and favorable endoscopic results. In these cases [12], a diagnosis of CRS can be obtained without resorting to more advanced imaging techniques.

In addition, a 2012 study conducted by Ferguson et al. indicated that nasal endoscopy has a sensitivity of 24% and a specificity of 100%, with mucopurulence only present in patients with positive CRS on CT [13]. Staging of allergic fungal sinusitis (AFS) has been shown to benefit extensively using diagnostic endoscopy. Based on nasal endoscopic results, Kupferberg-Kuhn classified AFS into four stages of the disease [14]. Endoscopy is the gold standard for collecting tissue samples and cultures and provides an objective inspection measure. However, study results have documented a greater than 90% correlation between endoscopically obtained cultures and maxillary sinus aspirates, making endoscopically guided cultures the current criterion standard. Historically, inferior meatal puncture was the diagnostic method used to identify pathogens in sinusitis [15, 16].

Researchers found that 90% of nasal endoscopy specimens yielded cultures with two or fewer bacterial isolates, while 55% lost a culture with a single isolate when used for microbiologic diagnosis [17]. These findings are more promising than those from a nasopharyngeal swab. Endoscopy plays a crucial function in the postoperative phase by allowing prompt debridement and monitoring for disease recurrence [3].

13.2.5 Technique

The nasal canals are numbed, and a decongestant is sprayed before the endoscope is inserted. Antifog solution is applied to a 3 mm 4 mm 0, or 30° scopes before insertion into the nasal cavity [3].

Then, the examiner makes three independent passages with the scope within each nostril (shown in the films below) [5, 18, 19]. The nasal mucosa and nasal cavity structures are inspected with each sweep. In particular, the examiner takes note of the nasal mucosa's color (pale vs. hyperemic), inflammation or hypertrophy of the mucosa, the presence of nasal polyps or secretions (purulent, thick, or thin), and the presence of any visible anatomic abnormalities (e.g., a septal deviation or spur, concha bullosa, or accessory ostia) [3].

13.2.5.1 First Pass

With the patient's head flexed, the scope is advanced along the floor of the nasal cavity and into the nasopharynx. The nasolacrimal duct and the inferior turbinates, where they drain, are inspected. The possibility of mucus or purulence draining into the nasopharynx is considered as the scope is moved posteriorly into the nasopharynx. The nasopharynx, including the eustachian tube openings and the fossa of Rosenmüller [3], is thoroughly inspected.

13.2.5.2 Second Pass

The second time around, the endoscope is inserted between the middle and inferior turbinates to look at the fontanelles and the inferior part of the middle meatus for supplementary maxillary Ostia. Next, the scope is advanced medially and posteriorly to the middle turbinate to investigate the sphenoethmoid depression lying medial to the middle and superior turbinates. During this passage, the superior turbinate can be used to see the oval or slit-shaped ostia of the sphenoid sinus [3].

The infundibulum, uncinate, and ethmoid bulla can be seen by withdrawing the scope and rotating it laterally under the middle turbinate. To insert the scope into the middle meatus, you may need to provide gentle medial pressure to the middle turbinate [3].

13.2.5.3 Third Pass

The third attempt typically calls for a 30° endoscope or a change in head position. The doctor can examine the olfactory cleft and detect any polyps or lesions. Due to the septum's curvature, it is usually only possible to thoroughly explore one side of the nose at a time [3].

13.2.6 Problems During the Procedure

In most cases, a rigid nasal endoscopy can be performed with minimal danger to the patient. Possible side effects of the surgery include sensitivity to the local anesthetic or decongestant, pain, discomfort, epistaxis, and vasovagal episodes. It is essential to confirm that the patient has no known allergies to the topical drugs before using them [3].

It is essential to exercise caution since nasal hemorrhage related to mucosal trauma can occur, especially in individuals at a higher risk for bleeding (such as those with a personal or familial history of bleeding disorders or who are presently using anticoagulants). Nasal biopsies taken from these patients also risk causing severe bleeding [3].

13.3 Flexible Laryngoscopy

The nasal cavity, sinuses, pharynx, and larynx can all be viewed using flexible laryngoscopy, which is becoming increasingly popular. The method requires a relatively modest diameter flexible endoscope and can be carried out in a doctor's office.

The nasal cavity is numbed and decongested beforehand for better visibility and comfort during the operation. In the technique, the examiner threads the end of the scope through the nasal opening down the floor of the nasal cavity. The examiner can see the inside of the nasal cavity to check for growths or lesions when the scope is inserted further. Direct visibility of the whole pharynx and larynx [2] is achieved by directing the scope inferiorly and advancing it gently as it nears the nasopharynx.

The fiberoptic telescope can be bent and swiveled in any number of directions, making it ideal for gaining insight into otherwise inaccessible spaces. However, flexible endoscopy is more challenging because it requires two hands to manipulate the equipment. Digital flexible endoscopes [3] have addressed the historical limitation of flexible endoscopy: poor visibility.

13.4 Direct Laryngoscopy

One of the benefits of direct laryngoscopy is that it can be used for diagnosis and treatment. General anesthesia is a subset of intubated anesthesia. The therapy provides a plain view of the pharynx and the larynx and permits the surgeon to do biopsies and remove tiny lesions. Simultaneously, the surgeon can palpate the oral cavity, oropharynx, and hypopharynx, which are difficult to palpate in a conscious patient [2].

The laryngoscope can be placed on a Mayo stand attached to the table (for hands-free use), and a microscope can be brought into focus to provide a more detailed view of the glottis and subglottis. Small lesions or topological anomalies can be better described and, if so desired, eliminated with a microscopic direct laryngoscopy. Vocal cord polyps, leukoplakia, intubation granulomas, contact ulcers, webs, nodules, hematomas, and papillomatosis are all lesions that can be diagnosed with a direct laryngoscopy. Furthermore, technological advancements make microlaryngoscopic examination of the vocal cords and CO_2 laser ablation or excision of small malignant tumors [2] possible.

13.5 Video Laryngoscopy

Direct laryngoscopy is different from the indirect laryngoscopy used in the clinic. Transnasal or transoral insertion of a fiberoptic or digital laryngoscope allows for vision of the larynx [20–22]. The movies below [20] show the distinction between direct and indirect laryngoscopy.

Images captured during video laryngoscopy can be viewed in real-time on a monitor by the doctor, patient, and other observers or saved for later review. Displaying images at a larger size on the screen enables a thorough inspection of the larynx. Fiberoptic intubation is predicated on video laryngoscopy [20].

Fiberoptic intubation includes threading an endotracheal (ET) tube over the shaft of a flexible fiberoptic scope. The patient's mouth or nose is used to insert the scope into the pharynx, and then the scope is advanced past the vocal folds and into the trachea. The ET tube is moved across the fiber optic cable into the patient's airway after visual confirmation of tracheal rings and carina. As soon as the tube is in position, the scope can be taken out, and the patient can begin to get ventilation [20].

The endoscopist will typically look via the scope's eyepiece as they execute a fiberoptic intubation. Hooking it up to a screen would be best to get the most out of the area. Showing the process to others in the room is a great learning tool [23, 24].

Video laryngoscopy is also utilized with stiff transoral laryngoscopy. Rigid laryngoscopes with built-in digital cameras are becoming increasingly common, with famous examples being the Airtraq laryngoscope (Prodol Meditec, Spain), the GlideScope (Verathon, Bothell, WA), and the Pentax-AWS (Pentax, Tokyo, Japan). Video laryngoscopy using a rigid laryngoscope, such as the GlideScope, has been found to provide a better image of the larynx than traditional laryngoscopy alone [25, 26].

13.5.1 Indications

Fiberoptic intubation can be performed on any patient who fits the intubation requirements. However, most doctors save fiberoptic intubation for patients with a challenging airway due to the specialized equipment required. The following conditions and patient types are more likely to have an unstable airway [27–30]:

- Micrognathia
- Mandibular fracture
- Partially obstructing laryngeal lesions such as papilloma or supraglottis
- A necessity for awake intubation
- Cervical spine injuries or cervical instability
- Rheumatoid arthritis (or patients unable to extend the neck)
- A history of head and neck radiation
- Trismus
- Craniofacial abnormalities

In January 2019, recommendations for intubation and extubation in the intensive care unit (ICU) were issued by the French Society of Anesthesia and Intensive Care Medicine (SFAR) and the French-Speaking Intensive Care Society (SRLF) [31].

For tracheal intubation guidance in patients with COVID-19, video laryngoscopy has been argued to be better than direct laryngoscopy [32, 33].

13.5.2 Contraindications

Airway (Cancer) (Highly Obstructive Pulmonary Disease (HNPPD) is a disease in which the lungs become obstructed with cancerous tissue). Patients with laryngeal trauma, especially those with a possible cricotracheal separation, are likewise advised against using it. In patients with craniofacial trauma actively bleeding into the oropharynx, fiberoptic intubation is relatively contraindicated and may be dangerous [20].

13.5.3 Outcomes

Blair et al. used medium-fidelity human simulators to simulate challenging airway scenarios (cervical spine immobilization and trismus) and found that video laryngoscopy significantly improved glottic exposure compared with direct laryngoscopy (97% Cormack-Lehane grade I or II vs. 51%) [34].

Lewis et al. conducted a Cochrane review comparing video laryngoscopy and direct laryngoscopy for adult tracheal intubation. They found that video laryngoscopy has several advantages over direct laryngoscopy, including a better glottic view and a decreased risk of laryngeal/airway trauma, especially in patients with a difficult airway [35]. Lowering the incidence of complication during a video bronchoscopy (bronchoscopy) (20%) and lowering the incidence of complication during a video bronchoscopy (20%).

Another Cochrane review comparing the two methods in children (excluding neonates) found that intubation took longer and intubation failure was more common when using video laryngoscopy compared to direct laryngoscopy. However, the quality of the evidence could have been better [36]. No firm conclusions could be drawn regarding the deleterious hemodynamic responses and other adverse effects of intubation in this cohort or whether video laryngoscopy may lead to an enhanced view of the vocal cords [20].

Video laryngoscopy did not improve intubation success rates over direct laryngoscopy in emergency and critically ill patients, according to a comprehensive study and meta-analysis by Jiang et al. [37]

13.5.4 Equipment

Equipment required for video laryngoscopy includes the following [20]:

- Fiberoptic bronchoscope with a light source
- Camera with the monitor if intubation is to be projected to the screen
- Lidocaine 4%
- Nasal trumpets, 28 and 36 French
- Glycopyrrolate 0.2 mg (to be administered intravenously (IV) before the start of the procedure)
- Endotracheal (ET) tubes (see Treatment for additional information)
- Warmed saline
- Syringe, 12 mL
- Oral airway
- Carbon dioxide detector
- Antifog solution or an alcohol pad
- Suction tubing
- Oxygen with cannula

13.5.5 Approach Considerations

Choosing the right endotracheal (ET) tube is crucial. The tube must snugly fit over the fiber optic scope. The ET tube's internal diameter should be 3 mm more significant than the scope's [38]. A significant distance between the scope and the tube can make threading the tube over the fiberoptic shaft difficult and increase the risk of the tube being entangled in the laryngeal tissues [38]. It is crucial to utilize an ET tube that is small enough to fit through the patient's nasal cavity if nasal intubation is to be conducted. A tube size of 7.0 or smaller is recommended for big males. When the patient is awake during intubation, the most painful part of the process is moving the tube through the nasal channel; therefore, getting the size right is crucial [20].

Fiberoptic intubation can be performed with the help of specialized ET tubes. Standard nasal anatomy is accommodated with a prefabricated Ring–Adair–Elwyn (RAE) tube (Covidien-Nellcor, Boulder, CO). To prevent damaging the fiberoptic channels of the bronchoscope, it is recommended to soak the nasal RAE tube in warm saline for 5 min before intubation [20].

Intubation with a Flexi-Tip tube is another option. This tube makes intubation and insertion of a bronchoscope into the airway much more straightforward than with a traditional line. The arytenoid cartilage is less likely to become trapped on the flexible tip, which points toward the lumen's center [39]. If the bronchoscope's tip mists over, touching the patient's mucosal surface will clear it immediately. To clean the tip, you could also ask the patient to swallow [20].

If the surgery needs to be done while the patient is awake, a thorough explanation of what will happen and why is essential for the patient's cooperation.

The arytenoids are a potential snare for the ET tube if the fiberoptic scope has difficulty passing through the vocal folds and into the airway. Repeat steps 20 and 21 with the ET tube retracted 1–2 cm and rotated 90 or 180°.

To facilitate movement, the bronchoscope should be held taut at all times by the bronchoscopist.

The larynx can be better seen if the patient moves their head or jaw forward [20].

References

1. Mitchell C. Endoscopic examination of the upper respiratory tract. In: Costa LRR, Paradis MR, editors. Manual of clinical procedures in the horse. Wiley; 2017. p. 210–5. https://doi.org/10.1002/9781118939956.ch20.
2. Jacobson AS. Urken ML, Teng MS. ACS surgery: principles and practice. Head and neck diagnostic procedures. Medscape. https://www.medscape.com/viewarticle/521712_7. Accessed 3 June 2023.
3. Mallen JR. Nasal endoscopy. In: Meyers AD, editor. Medscape. 2021. https://emedicine.medscape.com/article/1890999-overview. Accessed 3 June 2023.
4. Stammberger H. Functional endoscopic sinus surgery. Philadelphia: BC Decker; 1991.
5. Kennedy DW, Zinreich SJ, Rosenbaum AE, Johns ME. Functional endoscopic sinus surgery. Theory and diagnostic evaluation. Arch Otolaryngol. 1985;111(9):576–82.
6. Levine HL. The office diagnosis of nasal and sinus disorders using rigid nasal endoscopy. Otolaryngol Head Neck Surg. 1990;102(4):370–3.

7. Lanza DC. Diagnosis of chronic rhinosinusitis. Ann Otol Rhinol Laryngol Suppl. 2004;193:10–4.
8. Lund VJ, Kennedy DW. Quantification for staging sinusitis. The Staging And Therapy Group. Ann Otol Rhinol Laryngol Suppl. 1995;167:17–21.
9. Annamalai S, Davis J, Kubba H. How subjective is nasal endoscopy? A study of interrater agreement using the Lund and Mackay scoring system. Am J Rhinol. 2004;18(5):301–3.
10. Kuhn FA. Role of endoscopy in the management of chronic rhinosinusitis. Ann Otol Rhinol Laryngol Suppl. 2004;193:15–8.
11. Bhattacharyya N, Lee LN. Evaluating the diagnosis of chronic rhinosinusitis based on clinical guidelines and endoscopy. Otolaryngol Head Neck Surg. 2010;143(1):147–51.
12. Shargorodsky J, Bhattacharyya N. What is the role of nasal endoscopy in the diagnosis of chronic rhinosinusitis? Laryngoscope. 2013;123(1):4–6.
13. Ferguson BJ, Narita M, Yu VL, Wagener MM, Gwaltney JM Jr. Prospective observational study of chronic rhinosinusitis: environmental triggers and antibiotic implications. Clin Infect Dis. 2012;54(1):62–8.
14. Kupferberg SB, Bent JP 3rd, Kuhn FA. Prognosis for allergic fungal sinusitis. Otolaryngol Head Neck Surg. 1997;117(1):35–41.
15. Vogan JC, Bolger WE, Keyes AS. Endoscopically guided sinonasal cultures: a direct comparison with maxillary sinus aspirate cultures. Otolaryngol Head Neck Surg. 2000;122(3):370–3.
16. Benninger MS, Payne SC, Ferguson BJ, Hadley JA, Ahmad N. Endoscopically directed middle meatal cultures versus maxillary sinus taps in acute bacterial maxillary rhinosinusitis: a meta-analysis. Otolaryngol Head Neck Surg. 2006;134(1):3–9.
17. Nadel DM, Lanza DC, Kennedy DW. Endoscopically guided cultures in chronic sinusitis. Am J Rhinol. 1998;12(4):233–41.
18. Bolger WE, Kennedy DW. Nasal endoscopy in the outpatient clinic. Otolaryngol Clin N Am. 1992;25(4):791–802.
19. Lanza DC, Kennedy DW. Current concepts in the surgical management of nasal polyposis. J Allergy Clin Immunol. 1992;90(3 Pt 2):543–5; discussion 546.
20. Verma SP. Video laryngoscopy and fiberoptic-assisted tracheal intubation technique. In: Mosenifar Z, editor. Medscape. 2023. https://emedicine.medscape.com/article/110880-technique. Accessed 3 June 2023.
21. Pott LM, Murray WB. Review of video laryngoscopy and rigid fiberoptic laryngoscopy. Curr Opin Anaesthesiol. 2008;21(6):750–8.
22. Liao CC, Liu FC, Li AH, Yu HP. Video laryngoscopy-assisted tracheal intubation in airway management. Expert Rev Med Devices. 2018;15(4):265–75.
23. Howard-Quijano KJ, Huang YM, Matevosian R, Kaplan MB, Steadman RH. Video-assisted instruction improves the success rate for tracheal intubation by novices. Br J Anaesth. 2008;101(4):568–72.
24. Sowers N, Kovacs G. Use of a flexible intubating scope in combination with a channeled video laryngoscope for managing a difficult airway in the emergency department. J Emerg Med. 2016;50(2):315–9.
25. Rai MR, Dering A, Verghese C. The Glidescope system: a clinical assessment of performance. Anaesthesia. 2005;60(1):60–4.
26. Serocki G, Bein B, Scholz J, Dörges V. Management of the predicted difficult airway: a comparison of conventional blade laryngoscopy with video-assisted blade laryngoscopy and the GlideScope. Eur J Anaesthesiol. 2010;27(1):24–30.
27. Klock PA Jr. Airway assessment and prediction of the difficult airway. In: Hagberg CA, Artime CA, Aziz MF, editors. Hagberg and Benumof's airway management. 5th ed. Philadelphia: Elsevier; 2023. p. 195–207.
28. Green-Hopkins I, Werner H, Monuteaux MC, Nagler J. Using video-recorded laryngoscopy to evaluate laryngoscopic blade approach and adverse events in children. Acad Emerg Med. 2015;22(11):1283–9.
29. Sarkılar G, Sargın M, Sarıtaş TB, Borazan H, Gök F, Kılıçaslan A, et al. Hemodynamic responses to endotracheal intubation performed with video and direct laryngoscopy in patients scheduled for major cardiac surgery. Int J Clin Exp Med. 2015;8(7):11477–83.

30. Brown CA 3rd, Bair AE, Pallin DJ, Laurin EG, Walls RM. National Emergency Airway Registry (NEAR) investigators. Improved glottic exposure with the video Macintosh laryngoscope in adult emergency department tracheal intubations. Ann Emerg Med. 2010;56(2):83–8.
31. (Guideline) Quintard H, l'Her E, Pottecher J, Adnet F, Constantin JM, De Jong A, et al. Experts' guidelines of intubation and extubation of the ICU patient of French Society of Anaesthesia and Intensive Care Medicine (SFAR) and French-speaking Intensive Care Society (SRLF): in collaboration with the pediatric Association of French-speaking Anaesthetists and Intensivists (ADARPEF), French-speaking Group of Intensive Care and Paediatric emergencies (GFRUP) and Intensive Care physiotherapy society (SKR). Ann Intensive Care. 2019;9(1):13.
32. De Jong A, Pardo E, Rolle A, Bodin-Lario S, Pouzeratte Y, Jaber S. Airway management for COVID-19: a move towards universal videolaryngoscope? Lancet Respir Med. 2020;8(6):555.
33. Gómez-Ríos MÁ, Casans-Francés R, Abad-Gurumeta A, Esquinas A. The role of videolaryngoscopy in airway management of COVID-19 patients. Anaesthesiol Intensive Ther. 2020;52(4):344–5.
34. Bair AE, Olmsted K, Brown CA 3rd, Barker T, Pallin D, Walls RM. Assessment of the Storz video Macintosh laryngoscope for use in difficult airways: a human simulator study. Acad Emerg Med. 2010;17(10):1134–7.
35. Lewis SR, Butler AR, Parker J, Cook TM, Smith AF. Videolaryngoscopy versus direct laryngoscopy for adult patients requiring tracheal intubation. Cochrane Database Syst Rev. 2016;11:CD011136.
36. Abdelgadir IS, Phillips RS, Singh D, Moncreiff MP, Lumsden JL. Videolaryngoscopy versus direct laryngoscopy for tracheal intubation in children (excluding neonates). Cochrane Database Syst Rev. 2017;5:CD011413.
37. Jiang J, Ma D, Li B, Yue Y, Xue F. Video laryngoscopy does not improve the intubation outcomes in emergency and critical patients—a systematic review and meta-analysis of randomized controlled trials. Crit Care. 2017;21(1):288.
38. Ovassapian A. The flexible bronchoscope. A tool for anesthesiologists. Clin Chest Med. 2001;22(2):281–99.
39. Kristensen MS. The Parker flex-tip tube versus a standard tube for fiberoptic orotracheal intubation: a randomized double-blind study. Anesthesiology. 2003;98(2):354–8.

14 Upper Airway Evaluation: Diagnostic Clues from Upper Respiratory Tract

Sedef Narin Tongal, Adaeze Ayuk, and Hasan Yüksel

14.1 Upper Airways

Flexible bronchoscopy is frequently used for anatomical and functional evaluation of the upper and lower airways in childhood. The upper airway starts from the nasal cavity and continues to the extrathoracic part of the pharynx, larynx, and trachea.

1. Flexible airway endoscopy provides insight into the causes and appearance of **congenital and acquired anomalies** of the nasal cavity, pharynx, and larynx.
   (a) The nasopharyngeal region: Choanal stenosis and atresia, nasal masses, craniofacial abnormalities, adenotonsillar hypertrophy, and base of tongue lesions can be investigated using bronchoscopy.
   (b) The laryngeal region: Laryngomalacia, subglottic stenosis, subglottic edema, vocal cord paralysis, hemangioma, cyst, papillomatosis, web, cleft and vocal cord dysfunction, and upper respiratory tract disease associated with gastroesophageal reflux can be evaluated.

   In children, the airway diameter is narrower and the subglottic region is the narrowest. In addition, the larynx is softer and the epiglottis is omega-shaped in children. Flexible airway endoscopy provides insight into pathologies of the upper airways that lead to **airway obstruction**, although rare in newborns and early infancy and more common in older children. Obstruction can lead to the collapse of the extrathoracic airways. Early diagnosis and treatment is imperative as there is associated morbidity and mortality.

S. N. Tongal · H. Yüksel (✉)
Department of Pediatric Pulmonology, Manisa Celal Bayar School of Medicine, Manisa, Turkey

A. Ayuk
Department of Pediatrics, College of Medicine, University of Nigeria – Enugu Campus/University of Nigeria Teaching Hospital, Enugu, Nigeria

H. Yüksel et al. (eds.), *Pediatric Airway Diseases*, Comprehensive ENT,
https://doi.org/10.1007/978-3-031-74853-0_14

Bronchoscopic appearance of the upper airway: For ease of visualization of the upper airway, a face mask is used with sedation and flexible bronchoscopy is performed through the nose and advanced along the middle or lower meatus. If the patient is intubated under anesthesia or a laryngeal mask is applied during the bronchoscopy procedure, examination of the upper airway may not be possible. Using the facemask method, with the patient lying on his/her back, the base of the nose is observed above and the roof of the nose below. İn a normal anatomy, the turbinate should appear smooth and clean. No pathologies like polyps or purulent secretions should be seen obstructing the course of the bronchoscope. The upper turbinate is rarely seen in this procedure. In the presence of a deviated septum, the bronchoscope can be passed more easily from one side than the other. The opening of the Eustachian tube can be seen on the lateral wall of the nasopharynx in older children. Adenoidal tissue in the posterior part of the nasopharynx can also be seen, especially in preschool children while tonsillar tissue is best evaluated in oral procedures. The epiglottis and laryngeal opening should also be seen clearly.

Bronchoscopic appearance of the larynx: The larynx is best examined under light anesthesia with spontaneous breathing. Anatomically, there are marked differences between the larynx of children and adults. In young children, it is located anteriorly and superiorly, whereas it becomes more centralized and inferiorly positioned with increasing age. The larynx is also smaller and the lower end of the cricoid cartilage is at the middle level of C5 in the newborn and in the shape of a cone, while in adults it is at the lower level of C6.

During bronchoscopy, the vocal cords should move equally and converge centrally. The arytenoids are usually more mobile in infancy and their prolapse toward the laryngeal inlet may be normal in the early infancy period. If there is evidence of obstruction, surgical intervention should be considered. In the child, the cuneiform and corniculate cartilages may not be distinguished as separate structures. A cleft if present, may be visualized in the posterior laryngeal wall. Because it may be difficult to see this area with a flexible bronchoscope, it is technically more successful in visualizing anterior structures [1–3].

14.2 Indıcatıons for Upper Aırway Imagıng

14.2.1 Pathologıes of Upper Airway wıth Noisy Breathing

Diagnostic airway endoscopy is used in children with symptoms such as nasal congestion, sleeping with an open mouth, snoring, stridor, and hoarseness, who hitherto had not responded to medical treatment or have had an atypical course. Although it may sometimes be difficult to decide very young infants, evaluation of the airway should be performed without delay in children with persistent or recurrent stridor, especially if there are accompanying findings such as hoarseness, apnea, feeding difficulties, or growth retardation.

When children present with stridor, endoscopic examination can be performed, looking out for laryngomalacia and further excluding other possible differentials. For most procedures, the flexible endoscope is passed through the nose and this gives the opportunity for the upper airways to be examined in detail as the pharynx and larynx can be well observed with the head and neck in the neutral position.

Depending on the indication, in some cases where examination under anesthesia is planned for the upper airway, evaluation of the lower airway may also be required . Upper airway lesions may frequently coexist with lower airway lesions.

VCD can present with inspiratory sounds (stridor) and in children with suspected vocal cord dysfunction (VCD), the diagnosis is made by visualization of paradoxical narrowing of the anterior portion of the vocal cords during inspiration.

Upper airway endoscopy is also useful for the evaluation of patients with postextubation stridor. While reintubation may be required immediately in some patients. The development of scar tissues on extubation following prolonged intubation takes a longer time to develop; thus, initial endoscopic findings may be normal and reevaluation should be kept in view [4–10].

14.2.2 Nasopharyngeal-Related Pathologies (Congenital and Acquired)

Many of these disease entities may present as dysmorphic syndromes with attendant craniofacial abnormalities and associated mandibular or maxillary hypoplasia. In such patients, it may be difficult to provide airway stability due to concomitant micrognathia, glossoptosis, adenotonsillar hypertrophy, cleft palate, midface hypoplasia, or a narrowed nasopharynx associated with tongue hypertrophy [11].

(a) **Choanal Atresia:** This is the most common congenital anomaly of the nose. Coanal atresia is frequently associated with other anomalies, the association with CHARGE syndrome being the most common and serious [11, 12]. Unilateral atresia is more common and may not be detected until later in childhood. However, when bilateral, it can cause severe airway obstruction. The diagnosis can be confirmed using flexible endoscopy. Computed tomography CT scan of the head is usually necessary to determine the exact location of the obstruction and whether the defect is bony or membranous.

(b) **Congenital Masses of the Nasal Region:** These are rare, cystic structures or sometimes more solid masses such as hemangiomas, neurofibromas, and gliomas. Solid masses may be associated with midline defects such as cleft palate. If a polyp is visualized in a newborn, differentials to be considered include encephalocele or glioma until the definitive diagnosis is made [11, 13].

(c) **Adenotonsillar Hypertrophy:** This is a common cause of obstructive sleep apnea in children and may worsen airway obstruction in patients with pharyngeal collapse.

(d) **Cysts or mass lesions arising from the dorsal surface of the tongue** are rare and can cause significant airway obstruction, often with feeding difficulties [11].

14.2.3 Laryngeal Pathologies

(a) **Laryngomalacia:** This is the most common congenital laryngeal anomaly. It is uncertain if laryngomalacia develops due to an anatomical problem or delayed neuromuscular development. It is usually defined by the onset of inspiratory stridor in the first 4–6 weeks of life. Stridor increases during crying, agitation, feeding, and respiratory tract infections. Stridor tends to improve as the child grows. Surgical treatment is rarely required. It is frequently associated with other airway problems and gastroesophageal reflux [14, 15] (Fig. 14.1).

(b) **Subglotic Stenosis:** Membranous bilateral symmetrical stenosis may develop with the thickening of the soft tissues in the **subglottic area**, resembling the appearance of acute subglottic edema. Cartilaginous subglottic stenosis is due to malformation of the cricoid cartilage and causes variable stenosis that is not symmetrical in appearance. Children with subglottic stenosis may present with different clinical findings depending on the grade ranging from severe respiratory distress in the neonatal period to the development of inspiratory or biphasic stridor within the first few months of life. Thus the signs and symptoms depend on the severity of the stenosis; Myer et al. proposed a grading of the proportion of stenosis, (I to IV); with grade 1 having up to 50% obstruction of the lumen, grade 2 having 51–70% obstruction, grade 3 having more than 71% obstruction of the lumen, and grade 4 having no detectable lumen. Cases in which stenosis develops due to airway trauma caused by prolonged intubation and tracheostomy are more common than congenital ones [14, 16, 17] (Fig. 14.2).

(c) **Subglottic Edema:** This can be caused by infection, allergy, or trauma. Endoscopically, the subglottic area is symmetrically narrowed, often with supraglottic edema. It is the most common complication of rigid bronchoscopy.

(d) **Vocal Cord Paralysis and Dysfunction:** If due to traumatic causes are usually unilateral and especially affect the left side and can be visualized as the absence

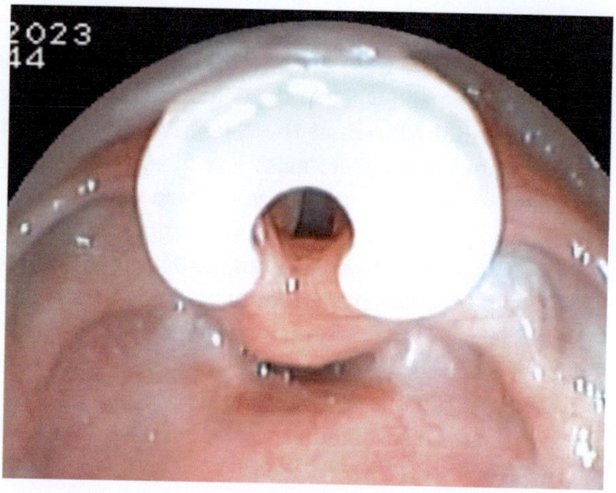

Fig. 14.1 Laryngomalacia

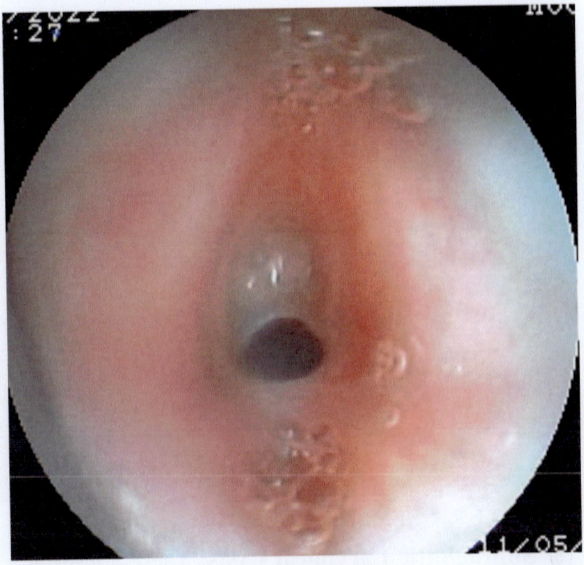

Fig. 14.2 Subglottic stenosis

of movement on the affected side. Unilateral vocal cord paralysis is difficult to diagnose. Bilateral paralysis may be due to a severe central nervous system malformation such as Arnold-Chiari malformation. In the more common abductor paralysis (closed appearance of the glottis), bilateral paralysis may present with stridor, hoarseness, and respiratory distress, whereas unilateral paralysis may be asymptomatic. Aphonia and aspiration may develop in the rarer adductor paralysis (open glottis). For optimal diagnostic evaluation, the movement of the vocal cords and arytenoids should not be evaluated under general anesthesia, but rather imaging while the patient is awake or under mild sedation/reawakening from anesthesia as it wears off [18]. Vocal cord dysfunction is characterized by paradoxical closure of the vocal cord during inspiration or during both inspiration and expiration. The resulting symptoms and signs include sudden onset of dyspnea, wheezing, inspiratory or biphasic stridor, and cough; with these findings, they can often be misdiagnosed as asthma. The diagnosis is usually difficult; it can be confirmed by laryngoscopy performed without sedation, and it is seen that the anterior part of the vocal cords is closed, leaving a narrow gap [19, 20].

(e) **Hemangiomas** are among the most common laryngeal masses seen in infancy. Infants may present with mild to moderate stridor or with sudden (biphasic) stridor and recurrent or atypical croup. They are more commonly found in the subglottic area and more rarely in the supraglottic area as an asymmetric mass. Subglottic hemangiomas are usually unilateral. Endoscopic diagnosis may be difficult because they may have a normal epithelial appearance. Cutaneous hemangiomas may also be seen simultaneously in some infants. These hemangiomas usually grow rapidly until about 6–10 months and then usually start to shrink at around 1.5 years of age [21] (Fig. 14.3).

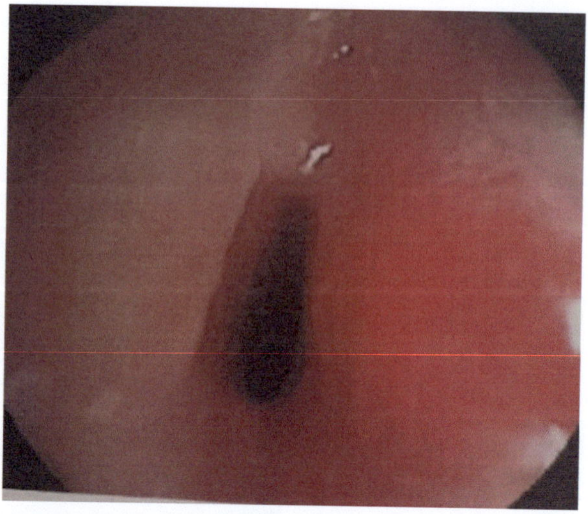

Fig. 14.3 Hemangioma

(f) **Supraglottic Laryngeal Cysts:** These are usually located in the aryepiglottic fold or epiglottis and are often congenital. They develop as a result of iatrogenic trauma such as intubation. Diagnosis is easy if the cysts are covered with thin mucosa, while others appear as a submucosal mass. Infants usually present with stridor, hoarseness, or aphonia and sometimes feeding difficulties [14].

(g) **Laryngeal Papillomatosis:** Although rare, it is the most common benign neoplasm of the larynx after infancy. It is caused by human papillomavirus types 6 and 11. It may regress spontaneously or may show a tendency to recur and spread all over the airways and lungs. The vocal cord is the most common site of lesions and they are typically multiple, irregular, and fragile masses. They usually present with hoarseness and stridor, less frequently with cough or respiratory distress [22].

(h) **Laryngeal Web (Vocal Folds):** They are usually seen at the level of the glottis, but may also be present in the supraglottic and subglottic regions. Webs can be classified as complete or incomplete. The presentation may vary from hoarseness and aphonia to (biphasic) stridor and respiratory distress [14] (Fig. 14.4).

(i) **Congenital Posterior Laryngeal Cleft:** This is a rare condition that develops between the larynx and hypopharynx; and in severe cases, it may extend inferior to the trachea. It may be associated with other anomalies of the trachea or esophagus and other congenital anomalies. It can be classified as type 1 supraglottic interarytenoid cleft not extending below the level of the vocal cord, type 2 cleft extending below the level of the vocal cord (partial involvement of the cricoid cartilage), type 3 cleft along the cricoid cartilage with or without extension into the cervical trachea, type 4 cleft extending into the thoracic trachea (may extend to the carina). Aspiration, cyanosis, and cough may occur with feeding. First suspicion is required for diagnosis. Rigid rather than flexible bronchoscopy is more ideal for detecting cleft. Bifid epiglottis and anterior cleft of the larynx are very rare; while bifid epiglottis is usually associated with other anomalies, anterior cleft may be found as an isolated defect [14, 23, 24] (Fig. 14.5).

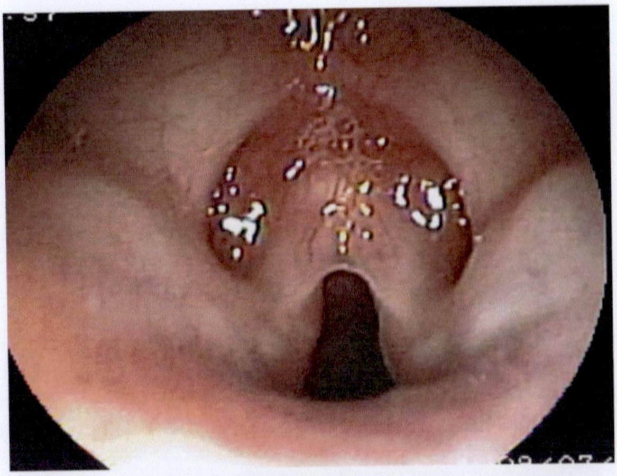

Fig. 14.4 Anterior laryngeal web

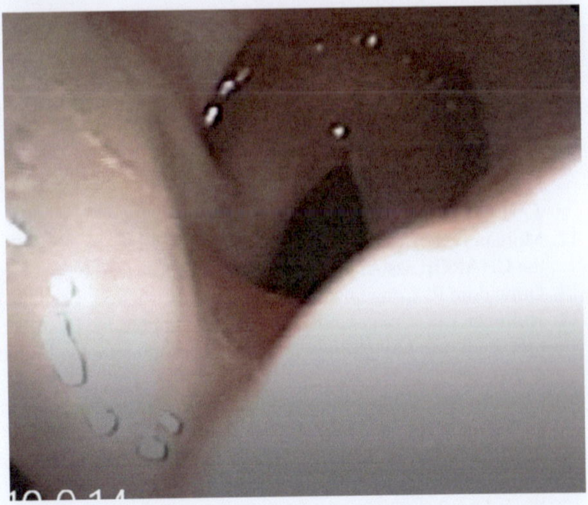

Fig. 14.5 Type 1 laryngeal cleft

(j) **Gastroesophageal Reflux Disease:** Though not an anatomical structural defect has been associated with many respiratory symptoms in infants and children, including hoarseness, chronic cough, stridor, and wheezing, and with chronic sinusitis, otitis media, chronic laryngitis, recurrent croup, and laryngomalacia. Endoscopic findings that may reveal granular changes in the epiglottis, erythema, and edema in the mucosa covering the arytenoid cartilage and posterior wall of the glottis (posterior laryngitis), vocal cord nodules, ulcers and granulation tissue, and rarely subglottic stenosis [25, 26].

In conclusion, endoscopy can be used to examine only the upper airway, but since upper and lower airway lesions can frequently be seen together, it should be preferred to visualize both upper and lower airways in the same procedure unless there is an exceptional situation for the child.

References

1. Adewale L. Anatomy and assessment of the pediatric airway. Paediatr Anaesth. 2009;19(suppl 1):1–8.
2. Dalal PG, Murray D, Messner AH, Feng A, McAllister J, Molter D. Pediatric laryngeal dimensions: an age-based analysis. Anesth Analg. 2009;108:1475–9.
3. Park S, Shin SW, Kim HJ, Byeon GJ, Yoon JU, Kim EJ, Kim HY. Choice of the correct size of endotracheal tube in pediatric patients. Anesth Pain Med (Seoul). 2022;17(4):352–60.
4. Wood RE. Spelunking in the pediatric airways: explorations with the flexible fiberoptic bronchoscope. Pediatr Clin N Am. 1984;31:785–99.
5. Midulla F, de Blic J, Barbato A, Bush A, Eber E, Kotecha S, Haxby E, Moretti C, Pohunek P, Ratjen F. Flexible endoscopy of paediatric airways. Eur Respir J. 2003;22:698–708.
6. Eber E, Zach M. Flexible fiberoptic endoscopy in children with upper airway obstruction. Monatsschr Kinderheilkd. 1996;144:43–7.
7. Zoumalan R, Maddalozzo J, Holinger LD. Etiology of stridor in infants. Ann Otol Rhinol Laryngol. 2007;116:329–34.
8. Gonzalez C, Reilly JS, Bluestone CD. Synchronous airway lesions in infancy. Ann Otol Rhinol Laryngol. 1987;96:77–80.
9. Masters IB, Chang AB, Patterson L, Wainwright C, Buntain H, Dean BW, Francis PW. Series of laryngomalacia, tracheomalacia, and bronchomalacia disorders and their associations with other conditions in children. Pediatr Pulmonol. 2002;34:189–95.
10. Chun R, Preciado DA, Zalzal GH, Shah RK. Utility of bronchoscopy for recurrent croup. Ann Otol Rhinol Laryngol. 2009;118:495–9.
11. Lusk RP. Nasal and pharyngeal lesions. In: Holinger LD, Lusk RP, Greene CG, editors. Pediatric laryngology and bronchoesophagology. Philadelphia: Lippincott-Raven; 1997. p. 117–35.
12. Morgan D, Bailey M, Phelps P, Bellman S, Grace A, Wyse R. Ear-nose-throat abnormalities in the CHARGE association. Arch Otolaryngol Head Neck Surg. 1993;119:49–54.
13. Dinwiddie R. Congenital upper airway obstruction. Paediatr Respir Rev. 2004;5:17–24.
14. Holinger LD. Congenital laryngeal anomalies. In: Holinger LD, Lusk RP, Greene CG, editors. Pediatric laryngology and bronchoesophagology. Philadelphia: Lippincott-Raven; 1997. p. 137–64.
15. Chandra RK, Gerber ME, Holinger LD. Histological insight into the pathogenesis of severe laryngomalacia. Int J Pediatr Otorhinolaryngol. 2001;61:31–8.
16. Schroeder JW Jr, Holinger LD. Congenital laryngeal stenosis. Otolaryngol Clin N Am. 2008;41:865–75.
17. Myer CM 3rd, O'Connor DM, Cotton RT. Proposed grading system for subglottic stenosis based on endotracheal tube sizes. Ann Otol Rhinol Laryngol. 1994;103:319–23.
18. Holinger PC, Holinger LD, Reichert TJ, Holinger PH. Respiratory obstruction and apnea in infants with bilateral abductor vocal cord paralysis, meningomyelocele, hydrocephalus, and Arnold-Chiari malformation. J Pediatr. 1978;92:368–73.
19. Noyes BE, Kemp JS. Vocal cord dysfunction in children. Paediatr Respir Rev. 2007;8:155–63.
20. King CS, Moores LK. Clinical asthma syndromes and important asthma mimics. Respir Care. 2008;53:568–80.
21. Rahbar R, Nicollas R, Roger G, Triglia J-M, Garabedian E-N, McGill TJ, Healy GB. The biology and management of subglottic hemangioma: past, present, future. Laryngoscope. 2004;114:1880–91.
22. Derkay CS, Wiatrak B. Recurrent respiratory papillomatosis: a review. Laryngoscope. 2008;118(7):1236–47.
23. Pezzettigotta SM, Leboulanger N, Roger G, Denoyelle F, Garabédian EN. Laryngeal cleft. Otolaryngol Clin N Am. 2008;41:913–33.
24. Benjamin B, Inglis A. Minor congenital laryngeal clefts: diagnosis and classification. Ann Otol Rhinol Laryngol. 1989;98:417–20.

25. Yellon RF, Goldberg H. Update on gastroesophageal reflux disease in pediatric airway disorders. Am J Med. 2001;111(suppl 8A):78S–84S.
26. Hoa M, Kingsley EL, Coticchia JM. Correlating the clinical course of recurrent croup with endoscopic findings: a retrospective observational study. Ann Otol Rhinol Laryngol. 2008;117:464–9.

Preschool Lung Function Testing and the Upper Respiratory Tract

15

Seda Tunca, Özge Yilmaz, and Enrico Lombardi

Abbreviations

GLI Global Lung Function Initiative
FOT Forced Oscillation Technique
FRC Functional residual capacity
Raw Resistance airway
RV Residual volüme
TLC Total lung capacity

15.1 Introduction

The essential anatomical and functional differences between the pediatric and adult airways contribute to understanding the various respiratory symptoms and the differences during disease. Knowing the essential features of pediatric airways is helpful in the prevention, management, and treatment of acute and chronic diseases of the respiratory tract. The developmental changes in the structure of respiratory tracts during childhood should also be paid attention to. The age-related variations should be taken into consideration in the evaluation of airway function in the light of united airway theory, and a combined evaluation should be performed considering anatomical, physiological, and chemical differences.

S. Tunca · Ö. Yilmaz (✉)
Department of Pediatric Allergy, School of Medicine, Manisa Celal Bayar University, Manisa, Türkiye

E. Lombardi
Pediatric Pulmonary Unit, Meyer Children's Hospital, Florence, Italy
e-mail: e.lombardi@meyer.it

H. Yüksel et al. (eds.), *Pediatric Airway Diseases*, Comprehensive ENT,
https://doi.org/10.1007/978-3-031-74853-0_15

Upper airways have a changing and developing structure with age, particularly in the preschool period and in younger children. Children have a relatively smaller oral cavity and larger tongue in the upper airway in comparisonto adults. This condition should be emphasized as an indicator of the fact that obstruction risk is higher and nasal obstruction may lead to more serious consequences in children. Epiglottis is longer and weaker, it may easily cause obstruction if it is edematous. Tonsil and adenoid tissues rapidly grow in childhood and may cause serious obstructions in case of infections resulting in edema. Since the larynx and glottis are located in the upper aspect of the neck in children, aspiration risk in children is higher than in adults. Similar differences between children and adults also apply to lower airways. Therefore, it is of utmost importance to take all these differences into consideration when measuring airway function in children and prefer the most appropriate airway measurement technique for the selected age group with respect to diagnosis and treatment.

The lower respiratory tract in children has many differences compared to adults. Since the wall thickness of the bronchi is thinner, it may cause easy collapse of the lumen during inspiration. On the other hand, the length of the trachea is shorter in children than in adults, which facilitates the access of inflammation to the lower airways. Abdominal breathing is predominant in children, especially in the newborn and early childhood, due to the weak intercostal muscles and the fact that the cartilaginous part of the thorax is more than the bony part. In addition, a significant increase in the number of alveoli is observed from newborn to adulthood until the age of eight to ten. Especially in newborns and early childhood, abdominal breathing is at the forefront in children due to the weak intercostal muscles and the fact that the cartilage part of the thorax is more than the bone part. There is also a marked increase in the number of alveoli from the newborn to adulthood, up to 8–10 years of age. After this age, a decrease in number is observed, while structural development comes to the fore. Lung surface area also increases from childhood to adulthood. All these differences show that the tests related to the lower airway in children should be evaluated by considering the appropriate percentile range and anatomical and physiological differences in the evaluation stages.

15.2 Airway Measurements

Since respiratory system diseases may progress with a high-risk clinical course for mortality and morbidity, respiratory function tests have an important role in diagnosis and follow-up. The evaluation of lung function is more difficult in infants and preschoolers compared with older children. Because of the lack of cooperation during measurements, several conditions such as lying during natural sleep or under sedation can be used in infants, while this is not feasible in preschool children.

In children aged over 5 years and adults, spirometry is the gold standard technique in the measurement of lung function [1]. However, spirometry cannot be performed very often by the younger age group, because of collaboration issues. On the other side, body plethysmography is the gold standard method in the determination of airway resistance and lung volumes [2]. Airway resistance is determined by lung volume and is expected to decrease as lung volume increases [3, 4]. Body plethysmography is performed by closing the patient into a cabin and asking the patient to perform respiratory maneuvers. Young children may experience difficulties in performing these maneuvers. Therefore, body plethysmography is preferably performed in older age groups for accurate diagnosis and treatment approach. Other techniques, like respiratory oscillometry and the interrupter technique, that only require tidal breathing and minimal collaboration from the subject, have proved to be more suitable for measuring airway resistance in preschool children [5]. Differently from the interrupter technique, oscillometry can also differentiate the upper airway component of respiratory impedance and give information about reactance, which can be interpreted as compliance (or distensibility) of the respiratory system (Table 15.1).

Table 15.1 Tests used in the evaluation of the lower airway

Test applied	Area of use	Measurements
Spirometry	Used to measure lung function in children over 6 years of age and adults	The relationship between volume and time and the relationship between flow and volume are shown
Pletismography	Used to determine airway resistance (raw) and lung volumes	Residual volume (RV), total lung capacity (TLC), and functional residual capacity (FRC) allow the measurement of all static and dynamic lung volumes
Airway occlusion techniques	In cases such as occlusion of the airways at the end of inspiration or expiration, it is used in the evaluation of passive respiratory system mechanics (respiratory system compliance, resistance)	The airflow interrupter technique (Rint) is a simple method of measuring airway resistance
Multiple breath helium dilution	It is an easily applicable method used for the determination of lung volumes, mostly FRC, during tidal breathing	Used for the determination of FRC (functional residual capacity)
Multiple breath wash test	Detection of ventilation disorders in small peripheral airways and early detection of lung disease in children with or without minimal clinical symptoms	Residual volume (RV), total lung capacity (TLC), and functional residual capacity (FRC) are determined
Forced oscillation technique	The forced oscillation technique (FOT) is a simple and noninvasive method that utilizes external sound/pressure waves generated by a loudspeaker	It enables the evaluation of the mechanical properties of the lung by measuring the change in pressure and flow
Impulse oscillometry	It is a type of forced oscillation technique. More detailed analyses of respiratory function are provided with square pressure waves generated regularly five times per second	Impedance (Z), resistance (R), reactance (X), resonance frequency (Fres), and reactance area (AX) can be measured with IOS. These values are measured and named at specific frequencies (5–35 Hz)

15.3 The Most Appropriate Lung Function Technique in Preschoolers

The answer to this question always depends on the clinical/research issue we are facing [6]. Oscillometry, also called Forced Oscillation Technique (FOT), is evaluated as one of the most suitable techniques regarding applicability in preschool children [5]. This technique requires no challenging expiration maneuvers and is diagnostically very precious when the difficulty in the clinical evaluation of lower airways increases as age decreases [7]. In the application of oscillometry, sound waves produced using a loudspeaker and transmitted to the lung cause changes in pressure and these changes result in differences in airflow. The measurement of these changes in pressure and airflow allows the determination of the mechanical properties of the lung by giving an estimate of respiratory impedance (Zrs), which includes resistance (Rrs, frictional losses of the respiratory system) and reactance (Xrs, elastic properties of the respiratory system at low frequencies and inertial forces of the air columns at higher frequencies) [8, 9].

Sinusoidal waves or impulses (impulse oscillometry, IOS) have been used, both as single-frequency or multiple-frequency signals, with frequencies 5–10 Hz being considered to reflect the mechanical properties of the total airways and higher frequencies giving an estimate of more proximal airways [8–10]. This is because high-frequency sound waves return from the large airways, while low-frequency sound waves progress through the peripheral system and also provide information about distal airways. Rrs increases at all frequencies in case of central airway obstruction, whereas low-frequency Rrs increases with no change in high-frequency Rrs in case of small airway obstruction.

Momentum through the airways transmitting the pressure waves and expansion capacity of the lung tissue constitutes Xrs. At low frequencies, the lung has a passive expansion, high elasticity, and high expansion capacity. As frequency increases, active stretching is passed, and amount of the distributed energy increases. At the transition frequency of passive expansion-active stretching, the required pressure and elastic expansion capacity become equal at a point. This frequency at which expansion capacity (reactance) becomes 0 is named resonant frequency (fres) and is associated with the anterior-posterior diameter and tissue structure of the chest. The fres values increase, because Xrs is more negative, at low frequencies in obstructive and restrictive cases [11]. The area under the curve of reactance (AX) is the area under the Xrs curve between the lowest frequency and fres; this index is reported to be more sensitive than Xrs itself in detecting changes in compliance of the respiratory system [9].

Oscillometry is often used in the acute and chronic stages of asthma or chronic lung disease of prematurity. In proximal obstruction, Rrs increases independently from frequency whereas Xrs is affected very little or none. In distal obstruction, low-frequency Rrs increases and Xrs decreases. Because of this frequency dependence, often evident in respiratory disease, the difference between Rrs measured at 5 Hz and Rrs measured at 20 Hz (Rrs5–20) is often used to describe the mechanics of peripheral airways. Rrs5–20 may actually also reflect other determinants of respiratory mechanics, including upper airway shunt (compliant zones proximal to the area of increased resistance) [9].

In children with asthma, Rrs5, AX, and fres increase whereas X5 decreases [12]. Shi et al. have compared essential spirometry and IOS indices in a study conducted on two groups of children with controlled and uncontrolled asthma. R5 and AX values were significantly different between the two groups whereas no difference was found between baseline spirometry values [13]. The other advantage of oscillometry compared with other techniques, besides the applicability in preschool children due to no requirement of extra effort by the patient during breathing, is the information of reactance and resistance at different frequencies even from nonhomogeneous regional areas in the lung structure. Its capability to detect even the little changes in the small or central airways seems very precious when it comes to early diagnosis in comparison with spirometry [14, 15].

Oscillometry is also a very precious technique for the evaluation of the long-term pulmonary function of children with bronchopulmonary dysplasia and preterm birth. A study comparing children with late preterm birth to healthy controls born at term using the IOS technique found that mean Rrs5 and Rrs10 values were higher in the late preterm group compared to the control group and that mean Rrs5, Rrs10, and Zrs5 values were higher in the late preterm children hospitalized for pulmonary infection compared to the control group [16]. Another study using a sinusoidal signal found that 5-year-old children born very preterm (<32 weeks of gestational age) had impaired Xrs8 and AX, but not Rrs8, when compared with their expected values, showing that the respiratory damage in these children is primarily due to decreased respiratory compliance [17].

Appropriate reference equations are crucial to distinguish the effects of the disease from the effects of growth and development in the preschool period. Information about repeatability, differential sensitivity, and specificity is also important to reliably interpret lung function results [6]. Several reference equations are available for oscillometry in adults and children [13]. The Global Lung Function Initiative (GLI, www.lungfunction.org) is also collecting reference data for oscillometry from worldwide laboratories to develop global reference equations for adults and children.

As a conclusion, measuring airway function in children should involve a different approach than in adults, taking into consideration both anatomical and physiological differences. It is very important to select the most appropriate respiratory function test routinely used in the diagnosis and follow-up of respiratory tract disease. Many pulmonary function techniques are very precious methods in the evaluation of lung disease, but not all of them are highly feasible in preschool children. In recent years, the development and implementation of novel techniques requiring minimum cooperation, such as oscillometry, allowed us to obtain more reliable and beneficial measurements in preschool children. Also, oscillometry can differentiate resistance from reactance and give information about the upper airway component of respiratory impedance. The selection of the most accurate technique for the appropriate patient group will, doubtlessly, increase the chance of diagnostic accuracy and, hopefully, treatment success.

References

1. Miller MR, Hankinson J, Brusasco V, et al. Standardisation of spirometry. Eur Respir J. 2005;26(2):319–38.
2. Kjaer BB, Jensen JS, Nielsen KG, et al. Lung function and bronchial responsiveness after mycoplasma pneumoniae infection in early childhood. Pediatr Pulmonol. 2008;43(6):567–75.
3. Klug B, Bisgaard H. Specific airway resistance, interrupter resistance, and respiratory impedance in healthy children aged 2-7 years. Pediatr Pulmonol. 1998;25(5):322–31.
4. Escobar H, Carver TW. Pulmonary function testing in young children. Curr Allergy Asthma Rep. 2011;11(6):473–81.
5. Rosenfeld M, Allen J, Arets BH, et al. An official American Thoracic Society workshop report: optimal lung function tests for monitoring cystic fibrosis, bronchopulmonary dysplasia, and recurrent wheezing in children less than 6 years of age. Ann Am Thorac Soc. 2013;10(2):S1–S11.
6. Beydon N, Davis SD, Lombardi E, et al. An official American Thoracic Society/European Respiratory Society statement: pulmonary function testing in preschool children. American journal of respiratory and critical care medicine. Am J Respir Crit Care Med. 2007;175(12):1304–45.
7. Fainardi V, Lombardi E. Lung function tests to monitor respiratory disease in preschool children. Acta Biomed. 2018;89(2):148–56.
8. King GG, Bates J, Berger KI, et al. Technical standards for respiratory Oscillometry. Eur Respir J. 2020;55(2):1900753.
9. Kaminsky DA, Simpson SJ, Berger KI, et al. Clinical significance and applications of oscillometry. Eur Respir Rev. 2022;31(163):210208.
10. Starczewska-Dymek L, Bozek A, Dymek T. Application of the forced oscillation technique in diagnosing and monitoring asthma in preschool children. Adv Respir Med. 2019;87(1):26–35.
11. Desiraju K, Agrawal A. Impulse oscillometry: the state-of-art for lung function testing. Lung India. 2016;33(4):410–6.
12. Kaminsky DA. What does airway resistance tell us about lung function? Respir Care. 2012;57(1):85–99.
13. Shi Y, Aledia AS, Galant SP, George SC. Peripheral airway impairment measured by oscillometry predicts loss of asthma control in children. J Allergy Clin Immunol. 2013;131(3):718–23.
14. Smith HJ, Reinhold P, Goldman MD. Forced oscillation technique and impulse oscillometry. In: Gosselink R, Stam H, editors. Lung function testing. European Respiratory Society Publications; 2005.
15. Bickel S, Popler J, Lesnick B, et al. Impulse oscillometry: interpretation and practical applications. Chest. 2014;146(3):841–7.
16. Er I, Gunlemez A, Uyan ZS, et al. Evaluation of lung function on impulse oscillometry in preschool children born late preterm. Pediatr Int. 2016;58(4):274–8.
17. Lombardi E, Fainardi V, Calogero C, et al. Lung function in a cohort of 5-year-old children born very preterm. Pediatr Pulmonol. 2018;53(12):1633–9.

Spirometry and Upper Respiratory Tract 16

Václav Koucký and Nazan Cobanoglu

16.1 Introduction

Spirometry is a fundamental lung function examination. It informs about lung volumes and inspiratory and expiratory flows, which reflect airway patency and stability. Forced vital capacity (FVC), forced expired volume in 1 s (FEV_1) and Tiffeneau index (FEV_1/FVC) are the most important spirometry parameters. These parameters are primarily intended to detect lower airway obstruction. Additionally, they may raise suspicion about restrictive disorder (which needs estimation of total lung capacity to confirm). Although the sensitivity and specificity of spirometry for upper airway pathology is limited, there are visual and quantitative criteria, which may help in detecting upper airway obstruction. Visual criteria are based on the evaluation of flow-volume loop shape both in inspiration and expiration. The 'knee' shape is one of the most typical findings. The quantitative criteria include the Empey index (ratio of FEV_1 and peak expiratory flow) and others that use parameters characterising inspiratory flows, expiratory flow at different levels of FVC and others. Nevertheless, spirometry is just supportive method for the first-line assessment of upper airway function and requires further confirmation. Spirometry may also inform on the concomitant lower airway pathology and trigger a more detailed investigation.

V. Koucký (✉)
Department of Paediatrics, 2nd Faculty of Medicine, Charles University and University Hospital Motol, Prague, Czech Republic
e-mail: Vaclav.koucky@fnmotol.cz

N. Cobanoglu
Division of Paediatric Pulmonology, Department of Paediatrics, Faculty of Medicine, Ankara University, Ankara, Turkey

H. Yüksel et al. (eds.), *Pediatric Airway Diseases*, Comprehensive ENT,
https://doi.org/10.1007/978-3-031-74853-0_16

16.2 Background

Spirometry is a fundamental lung function examination. It is widely available, quick to perform and well known among respiratory physicians. On the other hand, it requires the cooperation of the subject and is sensitive to the quality of manoeuvre (risk of falsely pathological results). Spirometry may be successfully performed in children aged 5 years and more, with experienced lab personnel even earlier (3-year-old children). For children under 3 years of age, there are special methods for lung function testing such as raised volume rapid thoracoabdominal compression [1]. This is a technically highly demanding method usually performed in chloralhydrate-induced sleep and is available in several centres worldwide. It may yield similar outcome parameters like spirometry in older children, but the clinical value needs further evaluation.

Forced spirometry is the most common version of spirometry. The manoeuvre consists of deep inspiration and forced and long expiration. Sufficient effort from the patient is crucial as it is necessary to reach residual volume (RV) and total lung capacity (TLC) levels during the manoeuvre. Only this will allow proper estimation of vital capacity (VC) (Fig. 16.1). Moreover, expiration must be forced to reach maximal flow and flow limitation. Otherwise, the patency of airways may be underestimated, and false-positive finding of airway obstruction is present.

Technical aspects of spirometry are described in several international documents published by the European Respiratory Society (ERS) and the American Thoracic Society (ATS) [2–4]. They state details on the technical requirements to the equipment and other considerations, the test procedure itself, within- and between-manoeuvre evaluation, describe outcome indices, quality control and many others. All physicians dealing with spirometry must be familiar with these recommendations. As they are beyond the scope of this text, we refer interested readers to the respective documents.

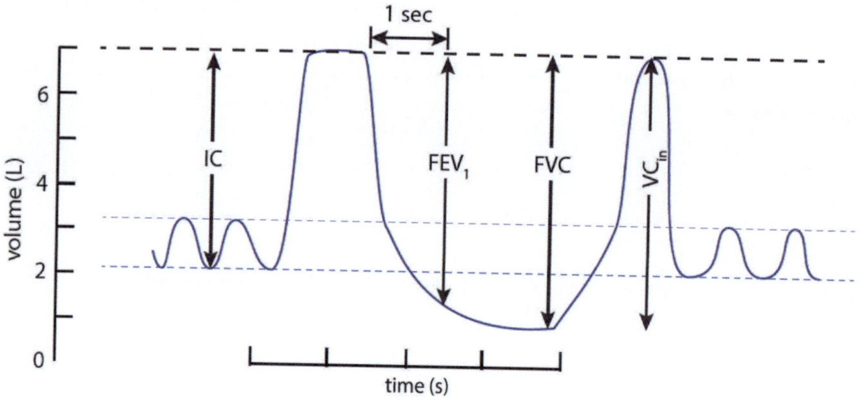

Fig. 16.1 Volume time tracing of the spirometry measurement

Forced spirometry is usually depicted by a flow-volume (FV) loop (Fig. 16.2). While on the x-axis volume (V) is shown, the y-axis represents flow (F). Inspiratory flow is negative (below the x-axis) and expiratory flow is positive (above the x-axis). Pathology (airway obstruction) localised outside the thorax (extra-thoracally—i.e. above the upper thoracic aperture, e.g. upper airway obstruction) will primarily manifest during inspiration. On the other hand, pathology localised intra-thoracally (i.e. under upper thoracic aperture—in the thorax, e.g. peripheral airway obstruction) will primarily affect the expiratory part of the FV loop. In case of severe and fixed obstruction of any localisation along the bronchial tree, both breath phases may be affected. This is a basic rule for the interpretation of spirometry results and follows from the physiology of the respiratory tract (see changes in the pressure in the airway during individual breath phases). Based on this fact, characteristic shapes of flow volume loops are described (see Fig. 16.3). Although they do not allow definitive diagnosis, they are very helpful in first-line evaluation and may give hints on the specific pathology—e.g. peripheral or central airway obstruction, large airway instability, premature termination of expiration, etc.

Beside FV loop shapes, different outcome parameters (indices) may be derived from the forced spirometry. They are summarised in Table 16.1 along with their definitions. These outcomes are usually expressed in absolute values (litres or litres per second) and related to the appropriate norm (reference values). Currently, multiethnic reference values derived within the GLI2012 initiative (Global Lung Initiative) [5] are usually used, although national or other specific reference values [6–8] may be preferred in some cases (e.g. availability of the reference for more outcome parameters, better suitability for the respective population, better comparability to the previous measurements in the respective patient, etc.).

The comparison of the measured (absolute) value of the respective outcome to the norm may be expressed in various ways. Historically, this was done as a

Fig. 16.2 Flow-volume loop. *PEF*, peak exspiratory flow; *FVC*, forced vital capacity; *MEF75*, maximum exspiratory flow at 75% of FVC; *MEF50*, maximum exspiraotry flow at 50% of FVC; *MEF25*, maximum exspiratory flow at 25% of FVC; *IRV*, inspiratory reserve volume; *Vt*, tidal volume; *ERV*, exspiratory reserve volume; *MIF50*, maximum inspiratory flow at 50% of FVC

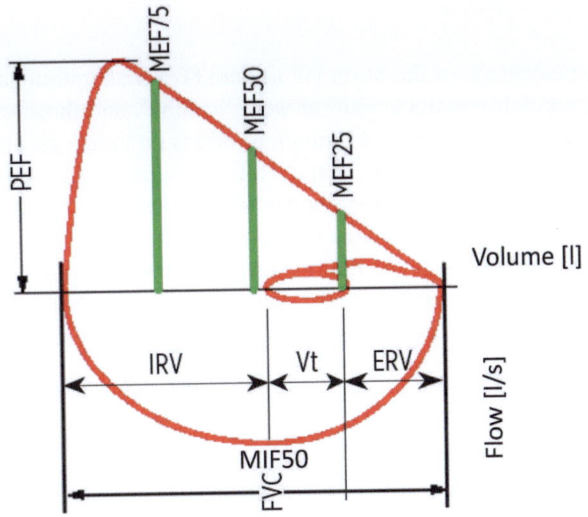

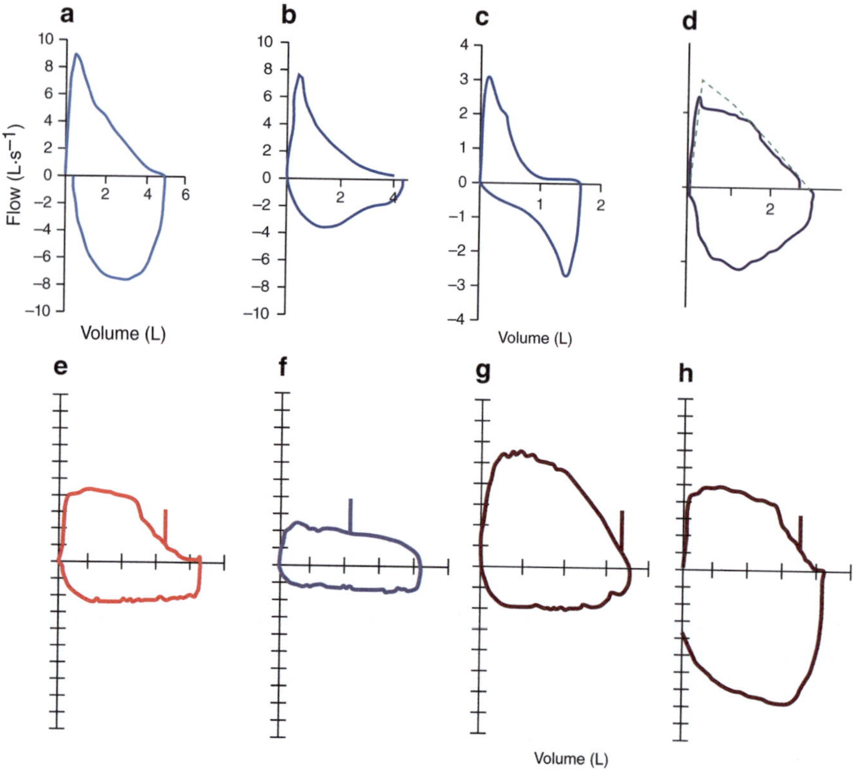

Fig. 16.3 Typical shapes of the flow-volume loops. (**a**) Normal flow volume loop; (**b**) peripheral airway obstruction; (**c**) one-sided main bronchus obstruction; (**d**) large (central) airway instability (tracheomalacia); (**e**) fixed upper airway obstruction (mild); (**f**) fixed upper airway obstruction (severe); (**g**) variable extrathoracic upper airway obstruction; (**h**) variable intrathoracic upper airway obstruction

percentage of the norm (% n), and 80% was traditionally considered as a level of normality (values >80% n were 'healthy', and those <80% were 'diseased'). This approach has several limitations and is no longer recommended [9]. The main reason for that is the fact that the reference data distribution of the respective outcomes is not uniform and the standard deviations differ for the respective outcomes. Thus, 80% may be still within the norm for one outcome but not for the other. Moreover, the classification of the impairment severity is not uniform for all the parameters (see example in Table 16.2, which is based on Zapletal's reference values) [8].

Currently, use of z-score is preferred. Z-score may be calculated as follows:

$$\mathrm{z-score} = \frac{\text{measured value} - \text{reference value}}{\text{standard deviation}}$$

Table 16.1 Forced spirometry outcome parameters

Parameter	Abbreviation (unit)	Definition
Forced vital capacity	FVC (L)	Maximal forcefully exhaled volume from maximal volume level (TLC) to minimal volume level (RV)
Forced volume exhaled in the first t-seconds	FEV_t (L)	Maximal forcefully exhaled volume during the first t-seconds (usually 0.5, 1 and 6 s)
Peak expiratory flow	PEF (L/s)	Maximal flow during exhalation
Maximal expiratory flow at 25%, 50% and 75% levels of FVC[a]	MEF_{25}, MEF_{50}, MEF_{75} (L/s)	Maximal expiratory flow when 25, 50, or 75% of FVC remains to be exhaled
Area under the curve	Aex (L*L/s)	Area under the expiratory part of the FV loop
Maximum inspiratory flow	MIF (L/s)	Maximal flow during inspiration
Maximum inspiratory flow at 50% level of FVC	MIF_{50} (L/s)	Maximal inspiratory flow when 50% of FVC has been inhaled

[a] Alternatively (typically in US), FEF_{XX} may be used. XX denotes how much of the FVC has already been exhaled. Thus, $MEF_{75} = FEF_{25}$, $MEF_{50} = FEF_{50}$, and $MEF_{25} = FEF_{75}$. We use MEF_{XX} in the text, which is preferred in Europe. TLC = total lu ng capacity

Table 16.2 Zapletal's classification of airway obstruction based on MEF_{25}, MEF_{50} and PEF for preschool children

		Peripheral airway		Central airway
		MEF_{25}	MEF_{50}	PEF
Degree	Description	% n		
1	Mild	70–60	75–66	80–72
2	Moderate	59–50	65–58	71–64
3	Severe	< 49	< 57	< 63

and when comparing to norm, it reflects also the variability of the reference population (standard deviation). Thus, there is just one level of normality for all the outcomes, which is usually set to 1.65 SD (Fig. 16.4). Moreover, the classification of the impairment severity is uniform for all outcomes (Table 16.3). Additionally, for the first-line evaluation of the results, lower and upper limits of norm (LLN and ULN) may be used. Limits of the norm are borderline values of the parameter, which are just in the norm. Everything, that is under (LLN) or above (ULN), is already pathologic. Limits of the norm may be used to simplify the interpretation of lung function results.

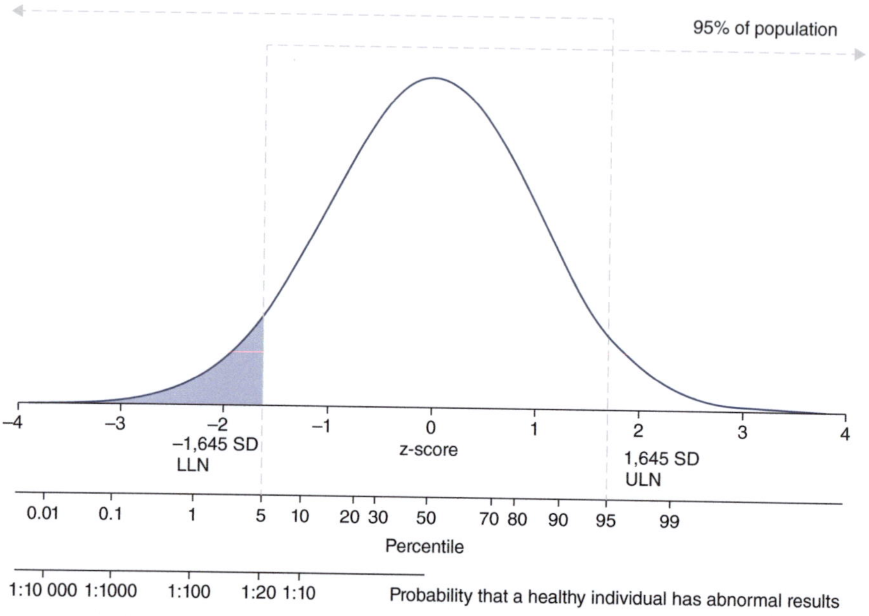

Fig. 16.4 Z-score, percentiles and impairment probability for normally-distributed. *SD* standard deviation; *LLN* lower limit of norm; *ULN* upper limit of norm

Table 16.3 Classification of impairment severity based on z-score for whatever parameter proposed by ERS 2022 [9]

Degree	Description	z-score[a]
1	Mild	−1.65 to −2.5 SD
2	Moderate	−2.5 to −4 SD
3	Severe	< −4 SD

SD standard deviation

[a] For whatever outcome parameter

16.3 Forced Spirometry and Upper Airway Pathology

Spirometry is not primarily intended to evaluate upper airway pathology. Other lung function methods such as rhinomanometry, body plethysmography (airway resistance measurement), etc., may be more helpful. The value of spirometry in assessing upper airway obstruction is based on the fact, that it is widely available and may raise suspicion about upper airway obstruction during the first-line lung function testing. The most common clinical scenarios, when upper airway obstruction may be present include laryngomalacia and tracheomalacia (airway instability—variable obstruction), fixed obstruction in laryngeal stenosis, (bilateral) vocal cord palsy, laryngeal oedema, tracheal stenosis—extraluminal (compression by great vessels, goitre), intraluminal (mucus stagnation, granulation tissue, foreign body, tumours) or intramural (complete cartilaginous rings). It is important to note, that both the specificity and sensitivity of spirometry for upper airway pathology are not very high. Other methods such as computed tomography or flexible endoscopy are necessary to confirm the suspicion.

The value of forced spirometry and FV loop for diagnosing upper airway obstruction has been evaluated previously and different criteria have been proposed. Upper airway obstruction may be suspected based on the shape of the FV loop (so-called visual criteria). Variable extrathoracic upper airway obstruction (e.g. laryngomalacia) is characterised by flow limitation during the inspiration, while the expiratory part of the FV loop is without alteration (Fig. 16.3g). In the case of variable intrathoracic upper airway obstruction, flow limitation is present during expiration, while the inspiratory part of the FV loop is without alteration (Fig. 16.3h). In fixed upper airway stenosis (e.g. laryngeal stenosis, subglottic stenosis, etc.), both inspiratory and expiratory flows at higher levels of FVC (more than 50%) are limited. Thus, PEF, MEF_{75} and MIF_{50} are reduced, while those at lower volume levels (MEF_{50} and MEF_{25}) may be normal. The typical FV loop shapes are shown in Fig. 16.3e, f. In upper airway obstruction, the lung volumes (FVC and others) are usually not affected. Typical shapes of FV curves in upper airway obstruction mentioned above have been described by different authors [10–13] and are usually called sawtooth (or knee) shape (Fig. 16.3d), FV loop with plateau, oscillations, etc.

Quantitative criteria to detect upper airway obstruction have been developed [10, 14–18]. The most frequently used criteria include:

1. Ratio of FEV_1 (in ml) to peak expiratory flow (PEF, in l/min) > 10 ml/(l/min)[1] (based on the criteria of Empey [14]).
2. Difference between PEF z-score and FEV_1 z-score ≤ −2 (based on the criteria of Zapletal [18]).
3. Ratio of $MEF_{50\%}$ to the flow at the mid-point of the forced inspiratory manoeuvre ($MIF_{50\%}$); an abnormal $MEF_{50\%}/MIF_{50\%}$ is defined as <0.30 or >1 (based on the criteria of [15]).
4. Ratio of FEV_1 to forced expiratory volume in the first 0.5 s ($FEV_{0.5}$) >1.5 (based on the criteria of Rotman et al. [17]).
5. $MIF_{50\%}$ < 100 L/min (based on the criteria of Rotman et al. [17]).

Although they are primarily intended for use in adults, some of them may be used even in children. Their sensitivity and specificity have been studied previously. Modrykamien et al. [19] examined spirometry in 475 adults, who had accepted-standard tests for upper airway obstruction available (bronchoscopy, laryngoscopy, neck CT and chest CT). The prevalence of upper airway obstruction was low (7.5%) in a population of patients referred for spirometry to a tertiary centre. The authors concluded that the diagnostic performance of the individual quantitative criteria for detecting upper airway obstruction from the flow-volume loop was poor. The sensitivity ranged from 5.5 to 47.2% and the specificity from 60.5 to 96.8%. There was a

[1] In children, the cut off value >8 mL/L/min was proposed by some authors to increase the sensitivity [22].

significant risk of undetecting upper airway obstruction when relying on spirometry alone. When aggregated, the diagnostic performance could be slightly improved: the sensitivity of the aggregated criteria (≥ 1 quantitative criterion) was 69.4% and specificity 30.2%; area under the receiver-operator characteristic curve for the aggregate criteria exceeded 0.6, while for the individual criteria, it ranged from 0.4 to 0.5.

Spirometry indices in children with tracheomalacia were studied by Boonjindasup et al. [20]. The 'knee' shape of the FV loop was common in children with tracheomalacia and PEF was significantly reduced in children with tracheomalacia. However, the Empey index was normal (8.21 ± 1.59, mean ± standard deviation) and could not be used to characterise tracheomalacia. In children with subglottic stenosis, the role of spirometry has been investigated by Abdullah et al. [21]. The Empey index ranged from 7.34 to 21.40 mL/L/min and significantly improved after dilation. It did not correlate with the severity of the stenosis. The authors concluded that spirometry might be a useful marker in following up patients with subglottic stenosis and a good indicator to determine intervention outcomes. Olbers et al. [22] studied spirometry results in children after surgical repair of oesophageal atresia with tracheoesophageal fistula. They found elevated Empey index (FEV_1/PEF > 8 mL/(L/min)) in 58% of cases. Recurrent pneumonias were more frequent in children with elevated Empey index (73% vs. 27%). About 87% of children with increased Empey index had respiratory symptoms of any kind.

Especially in children, special attention must be paid to the quality and reproducibility of the FV loop as improper technique may result in falsely pathological results. For instance, muscle weakness, collapsibility of the soft tissues in the upper airway, mouthpiece obstruction via tongue or improper position of mouthpiece may all result in findings mimicking upper airway pathology. For these reasons, repeated manoeuvres are helpful in distinguishing artefacts from true pathology. Development of the findings during follow-up may also be helpful.

In conclusion, different visual and quantitative criteria to detect upper airway obstruction from forced spirometry have been proposed. Their diagnostic value was studied in different clinical situations and seems to be limited. Despite this fact, they should not be neglected when spirometry is available as it may raise suspicion of upper airway pathology. Confirmation using other standard diagnostic tests (endoscopy, computed tomography) is required.

References

1. Lum S, Hülskamp G, Merkus P, Baraldi E, Hofhuis W, Stocks J. Lung function tests in neonates and infants with chronic lung disease: forced expiratory maneuvers. Pediatr Pulmonol. 2006;41:199–214.
2. Graham BL, Steenbruggen I, Barjaktarevic IZ, Cooper BG, Hall GL, Hallstrand TS, et al. Standardization of spirometry 2019 update an official American Thoracic Society and European Respiratory Society technical statement. Am J Respir Crit Care Med. 2019;200(8):E70–88.
3. Beydon N, Davis SD, Lombardi E, Allen JL, Arets HGM, Aurora P, et al. An official American Thoracic Society/European Respiratory Society statement: pulmonary function testing in preschool children. Am J Respir Crit Care Med. 2007;175(12):1304–45.

4. Miller MR, Hankinson J, Brusasco V, Burgos F, Casaburi R, Coates A, et al. Standardisation of spirometry. Eur Respir J. 2005;26(2):319–38.
5. Quanjer PH, Stanojevic S, Cole TJ, Baur X, Hall GL, Culver BH, et al. Multi-ethnic reference values for spirometry for the 3-95-yr age range: the global lung function 2012 equations. Eur Respir J. 2012;40(6):1324–43.
6. Quanjer PH, Tammeling GJ, Cotes JE, Pedersen OF, Peslin R, Yernault JC. Lung volumes and forced ventilatory flows. Eur Respir J. 1993;6(Suppl 16):5–40.
7. Zapletal A, Paul T, Samánek M. Significance of contemporary methods of lung function testing for the detection of airway obstruction in children and adolescents (author's transl). Z Erkr Atmungsorgane. 1977;149(3):343–71.
8. Zapletal A, Chalupová J. Forced expiratory parameters in healthy preschool children (3-6 years of age). Pediatr Pulmonol. 2003;35(3):200–7.
9. Stanojevic S, Kaminsky DA, Miller MR, Thompson B, Aliverti A, Barjaktarevic I, et al. ERS/ATS technical standard on interpretive strategies for routine lung function tests. Eur Respir J. 2022;60(1):2101499.
10. Miller RD, Hyatt RE. Obstructing lesions of the larynx and trachea: clinical and physiologic characteristics. Mayo Clin Proc. 1969;44(3):145–61.
11. Anzueto A, Levine SM, Tillis WP, Calhoon JH, Bryan CL. Use of the flow-volume loop in the diagnosis of bronchial stenosis after single lung transplantation. Chest. 1994;105(3):934–6.
12. Sanders MH, Martin RJ, Pennock BE, Rogers RM. The detection of sleep apnea in the awake patient. The "saw-tooth" sign. JAMA. 1981;245(23):2414–8.
13. Vincken W, Cosio MG. Flow oscillations on the flow-volume loop: a nonspecific indicator of upper airway dysfunction. Bull Eur Physiopathol Respir. 1985;21(6):559–67.
14. Empey DW. Assessment of upper airways obstruction. BMJ. 1972;3(5825):503–5.
15. Miller RD, Hyatt RE. Evaluation of obstructing lesions of the trachea and larynx by flow-volume loops. Am Rev Respir Dis. 1973;108(3):475–81.
16. Yernault JC, Englert M, Sergysels R, De Coster A. Upper airway stenosis: a physiologic study. Am Rev Respir Dis. 1973;108(4):996–1000.
17. Rotman HH, Liss HP, Weg JG. Diagnosis of upper airway obstruction by pulmonary function testing. Chest. 1975;68(6):796–9.
18. Alois Z, Milan Š, Tomáš P. Lung function in children and adolescents: methods, reference values, vol. 22. Basel; New York: Karger; 1987.
19. Modrykamien AM, Gudavalli R, McCarthy K, Liu X, Stoller JK. Detection of upper airway obstruction with spirometry results and the flow-volume loop: a comparison of quantitative and visual inspection criteria. Respir Care. 2009;54(4):474–9.
20. Boonjindasup W, Marchant JM, McElrea MS, Yerkovich ST, Thomas RJ, Masters IB, et al. Pulmonary function of children with tracheomalacia and associated clinical factors. Pediatr Pulmonol. 2022;57(10):2437–44.
21. Abdullah A, Alrabiah A, Habib SS, Aljathlany Y, Aljasser A, Bukhari M, et al. The value of spirometry in subglottic stenosis. Ear Nose Throat J. 2019;98(2):98–101.
22. Olbers J, Gatzinsky V, Jönsson L, Friberg LG, Abrahamsson K, Sillén U, et al. Physiological studies at 7 years of age in children born with esophageal atresia. Eur J Pediatr Surg. 2015;25(5):397–404.

Allergen Testing: Purpose, Procedure, Interpretation

17

Cansu Özdemiral and Ümit Murat Şahiner

Abbreviations

AECs	Allergen Exposure Chambers
BAT	Basophil activation test
CAMP	Childhood Asthma Management Program
CRD	Component resolved diagnosis
CCD	Cross-reactive carbohydrate determinants
EAACI	European Academy of Allergology and Clinical Immunology
EMA	European Medicines Agency
ECP	Eosinophilic cationic protein
FDA	Food and Drug Administration
FEV1	Forced expiratory flow in 1 s
GA²LEN	Global Allergy and Asthma European Network
ICDRG	International Contact Dermatitis Research Group
NAC	Nasal allergen challenge
nsLTP	Non-specific lipid transfer proteins
PNIF	Peak nasal inspiratory flow
RAST	Phadebas radioallergosorbent test
PAF	Platelet activating factor
PFAS	Pollen Food Allergy Syndrome
sAT	Serum acute tryptase
sBT	Serum baseline tryptase
SPT	Skin prick test
sIgE	Specific IgE

C. Özdemiral · Ü. M. Şahiner (✉)
Department of Pediatric Allergy and Asthma, Hacettepe University Faculty of Medicine, Ankara, Türkiye
e-mail: cansuozdemiral@hacettepe.edu.tr; umit.sahiner@hacettepe.edu.tr

H. Yüksel et al. (eds.), *Pediatric Airway Diseases*, Comprehensive ENT,
https://doi.org/10.1007/978-3-031-74853-0_17

TNSS	Total Nasal Symptom Score
VAS	Visual analog scale

17.1 Introduction

Allergic diseases exert a significant global burden, impact individuals across all age groups. Allergies to food, aeroallergens, drugs, and venom complicate patients' lives and, at sometimes pose life-threatening risks. Type 1 immediate hypersensitivity and Type 4 delayed hypersensitivity constitute major underlying mechanisms in allergic diseases. Clinical history takes a light for the allergist to make a diagnosis and frequently diagnosis is completed with the basic tests. Skin prick/puncture tests, intradermal tests, and patch tests are skin tests that have been utilized to diagnose allergic diseases. The SPT is the most frequently used method that is safe and reliable. SPT typically induces a wheal and flare reaction, indicative of Type 1 hypersensitivity. Positive SPT results are defined by wheal diameters ≥3 mm, taking into account the results of both positive and negative controls. In intradermal skin testing, allergen extracts are administered into the dermis at a concentration that is 100–1000 times less than that used in SPT. Patch tests are typically used for patients experiencing delayed-type hypersensitivity reactions. Nevertheless, conducting skin tests and accurately interpreting the results need adequate training and also involve the possibility of unexpected systemic responses. Total serum IgE measurement has limited utility in allergic diseases. Serum-specific IgE (sIgE) measurement, as a complementary or alternative diagnostic tool, is widespread. Component-resolved diagnosis might be beneficial in cases where polysensitization complicates the diagnosis, or when negative skin prick test (SPT) findings are obtained despite a potential history of allergy. The allergen provocation test could be used as a gold standard method in particular patients.

17.2 Tests

17.2.1 Skin Tests

Skin tests involve introducing an allergen through a break in the skin, which are could be utilized for detecting allergies to inhalants, food, insect venom, or drugs. When sensitivity to the relevant allergen exists, specific IgE molecules bound to mast cell surface receptors become cross-linked, triggering mast cells to degranulate and release histamine along with other mediators. Skin tests result in the formation of a wheal and flare response, which is indicative of Type 1 hypersensitivity [1]. In 1865, Charles H. Blackley, a physician suffering from allergic rhinitis, conducted the first skin test on himself. Using a lancet, he scratched a quarter-inch area of his skin and applied grass pollen grains placed on wet gauze to the scarred area, covering it with an occlusive bandage. This experimental procedure resulted in significant itching and a large cutaneous response [2]. Due to the increased pain, reduced repeatability, and possibility of maintaining several linear depigmented patches following scratch testing, as well as the higher risk of causing a systemic allergic response, it is no longer recommended to use scratch tests. Instead, skin prick/puncture tests, intradermal tests, and patch tests have been widely utilized in diagnosing allergic diseases [3].

Skin prick test (SPT): In 1959, H. Ebruster reported the identification of Type 1 hypersensitivity reactions through the use of the SPT [4]. Pepys modified the SPT at 1970, and it is still frequently utilized for allergy diagnosis today [5]. Both the EAACI (European Academy of Allergology and Clinical Immunology) and the US Council of Allergy Asthma and Immunology recommended the initial use of skin prick/puncture tests for individuals whose clinical histories suggest Type 1 hypersensitivity reactions to inhalant allergens [1, 6]. SPTs are minimally invasive, quick, inexpensive, reproducible, and reliable, exhibiting a strong correlation with symptoms [7]. The implementation of standardized procedures became imperative owing to variances in performing SPT, selecting allergens, and interpreting the results. The Global Allergy and Asthma European Network (GA2LEN) conducted a study across 17 centers in 14 countries, leading to the development of a standardized SPT protocol [8]. Standardized protocol, includes using Histamine dihydrochloride 0.1% as positive control, NaCl 0.9% as negative control, and an allergen panel

Table 17.1 Standard skin prick test panel [7]

Positive control	Histamindihydrochloride 0.1%
Negative control	NaCl 0.9%
Alder	*Alnus incana*
Birch	*Betula alba*
Cypress	*Cupressus sempervirens*
Grass mix	*Smooth meadow grass/Poa pratensis, cock's foot grass/Dactilis glomerata, perennial rye grass/Lolium prenne, timothy grass/Pheleum pratense, meadow fescue/Festuca pratensis, meadow oat grass/ Helictotrichon pretense*
Hazel	*Corylus avellana*
Mugwort	*Artemisia vulgaris*
Olive	*Olea europaea*
Parietaria	*Parietaria*
Plane	*Platanus vulgaris*
Ragweed	*Ambrosia artemisiifolia*
Dermatophagoides farinae	
Dermatophagoides pteronyssinus	
Blatella	*Blatella germanica*
Alternaria	*Alternaria alternata (tenuis)*
Aspergillus	*Aspergillus fumigatus*
Cladosporium	*Cladosporium herbarum*
Cat	
Dog	

involving common allergens, as detailed in Table 17.1 [7]. A minimal amount of an allergen extract containing particular components, both genuine and cross-reacting, is required for the test [9]. The allergen panel selection can be determined according to patients' age, clinic, and geographic area, typically encompassing 8–12 allergens, which is usually adequate [10, 11]. The allergen extracts must possess high potency and stability, while also considering their shelf life. The pricking device should be sterile and only be used once for each allergen. They are available in a variety of sizes (single or multiple puncture devices), shapes (lancet, needle, bifurcated lancet, with or without guard), materials (plastic or metal), and preparations (precoated with the allergen extract, or not) [9]. The examples of pricking devices are depicted in Fig. 17.1. No SPT device has been established as the gold standard in the literature [9]. SPT is conducted on the anterior arm or back and is limited to healthy skin [12]. To prevent cross-contamination, a minimum of 2 cm spacing between prick tests is recommended. The most commonly used SPT method involves applying a drop of the allergen extract to a marked area of the skin and then inserting the device through the drop at a 45–60° angle, ensuring it does not penetrate beyond the epidermis. If the device is inserted at a 90° angle, it is referred to as a skin puncture test, skin test methods are illustrated in Fig. 17.2 [12]. A different SPT technique was used, in which submerge the device into the allergen, then drop to the test area, and apply vertical pressure. Comparable results were found with less effort and expense [13]. It's important to note that performing the SPT should not cause bleeding [12]. The best outcomes can be anticipated by selecting a single prick/puncture tool and effectively training skin technicians in its use. Skin test proficiency protocols should be used to establish consistency in skin test performance among technicians in order to achieve quality assurance. Post-histamine control applications have been advised to adhere to proposed standards, such as a coefficient variation of less than 20% (as per EAACI) and less than 30% (as per Childhood Asthma Management Program—CAMP) [14, 15]. The peak reactivity of prick/puncture tests occurs between 15 and 20 min, then the diameters of the erythema and wheal should be measured in millimeters (mm) and compared with positive and negative controls. An example of the SPT is exhibited in Fig. 17.3. The wheal diameter is determinative while interpreting the test result. In clinical studies, wheal diameters ≥3 mm are considered positive in SPTs whereas less than 3 mm may be accepted positive in epidemiologic studies [16]. Although the severity of clinical symptoms is not always predicted by wheal size, larger wheal sizes may indicate a favorable positive response to nasal provocation. The correlation between wheal size and clinical symptoms may be

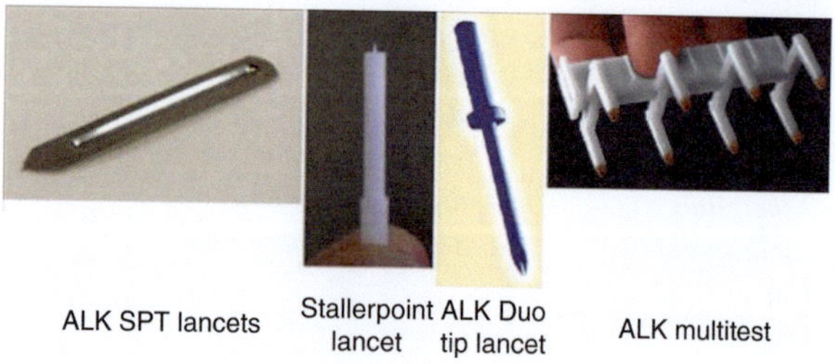

Fig. 17.1 The examples of skin prick test devices

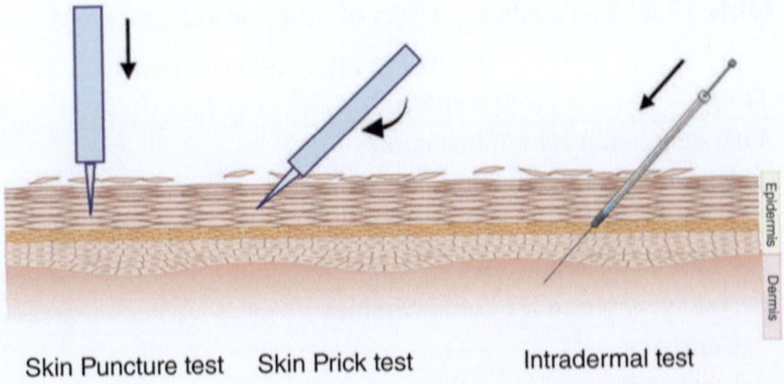

Fig. 17.2 Skin test methods

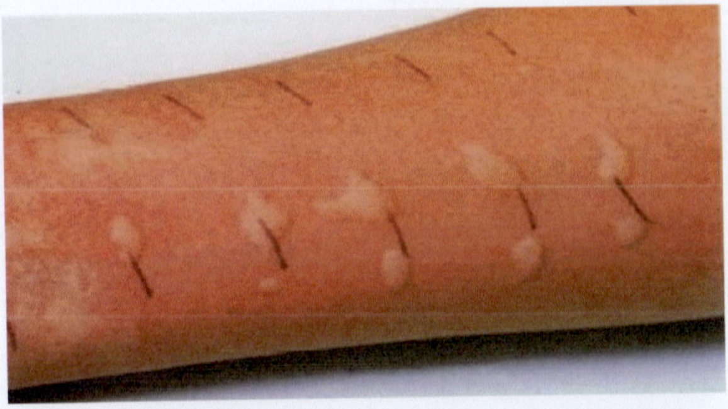

Fig. 17.3 An example of skin prick test

subject to variation depending on demographic characteristics and allergen extracts utilized [17]. Clinicians should note that false positive and false negative results are possible. False positive results can occur with excessive pressure, nonspecific enhancement due to nearby strong local reactions, or dermographism, where the wheal of the negative control measures ≥3 mm [18]. Several factors can lead to false-negative skin test results, including prior use of antihistamines or anxiolytics, inappropriate allergen extracts, poor technique, limited local production of allergen-specific IgE restricted to the nose or eye, conditions that attenuate skin response (such as renal failure, cancer, or UV-B radiation exposure), and performing the test weeks after a systemic allergic reaction [12, 19, 20]. Positive histamine responses may vary in individuals, that should not be attributed to allergic disease severity [12]. Table 17.2 provides a list of medications that can influence SPT results and the recommended avoidance period prior to the test [21]. Uncontrolled or severe asthma, severe or unstable cardiovascular disease, and pregnancy are contraindications for SPT [22]. SPT can be used in all ages; however, results must be interpreted carefully while performing on infants. Repeated SPT for children may be considered in the case of new symptoms related to recently introduced inhalant allergens [6, 23]. SPT has high sensitivity (70–95%) and specificity (80–97%) for diagnosing inhalant allergies [12]. SPT results should be interpreted in accordance with the clinical relevance. The type of allergen and the region where the patient resides determine whether a given sensitivity is likely to be clinically important. In the absence of clinical findings (patient history and/or physical examination), a positive SPT solely indicates sensitization rather than allergy. For individuals suspected of having allergies, additional tests such as nasal, eye, or bronchial provocation tests may be required for confirming the diagnosis.

Table 17.2 The inhibitory effect of drugs on skin prick test

Drugs	Degree of effect on histamine response	Avoidance time (day) prior the test
First generation H1 antihistamines		
Diphenhydramine	0/+	1–3
Hydroxyzine	+++	1–10
Chlorpheniramine	++	1–3
Second generation H1 antihistamines		
Cetirizine	++++	3–10
Levocetirizine	++++	3–10
Loratadine	++++	3–10
Desloratadine	++++	3–10
Fexofenadine	++++	3–10
Azelastine	++++	3–10
Bilastine	++++	3–10
Ebastine	++++	3–10
Ketotifen	++++	>5
H2 antihistamines		
Ranitidine	0/+	2
Cimetidine	0/+	2
Tricyclic antidepressants		
Imipramine	++++	Up to 21 days
Doxepin	++	3–11
Phenothiazine	++	Up to 10 days
Corticosteroids		
Inhaled	0	–
Systemic	0/++	
Topical	0/++	10–21
Montelukast	0	0
Omalizumab	++++	42–56 (up to 1 year)

Intradermal (ID) Skin Tests: ID tests may be utilized when a patient's medical history indicates an allergic disease yet the SPT is negative. However, allergies to Hymenoptera venom, drugs, and Alternaria stand as exceptions where ID tests can be used irrespective of SPT results [24]. These tests involve introducing allergen extracts, typically 100–1000 times less concentrated (0.02–0.05 mL), into the dermis using a disposable 0.5- or 1.0-mL syringe. After 10–15 min, erythema and wheal diameters are measured in millimeters. ID skin tests demonstrate higher sensitivity but lower specificity compared to SPT, especially in the context of certain drugs and insect venom. The clinical manifestations may not always align with the positive identification of the skin test results. There are concerns over the performance characteristics (sensitivity and specificity) of intradermal tests relative to SPT, therefore the role of intradermal testing for aeroallergen sensitivity is debatable [22]. The correlation between ID skin tests and inhalation challenge tests is less compared to SPTs [25]. Additionally, ID skin tests are more uncomfortable, time-consuming, expensive, and pose a greater risk of anaphylaxis than SPTs. In fact, deaths related to ID skin tests using food and drug extracts have been reported [26].

Prescreening with prick/puncture tests is a useful strategy to prevent potentially fatal ID skin test reactions. f prick/puncture test prescreening is not employed, considering preliminary intracutaneous serial threshold titrations, starting with high dilutions, becomes crucial [12].

Patch Test: The patch test, introduced by Jadassohn in 1895, remains a gold standard diagnostic method for diagnosing Allergic Contact Dermatitis [27]. Food and drug allergies linked with Type 4 hypersensitivity reactions could be diagnosed with patch tests. However, a primary limitation is the lack of standardized protocols for patch tests in diagnosing both food and drug allergies. Patch tests have superior diagnostic performance compared with SPT and in vitro sIgE measurement to dust mite allergy in patients in particularly have allergic rhinitis and atopic dermatitis [28]. Allergens are mixed with petrolatum or liquid transporter at established concentrations. It is applied to the back of the patient in patch test chamber then fixed. In individuals previously sensitized to specific allergens, a delayed type immunologic reaction, involving T-cell responses and proinflammatory cytokines, typically occurs 48 h after reintroduction. Therefore, patch tests are read at 48 h after performing. Figure 17.4 displays a patient underwent a patch test and its result after 48 h. According to International Contact Dermatitis Research Group (ICDRG) recommendations, positive results are defined by the presence of erythema, infiltration, papule, vesicle, or ulcer, while only faint erythema is considered a doubtful reaction [29]. If necessary late reading is performed at 72–96 h and occasionally 7 days later [30]. To ensure accurate results during patch testing, it's recommended to avoid systemic corticosteroids for at least 1 week before the test. Using prednisone more than 10 mg/day is typically contraindicated due to causing false negative results. Antihistamines have not effect on delayed hypersensitivity thus no restriction before patch testing [31].

17.2.2 Determination of IgE in Serum

Total IgE: Total IgE levels are the lowest among all immunoglobulins in the serum. The "normal value" for total IgE in children gradually rises until prepuberty, at the

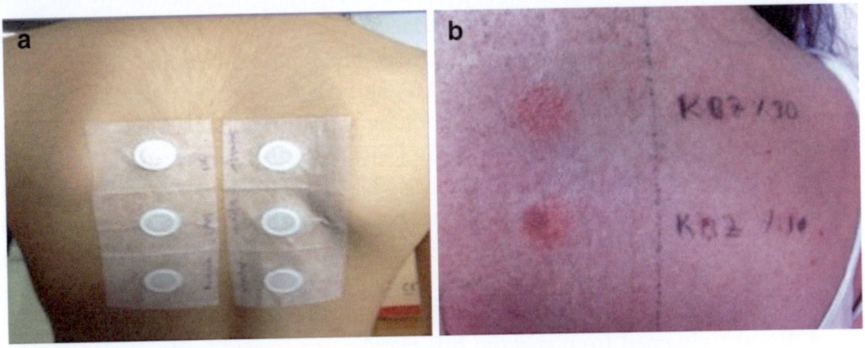

Fig. 17.4 A patient underwent a patch test (**a**) and its result after 48 h (**b**)

time it reaches adult levels. A Total IgE level ranging from 0 to 100 kU/L is often considered within the normal range. However, it was noted in 2014 that the range of normal total IgE levels is 2–214 kU/L. The utility of total serum IgE in clinical settings is limited. Increased total IgE levels can be detected at allergic disease nonetheless there are many diseases may cause increased total IgE level including various infections particularly parasitic infections, neoplasms, immunodeficiencies, Cystic fibrosis, hepatic disorders, etc. Moreover, a normal total IgE level does not rule out allergy, as approximately 25% of allergic patients may have normal total IgE levels [32]. While the measurement of total IgE levels is not recommended for allergy diagnoses [12], the ratio of specific IgE (sIgE) to total IgE holds significance in assessing effector cell activity and contributes to allergy diagnosis in clinical practice. While the measurement of total IgE levels is not recommended for allergy diagnoses [12], the ratio of specific IgE (sIgE) to total IgE holds significance in assessing effector cell activity and contributes to allergy diagnosis in clinical practice. Assessing the total IgE levels is valuable for identifying and monitoring patients with Allergic Bronchopulmonary Aspergillosis. It is also helpful in determining whether to start biologic therapies in individuals with severe asthma.

Specific IgE (sIgE): Various allergens, whether in food, aeroallergens, latex, venom, drugs, or occupational substances, can trigger the production of specific IgE (sIgE) in sensitive individuals, detectable through in vivo (skin tests) or in vitro tests. History-based diagnosis of allergic rhinitis, asthma, dermatitis, urticaria, angioedema, ocular inflammation, anaphylaxis, and food and venom allergies can be confirmed through allergen sIgE antibodies in serum. The most used in vitro test in the field of allergy is the sIgE assays. Unlike total IgE levels, sIgE measurement is reliable for allergy diagnosis. However, it's crucial to employ validated techniques when measuring sIgE levels. The initial assay developed for detecting sIgE antibodies was the Phadebas radioallergosorbent test (RAST) by Pharmacia in Uppsala, Sweden. In the RAST, the allergen is affixed to a solid phase, such as a paper disk, and is incubated with human serum containing allergen-specific IgE antibodies. Subsequently, unbound serum proteins are washed away using a buffer solution, and radiolabeled anti-human sIgE antibodies are introduced to bind to the bound sIgE. The remaining radioactivity on the disk correlates with the patient's sensitivity level, and the results are expressed as arbitrary units per milliliter of sIgE [33]. RAST was once a brand name, but it was frequently (and incorrectly) used to imply to any sIgE test. Thus, it is accepted more appropriate to use term "immunoassay". Immulite 2000, ImmunoCAP Systems, Hy-Tec E/A, Hitachi CLA multiple allergen test, CAP system, Hyor Turbo-MP, and Ala Stat are current commercial-specific IgE technologies. Multiallergen immunoassays, unlike ImmunoCAP, can simultaneously detect more than 30 sIgEs [34]. Nevertheless, it can only provide semiquantitative sIgE values, and its accuracy has been disputed. Any allergists and laboratories favor the Phadia ImmunoCap System (Phadia AB, Uppsala, Sweden) due to its automated nature, reproducibility, sensitivity, and specificity. To enhance allergen binding, cellulose sponge is employed instead of a paper disk, and a quantitative fluorescence enzyme immunoassay utilizing fluorescent anti-sIgE is utilized. Results obtained from specific IgE tests are calibrated to the WHO 75/502

Table 17.3 The classification according to specific IgE levels

Class	Specific IgE level (kUA/L)
0	<0.35
1	0.35–0.69
2	0.70–3.49
3	3.50–17.49
4	17.50–49.99
5	50–99.99
6	≥100

international human serum IgE reference preparation and are quantitatively presented within the range of 0.10–100 kU/L. Also results are reported by classes (0–VI) (Table 17.3). The positive sIgE is considered conventionally as >0.35 kU/L. For certain foods, 95% cutoff values of sIgE have been established using the ImmunoCap System to predict clinical reactivity, in children with food allergies. However, there are no established sIgE cutoff thresholds available for predicting clinical reactivity to aeroallergens. Patients with high sIgE levels are more likely to exhibit symptoms upon allergen exposure compared to those with lower sIgE levels. Nonetheless, it's crucial to note that high sIgE levels do not necessarily indicate the severity or intensity of the allergic reaction. The precise threshold quantities of allergens that may trigger clinical responses in patients have yet to be firmly established. Nevertheless ≥Class 3 levels provide facilitate to clinicians determining the culprit allergen, if consistent clinical history is available. Since <3 Class levels may be attributed to sensitivity in some individuals, who have no clinical findings. The sensitivity and specificity of immunoassays are influenced by the technology used and the quality of allergens employed. Generally, these assays exhibit a specificity and sensitivity range of 30–95% and 60–95%, respectively [12, 35]. The reported sensitivity of these immunoassays is approximately 75% when compared to prick/puncture skin testing [12]. One limitation of sIgE assessments is their tendency to detect varying sIgE positivity in individuals without accompanying clinical symptoms, particularly among patients with very high IgE levels. Currently, no established threshold of total IgE exists to determine false positivity in these cases. One of the benefits of using sIgE tests is that they are not influenced by the use of antihistamines, dermographism, or skin problems. Additionally, these assays may be conducted in individuals who are at a high risk of anaphylaxis due to SPT. The comparison of the SPT and sIgE assays is shown in Table 17.4 [36, 37]. While both SPT and sIgE testing are available, employing both in clinical practice might not always be necessary. The choice of diagnostic testing should be made on an individual basis to prevent unnecessary costs. These testing procedures should be reserved for situations where identifying additional allergic sensitizations would significantly influence the patient's treatment and overall well-being [38].

Table 17.4 The comparison of the SPTs and serum sIgE

	Skin prick test	Specific IgE assay
Sensitivity	Higher	High
Specificity	High	Higher
Requires healthy skin	Yes	No
Patients with dermographism	Not used	Used
Drug effects	Yes	No
Requires adequately trained staff	Yes	No
Cost	Low	High
A large number of allergens can be tested	Yes (including fresh foods)	Limited
Results interpretation	More subjective	More objective
False positivity in patients with elevated Total IgE	No	Possible
Results available time	Immediately	Several days-weeks

17.2.3 Component Resolved Diagnosis (CRD)

The ability to diagnose allergy disorders has significantly improved with the molecular analysis or CRD through development of microarray technology. CRD involves identifying specific IgE against purified native and recombinant allergenic compounds. CRD provides a detailed representation of the sensitization pattern in patients with multiple sensitivities, assists in identifying cross-reactivity and co-sensitization, and contributes to the rule-out allergy [39]. Allergens are classified into two subtypes: major allergens and minor allergens. A major allergen is defined as an allergen recognized by more than 50% of the sensitized population. Major allergens are primary triggers for the production of specific IgE and subsequently induce allergic reactions. Allergic reactions to minor allergens are frequent in regions with significant exposure to these allergens. Understanding a patient's sensitivities to both major and minor allergen components becomes crucial, especially in the context of considering immunotherapy. This is due to the fact that commercial extracts are typically well standardized only for major allergens. In the case of pollen allergy, CRD plays a pivotal role in identifying genuine allergenic molecules, aiding in the decision-making process for immunotherapy. A study from the European Community Respiratory Health Survey revealed that nearly a quarter of the patients were polysensitized with pollens, this has significant implication on deciding to prescribe immunotherapy [40]. Storage proteins, oleosins, defensins, nonspecific lipid transport proteins (nsLTP), PR-10 proteins, profilins, and cross-reactive carbohydrate determinants (CCD) are significant protein families to give rise allergy [41]. Cross-reactivity can occur when two molecules from different species share more than 70% similarity in their primary amino acid sequence. There are known cross-reactivities among pollen–pollen, plant food–plant food, pollen–plant food, and pollen–plant food latex [42]. Due to their similarity to the genuine molecule, cross-reactive allergenic molecules can only trigger an allergic reaction after prior interaction with the primary sensitizer [41]. Type 1 food allergens induce allergic reactions after being absorbed from gastrointestinal tract however type 2 allergens elicit allergic reactions once patient is being sensitized to inhalant allergens. When people with a pollen allergy especially with birch pollen (Bet v 1) consume fruits and vegetables, they may experience the Pollen Food Allergy Syndrome (PFAS). This syndrome triggers an acute and generally mild allergic response in the oral mucosa. Cross-reactivity between pollen allergens and fruit and/or vegetable allergens results in the formation of PFAS, which is associated with plant-related allergy components present in fruits and vegetables such as lipid transfer proteins, profilin, and PR-10 proteins [43]. In a small subset of patients with allergic rhinitis triggered by grass pollen allergy, sensitization to profilins, which are pan-allergens found in fruits, may occur. Profilins, along with Cross-Reactive Carbohydrate Determinants (CCD), exhibit high cross-reactivity with pollens, yet their clinical significance appears limited. Moreover, their quantification in Allergen Immunotherapy (AIT) extracts is generally not performed. Polysensitization to animal dander from cats, dogs, and horses is well-known and might be explained by cross-reactive lipocalins and albumins, detectable through CRD. CRD holds promise in predicting the risk of systemic reactions in food allergies among specific patients due to certain allergen components associated with severe allergic reactions. In the instance of peanuts, Ara h 2 (a storage protein) appears to be the best predictor of peanut allergy, decreasing the need for peanut challenges by at least 50%. Similarly, in hazelnut allergies, Cor a 9 and Cor A 14, and in soybean allergies, Gly m 5 and Gly m 6, have been identified as components linked to severe allergic reactions [44]. CRD emerges as a valuable tool in cases of anaphylaxis where the cause cannot be identified through medical history alone. However, when diagnostic tests, including SPT and sIgE, are inconclusive, the CRD can be utilized since it identifies more allergens than SPT and sIgE. Therefore CRD could be highly helpful in cases of anaphylaxis caused by hidden allergies [45]. Studies have shown that among patients experiencing idiopathic anaphylaxis, nearly half were found to have new allergenic sensitizations, with approximately 20% of these cases identifying the probable cause of the anaphylaxis [46]. Singleplex and multiplex assays are used in CRD. Singleplex tests assay the allergen selected based on the patient's medical history, clinical data, and skin prick test results. On the other hand, multiplex-microarray assays detect multiple specific IgEs against various allergens simultaneously. A multiplex CRD should generally be carried out for complex instances with multiple sensitizations to food and respiratory allergens as well as for idiopathic anaphylaxis. CRD exhibits a sensitivity ranging from 66 to 100% for food allergens, while its specificity varies from 0 to 95%. These results have been derived from studies utilizing food challenge tests as a gold standard method. However, there is no established gold standard method used to ascertain the sensitivity and specificity of CRD for inhalant allergens. Nevertheless, CRD results can be compared either with SPT outcomes or with specific IgE determination methods using allergenic extracts.

17.2.4 Tryptase

Tryptase is main biomarker of mast cells, which takes play a role in Type 1 hypersensitivity reactions. Strong activation signals, such as the cross-linking of FceRIgE

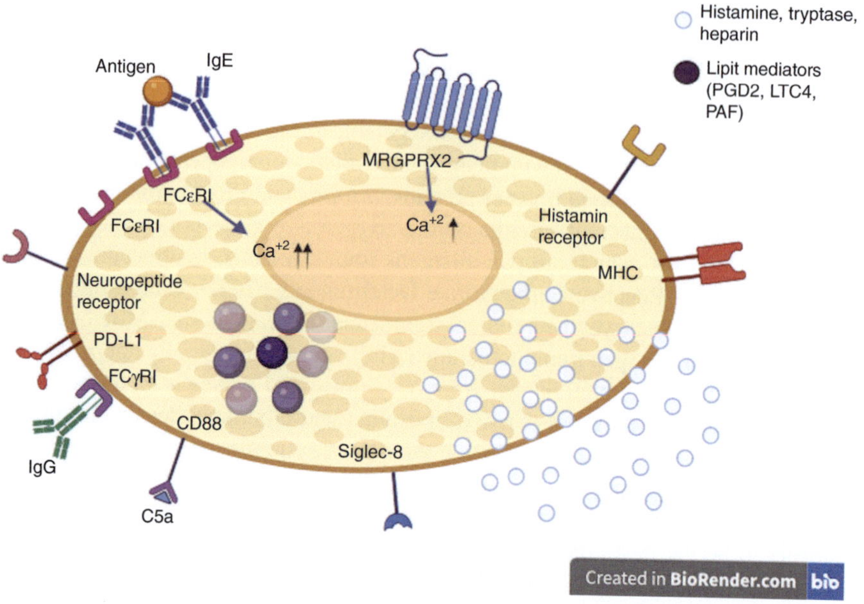

Fig. 17.5 Main receptors and ligands in mast cell activation. In Type 1 hypersensitivity reactions; the cross-linking of FceRIgE complexes following the interaction of cell-bound IgE with the homologous allergen cause mast cell degranulation. Preproduced histamine and tryptase are released immediately. PGD2, LTC4 and PAF are newly synthesized so released in late phase

complexes following the interaction of cell-bound IgE with the homologous allergen cause mast cell degranulation. It causes the release of preproduced histamine and tryptase in seconds to minutes. Newly synthesized molecules play a role in the late-phase response to the allergen; leukotrienes (LTC4, LTD4, LTE4), platelet-activating factor (PAF), and PGD2 are the main mediators. Mast cell and mediators of the activation are demonstrated in Fig. 17.5. In anaphylaxis, tryptase releasing leads to increased vascular permeability favoring vascular leak and thus hypotension, smooth muscle contraction, leukocyte recruitment, and induction of inflammation. Acute tryptase release in the bloodstream is detectable with a delay of 15–20 min after the onset of symptoms due to mast cells is tissue-resident cells and reaches peak at approximately 1 h and remains elevated 4–6 h. Serum baseline tryptase (sBT) can be detected 24 h after onset. The 95th percentile of serum baseline tryptase is demonstrated 8.4 μg/L at 2022; however, it was shown 7.2 μg/L in pediatric age group [47, 48]. Serum acute tryptase (sAT) over [2+ (1.2 × sBT)] μg/L supports mast cell degranulation even when sAT is within the normal reference range. However, increased sBT levels are seen in 5–10% of the healthy population. Moreover elevated sBT levels can be detected in Hereditary alpha tryptasemia, mast cell disorders (cutaneous or systemic), myeloid leukemia, chronic helminth infections, and chronic renal failure [49].

17.2.5 Basophil Activation Test (BAT)

Basophils contain cytoplasmic secretory granules which have similar functional properties with mast cells and participate in systemic allergic reaction. BAT is conducted via flow cytometry, that the expression of activation markers on the surface of blood basophils is assessed before and after stimulation with allergens or controls. Mast cells, a tissue-resident cell expresses FcRI but cannot be used for in vitro diagnostic testing, thus make basophils a particularly interesting option to research sIgE/FcRI-dependent degranulation. BAT holds a distinct advantage over merely quantifying allergen-specific IgE levels because it is a functional assay that involves the activation of live cells within fresh whole blood by specific allergens [50]. Basophils express several surface markers such as CD193, CD203, CD123, and HLA-DR. Upon exposure to an allergen, basophil activation can be identified by changes in certain surface proteins. Among these, CD63 stands out as the most commonly used activation marker, while CD203 upregulation is another indicator of basophil activation [51]. An example of BAT result is shown in Fig. 17.6. Histamine released into the cell supernatant is directly and significantly correlated with CD63 expression on basophils' surfaces [51]. However, it is known that basophils transiently do not respond to stimulation by FcRI in 10% of the individuals, even though they express normal levels of cell surface IgE and respond effectively to an IgE-independent stimulus by upregulating CD63. The use of BAT may reduce the necessity for in vivo procedures such intradermal testing and allergen challenges, which could result

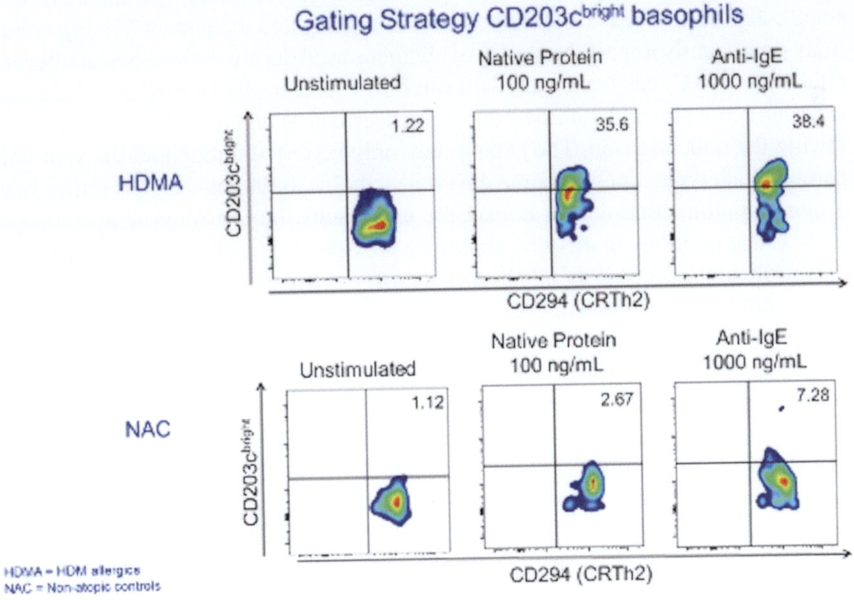

Fig. 17.6 An example of BAT result

in allergic responses with varying severity. Due to the insufficient validation and standardization in laboratories, BAT may be used when standard clinical (skin prick test) and laboratory (sIgE) tests are unclear, inconsistent with the anamnesis, or highly risky to carry out [52]. It is recommended to perform the BAT no later than 6–12 months following the clinical reaction. It is denoted that antihistamines have not any effect on BAT results, yet steroids and immunosuppressive drugs reduce activation [53].

17.2.6 Provocation Tests

The allergen provocation test has been used as a gold standard method for allergic disorders diagnose more than 50 years. Provocation tests may be used to make a diagnosis in cases when anamnesis and sensitization are inconsistent or sIgE is not detected. Nasal, conjunctival, and bronchoprovocation tests can be conducted with utilizing allergen extracts in order to elicit symptoms and clinically establish the relevance of IgE-mediated sensitization. Allergen provocation tests play a crucial role not just in diagnosis but also in deepening our understanding of the mechanisms underlying allergic diseases. They are fundamental in researching and developing new treatments for allergies. However, conducting provocation tests is a complex process. It demands well-trained staff, standardized conditions in testing rooms (including temperature and humidity control for aeroallergen provocations), and meticulous attention to detail. Moreover, the selection of allergens for these tests is critical and should be based on a comprehensive understanding of the patient's clinical history. Factors like the nature of symptoms (perennial or seasonal), exposure to pets or other potential allergens, and the patient's living conditions significantly impact the choice of allergens used during the test. **Nasal allergen challenge (NAC)** has been used with soluble or freezed-dry lyophylizated allergen extracts. NAC should be carried out using seasonal allergens at least 4 weeks following the pollen season. The patient may only be tested throughout the year with perennial allergens, such as home dust mites, molds, or animal dander, if they have minor symptoms that do not impact the test results. he test room temperature of 20.5 °C and humidity of 40–60% should be provided [54]. A baseline measurement, a control challenge, and an allergen challenge are the three measuring phases that constitute the actual challenge procedure. At each step, nasal breathing is both subjectively and objectively evaluated. After 15 min acclimating in test room, baseline measurements are conducted with symptom score assessment and an objective evaluation of nasal patency. The allergen aerosol is given to patient 10 min after seen no effect with control solution. The simplest and most reliable device is recommended as a pump-aerosol spray. Applying two puffs (50 μL per puff) of the allergen to each nostril, one in the inferior meatus and one on the direction of the middle turbinate, is advised. Spraying directly at the nasal septum should be avoided to reduce mechanical irritation. It is specifically recommended that inhalation deeply before applying the allergen, hold the breath throughout application, and exhale fully afterward. This method avoids a potential side effect of NAC, which is aerosol

Table 17.5 Recommendations for evaluating NAC as positive [55] (taken from EAACI Position paper on the standardization of nasal allergen challenges)

Method	Clearly positive	Moderately positive
Subjective measures		
Visual analog scale (VAS)	Symptoms ≥55 mm	Symptoms ≥23 mm
Lebel score	Increase of ≥5 points	Increase of ≥3 points
Linder score	Increase of ≥5 points	Increase of ≥3 points
Total symptom nasal score (TNSS)	Increase of ≥5 points	Increase of ≥3 points
Objective measures		
Peak nasal inspiratory flow (PNIF)	Flow decrease of ≥40%	Flow decrease of ≥20%
Acoustic rhinometry (AcRh)	CSA-2 decrease of ≥40%	Decrease in sum of 2–6 cm^3 ≥ 27% bilaterally
Active anterior rhinomanometry (AAR)	Flow decrease of ≥40% at 150 Pa	Flow decrease in ≥20% at 150 Pa
4-phase-rhinomanometry (4PR)	≥40% increase in logarithmic(lg) effective resistance	≥20% increase in lg effective resistance

penetration into the lower respiratory tract via the nasopharynx. NAC response is assessed with subjective evaluation through symptom ratings and an objective evaluation of nasal patency which is using the peak nasal inspiratory flow (PNIF), an acoustic rhinometer, an anterior rhinomanometry, or a 4-phase rhinomanometry. The increase of ≥30% for Total Nasal Symptom Score (TNSS) or visual analog scale (VAS) is frequently accepted as positive in subjective assessments. Objective NAC results are defined as positive when ≥40% decrease of flow is detected [55]. Evaluations of the NAC results are shown in Table 17.5 [55]. Although it has never been documented, a nasal allergen challenge can cause an anaphylactic reaction.

Allergen Exposure Chambers (AECs) are provocation tests with stable and reproducible priorities under standardized environmental circumstances. At 1987, Vienna Challenge Chamber was the first defined and Der P-1 and Grass antigens were used. In addition to Der P-1 and Grass antigens Ragweed and Japanese cedar pollen antigens were utilized with different devices over time. AECs offer the unique advantage of simulating real-world allergen exposures, testing the response of the entire patient rather than focusing solely on a specific target organ. This comprehensive approach includes exposure to both the upper and lower airways, along with the conjunctival mucosa. A correlation between the symptoms during AEC and at natural seasonal exposure was shown in a study [56]. FDA (Food and Drug Administration) underscores that AECs may be used in clinical assessment of allergic rhinitis however EMA (European Medicines Agency) determined the necessity of validation [57, 58].

Bronchial Provocation Tests (BPT): Abnormal bronchoconstrictor response of the airways due to specific or nonspecific stimuli is considered to be a characteristic pathophysiological feature of asthma. Detecting airway inflammation and airway hyperresponsiveness is important of asthma diagnose. BPT can provide significant information that could not be detected by noninvasive indicators of airway inflammation. BPT becomes particularly important when other diagnostic measures, such as spirometry or assessing bronchodilator response, yield inconclusive results. It's especially useful in identifying triggers related to exposure to environmental or occupational allergens. Moreover, BPT may play a significant role in assessing the efficacy of current asthma therapy. To evaluate airway responsiveness in patients BPT could be performed directly or indirectly methods. Direct BPT involves substances like methacholine or histamine that directly act on specific receptors on the bronchial smooth muscle cells. When these substances come into contact with these receptors, they trigger the contraction of the smooth muscles, leading to airway narrowing. Methacholine is a synthetic derivative of the neurotransmitter acetylcholine. Since histamine is linked to greater systemic adverse effects, such as headache, flushing, and hoarseness, methacholine is more frequently utilized. Indirect BPT, on the other hand, involves substances or stimuli like hypertonic saline, mannitol, adenosine monophosphate, cold air, or exercise. These agents trigger the release of various mediators within the airways, causing inflammation and, subsequently, airway constriction. Indirect methods are beneficial in assessing the overall response of the airways, involving not just smooth muscle cells but also various mediators, receptors, and cells within the airway walls. Thus, indirect BPT is considered to be more specific for asthma. Methacholine is available as dry crystalline powder (Provocoline®) has 100 mg vial. Methacholine solution is prepared with normal saline (0.9% sodium chloride) as the diluent of choice. The five-breath method and a dosage regimen employing methacholine concentrations of 0.0625, 0.25, 1, 4 and 16 mg/mL have been recommended by the American Thoracic Society [59]. Baseline spirometry is performed (FEV1 (forced expiratory flow in 1 s) >70%) then 2 mL of the first diluted solution is given with nebulizer which has a dosimeter to patient. The patient inhales five time from the nebulizer. The FEV1 at about 30 and 90 s after the fifth inhalation is measured. If the FEV1 decline is less than 20%, challenge test is continued subsequent concentration. If the FEV1 falls more than 20% from baseline or the highest concentration has been given methacholine challenge test is finished and considered to be positive. If the FEV1 does not decrease by at least 20% after the maximum dose (i.e., 16 mg/mL), the PC_{20} (provocative concentration causing a 20% fall in FEV1) should be documented as ">16 mg/mL". If PC_{20} is greater than 16 mg/mL, it is highly probable that the patient does not currently have asthma. However methacholine challenge testing has a higher negative predictive power than positive predictive power, it is more beneficial in eliminating an asthma diagnosis than in establishing one [59, 60].

In patients with asthma who have a history of experiencing dyspnea during or after exertion, exercise challenge test can be used to diagnose exercise induced bronchoconstriction. The motor-driven treadmill with adjustable speed and grade or the electromagnetically braked cycle ergometer are the preferred forms of exercise to challenge test. The exercise duration is typically 6 min for children under the age of 12 and 8 min for older children and adults. Both speed and grade begin at a low level and increase in difficulty until the heart rate (estimated as 220-age in years) reaches 80–90% of the predicted maximum. Exercise intensity may be measured by measuring ventilation rather than heart rate. Ventilation should reach 40–60% of the predicted maximum voluntary ventilation (estimated as FEV1x35). When the patient has exercised for at least 4 min at the target heart rate or breathing, the test is completed. Patients can terminate the test any time. Spirometry is used before and after exercise. After finishing exertion, spirometry should be performed 5, 10, 15, 20, and 30 min later. 10% of a decline is regarded as abnormal however more than 15% decline as more diagnostic for exercise induced bronchoconstriction [59].

17.2.7 Nasal sIgE

Nasal sIgE measurement has high specificity however low sensitivity for diagnosis of local allergic rhinitis. However the sensitivity, specificity, positive predictive value, negative predictive value, and diagnostic accuracy for local sIgE as a diagnostic tool for the diagnosis of local allergic rhinitis is founded in a small patient group 91%, 78%, 98%, 94%, respectively [61]. Although several samples (secretions, scraping, brushing, tissue homogenates, etc.) have been used to assess nasal sIgE, none of them have been validated [62].

17.2.8 Nasal Smear Eosinophilia

Eosinophils are recruited from blood to nasal mucosa due to Type 2 immunity and cytokines. More than 10% eosinophils are detected at nasal smear is frequently accepted as nasal eosinophilia. Nasal eosinophilia may seen in patients with AR, Nonallergic rhinitis with eosinophilia syndrome, and Chronic rhinosinusitis with nasal polyposis. A correlation is known between AR symptoms and nasal smear eosinophil counts [63].

17.2.9 Eosinophilic Cationic Protein (ECP)

The levels of the ECP in tissue and peripheral blood strongly linked with the amount of eosinophils. ECP may increase in allergic diseases including asthma, allergic rhinitis, and atopic dermatitis, also infections, and Hypereosinophilic syndrome. Elevated ECP may be detected at serum, sputum, nasal lavage, bronchoalveolar fluid, and skin. ECP and airway inflammation have a favorable correlation, but not with airway hyperresponsiveness. Nevertheless, it has been demonstrated to be useful in determining the severity of asthma, compliance with anti-inflammatory asthma therapy, and as a guide for reducing inhaled corticosteroid dosage [64].

17.3 Future Perspectives and Conclusion

The rising prevalence of allergies worldwide has indeed necessitated the development of more precise and specific diagnostic tests. In addition to the tests that have been performed safely and results are reliable for decades to diagnose or rule out allergy, there is still need for tests provide more specific and precise results. There is lack of evaluation and validation for sIgE cut off thresholds for inhalant allergens to predict clinical reactivity. RD promises hope to clinicians and patients for unresolved allergic circumstances and findings can significantly contribute to individualized approach to the patient, however time consuming and interpretation the results depends on specific training are among difficulties. Increased validation and standardization of the laboratories for BAT may reduce the necessity for in vivo procedures such intradermal testing and allergen challenges. Affording required standardized conditions make using AEC difficult, however it may provide results similar to the exposure in real life due to provoke with whole body.

In summary, while advancements in allergy testing offer promising prospects for more accurate diagnoses and personalized treatment approaches, challenges like standardization, interpretation, and practical application hinder their widespread adoption and effectiveness. Nonetheless, ongoing research and improvements aim to address these limitations for better management of allergic conditions in the future.

References

1. Dreborg S, Frew A. Position paper: allergen standardization and skin tests. Allergy. 1993;48(s14):49–54. https://doi.org/10.1111/j.1398-9995.1993.tb04756.x.
2. Blackley CH. Experimental researches on the causes and nature of Catarrhus aestivus (Hay fever or Hay-asthma), vol. 133. London, England: Balliere Tindall Cox; 1873. p. 181.
3. Indrajana T, Spieksma FTM, Voorhorst R. Comparative study of the intracutaneous, scratch and prick tests in allergy. Ann Allergy. 1997;29:639–50.
4. Ebruster H. The prick test, a recent cutaneous test for the diagnosis of allergic disorders. Wien Klin Wochenschr. 1959;71:551–4.
5. Pepys J. Skin testing. Br J Hosp Med. 1975;14:412–7.
6. Demoly P, Michel F, Bousquet J. In vivo methods for study of allergy. Skin tests, techniques and interpretation. In: Middleton E, Reed C, Ellis E, Adkinson N, Yunginger J, Busse W, editors. Allergy, principles and practice. 5th ed. Mosby Co: St Louis, MO; 1998. p. 530–9.
7. Heinzerling L, Mari A, Bergmann KC, et al. The skin prick test—European standards. Clin Transl Allergy. 2013;3:3. https://doi.org/10.1186/2045-7022-3-3.
8. Heinzerling LM, Burbach GJ, Edenharter G, et al. GA2LEN skin test study I: GA2LEN harmonization of skin prick testing: novel sensitization patterns for inhalant allergens in Europe. Allergy. 2009;64(10):1498–506. https://doi.org/10.1111/j.1398-9995.2009.02093.x.
9. Popov TA, Passalacqua G, González-Díaz SN, et al. Medical devices in allergy practice. World Allergy Organ J. 2020;13(10):100466. https://doi.org/10.1016/j.waojou.2020.100466.
10. Şahiner UM, Civelek E, Yavuz ST, Büyüktiryaki AB, Tuncer A, Şekerel BE. Skin prick testing to aeroallergen extracts: what is the optimal panel in children and adolescents in Turkey? Int Arch Allergy Immunol. 2012;157(4):391–8. https://doi.org/10.1159/000329870.

11. Newson RB, van Ree R, Forsberg B, et al. Geographical variation in the prevalence of sensitization to common aeroallergens in adults: the GA2LEN survey. Allergy. 2014;69(5):643–51. https://doi.org/10.1111/all.12397.
12. Bernstein IL, Li JT, Bernstein DI, et al. Allergy diagnostic testing: an updated practice parameter. Ann Allergy Asthma Immunol. 2008;100(3 Suppl 3):S1–148. https://doi.org/10.1016/s1081-1206(10)60305-5.
13. Buyuktiryaki B, Sahiner UM, Karabulut E, Cavkaytar O, Tuncer A, Sekerel BE. Optimizing the use of a skin prick test device on children. Int Arch Allergy Immunol. 2013;162(1):65–70. https://doi.org/10.1159/000350788.
14. Skin tests used in type I allergy testing position paper. Sub-committee on skin tests of the European Academy of Allergology and Clinical Immunology. Allergy. 1989;44(s10):11–59.
15. Oppenheimer J, Nelson HS. Skin testing. Ann Allergy Asthma Immunol. 2006;96(2 Suppl 1):S6–12. https://doi.org/10.1016/s1081-1206(10)60895-2.
16. Bousquet PJ, Chatzi L, Jarvis D, Burney P. Original article: assessing skin prick tests reliability in ECRHS-I. Allergy. 2008;63(3):341–6. https://doi.org/10.1111/j.1398-9995.2007.01581.x.
17. Nevis IF, Binkley K, Kabali C. Diagnostic accuracy of skin-prick testing for allergic rhinitis: a systematic review and meta-analysis. Allergy Asthma Clin Immunol. 2016;12(1):20. https://doi.org/10.1186/s13223-016-0126-0.
18. Bousquet J, Heinzerling L, Bachert C, et al. Practical guide to skin prick tests in allergy to aeroallergens. Allergy. 2012;67(1):18–24. https://doi.org/10.1111/j.1398-9995.2011.02728.x.
19. Rondón C, Romero JJ, López S, et al. Local IgE production and positive nasal provocation test in patients with persistent nonallergic rhinitis. J Allergy Clin Immunol. 2007;119(4):899–905. https://doi.org/10.1016/j.jaci.2007.01.006.
20. Leonardi A, Fregona IA, Gismondi M, Daniotti E, Carniel G, Secchi AG. Correlation between conjunctival provocation test (CPT) and systemic allergometric tests in allergic conjunctivitis. Eye (Lond). 1990;4(Pt 5):760–4. https://doi.org/10.1038/eye.1990.109.
21. Chiriac AM, Bousquet J, Demoly P. 70—In vivo methods for the study and diagnosis of allergy. In: Adkinson NF, Bochner BS, Burks AW, et al., editors. Middleton's allergy. 8th ed. W.B. Saunders; 2014. p. 1119–32. https://doi.org/10.1016/B978-0-323-08593-9.00071-1.
22. Wise SK, Lin SY, Toskala E, et al. International consensus statement on allergy and rhinology: allergic rhinitis. Int Forum Allergy Rhinol. 2018;8(2):108–352. https://doi.org/10.1002/alr.22073.
23. Cox L, Williams B, Sicherer S, et al. Pearls and pitfalls of allergy diagnostic testing: report from the American College of Allergy, Asthma and Immunology/American Academy of allergy, asthma and immunology specific IgE test task force. Ann Allergy Asthma Immunol. 2008;101(6):580–92.
24. Gendo K, Larson EB. Evidence-based diagnostic strategies for evaluating suspected allergic rhinitis. Ann Intern Med. 2004;140(4):278–89. https://doi.org/10.7326/0003-4819-140-4-200402170-00010.
25. Schwindt CD, Hutcheson PS, Leu SY, Dykewicz MS. Role of intradermal skin tests in the evaluation of clinically relevant respiratory allergy assessed using patient history and nasal challenges. Ann Allergy Asthma Immunol. 2005;94(6):627–33. https://doi.org/10.1016/S1081-1206(10)61319-1.
26. Lockey R, Benedict L, Turkeltaub P, Bukantz S. Fatalities from immunotherapy (IT) and skin testing (ST). J Allergy Clin Immunol. 1987;79(4):660–77. https://doi.org/10.1016/S0091-6749(87)80164-1.
27. Jadassohn J. Zur Kenntnis der medikamentoessen Dermatosen. In: Jarisch A, Neisser A, editors. Verhandlungen der Deutschen Dermatologischen Gesellschaft, V Kongress. Berlin: Julius Springer; 1895. p. 103–29.
28. Fuiano N, Incorvaia C. Utility of the atopy patch test in the diagnosis of allergic rhinitis. Iran J Otorhinolaryngol. 2016;28(86):169–75.
29. Lachapelle JM, Bruze M, Elsner PU, editors. Patch testing tips: recommendations from the ICDRG. Springer; 2014. https://doi.org/10.1007/978-3-642-45395-3.

30. Wilkinson DS, Fregert S, Magnusson B, et al. Terminology of contact dermatitis. Acta Derm Venereol. 1970;50(4):287–92. https://doi.org/10.2340/0001555550287292.
31. Garg V, Brod B, Gaspari AA. Patch testing: uses, systems, risks/benefits, and its role in managing the patient with contact dermatitis. Clin Dermatol. 2021;39(4):580–90. https://doi.org/10.1016/j.clindermatol.2021.03.005.
32. Kjellman NM, Johansson SG, Roth A. Serum IgE levels in healthy children quantified by a sandwich technique (PRIST). Clin Allergy. 1976;6(1):51–9. https://doi.org/10.1111/j.1365-2222.1976.tb01411.x.
33. Emanuel IA. In vitro testing for allergy diagnosis. Otolaryngol Clin N Am. 2003;36(5):879–93. https://doi.org/10.1016/S0030-6665(03)00051-3.
34. Lee JH, Park KH, Kim HS, et al. Specific IgE measurement using AdvanSure® system: comparison of detection performance with ImmunoCAP® system in Korean allergy patients. Clin Chim Acta. 2012;413(9–10):914–9. https://doi.org/10.1016/j.cca.2012.02.018.
35. Nolte H, DuBuske LM. Performance characteristics of a new automated enzyme immunoassay for the measurement of allergen-specific IgE. Summary of the probability outcomes comparing results of allergen skin testing to results obtained with the HYTEC system and CAP system. Ann Allergy Asthma Immunol. 1997;79(1):27–34. https://doi.org/10.1016/S1081-1206(10)63080-3.
36. Bao Y, Chen J, Cheng L, et al. Chinese guideline on allergen immunotherapy for allergic rhinitis. J Thorac Dis. 2017;9:4607–50. https://doi.org/10.21037/jtd.2017.10.112.
37. Robinson M, Smart J. Allergy testing and referral in children. Aust Fam Physician. 2008;37:210–3.
38. de Vos G. Skin testing versus serum-specific IgE testing: which is better for diagnosing aeroallergen sensitization and predicting clinical allergy? Curr Allergy Asthma Rep. 2014;14(5):430. https://doi.org/10.1007/s11882-014-0430-z.
39. Valenta L, Niederberger H, Kraft G. The recombinant allergen-based concept of component-resolved diagnostics and immunotherapy (CRD and CRIT). Clin Exp Allergy. 1999;29(7):896–904. https://doi.org/10.1046/j.1365-2222.1999.00653.x.
40. Bousquet PJ, Castelli C, Daures JP, et al. Assessment of allergen sensitization in a general population-based survey (European Community Respiratory Health Survey I). Ann Epidemiol. 2010;20(11):797–803. https://doi.org/10.1016/j.annepidem.2010.05.012.
41. Matricardi PM, Kleine-Tebbe J, Hoffmann HJ, et al. EAACI molecular allergology user's guide. Pediatr Allergy Immunol. 2016;27(Suppl 23):1–250. https://doi.org/10.1111/pai.12563.
42. Luengo O, Cardona V. Component resolved diagnosis: when should it be used? Clin Transl Allergy. 2014;4:28. https://doi.org/10.1186/2045-7022-4-28.
43. Carlson G, Coop C. Pollen food allergy syndrome (PFAS): a review of current available literature. Ann Allergy Asthma Immunol. 2019;123(4):359–65. https://doi.org/10.1016/j.anai.2019.07.022.
44. Klemans RJB, Otte D, Knol M, et al. The diagnostic value of specific IgE to Ara h 2 to predict peanut allergy in children is comparable to a validated and updated diagnostic prediction model. J Allergy Clin Immunol. 2013;131(1):157–63. https://doi.org/10.1016/j.jaci.2012.08.010.
45. Martín-Muñoz MF, Diaz-Perales A, Cannabal J, Quirce S. Anaphylaxis to hidden potato allergens in a peach and egg allergic boy. Eur Ann Allergy Clin Immunol. 2017;49(1):45–8.
46. Heaps A, Carter S, Selwood C, et al. The utility of the ISAC allergen array in the investigation of idiopathic anaphylaxis. Clin Exp Immunol. 2014;177(2):483–90. https://doi.org/10.1111/cei.12334.
47. Sahiner UM, Yavuz ST, Buyuktiryaki B, et al. Serum basal tryptase levels in healthy children: correlation between age and gender. Allergy Asthma Proc. 2014;35(5):404–8. https://doi.org/10.2500/aap.2014.35.3769.
48. Michel M, Klingebiel C, Vitte J. Tryptase in type I hypersensitivity. Ann Allergy Asthma Immunol. 2023;130(2):169–77. https://doi.org/10.1016/j.anai.2022.08.996.
49. Valent P, Bonadonna P, Hartmann K, et al. Why the 20% + 2 tryptase formula is a diagnostic gold standard for severe systemic mast cell activation and mast cell activation syndrome. Int Arch Allergy Immunol. 2019;180(1):44–51. https://doi.org/10.1159/000501079.

50. Santos AF, Douiri A, Bécares N, et al. Basophil activation test discriminates between allergy and tolerance in peanut-sensitized children. J Allergy Clin Immunol. 2014;134(3):645–52. https://doi.org/10.1016/j.jaci.2014.04.039.
51. Knol EF, Mul FP, Jansen H, Calafat J, Roos D. Monitoring human basophil activation via CD63 monoclonal antibody 435. J Allergy Clin Immunol. 1991;88(3 Pt 1):328–38. https://doi.org/10.1016/0091-6749(91)90094-5.
52. Santos AF, Alpan O, Hoffmann HJ. Basophil activation test: mechanisms and considerations for use in clinical trials and clinical practice. Allergy. 2021;76(8):2420–32. https://doi.org/10.1111/all.14747.
53. Ansotegui IJ, Melioli G, Canonica GW, et al. IgE allergy diagnostics and other relevant tests in allergy, a World Allergy Organization position paper. World Allergy Organ J. 2020;13(2):100080. https://doi.org/10.1016/j.waojou.2019.100080.
54. Dordal MT, Lluch-Bernal M, Sánchez MC, et al. Allergen-specific nasal provocation testing: review by the rhinoconjunctivitis committee of the Spanish Society of Allergy and Clinical Immunology. J Investig Allergol Clin Immunol. 2011;21(1):1–12; quiz follow 12.
55. Augé J, Vent J, Agache I, et al. EAACI position paper on the standardization of nasal allergen challenges. Allergy. 2018;73(8):1597–608. https://doi.org/10.1111/all.13416.
56. Jacobs RL, Harper N, He W, et al. Responses to ragweed pollen in a pollen challenge chamber versus seasonal exposure identify allergic rhinoconjunctivitis endotypes. J Allergy Clin Immunol. 2012;130(1):122–127.e8. https://doi.org/10.1016/j.jaci.2012.03.031.
57. Developing drug products for treatment guidance for industry. U.S. Food and Drug Administration. 2020. https://www.fda.gov/regulatory-information/search-fda-guidance-documents/allergic-rhinitis-developing-drug-products-treatment-guidance-industry. Accessed 24 July 2023.
58. Committee for Medicinal Products for Human Use (CHMP). Guideline on the clinical development of products for specific immunotherapy for the treatment of allergic diseases. November 2008
59. Crapo RO, Casaburi R, Coates AL, et al. Guidelines for methacholine and exercise challenge testing-1999. This official statement of the American Thoracic Society was adopted by the ATS Board of Directors, July 1999. Am J Respir Crit Care Med. 2000;161(1):309–29. https://doi.org/10.1164/ajrccm.161.1.ats11-99.
60. Hallstrand TS, Leuppi JD, Joos G, et al. ERS technical standard on bronchial challenge testing: pathophysiology and methodology of indirect airway challenge testing. Eur Respir J. 2018;52(5):1801033. https://doi.org/10.1183/13993003.01033-2018.
61. Meng Y, Wang Y, Lou H, et al. Specific immunoglobulin E in nasal secretions for the diagnosis of local allergic rhinitis. Rhinology. 2019;57(4):313–20. https://doi.org/10.4193/Rhin18.292.
62. Rondón C, Eguíluz-Gracia I, Shamji MH, et al. IgE test in secretions of patients with respiratory allergy. Curr Allergy Asthma Rep. 2018;18(12):67. https://doi.org/10.1007/s11882-018-0821-7.
63. Vanderhaegen T, Gengler I, Dendooven A, Chenivesse C, Lefèvre G, Mortuaire G. Eosinophils in the field of nasal polyposis: towards a better understanding of biologic therapies. Clinic Rev Allerg Immunol. 2022;62(1):90–102. https://doi.org/10.1007/s12016-021-08844-7.
64. Bystrom J, Amin K, Bishop-Bailey D. Analysing the eosinophil cationic protein—a clue to the function of the eosinophil granulocyte. Respir Res. 2011;12(1):1–20. https://doi.org/10.1186/1465-9921-12-10.

Smell Testing: Purpose, Procedure, Interpretation

18

Ali Türkcan, Nuray Bayar Muluk, and Philippe Rombaux

18.1 Introduction

Deterioration of the sense of smell can be either quantitative (a reduction in intensity) or qualitative (a change in quality or degree of distortion). To a greater extent than via history, olfactory testing can reveal quantitative impairment (such as distortion) [1].

Clinical olfactory testing presents a patient with an olfactory probe to his or her nose and records the individual's reaction. This type of evaluation is sometimes called "psychophysical testing" [2, 3]. Patients undergoing olfactory testing should be cooperative, able to follow directions, and articulate their preferences [2]. Odor identification and odor discrimination tests are examples of suprathreshold olfactory testing. Olfactory threshold tests fall into a similar category. Supranasal tests are more likely to evaluate the central processing of olfactory information. In contrast, odor threshold tests are more likely to evaluate the peripheral olfactory ability (such as the conductive and sensorineural function of the nose) [2, 4]. Consequently, olfactory testing [1] might consist of both odor threshold tests and suprathreshold tests.

A. Türkcan
Department of Otolaryngology, Van Research and Training Hospital, Van, Türkiye

N. Bayar Muluk (✉)
Department of Otorhinolaryngology, Faculty of Medicine, Kırıkkale University, Kırıkkale, Türkiye

P. Rombaux
Department of Otorhinolaryngology, and Institute of Neurosciences, Catholic University of Louvain, Saint Luc University Clinics, Brussels, Belgium
e-mail: Philippe.Rombaux@uclouvain.be

H. Yüksel et al. (eds.), *Pediatric Airway Diseases*, Comprehensive ENT,
https://doi.org/10.1007/978-3-031-74853-0_18

18.2 Possible Olfactory Disorder Diagnosis

18.2.1 Conductive Defects

Many problems with smell may be traced back to inflammation. Some examples include allergic rhinitis, acute rhinitis, and toxic rhinitis (caused by cocaine usage). Despite effective allergic, medicinal, and surgical treatment, the gradual mucosal illness caused by chronic rhinosinusitis frequently results in impaired olfactory function.

The olfactory epithelium may not receive odorants if a mass blocks the nasal cavity. Nasal polyps, inverted papilloma, and other nasal tumors are the most prevalent conditions [5].

Obstruction can also be caused by congenital disabilities, including encephaloceles and dermoid cysts [5].

Hyposmia is caused by decreased or eliminated nasal airflow and is common in patients with a laryngectomy or tracheotomy. Lack of early stimulation of the olfactory system [5] is a possible explanation for long-term difficulties with olfaction in children who have had tracheotomies and are subsequently decannulated.

18.2.2 Defects in the Central Nervous System or the Peripheral Nervous System

Infectious and inflammatory diseases exacerbate central abnormalities in olfaction and transmission. Although a viral URTI can cause a loss of smell because it replaces olfactory neuroepithelium with respiratory epithelium, research suggests that stem cells persist, opening the door to the possibility of olfactory epithelial regeneration in some cases. In these circumstances, restoring the sense of smell might take months, even years, and in rare cases, may never happen at all. The inability to smell is a symptom of several disorders, including multiple sclerosis, Wegener granulomatosis, and sarcoidosis (which affects brain structures). Although chronic rhinosinusitis was formerly assumed to be primarily a conductive problem due to mucosal edema and polyp development, recent research suggests that it also disrupts the neuroepithelium, leading to permanent loss of olfactory receptors due to upregulated apoptosis [5].

18.2.3 Inherited Disorders

Some congenital disorders have been linked to a decline in brain function. Genetic olfactory dysfunction, such as that seen in people with Kallmann syndrome, results from underdevelopment of the olfactory system and hypogonadotropic hypogonadism. One research showed that patients with Kallmann syndrome lacked the vomeronasal organ [5].

18.2.3.1 Hormonal Disturbances

Olfactory function may be impacted by endocrine disorders (such as hypothyroidism, hypoadrenalism, and diabetes mellitus) [5].

18.2.3.2 Systemic and Inhalant Drug Toxicity

Olfactory impairment may be caused by the toxicity of systemic or inhaled medicines (such as aminoglycosides or formaldehyde). Alcohol, nicotine, chemical solvents, and zinc salts applied topically are some drugs and molecules that might affect your sense of smell [6].

18.3 Anatomy of the Olfactory System

The olfactory neuroepithelium is found above the cribriform plate, the superior nasal septum, and the superior-lateral nasal wall of each nasal chamber. In this pseudostratified neuroepithelium, the primary olfactory receptors are located. This region is a thick neural sheet in newborns, but it is interdigitated with respiratory and olfactory tissues in adolescents and adults. Humans' olfactory neuron count declines with aging. The olfactory epithelium is made up of olfactory sensory neurons and includes basal cells that enable regeneration of the epithelium and the olfactory sensory neurons themselves [5, 7].

The ability to smell relies on olfactory receptor cells activated by volatile substances. The olfactory receptors can only be activated if molecules in the air touch them as they travel through the nasal canal on relatively turbulent air currents. Retronasal olfaction refers to the process by which odorants enter the nose from the back, through the nasopharynx, and then travel to the olfactory receptor. Flavor perception while eating and drinking is widely believed to be facilitated by this process. To reach the olfactory receptor [8], odorants must first penetrate the mucosal membrane. The intensity of an aroma is proportional to the time, volume, and speed with which it is inhaled [5].

There is a primary sensory bipolar neuron in each olfactory receptor cell. More than 100 million of these neurons are in the typical nasal cavity. In contrast to other neurons, olfactory neurons are continually produced by the underlying basal cells. Each new receptor cell is created on average every 30–60 days [5].

Each new receptor cell develops connections with mitral and tufted cells in the olfactory bulb [5] via an axon (CN I) sent to the central nervous system.

There is a lengthy central process on the bipolar olfactory neurons and a shorter peripheral process. The mucosal surface is covered in a thick mat of immobile cilia, and the peripheral process continues to the mucosa, where it terminates in an olfactory knob. Odorant interactions are mediated by receptors expressed in the cilia. G-protein coupled receptors (GPCRs) linked to adenylate cyclase comprise the odor receptor protein family. Linda Buck and Richard Axel won the Nobel Prize in 2004 [5] for discovering the genes that encode them in 1991.

The most prominent gene family in the human genome consists of over 900 members. Since each neuron in a mouse only expresses a single gene, odorants are identified by the intricate binding pattern they generate. It is safe to assume the same holds for people. It is fascinating that these genes have been found in unexpected places, including sperm and the digestive tract. Researchers are trying to figure out what these genes do besides aid with smell [8].

When an odorant connects to a receptor, a signaling cascade causes the neuron to depolarize and convey the signal along the neuron's axon. These axons eventually converge within the fila olfactory, a bundle of axons that extends deep into the epithelium [5].

These axons go ipsilaterally to the olfactory bulb via the cribriform plate. The olfactory receptor cells communicate with mitral and tufted cells in the olfactory bulb, clustered in glomeruli structures. Receptor-like neurons generate an early topographical odorant map by having their axon terminals connect inside the same glomeruli. The chemical makeup of an odor is assumed to trigger a specific set of odorant receptors. In response, the olfactory bulb's associated glomeruli get excited, resulting in a distinct excitation pattern for each odorant [5].

The olfactory bulb's central transmitter neurons are the glomerular cells. Axons from these cells travel to the olfactory cortex, which is divided into five parts, including [1] the anterior olfactory nucleus, connecting the two olfactory bulbs through the anterior commissure, [2] the olfactory tubercle, [3] the pyriform cortex, which is the central olfactory discrimination region, [4] the cortical nucleus of the amygdala, and [5] the entorhinal area, which projects to the hippocampus [5].

No thalamic relay is required for the olfactory pathway's cortical projections to occur. The conscious experience of scents likely involves relays from the olfactory tubercle and the pyriform cortex, which project to other olfactory cortical areas and the medial dorsal nucleus of the thalamus [5].

On the other hand, the limbic system's entorhinal region and the amygdala's cortical nucleus may have a role in the hedonic or emotional aspects of smells. When a highly unpleasant odorant is introduced, regional cerebral blood flow (as assessed by positron emission tomography) increases dramatically in the amygdala, and this rise is correlated with subjective assessments of perceived aversiveness [5].

The vomeronasal organ (VNO), or the Jacobson organ, is a membrane structure found on both sides of the nose, nestled deep inside the nasal respiratory mucosa and close to the septal perichondria. When the septal cartilage meets the bony septum, 2 cm from the nose, its opening may be seen in the nasal vestibule in 91–97% of adult individuals. Postnatal humans have not been discovered to have axons extending from the VNO [5], as seen in lower species.

18.4 Odor Threshold Tests

Odor threshold studies use the progressive presentation of phenyl ethyl alcohol or n-butanol probes at varying concentrations, sometimes in combination with odorless probes ("blanks") [2, 3]. Patients are required to respond (= forced-choice process) [2] even if they are unsure about whether or not they have experienced an odor. Once the threshold for detecting the odor probe has been crossed, the odor concentration gradually declines and increases throughout several iterations [3]. By averaging the reversals, as is done here, dependability is improved [3]. The Snap and Sniff [9] and the pen-like odor dispensing device [10] threshold tests are often employed in clinical practice.

18.5 Tests of Smell Sensitivity Above the Threshold

Suprathreshold testing employs patient-perceivable doses of odorants. The University of Pennsylvania Smell Identification Test (UPSIT) and odor identification tests using pen-like odor dispensing devices [11, 12] are the most frequently utilized suprathreshold tests. The forced-choice approach involves providing the patient with a list of possible responses in written or visual form and then having them smell an odor probe and select the one they believe is correct. The test's outcome is reported as the total number of correct responses. Due to cultural differences, the validity and reliability of the reported scents must be verified for each community studied [3]. Most of these exams come with normative data that may be used to place a person in a percentile range based on their gender and age [2, 3]. Odor discrimination tests, such as those done using pens that dispense odors, are another type of suprathreshold test. The patient is given a series of odor probes and instructed to memorize and discriminate between them; however, they are not required to provide particular names to the scents they smell. Once again, the test's outcome is recorded as the total number of correct responses. Compared to olfactory threshold testing, suprathreshold tests need higher levels of cognitive capacity, namely in executive function and semantic memory [13].

Hedonic value tests are another kind of suprathreshold olfactory test [2, 3]. These procedures incorporate emotional factors since they determine whether or not a specific odor is liked or disliked. In the medical field, hedonic tests are infrequently used [1].

18.6 Tests to Determine Gustatory Abilities

When patients experience a loss of smell, they typically also experience a loss of taste [2, 3]. This is because the retronasal pathway allows volatiles from meals to reach the olfactory receptors and trigger the olfactory receptors on the olfactory epithelium. Smells associated with food are misinterpreted as "taste," even when gustatory skill is unaffected. So, screening for gustatory functioning, including liquids applied to the tongue or the taste strip test [14, 15], should be a part of olfactory testing. The patient is asked to report if the probe feels salty, sour, bitter, or sweet when it is dropped or placed on the tongue. The score on the exam is determined by the total number of correct responses [1].

18.7 Personal Evaluation of Smell

The influence of olfactory cues (or the lack thereof) on our actions may not always be evident [2, 3]. Furthermore, patient self-assessments are negatively associated with objective tests of their sense of smell [16, 17]. However, a scale from zero (none) to ten (superb) may be employed for subjective reporting of olfactory abilities, such as in epidemiological investigations [18].

18.8 Clinical Measurement of Olfaction

When chemosensory dysfunction is the primary complaint, it is crucial to quantify the degree to which smell and taste are impaired. Sensory testing is performed primarily to evaluate chemosensory impairment [5].

Some commercially accessible tests aim to standardize and streamline the arduous clinical examination process. Testing one nostril at a time may be more successful in detecting an olfactory disease [19], even though it is common practice to test both simultaneously to save time. This is in contrast to other sensory systems, where testing in just one direction is routine for identifying pathology.

There are now olfactory function tests available that can evaluate a person's olfactory capacity by gauging their threshold for detecting and identifying odors. The butanol threshold test (Sensonics, Inc., www.sensonics.com), the University of Pennsylvania Smell Identification Test (UPSIT), and the Sniffin' Sticks test (Burghart Messtechnik GmbH, www.burghart-mt.de) are also examples of such assessments. Odor recognition tests and electrocorticographic (ECoG) measurements of the brain have been utilized in laboratories to assess abnormal smell in patients with neurological disorders [5].

18.8.1 Butanol Threshold Test

The butanol threshold test is a forced-choice procedure wherein one sniff vial contains an aqueous concentration of butyl alcohol, and the other has water. The patient is asked to choose which bottle contains the odorant; this is done independently for each nostril. If they get even one of the choices wrong, the concentration of butanol in the bottle is increased by a factor of 3, and so on, until they either get five answers right or are unable to choose the bottle containing 4% butanol.

The detection threshold is the lowest butanol concentration at which the patient responded affirmatively on five occasions. The patient's point is compared to that of a normative sample of subjects using the scoring system [5].

18.8.1.1 The Penn State University Odor Identification Exam

The UPSIT uses a scratch-and-sniff style with 40 microencapsulated scents and four different response options. The individual is given the exam alone and told to make an educated estimate if they get a question wrong [5].

Patients with anosmia often have a 10% accurate rate or lower (10/40). The data is examined by comparing the test results to age- and gender-specific norms. The reliability of this exam across administrations is relatively high [5].

A table compares scores from different patient groups, such as those with multiple sclerosis, those with Korsakoff syndrome, and those pretending to have anosmia. Those in the second category routinely post-test scores much below what would be predicted by random chance [5].

18.8.2 Cross-Cultural Smell Identification Test

A UPSIT variation that may be administered in 5 min was proposed for a speedy evaluation of smell. Input on odor recognition from several cultures went into creating the Cross-Cultural Smell Identification Test (CC-SIT), which consists of 12 items. These nations include China, Colombia, France, Germany, Italy, Japan, Russia, and Sweden.

Bananas, chocolate, cinnamon, gasoline, lemon, onion, paint thinner, pineapple, rose, soap, smoke, and turpentine are some of the odorants that may be found. Representatives from all countries most commonly detected these odorants [5].

Due to its speed and accuracy, this test is an excellent replacement for more time-consuming methods of assessing olfactory function in a clinical context.

The short duration of the test reduces its ability to pick up on small shifts in olfactory function [5].

18.8.3 Sniffin' Sticks

Three aspects of smell are tested using a set of reusable pens with built-in odor dispensers: (1) odor threshold using a single staircase method, (2) odor discrimination using forced choice between 3 of 16 commonly used odorants, and (3) odor identification using multiple forced choice from four verbal items. To get a complete picture of how well your sense of smell is working, add up your scores from all three tests to get a total score out of 5.

18.8.4 Olfactory-Evoked Response (Usually Reserved for Research Studies)

Electrodes placed on the scalp (EEG) and the eye (electrooculogram) measure olfactory-evoked potentials, normalizing the patient's sensitivity to eye movements. Maintaining focus requires a visual tracking job, but white noise played through headphones covers up any audible cues [5, 6].

Carbon dioxide (which has no smell but stimulates the trigeminal nerve) or hydrogen sulfide is supplied to the nose in a steady stream via an olfactometer. The initial negative peak, denoted by N1, is followed by a second positive trough, represented by P2. These two numbers (both 5) are used to calculate latencies.

The clinical use of olfactory evoked responses as a standard diagnostic tool is limited. The UPSIT outperformed olfactory evoked responses in identifying abnormalities in individuals with neurologic illness [5].

The authors have shown that the self-administered UPSIT test helps measure olfactory function in a busy clinical practice. A simple screening test with a typical alcohol pad can be performed instead if the olfactory tests mentioned above are unavailable. The patient is given the contents of the envelope after opening it. The pad is placed at the level of the umbilicus and is gradually pushed closer to the nose while the patient's eyes are closed. The patient must let the tester know when alcohol is discovered again. Patients with hyposmia [5] can be identified by a pad placement less than 20 cm from their nose.

References

1. Kronenbuerger M, Pilgramm M. Olfactory testing. In: StatPearls. Treasure Island, FL: StatPearls Publishing; 2023. https://www.ncbi.nlm.nih.gov/books/NBK565861/. Accessed 23 Oct 2023.
2. Hummel T, Whitcroft KL, Andrews P, Altundag A, Cinghi C, Costanzo RM, Damm M, Frasnelli J, Gudziol H, Gupta N, Haehner A, Holbrook E, Hong SC, Hornung D, Hüttenbrink KB, Kamel R, Kobayashi M, Konstantinidis I, Landis BN, Leopold DA, Macchi A, Miwa T, Moesges R, Mullol J, Mueller CA, Ottaviano G, Passali GC, Philpott C, Pinto JM, Ramakrishnan VJ, Rombaux P, Roth Y, Schlosser RA, Shu B, Soler G, Stjärne P, Stuck BA, Vodicka J, Welge-Luessen A. Position paper on olfactory dysfunction. Rhinology. 2016;56(1):1–30.
3. Doty RL. Psychophysical testing of smell and taste function. Handb Clin Neurol. 2019;164:229–46.
4. Whitcroft KL, Cuevas M, Haehner A, Hummel T. Patterns of olfactory impairment reflect underlying disease etiology. Laryngoscope. 2017;127(2):291–5.
5. Holbrook EH. Disorders of taste and smell. In: Meyers AD editor. Medscape. 2022. https://emedicine.medscape.com/article/861242-overview#a4. Accessed 23 Oct 2023.
6. Tuccori M, Lapi F, Testi A, Ruggiero E, Moretti U, Vannacci A, et al. Drug-induced taste and smell alterations: a case/non-case evaluation of an Italian database of spontaneous adverse drug reaction reporting. Drug Saf. 2011;34(10):849–59.
7. Schwob JE, Jang W, Holbrook EH, Lin B, Herrick DB, Peterson JN, et al. Stem and progenitor cells of the mammalian olfactory epithelium: taking Poietic license. J Comp Neurol. 2017;525(4):1034–54.
8. Patel RM, Pinto JM. Olfaction: anatomy, physiology, and disease. Clin Anat. 2014;27(1):54–60.
9. Doty RL, Wylie C, Potter M, Beston R, Cope B, Majam K. Clinical validation of the olfactory detection threshold module of the Snap & Sniff® olfactory test system. Int Forum Allergy Rhinol. 2019;9(9):986–92.
10. Hummel T, Sekinger B, Wolf SR, Pauli E, Kobal G. 'Sniffin' sticks': olfactory performance assessed by the combined testing of odor identification, odor discrimination and olfactory threshold. Chem Senses. 1997;22(1):39–52.
11. Doty RL, Shaman P, Dann M. Development of the University of Pennsylvania Smell Identification Test: a standardized microencapsulated test of olfactory function. Physiol Behav. 1984;32(3):489–502.
12. Kobal G, Hummel T, Sekinger B, Barz S, Roscher S, Wolf S. "Sniffin' sticks": screening of olfactory performance. Rhinology. 1996;34(4):222–6.
13. Hedner M, Larsson M, Arnold N, Zucco GM, Hummel T. Cognitive factors in odor detection, odor discrimination, and odor identification tasks. J Clin Exp Neuropsychol. 2010;32(10):1062–7.
14. Hummel T, Landis BN, Hüttenbrink KB. Smell and taste disorders. GMS Curr Top Otorhinolaryngol Head Neck Surg. 2011;10:Doc04.

15. Mueller C, Kallert S, Renner B, Stiassny K, Temmel AF, Hummel T, Kobal G. Quantitative assessment of gustatory function in a clinical context using impregnated "taste strips". Rhinology. 2003;41(1):2–6.
16. Adams DR, Wroblewski KE, Kern DW, Kozloski MJ, Dale W, McClintock MK, Pinto JM. Factors associated with inaccurate self-reporting of olfactory dysfunction in older US adults. Chem Senses. 2017;42(3):223–31.
17. Nordin S, Monsch AU, Murphy C. Unawareness of smell loss in normal aging and Alzheimer's disease: discrepancy between self-reported and diagnosed smell sensitivity. J Gerontol B Psychol Sci Soc Sci. 1995;50(4):P187–92.
18. Hoffman HJ, Ishii EK, MacTurk RH. Age-related changes in the prevalence of smell/taste problems among the United States adult population. Results of the 1994 disability supplement to the National Health Interview Survey (NHIS). Ann N Y Acad Sci. 1998;855:716–22.
19. Poupon D, Hummel T, Haehner A, Welge-Luessen A, Frasnelli J. Nostril differences in the olfactory performance in health and disease. Chem Senses. 2017;42(8):625–34.

Taste Testing: Purpose, Procedure, Interpretation

19

Ramazan Öcal, Nuray Bayar Muluk, and Desiderio Passali

19.1 Introduction

Several factors can contribute to adult taste and smell disorders, including metabolic and endocrine abnormalities, neurological disorders, inflammatory conditions of the nasal passages and paranasal sinuses, head trauma and surgery, infections, chemical exposures, medications, and normal aging. Flavor perception can be significantly impacted by problems with taste and smell, which can lower quality of life and make it difficult to obtain enough nourishment [1].

19.2 Definitions

Normogeusia and normosmia relate to having typical gustatory and olfactory capabilities. Flavor and odor problems include [1].

19.2.1 Taste Dysfunction Abnormalities

Disturbances of taste perception include the following:

R. Öcal
Department of Otolaryngology-Head and Neck Surgery, Faculty of Medicine, Ankara Research and Training Hospital, Health Sciences University, Ankara, Türkiye

N. Bayar Muluk (✉)
Department of Otorhinolaryngology, Faculty of Medicine, Kırıkkale University, Kırıkkale, Türkiye

D. Passali
Department of Medical, Surgical and Neuroscience Sciences, and Department of Otorhinolaryngology, University of Siena, Siena, Italy

H. Yüksel et al. (eds.), *Pediatric Airway Diseases*, Comprehensive ENT, https://doi.org/10.1007/978-3-031-74853-0_19

- *Hypogeusia*, in which something that would generally taste good feels bad;
- *Ageusia*, in which taste function is absent;
- *Dysgeusia*, in which taste sensations (of sweetness, sourness, saltiness, bitterness, or metallicity) change in response to a tastant stimulus.
- *Aliageusia*, in which something that would typically taste good feels bad;
- *Parosmia*, Abhorrent odor perception either with an odorant stimulus (troposmia or smell distortion) or without an odorant stimulus (phantosmia).
- *Dysosmia* is a general term for abnormalities in olfactory perception.

It includes conditions such as hyposmia (reduced smell function) and anosmia (the inability to detect odors), as well as parosmia (the perception of unpleasant odors in response to an odorant stimulus (troposmia or smell distortion) or in the absence of such a stimulus (phantosmia)).

19.3 Anatomy and Physiology of Taste

Different receptors and cerebral pathways are involved in gustation and olfaction, respectively; hence, their physiology and anatomy are distinct. Efferent taste, olfactory input, and other sensory data are necessary for accurate flavor perception [1].

The sense of taste is triggered when a chemical or other stimulus activates taste receptor cells, sending signals to the brain via afferent nerves [1].

Information regarding tastants (taste-stimulating chemicals or substances) is received by taste receptor cells (neuroepithelial cells) and transmitted to the central nervous system via afferent neurons. The typical lifespan of a taste receptor cell is 10 days [2].

The tongue's dorsal and lateral surfaces, as well as the soft palate, uvula, larynx, pharynx, epiglottis, and esophagus [3], are home to taste buds, each of which contains approximately 50–150 taste receptor cells. Taste pores, tiny apertures in the epithelial surface, are how tastants travel to the receptor cells within the taste buds.

Papillae are the structures that house taste buds on the tongue. The three types of papillae are as follows [1]:

The fungiform papillae can be seen throughout the first two-thirds of the tongue. The average number of papillae on a human tongue is 190, although this can range from 184 to 198. Eighty percent of the tongue's fungiform taste buds are found in the first 2 cm [4].

The tongue's foliate papillae are found on its dorsal and lateral posterior surfaces.

These papillae, known as the circumvallate papillae, are found toward the back of the tongue.

Twenty taste buds are packed into each fungiform papillae, whereas hundreds are packed into each circumvallate and foliate papillae [5].

The vagus nerve (cranial nerve X), glossopharyngeal nerve (cranial nerve IX), and facial nerve (cranial nerve VII) all provide innervation to areas of the brain that contain taste buds [1].

The chorda tympani is a branch of the facial nerve that supplies sensation to the front two-thirds of the tongue. The superficial petrosal nerve, another facial nerve branch, provides feeling to the palate.

The glossopharyngeal nerve supplies the back of the tongue with sensation.

The vagus nerve supplies the vocal cords and pharynx.

The solitary tract nucleus in the medulla is the site of synaptic connections made by primary afferent taste neurons. The primary gustatory cortex and thalamus receive taste information [6]. Due to the involvement of numerous cranial nerves in gustatory function [1], ageusia (total loss of taste) cases are sporadic.

The subjective gustation experience is influenced by more than just the afferent taste innervation of the tongue and taste buds. Other sensations, such as the burning and irritation given by hot peppers and the odors of ammonia, are accounted for by the branches of the trigeminal nerve (cranial nerve V), which innervate the inside of the mouth and nasal cavities. The nasal cavity and oropharynx are also supplied with sensory nerves from the anterior ethmoid, nasopalatine, posterior palatine, and buccal regions [1].

The tastants must pass through the mucous layer above the taste receptor neurons, and saliva plays a crucial part in this process. Water-soluble taste chemicals are easily transported to receptor cells, but insoluble tastants require carrier proteins [1].

By activating protein-coupled receptors, tastant administration leads to membrane alterations that open ion channels and neuron depolarization [7].

If there is an aberration in any of these components, it might lead to alterations in gustatory function. Causes of aberrant taste include abnormalities in the taste cell receptor proteins or ion channels [8–10] and changes in the makeup of saliva or mucous around the taste buds [11–14].

Sweet, sour, salty, and bitter are the four traditional taste qualities mentioned and commonly evaluated. In addition, umami (the glutamate taste) is discussed [15–17]. Due to the intricacy of the umami taste system, it has traditionally been more practical to examine only the original four taste qualities; however, umami is sometimes included in regular clinical evaluations of gustatory function [1].

19.4 Etiology of Gustatory Dysfunction

Many things that people think are flavor flaws are, in fact, the result of a problem with their sense of smell. The flavor is a multisensory experience originating from the food's aroma, taste, texture, and warmth. When food is introduced to the mouth, it stimulates several different taste buds [18].

Tongue movement can help spread the flavor over more taste buds, improving the overall flavor. Taste is the sense that adaptation has the most significant impact [18].

Taste dysfunction can have various causes, but the most common causes include a previous upper respiratory tract infection (URTI), a head injury, or idiopathic causes.

Impairment of gustation can be caused by damage to any part of the gustatory system, including the mucosa, taste buds, unmyelinated nerves, cranial nerves, or the brain stem [18].

Disorders of the oral cavity and mucosa, such as infections, inflammation, and radiation-induced mucositis, can diminish the ability to taste. Since taste buds are typically considered radioresistant [18], the microvilli of the taste buds are likely to be the site of harm during irradiation.

Hypogeusia and cacogeusia are often the result of neglectful dental care. Secondary taste bud involvement is a potential cause of taste abnormalities caused by infections with viruses, bacteria, fungi, and parasites [18].

It is not the loss of taste buds that causes average aging-related taste loss [19, 20] but alterations in taste cell membranes, including altered activity of ion channels and receptors.

Over two hundred drugs [21] have been linked to impaired taste. This is especially important for clinicians to remember when dealing with patients taking many medications.

Loss of appetite and loss of taste bud function are common side effects of head and neck cancer treatment [18].

Dentures and other palatal prostheses can reduce your ability to detect sour and bitter flavors, and cleaning your tongue can dull your sense of taste [18].

Taste can be temporarily or permanently altered through surgery. When the tongue or other parts of the mouth are removed, most often for cancer treatment, the number of taste buds in the mouth is reduced. Chemotherapy and radiation can impair one's sense of taste by damaging taste receptors and reducing saliva production. Temporary dysgeusia can occur after otologic surgery if the chorda tympani nerve is stretched or cut. Alternate innervation from the otic ganglion to the geniculate ganglion via the more significant superficial petrosal nerve [18] means that even a bilateral injury may not produce permanent taste abnormalities.

The senses of smell and taste could be negatively affected by gastric bypass. A total of 73% and 42% of 103 patients in a study by Graham et al. who underwent Roux-en-Y gastric bypass reported changes in taste and smell, respectively [3]. In contrast, patients appear to have less olfactory loss if the bypass is performed laparoscopically [22].

Flavor deviations are associated with nutritional deficits. Reduced amounts of zinc, copper, and nickel have been linked to unpleasant taste sensations. Anorexia, malabsorption, and excessive urine loss contribute to nutritional deficits [18].

Taste and olfactory abnormalities are often linked to endocrine issues. Sensitivity to taste may be diminished by diabetes mellitus, hypogonadism, Sjögren syndrome, and pseudohypoparathyroidism and enhanced by hypothyroidism and adrenal cortical insufficiency. Taste is also affected by hormonal shifts during menstruation and pregnancy [18].

A more significant detection threshold for glutamic acid and hydrochloride is observed in AIDS patients [23], and AIDS patients frequently report changes in their sense of taste.

A person's sense of taste might be affected by their genes. An inherited feature is the capacity to detect the bitter flavor of phenylthiourea and other molecules containing a -N-C = group. Caffeine, potassium chloride (KCl), and saccharin are all seen as more bitter by phenylthiourea tasters, according to studies. The inability to taste is a severe symptom of type I familial dysautonomia (Riley–Day syndrome) [18].

Taste sensitivity can be impaired by injuries to the central nervous system or peripheral nerves, such as in multiple sclerosis, facial paralysis, or thalamic or uncal lesions.

Diseases such as lichen planus, aglycogeusia, Sjögren syndrome, renal failure with uremia and dialysis, erythema multiforme, geographic tongue, and cirrhosis can all have an impact on a person's sense of taste [18].

19.4.1 Taste Dysfunction

Due to the redundancy in taste neuroanatomy, ageusia is uncommon, although dysgeusia and hypogeusia are more common [20]. Dysgeusia and hypogeusia can occur when there is a problem with the salivary glands, carrier proteins, or taste receptors [1], all of which are necessary for normal gustatory function.

- **Infectious and Inflammatory Causes**
- Dysgeusia and hypogeusia can be caused by infections and inflammatory disorders everywhere in the oropharynx, including the teeth, larynx, throat, tongue, taste buds, and salivary glands [1].
- **Infectious causes** [1]:
  - Dysgeusia may be caused by gingivitis, oropharyngeal candidiasis (thrush), or dental caries. Oropharyngeal infections can impair Gustatory function, reducing the blood supply to the tongue and taste buds. In addition, genetic polymorphisms in taste receptor proteins, which alter taste sensitivity and preferences for sweet tastes, may predispose individuals to developing dental caries by causing an increase in sugary food consumption [24].
  - In the context of influenza-like diseases, hypogeusia and dysgeusia can occur, possibly due to taste pore rupture and inflammatory cell infiltration into the lamina propria [25].
  - Ageusia and anosmia are often the first signs of coronavirus disease 2019 (COVID-19) in patients, appearing either before or after the beginning of other symptoms [26–30]. Sixty-three to eighty-five percent of patients experience taste and smell disturbances, with most experiencing symptoms within 4 days after becoming unwell [31–34].
- **Inflammatory causes:**
- Hypogeusia and dysgeusia can be caused by inflammation of the salivary glands, as seen in Sjögren's syndrome, other autoimmune illnesses, or systemic radioiodine therapy [35, 36]. Additionally, xerostomia (dry mouth) may boost the danger of tooth decay [37].

- If the tongue is inflamed (glossitis), the taste pores that allow tastants to reach the taste buds may close. Atrophic glossitis, where many or all of the lingual papillae and taste buds are lost, can be brought back to health by taking vitamin B-12 supplements [1].
- Direct harm to taste cells and damage to taste buds and salivary glands [38] can result from radiation therapy (or accidental exposure to ionizing radiation) to the head and neck, leading to impaired taste. Oropharyngeal infections, made more likely by reduced saliva production, can further diminish gustatory function [39]. Radiation dosage to the tongue significantly correlates with the severity of taste impairment. Since taste cells are constantly regenerated, taste impairment improves over time once radiation therapy is finished [38].
- Hypogeusia and dysgeusia can be caused by acid reflux, specifically laryngopharyngeal reflux [40–42], which can alter one's taste preferences and sensitivity [43].
- Direct tastant activity, effects on saliva, taste receptor cells, peripheral neurons, the central nervous system (CNS), and zinc levels, among other unknown products [1, 2], are just some of the processes by which medications might alter gustatory function.
- **Drugs**
- Some drugs that may cause adverse reactions in the sense of taste include [1]:
- Treatments for dysgeusia include the following:
  - ACE inhibitors, ARBs, dipyridamole, nitroglycerin, vandetanib, and vismodegib
  - Acetazolamide and methylphenidate for bitter dysgeusia
  - Drugs *such as allopurinol, baclofen, beta-lactam antibiotics (such amoxicillin and cephalexin), clarithromycin, metronidazole, ethambutol, flurazepam, interferon-gamma, levamisole, lithium, tetracycline, tocainide, and intravenous lidocaine have been shown to alleviate symptoms of metallic dysgeusia.*
  - Hypogeusia (to one or more tastants) or ageusia—angiotensin-converting enzyme (ACE) inhibitors, angiotensin receptor blockers (ARBs), amiloride, amphotericin B, amrinone, bleomycin, carbamazepine, carboplatin, cisplatin, chlorhexidine mouth rinse, dicyclomine, diltiazem.
  - Chemical, toxic, and metal exposure often result in dysgeusia and phantogeusia; ageusia is unusual [1].
- **Exposure to chemicals, toxins, and metals**—Exposure to chemicals, toxins, and metals typically causes dysgeusia and phantogeusia; ageusia is rare [1].
  - Taste bud morphology [44] and peripheral and central nervous system (CNS) signal transmission [45] can be altered by acute exposure to organophosphates, leading to impaired gustatory function. Ingesting contaminated air, water, or food exposes taste buds to pesticides.
  - Mercury, copper, zinc, chromium, arsenic, and lead are only some of the metals and metalloids that have been linked to altered taste. All seven adults reported a sweet metallic taste in a case series of occupational acute lead poisoning [46]. In addition to respiratory and systemic problems [47], a sweet,

metallic taste is a defining feature of metal-fume fever (occupational exposure to zinc oxide fumes in brass and steel foundry workers and welders).
- Short-term dysgeusia has been linked to acute solvent exposure [48, 49].

Due to the redundancy of the nerves involved in taste function, cases of complete ageusia caused by nerve injury are sporadic; similarly, chances of profound hypogeusia in the absence of substantial central neurologic impairment are equally uncommon. For instance, patients with a history of head trauma were shown to have a prevalence of 19% for dysgeusia but just 2% for total loss of taste [50].

However, mild hypogeusia is more common in the presence of nerve injury and is associated with regionalized loss of taste. For instance, the anterior two-thirds of the tongue on the affected side can be affected by taste loss or dysgeusia if the chorda tympani nerve is injured [51]. Third, molar extractions are associated with chorda tympani and lingual nerve risks [52, 53]. The lingual branch of the glossopharyngeal nerve [54] can be injured during bronchoscopy, laryngoscopy, or tonsillectomy, leading to impaired taste.

Zinc deficiency is linked to dysgeusia and hypogeusia [55, 56], and vitamin B-12 deficiency can impair taste function by inducing atrophic glossitis. Patients with taste disturbances at risk for zinc deficiency should have their zinc levels checked [57], including those with malnutrition, malabsorption, Crohn's disease, chronic liver disease, diabetes mellitus, sickle cell disease, and end-stage kidney disease.

Dysgeusia has been linked to several metabolic and endocrine problems, such as early onset polycystic kidney disease (ESKD), hypothyroidism, and diabetes mellitus (types I and II) [45].

Multiple factors contribute to the taste changes seen in ESKD [58, 59]. Fewer fungiform taste buds have been linked to ESKD [60], and hemodialysis patients with ESKD have lower saliva production and a different saliva composition [61]. Zinc deficiency may also occur in hemodialysis patients [62].

- Dysgeusia and hypogeusia are the most common taste impairments in diabetic patients, but other states exist. Patients with diabetes may experience hypogeusia to sweet taste, characterized by an elevated taste threshold for sweet flavors relative to healthy controls [63]. Dysgeusia may also be influenced by diabetic neuropathy [64].
- Dysgeusia may be related to hypothyroidism. In a cohort of 18 people with untreated primary hypothyroidism, for instance, more than 80% were found to show hypogeusia to one or more taste stimuli [65], even though only 50% of those people believed their sense of taste was impaired or altered. Multiple factors, including changes in saliva production, mucous membrane, and taste bud shape, likely contribute to taste disruption in hypothyroidism. However, the taste disturbance disappears if thyroid function is restored to normal [66].

Multiple sclerosis [67, 68], Parkinson's disease [69], and Alzheimer's disease [70] have all been linked to hypogeusia or dysgeusia as a symptom of their respective diseases.

Unknown in origin, burning mouth syndrome (BMS) primarily affects post-menopausal women and is characterized by chronic, fluctuating, burning intraoral discomfort without external evidence of inflammation [71, 72]. The exact pathophysiologic process is unclear, but it is thought to be related to peripheral and central nervous system dysfunction.

19.4.2 COVID-19

The 2019 coronavirus illness (COVID-19) is characterized by anosmia and dysgeusia. Anosmia, hyposmia, and dysgeusia should raise suspicion of COVID-19 infection, according to the American Academy of Otolaryngology-Head and Neck Surgery (AAO-HNS) [73–75]. This is especially true in patients who do not have other respiratory diseases, such as allergic rhinitis, acute rhinosinusitis, or chronic rhinosinusitis. After exposure to the COVID-19 virus (i.e., severe acute respiratory syndrome coronavirus 2 (SARS-CoV-2)), the CDC has added "new loss of taste or smell" to the list of symptoms that may appear 2–14 days later [76]. The WHO has included the inability to detect odors or flavors in the list of less common symptoms associated with COVID-19 [77].

In a study of 103 individuals with COVID-19, Speth et al. [78] showed that olfactory impairment was present in 61.2% of cases, with onset at median infection day 3. Loss of taste correlated strongly with the severity of olfactory impairment. Patients also reported significantly worse shortness of breath when they had olfactory impairment. Researchers also discovered that olfactory impairment was more common in women [78] and decreased with age.

Aziz et al. [79] conducted a literature review and found that over 50% of COVID-19 patients have impaired taste sense using pooled analysis; however, the frequency may be significantly more significant due to underreporting [79].

19.5 Taste Disorder Diagnosis

A taste or smell disorder can be diagnosed with a complete history and physical examination. Pay close attention to a patient's history of URIs, nasal or sinus pathology, trauma, other medical issues, and drugs [18].

Sinus CT scans should be ordered if the patient's history and physical examination do not fit a typical profile. Without central nervous system symptoms or an abnormal neurologic examination, an intracranial mass such as meningioma is unlikely to cause olfactory loss. A brain MRI is usually only advised when the history is complicated or additional neurologic symptoms or signs are present (for instance, a 50-year-old woman with a taste phantom that has persisted for 6 months). A typical laboratory panel is not indicated, although tests can be ordered to assess for allergies, diabetes, thyroid issues, kidney and liver health, hormone imbalances, and nutritional deficiencies. Biopsy of the olfactory epithelium is primarily employed as a research tool [18].

19.6 Taste Evaluation in the Clinic

Taste disorder evaluation has yet to progress as far as olfactory disorder evaluation. Specifically, thresholds of detection or recognition must be determined. Since only five primary taste sensations and only four of them are evaluated [18], there is no analogous strategy to odor identification tests.

The threshold evaluation is affected by the tongue's ability to produce saliva and by the size of the stimulated tongue area. Therefore, the results of such examinations tend to vary widely. There is no guarantee that a change in suprathreshold taste intensity will correlate with a shift in threshold detection. The extent of gustatory function or impairment cannot be determined only through taste threshold testing. After radiation therapy, a patient's recognition thresholds for the four taste attributes may return to normal, but the reported tastes may still be substantially diminished in magnitude [18].

19.6.1 Predicting the Threshold

It is possible to acquire a set of 16 taste strips (Burghart, Messtechnik, Germany) that have already been impregnated with four different taste qualities (sweet, sour, salty, and bitter) at four different concentrations. Sweet (0.4 g/mL sucrose), sour (0.3 g/mL citric acid), salty (0.2 g/mL sodium chloride), bitter (0.006 g/mL quinine hydrochloride), and umami (0.025 g/mL sodium chloride). There are published normative values [18] for these tapes.

19.6.2 Magnitude Matching

In suprathreshold testing, the patient's reactions to tastes with intensities beyond the threshold are evaluated. Magnitude matching [18] is a psychophysical technique to quantify this characteristic.

Numbers have been used in other studies of suprathreshold tastes, but a direct comparison between people is impossible. There is no psychological significance to round numbers such as 10 or 100 [18].

In contrast, the process [18] of magnitude matching makes use of one normal sensory modality (hearing) to compensate for a deficit in another modality (taste).

For the magnitude matching job, we supply a range of salt, sugar, acid, and alkaline tones (1000 Hz) and a range of sodium chloride, sucrose, citric acid, and quinine hydrochloric acid concentrations. While listening to the tones through headphones, the patient drinks each solution and attempts to expectorate it. The individual gives subjective ratings of stimulus intensity. By comparing the data to loudness functions, we can see that taste disorders manifest as subdued psychophysical responses. That is, in contrast to people without hypogeusia, those who suffer from this condition tend to equate higher concentrations of tastes with lower tones. The principal drawbacks of this testing method are that it requires normal hearing to function and is highly time-consuming to administer and interpret [18].

19.6.3 Spatial Test

The ability to taste in different parts of the mouth and tongue can be evaluated with a spatial test. Damage to any of the three major nerves that supply the gustatory system [18]—the glossopharyngeal nerve, the vagus nerve, and the chorda tympani branch of the facial nerve—or their ganglia can result in a disturbance of taste that can be assessed only by examining the anatomic areas supplied by those nerves.

Four pieces of standard-sized filter paper are saturated with high concentrations of the four fundamental flavors to conduct the tests. The sheets are distributed randomly throughout all eight tongue segments and both sides of the soft palate. Patients then used the same scale as in the whole-mouth assessment [18] to rate the intensity and quality of the flavor.

References

1. Lafreniere D. Taste and olfactory disorders in adults: anatomy and etiology. In: Deschler DG, Givens J, editors. UpToDate®; 2022.
2. Beidler LM, Smallman RL. Renewal of cells within taste buds. J Cell Biol. 1965;27:263.
3. Graham L, Murty G, Bowrey DJ. Taste, smell and appetite change after roux-en-Y gastric bypass surgery. Obes Surg. 2014;24:1463.
4. Miller IJ Jr. Variation in human fungiform taste bud densities among regions and subjects. Anat Rec. 1986;216:474.
5. Mistretta CM, Baum BJ. Quantitative study of taste buds in fungiform and circumvallate papillae of young and aged rats. J Anat. 1984;138(Pt 2):323.
6. Mistretta CM. Developmental neurobiology of the taste system. In: Getchell TV, Bartoshuk LM, Doty RL, et al., editors. Smell and taste in health and disease. New York: Raven Press; 1991. p. 35.
7. Kinammon S, Getchell TV. Sensory transduction in olfactor receptor neurons and gustatory receptor cells. In: Getchell TV, Bartoshuk LM, Doty RL, et al., editors. Smell and taste in health and disease. New York: Raven Press; 1991. p. 145.
8. Plata-Salaman CR, Scott TR, Smith-Swintosky VL. Gustatory neural coding in the monkey cortex: L-amino acids. J Neurophysiol. 1992;67:1552.
9. Taruno A, Vingtdeux V, Ohmoto M, et al. CALHM1 ion channel mediates purinergic neurotransmission of sweet, bitter and umami tastes. Nature. 2013;495:223.
10. Nishida K. Molecular mechanisms of taste disorder in oxaliplatin-administered rats. Yakugaku Zasshi. 2016;136:1017.
11. Christensen CM. Role of saliva in human taste perception. In: Neiselman HL, Rivlin RS, editors. Clinical measurement of taste and smell. New York: Macmillan Publishing Co.; 1986. p. 414.
12. Bartoshuk LM. The psychophysics of taste. Am J Clin Nutr. 1978;31:1068.
13. Dietlein M, Drzezga A. Taste dysfunction (dysgeusia) and radioiodine therapy of thyroid cancer—be aware of side effects by antidepressants and sedatives. Vorschädigung durch Antidepressiva und Sedativa beachten. Nuklearmedizin. 2017;56:125.
14. Pushpass RG, Daly B, Kelly C, et al. Altered salivary flow, protein composition, and rheology following taste and TRP stimulation in older adults. Front Physiol. 2019;10:652.
15. Heckmann JG, Heckmann SM, Lang CJ, Hummel T. Neurological aspects of taste disorders. Arch Neurol. 2003;60:667.
16. Stańska K, Krzeski A. The umami taste: from discovery to clinical use. Otolaryngol Pol. 2016;70:10.

17. Zhang Y, Venkitasamy C, Pan Z, et al. Novel umami ingredients: umami peptides and their taste. J Food Sci. 2017;82:16.
18. Holbrook EH. Disorders of taste and smell. In: Meyers AD, editor. Medscape. 2022. https://emedicine.medscape.com/article/861242-overview#a4. Accessed 3 June 2023.
19. Boesveldt S, Lindau ST, McClintock MK, Hummel T, Lundstrom JN. Gustatory and olfactory dysfunction in older adults: a national probability study. Rhinology. 2011;49(3):324–30.
20. Wylie K, Nebauer M. "The food here is tasteless!" food taste or tasteless food? Chemosensory loss and the politics of undernutrition. Collegian. 2011;18(1):27–35.
21. Wang T, Glendinning J, Grushka M, Hummel T, Mansfield K. From the cover: drug-induced taste disorders in clinical practice and preclinical safety evaluation. Toxicol Sci. 2017;156(2):315–24.
22. Zerrweck C, Gallardo VC, Calleja C, Sepulveda E, Guilber L. Gross olfaction before and after laparoscopic gastric bypass. Obes Surg. 2017;27(11):2988–92.
23. Feng P, Huang L, Wang H. Taste bud homeostasis in health, disease, and aging. Chem Senses. 2014;39(1):3–16.
24. Eriksson L, Esberg A, Haworth S, et al. Allelic variation in taste genes is associated with taste and diet preferences and dental caries. Nutrients. 2019;11(7):1491.
25. Henkin RI, Larson AL, Powell RD. Hypogeusia, dysgeusia, hyposmia, and dysosmia following influenza-like infection. Ann Otol Rhinol Laryngol. 1975;84:672.
26. Centers for Disease Control and Prevention. Coronavirus disease 2019 (COVID-19): symptoms of coronavirus. https://www.cdc.gov/coronavirus/2019-ncov/symptoms-testing/symptoms.html. Accessed 28 Apr 2020.
27. Beltrán-Corbellini Á, Chico-García JL, Martínez-Poles J, et al. Acute-onset smell and taste disorders in the context of COVID-19: a pilot multicentre polymerase chain reaction based case-control study. Eur J Neurol. 2020;27:1738.
28. Spinato G, Fabbris C, Polesel J, et al. Alterations in smell or taste in mildly symptomatic outpatients with SARS-CoV-2 infection. JAMA. 2020;323:2089.
29. Tong JY, Wong A, Zhu D, et al. The prevalence of olfactory and gustatory dysfunction in COVID-19 patients: a systematic review and meta-analysis. Otolaryngol Head Neck Surg. 2020;163:3.
30. Agyeman AA, Chin KL, Landersdorfer CB, et al. Smell and taste dysfunction in patients with COVID-19: a systematic review and meta-analysis. Mayo Clin Proc. 2020;95:1621.
31. Chiesa-Estomba CM, Lechien JR, Radulesco T, et al. Patterns of smell recovery in 751 patients affected by the COVID-19 outbreak. Eur J Neurol. 2020;27:2318.
32. Petrocelli M, Cutrupi S, Salzano G, et al. Six-month smell and taste recovery rates in coronavirus disease 2019 patients: a prospective psychophysical study. J Laryngol Otol. 2021;135:436.
33. Vaira LA, Hopkins C, Petrocelli M, et al. Smell and taste recovery in coronavirus disease 2019 patients: a 60-day objective and prospective study. J Laryngol Otol. 2020;134:703.
34. Boscolo-Rizzo P, Borsetto D, Fabbris C, et al. Evolution of altered sense of smell or taste in patients with mildly symptomatic COVID-19. JAMA Otolaryngol Head Neck Surg. 2020;146:729.
35. Napeñas JJ, Rouleau TS. Oral complications of Sjögren's syndrome. Oral Maxillofac Surg Clin North Am. 2014;26:55.
36. Negoro A, Umemoto M, Fujii M, et al. Taste function in Sjögren's syndrome patients with special reference to clinical tests. Auris Nasus Larynx. 2004;31:141.
37. Quilici D, Zech KN. Prevention and treatment options for medication-induced xerostomia. Gen Dent. 2019;67:52.
38. Deshpande TS, Blanchard P, Wang L, et al. Radiation-related alterations of taste function in patients with head and neck cancer: a systematic review. Curr Treat Options in Oncol. 2018;19:72.
39. Mossman K, Shatzman A, Chencharick J. Long-term effects of radiotherapy on taste and salivary function in man. Int J Radiat Oncol Biol Phys. 1982;8:991.
40. Kabadi A, Saadi M, Schey R, Parkman HP. Taste and smell disturbances in patients with gastroparesis and gastroesophageal reflux disease. J Neurogastroenterol Motil. 2017;23:370.

41. Suzuki M, Yokota M, Matsumoto T, et al. Proton pump inhibitor ameliorates taste disturbance among patients with laryngopharyngeal reflux: a randomized controlled study. Tohoku J Exp Med. 2019;247:19.
42. Altundag A, Cayonu M, Salihoglu M, et al. Laryngopharyngeal reflux has negative effects on taste and smell functions. Otolaryngol Head Neck Surg. 2016;155:117.
43. Shibata T, Nakamura M, Omori T, et al. Association between individual response to food taste and gastroesophageal symptoms. J Dig Dis. 2015;16:337.
44. Vij S, Kanagasuntheram R. Effect of tri-O-cresyl phosphate (TOCP) poisoning on sensory nerve terminations of slow loris (Nycticebus coucang coucang). Acta Neuropathol. 1972;20:150.
45. Reiter ER, DiNardo LJ, Costanzo RM. Toxic effects on gustatory function. Adv Otorhinolaryngol. 2006;63:265.
46. Kachru DN, Tandon SK, Misra UK, Nag D. Occupational lead poisoning among silver jewellery workers. Indian J Med Sci. 1989;43:89.
47. Gordon T, Fine JM. Metal fume fever. Occup Med. 1993;8:504.
48. Yu IT, Lee NL, Zhang XH, et al. Occupational exposure to mixtures of organic solvents increases the risk of neurological symptoms among printing workers in Hong Kong. J Occup Environ Med. 2004;46:323.
49. Gobba F. Occupational exposure to chemicals and sensory organs: a neglected research field. Neurotoxicology. 2003;24:675.
50. Cecchini MP, Cardobi N, Sbarbati A, et al. Post-traumatic taste disorders: a case series. J Neurol. 2018;265:836.
51. Jeppsson PH, Hallén O. The taste after operation for otosclerosis. Pract Otorhinolaryngol (Basel). 1971;33:215.
52. Blackburn CW, Bramley PA. Lingual nerve damage associated with the removal of lower third molars. Br Dent J. 1989;167:103.
53. Mott A, Shafer D, Miller D, et al. Gustatory function after oral maxillofacial surgery. Chem Senses. 1994;19:526–7.
54. Boenninghaus HG, Denecke U. Paralysis of the hypoglossal nerve after tonsillectomy? (author's transl). Laryngol Rhinol Otol (Stuttg). 1982;61:189.
55. Pisano M, Hilas O. Zinc and taste disturbances in older adults: a review of the literature. Consult Pharm. 2016;31:267.
56. Yagi T, Asakawa A, Ueda H, et al. The role of zinc in the treatment of taste disorders. Recent Pat Food Nutr Agric. 2013;5:44.
57. Braun LA, Rosenfeldt F. Pharmaco-nutrient interactions—a systematic review of zinc and antihypertensive therapy. Int J Clin Pract. 2013;67:717.
58. Fernström A, Hylander B, Rössner S. Taste acuity in patients with chronic renal failure. Clin Nephrol. 1996;45:169.
59. Ciechanover M, Peresecenschi G, Aviram A, Steiner JE. Malrecognition of taste in uremia. Nephron. 1980;26:20.
60. Astbäck J, Fernström A, Hylander B, et al. Taste buds and neuronal markers in patients with chronic renal failure. Perit Dial Int. 1999;19(Suppl 2):S315.
61. Bossola M. Xerostomia in patients on chronic hemodialysis: an update. Semin Dial. 2019;32:467.
62. Taki Y, Imai N, Shibagaki Y. Zinc deficiency anaemia in haemodialysis patients: often overlooked but a treatable cause of anaemia. Nephrology (Carlton). 2017;22:1037.
63. Khera S, Saigal A. Assessment and evaluation of gustatory functions in patients with diabetes mellitus type II: a study. Indian J Endocrinol Metab. 2018;22:204.
64. Borgnakke WS, Anderson PF, Shannon C, Jivanescu A. Is there a relationship between oral health and diabetic neuropathy? Curr Diab Rep. 2015;15:93.
65. McConnell RJ, Menendez CE, Smith FR, et al. Defects of taste and smell in patients with hypothyroidism. Am J Med. 1975;59:354.
66. Deniz F, Ay SA, Salihoglu M, et al. Thyroid hormone replacement therapy improves olfaction and taste sensitivity in primary hypothyroid patients: a prospective randomised clinical trial. Exp Clin Endocrinol Diabetes. 2016;124:562.

67. Hashimoto T, Doden T, Ono Y, Uematsu T. Bilateral hypogeusia caused by a small lesion in the lower midbrain tegmentum. BMJ Case Rep. 2012;2012:bcr2012006837.
68. Benatru I, Terraux P, Cherasse A, et al. Gustatory disorders during multiple sclerosis relapse. Rev Neurol (Paris). 2003;159:287.
69. Zlotnik Y, Balash Y, Korczyn AD, et al. Disorders of the oral cavity in Parkinson's disease and parkinsonian syndromes. Parkinsons Dis. 2015;2015:379482.
70. Kouzuki M, Suzuki T, Nagano M, et al. Comparison of olfactory and gustatory disorders in Alzheimer's disease. Neurol Sci. 2018;39:321.
71. Jääskeläinen SK. Pathophysiology of primary burning mouth syndrome. Clin Neurophysiol. 2012;123:71.
72. Klasser GD, Grushka M, Su N. Burning mouth syndrome. Oral Maxillofac Surg Clin North Am. 2016;28:381.
73. American Academy of Otolaryngology—Head and Neck Surgery. AAO-HNS: anosmia, hyposmia, and dysgeusia symptoms of coronavirus disease. AAO-HNS. 2020. https://www.entnet.org/content/coronavirus-disease-2019-resources. Accessed 23 Mar 2020.
74. Kaye R, Chang CWD, Kazahaya K, Brereton J, Denneny JC III. COVID-19 anosmia reporting tool: initial findings. https://www.entnet.org/sites/default/files/uploads/kaye_covid-19_anosmia_reporting_tool_initial_findings.pdf.
75. American Academy of Otolaryngology—Head and Neck Surgery. COVID-19 anosmia reporting tool. AAO-HNS. https://www.entnet.org/content/reporting-tool-patients-anosmia-related-covid-19. Accessed 21 Apr 2020.
76. Centers for Disease Control and Prevention. Symptoms of coronavirus. coronavirus disease 2019 (COVID-19). 2020. https://www.cdc.gov/coronavirus/2019-ncov/symptoms-testing/symptoms.html. Accessed 21 Apr 2020.
77. WHO. Q&A on coronaviruses (COVID-19). World Health Organization; 2020. https://www.who.int/emergencies/diseases/novel-coronavirus-2019/question-and-answers-hub/q-a-detail/q-a-coronaviruses. Accessed 6 May 2020.
78. Speth MM, Singer-Cornelius T, Obere M, Gengler I, Brockmeier SJ, Sedaghat AR. Olfactory dysfunction and sinonasal symptomatology in COVID-19: prevalence, severity, timing and associated characteristics. Otolaryngol Head Neck Surg. 2020;163(1):114–20.
79. Douglas D. About half of COVID-19 patients have altered sense of taste. Reuters Health Information; 2020.

Part III

Symptoms and Signs Related with Upper and Lower Respiratory Tract Diseases

Otalgia in Children

20

Yeşim Yüksel, Erdem Atalay Çetinkaya,
and Codrut Sarafoleanu

20.1 Introduction

Otalgia, a prevalent symptom in pediatric age groups, is one of the most common causes of hospital admissions. It is a highly distressing condition for both the child and the family, especially in kids below two who cannot articulate their pain. Otalgia may occur due to otologic or non-otologic causes. Otalgia due to otologic causes is termed primary while non-otologic otalgia is called secondary [1–3]. Primary otalgia with otologic causes is the most common in children. Otologic causes may originate from the auricle, external auditory canal, and middle ear. However, non-otologic conditions with oral, oropharyngeal, laryngeal, dentoalveolar, sinonasal, and musculoskeletal origins may also cause referred otalgia in childhood [3]. Therefore, when it comes to ear pain in children, otologic examination is not enough, other structures in the ear that may cause secondary otalgia should also be examined.

In this chapter, primary and secondary causes, clinical diagnosis, and evaluation of otalgia will be covered.

Y. Yüksel · E. A. Çetinkaya (✉)
Department of Otorhinolaryngology, University of Health Sciences, Antalya Training and Research Hospital, Antalya, Turkey

C. Sarafoleanu
Department of Otorhinolaryngology, Head and Neck Surgery, Carol Davila University of Medicine and Pharmacy, Santa Maria Hospital, Bucharest, Romania

H. Yüksel et al. (eds.), *Pediatric Airway Diseases*, Comprehensive ENT,
https://doi.org/10.1007/978-3-031-74853-0_20

20.2 Primary Otalgia Causes

20.2.1 Auricle

20.2.1.1 Infections

Infections such as cellulitis, perichondritis, and herpes zoster oticus (Ramsay Hunt syndrome) may affect the auricle, causing otalgia.

While cellulitis often occurs following trauma, insect bites, and piercings, perichondritis develops primarily due to blunt trauma. Both conditions entail pain, hyperemia, swelling, and tenderness; however, the ear lobe, which is noncartilaginous, is not affected in perichondritis [4].

Herpes zoster oticus, on the other hand, is a unilateral infection resulting from varicella. In this condition, vesicular lesions may involve the auricle and external auditory canal and cause pain, burning sensation, itching, and hyperesthesia [5, 6].

20.2.1.2 Trauma

Trauma to the auricle and external auditory canal may result in ecchymosis, abrasion, contusion, laceration, or hematoma depending on the severity of the trauma. Early recognition and treatment of these post-traumatic pathologies, especially hematomas, is highly crucial for an optimal cosmetic outcome [4, 6].

20.2.1.3 Allergic Angioedema

Allergic reactions following exposure to the relevant allergen in patients suffering from insect bites or contact dermatitis may lead to itching, swelling, mild pain, induration, or tenderness in the auricle [4].

20.2.1.4 Thermal Damage

Exposure to extreme cold can cause frostbite of the auricle. Initially, numb and pale in color, the auricle later becomes painful, edematous, and erythematous. If the damage progresses, arterial circulation is compromised, and thus necrotic changes may ensue [6].

In auricular burns, although there are different additional findings depending on the degree of burn, pain, which is initially persistent and severe and later becomes intermittent, is a highly unpleasant symptom [6].

The causes of otalgia originating from the auricle are as mentioned above; the patient's medical history is often enough to make a clinical diagnosis. Following the diagnosis, treatment should be planned in accordance with and aimed at the etiology.

20.2.2 External Auditory Canal

20.2.2.1 Otitis Externa

Otitis externa is an inflammation of the external auditory canal and is caused by swimming, excessive humidity, and localized trauma [6]. *P. aeruginosa*, *S. aureus*, and other gram-negative bacilli are the most common pathogens. The main symptoms in acute cases are pain and localized tenderness in the ear canal [7]. There may also be a feeling of fullness inside the ear, itching, and discharge. Fever is rarely concomitant. Physical examination findings include tenderness in the tragus and pain during otoscopy in most patients. The external auditory canal may be edematous, hyperemic, or macerated.

In particular, prolonged bacterial otitis externa or extended use of topical antibiotics may cause disturbance of the external auditory canal flora. This often leads to fungal otitis externa, or otomycosis, caused by pathogens such as Aspergillus and Candida. While these patients may have a feeling of fullness inside the ear, intense itching, and sometimes pain, they may also be asymptomatic [4].

20.2.2.2 Malignant Otitis Externa

Malignant otitis externa, which is extremely rare in pediatric patients, is a potentially fatal infection resulting from the spread of infection in the external auditory canal to adjacent structures through the bone. It is more common in immunocompromised, diabetic, and HIV-positive patients. Patients typically have a persistent earache that is quite deep and intense and lasts longer than 1 week. Depending on the spread of infection, complications such as chondritis, temporal bone and skull base osteomyelitis, meningitis, brain abscess, and facial paralysis may develop. Computed tomography and magnetic resonance imaging are critical in the diagnosis [8].

20.2.2.3 Eczematous Dermatitis

Especially in atopic children, some chemicals may have an irritant effect on the external auditory canal after the skin barrier is impaired due to different reasons such as excessive cleaning of this area. This leads to recurrent erythematous, edematous, painful, and itchy lesions. If the disease becomes chronic, the skin in and around the external auditory canal becomes atrophic and dry. Itching then occurs as the main symptom. In eczematous dermatitis, avoiding contact with water and chemicals is as important as medical treatment [4].

20.2.2.4 Furunculosis

Mainly caused by *S. aureus*, furunculosis is a local skin infection originating in the hair follicles and sebaceous and ceruminous glands located in the cartilaginous part of the external auditory canal. Increased ear pain with chewing is typical, and there is a tender, hyperemic swelling at the canal entrance. The main treatment is incisional drainage of the lesion together with antibiotherapy if needed [4, 6].

20.2.2.5 Foreign Body

One of the causes that should be considered in cases of children presenting with otalgia is the foreign body in the ear. Foreign bodies in the external ear canal are quite common in children because of children's tendency to insert small objects into their ears. Ear pain, aural fullness, and mild hearing loss are the main symptoms [4, 6]. If detected by otoscopic examination, the foreign body should be removed as soon as possible by an ENT physician using special instruments. It should be kept in mind that attempts to remove the foreign body by non-specialists or family members may lead to undesirable consequences such as external auditory canal injury and tympanic membrane perforation.

20.2.2.6 Cerumen Impaction

Cerumen, a mixture of the special secretion produced by the ceruminous glands in the external auditory canal, exfoliated epithelial cells, and the secretion of the pilosebaceous glands, is the most common cause of congestion and discomfort in the ear. It is so common that it occurs in one in ten children. Symptoms include itching, mild hearing loss, and pain due to movement of the cerumen, especially in case of contact with the tympanic membrane. Sometimes pain occurs when cerumen is attempted to be removed. Removal of the cerumen by curette or aspiration under the microscope relieves the symptoms [6, 8].

20.2.2.7 Tumors

Tumors of the external auditory canal are very rare in pediatric patients. Pain in and discharge from the ear is the most common reason for presentation. Rhabdomyosarcoma, lymphoma, and eosinophilic granuloma are the reported tumors of the external auditory canal in children. These patients have a granulomatous mass and bloody or serohemorrhagic discharge in the external auditory canal. It is of utmost importance that patients with otitis externa or perforated otitis media with frequent recurrences and persistent symptoms and signs be evaluated for possible tumors of the external auditory canal [4].

20.2.3 Middle Ear

20.2.3.1 Acute Otitis Media

Acute otitis media is the most common cause of primary otalgia in children and one of the most common diseases diagnosed by clinicians. Approximately 70% of children have at least one episode of acute otitis before the age of two. It peaks at 6–15 months of age and usually occurs following upper respiratory tract infections [3, 9, 10]. In infants and young children, the development of otitis media is facilitated by reasons such as shorter and wider Eustachian tube, higher occurrence of upper respiratory tract infections, immature immune system, and frequent adenoid hypertrophy, which has an obstructive effect and acts as a reservoir for pathogenic agents. The most common infectious agents are viruses (adenovirus, respiratory syncytial virus, influenza virus) and bacteria (*Streptococcus pneumoniae*, *Haemophilus influenzae*, *Moraxella catarrhalis*). However, approximately 60% of patients recover spontaneously within 24 h and 80% within 3 days without any treatment [10]. In acute otitis media, ear pain is initially milder but then turns into a pulsatile pain that is felt directly inside the ear and increases especially in the supine position. The pain decreases dramatically when the tympanic membrane is perforated [8]. Fever accompanies in some patients. Infants may show nonspecific symptoms such as restlessness, loss of appetite, and sleep disturbance. Following perforation of the tympanic membrane, some patients may experience otorrhea, and at times vomiting and lethargy may be observed [3, 4]. In patients with acute otitis media, a bulging tympanic membrane with decreased mobility is the most specific finding on otoscopic examination [11]. Depending on the opacity of the membrane and the color of the fluid behind the membrane, a yellow, white, or green reflex may be observed. In children with acute otitis media, appropriate analgesics should be given to reduce pain, especially in the first 24 h. In those whose symptoms do not resolve within 48–72 h, antibiotherapy is deemed appropriate.

In children, acute otitis media may progress with complications. Complications such as hearing loss and suppurative tympanic membrane perforation are more common while severe complications such as facial paralysis, mastoiditis, labyrinthitis, meningitis, intracranial abscess, and lateral sinus thrombosis are much rarer [3, 4]. In cases with symptoms such as fever, severe otalgia, headache, irritability, loss of appetite, otorrhea, vomiting, and lethargy that do not diminish despite medical treatment, more caution should be exercised and the patient should be evaluated for complications.

Bullous myringitis usually involves focal bullae on the tympanic membrane without fluid accumulation in the middle ear. Bacterial pathogens are frequently implicated, however, the condition may also develop due to trauma. Ear pain is the most distinctive symptom [4].

20.2.3.2 Otitis Media with Effusion

It is an inflammatory condition characterized by the accumulation of serous or mucoid fluid behind an intact tympanic membrane without signs of acute infection. It usually occurs as a result of the impairment of ventilation, drainage, or protective functions of the Eustachian tube due to nasal infection or allergy. Patients are usually asymptomatic. In symptomatic patients, however, the main complaint is hearing loss while some may have mild ear pain. On otoscopic examination, the tympanic membrane is opaque, retracted, and usually amber in color, its vascularity is elevated, and there is an air-fluid level behind the membrane [3, 4]. First, follow-up and medical treatment are recommended. In patients whose symptoms do not subside, surgical myringotomy with a ventilation tube should be performed.

20.2.3.3 Eustachian Tube Dysfunction

The Eustachian tube in children is anatomically different than in adults and reaches its adult form around the age of 7. Anatomical or physiologic dysfunction of the Eustachian tube may develop due to inflammatory causes such as upper respiratory tract infection or allergic rhinitis, or obstructive lesions of the nasopharynx and middle ear. Patients may experience ear pain, tinnitus, subjective sensation of ear fullness, or hearing loss. These complaints are especially pronounced while chewing, swallowing, and yawning. On otoscopic examination, everything may be normal, or tympanic membrane retraction may also be observed [4, 6, 9].

Current ENT guidelines consider otoscopy or otomicroscopy, tympanometry, Weber and Rinne tests or pure tone audiometry, nasopharyngoscopy to assess the pharyngeal opening of Eustachian tube to be the most essential assessment tools. Still, they have to be adapted to the patient age and compliance [12].

20.2.3.4 Cholesteatoma

Cholesteatomas are benign masses that develop from keratinized epithelium that should not normally be present in the middle ear cavity. It is locally invasive and its osteolytic effect worsens with infection. It is divided into three categories: congenital, acquired, and unclassifiable cholesteatoma. Acquired cholesteatomas are most common and result from retraction pockets of the tympanic membrane caused by permanent eustachian dysfunction. They may also result from perforation of the tympanic membrane, trauma, or iatrogenic causes. They can lead to bone erosion where they are located (Fig. 20.1).

Congenital cholesteatomas that develop behind the intact tympanic membrane without any history of infection or otitis are more common in boys. Most of them are recognized incidentally at the age of 4–5. There may be complaints such as ear pain or a sensation of fullness in the ear. Otoscopy reveals a whitish mass behind the intact tympanic membrane, often at the anterosuperior or around the manubrium. The CT scan of the ear completes the disease assessment.

The literature describes the Potsic staging system for congenital cholesteatoma: stage I—one single quadrant of the tympanic cavity affected; stage II—multiple quadrants are affected, but with no ossicular involvement or mastoid extension; stage III—presence of ossicular involvement; stage IV—mastoid extension. This classification system reflects a strong association between staging and recurrence of disease, ranging from a 13% recurrence rate in stage I to a 67% rate in stage IV [13]. Congenital cholesteatoma usually grows slowly and has no symptoms until the presence of secondary ossicular erosion, local infection, damage of the tympanic membrane, and otorrhea. Thus, in advanced stages of the disease, differentiating between acquired and congenital cholesteatoma may be impossible.

Given the high morbidity risk and complications, surgical treatment is ideal for cholesteatoma [13].

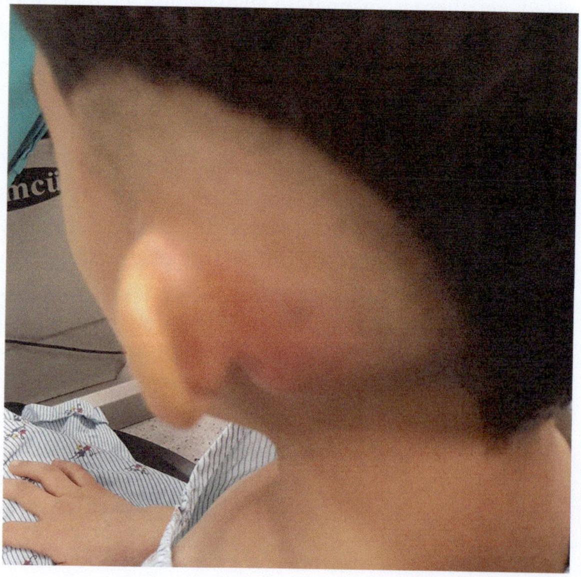

Fig. 20.1 Mastoid abscess due to cholesteatoma. (Picture taken from the archive of Prof Dr. Erdem Atalay Cetinkaya)

20.2.3.5 Trauma

Ear pain can be a symptom of severe trauma or skull base fractures affecting the middle ear. In addition to blunt and penetrating trauma, we may encounter cases of barotrauma.

Traumatic tympanic membrane perforation is the most common trauma-induced condition. It may be caused by penetrating objects or barotrauma. Patients experience severe ear pain during trauma, which may be accompanied by hearing loss and tinnitus.

After blunt trauma or barotrauma, blood accumulation may occur in the middle ear cavity called hemotympanum. Rarely, blood may accumulate in the middle ear through the Eustachian tube in children with profuse epistaxis [14]. On examination, the tympanic membrane is red or purple and may be bulging.

Another condition that may develop due to trauma is the ossicular chain anatomy disruption. In addition to ear pain, severe hearing loss may also be observed as a symptom. These patients should be evaluated with computed tomography.

Inner ear injuries are rare but severe in children. It should be suspected in the presence of tinnitus, hearing loss, and vertigo after trauma. Urgent surgical intervention may be required in some patients.

Ear pain is a significant symptom in fractures of the skull base that may result from blunt trauma to the ear region. Altered mental status, headache, and vomiting may be observed, or focal neurologic findings may be noted. Physical examination findings may include ecchymosis, swelling, tenderness, hemotympanum, tympanic membrane perforation, facial palsy, bloody or cerebrospinal fluid otorrhea, periorbital ecchymosis, cerebrospinal fluid rhinorrhea on the mastoid bone, and other parts of the temporal bone [4].

20.3 Secondary Otalgia Causes

In pediatric patients, while primary otalgia is frequently seen due to ear-related causes, sometimes referred to as ear pain, i.e., secondary otalgia, due to pathologies of the structures around the ear can be observed [15]. The ear has a rich sensory innervation. Sensory fibers from the V (trigeminal), VII (facial), IX (glossopharyngeal), X (vagus), and C2–C3 cervical nerves innervate the outer ear and middle ear. Due to the long course of these nerves, ear pain may also be a symptom in diseases of other structures they innervate. The inner ear structures, on the other hand, are innervated by the VIIIth cranial nerve (vestibulocochlear), which has no pain fibers; therefore, most inner ear pathologies do not present pain [2].

20.3.1 Oropharyngeal Infections

In pediatric patients, referred ear pain may occur after oral cavity conditions such as gingivitis, aphthous stomatitis, and glossitis, oropharyngeal infections such as pharyngitis and tonsillitis, and adenoidectomy and tonsillectomy operations.

Acute pharyngotonsillitis is the most common cause of secondary otalgia in children. Acute pharyngotonsillitis is quite common between the ages of 5–15. The most common causative agents are viruses; however, bacteria account for 15–30% of cases. Group A beta-hemolytic streptococci are mainly the most common bacterial agent. The disease has an acute onset. It may present a clinical picture ranging from mild sore throat to exudative tonsillitis with high fever. Patients have complaints such as fever over 38 °C, shivering, malaise, dysphagia, arthralgia, and ear pain. The pharynx and tonsils have a hyperemic and edematous appearance on physical examination. Exudation occurs on the tonsils as the condition progresses. There is tender lymphadenopathy in the neck. Patients usually respond well to medical treatment. Correct diagnosis and treatment of acute pharyngotonsillitis brings positive outcomes, including preventing complications such as acute rheumatic fever, acute glomerulonephritis, and peritonsillar abscesses, and reduction of acute morbidity associated with the disease [16].

20.3.2 Dental Causes

In children, referred ear pain is joint especially during the teething period. It usually occurs due to problems affecting mandibular molar teeth. The pain is mostly localized on the side of the problematic teeth. In children presenting with ear pain and normal otoscopy findings, a history of teething, infection, dental caries, trauma, and bruxism should be inquired [17]. During the oral cavity examination, swelling of the gingiva or face may be detected if there are dental pathologies, gingivitis, or dental abscesses. Patients with dental pathology should be referred to a dentist [3].

20.3.3 Auricular Lymphadenitis

Preauricular lymph nodes may be enlarged, often in response to ocular infections such as conjunctivitis or parotid diseases, and postauricular lymph nodes may be enlarged in response to external ear and mastoid skin pathologies, or infectious mononucleosis. If acute infection develops in these lymph nodes, redness and fluctuation may be observed in addition to pain. The pain may also be felt inside the ear [4].

20.3.4 Neck Abscess

Deep neck infections, which are rare in children, start as cellulitis-phlegmon in the soft tissues in the potential cavities of the neck and usually result in abscess development. Late diagnosis or inadequate treatment may lead to severe complications. Peritonsillar abscesses are more common in adolescents and older children, whereas retropharyngeal abscesses are observed more commonly in children under 5 years of age. Parapharyngeal abscesses, on the other hand, can be seen in all ages. Although studies differ, peritonsillar and parapharyngeal abscesses are encountered more frequently in clinical presentations, and these cause referred ear pain. Treatment of neck abscesses in children includes appropriate intravenous antibiotherapy, follow-up, and surgical drainage if necessary [18].

20.3.5 Parotitis

Parotid gland diseases involve localized pain in the inferior part of the ear. On examination, swelling, tenderness, and redness can be seen in this area. Most parotid gland infections in children are viral (such as mumps, parainfluenza, influenza A) [19, 20]. Parotid involvement is typically bilateral in these infections. Bacterial parotitis caused by *S. aureus* is rare and presents with high fever. Unilateral and erythematous parotid swelling, tenderness, and pus from Stensen's duct with parotid massage may be observed [21].

Sialolithiasis leading to obstruction of the parotid gland duct may cause swelling and pain in the glands and referred ear pain. However, this pathology is rarely found in pediatric population, which accounts for only 3% of cases [22].

Recurrent parotitis is a noninfectious inflammatory disease of the parotid gland characterized by repeated parotitis attacks. It can affect both glands. It requires no treatment other than analgesia and regular monitoring [3, 4].

20.3.6 Temporomandibular Joint Dysfunction

Temporomandibular joint dysfunction is more common in children over 10 years of age but is rare in younger age groups. The temporomandibular joint may be affected by rheumatoid arthritis, bruxism (teeth grinding), trauma, and infections. Patients may complain of ear pain, a sensation of fullness in the ear, and a clicking sound. The pain is exacerbated by opening the mouth or clenching the teeth. While no pathology is observed in the ear on examination, clicking, crepitation, preauricular tenderness, and malocclusion may be detected on joint examination. Appropriate analgesics should be used in treatment, soft food diet and heat application should be recommended, and joint pathologies should be investigated in patients [3, 17].

20.3.7 Sinusitis

Sinus infections, especially of the maxillary and ethmoid sinuses, may cause referred pain in the ear via the second branch of the trigeminal nerve [8]. In these patients, nasal obstruction is the most common symptom, and findings such as anterior or posterior nasal discharge and cough are present. The medical treatment given to patients with sinusitis findings determined by history and physical examination relieves the symptoms.

20.4 Differential Diagnosis

To make a clinical diagnosis in pediatric patients presenting with otalgia complaints, first, a thorough anamnesis should be taken, and the causes that may lead to otalgia should be inquired. In the anamnesis taken considering the child's age, the localization and spread of pain, factors that exacerbate pain (such as chewing), risk factors, and otologic and systemic concomitant factors should be questioned.

In terms of the diagnostic approach, it is essential to evaluate the information from the family regarding the etiology as part of the anamnesis by considering the age groups of the children. For example, acute otitis media is most frequently encountered in children up to 3 years of age, while tonsillitis is more common in the 5–15 age group. In a 10-month-old child presenting with ear pain and normal otoscopic findings, otalgia due to teething should be considered. In contrast, dental infection or temporomandibular joint dysfunction should be considered in a 10-year-old child. Having information about the history of foreign body, onset of complaints after swimming, environmental factors such as insect bites or exposure to heat or cold that may have caused thermal damage, presence of recurrent ENT-related chronic infections, history of surgical operations with the use of ventilation tube, presence of concomitant diabetes, immunodeficiency or atopic nature is highly significant in the differential diagnosis of otalgia in children. In addition to fever, otorrhea, and hearing loss, which are the cardinal symptoms usually accompanying the otalgia complaint, symptoms related to the causative pathology, such as itching, increased sensitivity, and pain with pressure on the tragus, a sensation of fullness in the ear, tinnitus, vertigo, rhinorrhea, headache, chewing and swallowing difficulties should also be evaluated. In younger children, nonspecific symptoms such as restlessness, loss of appetite, sleep disturbance, and excessive crying may accompany otalgia (Table 20.1).

Physical examination can quickly reveal signs of infection such as perichondritis, cellulitis, and herpes zoster related to the auricle; thermal damage and angioedema; auricle pushed forwards, which may be a sign of mastoiditis; abrasion, contusion, laceration, and ecchymosis in the ear due to ear and head trauma; ecchymosis in the periorbital area and on the mastoid bone skin; localized lymphadenopathy and lymphadenitis in the periauricular region; signs related to parotid diseases. In physical examination, the otoscopic examination should follow the inspection. In patients presenting normal findings in the ear examination, temporomandibular joint test, nasal examination, oral cavity, oropharynx, and neck examination are required to diagnose the pathologies causing secondary otalgia. Moreover, facial nerve examination is also crucial in children with suspected facial palsy. When it is deemed necessary about the etiology of otalgia in relevant patients, laboratory tests and radiological imaging should be requested, and audiometric and tympanometric examinations should be performed (Table 20.2). These examinations are needed for early diagnosis of complications, especially in patients with prolonged symptoms who do not respond to medical treatment for the etiology.

Ear pain in children is a complaint that should be heeded. Ear pain may have a simple cause, such as teething or a plug or foreign body in the ear, or it may as well be a symptom of a severe condition such as mastoiditis, meningitis, facial palsy, and brain abscess. Therefore, in pediatric presentations due to otalgia, a detailed history should be taken along with the physical examination and, if necessary, appropriate tests to make an accurate diagnosis. Then proper treatment and follow-up should be applied.

Table 20.1 Symptoms and examination findings consistent with the clinical diagnosis causing otalgia in children

Symptoms and examination findings/clinical diagnosis	Otalgia	Fever	Otorrhea	Hearing Loss	Other symptoms and findings
Primary otalgia					
Auricle					
Infection (perichondritis, cellulitis, H. zoster)	xx	+/–	–	–	Itching
Trauma	x/xx/xxx	–	–	–	Bleeding
Allergic angioedema	x/xx	–	–	–	–
Thermal damage	x/xx/xxx	–	–	–	–
External auditory canal					
Otitis externa	x/xx	+/–	+	–	Itching, tragal tenderness
Malignant Otitis externa	xxx	+/–	+	+	–
Eczematous dermatitis	x/xx	–	–	–	Itching
Furunculosis	x/xx	–	–	–	–
Foreign body	x/xx	–	+/–	+/–	–
Cerumen impaction	x	–	–	+/–	–
Tumors	xx/xxx	–	+	+/–	–
Middle ear					
Acute otitis media	xx/xxx	+	+/–	+/–	Restlessness, vomiting, headache
Otitis media with effusion	x/–	–	–	+	–
Eustachian tube dysfunction	x	–	–	+/–	Tinnitus
Cholesteatoma	x/xx	–	+/–	+	–
Trauma	x/xx/xxx	–	+/–	+/–	Rhinorrea, vertigo, tinnitus
Secondary otalgia					
Oropharyngeal infections	x/xx	+	–	–	Dysphagy, sore throat
Dental causes	x/xx	+/–	–	–	Toothache
Auricular lymphadenitis	x	+/–	–	–	–
Neck abscess	x/xx	+	–	–	Swelling, hyperemia
Parotitis	x/xx	+/–	–	–	–
Temporomandibular joint dysfunction	x	–	–	–	Difficulty chewing, clicking sound, malocclusion
Sinusitis	x	+/–	–	–	Nasal congestion, cough, nasal discharge

Otalgia severity x:mild, xx:moderate, xxx:severe; + presence; – absence

Table 20.2 Presence of examination, laboratory, and radiological findings consistent with the clinical diagnosis causing otalgia in children

Examination findings/ clinical diagnosis	Inspection findings	Otoscopic examination findings	Laboratory findings	Radiological findings (CT/ MR)
Primary otalgia				
Auricle				
Infection (perichondritis, cellulitis, H. zoster)	+	+/–	+/–	–
Trauma	+	+/–	–	+/–
Allergic angioedema	+	–	–	–
Thermal damage	+	+/–	–	–
External auditory canal				
Otitis externa	+/–	+	–	–
Malignant Otitis externa	+/–	+	+	+
Eczematous dermatitis	+	+	–	–
Furunculosis	+	+	+/–	–
Foreign body	+/–	+	–	–
Cerumen impaction	–	+	–	–
Tumors	+/–	+	+/–	+
Middle ear				
Acute otitis media	–	+	+	+/–
Otitis media with effusion	–	+	–	+/–
Eustachian tube dysfunction	–	+	–	–
Cholesteatoma	–	+	–	+
Trauma	+	+	–	+
Secondary otalgia				
Oropharyngeal infections	+	–	+	–
Dental causes	+/–	–	+/–	+
Auricular lymphadenitis	+	–	+/–	–
Neck abscess	+	–	+	+
Parotitis	+	–	+/–	–
Temporomandibular joint dysfunction	+/–	–	–	+/–
Sinusitis	–	–	+/–	+/–

References

1. Earwood JS, Rogers TS, Rathjen NA. Ear pain: diagnosing common and uncommon cause. Am Fam Physician. 2018;97(1):20–7.
2. Harrison E, Cronin M. Otalgia. Aust Fam Physician. 2016;45(7):493–7.
3. Majumdar S, Wu K, Bateman ND, Ray J. Diagnosis and management of otalgia in children. Arch Dis Child Educ Pract Ed. 2009;94:33–6.
4. Greenes D, Neuman MI, Wiley JF. Evaluation of earache in children. 2023. www.uptodate.com.
5. Kansu L, Yılmaz I. Herpes zoster oticus (Ramsay Hunt syndrome) in children: case report and literature review. Int J Pediatr Otorhinolaryngol. 2012;76:772.

6. Leung AKC, Fong JHS, Leong AG. Otalgia in children. U Natl Med Assoc. 2000;92:254–60.
7. Rosenfeld RM, Schwartz SR, Cannon CR, et al. Clinical practice guideline: acute otitis externa. Otolaryngol Head Neck Surg. 2014;150:S1–S24.
8. Neilan RE, Roland PS. Otalgia. Med Clin North Am. 2010;94(5):961–71.
9. Jamal A, Alsabea A, Tarakmeh M, Safar A. Etiology, diagnosis, complications, and management of acute otitis media in children. Cureus. 2022;14(8):e28019.
10. Büyükcam A, Kara A, Bedir T, Gülhan B, Özdemir H, Sütçü M, et al. Pediatricians' attitudes in management of acute otitis media and ear pain in Turkey. Int J Pediatr Otorhinolaryngol. 2018;107:14–20.
11. Lieberthal AS, Carroll AE, Chonmaitree T, et al. The diagnosis and management of acute otitis media. Pediatrics. 2013;131:e964.
12. Makuszewska M. Classification, diagnosis and treatment of Eustachian tube dysfunction–literature review. Polish Otorhinolaryngol Rev. 2021;10(4):22–8.
13. Levenson MJ, Parisier SC, Chute P, Wenig S, Juarbe C. A review of twenty congenital cholesteatomas of the middle ear in children. Otolaryngol Head Neck Surg. 1986;94(5):560–7.
14. Fontes Lima A, Carvalho Moreira F, Sousa Menezes A, Esteves Costa I, Azevedo C, Sá Breda M, Dias L. Is pediatric cholesteatoma more aggressive in children than in adults? A comparative study using the EAONO/JOS classification. Int J Pediatr Otorhinolaryngol. 2020;138:110170.
15. Hurtado TR, Zeger WG. Hemotympanums secondary to spontaneous epistaxis in a 7-year-old. J Emerg Med. 2004;26:61.
16. Conover K. Earache. Emerg Med Clin North Am. 2013;31:413.
17. Vicedomini D, Lalinga G, Lugli N, D'Avino A. Diagnosis and management of acute pharyngotonsillitis in the primary care pediatrician's office. Minerva Pediatr. 2014;66(1):69–76.
18. Ely JW, Hansen MR, Clark EC. Diagnosis of ear pain. Am Fam Physician. 2008;77(5):621–8.
19. Erbaş İC, Özlü C, Asrak HK, Güzin AÇ, Belet N. Deep neck infections in childhood. J Pediatr Inf. 2021;15(1):38–43.
20. Battle S, Laudenbach J, Maguire JH. Influenza parotitis: a case from the 2004 to 2005 vaccine shortage. Am J Med Sci. 2007;333:215.
21. Francis CL, Larsen CG. Pediatric sialadenitis. Otolaryngol Clin N Am. 2014;47:763.
22. Stong BC, Sipp JA, Sobol SE. Pediatric parotitis: a 5-year review at a tertiary care pediatric institution. Int J Pediatr Otorhinolaryngol. 2006;70:541.

Otorrhea in Children

21

Yavuz Sultan Selim Yıldırım, Nuray Bayar Muluk, and Chae-Seo Rhee

21.1 Introduction

Otorrhea refers to the discharge of fluid from the ear. It can occur due to issues in the external ear canal or middle ear problems involving a perforation in the tympanic membrane (TM). To discern the primary reasons behind otorrhea in children, a thorough examination and medical history are essential. The majority of children experiencing otorrhea are typically diagnosed with bacterial otitis externa or acute otitis media (AOM) featuring a perforated tympanic membrane. Also, button batteries require emergent removal because pressure necrosis and/or severe burns from residual electric current or leakage of caustic contents may rapidly lead to extensive damage to adjacent structures [1]. Patients who appear unwell or exhibit otorrhea following head trauma necessitate immediate and thorough efforts to diagnose and address potential life-threatening factors contributing to otorrhea, such as basilar skull fractures, necrotizing otitis externa, or infectious complications associated with acute otitis media.

Otorrhea presents a common challenge for otolaryngologists, with its causes ranging from relatively harmless to severe and life-threatening conditions. Consequently, an accurate determination of the underlying cause becomes paramount in establishing an effective treatment plan. In this discussion, we will focus

Y. S. S. Yıldırım
Clinic of Otorhinolaryngology, Elazig Fethi Sekin City Hospital, Elazig, Turkey

N. Bayar Muluk (✉)
Department of Otorhinolaryngology, Faculty of Medicine, Kırıkkale University, Kırıkkale, Turkey

C.-S. Rhee
Department of Otorhinolaryngology, Head and Neck Surgery, College of Medicine, Seoul National University, Seoul, South Korea
e-mail: csrhee@snu.ac.kr

H. Yüksel et al. (eds.), *Pediatric Airway Diseases*, Comprehensive ENT,
https://doi.org/10.1007/978-3-031-74853-0_21

on the most prevalent causes of otorrhea in children and provide guidance on decision-making for management based on a precise diagnosis.

21.2 Bacterial Otitis Externa

Acute otitis externa is a common condition characterized by inflammation of the ear canal. Bacterial infection, primarily driven by *Pseudomonas aeruginosa* and *Staphylococcus aureus*, is the main cause of the acute form. It manifests with the sudden onset of inflammation in the ear canal, leading to symptoms like ear pain, itching, swelling of the canal, redness, and discharge. Often, this condition arises after activities like swimming or minor injuries resulting from improper cleaning. A characteristic sign is tenderness when moving the tragus or pinna.

Upon examination, you will observe an ear canal that appears red, swollen, and contains cellular debris. Importantly, external otitis does not necessarily involve the middle ear, so there may not be any middle ear fluid buildup or a purulent middle ear infection. When visible, the eardrum (tympanic membrane or TM) typically exhibits redness or debris. In some cases, the swollen canal can make it challenging to see the eardrum clearly. The discharge is usually purulent, ranging from white to yellow and may dry to form a crust.

For uncomplicated cases, the preferred treatment options include topical antimicrobials or antibiotics like acetic acid, aminoglycosides, polymyxin B, and quinolones. These medications are available in formulations with or without topical corticosteroids, and the addition of corticosteroids can help expedite symptom relief. Oral antibiotics are reserved for situations where the infection has spread beyond the ear canal or in patients at risk of a rapidly worsening infection [2, 3].

21.3 Acute Otitis Media

Acute Otitis Media (AOM) is an infection of the middle ear, which can be caused by viruses and/or bacteria. It stands as the most common childhood infection for which antibiotics are prescribed in the United States. On occasion, during an episode of acute otitis media, the eardrum may rupture. This is often accompanied by ear pain and a relatively short-lived fever, followed by relief from pain coinciding with the onset of ear discharge. The drainage typically appears clear or white. The perforation may have healed by the time the patient seeks medical attention, but the discharge may persist for some time, especially if external otitis has developed.

Frequently, the perforation itself may not be visible during ear examination (otoscopy) due to the ear discharge obstructing the view of the tympanic membrane (TM). Alternatively, the perforation may have healed rapidly, as shown in Fig. 21.1. When it is visible, the TM typically exhibits an abnormal appearance and lacks mobility when assessed with pneumatic otoscopy. If the perforation is of recent origin, it generally heals spontaneously once the infection resolves [4, 5].

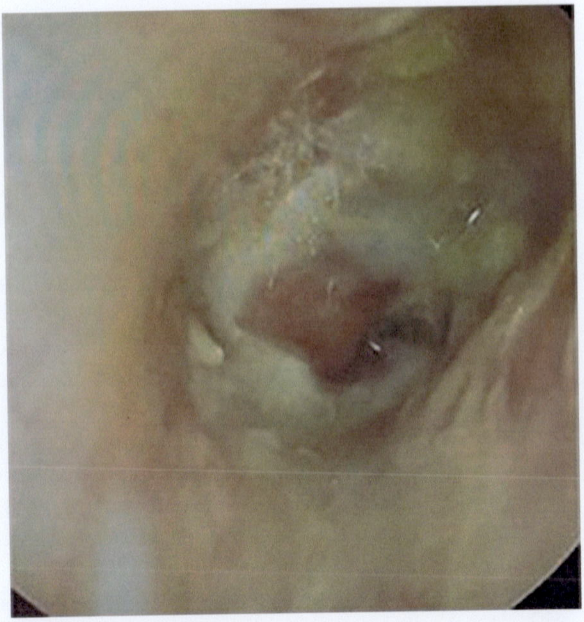

Fig. 21.1 Endoscopic view of suppurated acute otitis media

21.4 Chronic Suppurative Otitis Media

Chronic suppurative otitis media (CSOM), or mastoiditis, is an eardrum perforation with chronic drainage from the middle ear cleft [5]. This condition is more frequently seen in children who lack access to health care and, thus, do not have timely diagnosis and treatment of acute otitis media. It should not be confused with long-standing otitis media with effusion (OME, or "serous" otitis media) or persistent acute otitis media, which involve an intact tympanic membrane and no drainage.

CSOM is often painless. On examination, a debris-filled canal is noted. The discharge is often white to yellow and mixed with soft cerumen. Pseudomonas aeruginosa and Staphylococcus aureus are common pathogens. Treatment typically consists of topical antibiotic ear drops, with topical quinolones being the best-studied treatment choice. Parenteral antibiotic administration guided by culture of the ear discharge and/or tympanomastoidectomy may be necessary in refractory cases, though the evidence for the superiority of systemic antibiotics over topical quinolone antibiotics is mixed and not convincing [5, 6].

21.5 Foreign Body

The primary foreign objects encountered in cases are usually food, plastic toys, and small household objects. Identifying these cases can be challenging due to the often unnoticed nature of the incident, non-specific symptoms, and frequent initial misdiagnosis. In the majority of instances involving foreign objects lodged in the ear or nose, a trained physician can safely extract them within an office setting with minimal risk of complications. Typical removal techniques comprise the use of forceps, water irrigation, and suction catheters. Typical foreign bodies include:

- Toys or small objects placed in the ear by toddlers or placed into younger sibling's ears
- Insects, although they are often so irritating that removal occurs before otorrhea develops
- Food material, especially nuts with irritating oils that can cause a significant reaction
- Button batteries (often used in small electronic devices such as hearing aids)
- Expelled tympanostomy tube with granulation tissue and bloody otorrhea

Button batteries require **emergent removal** because pressure necrosis and/or severe burns from residual electric current or leakage of caustic contents may rapidly lead to extensive damage to adjacent structures [1].

Otoscopy serves as a diagnostic tool. However, the presence of either cerumen buildup or otorrhea may obstruct the visibility of the foreign body, necessitating cleaning before the object becomes visible (as depicted in Fig. 21.2). In cases where ear foreign bodies are present and do not lead to otorrhea, straightforward techniques can typically be employed for removal within an outpatient environment. However, if removal in the outpatient setting is not feasible, the foreign body should be extracted in an operating room while the patient is under sedation or general anesthesia. The initial attempt at removal is of paramount importance since the success rates significantly decrease after the first unsuccessful attempt. Consequently,

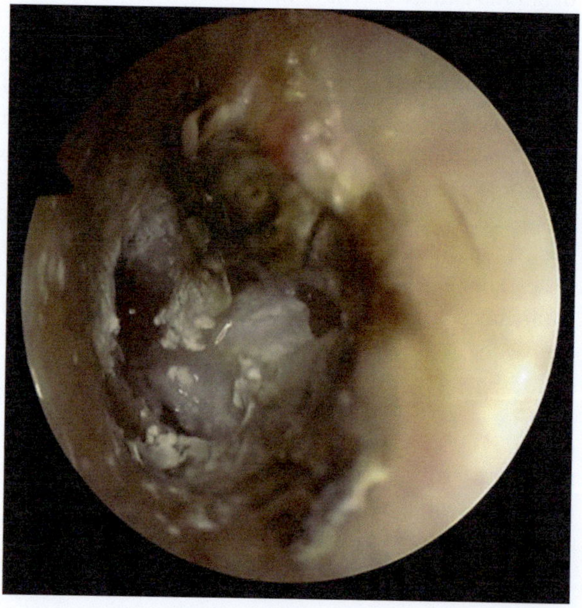

Fig. 21.2 Endoscopic view of foreign body in external ear canal

complications are more likely to arise as the number of failed removal attempts increases. These removal attempts can often be painful, lead to bleeding that limits visibility, and potentially push the foreign body further into the ear canal.

21.5.1 Cerumen

Annoying to many parents but generally harmless, some children have thin cerumen that can present as ear drainage. In general, cerumen is only a problem if it is impacted or precludes eardrum examination. Removal may be necessary in such cases, but precautions should be taken when instrumenting the ear canal [7].

21.5.2 Tympanostomy Tube Drainage

About 10–30% of children with tympanostomy tubes will have at least one episode of acute otorrhea while their tympanostomy tubes are in place immediately postoperatively or during an episode of acute otitis media (Fig. 21.3). The drainage is usually foul-smelling, mucoid, and may be mixed with blood. It is generally treated with antibiotic drops. Suction cleaning of the ear canal may be needed for slides to be effective. Rarely, systemic antibiotics or even mastoid surgery is required if the drainage is persistent.

In a patient with a history of trauma or compromised immune system, the presence of otorrhea can be a sign of a critical and potentially life-threatening condition.

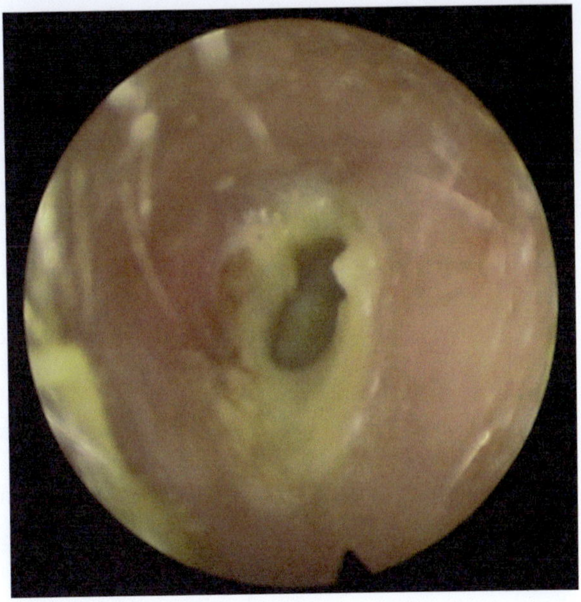

Fig. 21.3 Endoscopic view of infected ventilation tube with mucoid discharge

21.5.3 Traumatic Cerebrospinal Fluid Otorrhea

Trauma to the temporal bone can lead to immediate leaks through the fracture line or delayed leaks caused by obstructions in the cochlear aqueduct, typically due to soft tissue or bone. The presence of cerebrospinal fluid (CSF) otorrhea is a significant concern following head trauma. If there is any discharge from the ear noticed after a severe head injury, especially if it is clear or contains blood, it is essential to evaluate the patient for CSF otorrhea, which can originate from a basilar temporal skull fracture. Additionally, hemorrhagic otorrhea may result from middle ear trauma caused by a direct ear impact, auditory barotrauma, or the insertion of a foreign object into the external ear canal [8].

To assess the potential CSF leakage, a quick bedside test can be performed by placing a drop of ear drainage on absorbent material like a coffee filter or paper towel. A rapidly spreading "halo" or a ring of clear fluid around the area stained with red blood indicates a positive result. However, it is crucial to note that the halo test does not differentiate between CSF, saline, saliva, or other clear fluids and has not undergone formal clinical validation.

As an alternative, healthcare professionals may analyze the fluid coming from the ear or nose for the presence of beta2 transferrin, a variant of the transferrin protein primarily found in cerebrospinal fluid.

21.5.4 Complications of Acute Otitis Media

The mastoid air cells are linked to the far end of the middle ear through a narrow canal or antrum. Consequently, most instances of Acute Otitis Media (AOM) involve some degree of inflammation in the mastoid. In exceptional cases, the mastoid infection does not resolve, leading to the development of acute mastoiditis, characterized by the accumulation of pus within the mastoid air cells. The child with mastoiditis will have painful swelling behind the ear that typically pushes the pinna forward.

Other infratemporal complications that occur by contiguous spread of infection include petrositis (Gradenigo syndrome with sixth nerve palsy) and labyrinthitis.

Intracranial complications arising from Acute Otitis Media (AOM) are of special concern when dealing with children who exhibit signs of illness. These complications can encompass conditions such as "meningitis, epidural abscess, brain abscess, lateral sinus thrombosis, cavernous sinus thrombosis, subdural empyema, and carotid artery thrombosis" [9, 10]. Patients experiencing these complications typically present with fever and gradually develop a toxic appearance. Some may also display cranial nerve deficits, with cranial nerve VII (facial nerve) being the most commonly affected, and less frequently, cranial nerve VI [9, 10].

21.5.5 Necrotizing Otitis Externa (Malignant External Otitis)

Malignant external otitis is a condition primarily affecting children who have chronic illnesses or are immunosuppressed. Clinicians should be on the lookout for signs such as severe and persistent ear pain, ear discharge containing *Pseudomonas aeruginosa*, a significantly elevated erythrocyte sedimentation rate, and evidence of bone damage on a computed tomography scan, especially when dealing with these vulnerable populations. The infection typically starts with a skin infection and can progress to involve deeper structures like cartilage, tissue, and bone. As the infection advances, it can lead to complications such as osteomyelitis at the base of the skull, osteomyelitis of the temporomandibular joint, the formation of brain abscesses, and the development of generalized bacterial sepsis. Culture of the external ear canal in otorrhea is rarely helpful, as Pseudomonas species are commonly identified with or without local infection. It is also quite difficult to obtain samples from the middle ear that are not contaminated by external canal flora. In addition, culture rarely changes management decisions in children with otorrhea.

Indications for culture of ear drainage include:

- Suspected necrotizing otitis externa
- Otitis media with chronic drainage, where previous treatment has failed

Patients with malignant external otitis classically present with otorrhea and exquisite otalgia which are not responsive to topical measures used to treat simple external otitis. The pain is generally more severe than that found in simple external otitis, although the two may be difficult to distinguish in their early stages. The pain in malignant external otitis tends to extend into the temporomandibular joint, resulting in pain with chewing [11].

On physical examination, purulent otorrhea is seen in more than half of cases, and ipsilateral lower motor neuron facial nerve palsy can also be present. Granulation tissue may be visible in the inferior portion of the external auditory canal at the bone–cartilage junction (at the site of Santorini's fissures). This finding may be absent in atypical patients (e.g., HIV-infected patients and children). Early empiric antibiotic therapy and, if needed, surgery are essential to good outcomes [12].

21.5.6 Neoplasms

Cancer is an uncommon source of otorrhea in childhood; however, it should be taken into consideration in cases where there is abnormal tissue growth in the ear canal or when extended treatment for external otitis does not yield the expected results.

Ear canal cancer is a less frequent occurrence compared to cancer in the outer ear (auricular cancer), but it tends to present with more aggressive characteristics. During the initial stages, it may be challenging to distinguish it from external otitis.

Furthermore, it is worth noting that rhabdomyosarcoma and neuroblastoma can also present as tumors within the auditory canal in children [13].

Less commonly, otorrhea may arise from the following conditions:

Contact Dermatitis
Topical medications or cosmetics may cause local irritation and inflammation with ear drainage. A typical history reveals the offending agent being used, often for a pre-existing condition such as otitis externa or cerumen impaction. Pruritus, pain, and inflammation on examination accompany the otorrhea. Treatment consists of topical corticosteroids and avoidance of the allergen.

Bullous Myringitis
Often associated with respiratory symptoms or acute otitis media, bullous myringitis describes serous liquid-filled blisters, or "bullae," on the tympanic membrane. When the bullae rupture, thin bloody otorrhea may occur, and pain is often relieved. The external ear canal is not typically involved.

Granulation Tissue
Granulation tissue can develop in several conditions and can be associated with otorrhea. As mentioned, this tissue can accumulate around a foreign body (such as a tympanostomy tube). It can also be seen in granulomatous disease (such as Langerhans cell histiocytosis) or chronic inflammatory conditions (such as chronic otitis media). The rich vascular supply can also lead to leakage of lymphatic fluid [14].

21.5.7 Polyps

Polyps within the ear canal's external region can develop as a reaction to inflammation or infections, such as chronic otitis media, cholesteatoma, or the presence of a foreign body (e.g., a dislodged tympanostomy tube). In rare instances, they might originate from a tumor, such as Langerhans Cell Histiocytosis, teratoma, or a neoplasm. These polyps often result in the discharge of bloody or serous fluid from the ear, particularly when manipulated, displaying characteristics akin to granulomas. Treatment for ear polyps can lead to rapid resolution through the application of topical antibiotics and/or anti-inflammatory therapy [15].

21.5.8 Otomycosis

Otomycosis is a fungal infection of the external auditory canal and a common reason for external otitis treatment failure, usually caused by Aspergillus species. Patients with fungal external otitis commonly report itching, discomfort, discharge, discomfort, and feeling that something is in the ear canal. Otorrhea is generally thick and purulent. Deep-seated itching is the most troublesome symptom; pain is less intense than bacterial otitis externa. Fungal organisms have a very characteristic appearance in the ear canal, especially under magnified vision [16]. Topical antifungals are given, and thorough suction cleaning of the meatus is performed. And meautus should kept dry. In persistent infections, oral antifungals like Itraconazole may be prescribed.

21.5.9 First Branchial Cleft Cysts

The first branchial pouch originates within the pharynx and extends outwards and upwards to connect with the first branchial cleft, ultimately giving rise to the eustachian tube. Rarely, congenitally anomalous first branchial cleft cysts may drain into the external ear canal. A mass in the periauricular region may suggest this diagnosis in the face of chronic drainage with a normal tympanic membrane.

21.5.10 Cholesteatoma

A cholesteatoma is an anomalous development of squamous epithelial tissue. These growths can manifest within the middle ear and mastoid region (referred to as middle ear cholesteatoma) or, less frequently, within the ear canal itself (termed external ear canal cholesteatoma). Over time, a cholesteatoma may progressively expand, encompassing, and damaging the ossicles, which can result in conductive hearing impairment. Hearing loss may also occur if the cholesteatoma blocks the orifice of the eustachian tube, leading to the accumulation of fluid in the middle ear. Typically, surgical intervention is necessary for the treatment of most cholesteatomas [17, 18].

21.5.11 Spontaneous Cerebral Spinal Fluid Otorrhea

Apart from basilar skull fractures resulting from head injuries, spontaneous cerebrospinal fluid (CSF) otorrhea can also originate from defects in the tegmen tympani, located in the floor of the temporal bone. The possibility of these defects should be considered in situations where otorrhea persists after ruling out more typical causes, or in cases involving a child who has experienced multiple episodes of meningitis. A noninvasive approach to diagnosis involves utilizing high-resolution computed tomography (CT) with thin slices through the temporal bone [19].

References

1. Schulze SL, Kerschner J, Beste D. Pediatric external auditory canal foreign bodies: a review of 698 cases. Otolaryngol Head Neck Surg. 2002;127:73–8.
2. Macfadyen CA, Acuin JM, Gamble C. Systemic antibiotics versus topical treatments for chronically discharging ears with underlying eardrum perforations. Cochrane Database Syst Rev. 2006;(1):CD005608.
3. Boyce TG. Otitis externa and necrotizing otitis externa. In: Long SS, Pickering LK, Prober CG, editors. Principles and practice of pediatric infectious diseases. 4th ed. Edinburgh: Elsevier Saunders; 2012. p. 220–2.

4. Heikkinen T, Ruuskanen O. Signs and symptoms predicting acute otitis media. Arch Pediatr Adolesc Med. 1995;149(1):26–9.
5. Mansour S, Magnan J, Nicolas K, Haidar H. Chronic Suppurative otitis media (CSOM): a middle ear mucosal disease. In: Middle ear diseases. Cham: Springer; 2018. https://doi.org/10.1007/978-3-319-72962-6_6.
6. Yorgancılar E, Yildirim M, Gun R, Bakir S, Tekin R, Gocmez C, et al. Complications of chronic suppurative otitis media: a retrospective review. Eur Arch Otorrinolaringol. 2013;270:69–76.
7. Chai TJ, Chai TC. Bactericidal activity of cerumen. Antimicrob Agents Chemother. 1980;18:638–41.
8. Magliocca KR, Vivas EX, Griffith CC. Idiopathic, infectious and reactive lesions of the ear and temporal bone. Head Neck Pathol. 2018;12:328.
9. Ceylan A, Bayazit Y, Yilmaz M, Celenk F, Bayramoglu I, Uygur K, et al. Extracranial complications of chronic otitis media. Int Adv Otol. 2009;5:51–5.
10. Wu JF, Jin Z, Yang JM, Liu YH, Duan M. Extracranial and intracranial complications of otitis media: 22-year clinical experience and analysis. Acta Otolaryngol. 2012;132:261–5.
11. Rubin J, Yu VL, Stool SE. Malignant external otitis in children. J Pediatr. 1988;113(6):965–70. https://doi.org/10.1016/s0022-3476(88)80564-x.
12. Roland PS, Stroman DW. Microbiology of acute otitis externa. Laryngoscope. 2002;112:1166–77.
13. Janz TA, Camilon PR, Cheung AY, Nguyen SA, White DR, Weber PC. A review of pediatric middle ear tumors and analysis of the demographics, management, and survival of pediatric rhabdomyosarcomas of the middle ear. Int J Pediatr Otorhinolaryngol. 2018;112:109–12. https://doi.org/10.1016/j.ijporl.2018.06.017. Epub 2018 Jun 12
14. Harris KC, Conley SF, Kerschner JE. Foreign body granuloma of the external auditory canal. Pediatrics. 2004;113:e371.
15. Gliklich RE, Cunningham MJ, Eavey RD. The cause of aural polyps in children. Arch Otolaryngol Head Neck Surg. 1993;119:669.
16. Anwar K, Gohar MS. Otomycosis; clinical features, predisposing factors and treatment implications. Pak J Med Sci. 2014;30(3):564–7. https://doi.org/10.12669/pjms.303.4106.
17. Persaud RA, Hajioff D, Thevasagayam MS, et al. Keratosis obturans and external ear canal cholesteatoma: how and why we should distinguish between these conditions. Clin Otolaryngol Allied Sci. 2004;29:577.
18. Shire JR, Donegan JO. Cholesteatoma of the external auditory canal and keratosis obturans. Am J Otol. 1986;7:361.
19. Rao AK, Merenda DM, Wetmore SJ. Diagnosis and management of spontaneous cerebrospinal fluid otorrhea. Otol Neurotol. 2005;26:1171.

22 Nasal Congestion in Children

Murat Gümüşsoy and İbrahim Çukurova

22.1 Introduction

Nasal congestion is common in newborns, infants, and older children and is a significant problem. It is one of the most common reasons for consultation in ear, nose, and throat (ENT) practice, where it is requested to be evaluated by pediatricians under outpatient clinic conditions. Although the subjective perception of difficulty or difficulty breathing through the nose and expressing this situation as disturbing is defined as nasal congestion, the problem is slightly different for children. It should not be forgotten that nasal congestion, considered a simple finding, can cause serious, life-threatening consequences such as malnutrition, respiratory distress, and sleep apnea, especially in the neonatal period [1].

The first 3 months are when the newborn's air needs are met only through nasal breathing. Partial or complete nose obstruction as an entrance to the upper respiratory tract causes the child to experience respiratory failure. While both nasal obstructions inevitably result in emergency airway obstruction, partial or single nasal obstruction clinically results in more difficulty in feeding. Both situations may require a critical and urgent approach. For older age groups, a blocked nose is more likely to result in poor quality of life rather than an emergency approach and constitutes a substantial patient group in ENT practice [2].

The history taken from the families regarding nasal congestion is significant for diagnosis. In the past, children's day and night findings should be questioned in detail, especially the child's feeding, sucking, sleep, and wakefulness status provide clues for the approach to nasal congestion. Additionally, runny nose, bleeding, and snoring are other findings that should be questioned [3].

M. Gümüşsoy · İ. Çukurova (✉)
Health Sciences University Izmir Tepecik SUAM ENT Clinic, Izmir, Turkey

Department of Otolaryngology-Head and Neck Surgery, Izmir Tepecik Training and Research Hospital, University of Health Sciences, Izmir, Turkey

H. Yüksel et al. (eds.), *Pediatric Airway Diseases*, Comprehensive ENT,
https://doi.org/10.1007/978-3-031-74853-0_22

ENT examination should be performed as thoroughly and completely as possible in pediatric patients. Anatomical structures, especially those involving the upper airway, should be evaluated in detail with rigid or flexible endoscopy. Although radiological imaging methods are not routine after endoscopic evaluation with the preliminary diagnosis of nasal obstruction in children, they can be used when necessary in suitable patients. Imaging in children may be limited for different reasons, especially compliance problems. In addition, it is almost impossible to apply nasal airflow tests, acoustic rhinometry, rhinomanometry, and similar methods in children, which we can use for nasal congestion in adult patients [1–3].

Nasal congestion in children can generally occur due to congenital or acquired anatomical disorders, mucosal pathologies, and many different and various diseases that block air passage due to the mass effect. In addition, the obstruction may be unilateral, bilateral, permanent, or temporary (during the day). The most crucial difference is that the causes of nasal congestion in children may differ etiologically depending on the child's age. While physiological and congenital causes cause nasal congestion in the newborn period, infectious causes come to the fore as the child grows. For all these reasons, it can be challenging to focus on the problem in children who complain of nasal congestion. Therefore, detailed history, ENT examination, and endoscopic examination contain important clues for diagnosis. Radiological imaging, even a biopsy, may sometimes be required for diagnostic purposes [4, 5].

22.2 Nasal Breathing in the Neonatal Period

Especially in children, the first 12 weeks following birth are critical in terms of the need for mandatory nasal breathing. Any obstacle in nasal breathing can cause severe and life-threatening problems in the child. Anatomical structures in the neonatal period differ between infants and children. Inside the mouth, the tongue is more extensive, complicated, and attached to the soft palate than the oropharynx opening. The epiglottis is located above the level of the soft palate. Placing the epiglottis and larynx in a higher position than usual allows the newborn to feed and breathe air simultaneously. Therefore, nasal congestion negatively affects breathing and nutrition [4–6].

The nasal cavity contributes approximately half of the total resistance of commonly inhaled air. Therefore, the degree of obstruction and the findings are at the forefront. As a sign of respiratory distress, the nasal flap participates in breathing, trying to balance breathing by reducing inspiratory airflow resistance. However, due to the degree of obstruction and increased air resistance, rapid desaturation and respiratory difficulty will occur for newborns with nasal obstructions following birth. The situation is urgent and fatal if left untreated. Airway patency should be ensured quickly, and the newborn should be intubated. If intubation cannot be performed, tracheotomy should be performed in emergencies. Unilateral nasal obstruction occurs in later periods in direct proportion to the degree to which it affects breathing and nutrition [5, 6].

Several physiological changes from the neonatal period and childhood can trigger nasal congestion. The physiological mechanism controlled by the autonomic nervous system on both sides of the nasal cavity, which we call the nasal cycle, ensures the nasal airflow resistance remains balanced. The nasal cycle is increased on one side of the nose by the erectile properties of the turbinates and decreased on the other, resulting in physiological nasal congestion that may last between 30 min and 6 h. In addition, positionally, nasal congestion may occur due to congestion in the underlying nasal cavity when the child is laid on its side. In the first year of life, nasal congestion is expected due to physiological reasons, especially nasal congestion, and affects sleep quality. Nevertheless, with the rapid growth pattern of the newborn and the nasal volume approximately doubling in the first 6 months of life, a significant improvement in the symptoms of nasal congestion is observed [6, 7].

Evaluation of a newborn with nasal congestion begins with a history taken from the mother, father, and relatives. In addition to nasal congestion, it is learned whether symptoms such as runny nose, wheezing, or feeding problems are accompanied. It is essential when the findings are noticed and whether they are intermittent or continuous. The diseases the mother had during pregnancy, the medications she used, familial genetic disorders, and conditions detected before birth should be questioned in detail. Learning the details of the labor process and its aftermath (early birth, prematurity, prolonged labor time, difficult birth, birth trauma, postnatal resuscitation, or intubation history) may be helpful in diagnosis [8]

After the newborn has an adequate airway after birth, a detailed physical examination should be performed to investigate the presence of deformity, asymmetry, and skin lesions in the newborn's body. Afterward, nasal patency should be evaluated. The most commonly used practical and easy method to assess nasal patency is to evaluate the patency by advancing from the tip of the nose towards the nasopharynx with a plastic catheter or cannula. However, today, the most valid method for nasal obstruction is direct examination and examination of the nasal cavity up to the nasopharynx using flexible or rigid endoscopy. After endoscopic examination, pathology is detected, and radiological evaluation (Computed Tomography (CT) and Magnetic Resonance Imaging (MRI)) is performed. CT is more valuable for evaluating bone structures such as choanal atresia and piriform aperture stenosis, and MRI is more practical for soft tissues and intracranial extension and connections. In the presence of an obstructive lesion, biopsy should also be considered. However, a biopsy should only be performed with radiological evaluation [9].

22.3 Etiology of Nasal Congestion in Children

The complaint of nasal congestion, which we frequently encounter in children from birth to adulthood, is the most important of the clinical problems that sleep disturbance, snoring, OSAS findings, and regression in growth, development, and learning abilities can accompany.

Nasal and paranasal symptoms may accompany nasal congestion. These are the basics of common diseases, such as allergic rhinitis, rhinosinusitis, septal deviation, adenoid hypertrophy, or nasal trauma.

It may be a symptom. In addition, lung-related pathologies such as asthma may also accompany it.

Different classifications have been used in the literature for the etiology of nasal congestion in children. Nasal congestion is a comprehensive issue that can be seen due to congenital or acquired anatomical disorders, mucosal level, or structural disorders that can block the nasal passage due to mass effects, trauma, and iatrogenic reasons. The obstruction may be bilateral or unilateral, or it may be permanent or temporary.

This section will discuss the etiological causes of nasal congestion, their prevalence according to age, and their diagnosis and treatment [7–10].

Nasal congestion in children can be evaluated in two groups according to age.

1. Causes of nasal congestion in newborns and babies.
   (a) Physiological (Nasal cycle and positional congestion).
   (b) Neonatal rhinitis.
   (c) Congenital.
   (d) Trauma.
   (e) Neoplasia (benign, malignant).
2. Causes of nasal congestion in children.
   (a) Inflammatory/infectious.
   (b) Adenoid hypertrophy.
   (c) Foreign body (unilateral obstruction).
   (d) Septal deviation.
   (e) Neoplasia (benign, malignant).
   (f) Systemic diseases.

Generally, the etiological causes of nasal congestion in children are classified in Table 22.1.

Table 22.1 Causes of nasal congestion in children

1. Physiological
2. Congenital
(a) Choanal atresia
(b) Pyriform aperture stenosis
(c) Nasal dermoid
(d) Nasal glioma
(e) Encephalocele
(f) Nasolacrimal duct cysts
3. Infectious
(a) Neonatal rhinitis
(b) Infectious rhinitis (rhinosinusitis)
(c) Adenoid hypertrophy
4. Inflammatory
(a) Allergic rhinitis
(b) Nonallergic rhinitis
(c) Nasal polyp-Antrochoanal polyp
(d) Inferior turbinate hypertrophy
5. Neoplasia
(a) Benign
• Juvenile nasopharyngeal angiofibroma
• Nasopharyngeal teratoma
(b) Malignant
• Adenocarcinoma
• Esthesioneuroblastoma
• Lymphoma
• Metastatic disease
• Nasopharynx carcinoma
• Rhabdomyosarcoma
• Squamous cell carcinoma
6. Systemic
(a) Cystic fibrosis
(b) Primary ciliary dyskinesia
7. Trauma/iatrogenic
(a) Septal hematoma
(b) Septum deviation
(c) Foreign body in the nose

22.4 Congenital Causes

22.4.1 Choanal Atresia

Many congenital facial deformities in childhood can cause nasal congestion. The most common is choanal atresia, in which the opening between the nasal cavity and the nasopharynx is impaired due to one or bilateral atresia obstruction in the posterior part of the nasal cavity (Fig. 22.1). In 30% of the cases, it is bilateral, and in 70% of the cases, bone and membranous components are seen together. Its

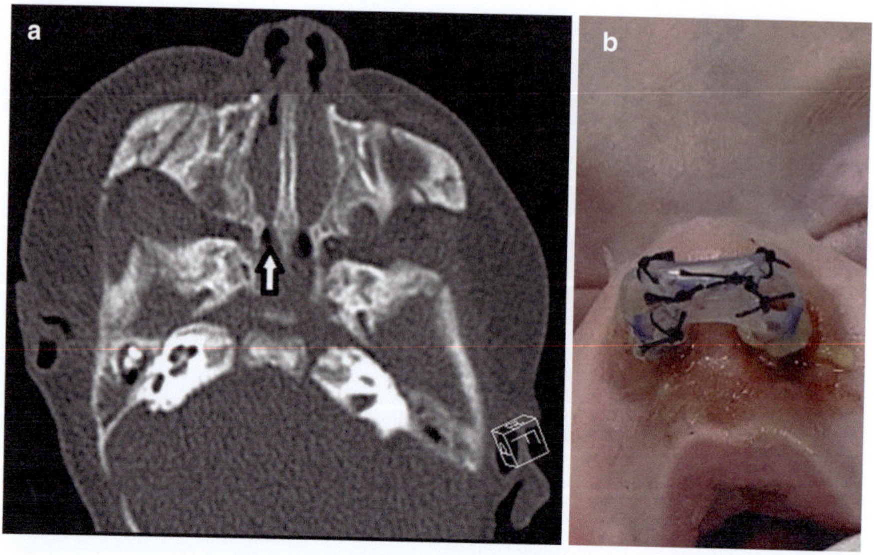

Fig. 22.1 The newborn was evaluated for respiratory distress. (**a**) Paranasal axial CT, white arrow, bone atretic plaque in the choanal region, (**b**) Silicone tube stent placed in both noses after surgery

incidence is 1/5000–7000 births. Regarding gender, the female/male ratio is 2/1, it is unilateral, and the right side is predominant. It may be accompanied by additional congenital anomalies in approximately 40–60% of cases. Choanal atresia and CHARGE syndrome [C: "coloboma," H: "heart defects (congenital heart disease)," A: "atresia (choanal)," R: "retardation (mental)," G: "genital hypoplasia," E: "ear abnormalities/deafness"] is more common than other anomalies [11] (Fig. 22.1).

For the newborn, bilateral choanal atresia is a vital condition accompanied by immediate respiratory failure and cyanosis. In unilateral atresia, the diagnosis may be made late. Children may be asymptomatic or apply to the clinic with complaints of runny nose, sleep disorders, and feeding problems. Atresia is often noticed when the nasogastric tube cannot be passed through the nose. Diagnosis can be made by ENT examination and flexible endoscopic nasal examination. Radiological analysis should be performed to evaluate the atresia's location, position, and anatomical structures. Paranasal CT in the axial-coronal plane should be the first choice. Before radiological imaging, aspiration of both nasal cavities should be performed in a child with suspected choanal atresia to evaluate CT more efficiently [12].

22.4.1.1 Points to Consider in Axial-Coronal Paranasal CT

1. Unilateral or bilateral atresia, bone and membranous association, and thickness of atresia.
2. In axial imaging, the portion of the airway opening to the nasopharynx is less than 3 mm; that is, it shows narrowing, evident in the posterior part of the nasal cavity.
3. Monitoring the air-liquid level above the obstruction level.

4. Thickening in the vomer.
5. Hypertrophic inferior turbinates are findings that can be determined radiologically.

The treatment of choanal atresia is surgery, and today, transnasal endoscopic surgery is the most frequently preferred approach. Surgery aims to eliminate the atresic plaque. Different studies have reported that transnasal endoscopic surgery success rates are between 70 and 90%. After nasal passage patency, silicone tube stents are placed and kept for at least 3 weeks (Fig. 22.1). Re-occlusion of the atresia area opened in choanal atresia surgery is still the biggest obstacle to success. Risk factors include gastroesophageal reflux, bilateral bone atresia, and age at surgery less than 10 years old. Since bilateral nasal passage obstruction is an airway emergency in children, it should be treated surgically as soon as possible. In necessary patients, the patient should be provided with an oral airway until surgical treatment. In unilateral patients, it can wait until 18–24 months at the earliest or often until school age. Children with feeding difficulties can benefit from McGovern pacifiers until surgical intervention [13, 14].

22.4.2 Pyriform Apertura Stenosis

Also known as stenosis of the front part of the nose, it is a rare congenital anomaly that occurs as the pyriform aperture of the maxillary bone, which forms the entrance to the nose, grows more than usual towards the medial or becomes ossified, resulting in a narrowing of the aperture. In children, symptoms similar to children with bilateral choanal atresia are observed, with feeding difficulties and cyanosis attacks. It may be accompanied by anomalies such as prominent central incisors, hypoplastic maxillary sinuses, or holoprosencephaly. Diagnosis is made by showing on CT that the maxillary aperture in the front of the nose is narrower than usual. Airway management is the most critical aspect of treatment [15].

Medical interventions include McGovern pacifiers, oral airway, or endotracheal intubation. Publications state that surgical intervention will be necessary when the distance between piriform openings is less than 5.7 mm. The transnasal sublabial approach is the preferred surgical method. With the sublabial approach, the bone is opened laterally and downwards, gaining a wide airway. Particular attention should be paid to tooth buds. It is recommended that nasal stents be retained for 4–6 weeks following surgery [16].

22.4.3 Nasal Midline Congenital Masses

22.4.3.1 Nasal Dermoid Cyst

It is the most common congenital midline nasal lesion. Nasal dermoid cysts refer to cystic congenital anomalies lined with squamous epithelium, which is located on the midline nasal dorsum and has a channel that can pass through the skin, through the septum, through the cribriform plate, and extend to the skull base and even to the dura. They can be somewhere between the glabella and columella. Cystic expansion of the duct is defined as a dermoid cyst [17].

Nasal dermoid cysts may contain skin appendages (mesodermal). About 60% of the cysts are seen outside the nose, 30% are inside the nose, and the remaining 10% are of mixed type. Radiological examination is vital for diagnosis. CT is used for bone structures and relationships, and MRI with Gadolinium is used to evaluate intracranial extension and soft tissue. The treatment is surgical, and total excision is essential. Inadequate surgery may result in recurrence [18].

22.4.3.2 Nasal Glioma

Nasal gliomas are craniofacial masses developed from remnants of congenital benign neuro-glial tissues. Although they are perceived as tumors, they are accumulations of glial tissue in the extradural region. These are abnormal connections between the embryonic ectodermal and neuroectodermal parts due to the incomplete closure of the anterior fontanelle between the nasal and frontal bones. About 30% of nasal gliomas are intranasal, and 15–20% have an intracranial connection with a fibrous band. On examination, it is smooth, not compressed by pressure; the overlying skin may be discolored or telangiectatic, and the mass is not attached to the mobile skin. Gliomas that have grown inside the nose can cause septal deviation. Sometimes, they can look like antrochoanal polyps. They may protrude from the anterior or posterior nasal cavity as pink-red polypoid masses. In MRI evaluation, detailed information about the intracranial distance can be obtained, and it also provides differentiation from other midline anomalies (encephalocele, dermoid cyst, etc.). Gliomas appear isointense on T1 and heterogeneous on T2 and do not capture contrast material. Treatment involves total excision of the mass [19, 20].

22.4.3.3 Encephalocele (Encephalo-Meningocele)

They are considered congenital neural tube defects. They always appear as extracranial herniation of meninges and brain tissue in the cranial defect area. They can be meninges (encephalocele), brain, and meninges (encephalo-meningocele). In nasal encephalocele formation, there is a bone defect between the frontal and ethmoid bones. The mass can be seen to grow with crying or with pressure on the jugular vein (Furstenberg test). Fronto-ethmoid encephaloceles are observed as compressible masses that give intranasal translucency. Clinically, they may present with nasal congestion, cerebrospinal fluid rhinorrhea, or recurrent attacks of meningitis [21].

CT and MRI examinations are required for diagnosis. While CT is used to show the location of the bone defect at the skull base, MRI provides information about the sac content and intracranial extension (Fig. 22.2). In cases where encephalocele is suspected, biopsy is not recommended due to intracranial relationship. When diagnosed in the first months of life, surgery should be planned to avoid the risk of meningitis and cosmetic deformity due to the growth of the mass. Treatment includes total removal of the group and repair of the dura [22, 23] (Fig. 22.2).

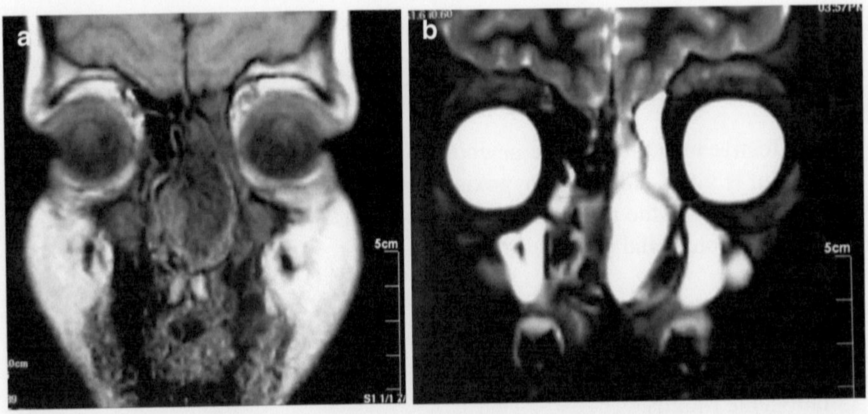

Fig. 22.2 A 6-year-old girl complains of long-term nasal congestion and snoring. (**a**) Encephalocele extending to the inferior of the left frontal lobe with a fibrous band in the coronal MRI T1 section of the patient. (**b**) T2 section Coronal MRI imaging of the case

Differential Diagnosis

(a) Nasal glioma and dermoid cysts do not shrink upon examination, whereas encephalocele is consistently soft and shrinks when pressed.
(b) Unlike nasal glioma and dermoid cysts, encephalocele may show transillumination.
(c) The formation associated with cerebrospinal fluid is encephalocele (herniation of the meninges).
(d) Nasal glioma has no connection with the intracranial region.
(e) Encephalocele is pulsative (positive Furstenberg).
(f) There is no pulsation in nasal glioma and dermoid cysts (negative Furstenberg).
(g) Radiological imaging is sufficient for diagnosis.
(h) Preoperative biopsy should not be performed.
(i) While cranial bone defects are seen radiologically in encephalocele and dermoid cysts, CT, and MRI, they are not seen in nasal glioma.

22.4.3.4 Nasolacrimal Duct Cyst (Dacryocystocele)

A nasolacrimal duct cyst develops due to incomplete canalization of the nasolacrimal duct during fetal development and can cause significant nasal obstruction in the newborn. Clinically, it is usually seen unilaterally, and the most common finding is epiphora. It is typical to see a bluish cystic lesion located in the medial canthus or an intranasal cystic mass [24].

Congestion in both noses occurs in 14% of cases and can close the nasal cavity and cause severe respiratory distress. CT is the method of choice for diagnosis. On CT, it can be seen as a cystic mass in the medial canthus region, expansion of the nasolacrimal duct, and a cystic mass filling the nasal passage at the level of the inferior turbinate. Its treatment is surgery [25].

22.5 Infectious Causes

22.5.1 Rhinitis in the Neonatal Period

Since effective breathing for the newborn is only possible with an open nose, nasal congestion is vital, and severe hypoxia can have serious consequences. In the differential diagnosis, the most common cause of nasal congestion, apart from physiological and congenital causes, is rhinitis [4–6].

22.5.1.1 Rhinitis Etiology

1. Neonatal rhinitis.
2. Bacterial or viral rhinitis.
3. Iatrogenic rhinitis.

22.5.2 Neonatal Rhinitis

It is the most common cause of nasal congestion in the neonatal period. Regardless of the causative pathology, it is observed as runny nose and congestion in children under 3. Although its etiology is unknown, many causes have been blamed: viral, inflammatory, vascular, drug-related, traumatic, hormones and drugs transmitted from the mother, etc. Nasal examination reveals bilateral nasal mucosa edema and mucoid nasal discharge. A regression in symptoms is observed after nasal lavage with physiological saline. Rhinitis symptoms resolve spontaneously over time [5, 26].

22.5.3 Bacterial or Viral Rhinitis

The causative agent is often bacteria such as maternal streptococci, staphylococci, chlamydia, gonorrhea, and syphilis, and less frequently, viral agents, especially respiratory syncytial virus. The clinical picture is nasal congestion after nasopharyngitis and rhinitis [27, 28].

22.5.4 Iatrogenic Rhinitis

Iatrogenic rhinitis is due to secondary infection, trauma, nasal catheterization, or uncleaned residues such as meconium remaining in the nose. Another factor associated with rhinitis findings in the neonatal period is gastroesophageal reflux. Nasal congestion causes an increase in negative intralaryngeal pressure during inspiration, thus facilitating reflux. Therefore, in the presence of a persistent nasal obstruction in the neonatal period, the possibility of gastroesophageal reflux should be investigated and treated [27–29].

22.5.5 Infectious Rhinitis (Rhinosinusitis)

Infectious rhinitis is often seen in childhood as inflammation of the nose and sinuses due to viral, bacterial, and less fungal reasons. Acute upper respiratory tract infections (rhinovirus) are infections of viral origin that are transmitted via droplets. Rhinitis clinically manifests with complaints of local itching and sneezing, congestion, and discharge (serous) in the nose, along with systemic symptoms such as chills, weakness, and fever. Flu (influenza) has a more severe course than rhinovirus. It causes more serious damage to the upper respiratory tract, often leading to secondary infection. The incidence of sinusitis increases in children after rhinovirus or influenza is the causative agent of rhinitis. Sinusitis is seen in 5–10% of children due to upper respiratory tract infections, especially between 6 and 8. It is more appropriate to call this condition, which clinically concerns both the nose and sinuses, rhinosinusitis rather than sinusitis [30, 31].

When we examine it physiopathologically, viral infections disrupt nasal mucociliary activity, cause mucosal edema, and narrow the sinus ostium, thus preparing the ground for the development of sinusitis. Due to the anatomical neighborhood of the sinuses with the nasal cavity, colonized Streptococcus pneumoniae, Haemophilus influenzae, and Moraxella catarrhalis can pass into the sinuses. The mechanism can be summarized as ostium occlusion, negative sinus pressure, and infection. Impaired sinus circulation, mucus, and bacterial colonization in the sinus can easily result in acute bacterial rhinosinusitis. The most common viral agent that disrupts this defense mechanism is rhinoviruses. Rhinoviruses have a very high infection capacity [32].

Rhinosinusitis is more straightforward to develop in children in two ways. The first reason is that the sinuses are small in volume, and their physiological defense mechanisms are not as fully developed as in adults due to their incomplete development.

Second, they experience frequent viral infections during childhood. The most critical risk factor for frequent infections is that the child goes to nursery or school. In the clinic of acute bacterial rhinosinusitis in children, nasal congestion, runny nose, posterior nasopharyngeal drainage, fever, cough, pain, especially on the side of the face where sinusitis occurs, edema, and halitosis (bad breath) are observed. ENT examination, especially nasal anterior rhinoscopy and endoscopic examination, is vital for diagnosis. Nasal endoscopic examination is essential for evaluating many different structures, such as anatomical structures (septum deviation, turbinate hypertrophy), adenoid hypertrophy, and foreign bodies. Additionally, nasal endoscopy provides essential clues to show allergic rhinitis, nasal polyps, mucosal edema, scarring, discharge, and crusting within the nose [33].

In children under age 6, clinical findings compatible with rhinosinusitis, history, and ENT examination are sufficient for diagnosis, and radiological evaluation is unnecessary. Radiological evaluation is useless, especially in children younger than 1 year old. It cannot be evaluated because it is not radiologically developed except for the ethmoidal and maxillary sinuses. Ethmoid and maxillary sinuses are present at birth. The remaining sinuses begin to ventilate after age four and reach adult size by age twelve.

In summary, maxillary and ethmoid sinusitis may occur in the neonatal and infant period. The most frequently requested plain radiograph is the Waters radiography. However, its contribution is limited; no radiological evaluation alone can diagnose rhinosinusitis. Clinical findings are always more valuable. The diagnosis of uncomplicated rhinosinusitis can be made based on history and clinical findings. In radiological evaluation, CT and MRI are useful in evaluating cases with chronic or recurrent sinusitis that are clinically considered complications [31–34].

Rhinosinusitis treatment in children is applied as antimicrobial treatment and supportive treatment for the causative agent. In treating rhinosinusitis, antimicrobial therapy shortens the duration of clinical recovery, especially for the causative agent, and prevents possible complications. In case of antibiotic resistance during treatment, it may be necessary to reconsider the following criteria in the history. Suppose the child goes to kindergarten or nursery, has received antibiotic treatment in the last 3 months, is less than 2 years old, has recently been hospitalized, and has received antibiotic treatment. In that case, there is a high probability of being infected with a Streptococcus pneumoniae strain that has reduced sensitivity to penicillin, especially amoxicillin. If these risks do not exist, amoxicillin is started orally at 45 mg/kg/day. However, if these risks exist, the amoxicillin dose is increased to 80–90 mg/kg/day [35].

As a supportive treatment, the main goal is to reduce edema in the nasal mucosa, open the Ostia, facilitate sinus drainage, and reduce fever. Decongestants, nasal steroids, nasal lavage, and mucolytic drugs are used for these purposes. However, no significant advantage of these drugs over placebo has been demonstrated. It should not be forgotten that long-term use of decongestant medications can cause rhinitis medicomentosa. The effectiveness of topical steroids in the treatment has been investigated, and it is stated that they may be beneficial only for rhinosinusitis caused by allergy. Nasal lavage is helpful in moistening and mechanical cleaning of the mucosa. However, it is challenging to apply to children under two. Pressure nasal lavage should be used cautiously, especially in children under six. Care should be taken in case of acute otitis media because the nasal flora passes to the middle ear via the eustachian tube [33–37].

22.6 Adenoid Hypertrophy

Adenoid hypertrophy is essential for nasal congestion and rhinosinusitis in children, especially between the ages of 2 and 6. Adenoid is anatomically located in the posterior nasopharynx and is an important member of the Waldeyer Ring. It is essential in developing and maturing non-immune B-lymphocytes, especially in the neonatal period, against environmental antigens during infection processes from the oral cavity and pharynx. Adenoid tissue grows in volume until age 6–7 and shrinks and atrophy during early puberty [38].

The presence of nasal congestion, purulent nasal discharge, postnasal discharge, fever, and cough suggests adenoid hypertrophy and infection. Rhinosinusitis and otitis media may often accompany the condition. Nasal congestion impairs orofacial facial development in the child, causing the typical appearance referred to as an adenoid face. This condition is a result of prolonged nasal congestion. A characteristic adenoid facial appearance with an open mouth appearance, short upper lip, widened nasal dorsum, dome palate, and retrognathic mandible formation can be mentioned in a child who breathes through the mouth instead of the nose [39, 40].

Adenoid hypertrophy in children causes eustachian tubal dysfunction and ear pathologies (serous and recurrent otitis media). In advanced cases, proportional to the degree of nasal obstruction, sleep-disordered breathing and regression in attention and learning skills may be added to the clinical picture [41].

The diagnosis is easily made by history and endoscopic examination (Fig. 22.1). Direct radiography has no place in diagnosis; it causes the child to receive unnecessary radiation. Instead, adenoid hypertrophy can be quickly evaluated with nasal and nasopharyngeal endoscopy. Treatment is surgical removal of adenoid tissue [39–41].

22.7 Inflammatory Causes

22.7.1 Allergic Rhinitis

It is one of the most common causes of nasal congestion in children, as a type 1 hypersensitivity reaction mediated by immunoglobulin E due to exposure of the nasal mucosa to the allergen, seen in 6–18% of children [42].

In its physiopathology, it is a picture of inflammatory origin, clinically characterized by watery eyes, itching, nasal discharge (serous), sneezing, and nasal congestion, as a result of the nasal mucosa, which has been previously sensitized, that is, encountered with the antigen, facing the same antigen. If the child is not treated early, maxillofacial anomalies may develop due to open-mouth breathing and nasal congestion. While questioning the history, the time when the symptoms appeared, whether they continue seasonally or throughout the year, accompanying cough, sleeping with the mouth open, snoring, sleep quality, growth and development, and nutritional status should be learned. In addition to the findings, whether there are frequent complaints of acute or serous otitis media or rhinosinusitis should be investigated. Pets and conditions that may cause allergies should be noted [43].

The most common symptom of allergic rhinitis in children is the allergic salute gesture. In this movement, the nose tip is involuntarily pressed upward with the palm to relieve nasal itching and ease nasal breathing. In addition, allergic shiners, which are characterized by the appearance of dark circles on the lower eyelid skin that turn into permanent pigmentation over time, and small half-moon-shaped lines (Dennie-Morgan lines) that appear on the lower eyelid are typical for allergic rhinitis. Endoscopic nasal examination is critical in the diagnosis of the disease. In endoscopy, mucosa and turbinates are pale, serous discharge is present, and inferior turbinate hypertrophy may also accompany. Additionally, adenoid hypertrophy, antrochoanal polyp, nasal polyp, acute otitis media, serous otitis media, and rhinosinusitis findings may also occur [44].

Clinical and anamnesis information is usually sufficient for the diagnosis of allergic rhinitis. Diagnosing and confirming allergy in children, considered in the history and examination, is possible with allergic skin tests. The sensitivity reaction to a specific antigen applied to the skin is measured. In this way, it is determined whether immunotherapy can be used or not [45].

The main goal in treating allergic rhinitis is to protect and stay away from allergens. If this is not possible, medical treatment, immunotherapy, and surgical treatment can be applied. Surgical treatment aims to include anatomical pathologies such as turbinate hypertrophy, where medical therapy fails, and septum deviation, where it is ineffective [42–45].

22.7.2 Nonallergic Rhinitis

This group includes all rhinitis in the absence of non-IgE-related immunological mechanisms. It is less common in children and occurs in 70% of adult patients after age twenty [45].

22.7.3 Eosinophilic Nonallergic Rhinitis (NARES)

Nasal congestion and runny nose are the most common symptoms. Although the disease occurs throughout the year, it is more common in autumn and winter, when the temperature difference between home and outdoor environments is highest. Sneezing, watery serous runny nose, itching, and symptoms such as nasal congestion are observed. It is a condition in which eosinophils are more than 20% in the smear. Additionally, this disease is characterized by the negativity of the prick skin test and the absence of serum IgE antibodies. It may occur alone or in association with nasal polyps, non-IgE-dependent asthma, or aspirin sensitivity. Corticosteroids are the most critical drug group in treatment [46].

22.7.4 Nasal Polyp

It is a chronic inflammatory disease whose etiology is not fully explained and is less common in children than antrochoanal polyps. It is often observed on both sides of the nose. Complaints of nasal congestion, runny nose, rhinosinusitis, or allergic rhinitis may accompany patients. Nasal polyps are more common in allergies, asthma, aspirin/nonsteroidal anti-inflammatory sensitivity, and cystic fibrosis (CF) patients. Therefore, nasal polyps in children are a clinical warning sign to investigate cystic fibrosis [47].

Nasal polyps are seen as pale, transparent, and smooth-surfaced mass lesions during endoscopic nasal examination. Approximately one-third have a unilateral antrochoanal polyp, another third have polyps secondary to the infective process associated with mucus retention that occurs in cystic fibrosis (CF), and the remainder are associated with a range of inflammatory conditions, although most remain idiopathic. Nasal examination and CT are sufficient for diagnosis and treatment planning. A prick skin test can be performed if there is a history of allergy. Although its treatment is planned medically and surgically, it is sometimes tricky. Corticosteroids are the most critical agents in medical treatment. Endoscopic sinus surgery is preferred in surgical treatment. Management of pediatric polyposis is often disappointing because the recurrence rate is high, except in those with antrochoanal polyps. Therefore, some authors recommend treatment with topical steroids as a routine approach in treating nasal polyps and resort to surgery only in case of failure [48, 49] (Fig. 22.3).

22.7.5 Antrochoanal Polyp

They are inflammatory polyps that originate from the mucosa of the maxillary sinus and extend from the maxillary ostium to the nasal cavity and often to the nasopharynx. It has two components: cystic and solid. Antrochoanal polyps are rare in children but occur at a higher rate than in the adult population. While antrochoanal polyps constitute 4–6% of all nasal polyps, they constitute 33% of the pediatric population. Although it is thought to develop as a complication of chronic inflammatory sinus disease in its physiopathology, studies in the pediatric population have reported that it creates an allergic basis in approximately half of the patients. Unlike adults, allergic polyps are more common than inflammatory polyps among children.

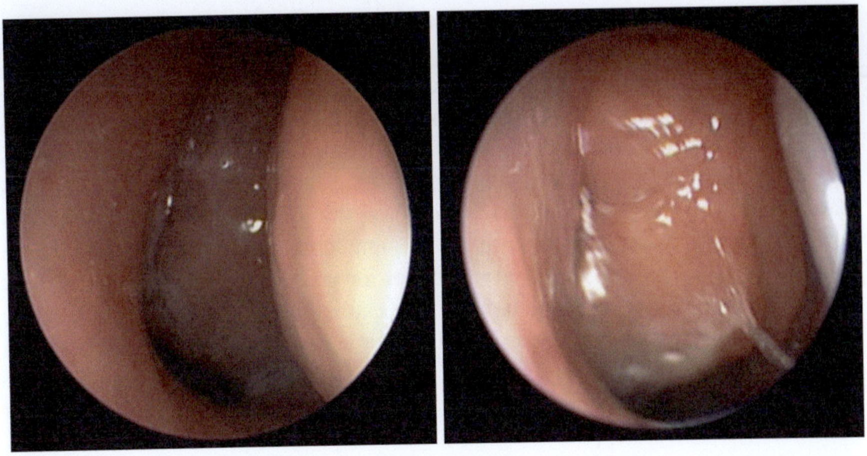

Fig. 22.3 Visualization of hypertrophic adenoid tissue from the nasal cavity with flexible endoscopy

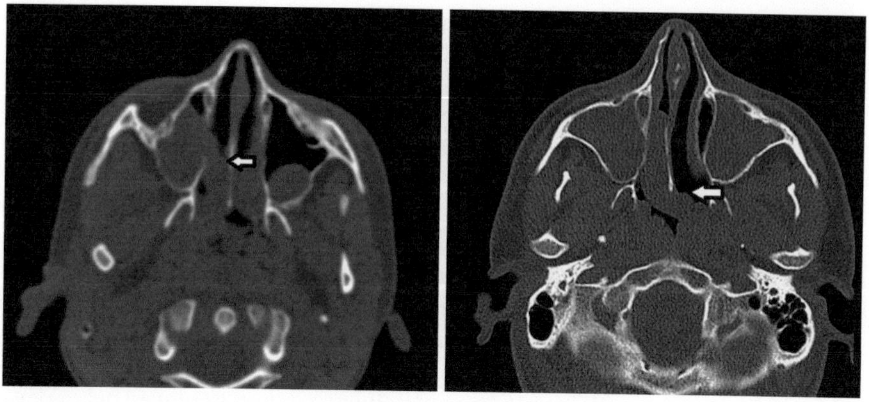

Fig. 22.4 Antrochoanal polyp originating from the left maxillary sinus extends to the middle meatus and then to the nasopharynx on paranasal axial CT

Although they often originate from the maxillary sinus, they may also arise from the septum, sphenoid sinus, ethmoid sinus, hard and soft palate, and turbinates. Although they are primarily unilateral, bilateral patients have been reported. They are frequently observed in children and young adults. The main symptoms are unilateral nasal congestion, runny nose, and postnasal drip. Computed tomography is the radiological evaluation of choice for evaluating antrochoanal polyps. Classically, they are considered as an opaque hypodense mass originating from the maxillary sinus and extending from the middle meatus to the nasal cavity (Fig. 22.4). The treatment is surgery, and endoscopic sinus surgery is preferred. To reduce recurrence rates, it is necessary to remove altogether the mucosa from which the polyp originates in the maxillary sinus [50, 51] (Fig. 22.4).

22.7.6 Inferior Turbinate Hypertrophy

Turbinates are functional anatomical structures important in humidifying and warming the inhaled air. The autonomic nervous system changes the size of the erectile turbinates with sympathetic and parasympathetic stimulation according to physiological needs. Inferior turbinate hypertrophy often occurs due to infection or inflammation caused by allergic rhinitis, vasomotor rhinitis, or infectious rhinitis. In physiopathology, acute or chronic mucosal-submucosal hypertrophy occurs due to congestion. This situation causes nasal congestion and negatively affects the child's quality of life. Inferior turbinate hypertrophy causes runny nose, nasal congestion, mouth breathing, obstructive sleep apnea, and craniofacial development disorder in children [52, 53].

The endoscopic nasal examination is sufficient to evaluate the hypertrophic inferior turbinates and the appearance of the mucosa (pale or hyperemic). As an imaging method, paranasal CT is preferred when medical treatment is inadequate, and surgery is considered [54].

In inferior turbinate hypertrophy, nasal steroids, antihistamines, and decongestants are used in medical treatment. Long-term drug use in children is challenging and reduces the effectiveness of treatment due to compliance problems. There is no definitive consensus for inferior turbinate surgery in children. Surgery aims to preserve the bone and erectile submucosa of the turbinate while preserving the inferior turbinate mucosa and to maximize nasal airflow by reducing nasal tissue [55].

Various surgical options have been recently described for treating medically resistant inferior turbinate hypertrophy in children, including laser ablation, submucosal microdebrider, and radiofrequency methods. Pediatric otolaryngologists have turned to mucosal protective procedures such as submucosal microdebrider turbinectomy and RF instead of turbinectomy, the preferred surgical method [52–55].

22.8 Neoplasia

22.8.1 Benign Tumors (Juvenile Nasopharyngeal Angiofibroma)

It manifests only in males and typically during adolescence, with recurrent nosebleeds and unilateral nasal obstruction. Although this is considered a benign tumor, it can be locally invasive. In nasal endoscopy, it is observed as a vascular mass in the posterior lateral part of the middle turbinate at the level of the sphenopalatine foramen. On endoscopy, it is seen as a light pinkish mass with a superficial vascular structure. Endoscopic nasal examination and radiological evaluation are essential in diagnosis. In cases of clinical suspicion of angiofibroma, biopsy is contraindicated due to the risk of bleeding. It is recommended that CT and MRI be evaluated together in imaging. CT is significant in assessing bone structures. A lobulated, unencapsulated soft tissue mass is typically centered over the sphenopalatine foramen. The posterior wall of the maxillary sinus may bend anteriorly (Holman-Miller sign). MRI is critical in evaluating the orbital and intracranial spread of the lesion. Treatment consists of primary embolization followed by surgical resection within 48 h, usually via an endonasal approach. Recent advances in radiological imaging, embolization, and endonasal surgical techniques and instruments have greatly improved the prognosis [56, 57].

22.8.2 Malignant Tumors

Although malignant nasal masses are rare, they are most commonly seen with nasal congestion and other symptoms such as a change in smell, nosebleeds, nasal/facial pain, nasal asymmetry, swelling, or numbness. Rhabdomyosarcoma, esthesioneuroblastoma, lymphoma, and squamous cell carcinoma can rarely be seen among other malignant nasal masses with minor salivary glands (adenocarcinoma or adenoid cystic adenomas), which can lead to the development of salivary gland tumors in the nasal cavity mucosa [58].

22.9 Systemic Causes

22.9.1 Cystic Fibrosis

It is the most common autosomal recessive genetic disease in Caucasians. Water and salt transport in the cell membrane is disrupted, and there is a change in the composition of the fluid secreted from the respiratory tract, pancreas, gastrointestinal tract, sweat glands, and other exocrine tissues. Because cystic fibrosis is a disease that affects more than one system, it manifests itself with very different clinical signs and symptoms. Recurrent lung infections during childhood and adolescence, purulent sputum production, nasal congestion, nasal polyposis, chronic and persistent rhinosinusitis, asthma, clubbing of fingers, hemoptysis, biliary cirrhosis, meconium ileus, diabetes mellitus, delayed puberty, and infertility are among the findings suggestive of cystic fibrosis. In addition to these clinical findings, measuring 100 mg of sweat chloride concentration above 60 mEq/L in three separate periods confirms the diagnosis. Its treatment can be achieved with a multidisciplinary approach. Medical treatment (corticosteroids) and surgical treatment may be required in patients with polyps in the nasal cavity. The monitoring and treatment team should include a pulmonologist, gastroenterologist, metabolism and nutrition specialist, dietitian, physiotherapist, and microbiologist. Depending on the complications that arise, assistance from other branches is provided, thus prolonging the patients' quality and duration of life [59–61].

22.9.2 Primary Ciliary Dyskinesia

It is characterized by chronic sinopulmonary infections starting from the neonatal period due to disorders in the structure and functions of cilia. It is characterized by ciliary immotility and ciliary dyskinesia. It is an autosomal recessive disease. There is a congenital disability in the structure and function of motile cilia. An increased incidence of infertility and situs in versus characterizes impairment in mucociliary filtration. Increased mucus and bacterial load in the airways is typical. While the diagnosis of cystic fibrosis can often be made at the age of one, in primary ciliary dyskinesia, if there is cardiac pathology, it may be delayed until the age of four or six if there is no [62].

For a definitive diagnosis, the nasal biopsy sample should be evaluated by video microscopy for cilia function and by electron microscopy for ultrastructural cilia defect. The diagnosis must be confirmed by genetic evaluation. It is essential to have a history of recurrent respiratory tract infections, sinusitis and otitis attacks, cardiac pathology with bronchiectasis, or a history of a relative diagnosed with primary ciliary dyskinesia. In cases where nasal polyps are seen together with chronic rhinosinusitis in children, the most common differential diagnosis is cystic fibrosis and rarely direct rhinosinusitis. Ciliary dyskinesia should be considered [63].

22.10 Trauma/Iatrogenic Causes

22.10.1 Nasal Trauma-Septal Hematoma

Septal deformity in children is often seen after trauma and can occur anytime. The nose and mandible are the facial bones most frequently traumatized. During newborns and childhood, fractures are not seen as often as in older children since most of the nasal skeleton has not developed and is cartilaginous. Therefore, nasal fractures are very rare in children under five. Instead of fractures in the nasal bones, septal hematoma, abscess, or septum deviation are more common. Septal hematoma can be defined as bleeding between the mucoperichondrium, which vascularly supplies the septum cartilage, and the septal cartilage, and the separation of the mucoperichondrium from the septum. This condition blocks blood flow to the nasal septum and causes avascular cartilage necrosis. The collected blood and necrotic tissue become an excellent focus for infection of the nasal mucosa, and an abscess forms. Septal hematoma clinic manifests itself with nasal obstruction, and if not intervened, septal necrosis occurs, resulting in septal perforation and irreversible nasal deformities (Fig. 22.5). Therefore, septal hematoma is a critical ENT emergency requiring early childhood diagnosis and treatment [64].

Examination of children after nasal trauma is more complex than for adults. Nasal palpation, deformity, and crepitation are problematic in pediatric patients. Endoscopic nasal examination is the gold standard. As an imaging modality, CT is the gold standard for imaging craniofacial and nasal fractures. Plain radiographs do not help diagnose nasal fractures in children. Signs and symptoms of septal hematoma after nasal trauma may develop within 24–72 h after the injury.

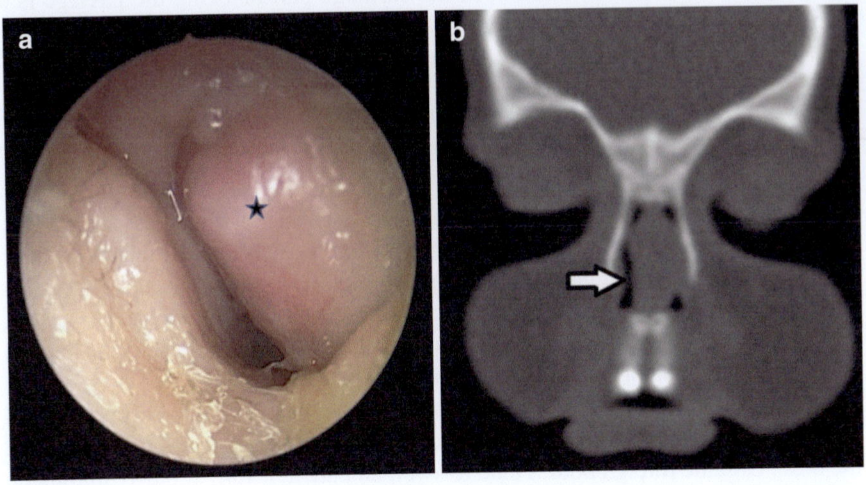

Fig. 22.5 (**a**) Septal hematoma anterior rhinoscopy nasal examination image, black star septal hematoma. (**b**) White arrow, septal hematoma image on paranasal coronal CT

For this reason, if nasal congestion occurs after nasal trauma, it should be shared with the children's families that it may be caused by septal hematoma. Septal hematoma and abscess treatment is performed under general anesthesia with incision, drainage, and tampons placed in the nose. Antibiotics and nasal care should be recommended to patients. The nasal tampon is usually left on for 2–3 days. It may be difficult for children to tolerate tampons [65].

22.10.2 Septum Deviation

While some authors mention that birth trauma is an essential factor in forming septum deviation in children, it has been reported that it can occur without birth trauma. As a result, septal deviation can cause nasal congestion in children and adults, whether congenital or acquired. The diagnosis of septum deviation can be easily made by endoscopic nasal examination. Its treatment is surgery, and its clinical indications must be based on solid foundations. These relate to the severity of the child's nasal congestion, such as sleeping with an open mouth, sleep-disordered breathing, and craniofacial anomalies. Septoplasty is possible at any age but rarely performed before age seven. The reason is that septoplasty may negatively affect the development of the nose and face. This view stems from the fact that, anatomically, the story of the septal cartilage continues until the age of five to six, and the vomer and perpendicular lamina continue until adolescence. On the other hand, waiting instead of surgically correcting a septum deviation that causes nasal congestion in a pediatric patient may be more harmful, considering the complications that may occur. Radiologically, paranasal CT is necessary for planning surgery [66, 67].

Surgically, to avoid disrupting the development of the nose and face, rearranging the septum with minimal resection of the cartilage part blocking the passage is a correct approach. In children, active growth foci should not be touched, and the bony septum should not be removed to avoid changes in facial development [68].

22.10.3 Nasal Foreign Bodies

Nasal foreign bodies are frequently encountered in children under the age of five. The most important reason is that children in this age group put objects in their hands into their noses while crawling or playing on the ground. We can divide foreign objects into two parts: living and non-living. Inanimate objects such as grains, beads, or buttons are more commonly seen in children. They often fall on the kitchen floor during cooking or are found by children at home [69].

When organic foreign bodies (chickpeas, beans, peas, etc.) come into contact with the nasal mucosa, they swell and become difficult to remove as they remain in the nose. Organic foreign bodies tend to swell and are generally more symptomatic than inorganic ones. For this reason, one should not wait for the removal of such foreign bodies and should be removed as soon as possible. Button batteries are attractive to children because of their small size and bright appearance; they are often inserted into the nose, ear, or mouth. Early diagnosis and urgent removal are essential. Any delay may lead to necrosis of the nasal mucosa and septal perforation [70].

The most critical complaints of patients with foreign bodies in the nose are nasal congestion and foul-smelling nasal discharge. It may also cause symptoms such as nosebleeds, facial pain, nasal regurgitation, facial swelling, nasal crusting, and cough. Objects can be located in any nasal cavity region, inferior to the inferior turbinate or anterior to the middle turbinate. Sometimes, the foreign body is not visible on nasal examination. When in doubt, the ideal method is rigid or flexible nasal endoscopy (Fig. 22.6). Edema, inflammation, or bleeding around the foreign body may prevent the foreign body from being seen. Foreign body and unilateral choanal atresia, nasal tumor, nasal polyp, septal abscess, and septal hematoma should be considered in the differential diagnosis in pediatric patients presenting with unilateral nasal obstruction or foul-smelling, purulent nasal discharge. In diagnosing nasal and paranasal sinus foreign bodies, the most important diagnostic methods besides examination are plain radiographs, CT, and MRI [71].

In immobile patients with full cooperation, foreign bodies can usually be removed using appropriate tools without leaking into the nasopharynx, esophagus, or trachea. Organic foreign objects that do not have corners are round (balls, beads, etc.) or may break apart when held. They should be removed by going behind the thing and pulling it forward with a curved tool such as an Itard probe or an angled hook. No attempt should be made to grasp or remove round foreign objects from the front with a bayonet or forceps. Meanwhile, the foreign body may return to the

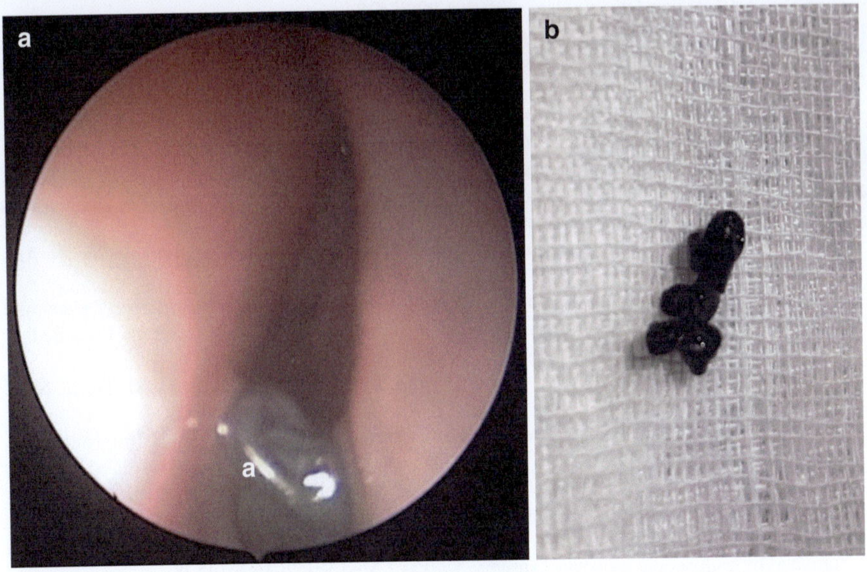

Fig. 22.6 (**a**) The foreign body is in front of the middle turbinate during an endoscopic examination of the left side of the nose. (**b**) The foreign body (plastic toy part) was removed from the nose

nasopharynx, trachea, or esophagus. Suppose the foreign body is angular and prominent. In that case, it can be removed by grasping it with special tools such as bayonet Hartman forceps, and if it is angular and small, alligator forceps. In cases where the nasal foreign body cannot be seen or retained, a balloon catheter can be applied [69–71].

References

1. Esmaili A, Acharya A. Clinical assessment, diagnosis and management of nasal obstruction. Aust Fam Physician. 2017;46:499–503.
2. Van Cauwenberge P, et al. Anatomy and physiology of the nose and the paranasal sinuses. Immunol Allergy Clin N Am. 2004;24(1):1–17.
3. Jones N. The nose and paranasal sinuses physiology and anatomy. Adv Drug Deliv Rev. 2001;51(1):5–19.
4. Valero A, Navarro AM, Del Cuvillo A, et al. Position paper on nasal obstruction: evaluation and treatment. J Investig Allergol Clin Immunol. 2018;28:67–90.
5. Leboulanger N. Nasal obstruction in children. Eur Ann Otorhinolaryngol Head Neck Dis. 2016;133(3):183–6.
6. Trabalon M, Schaal B. It takes a mouth to eat and a nose to breathe: abnormal oral respiration affects neonates' oral competence and systemic adaptation. Int J Pediatr. 2012;2012:207605.
7. Smith MM, Ishman SL. Pediatric nasal obstruction. Otolaryngol Clin N Am. 2018;51(5):971–85. https://doi.org/10.1016/j.otc.2018.05.005.
8. Lale A, Mason J, Jones N. Mucociliary transport and its assessment: a review. Clin Otolaryngol. 1998;23(5):388–96.
9. Neskey D, Eloy JA, Casiano RR. Nasal, septal, and turbinate anatomy and embryology. Otolaryngol Clin N Am. 2009;42(2):193–205.
10. Patel VA, Carr MM. Congenital nasal obstruction in infants: a retrospective study and literature review. Int J Pediatr Otorhinolaryngol. 2017;99:78–84.
11. Teissier N, Kaguelidou F, Couloigner V, Francois M, Van Den Abbeele T. Predic-tive factors for success after transnasal endoscopic treatment of choanal atresia. Arch Otolaryngol Head Neck Surg. 2008;134(1):57–61.
12. Blake KD, Prasad C. CHARGE syndrome. Orphanet J Rare Dis. 2006;1:34.
13. Strychowsky JE, Kawai K, Moritz E, et al. To stent or not to stent? A meta-analysis of endonasal congenital bilateral choanal atresia repair. Laryngoscope. 2016;126(1):218–27.
14. Willging JP. Transpalatal repair of choanal atresia. In: Potsic WP, Cotton RT, Handler SD, et al., editors. Surgical pediatric otolaryngology; 2016. p. 193–215.
15. Tate JR, Sykes J. Congenital nasal pyriform aperture stenosis. Otolaryngol Clin N Am. 2009;42:521–5.
16. Wormald R, Hinton-Bayre A, Bumbak P, et al. Congenital nasal pyriform aperture stenosis 5.7 mm or less is associated with surgical intervention: a pooled case series. Int J Pediatr Otorhinolaryngol. 2015;79(11):1802–5.
17. Zapata S, Kearns DB. Nasal dermoids. Curr Opin Otolaryngol Head Neck Surg. 2006;14:406–11.
18. Paradis J, Koltai PJ. Pediatric teratoma and dermoid cysts. Otolaryngol Clin North Am. 2015;48(1):121–36.
19. Bonne NX, Zago S, Hosana G, Vinchon M, Van den Abbeele T, Fayoux P. Endonasal endoscopic approach for removal of intranasal nasal glial heterotopias. Rhinology. 2012;50:211–7.
20. Özgür A, Dursun E, Şehitoğlu İ, Özergin Z, Çelebi Ö, Terzi S. Two cases of nasal glioma treated by endoscopic transnasal surgery. Kafkas J Med Sci. 2016;6:145–8.
21. Cukurova I, Gumussoy M, Yardim BG, Imamoglu T, Yigitbasi OG. Transnasal endoscopic approach for the treatment of the nasal encephalocele causing respiiratory distress. Nobel Med. 2011;7(2):117–2.

22. Gumussoy M, Ugur O, Cukurova I, Uluyol S. Recurrent meningitis and frontal encephalocele as delayed complications of craniofacial trauma. J Craniofac Surg. 2014;25(2):529–30.
23. Cukurova I, Gumussoy G, Yaz A, Bayol B, Yigitbasi OG. A benign teratoma presenting as an obstruction of the nasal cavity: a case report. J Med Case Rep. 2012;6(1):1–4.
24. Lecavalier M, Nguyen LH. Bilateral dacryocystoceles as a rare cause of neonatalrespiratory distress: report of 2 cases. Ear Nose Throat J. 2014;93(1):26–8.
25. Barham HP, Wudel JM, Enzenauer RW, et al. Congenital nasolacrimal duct cyst/dacryocystocele: an argument for a genetic basis. Allergy Rhinol (Providence). 2012;3(1):e46–9.
26. Mallol J, Crane J, von Mutius E, et al. The international study of asthma and allergies in childhood (ISAAC) phase three: a global synthesis. Allergol Immunopathol. 2013;41:73–85.
27. Workowski KA, Berman S, Centers for Disease C, Prevention. Sexually transmitted diseases treatment guidelines, 2010. MMWR Recomm Rep. 2010;59:1–110.
28. Gumuşsoy M, Gumuşsoy S, Çukurova I. The most frequently encountered rhinologic problems during pregnancy: appropriate approaches in diagnosis and therapy. J Tepecik Educ Res Hosp. 2017;27:13–9. https://doi.org/10.5222/terh.2017.013.
29. Cingi C, Özdoğanoğlu T, Songu M. Nasal obstruction as a drug side effect. Ther Adv Respir Dis. 2011;5:175–82.
30. Wallace DV, Dykewicz MS, Bernstein DI, Blessing-Moore J, Cox L, Khan DA, et al. The diagnosis and management of rhinitis: an updated practice parameter. J Allergy Clin Immunol. 2008;122(2):S1–84. https://doi.org/10.1016/j.jaci.2008.06.003.
31. Catlı T, Atilla H, Miller EK. Acute viral rhinitis. All around the nose. Heidelberg: Springer; 2019. p. 199–202. https://doi.org/10.1007/978-3-030-21217-9_23.
32. Monto AS. Epidemiology of viral respiratory infections. Am J Med. 2002;112(Suppl 6A):4s–12s.
33. Settipane RA, Charnock DR, Baraniuk JN, Shusterman D, et al. Epidemiology of rhinitis: allergic and nonallergic. Nonallergic rhinitis. New York, NY: Informa; 2007. p. 23–34.
34. Jeffe JS, Bhushan B, Schroeder JW Jr. Nasal saline irrigation in children: a study of compliance and tolerance. Intern J Pediatr Otorhinolaryngol. 2012;76:409–13.
35. Shaikh N, Wald ER, Pi M. Decongestants, antihistamines and nasal irrigation for acute sinusitis in children. Cochrane Database Syst Rev. 2012;(9):CD007909.
36. Shapiro DJ, Gonzales R, Cabana MD, Hersh AL. National trends in visit rates and antibiotic prescribing for children with acute sinusitis. Pediatrics. 2011;127(1):28–34.
37. Revai K, Dobbs LA, Nair S, Patel JA, Grady JJ, Chonmaitree T. Incidence of acute otitis media and sinusitis complicating upper respiratory tract infection: the effect of age. Pediatrics. 2007;119(6):e1408.
38. Feres MF, Hermann JS, Cappellette M, Pignatari SS. Lateral X-ray view of theskull for the diagnosis of adenoid hypertrophy: a systematic review. Int J Pediatr Otorhinolaryngol. 2011;75(1):1–11.
39. Brietzke SE, Brigger MT. Adenoidectomy outcomes in pediatric rhinosinusitis: a meta-analysis. Int J Pediatr Otorhinolaryngol. 2008;72(10):1541–5.
40. Ramadan HH, Cost JL. Outcome of adenoidectomy versus adenoidectomy with maxillary sinus wash for chronic rhinosinusitis in children. Laryngoscope. 2008;118(5):871–3.
41. Almac A, Elicora SS, Yumuk Z, Dundar V, Willke A. The relationship between chronic otitis media with effusion and surface and deep flora of hypertrophic adenoids. Int J Pediatr Otorhinolaryngol. 2009;73(10):1438–40. https://doi.org/10.1016/j.ijporl.2009.07.014.
42. Orlandi RR, Kingdom TT, Hwang PH, Smith TL, Alt JA, Baroody FM, et al. International consensus statement on allergy and rhinology: rhinosinusitis. Int Forum Allergy Rhinol. 2016;6:S22–S209.
43. Tharpe CA, Kemp SF. Pediatric allergic rhinitis. Immunol Allergy Clin N Am. 2015;35(1):185–98.
44. Gentile D, Bartholow A, Valovirta E, et al. Current and future directions in pediatric allergic rhinitis. J Allergy Clin Immunol. 2013;1:214–26.
45. Smart BA. The impact of allergic and nonallergic rhinitis on pediatric sinusitis. Curr Allergy Asthma Rep. 2006;6:221–7.

46. Ellis AK, Keith PK. Nonallergic rhinitis with eosinophilia syndrome. Curr Allergy Asthma Rep. 2006;6(3):215–20. https://doi.org/10.1007/s11882-006-0037-0.
47. Fokkens WJ, Lund VJ, Mullol J, et al. EPOS 2012: European position paper on rhinosinusitis and nasal polyps 2012. A summary for otorhinolaryngologists. Rhinology. 2012;50:1–12.
48. Weber SAT, Ferrari GF. Incidence and evolution of nasal polyps in children and adolescents with cystic fibrosis. Braz J Otorhinolaryngol. 2008;74(1):16–20. https://doi.org/10.1016/S1808-8694(15)30745-X.
49. Fokkens W, Lund V, Bochert V, Clement P, Hellings P, Holmstrom M, et al. EAACI position paper on rhinosinusitis and nasal polyps executive summary. Allergy. 2005;60:593–601.
50. Bakshi SS, Vaithy KA. Antrochoanal polyp. J Allergy Clin Immunol Pract. 2017;5:806–7.
51. Yaman H, Yilmaz S, Karali E, Guclu E, Ozturk O. Evaluation and management of antrochoanal polyps. Clin Exp Otorhinolaryngol. 2010;3:3.110-114.
52. Jiang ZY, Pereira KD, Friedman NR, Mitchell RB. Inferior turbinate surgery in children: a survey of practice patterns. Laryngoscope. 2012;122(7):1620–3. https://doi.org/10.1002/lary.23292.
53. Arganbright JM, Jensen EL, Mattingly J, et al. Utility of inferior turbinoplasty for the treatment of nasal obstruction in children: a 10-year review. JAMA Otolaryngol Head Neck Surg. 2015;141(10):901–4.
54. Kaya E, Özüdoğru E, Nogueira JF. Surgical management of the turbinates. All around the nose; 2020. p. 469–87. https://doi.org/10.1007/978-3-030-21217-9.
55. Komshian SR, Cohen MB, Brook C, Levi JR. Inferior turbinate hypertrophy: a review of the evolution of management in children. Am J Rhinol Allergy. 2018;33:212–9. https://doi.org/10.1177/1945892418815351.
56. Cloutier T, Pons Y, Blancal JP, Sauvaget E, Kania R, Bresson D, et al. Juvenilenasopharyngeal angiofibroma: does the external approach still make sense? Otolaryngol Head Neck Surg. 2012;147(5):958–63.
57. Gerth DJ, Tashiro J, Thaller SR. Pediatric sinonasal tumors in the United States:incidence and outcomes. J Surg Res. 2014;190(1):214–20.
58. Yi JS, Cho GS, Shim MJ, Min J-Y, Chung Y-S, Lee B-J. Malignant tumors of the sinonasal tract in the pediatric population. Acta Otolaryngol. 2012;132:21–6. https://doi.org/10.3109/00016489.2012.660730.
59. Sarafoleanu C, Manea C. Nasal manifestations of systemic diseases—a literature review. Romanian J Rhinol. 2014;4:81–92.
60. De Vincentiis GC, Sitzia E, Botteroa S, Giuzioa L, Simonetti A, Rossi P. Otolaryngologic manifestations of pediatric immunodeficiency. Int J Pediatr Otorhinolaryngol. 2009;73:S42–8.
61. Lahiri T, Hempstead SE, Brady C, Cannon CL, Clark K, Condren ME, Guill MF, Guillerman RP, Leone CG, Maguiness K, Monchil L, Powers SW, Rosenfeld M, Schwarzenberg SJ, Tompkins CL, Zemanick ET, Davis SD. Clinical practice guidelines from the cystic fibrosis foundation for preschoolers with cystic fibrosis. Pediatrics. 2016;137(4):e20151784. https://doi.org/10.1542/peds.2015-1784.
62. Lucas JS, Burgess A, Mitchison HM, Moya E, Williamson M, Hogg C. Diagnosis and management of primary ciliary dyskinesia. Arch Dis Child. 2014;99(9):850–6. https://doi.org/10.1136/archdischild-2013-304831.
63. Guo Z, Chen W, Wang L, Qian L. Clinical and genetic Spectrum of children with primary ciliary dyskinesia in China. J Pediatr. 2020;225:157–165.e5. https://doi.org/10.1016/j.jpeds.2020.05.052.
64. Wright RJ, Murakami CS, Ambro BT. Pediatric nasal injuries and management. Facial Plast Surg. 2011;27(5):483–90. https://doi.org/10.1055/s-0031-1288931.
65. Cakabay T, Ustun BS. Pediatric nasal traumas: contribution of epidemiological features to detect the distinction between nasal fractures and nasal soft tissue injuries. J Craniofac Surg. 2018;29(5):1334–7. https://doi.org/10.1097/SCS.0000000000004550.
66. Reitzen SD, Chung W, Shah AR. Nasal septal deviation in the pediatric and adult populations. Ear Nose Throat J. 2011;90(3):112–5.

67. Lawrence R. Pediatric septoplasy: a review of the literature. Int J Pediatr Otorhinolaryngol. 2012;76(8):1078–81.
68. Cristophel JJ, Gross CW. Pediatric septoplasty. Otolaryngol Clin N Am. 2009;42:287–94.
69. Abou-Elfadl M, Horra A, Abada RL, Mahtar M, Roubal M, Kadiri F. Nasal foreign bodies: results of a study of 260 cases. Eur Ann Otorhinolaryngol Head Neck Dis. 2015;132:343–6.
70. Regonne PE, Ndiaye M, Sy A, Diandy Y, Diop AD, Diallo BK. Nasal foreign bodies in children in a pediatric hospital in Senegal: a three-year assessment. Eur Ann Otorhinolaryngol Head Neck Dis. 2017;134:361–4.
71. Cetinkaya EA, Arslan İB, Cukurova İ. Nasal foreign bodies in children: types, locations, complications and removal. Int J Pediatr Otorhinolaryngol. 2015;79(11):1881–5. https://doi.org/10.1016/j.ijporl.2015.08.036.

Nasal Itching and Sneezing in Children 23

Nurullah Türe and Fatih Oğhan

23.1 Introduction

Nasal itching and sneezing occur after neural activation stimulation by environmental irritants and biological agents released during the local inflammation process. In particular, sneezing protects the body by playing an essential role in protecting and clearing the airway from irritating substances. A runny nose, nasal itching, and nasal congestion often accompany sneezing. This condition is generally observed due to rhinitis seen in allergies and viral upper respiratory tract infections.

Rhinitis is inflammation of the nasal mucosa. In rhinitis, nasal itching, sneezing, runny nose, and nasal congestion are observed. Along with rhinitis symptoms, accompanying complaints in the eyes, ears, and throat may be observed. Rhinitis is generally classified as allergic and non-allergic rhinitis [1, 2].

Regarding complaints, there is no significant difference between allergic and non-allergic rhinitis. For this reason, most pediatric patients presenting with rhinitis complaints are diagnosed with allergic rhinitis. Treatment management is carried out according to this diagnosis. Sometimes, differential diagnosis can be difficult in pediatric patients due to overlapping conditions. It is difficult to determine its incidence epidemiologically due to the need for more data on the prevalence of nasal itching and sneezing in allergic and non-allergic rhinitis in pediatric patients.

This chapter explains the pathophysiology and etiology of nasal itching and sneezing in children, the differential diagnosis of co-occurring diseases, and appropriate treatment options.

N. Türe · F. Oğhan (✉)
Kütahya Health Sciences University, Evliya Çelebi Training and Research Hospital, Izmir, Turkey
e-mail: fatih.oghan@ksbu.edu.tr

H. Yüksel et al. (eds.), *Pediatric Airway Diseases*, Comprehensive ENT,
https://doi.org/10.1007/978-3-031-74853-0_23

23.2 Pathophysiology

Itching is a nociceptive primitive defense mechanism that stimulates avoidance of inhaling harmful substances involving innate and adaptive immune mechanisms [3]. On the other hand, sneezing is caused by neural activation triggered by external environmental stimuli (irritants) or biological products formed in a local inflammatory process. Sneezing is a central reflex whose afferent arm begins in the nasal mucosa and whose efferent arm includes the nerves innervating the diaphragm, accessory respiratory muscles, and larynx. Sensory nerves in the nasal mucosa originate from the ophthalmic and maxillary branches of the trigeminal nerve [4].

Terminal sensory nerve endings are mostly unmyelinated nociceptor C fibers. Sometimes Aδ fibers (Aβ fibers) are also included [5, 6]. Nociceptor nerves respond to noxious external and internal stimuli through a series of receptors, such as transient receptor potential vanilloid type 1 (TRPV1) and transient receptor potential ankyrin type 1 (TRPA1) [7].

Nasal nerve endings contain receptors for chemicals such as the Histamine 1 (H1) receptor or the cysteinyl leukotriene 1 receptor (CysLTR1) [8, 9].

While H1 receptors in nasal sensory nerve endings explain the sneezing that occurs during exposure to allergens, transient receptor channels explain the sneezing and itching that occur when exposed to non-antigenic irritating substances [10].

Many pruritogens and receptors mediate itching, which occurs due to allergic rhinitis. After stimulation of nerve fibers in the nasal mucosa and activation of mast cells, histamine is released, which causes nasal itching [11]. Histamine increased in the nasal lavage fluid of allergic patients, but no increase was observed in non-allergic patients [12]. Neuropeptides such as substance P, CGRP, and vasoactive intestinal polypeptide (VIP) have been reported to be increased in the nasal lavage wash of patients with allergic rhinitis, which are thought to play a role in nasal itching. Furthermore, nerve growth factor (NGF) is expressed in the nasal epithelium and peripheral nerves in the nasal mucosa, and the expression of this neuropeptide is significantly increased after nasal allergen challenge in patients with allergic rhinitis compared to controls [13, 14]. House dust mites are affected by protease-activated receptor 2 (PAR2).

It has been shown to induce the release of inflammatory cytokines and ultimately cause nasal itching [15]. Additionally, it has been reported that nasal itching increases when a TRPV1 activator such as capsaicin is administered to patients with allergic rhinitis during seasonal allergen exposure [16]. Nerve expression of TRPV1 is also increased in patients with non-allergic rhinitis [17]. This phenomenon suggests inflammatory cytokines such as histamine and bradykinin cause nasal itching through TRPV1 receptors [18].

Physicians should know its close relationship with other allergic diseases, such as allergic conjunctivitis and asthma. Interestingly, pruritus has been reported as a preliminary symptom in patients with asthma [19]. Additionally, in a study investigating non-respiratory symptoms of acute asthma, nasal itching was observed before the asthma attack [20].

Mechanical trauma caused by nose scratching can release inflammatory molecules that further increase itching, creating a vicious circle [21].

23.3 Allergic Rhinitis

Allergic rhinitis is IgE-mediated inflammation of the nasal mucosa that develops against specific allergens such as pollen, mold, feather, and house dust mites. Symptoms occur after the release of inflammatory mediators. Clinical findings such as runny nose, sneezing, nasal itching, and congestion are usually observed. Symptoms such as itching, redness, and swelling in the eyes are often observed together. Additional diseases such as rhinosinusitis, otitis, and asthma can sometimes be observed [22].

Observation of symptoms for more than 1 h a day for 2 weeks and two or more additional symptoms suggests the diagnosis of allergic rhinitis in the child [23]. The mentioned symptoms are not observed with the same intensity in every patient. Some symptoms may seem more dominant than others.

Allergic rhinitis is the most common allergic disease in children [24]. Allergic rhinitis is observed in approximately 40 percent of children [25]. It was observed that the prevalence of allergic rhinitis in children in the United States increased from 13.4% in 1994 to 19.1% in 2003 [26]. In recent studies, the prevalence of allergic rhinitis in children was 13% [27]. Although the number of boys with allergic rhinitis was observed to be higher than girls at the ages of 6–7, it was observed that the number of girls was higher than boys at the ages of 13–14 [28]. Allergic rhinitis is the most common atopic disease under the age of 18 and is one of the leading chronic conditions [29]. Most patients develop symptoms of AR before age 20, and approximately half of these patients become symptomatic by age 6. If there is a history of allergy in the family on both the mother's and father's side, symptoms usually appear before adolescence. In the presence of a unilateral family history, symptoms are observed at older ages [30]. AR is rare in children younger than 2 years of age because it usually requires several years of allergen exposure to develop [31].

In children, sensitivity (presence of specific IgE) develops first to allergens (dust mites) constantly in the air. It has been observed that sensitivity to pollens and other seasonal allergens develops before clinical complaints appear [32].

When symptoms of allergic rhinitis are evaluated in terms of time, they are classified as intermittent if they occur after specific exposures, seasonal if they occur at certain times of the year, or perennial if the symptoms persist throughout the year [33]. Allergic rhinitis affects the upper respiratory tract and can be seasonal or year-round. In seasonal allergic rhinitis, symptoms usually occur in spring, summer, or fall and are often associated with pollen from trees, grass, and weeds. The number and type of pollen varies according to geographical regions. Even within a given area, weather patterns can cause annual changes in pollen count and the overall prevalence and severity of allergic rhinitis. Exposure to indoor and outdoor air pollutants, pet dander, cockroaches, dust mites, molds, and others must be considered in perennial allergic rhinitis. In some children, seasonal allergies may overlap and cause persistent symptoms [34]. Allergic rhinitis: Patients' daily activities, sleep, and school routines are classified as mild, moderate, or severe (persistent or intermittent) according to the duration of symptoms [35].

It negatively affects the child's quality of life and aggravates other allergic diseases, such as asthma [36]. At the same time, it disrupts the child's quality of life by negatively affecting their social activities, school performance, sleep status, and psychosocial communication [37]. It has been reported that approximately two million school days are lost every year due to allergic rhinitis [38].

Young children suffer from acute infective rhinitis very frequently every year, making it difficult to distinguish the condition from allergic rhinitis. If the condition lasts longer than 2 weeks and there are other accompanying allergic symptoms, allergic rhinitis, such as nasal itching, should be considered [39].

Allergic rhinitis can occur at any age, but patients with allergic rhinitis have been reported to experience symptoms in childhood or young adulthood. Nasal itching is very useful in distinguishing allergic rhinitis from other forms of rhinitis. Children generally do not complain of nasal itching but show it through various nose-wiping methods [40]. In patients, an "allergic salute" can typically be observed, which is observed as a horizontal wrinkle on the nasal dorsum and occurs when the nose is rubbed upwards with the palm [41].

Evaluation of AR requires a detailed history, including physical examination and laboratory evaluation, in addition to questioning the patient's environment and diet and the presence of allergies in the family. History and laboratory findings provide clues to provoking factors. Symptoms such as sneezing, runny nose, nasal itching, congestion, and laboratory findings of high IgE and sIgE antibodies and positive allergy skin test results indicate AR [42].

23.4 Non-allergic Rhinitis

The pathophysiology of networked conditions needs to be clearly defined. It is a situation where the true incidence of the disease is unknown. Current treatment is based on studies on adult individuals. There is no epidemiological data on the age at which non-allergic rhinitis occurs in children. In addition, the gender and age distribution of non-allergic rhinitis in the pediatric age group are unknown. In summary, only some aspects of pediatric non-allergic rhinitis in children have been explained, and its pathophysiology has yet to be fully explained. The lack of accurate diagnosis and appropriate treatment algorithms in managing the disease is noteworthy [43].

Non-allergic rhinitis is a disease that causes many clinical complaints with different etiologies and pathophysiologies.

Diagnosing non-allergic rhinitis in children is challenging due to disagreements on the classification of different forms of non-allergic rhinitis and the need to elucidate its pathophysiology. This problem is clinically diagnosed as non-allergic rhinitis. The common denominator of the clinical conditions under this umbrella diagnosis is the absence of systemic allergic sensitivity. Non-allergic rhinitis causes infrequent symptoms. Sneezing and nasal itching are less common in non-allergic rhinitis than in allergic rhinitis but can be seen in the NARES subtype of non-allergic rhinitis.

Non-allergic rhinitis at age four was reported to be 8.1%, and the prevalence at age eight was reported to be 6.3% [32]. Another study reported that NAR was observed in 24.9% of 6600 children with rhinitis symptoms. It has been reported that NAR is more common than AR in children under the age of 6, that the diagnosis of AR increases with age, and that NAR decreases to 10–15% in older children [44].

Under the non-allergic umbrella, conditions such as infectious rhinitis, non-allergic rhinitis with eosinophilia, vasomotor rhinitis, atrophic rhinitis, rhinitis due to structural and mechanical factors, rhinitis medicamentosa, neoplasms, vasculitis, and granulomatous disorders are included.

Children complain of runny nose, nasal congestion, and sneezing in infectious rhinitis. The complaints usually disappear within the first week, and the causative agent is mostly rhinoviruses [25].

In non-allergic rhinitis, where high eosinophilia is observed, the symptomatology of the disease and response to treatment is similar to allergic rhinitis. Still, unlike high IgE antibodies, high IgE antibodies are not observed [42].

Vasomotor rhinitis is characterized by the excessive response of the nasal mucosa to physical stimuli [42]. In vasomotor rhinitis, intermittent nasal congestion and runny nose are observed. A significant increase in complaints is observed, especially after exposure to air pollution and cold weather [45].

Atrophic rhinitis is a rare clinical condition that begins with puberty and results in slow and progressive atrophy of the nasal mucosa. It is typical for a crust to form in the nose and a foul odor [46].

23.5 Infectious Rhinitis

The most common form of non-allergic rhinitis in children is infectious rhinitis, which can be acute or chronic. Infectious rhinitis, commonly known as the common cold, is an acute and self-limiting disease. The most common cause is rhinoviruses. Children experience runny nose, nasal congestion, and sneezing, and the complaints usually disappear within the first week [47, 48]. Around 36% of patients have sneezing on the first day of the disease, and sneezing continues on the fifth day in more than 35% [49].

Other symptoms, such as cough and sore throat, are more prominent in infective rhinitis. Acute bacterial rhinosinusitis is a situation in which complaints sometimes continue in viral rhinitis, and the sinuses are additionally included in the clinical picture. Acute symptomatic bacterial sinusitis develops in approximately 0.5–2% of viral upper respiratory tract infections in children [25].

Acute bacterial sinusitis presents similarly to an upper respiratory tract infection, with a runny nose, congestion, cough, and sometimes fever and headache. Edema and erythema are common in the nasal mucosa. Because sinusitis can develop as a complication of an upper respiratory tract infection, a prior upper respiratory tract infection is commonly reported. Unlike an upper respiratory tract infection, patients with acute sinusitis experience signs and symptoms that worsen after 10 days; purulent nasal discharge and halitosis are typical [50, 51].

In the presence of a chronic mucopurulent discharge, pathologies such as adenoid hypertrophy, anatomical abnormalities, primary immunodeficiency, primary ciliary dyskinesia, or cystic fibrosis should be considered [48].

Sometimes, allergic rhinitis and infectious rhinitis are observed together in children. In cases where these two conditions overlap, differential diagnosis becomes difficult. It has been observed that an exaggerated response to viral upper respiratory tract infection is observed in atopic children [52]. Allergic rhinitis symptoms in children are often confused with infectious rhinitis symptoms. If symptoms last longer than 2 weeks, a cause other than infection should be sought. When diagnosis cannot be made by history and physical examination, a nasal swab can be taken, which is helpful in differential diagnosis. Detection of more than 5% of eosinophils in the nasal swab suggests allergy, and neutrophil predominance suggests infection [47].

23.6 NARES (Non-allergic Rhinitis with Eosinophilia Syndrome)

In Non-allergic Rhinitis with Eosinophilia Syndrome (NARES), which is evaluated under the table of non-allergic rhinitis, the dominant symptoms are continuous sneezing and excessive nasal discharge. Sometimes, it is accompanied by nasal congestion, itching, and a decreased sense of smell. The presence of increased eosinophils in the nasal swab, useful in differential diagnosis, is noteworthy. Failure to monitor systemic sensitivity helps differentiate it from allergic rhinitis. The skin prick test is negative. Specific IgE is not monitored. Its pathophysiology needs to be clearly understood. The hypothesized view is that nasal neural dysfunction causes symptoms [53].

23.6.1 Vasomotor Rhinitis

Vasomotor rhinitis is a diagnosis of exclusion. Common symptoms are primarily nasal congestion and runny nose but can also include nasal itching and sneezing. The pathophysiology of vasomotor rhinitis is not well understood but is believed to be due to autonomic dysregulation resulting in an imbalance in sympathetic and parasympathetic activity. In vasomotor rhinitis, symptoms begin suddenly and disappear quickly when the triggering factor is removed. The allergy test is negative. Symptoms may change depending on weather changes [54, 55].

Finally, it should not be forgotten that nonallergic, noninfectious rhinitis conditions occur due to exposure to irritants, hormonal dysfunction, and specific drugs. This should be considered in the differential diagnosis.

23.7 Evaluation

The ear, nose, and throat physical examination begins after the pediatric patient complaining of nasal itching and sneezing states their first complaint. Evaluation should always start by taking a comprehensive medical history. During the interrogation, attention should be paid to what the patient does not say and specific situations such as mouth breathing, dry mouth, and speaking. Detecting an allergic or infectious cause in children may be challenging, mainly when rhinitis is frequently observed. Therefore, other distinctive physical examination findings of allergic rhinitis should be questioned.

One of the characteristically noticeable findings of allergic rhinitis in children is the horizontal scar observed in the nose tip area. This is an important examination finding that is observed as a result of repeating the movement called allergic salute, which is performed by lifting the tip of the nose upwards with the palm of the hand, for at least 2 years to increase nasal breathing and reduce the feeling of itching. With advancing age and adolescence, this movement can be observed as facial grimacing [56, 57].

Notably, findings in neighboring organs should be noticed. Venous pooling occurs around the eyes secondary to inflammation in the nasal mucosa. The pigmentation observed on the lower eyelid skin due to hemosiderin accumulated under the skin during ponding is called allergic glitter. Venous pooling causes constant muscle spasms in the lower eyelid. Spasm in the Müller muscle causes small scars called Dennie-Morgan lines on the lower eyelid skin. Long and silky eyelashes sometimes accompany allergic rhinitis complaints [56].

Anterior rhinoscopy provides valuable information about the septum and lateral nasal wall. In allergic rhinitis, the nasal mucosa and turbinates may appear normal but are usually edematous and pale. At the same time, the color of the discharge in the nasal passage is helpful in distinguishing its fluidity. In contrast, the color of the nasal mucosa in patients with non-allergic rhinitis is usually standard, and acute viral rhinosinusitis has a red appearance. In current practice, every otolaryngologist successfully applies flexible nasopharyngoscopy and endoscope, which allows the anterior and posterior nasal structures to be distinguished more specifically than anterior rhinoscopy. Although nasal endoscope application is complex in young children, its benefit in clarifying nasal pathologies is excellent [58].

When the palate feels itchy, children may click while moving their tongue towards the palate to relieve this itching feeling [59]. Depending on the timing of allergen exposure, symptoms may be present year-round or seasonally [56].

Non-allergic rhinitis symptoms usually occur throughout the year. However, seasonal exacerbations can occur due to changes in humidity, temperature, and pressure. Differential diagnosis becomes difficult since these complaints overlap with allergic rhinitis complaints in autumn and spring. The absence of eye and palate symptoms is important in non-allergic rhinitis [60].

In non-allergic rhinitis, nasal secretions are generally normal except for edematous erythematous conchas. Nasal secretions can be observed as mucoid or transparent [61].

Both nasal passages should be examined, and attention should be paid to the color and consistency of the discharge detected in the nasal passage, the degree of edema in the mucosa, and the presence of turbinate hypertrophy. Examination of the oropharynx should also be included, and a postnasal drip should be noted. In addition, an ear examination should be performed, and the color and mobility of the tympanic membrane and the presence of fluid behind the membrane should be noted.

Perinatal infections such as Chlamydia can present as persistent rhinitis. In adolescence, inquiries about the onset of puberty may be helpful, as hormonal changes may cause nasal congestion [62].

It is essential to determine whether the patient is also sexually active. In some cases, syphilis may occur with chronic rhinitis [63]. All patients' previous sinus surgeries should be questioned.

Assessment of the chronicity of rhinitis is critical. Intermittent nasal congestion is more closely associated with self-limiting rhinovirus infections. Chronic persistent nasal congestion may indicate more complicated conditions such as adenoid hypertrophy or immobile cilia syndrome. Investigating all possible etiological factors is very important to make the correct diagnosis. Inquiry regarding exposure to potential triggers commonly associated with nasal hyperreactivity, such as odors, drafts, cold air, temperature changes, fatigue, stress, and spicy foods, will help the clinician confirm the etiology of the patient's chronic rhinitis. Reviewing past medication use and effectiveness may also help confirm the diagnosis [43].

Finally, nasal itching and sneezing symptoms are not sensitive or specific enough to distinguish between bacterial sinusitis and allergic or viral rhinitis. This often leaves patients in situations where the two conditions overlap.

23.8 Diagnosis

It is essential to question nose itching and other symptoms accompanying sneezing. Use diagnostic tools according to etiology. Allergic rhinitis, infectious rhinitis, and non-allergic, non-infectious rhinitis should be considered in the differential diagnosis of pediatric patients complaining of nasal itching and sneezing. Although almost all patients who applied to health institutions with rhinitis complaints were diagnosed with allergic rhinitis, it is worth emphasizing that in studies conducted, allergy could not be identified as the etiology in 40–64% of these patients. For this reason, after a preliminary diagnosis of rhinitis is made in patients presenting with sneezing, diagnostic tests should be used appropriately, and differential diagnosis should be made carefully.

Diagnosing allergic rhinitis in children is made by specific allergic complaints in the history and diagnostic tests.

In the preliminary diagnosis, allergy tests are performed for this purpose in the pediatric patient in whom allergy is suspected. Allergy tests to confirm the initial diagnosis include a skin prick test and serum-specific IgE. Skin prick test is frequently preferred in children because it is easy to apply, gives results quickly, can be used in office conditions, and has reasonable specificity and sensitivity. Serum-specific IgE is as sensitive as skin prick tests, which show the patient's complaints are due to allergies. Specific IgE is safely preferred, especially in patients who do not have a systemic reaction, have had a systemic reaction before, and have skin diseases where objective data must be provided [25].

When an infection is suspected, complete blood count, white cell count, and C-reactive protein (CRP) are helpful in differential diagnosis [1].

Nasal cytology is not a frequently used diagnostic method because it cannot be standardized, its results are highly variable, and its results have different sensitivity and specificity. Despite this, eosinophils in the nasal swab indicate inflammation and can help predict corticosteroid response [1].

Radiology for rhinitis is not routinely recommended. However, if rhinosinusitis or nasal polyposis is suspected, especially if it does not respond to medical treatment, a Computed Tomography scan is helpful. However, remember that radiation exposure in pediatric patients should be kept as low as possible [1].

Allergic rhinitis is often accompanied by eye symptoms (itchy and watery eyes), and many patients have a positive family history of allergic rhinitis [64].

Sinusitis is primarily a clinical diagnosis; imaging is used to confirm it and evaluate its complications when necessary. A CT scan compatible with sinusitis shows clouding, opacity, thickening of the mucosal interface, and air-fluid levels in the affected sinus [65].

Patients with non-allergic rhinitis often complain of nasal congestion and rhinorrhea, but they also complain less about sneezing and itching [66].

Blind cultures of the nasopharynx in children with rhinitis have little clinical value because pathogenic bacteria are present in the normal flora in 92% of asymptomatic healthy children [25].

A careful history and physical examination are the most effective diagnostic maneuvers in identifying allergic rhinitis in children. The distinction is sometimes tricky as allergic and non-allergic rhinitis often cannot be distinguished based on symptoms and require different management strategies and pharmacological treatments. Clinicians should perform specific diagnostic tests on pediatric patients when indicated.

23.9 Treatment

The aim of treating Allergic Rhinitis, which is considered the main culprit in nasal itching and sneezing and comes to mind first in the differential diagnosis in children, is to control the patients' symptoms, increase their quality of life and school success, and prevent the development of complications.

The best treatment for nasal itching and sneezing due to allergic rhinitis is allergy avoidance. Medical treatment is resorted to in pediatric patients who cannot achieve sufficient success despite protection and rearrangement of the environment. Immunotherapy is helpful in cases that fail medical treatment. Treatment includes environmental control, allergen avoidance, pharmacotherapy, and allergen-specific immunotherapy [33].

Informing families about avoiding allergen exposure is very important in managing pediatric patients. Although it does not seem possible to avoid allergens despite all restrictions, it has been reported that this method reduces allergen load [25].

Simple practices such as not being outdoors during pollen periods, using filters in motor vehicles, using glasses and hats outdoors, and washing hands and face are recommended [67].

To reduce contact exposure in managing allergic rhinitis caused by house dust mites, the environment should be ventilated frequently, dust should be removed often, items should be washed at temperatures higher than 55 °C, and carpets with less pile should be preferred. All the methods listed have been reported to relieve the symptoms of allergic rhinitis caused by house dust mites. Oral antihistamines and nasal steroids are both effective on sneezing and nasal itching.

23.10 Prognosis

In allergic rhinitis, where nasal itching and sneezing are frequently observed, the positive impact on the child's quality of life is excellent when compliance with the treatment is ensured. It is expected to produce specific drugs based on genetic sequences that target the cells, nerves, and cytokines involved in nasal itching and sneezing and treat these two conditions as a systemic process.

23.11 Conclusion

Every child who complains of nasal itching and sneezing should undergo a detailed history and physical examination, and other accompanying symptoms should be questioned. Further assessment and treatment should be performed for differential diagnosis of diseases in which nasal itching and sneezing occur together. Despite the high prevalence of allergic rhinitis in the pediatric population, this disease is often overlooked or undertreated.

Untreated allergic rhinitis impairs the child's and his parents' quality of life. Accurate and timely diagnosis of allergic rhinitis in children depends on awareness of the symptoms and signs of the disease and comorbidities, including asthma, sinusitis, and otitis media. Rhinitis complaints can be reduced, especially with simple measures, and they contribute positively to quality of life and school performance.

Physicians should differentially diagnose nasal itching and sneezing in children and perform specific diagnostic tests when necessary. Intranasal corticosteroids and non-sedating antihistamines are successfully used in the treatment.

References

1. Scadding GK, Kariyawasam HH, Scadding G, et al. BSACI guideline for the diagnosis and management of allergic and non-allergic rhinitis (revised edition 2017; first edition 2007). Clin Exp Allergy. 2017;47:856–89. https://doi.org/10.1111/cea.12953.
2. Öztürk Z, Bayar Muluk N, Oğuz O, Pinarbaşli MÖ, Güngör E, Arik D, Bal C, Cingi C. Investigation of the effects of allicin on the nasal mucosa. Ear Nose Throat J. 2024:1455613241257354. https://doi.org/10.1177/01455613241257354.

3. Widdicombe JG. Nasal pathophysiology. Respir Med. 1990;84:3–10. https://doi.org/10.1016/S0954-6111(08)80001-7.
4. Cauna N. Blood and nerve supply of the nasal lining. In: The nose. Upper airway physiology and the atmospheric environment; 1982. p. 45–70.
5. Cauna N, Hinderer KH, Wentges RT. Sensory receptor organs of the human nasal respiratory mucosa. Am J Anat. 1969;124:187–209. https://doi.org/10.1002/aja.1001240205.
6. Wallois F, Gros F, Condamin M, Macron JM. Postnatal development of the anterior ethmoidal nerve in cats: unmyelinated and myelinated nerve fiber analysis. Neurosci Lett. 1993;160:221–4. https://doi.org/10.1016/0304-3940(93)90418-K.
7. Alenmyr L, Herrmann A, Högestätt ED, et al. TRPV1 and TRPA1 stimulation induces MUC5B secretion in the human nasal airway in vivo. Clin Physiol Funct Imaging. 2011;31:435–44. https://doi.org/10.1111/j.1475-097X.2011.01039.x.
8. Taylor-Clark TE, Kollarik M, MacGlashan DW, Undem BJ. Nasal sensory nerve populations responding to histamine and capsaicin. J Allergy Clin Immunol. 2005;116:1282–8. https://doi.org/10.1016/j.jaci.2005.08.043.
9. Taylor-Clark TE, Nassenstein C, Undem BJ. Leukotriene D 4 increases the excitability of capsaicin-sensitive nasal sensory nerves to electrical and chemical stimuli. Br J Pharmacol. 2008;154:1359–68. https://doi.org/10.1038/bjp.2008.196.
10. Smith PK, Nilius B. Transient receptor potentials (TRPs) and anaphylaxis. Curr Allergy Asthma Rep. 2013;13:93–100. https://doi.org/10.1007/s11882-012-0301-4.
11. Pipkorn U, Karlsson G, Enerbäck L. Secretory activity of nasal mucosal mast cells and histamine release in hay fever. Int Arch Allergy Immunol. 1988;87:349–60. https://doi.org/10.1159/000234700.
12. Krayenbuhl MC, Hudspith BN, Brostoff J, et al. Nasal histamine release following hyperosmolar and allergen challenge. Allergy. 1989;44:25–9. https://doi.org/10.1111/j.1398-9995.1989.tb00441.x.
13. Raap U, Fokkens W, Bruder M, et al. Modulation of neurotrophin and neurotrophin receptor expression in nasal mucosa after nasal allergen provocation in allergic rhinitis. Allergy. 2008;63:468–75. https://doi.org/10.1111/j.1398-9995.2008.01626.x.
14. Wu XQ, Myers AC, Goldstone AC, et al. Localization of nerve growth factor and its receptors in the human nasal mucosa. J Allergy Clin Immunol. 2006;118:428–33. https://doi.org/10.1016/j.jaci.2006.04.037.
15. Lee NR, Baek SY, Gu A, et al. House dust mite allergen suppresses neutrophil apoptosis by cytokine release via PAR2 in normal and allergic lymphocytes. Immunol Res. 2016;64:123–32. https://doi.org/10.1007/s12026-015-8730-5.
16. Alenmyr L, Högestätt ED, Zygmunt PM, Greiff L. TRPV1-mediated itch in seasonal allergic rhinitis. Allergy. 2009;64:807–10. https://doi.org/10.1111/j.1398-9995.2009.01937.x.
17. Van Gerven L, Alpizar YA, Wouters MM, et al. Capsaicin treatment reduces nasal hyperreactivity and transient receptor potential cation channel subfamily V, receptor 1 (TRPV1) overexpression in patients with idiopathic rhinitis. J Allergy Clin Immunol. 2014;133:1332. https://doi.org/10.1016/j.jaci.2013.08.026.
18. Mosimann BL, White MV, Hohman RJ, et al. Substance P, calcitonin gene-related peptide, and vasoactive intestinal peptide increase in nasal secretions after allergen challenge in atopic patients. J Allergy Clin Immunol. 1993;92:82–8. https://doi.org/10.1016/0091-6749(93)90041-D.
19. Jones RS, Asthma in children. Harcourt Health Sciences. 1976
20. Shneerson J, Shneerson JM. Non-respiratory symptoms of acute asthma. Thorax. 1986;41:701–2. https://doi.org/10.1136/thx.41.9.701.
21. Hon KLE, Lam MCA, Leung TF, et al. Nocturnal wrist movements are correlated with objective clinical scores and plasma chemokine levels in children with atopic dermatitis. Br J Dermatol. 2006;154:629–35. https://doi.org/10.1111/j.1365-2133.2006.07213.x.
22. Leung DY, Sampson HA, Bonilla FA, et al. Pediatric allergy, principles and practice. 3rd ed; 2015.

23. Scadding GK, Scadding GW. Diagnosing allergic rhinitis. Immunol Allergy Clin N Am. 2016;36:249–60. https://doi.org/10.1016/j.iac.2015.12.003.
24. Selnes A, Nystad W, Bolle R, Lund E. Diverging prevalence trends of atopic disorders in Norwegian children. Results from three cross-sectional studies. Allergy. 2005;60:894–9. https://doi.org/10.1111/j.1398-9995.2005.00797.x.
25. Dykewicz MS, Wallace DV, Amrol DJ, et al. Rhinitis 2020: a practice parameter update. J Allergy Clin Immunol. 2020;146:721–67. https://doi.org/10.1016/j.jaci.2020.07.007.
26. Asher MI, Montefort S, Björkstén B, et al. Worldwide time trends in the prevalence of symptoms of asthma, allergic rhinoconjunctivitis, and eczema in childhood: ISAAC phases one and three repeat multicountry cross-sectional surveys. Lancet. 2006;368:733–43. https://doi.org/10.1016/S0140-6736(06)69283-0.
27. Meltzer EO, Blaiss MS, Naclerio RM, et al. Burden of allergic rhinitis: allergies in America, Latin America, and Asia-Pacific adult surveys. Allergy Asthma Proc. 2012;33(Suppl 1):113–41. https://doi.org/10.2500/aap.2012.33.3603.
28. Mallol J, Crane J, von Mutius E, et al. The international study of asthma and allergies in childhood (ISAAC) phase three: a global synthesis. Allergol Immunopathol. 2013;41:73–85. https://doi.org/10.1016/j.aller.2012.03.001.
29. Newacheck PW, Stoddard JJ. Prevalence and impact of multiple childhood chronic illnesses. J Pediatr. 1994;124:40–8. https://doi.org/10.1016/S0022-3476(94)70252-7.
30. Meltzer EO, Blaiss MS, Derebery MJ, et al. Burden of allergic rhinitis: results from the pediatric allergies in America survey. J Allergy Clin Immunol. 2009;124:S43–70. https://doi.org/10.1016/j.jaci.2009.05.013.
31. Kulig M, Klettke U, Wahn V, et al. Development of seasonal allergic rhinitis during the first 7 years of life. J Allergy Clin Immunol. 2000;106:832–9. https://doi.org/10.1067/mai.2000.110098.
32. Ramavaram S, Jones SM. Natural course and comorbidities of allergic and nonallergic rhinitis in children. Pediatrics. 2012;130:S23–4. https://doi.org/10.1542/peds.2012-2183KK.
33. Brożek JL, Bousquet J, Agache I, et al. Allergic rhinitis and its impact on asthma (ARIA) guidelines—2016 revision. J Allergy Clin Immunol. 2017;140:950–8. https://doi.org/10.1016/j.jaci.2017.03.050.
34. Wheatley LM, Togias A. Clinical practice. Allergic rhinitis. N Engl J Med. 2015;372:456–63. https://doi.org/10.1056/NEJMcp1412282.
35. Pawankar R, Bunnag C, Khaltaev N, Bousquet J. Allergic rhinitis and its impact on asthma in Asia Pacific and the ARIA update 2008. World Allergy Organ J. 2012;5:S212–7. https://doi.org/10.1186/1939-4551-5-s3-s212.
36. Gelfand EW. Pediatric allergic rhinitis: factors affecting treatment choice. Ear Nose Throat J. 2005;84:163–8. https://doi.org/10.1177/014556130508400314.
37. Pawankar R. Allergic diseases and asthma: a global public health concern and a call to action. World Allergy Organ J. 2014;7:12. https://doi.org/10.1186/1939-4551-7-12.
38. Sampson HA. Mount Sinai expert guides: allergy and clinical immunology. 1st ed. John Wiley & Sons, Ltd.; 2015.
39. Hellings PW, Fokkens WJ. Allergic rhinitis and its impact on otorhinolaryngology. Allergy. 2006;61:656–64.
40. Meltzer EO, Nathan R, Derebery J, et al. Sleep, quality of life, and productivity impact of nasal symptoms in the United States: findings from the burden of rhinitis in America survey. Allergy Asthma Proc. 2009;30:244–54. https://doi.org/10.2500/aap.2009.30.3230.
41. Skoner DP. Allergic rhinitis: definition, epidemiology, pathophysiology, detection, and diagnosis. J Allergy Clin Immuno. 2001;108(1):S2–8.
42. Kliegman RM, St. Geme J. Nelson textbook of pediatrics. 21st ed. Elsevier; 2019.
43. Berger WE, Schonfeld JE. Nonallergic rhinitis in children. Curr Allergy Asthma Rep. 2007;7:112–6. https://doi.org/10.1007/s11882-007-0008-0.
44. Chiang WC, Chen YM, Tan HKK, et al. Allergic rhinitis and non-allergic rhinitis in children in the tropics: prevalence and risk associations. Pediatr Pulmonol. 2012;47:1026–33. https://doi.org/10.1002/ppul.22554.

45. Kaliner MA. Classification of nonallergic rhinitis syndromes with a focus on vasomotor rhinitis, proposed to be known henceforth as nonallergic rhinopathy. World Allergy Organ J. 2009;2:98–101. https://doi.org/10.1097/wox.0b013e3181a9d55b.
46. Dutt SN, Kameswaran M. The aetiology and management of atrophic rhinitis. J Laryngol Otol. 2005;119:843–52. https://doi.org/10.1258/002221505774783377.
47. Gentile DA, Pleskovic N, Bartholow A, Skoner DP. Allergic rhinitis. In: Pediatric allergy: principles and practice. 3rd ed. Elsevier Inc.; 2016. p. 210–218.e2.
48. Fokkens WJ, Lund VJ, Mullol J, et al. European position paper on rhinosinusitis and nasal polyps 2012. Rhinol Suppl. 2012;50(suppl. 23):1–298.
49. Pappas DE, Hendley JO, Hayden FG, Winther B. Symptom profile of common colds in school-aged children. Pediatr Infect Dis J. 2008;27:8–11. https://doi.org/10.1097/INF.0b013e31814847d9.
50. Rose AS, Thorp BD, Zanation AM, Ebert CS. Chronic rhinosinusitis in children. Pediatr Clin N Am. 2013;60:979–91. https://doi.org/10.1016/j.pcl.2013.04.001.
51. Short S, Bashir H, Marshall P, et al. Diagnosis and treatment of respiratory illness in children and adults. Institute for Clinical Systems Improvement.
52. Corne JM, Lau L, Scott SJ, et al. The relationship between atopic status and IL-10 nasal lavage levels in the acute and persistent inflammatory response to upper respiratory tract infection. Am J Respir Crit Care Med. 2001;163:1101–7. https://doi.org/10.1164/ajrccm.163.5.9902047.
53. Ellis AK, Keith PK. Nonallergic rhinitis with eosinophilia syndrome and related disorders. Clin Allergy Immunol. 2016;19:87–100.
54. Wilson KF, Spector ME, Orlandi RR. Types of rhinitis. Otolaryngol Clin N Am. 2011;44:549–59. https://doi.org/10.1016/j.otc.2011.03.016.
55. Sin B, Togias A. Pathophysiology of allergic and nonallergic rhinitis. Proc Am Thorac Soc. 2011;8:106–14. https://doi.org/10.1513/pats.201008-057RN.
56. Schuler CF IV, Montejo JM. Allergic rhinitis in children and adolescents. Pediatr Clin N Am. 2019;66:981–93. https://doi.org/10.1016/j.pcl.2019.06.004.
57. Tarkan Ö, Sürmelioğlu Ö, Tuncer Ü. Alerjik Rinitte Güncel Tanı ve Tedavi Yaklaşımları. Arşiv Kaynak Tarama Dergisi. 2009;18:156–70.
58. Hughes RGM, Jones NS. The role of nasal endoscopy in outpatient management. Clin Otolaryngol Allied Sci. 1998;23:224–6. https://doi.org/10.1046/j.1365-2273.1998.00131.x.
59. Ng ML, Warlow RS, Chrishanthan N, et al. Preliminary criteria for the definition of allergic rhinitis: a systematic evaluation of clinical parameters in a disease cohort (I). Clin Exp Allergy. 2000;30:1314–31. https://doi.org/10.1046/j.1365-2222.2000.00853.x.
60. Mølgaard E, Thomsen SF, Lund T, et al. Differences between allergic and nonallergic rhinitis in a large sample of adolescents and adults. Allergy. 2007;62:1033–7. https://doi.org/10.1111/j.1398-9995.2007.01355.x.
61. Lieberman P, Pattanaik D. Nonallergic rhinitis. Curr Allergy Asthma Rep. 2014;14:439. https://doi.org/10.1007/s11882-014-0439-3.
62. Scadding GK. Non-allergic rhinitis: diagnosis and management. Curr Opin Allergy Clin Immunol. 2001;1:15–20. https://doi.org/10.1097/01.all.0000010979.45992.0f.
63. Alobid I, Guilemany JM, Mullol J. Nasal manifestations of systemic illnesses. Curr Allergy Asthma Rep. 2004;4:208–16. https://doi.org/10.1007/s11882-004-0028-y.
64. Rotiroti G, Roberts G, Scadding GK. Rhinitis in children: common clinical presentations and differential diagnoses. Pediatr Allergy Immunol. 2015;26:103–10. https://doi.org/10.1111/pai.12339.
65. Brook I. Acute and chronic bacterial sinusitis. Infect Dis Clin N Am. 2007;21:427–48. https://doi.org/10.1016/j.idc.2007.02.001.
66. Manole F, Bayar Muluk N, Oğuz O, Ulusoy S, Scadding GK, Prokopakis E, Kalogjera L, Rombaux P, Cingi C. Local allergic rhinitis—a narrative review. Eur Rev Med Pharmacol Sci. 2024;28(3):1077–88. https://doi.org/10.26355/eurrev_202402_35344.
67. Oğuz O, Manole F, Bayar Muluk N, Cingi C. Facial mask for prevention of allergic rhinitis symptoms. Front Allergy. 2023;4:1265394. https://doi.org/10.3389/falgy.2023.1265394. PMID: 38125295; PMCID: PMC10731048

Rhinorrhea: Pathogenesis, Diagnosis, and Treatment

24

İlker Burak Arslan and İbrahim Çukurova

24.1 Introduction

Rhinorrhea is the free, watery nasal discharge from one or both nares. Although rhinorrhea refers to a thin, mostly clear nasal discharge, this secretion may be a light, clear fluid, thick mucus, or something in between. The drainage may run out of your nose, down the back of your throat, or both. This condition occurs relatively frequently and may be recurrent or chronic. Synonyms are runny nose and nasal drip.

Rhinorrhea can be seen in any age group and is generally self-limited, but it may indicate a more severe illness. A mild nasal discharge after a simple emotional moment to cerebrospinal fluid that can threaten life. Both paranasal sinuses and nasal cavities' membranes secrete mucus regularly. Usually, the mucus is swallowed with saliva. However, the mucus starts dripping if its production increases.

The rhinorrhea could be anterior or posterior. The discharge draining from the nares is called anterior rhinorrhea. The anterior nasal drip is generally associated with allergic or viral rhinitis. The phlegm dripping into the throat from the nose is referred to as posterior nasal drip (posterior rhinorrhea).

24.2 Pathogenesis

Pathogenesis of rhinorrhea includes:

(a) Excessive production of mucus by the mucous membranes that line the nasal cavities.

İ. B. Arslan · İ. Çukurova (✉)
İzmir University of Health Sciences, Tepecik Training and Research Hospital, Section of Otorhinolaryngology, Izmir, Turkey

H. Yüksel et al. (eds.), *Pediatric Airway Diseases*, Comprehensive ENT,
https://doi.org/10.1007/978-3-031-74853-0_24

(b) Obstruction of nasal passage and cessation of posterior traveling of nasal secretions.
(c) A track from the nose to the brain produces cerebral spinal fluid leakage.

Potential sources of nasal discharge include the water condensed from humid expired air, serous and seromucous gland secretions, epithelial cells, goblet cells, and fluids from the mucosal microcirculation.

Rhinorrhea is a common symptom of allergic rhinitis and viral infections, such as the common cold [1]. In allergic Rhinitis, rhinorrhea is caused by IgE-mediated reactions against inhaled allergens and involves mucosal inflammation driven by type 2 helper T (Th2) cells. The inflammatory cascade of the immune system triggers the underlying mechanism of rhinorrhea in upper respiratory infection (URI). Active transport of chloride ions causes water flow from epithelial cells in response to mediators. Glandular secretions contribute to the rhinorrhea stimulated by mediators and neural reflexes [2]. Action potentials traveling through parasympathetic efferent nerves can lead to epithelial activation, rhinorrhea, and some vasodilatation.

Secondary to nasal congestion, rhinorrhea can also occur secondary to structural causes, such as septal deviation, choanal atresia, concha bullosa, cleft palate, adenoid hypertrophy, and neoplasia [3].

CSF rhinorrhea commonly occurs following head trauma, after intracranial or intranasal surgery, or due to destructive lesions. CSF fistula between the dura and the skull base causes discharge of CSF from the nose.

24.3 Diagnosis

24.3.1 History

It is essential to enquire some questions about rhinorrhea, including duration, periodicity, nocturnal variation, seasonal effects, one or two sides, association with trauma or prior surgery, and whether any are alleviating or provoking factors, one-sided or bilateral discharge.

Characteristics of rhinorrhea, such as watery, mucoid, color, and blood-tinged discharge should be asked. Previous and current therapeutic trials of medication and their efficacy, systemic disease, and recent psychological aspects of active or passive smoking should be recorded. Past medical and familial history should reveal allergic disorders and systemic diseases.

Physicians should seek symptoms of possible causes, including fever, sore throat, malaise, cough, and facial pain.

24.3.2 Examination

Physical examination begins with measuring vital signs, including temperature, respiratory rate, and oxygen saturation. The patient's conscious and neurological findings are needed to be checked. All patients should have thorough head and neck examination.

Nose: Examination of the nose should begin with examining the face. Skin scar, bone or cartilage deformity, allergic conjunctivitis, and sometimes an allergic crease may be seen on the patient's nose. Palpation of the nasal bones and alar cartilage may give additional information. The degree of alar collapse is observed in routine and forced inspiration.

Anterior rhinoscopy will allow an assessment of the nasal passage and mucosa. Color and state of the nasal mucosa, presence of nasal discharge, and differences of both nasal cavities should be noted. The effect of adenoid enlargement should be kept in mind. Inferior turbinate and internal nasal valve evaluated on each side.

Nasal endoscopy using a three-pass technique is best performed after applying a decongestant combined with a local anesthetic. The inferior meatus, middle meatus, superior meatus, spheno-ethmoidal recess, olfactory cleft, septal areas, and the nasopharynx should be visualized with narrow and angled nasal endoscopes.

Imaging is undertaken if there is any suspicion of severe disorders such as malignancy, encephalocele, and cerebrospinal fluid (CSF) leakage.

Ear: Nasal inflammation and nasal drainage may plug up the eustachian tube between the nose and the ear, causing an ear infection and pain. Usually, it begins with fullness in the ear and may progress to serous otitis or acute otitis due to the pathogen and duration of tubal occlusion.

Pharynx: Postnasal drip should be visualized as an indication of rhinitis. Hypertrophy or hyperemia of one or both palate-pharyngeus should also be a warning for viral upper airway infection. Tonsil size and obstruction of the oropharynx are also noted for acute and chronic disease. Diffuse pharyngeal hyperemia may be an alert for irritant exposure.

Neck: Cervical lymph nodes are a drainage site for the nose and nasopharynx. Palpable anterior cervical lymphadenopathy would not be an unusual finding in the infectious cause of rhinorrhea. Painless, fixed, and growing lymphadenopathies suggest nasal-nasopharyngeal malignancies.

Eyes: Evaluate for conjunctiva injection or erythema, which might indicate irritation and inflammation. Dennie-Morgan fold lines (creases originating at the inner canthus and running parallel to the lower lid margin) indicate an allergic response. Patients with a CSF leak and benign intracranial hypertension may also display bilateral papilledema.

Neurologic examination: Patients presenting with unilateral clear nasal discharge associated with nonspecific headache symptoms raise suspicions of rhinorrhea of cerebrospinal origin. Patients can also present with mental status changes, seizures, and meningitis.

24.4 Differential Diagnoses

Rhinorrhea should be divided into two subcategories: Physiological and pathological.

1. Physiological rhinorrhea.
   (a) Emotional rhinorrhea (Crying).
   (b) Hormonal (menstrual cycle, pregnancy) rhinorrhea.

   (c) Exercise-induced rhinorrhea.
   (d) Cold air-induced rhinorrhea.
2. Pathological rhinorrhea.
   (a) Allergic rhinitis.
   (b) Non-allergic rhinitis (vasomotor rhinitis).
   (c) Infectious rhinitis (Viral URI-bacterial URI).
   (d) Nasal foreign body.
   (e) Occupational rhinitis.
   (f) Eye irritation.
   (g) Systemic disease (Hypothyroidism, Wegener's granulomatosis, Sarcoidosis, Sjögren's syndrome, Systemic lupus erythematous).
   (h) Drug-induced rhinorrhea (Rhinitis medicomentosa, estrogen, progesterone, aspirin, NSAIDs, clonidine, prazosin, doxazosin, beta-blockers, calcium channel blockers, thiazides, ACE inhibitors, Amitriptyline, risperidone, gabapentin, cocaine).
   (i) Structural or mechanical conditions (Enlarges adenoids, choanal atresia, deviated septum, hypertrophic turbinates, tooth extending into the nasal passage, and congenital nasal vestibule cyst).
   (j) Cystic fibrosis, nasal polyposis.
   (k) Gustatory rhinitis.
   (l) Atrophic rhinitis.
   (m) Reflux-induced rhinitis or gastroesophageal reflux disease.
   (n) CSF.
   (o) Nasal tumors.

24.5 CSF Rhinorrhea

24.5.1 CSF Physiology

CSF is the end product of active and passive plasma filtration at the choroid plexus with minor contributions from ependymal cells and parenchymal capillaries. Most CSF production (80–90%) occurs in the choroid plexus of the lateral ventricles and the third and fourth ventricles. After circulation through the subdural space, CSF is reabsorbed into the venous system by arachnoid granulations in the dural surface of the superior sagittal sinus. Arachnoid villi use 1-way valves that rely on hydrostatic pressure to resorb CSF flowing in a pulsatile manner into the venous system. Resorption occurs when intracranial pressure is 1.5–7.0 cm H_2O greater than central venous pressure [4] (Table 24.1).

24.5.1.1 Pathogenesis

Cerebrospinal fluid (CSF) rhinorrhea refers to the loss of CSF through the nasal cavity via an abnormal communication between the subarachnoid space and the sinonasal tract. CSF usually discharges from the anterior nares. But posterior discharge may develop depending on the fistula's location at the skull base. CSF can

Table 24.1 Normal composition of CSF

	Normal range
Specific gravity/pH	1.006–1.007/7.4
CSF proteins	15–40 mg/dL
CSF lactate	1–3 mmol/L
CSF glucose	**50–80 mg/dL** (two thirds of blood glucose)
WBC count	Lymphocytes 0–5 (up to 30 in neonates)

occur due to a defect in either the skull base, paranasal sinuses, or the temporal bone through the eustachian tube. It usually occurs due to a breach in the bone, dura, and arachnoid meningeal layers. Persistent CSF rhinorrhea necessitates surgical intervention because of the risk of meningitis, which has been reported to range from 10% to 37% during conservative management. Another concern associated with CSF fistulae is the development of pneumocephalus.

Cerebrospinal fluid rhinorrhea can be classified based on etiology, anatomical location, age of the patient, timing of the diagnosis, type and extent of skull defect, duration of symptomatology, and the possible timing and type of repair to be undertaken. The causes of CSF rhinorrhea can also be classified as spontaneous or non-spontaneous. Approximately 80–90% of all cases of CSF rhinorrhea are caused by head injuries. The most frequently used type of classification is traumatic or non-traumatic [5–7]. The traumatic group can be divided into accidental (60–70%) and iatrogenic (20–30%). Common locations of head injury include ethmoid roof and cribriform plate where olfactory neurons, surrounded by dura and arachnoid, penetrate the nasal cavity. Iatrogenic causes of CSF leaks compromise the second most common etiology. Surgical procedures associated with this risk include endoscopic or open sinus surgery, transphenoidal pituitary surgery, and resection of skull base tumors. The two most common sites injured during endoscopic sinus surgery (ESC) are the lateral lamella of the cribriform plate and the posterior ethmoid roof near the face of the sphenoid [8].

The non-traumatic group is associated with brain tumors (intracranial and extracranial tumors, cholesteatoma, or tuberculoma are known to erode the bone directly), skull base congenital disabilities (congenital encephalocele, persistent cricopharyngeal canal, meningoceles, or meningoencephalocles) related to the temporal bone, skull base, or dura mater, or exposure to radiation therapy involving the base of the skull and spontaneous with or without an associated increased intracranial pressure.

Intranasal, intracranial, or metastatic tumors may cause CSF leaks via direct skull base erosion. Also, treating these tumors by surgery, radiotherapy, or chemotherapy may cause CSF fistula. Tumors may obstruct normal CSF flow and cause non-communicating hydrocephalus with constant, elevated intracranial pressure, leading to eventual bony dehiscence with CSF leak [8].

Congenital encephaloceles, meningoceles, or meningoencephalocles may lead to CSF fistula. The nasofrontal and nasoethmoidal subtypes of sincipital encephaloceles arise from a patent fonticulus nasofrontalis and foramen cecum, respectively, and present externally along the glabella or dorsum of the nose. The transethmoidal, sphenoethmoidal, and transsphenoidal subtypes of basal encephaloceles show intranasally and result from a defect along the cribriform plate, ethmoid roof, or sphenoid [8].

Care should be taken to evaluate the temporal bone and anterior skull base for the possibility of CSF otorrhea, as it can present as CSF rhinorrhea when the tympanic membrane is intact.

24.6 Diagnosis

Differentiating CSF rhinorrhea from other nasal secretions is not easily accomplished in every CSF leakage. Intermittent or late rhinorrhea after injury makes diagnosis more complicated. Past medical history reveals rhinorrhea seconder to accidental or iatrogenic trauma.

In the acute phase following the traumatic event, patients may present with epistaxis, nasal discharge, periorbital ecchymosis, chemosis, oculomotor impairment, anosmia, motor deficit, open-head injury with CSF leakage, loss of vision, cranial nerve deficits (most frequently, first–third and fifth–seventh cranial nerve injuries), meningitis, and pneumocephalus. In the chronic phase, patients may present with recurrent meningitis, intermittent nasal discharge, headaches, salty or sweet taste in the retropharyngeal space, hyposmia, and brain abscess [7].

Localization of the leak CSF may be accomplished by direct visualization with diagnostic nasal endoscopy. Encephalocele or skull base mass are also observed under endoscopic examination.

Rhinorrhea can be provoked by placing the patient's face downward (Reservoir sign) and observing for leakage for several minutes. The Vasalva maneuver can increase the intensity of the rhinorrhea in this position, making it easier to detect.

CSF combined with blood can leave a ring or a halo, "Target sign" refers to the ability of CSF to migrate further, creating a bull's-eye stain with blood in the center, on a filter paper or gauze. This has been discussed as the first clue of a CSF leak, especially in a trauma patient [9].

Intrathecal injection of a sodium fluorescein solution following a thorough endoscopic examination has been used to establish the diagnosis of CSF rhinorrhea. Also, it may be used for the exact location of the leak intraoperatively. A mixture of 0.1 mL 10% fluorescein and 9.9 sterile saline is injected into the intrathecal space during lumbar puncture. Its distinguishing yellow-green color helps detect CSF drainage, and a blue light filter further enhances detection. Reported complications of the fluorescein solution's injection, and thus limitations to its use, have ranged from mild tinnitus, headache, nausea and vomiting, transient pulmonary edema, confusion, seizures, and coma to death.

24.6.1 Chemical Diagnosis

Chemical analysis of rhinorrhea is the most frequently used method of diagnosing CSF leaks. The concentration of glucose is the oldest method of diagnosing CSF leaks. The glucose concentration in nasal secretions is 10 mg/dL or less. The glucose concentration in CSF exceeds 50% of the serum concentration except during meningitis, subarachnoid hemorrhage, or other unusual circumstances. Glucose detection using Gluco-stix test strips is not recommended as a confirmatory test due to its lack of specificity and sensitivity [10].

Beta-2 transferrin is a carbohydrate-free isoform of transferrin, which is almost exclusively found in the CSF, and blood or nasal secretion does not disturb the test. Beta-2 transferrin is absent in blood, nasal mucus, tears, or mucosal discharge. Beta-2 transferrin was reported to have a sensitivity of nearly 100% and a specificity of about 95% in a large retrospective study [11].

Another protein proposed as a potential marker for diagnosing CSF rhinorrhea is *beta* trace protein or *beta* TP. It is the second most abundant protein in human CSF following albümin and is mainly produced in the epithelial cells of the choroid plexus and in the leptomeninges. The CSF concentration of beta TP is approximately 35-fold higher than in plasma. It is also found in nasal secretions and other body fluids, but in very low concentrations [7]. Beta-trace test has a sensitivity of 97.3% and a specificity of nearly 100% [12].

24.6.2 Imaging Diagnosis

Once the presence of CSF leakage has been established, specific localization of the leak is essential for successful treatment. X-ray radiography is not used in CSF assessment or treatment. Nowadays, CT, MRI, and nuclear medicine are used in CSF leakage.

Significant osseous defects can be visualized on plain CT. Our clinic uses axial coronal and sagittal planes with 0.6 mm slice thickness. High-resolution CT (HRCT) of the skull base can identify the site of the CSF fistula as a dural and osseous defect. A 3-dimensional reconstruction of the bone should aid the evaluation of congenital or spontaneous defects to permit an in-depth analysis of the floor of the anterior or middle cranial fossa. The dural defect may not be identified, but the bone defect with fluid opacification of adjacent sinuses and a bone defect on CT with air communicating from the paranasal sinuses intracranially are clinching points in the diagnosis of CSF leak. CT is less valuable in identifying nontraumatic CSF leaks, such as those associated with the meningocele and meningoencephalocele [13].

In CT cisternography, contrast pooling in a sinus is considered to be a positive study. The ability of CT cisternography to accurately identify the culprit skull base defect depends on performing the procedure while CSF is actively leaking. Therefore, the overall sensitivity could be better because intermittent leaks will be missed. Sensitivity approaches 92% during active leaking, but it drops significantly to 40% when the CSF leak is intermittent. CT cisternography carries some low risk, including infection, bleeding at the puncture site, and lumbar CSF leaks, resulting in low-tension headaches.

MRI details the intracranial anatomy and pathology in multiple planes relatively quickly. The main disadvantage of MRI is its poor spatial resolution and lack of bony details. Imaging characteristics of MRI that were considered diagnostic of CSF leak were a CSF column extending extracranially from the subarachnoid space and herniation of brain tissue/meninges extracranially.

MR cisternography, typically consisting of multiplanar heavily T2-weighted sequences, is reported to be a susceptible and specific (85% and 100%, respectively) technique in localizing CSF leaks by demonstrating high signal intensity extending from the subarachnoid compartment into the sinonasal spaces. Success with MR cisternography does not seem to depend on an active CSF leak but, like high-resolution CT, is an anatomic study. MR cisternography also identifies associated meningoencephaloceles and secondary parenchymal changes in signal intensity that reflect underlying CSF leaks without exposing patients to lumbar puncture. However, MR cisternography does not provide the fine bony detail necessary for planning minimally invasive endoscopic repair. In our experience, all patients with positive results on an MR cisternogram, usually obtained after the CT scan to exclude a meningocele, have already had a high-resolution skull base CT for the surgical repair to be planned [14].

Radionuclide cisternography is rarely performed nowadays. The most ideal radiotracer is Technetium (Tc) 99 m labeled diethylenetriamine pentaacetic acid. Active CSF leakage should be present during study time for accurate diagnosis. The Tc-99 m radionuclide study poorly demonstrates intermittent CSF leaks. In such cases, a prolonged cisternography can be performed with a radiotracer having a longer biological half-life, such as the Indium (In) 111 diethylenetriamine pentaacetic acid. Delayed imaging can be performed with this radionuclide for up to 72 h to diagnose intermittent CSF leaks [13].

24.7 Treatment

Because of the meningitis risk, pneumococcal vaccination is recommended for patients having CSF fistula or who have undergone repair.

The surgical management of CSF rhinorrhea is usually warranted only after a conservative management trial in cases of immediate-onset CSF rhinorrhea following accidental trauma. Conservative management consists of a 7–10 days bed rest trial with the bed head elevated at approximately 30°. This inclination angle is sufficient to reduce the CSF pressure at the basal cisterns. Coughing, sneezing, nose blowing, and heavy effort should be avoided as much as possible. Diet and medicine, if necessary, to prevent constipation is also kept in mind. A subarachnoid lumbar drain may be placed to drain approximately 5–10 mL of CSF per hour. Continuous drainage is recommended over intermittent drainage to avoid spikes in CSF pressure. Although controversial, diuretics and acetazolamide can be used to lower intracranial pressure.

Surgical management is considered only after the failure of conservative management. The surgical management consists of either an intracranial or an extracranial approach. In some instances both approaches are combined. The traditional repair route is through a frontal craniotomy with the repair of the defect from the superior aspect.

Due to the rapid progress in endoscopic surgery, especially in the last two decades, the first choice for surgical treatment of CSF rhinorrhea is the endoscopic transnasal approach. Nasal endoscopy has received particular attention in pediatric patients. This is due to various factors, including the following: these patients need general anesthesia, their nasal passages are narrow, there is a higher incidence of nasal obstruction, and anatomic differences compared to adults due to the appearance and sizes of air sinuses and the presence of adenoids [15]. The possibility of treating encephaloceles (congenital) as a cause is also high, making the endoscopic approach much more complex [16].

24.7.1 Surgical Technique

Pediatric patients are operated in a supine position with a 15°–20° head end elevation under general anesthesia. Nasal cavities were decongested with lidocaine hydrochloride 2% with 0.0125 epinephrine. If the leak site was not confirmed preoperatively, induced positive pressure ventilation should reveal the CSF leak. 2.7 mm 0° and 30° endoscopes were used for the surgery. 4 mm 0°, 30°, and 45° endoscopes can be used in patients with wide nasal cavities, like adult patients. Otological instruments are more useful for children under 5 years old child.

Anatomical structures or nasal pathologies, such as middle turbinate nasal septal deviation that prevents surgical instruments' leading, should be resected. Meningocele or encephalocele prolapsed from the skull base defect, cauterized by bipolar cautery until the overhanging tissue is vaporized. The defect was identified, margins freshened, and the defect closed in multiple layers using fascia, cartilage, and gel foam. We prefer fascia lata due to its less morbidity and ease of accessibility. First, we package fascia lata, nearly two times bigger than skull base defect under the dura-over skull base. Then a little cartilage fitted defect smoothly. Another fascia lata layer is spread under bone defect. Fat tissue, muscle, artificial dura, and oxidized regenerated cellulose are used other materials for used materials according to the literature. Fibrin glue is used over the cartilage and second fascia layer. Geloams are placed and fixed with fibrin glue. Anterior nasal packing with nonabsorbable material was done in all cases. Nonabsorbable pack removal was done on the third postoperative day. Given the discomfort and non-compliance expected in pediatric patients, the Lumbar drain was not utilized in any cases contrary to adult cases. Acetazolamide was confined to bed rest for 4–6 weeks, along with I.V. antibiotics, antihistamines, stool softeners, and cough suppressants. All the cases were followed up for a minimum period of 12 months.

References

1. Knight A. The differential diagnosis of rhinorrhea. J Allergy Clin Immunol. 1995;95:1080–3.
2. Myint S, Taylor-Rabinson D. Viral and other infections of the human respiratory tract. In: Akerlund A, Bende M, editors. Section 5 pathophysiology of viral respiratory tract infections. Dordrecht: Springer; 1996. p. 83–104.

3. Naclerio RM, Bachert C, Baraniuk JN. Pathophysiology of nasal congestion. Int J Gen Med. 2010;3:47–57.
4. Mathias T, Levy J, Fatakia A, McCoul ED. Contemporary approach to the diagnosis and management of cerebrospinal fluid rhinorrhea. Ochsner Journal. 2016;16:136–42.
5. Oakley GM, Alt JA, Schlosser RJ, Harvey RJ, Orlandi RR. Diagnosis of cerebrospinal fluid rhinorrhea: an evidence-based review with recommendations. Int Forum Allergy Rhinol. 2016;6(1):8–16.
6. Boppana HK, Welch T, Calderon C. Spontaneous cerebrospinal fluid rhinorrhea: a case report. Cureus. 2020;12(7):e9401. https://doi.org/10.7759/cureus.9401.
7. Zıu M, Savage JG, Jimenez DF. Diagnosis and treatment of cerebrospinal fluid rhinorrhea following accidental traumatic anterior skull base fractures. Neurosurg Focus. 2012;32(6):E3.
8. Stucker FJ, Souza CD, Kenyon GS, Lian TS, Draf W, Schick B. Rhinology and facial plastic surgery. In: LaCour JB, Senior BA, editors. Chapter 42: diagnosis, evaluation and management of CDF rhinorrhea. Berlin Heidelberg: Springer-Verlag; 2009. p. 477–84.
9. Cukurova I, Cetinkaya EA, Aslan IB, Ozkul D. Endonasal endoscopic repair of ethmoid roof cerebrospinal fluid fistula by suturing the dura. Acta Neurochir. 2008;150:897–900.
10. Chan DT, Poon WS, Ip CP, Chiu PW, Goh KY. How useful is glucose detection in diagnosing cerebrospinal fluid leak? The rational use of CT and Beta-2 transferrin assay in detection of cerebrospinal fluid fistula. Asian J Surg. 2004;27:39–42.
11. Cerebrospinal fluid rhinorrhoea. Diagnosis and management. Med Oral Patol Oral Cir Bucal. 2007;12:E397–400.
12. Bachman G, Achtelik R, Nekic M, Michel O. Beta-trace-protein in der Diagnostik der Liquorfistel. HNO. 2000;48:496–500.
13. Vemuri NV, Karanam LSP, Manchikanti V, Dandamudi S, Puvvada SK, Vemuri VK. Imaging review of cerebrospinal fluid leaks. Indian J Radiol Imaging. 2017;27(4):441–6.
14. La Fata V, McLean N, Wise SK, DelGaudio JM, Hudgins PA. CSF leaks: correlation of high-resolution CT and multiplanar reformations with intraoperative endoscopic findings. Am J Neuroradiol. 2008;29(3):536–41. https://doi.org/10.3174/ajnr.A0885.
15. Husain M, Jha D, Husain N, Gupta RK. Neuroendoscopic treatment of paediatric cerebrospinal fluid rhinorrhoea. Pediatr Neurosurg. 2002;37:295–7. https://doi.org/10.1159/000066308.
16. Chappity P, Alok T, Rohit V. Endonasal endoscopic approach in management of paediatric CSF rhinorrhoea cases. Indian J Otolaryngol Head Neck Surg. 2015;67(1):88–92. https://doi.org/10.1007/s12070-014-0795-2.

Tonsillary Hypertrophy in Children

25

Abdullah Kınar, Cemal Cingi, and Tania Sih

25.1 Introduction

The palatine tonsils and adenoids are tissues of the Waldeyer ring, a group of lymphoepithelial tissues that includes tubal tonsils in the nasopharynx and the lingual tonsil. Collectively, these tissues participate in the mucosal immune system of the pharynx.

25.1.1 Waldeyer Ring

The German anatomist Heinrich von Waldeyer is noted for his anatomic description of the lymphoid tissue in the posterior nasopharynx and oropharynx. As mentioned previously, the Waldeyer ring consists of palatine (faucial) tonsils (the tonsils), pharyngeal tonsils (the adenoids), lingual tonsils, and tubal tonsils.

They are positioned strategically at the entrance of the gastrointestinal and respiratory tracts. The tonsils and adenoid serve as secondary lymphoid organs, initiating immune responses against antigens entering the body through the mouth or nose [1–4].

A. Kınar
Department of Otorhinolaryngology, Afyonkarahisar State Hospital, Afyonkarahisar, Turkey

C. Cingi (✉)
Medical Faculty, Department of Otorhinolaryngology, Eskişehir Osmangazi University, Eskisehir, Turkey

T. Sih
Department of Pediatric Otolaryngology, School of Medicine, University of São Paulo, São Paulo, Brazil
e-mail: tsih@amcham.com.br

H. Yüksel et al. (eds.), *Pediatric Airway Diseases*, Comprehensive ENT,
https://doi.org/10.1007/978-3-031-74853-0_25

25.2 Embryology of Tonsils

During the fourth fetal month, epithelial crypts grow into the epithelial connective tissue and are infiltrated by lymphoid cells. In the fifth month, the first primary follicles are seen. The palatine tonsils are first seen in the third month and are derived from the ventral portion of the second pharyngeal pouch. During the fourth month, ten solid epithelial (endodermal) buds entwine within the mesenchyme around the pharyngeal wall, and canalization occurs via programmed cell death. By the third trimester, organized lymph follicles are noted [1–4].

25.3 Anatomy

Palatine Tonsils Boundaries

- Anterior: Palatoglossus muscle.
- Posterior: Palatoglossus muscle.
- Lateral: Superior constrictor muscle.

Vascular Supply of Palatine Tonsils

- Tonsillar artery.
- Ascending pharyngeal artery.
- Tonsil branch of the facial artery.
- Dorsal lingual branch of the lingual artery.
- Ascending palatine branches of the facial artery.

Venous Drainage of Palatine Tonsils

- Peritonsillar plexus to the pharyngeal plexus, pterygoid plexus, and ultimately into the internal jugular and facial veins.

A meaningful anatomic relationship to note surgically is that the internal carotid artery is approximately 2.5 cm posterolateral to the tonsil. The tonsil drains into the tonsillar veins and the external palatine, pharyngeal, and facial veins. Another important surgical note is that the palatine veins are the most common cause of postoperative tonsillectomy bleeding.

25.3.1 Lymphatic Drainage

These are unique because they contain only efferent and no afferent lymphatic circulation; thus, lymph is not filtered through the tonsillar nodules. Drainage is directly to jugulodigastric nodes, upper deep cervical lymph nodes, and indirectly through retropharyngeal lymph nodes.

Efferent lymphatic drainage flows from the retropharyngeal lymph nodes to the upper deep cervical lymph nodes, especially the posterior triangle nodes.

25.3.1.1 Nerve Supply

- Tonsillar branches of the maxillary nerve and glossopharyngeal nerve.

  The glossopharyngeal nerve and styloid process descend almost vertically on the lateral surface of this musculature. These tonsils are preserved via the pterygopalatine (sphenopalatine) ganglion through the lesser palatine nerves and from the glossopharyngeal nerve. Pediatric patients often complain of ear pain after tonsillectomy.

  This is referred to as pain via the glossopharyngeal nerve, which also supplies the middle-ear cavity, including the medial wall of the tympanic membrane. The blood supply to these tonsils includes the facial artery (tonsillar branch and ascending palatine branch), ascending pharyngeal artery, dorsal lingual branch of the lingual artery, and internal maxillary artery (descending palatine artery, more significant palatine artery) [2, 3].

25.4 Histology of Waldeyer Ring

The epithelial covering of the palatine tonsils is stratified squamous epithelium, which invaginates into the crypts. The palatine tonsils contain 10–20 crypts, which penetrate the surface to reach various depths and may penetrate the entire tonsil to reach the fibrous capsule and blends with the mesenchymal structures. Growth of the palatine tonsils continues postnatally, and the palatine tonsil is active until age 15 years [2].

After puberty, the tonsillar tissue tends to involute, and more fibrosis appears.

In contrast to other oronasal lymphoid tissues, the palatine tonsils are covered with a pharynx basilar capsule fascia. The capsule is separated from the underlying musculature by loose connective tissue. Pus can collect here and cause a peritonsillar abscess.

25.5 Immune Function of Waldeyer Rings

The tonsils are the first lymphoid aggregates to encounter pathogens that enter the host via the upper respiratory and gastrointestinal tracts and thus are believed to play a role in host immunity to pathogens.

Stimulation of the immune system begins shortly after birth [1–4]. Terminally differentiated plasma cells can be seen around 2 weeks of age. This results in the development of secondary follicles. They also produce lymphocytes in a complete sequence of lymphopoiesis and are related immunologically to the gut-associated lymphoid system in humans [1–4].

Tonsils contain three other lymphoid compartments participating in immune functions beneath the epithelium. The lymphoid follicles have two compartments: the mantle zone and the germinal center (GC). The GC has a significant B cell concentration and is the center of B-cell responses that include the clonal expansion of B cells, the selection of B cells capable of receiving antigen-specific signals, the subsequent differentiation into B memory cells and plasma cells of various isotypes, and the induction of the gene encoding the J-chain carbohydrate. The follicles also contain a network of follicular dendritic cells (FDC) and a particular subset of germinal center dendritic cells that activate the GC T cells. The FDC can retain high amounts of immune complexes on their plasma membranes for long periods and thereby act as antigen-presenting cells, promoting the proliferation and differentiation of GC B cells [4].

The third or extrafollicular compartment contains T cells (primarily CD4+ helper cells), interdigitating dendritic cells (IDC), macrophages, and high-endothelial venules that facilitate the entry of T cells and B cells from the blood into the tonsils. The region is also a center of cytokine and antibody production.

After passing through the crypt epithelium, M cells can initiate immunologic responses, introducing foreign antigens to lymphocytes and antigen-presenting cells (APCs).

Tonsils lack afferent lymphatics; however, the epithelium contains a system of specialized channels lined by M cells that take up antigens into the vesicles and transport them to the intra- and subepithelial spaces, where they are presented to lymphoid cells. This transport function of M cells also serves as a portal for mucosal infections and immunizations. In addition to their transport function, the M cells initiate an immunologic response within the epithelium, bringing together high concentrations of foreign antigens with lymphocytes and antigen-presenting cells, such as macrophages and dendritic cells.

After passing through the crypt epithelium, inhaled or ingested antigens reach the extrafollicular region or lymphoid follicles. IDC and macrophages process the antigens in the extrafollicular area and present them to CD4+ T lymphocytes. Helper T cells then stimulate the proliferation of follicular B lymphocytes and their development into either antibody-expressing B memory cells capable of migration to the nasopharynx and other sites or plasma cells that produce antibodies and release them into the cryptlumen. Tonsillar plasma cells can have all five immunoglobulin (Ig) classes, helping to combat and prevent infection. Among the Ig isotypes, IgA may be considered the most essential product of the adenotonsillar immune system. In its dimeric form, IgA can attach to the transmembrane secretory component (SC) to form secretory IgA (SIgA), a critical part of the mucosal immune system of the upper airway. This component is necessary for binding IgA monomers to each other and the SC and is an essential product of B cell activity in the tonsil follicles. While the tonsils produce immunocytes bearing the J (joining) chain carbohydrate, the SC is produced only in the adenoid and extra tonsillar epithelium, and therefore, only the adenoid possesses a local secretory immune system [2–4].

25.6 Tonsillary Hypertrophy

The size of the tonsils appears to correlate with their level of immunologic activity, peaking between the ages of 3 and 10 years and demonstrating age-dependent involution. There is also some evidence that their size increases with bacterial load.

The tonsils and the adenoid are sites of continuous stimulation of the lymphoid cells. The most excellent immunological activity of the tonsils is found between the ages of 3 and 10 years; the tonsils are most prominent during this childhood period and subsequently demonstrate age-dependent involution. There is some evidence that their size increases with the bacterial load and the population of B and T cells [2–5].

At birth, the palatine tonsils are approximately 5 mm in anteroposterior diameter and 3.5 mm in vertical diameter, weighing about 0.75 g. During childhood, the palatine tonsils descend within their fossae as their vertical diameter grows faster than their anteroposterior diameter. When lymphoid tissue occupies disproportionate space in the pharynx, the upper airway becomes compromised.

Adenotonsillar disorders in children can be caused by various factors, including pathogens, allergies, genetic predisposition, and, rarely, neoplastic proliferation. Unilateral tonsillar hypertrophy should always raise suspicion of a tumor to physicians. Hyperplasia is a natural consequence of immune activity within these tissues but may become problematic when tissue size becomes excessive for the pharyngeal space they occupy. Infection of the tonsils and adenoids is common in this age group because they participate in immune processes and continuous exposure to inhaled and ingested antigens [5–10].

In immunologic disorders like X-linked agammaglobulinemia (XLA; Bruton-type agammaglobulinemia), it is a primary humoral immunodeficiency characterized by recurrent bacterial infections of the respiratory tract and increased susceptibility to enteroviral infection. The characteristic physical finding of XLA is the absence, or near lack, of the tonsils and adenoids, although they may be present if T cell areas are hypertrophied. The respiratory tract is the most common site of bacterial infections in XLA [11].

Activation-induced cytidine deaminase (AID) deficiency is a lack of lymphoid and tonsillar tissue. Tonsillar hypertrophy is often prominent and may prompt tonsillectomy [11].

In Mucopolysaccharide storage disorders, thickening in the nose and pharynx and hypertrophy of the tonsils and adenoids due to storage of glycosaminoglycans (GAGs) in these tissues can be seen [7–10, 12, 13].

Feenstra B et al. identified and replicated a genetic association with the variant rs2412971, intronic in *HORMAD2*at 22q12.2 with tonsillectomy. They also found that the risk allele for tonsillectomy corresponded to an increased risk of IgA nephropathy [14].

25.7 Physical Examination

Tonsil size is best determined in a neutral state (i.e., without the child gagging on a tongue depressor) to accurately estimate the volume of the pharynx they occupy—the Brodsky scale for clinical tonsil grading in children. Tonsil hyperplasia is graded visually, most commonly using a scale of 1 to 4. Tonsillar size is often described on a scale from 0 to 5 [15].

- **0:** Tonsils are entirely within the tonsillar pillar or previously removed by surgery.
- **1+:** Tonsils occupy 0–25% of the posterior pharynx or tonsils hidden within tonsil pillars.
- **2+:** Tonsils occupy 26–50% of the posterior pharynx or tonsils extending to the pillars.
- **3+:** Tonsils occupy 51–75% of the posterior pharynx or tonsils are beyond the pillars.
- **4+:** Tonsils occupy 76–100% of the posterior pharynx, or tonsils extend to the midline. "Kissing tonsils" could be seen in severe hyperplasia.

25.8 Symptoms of Hyperplasia of Tonsils in Childhood

Obstructive sleep Apnea or sleep disturbances.
Failure to thrive.
Abnormal dentofacial growth.
Dental abnormalities.
Cardiac or pulmonary disease exacerbated by upper airway obstruction.
Eating or swallowing disorders.
Speech impairment.
Halitosis.

In children, hyperplasia of the tonsils and adenoids is commonly associated with pharyngeal obstruction. During the daytime, children with an enlarged adenoid demonstrate mouth breathing, rhinorrhea, and hyponasal speech, while those with tonsil hyperplasia may exhibit a muffled, "hot potato" voice. However, the obstruction is even more apparent during sleep, when pharyngeal musculature relaxation exacerbates airflow resistance.

25.8.1 Obstructive Sleep Apnea

Obstructive sleep apnea is one of the most common reasons for adenotonsillectomy-related adenotonsillar hypertrophy. Children with obesity (especially if severe) are far more likely than lean children to have OSA, with reports of prevalence ranging from 13% to 59% [16, 17].

Nocturnal Polysomnography PSG (overnight PSG) is considered the gold standard for diagnosis of OSA, as it is the only method able to definitively identify the presence of obstructive events and quantify the severity of OSA, including gas-exchange abnormalities and sleep disruption.

Obstructive sleep apnea increased in children <2 years of age and children with obesity (especially if severe), Down syndrome, craniofacial abnormalities, neuromuscular disorders, sickle cell disease, or mucopolysaccharidoses obesity, achondroplasia, mucopolysaccharidoses, or craniofacial syndromes, or by dynamic collapse such as occurs in the supine position and under conditions of diminished neuromuscular tone such as sleep, Down syndrome, and cerebral palsy with prevalence estimates of 30–100% in Down syndrome, 15% in cerebral palsy, 85% in Pierre-Robin sequence, and over 50% in children with achondroplasia [18–20].

Severity is generally quantified based on the obstructive apnea-hypopnea index (OAHI). The OAHI is the total number of obstructive apneas and hypopneas divided by the entire sleep duration in hours. Although there is no consensus on the definition of OSAS in children, an OAHI of ≤1 is considered within normal limits. An OAHI of 1–5 is very mildly increased; 5–10 is mildly increased; 10–15 is moderately increased; and greater than 15 is severely abnormal. Unfortunately, polysomnography is expensive, time-consuming, and often unavailable. Other assessment techniques, such as audiotaping, videotaping, and home and abbreviated polysomnography, may be helpful but must be more accurate.

Studies suggest that children with even mild OSAS demonstrate a morning blood pressure surge, and those with OAHI greater than five show increased blood pressure load and 24-h ambulatory blood pressure, leading to cardiac hypertrophy. An association with enuresis has also been demonstrated in up to 50% of children with sleep disturbances. The mechanism of this is not established, but theories include alterations in normal arousal and self-alerting mechanisms, hormonal changes (lower levels of antidiuretic hormone), and increased intra-abdominal pressure. In behavioral studies, children with SRBD demonstrate significantly higher prevalence rates of problematic behaviors, including internalized (e.g., withdrawal, shyness, anxiety) and externalized (e.g., emotional lability, impulsivity, hyperactivity, aggressiveness, oppositional personality, somatic complaints, social problems) behaviors, compared with controls. The strongest, most consistent associations are for externalizing, hyperactive-type behaviors. Even children with primary snoring and OAHI less than five have been found to perform worse than controls on measures related to attention, social problems, and anxious or depressive symptoms, as well as overall cognitive abilities and some language and visuospatial functions. As a result, the polysomnographic level at which intervention should be considered for children with sleep disturbances and problem behaviors remains unclear. Neurocognitive impairment is also noted in children with OSAS and appears more severe in children with OSAS than in those with primary snoring. Several studies have established a lower level of school performance among children with OSAS, and children with poor academic performance are also more likely to demonstrate sleep disturbances [15, 21, 22].

References

1. Nave H, Gebert A, Pabst R. Morphology and immunology of the human palatine tonsil. Anat Embryol. 2001;204:367–73.
2. Isaacson G, Parikh T. Developmental anatomy of the tonsil and its implications for intracapsular tonsillectomy. Int J Pediatr Otorhinolaryngol. 2008;72:89–96.
3. Handelman CS, Osborne G. Growth of the nasopharynx and adenoid development from one to eighteen years. Angle Orthod. 1976;46:243–59.
4. Brandtzaeg P. Immunology of tonsils and adenoids: everything the ENT surgeon needs to know. Int J Pediatr Otorhinolaryngol. 2003;67(suppl 1):S69–76.

5. Lindroos R. Bacteriology of the tonsil core in recurrent tonsillitis and tonsillar hyperplasia—a short review. Acta Otolaryngo Suppl. 2000;543:206–8.
6. Jeong JH, Lee DW, Ryu RA, et al. Bacteriologic comparison of tonsil core in recurrent tonsillitis and tonsil hypertrophy. Laryngoscope. 2007;117:2146–51.
7. Harley EH. Asymmetric tonsil size in children. Arch Otolaryngol Head Neck Surg. 2002;128:767–9.
8. Berkowitz RG, Mahadevan M. Unilateral tonsillar enlargement and tonsillar lymphoma in children. Ann Otol Rhinol Laryngol. 1999;108:876–9.
9. Syms MJ, Birkmire-Peters DP, Holtel MR. Incidence of carcinoma in tonsil asymmetry. Laryngoscope. 2000;110:1807–10.
10. Sunkaraneni VS, Jones SE, Prasai A, Fish BM. Is unilateral tonsillar enlargement alone an indication of tonsillectomy? J Laryngol Otol. 2006;120:E21.
11. Aghamohammadi A, Parvaneh N, Rezaei N, et al. Clinical and laboratory findings in hyper-IgM syndrome with novel CD40L and AICDA mutations. J Clin Immunol. 2009;29:769.
12. Semenza GL, Pyeritz RE. Respiratory complications of mucopolysaccharide storage disorders. Medicine (Baltimore). 1988;67:209.
13. Bredenkamp JK, Smith ME, Dudley JP, et al. Otolaryngologic manifestations of the mucopolysaccharidoses. Ann Otol Rhinol Laryngol. 1992;101:472.
14. Feenstra B, Bager P, Liu X, Hjalgrim H, Nohr EA, Hougaard DM, Geller F, Melbye M. Genome-wide association study identifies variants in HORMAD2 associated with tonsillectomy. J Med Genet. 2017;54(5):358–64. https://doi.org/10.1136/jmedgenet-2016-104304. Epub 2016 Dec 9
15. Brodsky L. Modern assessment of tonsils and adenoids. Pediatr Clin N Am. 1989;36(6):1551–69. https://doi.org/10.1016/s0031-3955(16)36806-7. PMID: 2685730
16. Katz ES, D'Ambrosio CM. Pediatric obstructive sleep apnea syndrome. Clin Chest Med. 2010;31:221.
17. Bixler EO, Vgontzas AN, Lin HM, et al. Sleep-disordered breathing in children in a general population sample: prevalence and risk factors. Sleep. 2009;32:731.
18. Shott SR, Amin R, Chini B, Heubi C, Hotze S, Akers R. Obstructive sleep apnea: should all children with down syndrome be tested? Arch Otolaryngol Head Neck Surg. 2006;132(4):432–6. https://doi.org/10.1001/archotol.132.4.432. PMID: 16618913
19. Daniel M, Bailey S, Walker K, Hensley R, Kol-Castro C, Badawi N, Cheng A, Waters K. Airway, feeding and growth in infants with Robin sequence and sleep apnoea. Int J Pediatr Otorhinolaryngol. 2013;77(4):499–503. https://doi.org/10.1016/j.ijporl.2012.12.019. Epub 2013 Jan 11
20. Afsharpaiman S, Sillence DO, Sheikhvatan M, Ault JE, Waters K. Respiratory events and obstructive sleep apnea in children with achondroplasia: investigation and treatment outcomes. Sleep Breath. 2011;15(4):755–61. https://doi.org/10.1007/s11325-010-0432-6. Epub 2011 Jan 13. PMID: 21225355
21. Urschitz MS, Wolff J, Sokollik C, et al. Nocturnal arterial oxygen saturation and academic performance in a community sample of children. Pediatrics. 2005;115:e204–9.
22. Friedman BC, Hendeles-Amtai A, Kozimsky E, et al. Adenotonsillectomy improves neurocognitive function in children with obstructive sleep apnea syndrome. Sleep. 2003;26:999–1005.

Halitosis Due to Pediatric Ear, Nose, and Throat Field Infections

26

İlyas Dişikırık and Mahmut Alper Kanmaz

26.1 Introduction

Halitosis is a general term used to describe the unpleasant odor in the breath due to oral or non-oral reasons. It appears as a condition that can cause psychological problems in children and their families. It has a multifactorial pathology. Although it can occur due to intraoral and extraoral reasons, in 50% of patients in 90 cases, the cause is intraoral [1].

Halitosis that originates from the mouth is called oral malodor [2]. It occurs due to proteolytic destruction of organic substances in the mouth, especially by anaerobic bacteria found in the tongue coating [3]. Therefore, it is recommended to evaluate and reduce the microbial structure in the mouth in treatment [4].

The fissured structure of the tongue prepares the ground for bacteria to multiply there [5, 6]. Thus, this fissured structure creates a basis for the proliferation and growth of bacteria while also protecting these pathogens from the washing effect of saliva.

The accumulation of food residues, epithelial residues, and bacteria on the tongue dorsum as a coating is called tongue coating. It is stated that there is a close relationship between tongue coating and lousy breath [3, 5]. For this reason, the primary source of bad breath is accepted as the tongue dorsum [2, 3, 5].

Very few studies exist on the etiology and treatment of halitosis in children [7, 8].

Although halitosis occurs at different rates in different societies, the average incidence is 5–33%.

İ. Dişikırık
Medical Faculty, Department of Otorhinolaryngology, Sanko University, Gaziantep, Turkey

M. A. Kanmaz (✉)
Department of Otorhynolaryngology, Gaziantep Nizip State Hospital, Gaziantep, Turkey

H. Yüksel et al. (eds.), *Pediatric Airway Diseases*, Comprehensive ENT,
https://doi.org/10.1007/978-3-031-74853-0_26

26.2 History of Halitosis

The history of halitosis dates back to ancient times. Some sources mention halitosis in Greek, Roman, and Jewish cultures [9]. Halitosis was accepted as a clinical finding after Howe, one of the pioneers of halitosis research, described this symptom in 1874 [10].

In 1934, Fair and Wells developed a device to measure odor. Later, in 1940 and 1950, Fosdic and his colleagues conducted various studies on the etiology of halitosis using this device [3]. In the 1960s, Tonzetich and his colleagues introduced the gas chromatography method that measured volatile sulfur compounds (VSCs) in breath and saliva [11].

26.3 Epidemiology of Halitosis

In the few studies investigating the prevalence of halitosis in the general population, this rate varies between 22 and 50% [12]. Miyazaki et al. [13] found this rate to be 28% in Japan's 18–64 years age group. They found no difference in the amount of VSC between men and women and that age was not a risk factor for increased VSC. In their study, Liu et al. [14] stated that this rate was 27.5% in the Chinese population. In their research, Al-Ansari et al. [15] found this rate to be 23.3%.

In their study in Sweden, Soder et al. [16] evaluated lousy breath and periodontal disease and reported that 2.4% had severe bad breath.

Some studies have found no difference between the incidence and severity of halitosis between men and women [17, 18].

26.4 Classification of Halitosis

The most common classification for halitosis is the classification made by Miyazaki et al. According to this classification, halitosis is categorized as

1. True Halitosis.
2. Pseudo Halitosis.
3. Halitophobia is examined in three categories.

Genuine halitosis is a terrible breath problem easily diagnosed by organoleptic and chemical means. Pseudohalitosis is a condition in which the patient believes he has bad breath, even though he does not have bad breath. A state in which the patient still believes that they have terrible breath despite being treated, whether it is real or pseudohalitosis, is called Halitophobia [19].

Genuine halitosis is divided into physiological (temporary) and pathological. Physiological halitosis describes lousy breath due to temporary conditions such as dry mouth, hunger, stress, and consumption of smelly foods such as garlic and onions. Bad morning breath is the most common example of temporary halitosis because salivary secretion decreases during the night, the washing effect of saliva decreases, and anaerobes are prevented. VSC production increases, resulting in bad breath. This condition is not pathological and does not require treatment [9]. Again, hunger odor is one of the causes of temporary halitosis and occurs due to the decomposition of pancreatic fluid in the stomach during fasting.

Pathological halitosis is a condition that causes social problems that do not go away despite oral hygiene and treatment.

26.5 Halitosis Physiopathology

Oral malodor: Saliva is formed by the proteolytic destruction of organic substances, such as gingival crevicular fluid, interdental plaque, shed epithelial residues, postnasal discharge, and blood, such as glucose, mucin, peptide, and protein, by microorganisms in the mouth, and as a result, the formation of VSC. VSC is the most common cause of bad breath. These are hydrogen sulfide (H_2S), methyl mercaptan, and dimethyl sulfide [3]. On the other hand, diamines (putrescine, cadaverine), phenol compounds (indol, skatole, pyridine), short-chain fatty acids (butyric acid, propionic acid, valeric acid), alcohols, alkynes, ketones, and nitrogen-containing compounds are also among the factors that can cause bad breath [20–22].

The microorganisms responsible for the hydrolysis of peptides and proteins and the resulting VSC production are gram (−) proteolytic anaerobes [3, 23, 24]. The bacteria responsible for VSC production are shown in Table 26.1 [3, 23, 25].

The most important source region for VSC is the dorsoposterior region of the tongue [26, 27]. Because this area is the largest surface area of the tongue, the tongue papillae located here are protected from the proteolytic anaerobes accumulated between the taste buds from the washing effect of saliva, and these anatomical structures also provide the anaerobic environment necessary for the reproduction of bacteria. VSC concentration increases as you move from the tip of the tongue to the root of the tongue.

These bacteria found in the subgingival area are significantly associated with chronic periodontitis and gingivitis and cause VSC formation in the periodontal pocket and gingival crevicular fluid [28]. The same microorganisms settle on the tongue dorsum in individuals with a tongue coating. The papillary structure of the

Table 26.1 The bacteria responsible for VSC production

Actinobacillus actinomycetemcomitans	Campylobacter rectus	Porphyromonas endodontalis
Actinomyces species	Desulfovibrio species	Porphyromonas gingivalis
Atopobium parvulum	Eikenella corrodens	Prevotella species
Atopobium parvulum	Eubacterium sulci	Solobacterium moorei
Atopobium parvulum	Fusobacterium species	Tannerella forsythia (Bacteriodes forsythus/Tannerella forsythensis)
Atopobium parvulum	Peptostreptococcus micros	Treponema denticola

tongue dorsum provides the necessary anaerobic environment to reproduce these microorganisms. The microorganisms multiply here, and the production of VSCs, which causes bad breath, increases. Amino acids such as cysteine, and methionine, which are necessary for VSC production and contain sulfur, are found in saliva and gingival crevicular fluid. Research shows that oral malodor may be associated with gram (−) anaerobic bacteria in the saliva and dorsum of the tongue [28, 29].

There is a close relationship between oral malodor and the amount of saliva. Factors that reduce the flow rate of saliva may cause halitosis.

In the mechanism of halitosis caused by non-oral causes, volatile sulfur compounds formed from mouth breathing, affecting the salivary glands, and therefore eliminating the washing effect of saliva play a role. Halitosis can also be seen in gastroesophageal reflux due to the change in the acidity of the oral environment [30]. In other systemic diseases, bad breath may occur due to changes in the oral microflora due to the medications' effects.

26.6 Etiology of Halitosis

We can examine halitosis by dividing it into oral and non-oral causes.

26.6.1 Oral Halitosis (Intraoral Halitosis, Oral Malodor)

Bad breath is related to the condition of the oral cavity. Delanghe et al. [31] reported that the cause of approximately 87% of halitosis was intraoral. 51% originate from the tongue, 17% from gingivitis, 15% from periodontitis, and 17% from a mixture [32]. Oral causes include periodontal diseases, implant diseases, caries, necrotic dental pulps, mucosal ulcers, faulty restorations, 20-year pericoronitis, lack of salivation, presence of food residues, aphthous sores, dental abscesses, herpetic infections, candidiasis, xerostomia, poor oral hygiene. Causes such as peritonsillar abscess, mouth breathing, all unpolished surfaces in the mouth, dorsal part of the tongue being covered with plaque (large surface area of the tongue, papillary structure, and irregular and deeply fissured surface) can be listed as reasons.

26.6.1.1 Periodontal Infections

Bacteria associated with gingivitis and periodontitis are mostly gram (−) bacteria, and these bacteria are responsible for VSC production. This explains why the VSC level in the mouth has a positive relationship with the periodontal pocket depth and why the amount of VSC increases as the number and depth of periodontal pockets increase [5, 33, 34]. Low oxygen pressure in the deep periodontal pockets causes the pH there to decrease and an anaerobic environment to form, activating the decarboxylation of amino acids (such as lysine ornithine) to cadaverine and putrescine, two malodor diamines. This explains that VSC and other molecules may be essential in bad breath in gingivitis or periodontitis infections [35].

VSC causes thinning of periodontal pockets and mucosal epithelium, thereby increasing the permeability of the epithelium, and the connective tissue beneath the epithelium is exposed to bacterial metabolites, thereby accelerating the process of periodontitis. Also, methyl mercaptan causes connective tissue destruction by increasing collagenase production, interleukin-1, and cathepsin B production [6]. Additionally, methyl mercaptan affects the cytoskeleton of gingival fibroblasts. Methyl mercaptan alters cell proliferation and migration. Based on these data, VSC plays a role in the pathogenesis of gingivitis and periodontitis.

Tooth decay in children occurs due to the interaction of dietary carbohydrates with bacteria in the mouth, especially Streptococcus Mutans, on the tooth surface. Organic acids produced by bacteria fermenting carbohydrates demineralize the tooth surface, causing tooth decay. This is a significant cause of bad breath in children. If left unchecked, the decay progresses to the tooth's inner layers, and the inflammation reaches the alveolar bone, resulting in dental abscesses. The most effective way to prevent caries is to use fluoride water at a rate of 1 ppm. In addition, reducing carbohydrate intake through food is an essential method in caries prevention. Children should start brushing their teeth from the age of three and should be brought for dental check-ups.

26.6.1.2 Tongue Oriented Halitosis

The dorsal surface of the tongue has an irregular structure due to fissures and mucosal papillae. This distinctive, rough structure creates a suitable environment for the growth of bacteria [35, 36]. While approximately 25 bacteria can adhere to a single cell in other parts of the mouth, about 100 bacteria can attach to a single epithelial cell in the dorsum of the tongue. The irregular dorsal surface structure of the tongue causes microorganisms in the tongue to escape the washing effect of saliva and multiply. This tongue dorsum structure also provides low oxygen levels, driving anaerobic to increase [13]. A coating is formed by accumulating food residues, epithelial residues, and bacteria on the tongue dorsum. This is called tongue coating. VSC occurs when this tongue coating cannot be removed due to the irregular anatomical structure, which creates bad breath. A high correlation has been reported between tongue coating and halitosis formation [18, 35, 36]. For this reason, the tongue dorsum is considered the primary source of bad breath [14, 33, 35, 37].

In people with periodontal disease, hydrogen sulfide (H_2S) and methyl mercaptan (CH_3SH) production is predominant in the tongue dorsum [5, 18, 37, 38]. In people with good oral hygiene and who do not have periodontal disease, the source of halitosis is usually the tongue dorsum [39].

26.6.1.3 Peritonsillar Abscess

Peritonsillar abscess is one of the most common causes of bad breath in the pediatric age group. It usually develops after suppurative infection of the tonsils. It occurs due to the condition in the tonsil spreading to the peritonsillar area by perforating the tonsillar capsule, often from the upper pole, and the infection may remain there or apply to neighboring areas along the constrictor muscle. It may be caused by acute tonsillitis, but studies show anaerobes mainly cause it. Peritonsillar abscess is usually unilateral. There is fever, odynophagia, dysphagia, trismus, and neck lymphadenopathy.

The patient speaks as if there was a hot potato in his mouth. The patient cannot swallow his saliva due to pain, so his mouth becomes watery, and his breath smells. In physical examination (FM), the tonsil is pushed downward and medially, and the uvula is displaced to the opposite side. In the treatment, first of all, abscess drainage is performed. The patient is hospitalized if possible, and parenteral antibiotic treatment is started.

Candidiasis, which occurs due to weakening of the immune system seen in patients with long-term antibiotic use or corticosteroid treatment, chemotherapy or radiotherapy, and diabetic patients, is also a cause of halitosis in the pediatric age group and is cured by the use of antifungal drugs. Children with leukemia who receive radiotherapy and chemotherapy are also more prone to tissue destruction, infection, and bleeding. In this case, since protein degradation provides a suitable environment for accumulation of anaerobic bacteria, the production of odor-forming VSCs increases, and this causes bad breath.

Oroantral fistula, abscessed teeth, dental caries, open ulcers, fistulas, and papillary losses can also cause halitosis by causing accumulation of food residues and desquamated tissues.

In cases affecting the oral mucosa, such as herpetic gingivostomatitis, Vincent's stomatitis, measles, diphtheria, and herpangina, it is one of the causes of bad breath by causing tissue destruction, changes in salivary flow, and putrification.

26.7 Paranasal Sinus Diseases

They have a share of 5% in the causes of halitosis in children. These diseases can cause bad breath (postnasal drip), causing inflammation and increased mucus secretion. Nasal obstruction may also lead to mouth breathing and disrupt oral hygiene [10].

Sinusitis is a suppurative infection of the paranasal sinuses and is often a complication of colds and allergic rhinitis. Besides this, sinusitis is high in patients with cyanotic heart disease, cystic fibrosis, immunoglobulin deficiency, immobile cilia syndrome, and dental infection. Maxillary ethmoid and sphenoid sinuses are present at birth. The frontal sinus develops in the first year of life. The frontal sinuses may only appear as airy spaces at age 10.

In its etiology, preventing mucociliary flow paves the way for bacterial proliferation. The causative agents are generally pneumococci, H. influenza, M. catarrhalis, anaerobic bacteria, and rarely Streptococci and Staphylococci. Sinusitis may develop as a result of Aspergillus or Zygomycete infections in immunocompromised patients and patients with neutropenia. The patient may experience mucopurulent rhinorrhea, cough, sniffling, nasal voice, facial swelling, tenderness, headache, and postnasal drip.

Diagnosis can be easily made with paranasal CT and direct films. Amoxicillin-clavulanic acid, trimethoprim, and Cefaclor are generally effective in treating acute sinusitis. Complications are treated by drainage and parenteral route.

26.8 Adenoid Vegetation

Adenoid vegetation is another cause of pediatric halitosis. Adenoids are masses of normal lymphoid tissue in the nasopharynx. It reaches its maximum size until the age 3–7, spontaneously regresses, and becomes smaller after puberty. Adenoid hypertrophy and frequent infections may obstruct the mouth of the Eustachian tube, thus causing frequent middle ear infections or sinus infections by blocking the posterior sinus ostia. Chronic sinusitis causes constant irritation and hypertrophy of the adenoid tissue due to chronic inflammation and post-nasal discharge.

In addition, allergic reactions also cause adenoid hypertrophy. It most commonly causes complaints of sleeping with the mouth open, snoring, hearing loss, and halitosis in children.

Adenoids are most often involved during throat infections affecting the lymphoid tissues in the tonsil and lateral pharyngeal wall. Viral factors such as rhinovirus, adenovirus, influenza, and bacterial factors such as Group A Beta-Hemolytic Streptococci (GABHS) play a role in developing the disease. Various studies have shown that microorganisms that play a role in tonsil infection also cause adenoiditis [12]. The treatment is adenoidectomy.

26.9 Chronic Pharyngitis

Factors that irritate are of great importance in the chronicity of pharyngitis. Predisposing factors include acidic foods, smoking, spicy foods, environmental pollution, mouth breathing due to nasal congestion, and an atopic constitution.

Patients may apply to the ENT clinic complaining of a foreign body feeling in their throat, a raspy cough, tingling, and bad breath. Treatment is symptomatic in the acute phase. If there is a granular appearance, treatment can be made with the Mandel solution. However, the most crucial thing in medicine is the removal of predisposing factors. Polyps causing nasal obstruction, septal perforation, and adenoid vegetation are other conditions that may cause halitosis in children.

Foreign bodies in the nose or oropharynx can cause infection and lousy odor secondary to inflammation. Many foreign objects may have accidentally gotten into the nose and remained neglected for a long time. This situation should not be ignored, especially in children.

26.10 Chronic Tonsillitis

Chronic tonsillitis is a chronic inflammation of the tonsils after recurrent acute or subclinical infections. During acute tonsillitis, if a small abscess focused within the follicles is not treated adequately, it will continue and cause the next tonsillitis attack. Again, inflammatory rashes within the crypts may cause subclinical infection and cause acute tonsillitis attacks. The causative agent is mostly gram (+) bacteria. Among these bacteria, GABHS are the organisms most commonly seen in chronic tonsillitis.

Although chronic tonsillitis is common between the ages of 6–15, it can be seen at any age.

As a result of recurrent acute or subclinical infections in chronic tonsillitis, deep crypts form in the tonsils. Saliva, food, and necrotic waste can fill these crypts. If natural mechanisms cannot clear these, magma accumulates in the form of tonsil stones. In this case, halitosis will occur along with chronic inflammation [11]. Patients may have complaints such as recurrent sore throat and systemic complaints such as fever, joint pain, malaise, bad breath, and bad taste in the mouth.

Diagnosis of chronic tonsillitis is made by history and examination. antistreptolysin O (ASO), C-reactive protein (CRP), and sedimentation examination are requested to investigate GABHS. The definitive treatment for tonsillitis is tonsillectomy if there is an indication. Otherwise, if a bacterial agent is suspected, antibiotic treatment is recommended.

26.11 Tonsillolith

Tonsillolith is the formation of stones within the tonsil tissue. Fibrosis develops due to recurrent inflammation where the crypts are opened. Bacteria and epithelial residues accumulate in these crypts. Calcification occurs by depositing organic salts such as calcium phosphate or magnesium carbonate. It may cause bad breath and ulcerations. Complaints of sore throat, foreign body sensation in the back of the throat and otalgia may occur. Tonsillectomy is indicated in cases with severe clinical complaints that do not resolve with symptomatic treatment. One of the causes of pediatric halitosis is xerostomia. Xerostomia is a clinical condition we call capitalism or dry mouth syndrome. Many reasons can be listed in its etiology, and we can summarize them as follows: Aplasia of the salivary gland is an infrequent condition.

Innervation disorders of the salivary glands and many drugs can affect this innervation: antidepressants, antihistamines, diuretics, ganglion blockers, and parasympatholytic agents. Recurrent parotitis, defects in the histological structure of the salivary glands, the scarcity or absence of acinar cells, and the irreversible changes caused by radiotherapy to the salivary glands in the gland parenchyma tissue may also result. Xerostomia can be seen in some metabolic diseases, diabetes mellitus (DM), dehydration, and chronic renal failure syndrome. In addition, in cases such as liver disorders and systemic lupus erythematosus (SLE). Tooth decay, halitosis, and periodontitis are common pathologies in children with xerostomia. Treatment of xerostomia is directed toward the cause. Saliva secretion can be increased by treating metabolic diseases, especially dehydration. If it is related to the medications used, medication use is terminated. The mouth and teeth are cleaned with an antiseptic mouthwash at least twice daily.

26.12 Non-Oral Halitosis

The prevalence of bad breath due to non-oral causes is 13%. 4% of these originate from ear-nose-throat, 3% from oral and ear-nose-throat, and 1% from the digestive system [12]. Zenker's diverticulum, helicobacter pylori, gastritis, gastroesophageal reflux, and malabsorption syndromes can be mentioned regarding the digestive system. In the study by Delanghe et al. [31], ear-nose-throat problems were stated as the reason for halitosis in only 5–8% of the patients. Non-oral causes are generally systemic diseases (DM, kidney failure increases the uric acid level, causing an ammonium-like odor in the breath) foods. Vegetarians have less halitosis than a person who eats a lot of meat. Because the degradation products of protein substances in vegetables are very low. Meat usually contains fat, and the volatile fatty acids formed are absorbed through the veins and excreted in the breath. Bad smell occurs when substances such as garlic, onion, leek, alcohol, etc., are first absorbed in the circulatory system and then released from the lungs as air. In addition, upper respiratory tract diseases, pathological or physiological disorders in the nose and sinuses, tonsils, pharynx and digestive organs, vitamin and mineral deficiency (vitamin A, vitamin B12, and iron or zinc deficiency), diabetic ketoacidosis, liver failure, renal failure, uremia, radiation therapy, some lung diseases, Von Willebrand disease, Helicobacter pylori (bad breath disappeared in around 60% of cases after treatment by increasing VSC), aplastic anemia, leukemia, bleeding diseases such as thrombocytopenia, diphtheria, measles, pneumonia, syphilis, eosinophilic granuloma and Lettere diseases such as Siwe, high fever, precipitation of drugs, hunger, and stress can be shown (as they cause dryness in the mouth) [40–43]. At the same time, psychological factors such as anxiety and depression and some personality traits such as stress are risk factors for subjective halitosis [44]. Some parasites and their larvae (Ascaris lymbricoides, Trichuris trichura) pass through the lungs and cause infection. Parasitosis increases the amount of gas in the intestine. In a study conducted in the USA, the parasitic infestation rate in children with halitosis was 19% [45]. In another study, halitosis disappeared in 64% of 28 children with parasitosis with mebendazole treatment [46]. Trimethylaminuria (fish odor syndrome), a genetic metabolic disorder, causes an excessive increase in trimethylamine levels in the blood and lousy odor in the body. Hypermethioninemia is another metabolic disorder that causes oral halitosis. Cystinosis is a rare autosomal recessive disease characterized by intralysosomal cystine accumulation, and these patients' methionine levels in the blood and urine are very high. In infants, sleepiness is manifested by symptoms of distinctive urine, sweat and breath odor, bleeding tendency, and hypoglycemia.

26.13 Gastroesophageal Reflux

Gastroesophageal reflux, one of the causes of bad breath in children, is a common condition in babies up to 1-year-old. Single or several factors may be responsible at the same time. Factors such as decreased lower esophageal sphincter pressure, insufficient relaxation of this sphincter, large hiatus hernia, and delayed gastric emptying play a role. Babies have regurgitation, vomiting, and irritability. In older children and teenagers, regurgitation causes retrosternal inflammation, dysphagia, or severe asthma. Barium radiography is performed for diagnosis, but the result is expected in 30% of children. The most accurate results are obtained from studies in which 24-h esophageal pH is measured.

Reflux stops spontaneously when babies reach 18 months. If it persists and causes esophagitis, H2 blockers, antacids, and sucralfate suspensions can be given. Surgical intervention is required in cases of recurrent pneumonia, severe esophagitis, severe apnea, and failure to respond to 4–6 weeks of drug therapy.

26.14 Diagnosis

The methods used to diagnose halitosis can be divided into two groups: direct and indirect.

Direct methods:
1. Organoleptic.
2. Sulfur monitoring.
3. Gas chromatography.

Indirect method:
1. Indirect methods are based on detecting the microorganisms that produce VSC or evaluating the products produced by these microorganisms in vitro. Indirect methods include bacterial culture, smear, and enzyme studies [2].

26.14.1 Organoleptic Measurement

Patients exhale through a 2.5 cm diameter tube placed in their mouth, approximately 10 cm away from the nose of the physician performing the measurement [47]. In addition, in this method, the patient licks his wrist, waits for the licked area to dry, and smells it. Before organoleptic evaluation, patients should avoid antibiotics for 3 weeks before the procedure. It is necessary to avoid smoking, alcohol consumption, onion, garlic, and spicy foods 12 h before the process, and oral care procedures and consumption of food and beverages 2 h before the system [48]. A plastic spoon is placed on the tongue's surface to evaluate whether the odor originates from the tongue. Scraping is done with the tester, and the evaluation is made at a distance of 5 cm from the nose of the person doing the test.

This test is evaluated as follows: 0 = no odor, 1 = hardly detectable odor, 2 = slight but detectable odor, 3 = medium odor, 4 = strong bad odor, and 5 = extreme bad odor [49]. Organoleptic evaluation is the reference in the diagnosis of halitosis [50]. Gas chromatography and portable sulfite monitors can evaluate bad breath more objectively. Oho et al. [51] found a significant correlation between the results obtained by organoleptic testing, gas chromatography, and sulfite monitoring. Gas chromatography is based on separating gases with different molecular weights and boiling points in an environment. It is a method based on measuring the concentration of VSCs in oral air. This method is quite expensive and requires experienced personnel [3, 34, 52, 53]. For this reason, it is used mainly for research purposes (Table 26.2).

26.14.2 Sulfur Monitoring

A portable monitor that can measure oral volatile sulfur compounds (VSC) evaluates VSC concentrations together but does not provide information on their types. VSC measurement in the mouth is done as follows: A pipette is placed in the patient's mouth and he is asked to breathe through the nose by keeping his mouth closed. As a result of the electrochemical reactions between the VCS compounds in the breath, an electric current is generated proportional to the amount of VCS. This value is expressed numerically as ppb (parts per billion) [17, 55].

In some studies, the relationship between the organoleptic method and sulfur measurements was evaluated, and while organoleptic evaluation gave high scores in patients, sulfur measurements were found to be normal in patients. This is because substances or compounds that cause bad breath other than VSC (volatile short-chain fatty acids, polyamines, alcohols, phenyl compounds, alkanes, ketones, and nitrogen compounds) cannot naturally be detected by the sulfur monitor [21, 56, 57]

26.14.2.1 Indirect Methods

A different strategy in determining bad breath is the detection of VSC-producing microorganisms or their enzymes. Proteolytic obligate gram-negative anaerobes found in the subgingival plaque and tongue dorsum can be detected by the BANA test. BANA is a synthetic trypsin substrate that can be hydrolyzed by VSC-producing oral anaerobic bacteria [2]. When this strip is treated with saliva, if there is a VSC-producing microorganism in the saliva, the BANA molecule on the strip turns into β-naphthylamide and appears in blue. The BANA test is a practical and easy-to-use method. Still, its disadvantage is that it cannot identify different types of bacteria that do not produce VSCs responsible for halitosis [21, 58, 59]. Some studies have shown that while there is a statistically significant relationship between BANA scores and organoleptic measurements, it has a weak relationship with sulfur monitoring measurements [2].

Table 26.2 14 volatile sulfur compounds identified (VSB) [54]

Acetone	2-Butanone
2-Pentanone	Indole
Skatole	Dimethyl selenide
1-propanol	Dimethyl sulfide
Dimethyl disulfide	Dimethyl trisulfide
Allyl methyl sulfide	Carbon disulfide
Hydrogen sulfide	Methyl mercaptan

Rodriguez-Fernandez et al. [60] developed a fluorimetric sensor for measuring VSC and suggested that this method could be an alternative to commercial systems such as Halimeter. It is shown that the VSC monitor with the zinc oxide semiconductor sensor they developed could be used to diagnose halitosis [45]. They made a comparison with organoleptic evaluation in patients with severe halitosis. They stated that this monitor could be used in routine clinical studies and oral-dental screenings, as they found a high correlation. Hanada et al. [61] developed a portable GC system using a high-sensitivity indium oxide semiconductor gas sensor as a detector. In their study, Amano et al. [62] found a statistically significant relationship when they measured the VSC level by gas chromatography and the ammonia level by ammonia monitoring in 25 patients.

26.14.2.2 Measurement of Galactosidase Activity

Deglycosylation of glycoproteins is considered the initial stage in forming lousy breath. β-Galactosidase is one of the essential enzymes in deglycosylation. In this method, which is based on measuring the activity of this enzyme, the color change caused by the saliva sample taken on a paper disk is scored as 0: No color change, 1: Light blue color, and 2: Dark blue color. Some studies have found a significant relationship between β-Galactosidase test scores and organoleptic scores [63, 64].

26.14.2.3 Ammonia Monitoring

Ammonia produced by bacteria in the mouth can cause bad breath. Therefore, a portable monitor was developed to measure ammonia. Patients are asked to rinse their mouths with urea solution and measurements are made with a disposable piece placed in the mouth and connected to the gas detector. The air in the patient's mouth is transferred to the detector with the help of a pump, and the ammonia concentration produced by the bacteria can be seen on a scale.

26.14.2.4 Polymerase Chain Reaction (PCR)

This method is used for quantitative analysis of VSCs produced by oral bacteria. In this method, the amount of bacterial DNA forming VSC is determined by the amount of fluorescent dye formed on the DNA probe [23, 65].

26.15 Physical Examination

After physiological halitosis and halitophobia are ruled out, physical examination begins. A meticulous oral and otolaryngological examination is performed. 90% of the cause of bad breath originates from inside the mouth, increasing oral examination's importance. It is essential in the subgingival and proximal regions. Causes such as periodontal pockets, rotten teeth, tonsils, adenoid examination, tongue structure, whether there is a cleft tongue, aphthous lesions in the mouth, ulcerations, gum diseases, tongue coating, or post-nasal discharge can be easily noticed.

In people with good oral hygiene and dental health and a healthy periodontium, although the front part of the back of the tongue usually smells good, the real cause of the odor may be the back part of the tongue, that is, the tongue root. This area can be examined by scraping with a tongue depressor. This material usually results from postnasal discharge. Although the discharge is not initially foul-smelling when it reaches the tongue, it may cause a foul odor as it accumulates in the future. A conclusion can be drawn by comparing the scraping taken with a tongue depressor and bad breath.

One way to understand that the smell is coming from the mouth is to compare the smell coming from the mouth with the smell coming from the nose. If the smell comes from the mouth, the place to be investigated is the mouth. The odor may intensify during sleep, under stress, when the mouth is dry due to long conversations and side effects of medications, and in such cases, gum can be chewed for a few minutes to increase saliva secretion and to see whether the odor decreases. If we think that the odor is caused by oral etiology, the patient is told to gargle for a week and pay attention to dental cleaning (brushing, flossing). If the odor disappears, it is understood that it is caused by oral etiology [45]. If the odor originates from the nasal passage, lungs, or stomach, it will not disappear with mouthwash and teeth cleaning.

Another way to understand bad breath is to stick out the tongue thoroughly, hold the tip of the tongue with gauze, and scrape the base with another gauze for 45 s, Wait, and then smell. If an unpleasant odor is detected after these waiting periods, there is a halitosis problem [45].

Some people's bad breath worsens when they start talking when it does not normally exist. Therefore, in addition to exhaling through the mouth and nose, the patient should be asked to count out loudly 20 and simultaneously smell.

It is also essential to detect a fissured tongue (scrotal tongue) during physical examination. Enzymes such as lysozyme, myeloperoxidase, and immunoglobulin are higher in fissured tongues than in non-fissured tongues. When the fissured tongue becomes ulcerated and the rust is removed, saliva leaks. Excessive bacterial growth causes inflammation and odor occurs [45].

26.16 Treatment of Halitosis

A treatment plan is made to eliminate the cause and improve oral health. Although there are many factors in the etiology of bad breath, it is primarily due to oral causes. Therefore, it is aimed to reduce the amount of intraoral bacteria and convert persistent VSCs into non-volatile substrates. The treatment methods are listed below:

1. **Using masking products**
   Masking products alone do not treat halitosis. These are mints, toothpaste, mouthwashes, sprays, lozenges, and gums [4].
2. **Mechanical reduction of microorganisms and their substrates**
   It is possible by consuming breakfast, increasing saliva secretion, chewing gum, brushing teeth, using dental floss, toothpicks, tongue cleaning, and professional oral care [4].

Bad breath, which is intense in the morning as a result of the proliferation of microorganisms found in food residues and releasing proteins as a result of not washing the tongue as a result of fasting throughout the night and food residues accumulating on the tongue and decreasing saliva secretion, will be eliminated by eating solid foods and bad breath will decrease [66]. In a study, a 60% decrease in the hydrogen sulfide concentration and an 83% decrease in the methyl mercaptan concentration, which causes bad breath, was observed in people with bad morning breath despite no oral cleaning performed 1 h after breakfast [52]. Even just eating dry bread has been shown to reduce VSC concentration without any other action [67].

3. **Brushing teeth**

   It reduces the amount of bacteria in the mouth [68, 69], but studies have shown that tooth brushing alone is ineffective in eliminating bad breath [70, 71].

4. **Tongue brushing**

   Brushing the tongue reduces the tongue coating and, therefore, the number of microorganisms and the amount of substrates on the tongue [37, 72, 73]. The tongue coating should be removed during tongue brushing, especially on the posterior part of the tongue. In one study, brushing the tongue dorsum with toothpaste was more effective than brushing your teeth.

The clinician must find the source of the odor before starting treatment. It often requires dental treatment. The most effective method in the treatment of halitosis is to reduce anaerobes that cause VSC production by correcting periodontal disease with oral hygiene and primary dental care. An effective mouthwash should be added if bad breath persists despite good oral hygiene. Mouthwashes eliminate lousy breath by chemically reducing the number of microorganisms in the mouth [74]. Active agents frequently used in these products are chlorhexidine, triclosan, essential oils, and cetylpyridinium chloride (CPC). Other effective chemical agents are allylpyrocatechol, L-trifluoromethionine, and dehydroascorbic acid [4].

Chlorhexidine, the most commonly used of these, damages the bacterial cell membrane, increasing membrane permeability and, as a result, causes cell lysis and cell death [75].

In their study, [49] reported that the 0.2% chlorhexidine regimen provided a 43% decrease in VCS values and a more than 50% decrease in organoleptic scores [49]. However, long-term use of chlorhexidine also has disadvantages, such as causing bad taste in the mouth and discoloration of teeth [75, 76].

Many essential oils used to eliminate bad breath have strong antimicrobial properties. Olshan et al. [77] reported in their clinical study that toothpaste containing essential oil and 1% zinc citrate and essential oil effectively reduced bad breath for 1.5–2 h. Cetylpyridinium Chloride (CPC), also used to eliminate bad breath, prevents bacterial growth [78]. Yaegaki and Sanada [70] reported in their study that mouthwash containing CPC was 80% effective in reducing VSC for 3.5 h. L-trifluoromethionine, which is also recommended in the treatment of halitosis, works by inhibiting the production of methyl mercaptan, which occurs as a result of bacteria metabolizing methionine and causes bad breath.

Toothpaste, mouthwashes, lozenges, and other products reduce halitosis by chemically neutralizing odor compounds, including VSC. Common active ingredients of these products are metal ions and oxidizing agents. Metals such as zinc, sodium, tin and magnesium are thought to interact with sulfur. Zinc, one of these products, has advantages such as being non-toxic, non-cumulative, and not causing coloration compared to other metal ions. For this reason, it is one of the most preferred substances for controlling bad breath [79].

Sodium bicarbonate is frequently used in teeth cleaning in Japan and North America. It was reported in the studies of Brunette et al. [80] that toothpastes containing sodium bicarbonate were effective in reducing VSC levels.

Oxidizing tablets are thought to reduce bad breath due to the activity of dehydroascorbic acid, which is formed by the peroxide-based oxidation of ascorbate.

On the other hand, probiotics are among the recommended treatment options. Probiotics strengthen the host's immune system by producing the antimicrobial substance necessary to destroy or inhibit pathogenic microorganisms [81].

In their study, Suzuki et al. reported that daily consumed acid-resistant probiotic lactobacilli would play an essential role in the regression of lousy breath and odor-related factors, along with ensuring oral care and hygiene [82].

If we consider a diagnosis of Halitophobia after all organic causes have been excluded, the patient should be referred to the relevant branch for evaluation by a psychiatrist.

References

1. Armstrong BL, Sensat ML, Stoltenberg JL. Halitosis: a review of current literature. J Dent Hyg. 2010;84(2):65–74.
2. van den Broek AM, Feenstra L, de Baat C. A review of the current literature on aetiology and measurement methods of halitosis. J Dent. 2007;35(8):627–35.
3. Tonzetich J. Production and origin of oral malodor: a review of mechanisms and methods of analysis. J Periodontol. 1977;48(1):13–20.
4. van den Broek AM, Feenstra L, de Baat C. A review of the current literature on management of halitosis. Oral Dis. 2008;14(1):30–9.
5. Yaegaki K, Sanada K. Volatile sulfur compounds in mouth air from clinically healthy subjects and patients with periodontal disease. J Periodontal Res. 1992;27(4 Pt 1):233–8.
6. Lancero H, Niu J, Johnson PW. Exposure of periodontal ligament cells to methyl mercaptan reduces intracellular pH and inhibits cell migration. J Dent Res. 1996;75(12):1994–2002.
7. Amir E, Shimonov R, Rosenberg M. Halitosis in children. J Pediatr. 1999;134(3):338–43.
8. Paryavi-Gholami F, Minah GE, Turng BF. Oral malodor in children and volatile sulfur compound-producing bacteria in saliva: preliminary microbiological investigation. Pediatr Dent. 1999;21(6):320–4.
9. Sanz M, Roldan S, Herrera D. Fundamentals of breath malodour. J Contemp Dent Pract. 2001;2(4):1–17.
10. Rosenberg M. Clinical assessment of bad breath: current concepts. J Am Dent Assoc. 1996;127(4):475–82.
11. Dal Rio AC, Nicola EM, Teixeira AR. Halitosis—an assessment protocol proposal. Braz J Otorhinolaryngol. 2007;73(6):835–42.
12. Cortelli JR, Barbosa MD, Westphal MA. Halitosis: a review of associated factors and therapeutic approach. Braz Oral Res. 2008;22(Suppl 1):44–54.

13. Miyazaki H, Sakao S, Katoh Y, Takehara T. Correlation between volatile sulphur compounds and certain oral health measurements in the general population. J Periodontol. 1995;66(8):679–84.
14. Liu XN, Shinada K, Chen XC, Zhang BX, Yaegaki K, Kawaguchi Y. Oral malodor-related parameters in the Chinese general population. J Clin Periodontol. 2006;33(1):31–6.
15. Al-Ansari JM, Boodai H, Al-Sumait N, Al-Khabbaz AK, AlShammari KF, Salako N. Factors associated with self-reported halitosis in Kuwaiti patients. J Dent. 2006;34(7):444–9.
16. Soder B, Johansson B, Soder PO. The relation between foetor ex ore, oral hygiene and periodontal disease. Swed Dent J. 2000;24(3):73–82.
17. Rosenberg M, Kulkarni GV, Bosy A, McCulloch CA. Reproducibility and sensitivity of oral malodor measurements with a portable sulphide monitor. J Dent Res. 1991;70(11):1436–40.
18. Iwakura M, Yasuno Y, Shimura M, Sakamoto S. Clinical characteristics of halitosis: differences in two patient groups with primary and secondary complaints of halitosis. J Dent Res. 1994;73(9):1568–74.
19. Yaegaki K, Coil JM. Examination, classification, and treatment of halitosis; clinical perspectives. J Can Dent Assoc. 2000;66(5):257–61.
20. Loesche WJ, Kazor C. Microbiology and treatment of halitosis. Periodontol. 2002;2000(28):256–79.
21. Goldberg S, Kozlovsky A, Gordon D, Gelernter I, Sintov A, Rosenberg M. Cadaverine as a putative component of oral malodor. J Dent Res. 1994;73(6):1168–72.
22. Amano A, Yoshida Y, Oho T, Koga T. Monitoring ammonia to assess halitosis. Oral Surg Oral Med Oral Pathol Oral Radiol Endod. 2002;94(6):692–6.
23. Kato H, Yoshida A, Awano S, Ansai T, Takehara T. Quantitative detection of volatile sulfur compound-producing microorganisms in oral specimens using real-time PCR. Oral Dis. 2005;11(Suppl 1):67–71.
24. Washio J, Sato T, Koseki T, Takahashi N. Hydrogen sulfide producing bacteria in tongue biofilm and their relationship with oral malodor. J Med Microbiol. 2005;54(Pt 9):889–95.
25. Kazor CE, Mitchell PM, Lee AM, Stokes LN, Loesche WJ, Dewhirst FE, ve diğerleri. Diversity of bacterial populations on the tongue dorsa of patients with halitosis and healthy patients. J Clin Microbiol. 2003;41(2):558–63.
26. Waler S. On the transformation of sulfur-containing amino acids and peptides to volatile sulfur compounds (VSC) in the human mouth. Eur J Oral Sci. 1997;105:534–7.
27. Kojima K. Clinical studies on the coated tongue. Jpn J Oral Maxillofac Surg. 1985;31:1659–76.
28. Loesche WJ. The effects of antimicrobial mouthrinses on oral malodor and their status relative to US Food and Drug Administration regulations. Quintessence Int. 1999;30:311–8.
29. Morita M, Wang HL. Association between oral malodor and adult periodontitis: a review. J Clin Periodontol. 2001;28:813–9.
30. Hoshi K, Yamano Y, Mitsunaga A, et al. Gastrointestinal diseases and halitosis: association of gastric Helicobacter pylori infection. Int Dent J. 2002;52(Suppl3):207–11.
31. Delanghe G, Ghyselen J, Bollen C, van Steenberghe D, Vandekerckhove BN, Feenstra L. An inventory of patients_response to treatment at a multidisciplinary breath odor clinic. Quintessence Int. 1999;30:307–10.
32. Aydın M. Ağız Kokusu TeÇhisi ve Tedavisi. Dentalife. 2005;14:26–9.
33. Coli JM, Tonzetich J. Characterization of volatile sulphur compounds production at individual gingival crevicular sites in humans. J Clin Dent. 1992;3(4):97–103.
34. Persson S. Hydrogen sulfide and methyl mercaptan in periodontal pockets. Oral Microbiol Immunol. 1992;7(6):378–9.
35. Bosy A, Kulkarni GV, Rosenberg M, McCulloch CA. Relationship of oral malodor to periodontitis: evidence of independence in discrete subpopulations. J Periodontol. 1994;65(1):37–46.
36. Yaegaki K, Sanada K. Biochemical and clinical factors influencing oral malodor in periodontal patients. J Periodontol. 1992;63(9):783–9.
37. De Boever EH, Loesche WJ. Assessing the contribution of anaerobic microflora of the tongue to oral malodor. J Am Dent Assoc. 1995;126(10):1384–93.
38. Quirynen M, Mongardini C, van Steenberghe D. The effect of a 1-stage full-mouth disinfection on oral malodor and microbial colonization of the tongue in periodontitis. A pilot study. J Periodontol. 1998;69(3):374–82.

39. Danser MM, Gomez SM, Van der Weijden GA. Tongue coating and tongue brushing: a literature review. Int J Dent Hyg. 2003;1(3):151–8.
40. Madhushankari GS, Yamunadevi A, Selvamani M, Mohan Kumar KP, Basandi PS. Halitosis—an overview: part-I—classification, etiology and pathophysiology of halitosis. J Pharm Bioallied Sci. 2015;7:339–43.
41. Scully C, Porter R, Greenman J. What to do about halitosis? Br Med J. 1994;308:217–8.
42. Young K, Oxtoby A, Field EA. Halitosis: a review. Dent Update. 1993;20:57–61.
43. Yilmaz AE, Bilici M, Tonbul A, Karabel M, Dogan G, Tas T. Paediatric halitosis and helicobacter pylori infection. J Coll Physicians Surg Pak. 2012;22:27–30.
44. Vali A, Roohafza H, Keshteli AH, Afghari P, Javad Shirani M, Afshar H, et al. Relationship between subjective halitosis and psychological factors. Int Dent J. 2015;65:120–6.
45. Güngör A, Cıncık H, Çekin E, Cunda H. Ağız kokusu, GATA Ayın Kitabı, GATA Basımevi; 2005;66.
46. Rocha EM, Carvalho CR, Saad MJ, Velloso LA. The influence of ageing on the insülin signalling system in rat lacrimal and salivary glands. Acta Ophthalmol Scand. 2003;81:639–45.
47. Oho T, Yoshida Y, Shimazaki Y, Yamashita Y, Koga T. Characteristics of patients complaining of halitosis and the usefulness of gas chromatography for diagnosing halitosis. Oral Surg Oral Med Oral Pathol Oral Radiol Endod. 2001;91(5):531–4.
48. Quirynen M, Steenberghe DV. Oral malodor. In: Newman M, Taeki H, Klokkevold P, Carranza F, editors. Carranza's clinical periodontology. 11th ed. Iowa: Elsevier; 2011.
49. Rosenberg M, Kulkarni GV, Bosy A, McCulloch CAG. Reproducibility and sensitivity of oral malodor measurements with a portable sulfide monitor. J Dent Res. 1991;11:1436–40.
50. Laleman I, Dadamio J, De Geest S, Dekeyser C, Quirynen M. Instrumental assessment of halitosis for the general dental practitioner. J Breath Res. 2014;8:017103.
51. Oho T, Yoshida Y, Shimazaki Y, Yamashita Y, Koga T. Characteristics of patients complaining of halitosis and the usefulness of gas chromatography for diagnosing halitosis. Oral Surg Oral Med Oral Pathol Oral Radiol Endod. 2001;91:531–4.
52. Tonzetich J, Ng SK. Reduction of malodor by oral cleansing procedures. Oral Surg Oral Med Oral Pathol. 1976;42(2):172–81.
53. Murata T, Yamaga T, Iida T, Miyazaki H, Yaegaki K. Classification and examination of halitosis. Int Dent J. 2002;52(Suppl 3):181–6.
54. Van den Velde S, Quirynen M, van Hee P, van Steenberghe D. Halitosis associated volatiles in breath of healthy subjects. J Chromatography B. 2007;853:54–61.
55. Kozlovsky A, Goldberg S, Natour I, Rogatky-Gat A, Gelernter I, Rosenberg M. Efficacy of a 2-phase oil: water mouthrinse in controlling oral malodor, gingivitis, and plaque. J Periodontol. 1996;67(6):577–82.
56. Greenstein RB, Goldberg S, Marku-Cohen S, Sterer N, Rosenberg M. Reduction of oral malodor by oxidizing lozenges. J Periodontol. 1997;68(12):1176–81.
57. Furne J, Majerus G, Lenton P, Springfield J, Levitt DG, Levitt MD. Comparison of volatile sulfur compound concentrations measured with a sulfide detector vs. gas chromatography. J Dent Res. 2002;81(2):140–3.
58. Kozlovsky A, Gordon D, Gelernter I, Loesche WJ, Rosenberg M. Correlation between the BANA test and oral malodor parameters. J Dent Res. 1994;73(5):1036–42.
59. Loesche WJ, Lopatin DE, Giordano J, Alcoforado G, Hujoel P. Comparison of the benzoyl-DL-arginine-naphthylamide (BANA) test, DNA probes, and immunological reagents for ability to detect anaerobic periodontal infections due to Porphyromonas gingivalis, Treponema denticola, and Bacteroides forsythus. J Clin Microbiol. 1992;30(2):427–33.
60. Rodriguez-Fernandez J, Costa JM, Pereiro R, Sanz-Medel A. Simple detector for oral malodour based on spectrofluorimetric measurements of hydrogen sulphide in mouth air. Anal Chim Acta. 1999;398:23–31.
61. Hanada M, Koda H, Onaga K, Tanaka K, Okabayashi T, Itoh T, et al. Portable oral malodor analyser using highly sensitive In2O3 gas sensor combined with a simple gas chromatography system. Anal Chim Acta. 2003;475:27–35.
62. Amano A, Yoshida Y, Oho T, Koga T. Monitoring ammonia to assess halitosis. Oral Surg Oral Med Oral Pathol Oral Radiol Endod. 2002;94:692–6.

63. Sterer N, Greenstein RB, Rosenberg M. Beta-galactosidase activity in saliva is associated with oral malodor. J Dent Res. 2002;81(3):182–5.
64. Sterer N, Rosenberg M. Effect of deglycosylation of salivary glycoproteins on oral malodour production. Int Dent J. 2002;52(Suppl 3):229–32.
65. Suzuki N, Yoshida A, Nakano Y. Quantitative analysis of multispecies oral biofilms by TaqMan real-time PCR. Clin Med Res. 2005;3(3):176–85.
66. Kleinberg I, Wolff MS, Codipilly DM. Role of saliva in oral dryness, oral feel and oral malodour. Int Dent J. 2002;52(Suppl 3):236–40.
67. Suarez FL, Furne JK, Springfield J, Levitt MD. Morning breath odor: influence of treatments on sulfur gases. J Dent Res. 2000;79(10):1773–7.
68. Coil JM, Yaegaki K, Matsuo T, Miyazaki H. Treatment needs (TN) and practical remedies for halitosis. Int Dent J. 2002;52(Suppl 3):187–91.
69. Tanaka M, Anguri H, Nishida N, Ojima M, Nagata H, Shizukuishi S. Reliability of clinical parameters for predicting the outcome of oral malodor treatment. J Dent Res. 2003;82(7):518–22.
70. Yaegaki K, Sanada K. Effects of a two-phase oil-water mouthwash on halitosis. Clin Prev Dent. 1992;14(1):5–9.
71. Kleinberg I, Codipilly DM. Cysteine challenge testing: a powerful tool for examining oral malodour processes and treatments in vivo. Int Dent J. 2002;52(Suppl 3):221–8.
72. Gilmore EL, Bhaskar SN. Effect of tongue brushing on bacteria and plaque formed in vitro. J Periodontol. 1972;43(7):418–22.
73. Ralph WJ. Oral hygiene--why neglect the tongue? Aust Dent J. 1988;33(3):224–5.
74. Brading MG, Marsh PD. The oral environment: the challenge for antimicrobials in oral care products. Int Dent J. 2003;53(6 Suppl 1):353–62.
75. Jones CG. Chlorhexidine: is it still the gold standard? Periodontol. 1997;15:55–62.
76. Young A, Jonski G, Rolla G. Inhibition of orally produced volatile sulfur compounds by zinc, chlorhexidine or cetylpyridinium chloride—effect of concentration. Eur J Oral Sci. 2003;111(5):400–4.
77. Olshan AM, Kohut BE, Vincent JW, Borden LC, Delgado N, Qaqish J, Sharma NC, McGuire JA. Clinical effectiveness of essential oil-containing dentifrices in controlling oral malodor. Am J Dent. 2000;13.(Spec No:18C–22C.
78. Xiong H, Li Y, Slavik MF, Walker JT. Spraying chicken skin with selected chemicals to reduce attached salmonella typhimurium. J Food Prot. 1998;61(3):272–5.
79. Young A, Jonski G, Rolla G, Waler SM. Effects of metal salts on the oral production of volatile sulfur-containing compounds (VSC). J Clin Periodontol. 2001;28(8):776–81.
80. Brunette DM. Effects of baking-soda-containing dentifrices on oral malodor. Compend Contin Educ Dent Suppl. 1996;17(19):S22–32.
81. Maden EA, Altun C. Probiyotikler ve Ağız Sağlığı. Atatürk Üniv Diş Hek Fak Derg. 2012;22:334–9.
82. Suzuki N, Yoneda M, Tanabe K, et al. Lactobacillus salivarius WB21-containing tablets for the treatment of oral malodor: a double-blind, randomized, placebo-controlled crossover trial. Oral Surg Oral Med Oral Pathol Oral Radiol. 2014;117:462–70.

Dysphonia in Children

27

İbrahim Çukurova and İlter Denizoğlu

27.1 Introduction

Communication in the childhood has a crucial role in personal and social development. Pediatric dysphonia creates serious communication problems and restrictions in social and emotional functioning with improper voice quality, pitch and loudness, and voice breaks [1, 2]. A dysphonic child will be negatively affected (aggressive, sad, frustrated) emotionally and perceived more negatively (angry and noisy) by peers and adults [1, 3, 4]. They also report frustration and limited participation in important events due to their vocal inabilities [1].

Diagnosis, treatment, and follow-up in pediatric dysphonia must be considered with continuously changing structural and developmental biomechanical factors. Laryngeal position, vocal tract length (vertically short), histoanatomical structure, and functions of the larynx change throughout childhood. The vocal fold length is only 2.5–3.0 mm in the newborn and it reaches adult dimensions (female 11–15 mm and male 17–21 mm around 10–14 years of age) [5]. Lamina propria in the newborns is loose and pliable and does not have a layered structure. Vocal ligament appears between 1 and 4 years and the three-layered lamina propria is not clear until 15 years of age [6].

İ. Çukurova (✉)
İzmir University of Health Sciences, Tepecik Training and Research Hospital, Section of Otorhinolaryngology, Izmir, Turkey

İ. Denizoğlu
Department of Speech Language Therapy, Tinaztepe University Faculty of Health Sciences, Izmir, Turkey

H. Yüksel et al. (eds.), *Pediatric Airway Diseases*, Comprehensive ENT,
https://doi.org/10.1007/978-3-031-74853-0_27

27.2 Epidemiology

It is not easy to estimate the real prevalence of pediatric dysphonia because the pediatric dysphonia remains undiagnosed mostly. However, studies show a range between 1.4% and 23.9% [7–11]. These values increase in school age children from 6% to 38% [1, 9, 12]. Boys are more affected than girls between 7 and 12 years of age, while dysphonia is more frequent in girls after puberty [13]. Benign vocal fold lesions tend to be the most common etiology in childhood [14, 15]. Vocal fold nodules have been reported to have an incidence of 17–30% in the pediatric population [16, 17].

27.3 Etiology and Pathogenesis

Various etiologies can be defined in pediatric dysphonia: traumatic, infectious, inflammatory, iatrogenic, congenital, metabolic, and psychogenic [18, 19]. The most common reason for pediatric admission to the voice clinic is children who shout a lot and develop irritative chronic laryngitis and prenodular edema or nodules due to vocal trauma. Risk factors include childhood hearing problems, frequent upper respiratory tract problems, and family dynamics. Differential diagnosis of lesions such as vergeture that accompany and cause nodules is also important in treatment strategy.

Vocal fold nodule is a mucosal reaction to mechanical trauma. The glottic gaps (hourglass-shape, posterior gaps, etc.) create higher mucosal impact pressure on smaller parts of the vocal fold mucosa. The child tries to express him/herself by increasing the phonatory effort, and this vicious circle results with mucosal inflammatory response that continues with epithelial thickening.

The mucosal trauma creates a chronic tissue reaction, which restrains low-loudness phonation. Since low-pressure glottic closure will not be possible due to the nodular masses in between, the perception that "our boy always talks shouting" settles in the family as if it were a way of behavior. These patients develop a new type of glottic closure and breathing to compensate for this condition. Less common reasons may be congenital anomalies, laryngopharyngeal reflux, chronic sinonasal infections or allergies, papillomatosis, polyps, webs, cysts, sulci, laryngeal tumors, and metabolic and hormonal disorders.

Puberphonia is a functional dysphonia that affects mainly boys during puberty. Its prevalence is reported as 2–3% [20]. Physioanatomical alterations at the phonatory apparatus are under the effect of abrupt hormonal changes [21], the mean fundamental frequency decreases (1 octave in males and 3–5 semitones in females), and reaches the adult levels [20]. Puberphonia is a register shift between chest and falsetto registers. The child cannot adapt to the physioanatomical changes and uses the falsetto register that resembles the prepubertal pitch. The vocal output becomes a high-pitched metallic sound in addition to vocal instability, poor voice control, pitch breaks, breathiness, effortful phonation, and monotonous speech [22].

27.4 Diagnosis

Diagnosis and management of pediatric dysphonia require multidimensional thinking and a strategic approach. Coinciding pathologies such as nasal obstruction, attention deficit, and hyperactivity disorder (ADHD) should be considered. Hyperactivity, various communication disorders, aggression, academic success problems, and personality problems must be consulted with child and adolescent psychiatrists. Children are generally less aware of the problem and are referred by their families. This condition may not create a need for a definitive treatment, but providing a better voice for communication can satisfy the family and the patient. Children may not be able to provide sufficient anamnesis. Family and school environments provide important clues about pediatric dysphonia. In this context, when taking anamnesis, family members as well as responsible teachers at the school can be contacted.

27.5 Signs and Symptoms

The family or teacher often notices voice problems in children. They are referred to the clinic primarily for shouting behaviors, changes in vocal timbre, limitation of vocal communication abilities, and discomfort in the neck and face during speech.

27.5.1 Clinical Assessment

Evaluation for dysphonia in children usually involves laryngoscopy to evaluate for vocal fold lesions and vocal fold mobility [23]. Videolaryngostroboscopic evaluation is not as easy as in adults, but it is still a golden standard in children. It can be applied quickly by rigid or flexible endoscopes, assessment through general anesthesia may be a choice in some cases.

Acoustic evaluation can be made by voice analysis and perceptual (patient and/or clinician-based) questionnaires. Improvements during and after treatment in self-reported quality of life scales [24–26] may indicate that patients feel less limited by their voices in their social environments. Although auditory-perceptual evaluation may not give objective results [27–29], the clinician's ears are the most delicate tool for dysphonia.

Acoustic and aerodynamic voice analysis may also help for diagnostic and follow-up measures [30–32]. Voice therapy was shown to reveal improvements in cycle-to-cycle variation in frequency and amplitude (jitter, shimmer) as well as decreased noise in the voice signal (harmonic-to-noise ratio) [33, 34]. The aerodynamic improvement can be analyzed by phonation threshold pressure [35, 36] that also indicates vocal fold biomechanical changes (increased laryngeal pliability and decreased vocal fold viscosity) following therapy [2]. Acoustic-aerodynamic analysis may also give clues about the changes at vocal fold mass [24] but they never substitute endoscopic visualization.

27.6 Treatment

Treatment of pediatric dysphonia should be managed in a dynamic approach [25]. Although pediatric dysphonia may be expected to disappear after puberty [37], they may lead to severe communicative, psychosocial, and organic problems if neglected. So, verifying and explaining the situation to the child and family is necessary. Laryngopharyngeal reflux, sinonasal infections and allergies, ADHD, and other pathologies must also be considered.

Although nodules are known to respond to voice therapy well, Rosen 2012 treatment strategies may change according to duration and severity of symptoms. Needs of the individual child, especially if the communication problem affects social, academic, and personal well-being, define treatment process. Phonomicrosurgery may be the choice of treatment in recalcitrant nodules [38]. Pediatric vocal fold nodules generally resolve spontaneously at puberty [39]. On the other hand, if patients with puberphonia are not treated, they may continue with similar voice problems to adulthood.

27.6.1 Voice Therapy

Voice therapy in childhood is not the same with adults because it is not easy to communicate with children in a therapeutic sense. The motivational interview is the most crucial step in the treatment of pediatric dysphonia in the beginning. This increases awareness and adherence to therapy. Counseling should explain how to breathe quietly and give a comfortable, calm, easy-to-extract sound. The practice and exercises must be regarded as a play instead of homework. Anna Freud's words "play is the business for the child" shed light on the clinicians to add curiosity and play into therapy exercises. Anything can be transferred into a play; the clinician must be flexible and provide a playground within the therapy process.

Children prefer to be active and determined through the therapy process. It is not easy to make them passively obey the rules and do the homework exercises. So, it is better to make them feel independent, actively participate, and use their creativity; otherwise, a constructive relationship a friendship cannot be constituted. Every success must be celebrated together. The clinician must not be in a dictating, punishing state, which decreases motivation and therapy adherence.

Awareness of the child and family about vocal hygiene should be increased. Collaboration with the school and teacher is essential. Excessive crying, yelling in the play (football), cough, and throat clearing habits (attention should be paid to differential diagnoses such as laryngopharyngeal reflux, allergy, sinusitis, etc.) can be explained with examples. While exemplifying a child with a complex glottic attack and vocal abuse, it can be said to clap with his hands, for example, to explain that the same situation will also happen to the vocal folds by showing the redness and discomfort of their hands when the intensity of the applause increases gradually. Somatization of therapy exercises as much as possible will also help by using devices (e.g., tube phonation) associated with the play and the toy [40].

Empathy and being a playmate are critical skills for clinicians who are interested in pediatric dysphonia. Indirect conversations with puppets (finger puppets are a practical solution) can be made to make puppets give vocal hygiene suggestions. By using prosody, the child can feel the sense of music in the sound. For this, the stressed phonemes in a sentence can be represented by lines by doing the exercise of "drawing the sound" [41]. Various interactive cartoon programs, pictures, and toys prepared for pediatric voice therapies can be used.

The family must be included in therapy. Eliminating the environments where the child will shout and preventing the family from talking too loudly in the home environment affects the child. It is a fact that telling the child not to shout is a suggestion that cannot be realized. Shouting is a normal behavior, especially during the play with his/her peers. The child must either learn to shout correctly or find something that can be put in place to identify him/herself. For example, he can blow a whistle hanging on his neck when angry and shouting. However, it is necessary to arrange proper place and time; otherwise blowing a whistle in an unlikely place (e.g., in a school canteen) will not be acceptable.

Duration and number of sessions of voice therapy are another issues in pediatric dysphonia treatment. Pediatric voice therapy addressing benign vocal fold lesions and laryngeal edema was reported to require an average of 7.54 sessions [30]. Duration and time between sessions are adjusted according to child's compliance.

In puberphonia, patients can shift quickly to chest register from falsetto. The voice may improve in a few sessions, but the change at the vocal personality must be considered well. The therapy does not end when chest register is obtained; but when the patient can use the chest register properly in speech and singing activities [22].

27.7 Phonosurgery

The developing physioanatomy of the vocal fold structure makes surgical interventions more challenging to decide in the pediatric group. The dimensions of the surgical site are extremely smaller than adult larynx. The developing layers of the vocal fold mucosa are also critical. Because of the high risk of scar formation and trauma to the anterior and posterior macula flavas, microsurgical principles including technique and instruments must be considered carefully. Treatment of cysts and mature polyps usually requires surgery, but the surgical decision can be made according to impairments of the dysphonia on social and personal communication skills. The decision for surgery may be postponed for a while, provided that the patient is closely monitored.

Results should be interpreted cautiously due to the heterogeneity of the studies, techniques, and surgeries used. However, a systematic review and meta-analysis did find that pediatric patients with vocal fold nodules may see a reduction in dysphonia following surgery [17].

It should be noted that surgery, no matter how well it is performed, will not change the phonation patterns in motor memory. Before, and more importantly after surgery, it is essential to add voice therapy to the treatment. Patients and their relatives should be informed that surgery is only a part of the treatment and should be made aware of the importance of voice therapy. It is clear that the best treatment results will be obtained when surgery and therapy are combined to promote safe and economic voice use and prevent future injury [42].

References

1. Connor NP, Cohen SB, Theis SM, et al. Attitudes of children with dysphonia. J Voice. 2008;22(2):197–209.
2. Hoffman MR, Scholp AJ, Hedberg CD, Lamb JR, Braden MN, McMurray JS, Jiang JJ. Measurement reliability of phonation threshold pressure in pediatric subjects. Laryngoscope. 2019;129(7):1520–6. https://doi.org/10.1002/lary.27418.
3. Lass NJ, Ruscello DM, Bradshaw KH, Blankenship BL. Adolescents' perceptions of normal and voice disordered children. J Commun Disord. 1991;24(4):267–74. https://doi.org/10.1016/0021-9924(91)90002-Z.
4. Ma EP-M, Yu CH-Y. Listeners' attitudes toward children with voice problems. J Speech Lang Hear Res. 2013;56(5):1409–15. https://doi.org/10.1044/1092-4388(2013/11-0242).
5. Hirano M, Kurita S, Nakashima T. Growth development and aging of vocal folds. In: Bless DM, Abbs JH, editors. Vocal fold physiology: contemporary research and clinical issues. San Diego, CA: College-Hill Press; 1981. p. 22–43.
6. Prakash M, Johnny JC. What's special in a child's larynx? J Pharm Bioallied Sci. 2015;7(Suppl 1):S55–8. https://doi.org/10.4103/0975-7406.155797.
7. Baynes RA. An incidence study of chronic hoarseness among children. J Speech Hear Disord. 1966;31(2):172–6. https://doi.org/10.1044/jshd.3102.172.
8. Bhattacharyya N. The prevalence of pediatric voice and swallowing problems in the United States. Laryngoscope. 2015;125(3):746–50. https://doi.org/10.1002/lary.24931.
9. Carding PN, Roulstone S, Northstone K, ALSPAC study team. The prevalence of childhood dysphonia: a cross-sectional study. J Voice. 2006;20:623–30.
10. Johnson CM, Anderson DC, Brigger MT. Pediatric dysphonia: a cross-sectional survey of subspecialty and primary care clinics. J Voice. 2020;34(2):301.e1–5. https://doi.org/10.1016/j.jvoice.2018.08.01711.
11. Powell M, Filter MD, Williams B. A longitudinal study of the prevalence of voice disorders in children from a rural school division. J Commun Disord. 1989;22(5):375–82. https://doi.org/10.1016/0021-9924(89)90012-9.
12. Wilson DK. Voice problems in children. 3rd ed. Philadelphia, PA: Williams and Wilkins; 1987.
13. Garcia Martins RH, do Amaral HA, Tavares EL, et al. Voice disorders: etiology and diagnosis. J Voice. 2015;26(1):1–5.
14. Kılıç MA, Okur E, Yildirim I, Güzelsoy S. The prevalence of vocal fold nodules in school age children. Int J Pediatr Otorhinolaryngol. 2004;68(4):409–12. https://doi.org/10.1016/j.ijporl.2003.11.005.
15. Gramuglia ACJ, Tavares ELM, Rodrigues SA, Martins RHG. Perceptual and acoustic parameters of vocal nodules in children. Int J Pediatr Otorhinolaryngol. 2014;78(2):312–6. https://doi.org/10.1016/j.ijporl.2013.11.032.
16. Hseu A, Ongkasuwan J. Beyond nodules-diagnostic and treatment options in pediatric voice disorders. Otolaryngol Clin. 2019;52(5):949–56. https://doi.org/10.1016/j.otc.2019.06.006.
17. Ongkasuwan J, Friedman EM. Is voice therapy effective in the management of vocal fold nodules in children? Laryngoscope. 2013;123(12):2930–1. https://doi.org/10.1002/lary.23830.

18. Martins RH, Hidalgo Ribeiro CB, Fernandes de Mello BM, Branco A, Mendes Tavares EL. Dysphonia in children. J Voice. 2012;26:e17–20.
19. Cohen SR, Geller KA, Thompson JW, Birns JW. Voice change in the pediatric patient. A differential diagnosis. Ann Otol Rhinol Laryngol. 1983;92:437443.
20. Hammarberg B. Pitch and quality characteristics of mutational voice disorders before and after therapy. Folia Phoniat. 1987;39:204–16.
21. Hacki T, Heitmuller S. Development of the child's voice: premutation, mutation. IntJ Pediatr Otorhinolaryngol. 1999;5:141–4.
22. Denizoglu İ, Şahin M, Bayrak S, Uygun MN. Efficacy of doctorvox voice therapy technique for mutational falsetto. J Voice. 2019;33(6):950.e1–8. https://doi.org/10.1016/j.jvoice.2018.05.012.
23. Stachler RJ, Francis DO, Schwartz SR, et al. Clinical practice guideline: hoarseness (dysphonia) (update). Otolaryngol Neck Surg. 2018;158(Suppl1):S1–S42. https://doi.org/10.1177/0194599817751030.
24. Hartnick C, Ballif C, De Guzman V, Sataloff RT, Campisi P, Kerschner J, Shembel A, Reda D, Shi H, Sheryka Zacny E, Bunting G. Indirect vs direct voice therapy for children with vocal nodules: a randomized clinical trial. JAMA Otolaryngol Head Neck Surg. 2018;144(2):156–63. https://doi.org/10.1001/jamaoto.2017.2618.
25. Connelly A, Clement WA, Kubba H. Management of dysphonia in children. J Laryngol Otol. 2009;123(6):642–7.
26. So YK. Efficacy of voice therapy for children with vocal nodules. J Clin Otolaryngol Head Neck Surg. 2018;29(2):229–34. https://doi.org/10.35420/jcohns.2018.
27. Eadie T, Sroka A, Wright DR, Merati A. Does knowledge of medical diagnosis bias auditory-perceptual judgments of dysphonia? J Voice. 2011;25(4):420–9. https://doi.org/10.1016/j.jvoice.2009.12.009.
28. Eadie TL, Kapsner-Smith M. The effect of listener experience and anchors on judgments of dysphonia. J Speech Lang Hear Res. 2011;54(2):430–47. https://doi.org/10.1044/1092-4388(2010/09-0205).
29. Kreiman J, Gerratt BR. Sources of listener disagreement in voice quality assessment. J Acoust Soc Am. 2000;108(4):1867–76. https://doi.org/10.1121/1.1289362.
30. Fujiki RB, Thibeault SL. Pediatric voice therapy: how many sessions to discharge? Am J Speech Hear Res. 2022;31:2663–74. https://doi.org/10.1044/2022_AJSLP-22-00111.
31. Tezcaner CZ, Ozgursoy SK, Sati I, Dursun G. Changes after voice therapy in objective and subjective voice measurements of pediatric patients with vocal nodules. Eur Arch Otorrinolaringol. 2009;266(12):1923–7. https://doi.org/10.1007/s00405-009-1008-6.
32. Senkal OA, Ciyiltepe M. Effects of voice therapy in school-age children. J Voice. 2013;27(6):787–e19. https://doi.org/10.1016/j.jvoice.2013.06.007.
33. Glaze LE, Bless DM, Milenkovic P, Susser RD. Acoustic characteristics of children's voice. J Voice. 1988;2(4):312–9. https://doi.org/10.1016/S0892-1997(88)80023-7.
34. Jotz GP, Cervantes O, Abrahão M, Settanni FAP, de Angelis EC. Noise-to-harmonics ratio as an acoustic measure of voice disorders in boys. J Voice. 2002;16(1):28–31. https://doi.org/10.1016/S0892-1997(02)00068-1.
35. Braden M, Thibeault SL. Outcomes of voice therapy in children with benign vocal fold lesions. Int J Pediatr Otorhinolaryngol. 2020;136:110121. https://doi.org/10.1016/j.ijporl.2020.110121.
36. Fisher K, Swank P. Estimating phonation threshold pressure. J Speech Lang Hear Res. 1997;40(5):1122–9. https://doi.org/10.1044/jslhr.4005.1122.
37. Hakansson BA, Kitzing P. Do hoarse children get voice problems in adulthood? Acta Otolaryngol (Stockholm). 1984;412:4345.
38. Wu SS, Onakasuwan J, Anne S, Appachi S. Voice outcomes following surgical treatment for pediatric vocal fold nodules: a systematic review and meta-analysis. Int J Pediatr Otorhinolaryngol. 2023;166:111461. https://doi.org/10.1016/j.ijporl.2023.111461.

39. Song BH, Merchant M, Schloegel L. Voice outcomes of adults diagnosed with pediatric vocal fold nodules and impact of speech therapy. Otolaryngol Head Neck Surg. 2017;157(5):824–9. https://doi.org/10.1177/0194599817726285.
40. Denizoğlu. Textbook of clinical vocology (in Turkish) 2020. Ankara: Karaca Publishing; 2020.
41. Ross-Kugler L. Voice drawing. In: Behrman A, Haskell J, editors. Exercises for voice therapy. Plural Publishing; 2008. p. 121–2.
42. Murry T, Woodson G. A comparison of three methods for the management of vocal fold nodules. J Voice. 1992;6(3):271–6. https://doi.org/10.1016/S0892-1997(05)80153-5.

Dysphagia in Children

28

Dogan Barut, Grazia Fenu, and Funda Cetin

28.1 Introduction

Dysphagia, a condition characterized by difficulty in swallowing, comprises a range of challenges that impede safe, efficient, and sufficient food transport to the stomach [1, 2].

While the name "dysphagia" adequately characterizes the problem in adults, it fails to encompass the full complexity of the condition when it occurs in the pediatric population. The act of swallowing, considered one of the fundamental physiological processes in humans, initiates during the early stages of gestation and undergoes further development and variations following birth [3]. Given that swallowing is a dynamic and ongoing process, pediatric dysphagia (PD) exhibits diverse, intricate symptoms and indications similar to those observed in adults [1–3].

D. Barut
Division of Gastroenterology, Hepatology and Nutrition Disease, Department of Pediatrics, Medical School of Ege University, Izmir, Turkey

G. Fenu
Pulmonology Unit, Meyer Children Hospital, IRCCS, Florence, Italy
e-mail: grazia.fenu@meyer.it

F. Cetin (✉)
Division of Gastroenterology, Hepatology and Nutrition Disease, Department of Pediatrics, Medical School of Ege University, Izmir, Turkey

H. Yüksel et al. (eds.), *Pediatric Airway Diseases*, Comprehensive ENT, https://doi.org/10.1007/978-3-031-74853-0_28

28.2 Epidemiologic Characteristics

The reported prevalence of PD varies significantly, with estimates ranging from 0.9% to 80% [4]. This variation might be attributed to differences in the definition of dysphagia, the specific population under study, and the methodologies employed in the research [4, 5]. Feeding and swallowing dysfunction are diagnosed more frequently in children with preterm, neuromuscular abnormalities, cardiac diseases, anatomic malformations of the upper aerodigestive tract, and gastrointestinal tract issues [6, 7]. Children's swallowing difficulties must be managed with an early diagnosis and multidisciplinary team intervention [3].

28.3 Swallowing Physiologic Phases

The preparation phase, the oral phase, the pharyngeal phase, and the esophageal phase are the four traditional phases of a typical swallow. During the preliminary stage, the ingestion of food occurs in the oral cavity, where it is moistened with saliva, chewed, and shaped into a bolus using the oral tongue and hard palate. At around 6 months of age, this period begins to develop. Sucking from a nipple constitutes the preliminary stage before 6 months. Thc oral phase involves the oral tongue propelling the food bolus into the oropharynx and inducing the swallow reflex. The elevation of the soft palate prevents food's regurgitation into the nasopharynx.

The food bolus travels through the oropharynx and hypopharynx toward the esophagus using synchronized muscle contractions during the pharyngeal phase. The tongue and pharyngeal muscles propel the bolus into the pharynx. As the velum approaches the pharyngeal muscles, the larynx rises, and the vocal folds adduct [3, 8]. During the pharyngeal phase, breathing stops; when eating, breathing becomes faster and more erratic than during tidal breathing [9]. In the esophageal phase, the cricopharyngeus relaxes to allow the food bolus to enter the esophagus, and then the bolus is passed into the stomach by synchronized smooth muscle peristalsis [3–10]. Beginning in pregnancy, as early as gestational week 10 or 11, the suck and swallow develop. Most children typically begin to develop oral feeding proficiency and tolerance between weeks 34 and 38 of pregnancy. Involuntary reflexes in babies control all four phases. The preliminary and oral stages are controlled voluntarily in children and adults, but the pharyngeal and esophageal phases are still involuntary [6].

Dysphagia can be further classified into other categories based on the affected swallowing phase. Signs indicative of oral dysphagia include uncoordinated biting and chewing, underdeveloped or absent sucking, and inadequate manipulation of the food bolus. Laryngeal penetration, aspiration, food ingress into the airway below the vocal folds, asphyxiation, airway obstruction due to food, pharyngeal reflux, and nasopharyngeal reflux are all indicative manifestations of pharyngeal dysphagia. Esophageal dysphagia is caused by either a blockage in the esophagus that prevents food from passing through or poorly coordinated esophageal muscle contractions [2].

28.3.1 The Etiology of Dysphagia

The etiology of dysphagia can be a single medical problem, but it is typically complex and brought on by a combination of diseases and comorbidities. Table 28.1 lists some typical causes of swallowing difficulties. To choose the best solution, it is essential to establish the etiology of dysphagia.

28.3.1.1 Prematurity

Infants' dysphagia is frequently brought on by prematurity. The prevalence of feeding issues was shown to be 10.5% in premature children born at fewer than 37 weeks gestation and to increase to 24.5% in infants born with a very low birth weight of less than 1500 g, according to a significant population-based cohort study [11]. Delays in developing head control, tongue movement, palate function, gag reflex, and laryngeal feeling can cause poor swallowing. Dysphagia is more distinct and complex because of the common comorbidity of pulmonary and central nervous system disorders in premature newborns. The formation of a normal swallow can be further complicated and delayed by anomalies of the aerodigestive system, such as laryngomalacia, or iatrogenic damage brought on by respiratory assistance, such as prolonged intubation or tracheostomy [12].

28.3.1.2 Neuromuscular

The intricate coordination of sensory and motor activities required for a secure swallow is disrupted by neuromuscular diseases—dysphagia results from delayed reflexes, hypotonia, and generalized incoordination. The degree of the central nervous system injury and whether it is static or progressive affect the presentation and clinical course of the dysphagia [7]. Several medical diseases can have a significant impact on swallowing. These include cerebral palsy, congenital viral infections, Arnold-Chiari malformation, microcephaly, hydrocephalus, intraventricular hemorrhage, periventricular leukomalacia, traumatic brain injury, muscle dystrophies, seizure disorders, and malignancies. Cerebral palsy is the neurologic disorder most commonly associated with dysphagia in pediatric populations [3, 13].

28.3.1.3 Abnormalities of the Aerodigestive Tract's Anatomy

Anatomical anomalies of the upper aerodigestive tract might disrupt the intricate coordination needed for a good swallow. Common causes are listed in Table 28.1 by anatomical subsite and frequently change based on the patient's age [6, 7].

28.3.1.4 Disorders of the Gastrointestinal Tract

In healthy infants, gastroesophageal reflux, the flow of stomach contents back into the esophagus with or without regurgitation or vomiting, is a normal physiological process. The condition is referred to as gastroesophageal reflux disease (GERD) when accompanied by symptoms or consequences and is regarded as pathologic. A newborn with GERD typically exhibits signs of irritability, inability to thrive, unwillingness to eat, posturing, cough, stridor, and hoarseness. The youngster may experience epigastric pain, dysphagia, odynophagia, tooth erosion, and chest pain

Table 28.1 Disorders that predispose children to swallowing difficulties and dysphagia

Prematurity
• Low gestational age at birth
• Low birth weight
Respiratory and cardiac disorders
• Respiratory distress syndrome
• Bronchopulmonary dysplasia (chronic pulmonary disease)
• Laryngo–/tracheo–/bronchomalacia
• Cyanotic and acyanotic heart defects
Gastrointestinal disorders
• Tracheoesophageal fistula and esophageal atresia
• Congenital diaphragmatic hernia
• Gastroesophageal reflux disease (GERD) and achalasia
• Eosinophilic esophagitis
• Food allergies and intolerances
Neurological disorders
• Microcephaly
• Hydrocephalus
• Intraventricular hemorrhage
• Periventricular leukomalacia
• Birth asphyxia and cerebral palsy
Congenital abnormalities
• Tongue tie
• Cleft lip/palate
• Moebius syndrome
• Down syndrome
Iatrogenic complications
• Tube feeding
• Tracheostomy
• Certain medications (especially those that affect arousal, muscle tone)
Ingestional (caustic) injuries
• Cleaning agents, battery

as they get older. In older kids, frequent vomiting and regurgitation are not thought to be physiological. By lessening the upper aerodigestive tract's mucosal feeling, GERD can cause oropharyngeal dysphagia [13].

Eosinophilic esophagitis is an additional inflammatory disorder of the gastrointestinal tract that can impact the swallowing process in pediatric patients. Eosinophilic esophagitis (EoE) is a pathological condition characterized by immune system involvement associated with food allergies, genetic susceptibility, and several environmental variables. Children often appear with failure to thrive, vomiting during meals, dysphagia to both liquids and solids, retrosternal discomfort, and food impaction. During an esophagogastroduodenoscopy and biopsy, eosinophilic esophagitis is identified. Endoscopy frequently reveals esophageal edema and inflammation along with a lack of vascularity. Linear furrows, concentric rings (also known as trachealization), and white flecks on the mucosa can all be found inside the esophagus. The diagnosis made after a biopsy sample and more than 15 intraepithelial eosinophils per high-power field indicate eosinophilic esophagitis [14].

A rare cause of dysphagia in young children is cricopharyngeal achalasia. The symptoms of cricopharyngeal achalasia include coughing, choking, gagging, and nasal regurgitation. It leads to pharyngeal phase dysphagia. Due to a higher risk of laryngeal penetration, patients with cricopharyngeal achalasia may find it more difficult to swallow liquids. A tonically constricted upper esophageal sphincter that occasionally relaxes is a pathophysiologic feature of cricopharyngeal achalasia. A modified barium swallow study that identifies a typical bar in the cricopharyngeus region is frequently used to determine the disease. Esophageal manometry demonstrates that the cricopharyngeal muscles cannot relax [15].

28.3.1.5 Cardiopulmonary Disease

Premature and term infants with complex medical conditions, such as congenital heart disease and bronchopulmonary dysplasia, are at risk for swallowing dysfunction. Based on available reports, it has been shown that newborns who undergo heart repair surgery have a higher likelihood of experiencing dysphagia, with prevalence rates ranging from 22% to 50%. Dysphagia associated with cardiac defects and cardiac surgery can arise from various factors, including abnormal thoracic anatomy, iatrogenic injury such as damage to the recurrent laryngeal nerve, the need for prolonged intubation, ventilation or respiratory support, as well as the influence of anesthetics and narcotics [16].

28.4 Symptoms

Depending on the underlying etiology of the dysphagia, different children present with varying symptoms of swallowing difficulty. A caregiver should seek evaluation for feeding problems if a child exhibits symptoms like prolonged feeding times, little interest in feeding, or food refusal; postural changes like back arches and neck extensions; failure to thrive; nasal regurgitation; coughing; choking; wet respirations during and after feeding; and increased work of breathing. It is possible to have laryngeal penetration and aspiration without the typical eating symptoms [17].

The occurrence of laryngeal penetration and aspiration may manifest even in the absence of typical feeding signs. The term "silent aspiration" refers to the occurrence of aspiration without the presence of coughing or deliberate efforts to remove the food bolus from the airway. The stimulation of the laryngeal cough reflex is absent. Silent aspiration is believed to be associated with reduced laryngopharyngeal sensation, neurological weakness or lack of coordination in the pharyngeal musculature, or a weak cough. It is recommended that children who experience recurrent respiratory tract infections in the absence of any apparent indicators of swallowing difficulty should be subjected to an evaluation for dysphagia [18]. A comprehensive history and physical examination by a doctor are the first steps in evaluating a child for swallowing difficulties. Children with feeding difficulties are

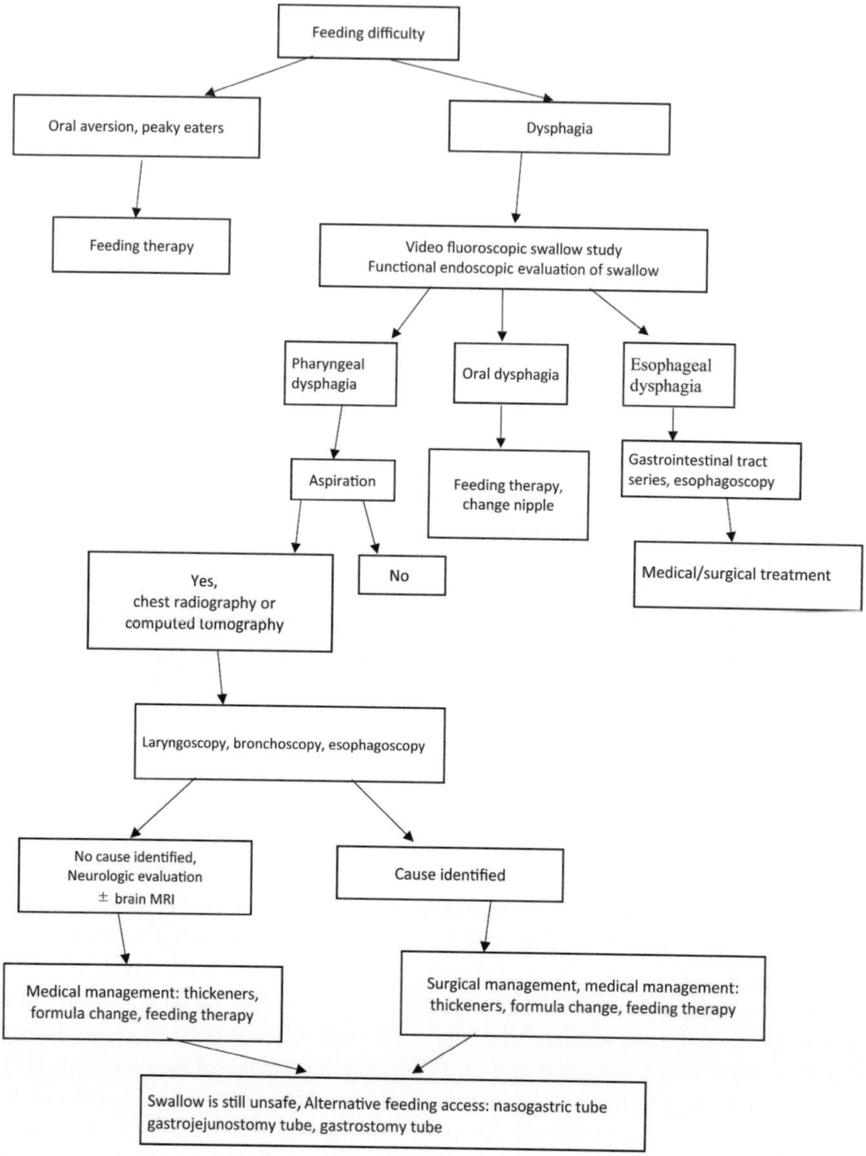

Fig. 28.1 Algorithm for evaluation and management of pediatric dysphagia

not uniformly evaluated. Although they exist for certain disease groups, no validated dysphagia screening tests exist for children. Figure 28.1 displays a strategy for diagnosing and treating pediatric dysphagia. The objectives of the subsequent tests include identifying a secure method of nutritional intake and the cause of the dysphagia [7].

28.5 Clinical Feeding Assessment

A speech-language pathologist (SLP) will frequently utilize a bedside swallow examination as one of their initial methods of assessing a child who may have dysphagia. The patient is given a food bolus in this clinical test, and the clinician watches the patient swallow. Only water is injected in some tests, while samples of various consistencies could be tested in others. A progressive volume challenge or a series of sips might introduce the water. The SLP can frequently identify whether the dysfunction occurs during the preparation phase, oral phase, pharyngeal phase, or a mixture of these phases. The SLP can determine the child's participation ability and the safety of continuing with more swallowing assessments. The bedside swallow is an adequate aspiration screening technique. However, it cannot pick up on silent aspiration [19].

28.6 Fluoroscopic Swallow Study in Video

The most popular test to assess patients with dysphagia is the videofluoroscopic swallow study, often known as the modified barium swallow study. The patient consumes food boluses ranging in viscosity from thin liquids to solids with infused radiographic dye. When swallowing varied consistencies, fluoroscopy checks for any penetration or aspiration into the airway. To examine all four phases of swallowing, the child is placed as close to their natural feeding position as is physically possible. This is done using a lateral radiography image. This procedure is the only method that can definitively prove penetration and aspiration. This examination cannot determine safe swallowing when nursing. The patient is exposed to radiation during the videofluoroscopic swallow study, and the time spent getting the test increases the exposure to the youngster [8].

28.7 Flexible Endoscopic Swallowing Evaluation

Though some SLPs undertake this examination alone, an otolaryngologist and an SLP typically perform a flexible endoscopic evaluation of swallowing. Examining the nasopharynx, oropharynx, hypopharynx, supraglottis, and glottis requires a flexible nasopharyngoscope. This test gives the examiners a detailed analysis of the patient's upper aerodigestive tract anatomy. Then, food boluses are provided, and it is possible to see them enter the airway as they are swallowed. The ability to analyze a nursing infant and the lack of radiation exposure are two advantages of this evaluation. Complete swallows can be evaluated more than once without putting the patient at greater risk. The inability to see the oral phase of swallowing, "white out" during swallowing, where tissues contract and may obstruct that examination, the failure to detect microaspiration, and the subjective nature of the evaluation are some limitations of flexible endoscopic evaluation of swallowing [7].

28.8 Imaging

The upper gastrointestinal tract series involves a radiographic examination of the esophagus, stomach, and duodenum while a food bolus impregnated with barium is swallowed. This examination can assess the structural anatomy and the esophageal swallowing phase. Chest radiography may be a crucial component of the workup in children with concerns about recurrent aspiration or pneumonia. Chest radiography could show signs of aspiration pneumonia or persistent lung disease. When choanal atresia, micrognathia, and vascular anomalies are detected, computed tomography or magnetic resonance imaging of the head, neck, and chest may also be recommended to assess suspected aberrant anatomy and further preoperative planning. Additionally, the effects of chronic aspiration, such as bronchiectasis, can be shown on chest computed tomography images.

28.9 Endoscopic Assessments

The comprehensive evaluation of a patient with pharyngeal or esophageal dysphagia and suspected penetration and aspiration must include direct laryngoscopy, bronchoscopy, and esophagoscopy.

Endoscopies might not be necessary if oral dysphagia is isolated. The otolaryngology, pulmonology, and gastrointestinal teams can frequently coordinate the evaluations with the same surgical procedure. By employing the direct laryngoscopy technique, the specialist in the field of otolaryngology can assess the presence of structural irregularities within several regions of the upper airway, including the oral cavity, oropharynx, glottis, and subglottis. It is feasible to diagnose airway anomalies, including vallecular cysts, laryngomalacia, vocal fold immobility, and laryngotracheoesophageal aperture [20, 21].

Diagnoses for tracheomalacia, tracheal stenosis, and tracheoesophageal fistula can be made with a tracheoscopy. The bronchoscopy can check for bronchomalacia, bronchiectasis, signs of persistent aspiration, and pneumonitis. The endoscopy can be supplemented with further testing like biopsies, bronchial washing, pepsin, and lipid-laden macrophage indices. An examination of the esophagus and, occasionally, distal tissues like the stomach and duodenum is possible during an esophagoscopy. It is possible to see mucosal alterations and extrinsic compression. To check for eosinophilic esophagitis and GERD consequences, biopsies may be done. A multichannel intraluminal impedance probe may be inserted to prevent acid and nonacid reflux [22].

28.9.1 High-Resolution Manometry

Esophageal dysphagia is a common complaint about referral for investigations of esophageal motility after the exclusion of obstructive lesions by endoscopy and histology. High-resolution manometry (HRM) with esophageal pressure topography analysis is now the method for evaluating esophageal contractility [23]. In addition, the dysfunction of bolus movement can lead to dysphagia, so evaluating bolus transit is of great importance for a better understanding of esophageal dysphagia [24, 25].

HRM uses a solid-state catheter assembly with closely spaced pressure sensors (typically 1-cm spacing intervals) positioned to traverse the entire length of the esophagus. Software interpolating this pressure data to esophageal pressure topography (EPT) allows visualization of esophageal motor function along a space-time-pressure continuum. In addition, the development of esophageal pressure topography (EPT) metrics aimed to provide a quantitative assessment of many aspects of esophageal motor function. These metrics include the measurement of deglutitive lower-esophageal sphincter (LES) relaxation using the integrated relaxation pressure (IRP) and the evaluation of peristaltic vigor using the distal contractile integral (DCI) [26, 27]. These EPT metrics and recognition of pressurization patterns on EPT facilitated the development of a hierarchical classification scheme of esophageal motility disorders: the Chicago Classification [28]. The Chicago classification provides a standard terminology for describing esophageal motility disorders and is used worldwide.

28.10 Medical Management

The care of a multidisciplinary team with expertise in pediatric swallowing difficulties is beneficial for children with dysphagia. Pediatricians, developmental pediatricians, neurologists, otolaryngologists, pulmonologists, and gastroenterologists could make up this team. When no other abnormalities are discovered during a thorough examination, including endoscopies, children with dysphagia should receive special consideration from a neurologic specialist. Accurately identifying the underlying etiology is crucial for effectively managing dysphagia [3, 12, 29].

Feeding therapy, performed by an experienced SLP, is often the first-line treatment for infants and children with dysphagia. To improve the suck-swallow-breathe sequence, this therapy may involve adjusting the method of food delivery, such as the nipple flow or spoon, feeding position, or feeding pace. The strength, mobility, and coordination of the lips, tongue, jaw, soft palate, and pharyngeal muscles are enhanced by sensory and motor exercises administered by a certified speech-language pathologist. Only if it is determined that the child is safe to try oral intake may feeding treatment be tried [3, 29].

A study may also test other formulations to see if the patient tolerates them better. The nutritional value of feeds may be improved by increasing their caloric content if a child can consume some oral meals. It might be essential to consult a pediatric dietitian to maintain proper nutritional intake. If modifying the formula doesn't work, the food bolus' consistency may need to be thickened. Thickened feeds might lessen or treat GERD, aspiration, and laryngeal penetration. By decreasing bolus transit and enhancing bolus cohesiveness during a swallow, thickeners have also been proven to alter swallowing mechanics and improve feeding pacing [29, 30].

Based on GERD clinical symptoms, reflux regimens, such as proton pump inhibitors and histamine H2 receptor antagonists, are frequently given. Numerous dysphagia symptoms resemble GERD symptoms, leading to the misuse of pharmaceutical treatment. In 1–2 years, many infants with aspiration will improve with time and prudent management [31, 32].

28.11 Surgical Management

The surgical treatment of dysphagia in pediatric patients is recommended when a structural anomaly is determined to be the underlying cause of the swallowing difficulty.

28.11.1 Ankyloglossia

Ankyloglossia, commonly referred to as tongue-tie, is a subject that has garnered significant attention and generated considerable debate within the field of feeding research. Frenotomy refers to the surgical procedure involving the division of the lingual frenulum and improves feeding in many patients with ankyloglossia and restricted tongue range of motion. The surgery is often associated with a low level of risk, with rare occurrences of problems such as bleeding, infection, harm to the salivary ducts, and the potential necessity for correction. Nevertheless, there is an increasing apprehension regarding the potential overdiagnosis and overtreatment of ankyloglossia. A constricted lingual frenulum is frequently recognized as contributing to breastfeeding challenges. However, it is essential to acknowledge that the underlying issue is typically more complex, involving various factors such as the positioning of the jaw, the characteristics of the maternal nipple, and the coordination of oral movements [33].

28.11.2 Laryngomalacia

Laryngomalacia is a medical condition characterized by the abnormal softening of the tissues. The presence of swallowing difficulty in individuals with laryngomalacia is believed to be caused by multiple factors. The prevalence of dysphagia in individuals diagnosed with laryngomalacia has been documented to range from 50% to 86%, regardless of any additional medical comorbidities. The disability could be associated with reduced sensory perception and neuromuscular control of the pharynx and larynx inherent to laryngomalacia. The physically restricted larynx imposes a more significant workload on breathing during feeding, disrupting the typical sequence of suck-swallow-breathe. Supraglottoplasty is a microlaryngeal procedure that divides the aryepiglottic folds and removes redundant supra-arytenoid tissue using cold steel, laser, or microdebride [34, 35].

28.11.3 Laryngeal Cleft

The laryngeal cleft is another area of significant study and controversy in the otolaryngology literature. The condition known as laryngeal cleft can be classified into four distinct degrees based on the extent of the interarytenoid cleft. Type 1 involves an extension of the cleft up to the level of the vocal folds, while type 2 extends beyond the vocal folds and into the cricoid cartilage. Type 3 is characterized by an extension of the aperture into the cervical trachea, and type 4 involves an extension into the thoracic trachea. The prevailing consensus in the field acknowledges that cleft types 2–4 are classified as anatomical anomalies and necessitate surgical intervention for healing. The laryngeal cleft is diagnosed on direct laryngoscopy with palpation of the interarytenoid groove [36].

28.12 Conclusions

Dysphagia is a disease that is becoming more prevalent among pediatric patients, mainly due to advancements in healthcare that have led to increased survival rates among premature and medically complicated children. Dysphagia can arise from diverse causes, frequently exhibiting a multifactorial nature. Utilizing a multidisciplinary team for evaluation purposes can enhance the precision of diagnoses and provide valuable guidance for effective management strategies.

References

1. Gosa MM, Carden HT, Jacks CC, Threadgill AY, Sidlovsky TC. Evidence to support treatment options for children with swallowing and feeding disorders: a systematic review. J Pediatr Rehabil Med. 2017;10:107–36.
2. Dodrill P, Gosa MM. Pediatric dysphagia: physiology, assessment, and management. Ann Nutr Metab. 2015;66:24–31.
3. Kakodkar K, Schroeder JW Jr. Pediatric dysphagia. Pediatr Clin N Am. 2013;60:969–77.
4. Bhattacharyya N. The prevalence of pediatric voice and swallowing problems in the United States. Laryngoscope. 2015;125:746–50.
5. Benfer KA, Weir KA, Bell KL, Ware RS, Davies PS, Boyd RN. Oropharyngeal dysphagia in preschool children with cerebral palsy: oral phase impairments. Res Dev Disabil. 2014;35:3469–81.
6. Raol N, Schrepfer T, Hartnick C. Aspiration and dysphagia in the neonatal patient. Clin Perinatol. 2018;45(4):645–60. https://doi.org/10.1016/j.clp.2018.07.005.
7. Durvasula VSPB, O'Neill AC, Richter GT. Oropharyngeal dysphagia in children: mechanism, source, and management. Otolaryngol Clin North Am. 2014;47(5):691–720. https://doi.org/10.1016/j.otc.2014.06.004.
8. Delaney AL, Arvedson JC. Development of swallowing and feeding: prenatal through the first year of life. Dev Disabil Res Rev. 2008;14(2):105–17. https://doi.org/10.1002/ddrr.16.
9. McFarland DH, Lund JP. Modification of mastication and respiration during swallowing in the adult human. J Neurophysiol. 1995;74(4):1509–17. https://doi.org/10.1152/jn.1995.74.4.1509.
10. Miller CK, Willging JP. Advances in the evaluation and management of pediatric dysphagia. Curr Opin Otolaryngol Head Neck Surg. 2003;11(6):442–6. https://doi.org/10.1097/00020840-200312000-00006.

11. Motion S, Northstone K, Emond A, et al. Persistent early feeding difficulties and subsequent growth and developmental outcomes. Ambul Child Health. 2001;7(3/4):231–7. https://doi.org/10.1046/j.1467-0658.2001.00139.x.
12. Durvasula VSPB, Lawson BR, Bower CM, Richter GT. Supraglottoplasty outcomes in neurologically affected and syndromic children. JAMA Otolaryngol Head Neck Surg. 2014;140(8):704–11. https://doi.org/10.1001/jamaoto.2014.983.
13. Rosen R, Vandenplas Y, Singendonk M, et al. Pediatric gastroesophageal reflux clinical practice guidelines: joint recommendations of the North American Society for Pediatric Gastroenterology, Hepatology, and Nutrition and the European Society for Pediatric Gastroenterology, Hepatology, and Nutrition. J Pediatr Gastroenterol Nutr. 2018;66(3):516–54. https://doi.org/10.1097/MPG.0000000000001889.
14. Noel RJ, Putnam PE, Rothenberg ME. Eosinophilic esophagitis. N Engl J Med. 2004;351(9):940–1. https://doi.org/10.1056/NEJM200408263510924.
15. Mohan S, Bowe SN, Hirner LM, Zar-Kessler C, Hartnick CJ. Modified approach for pediatric external cricopharyngeal myotomy. Int J Pediatr Otorhinolaryngol. 2018;105:111–4. https://doi.org/10.1016/j.ijporl.2017.12.019.
16. Malkar MB, Jadcherla S. Neuromotor mechanisms of pharyngoesophageal motility in dysphagic infants with congenital heart disease. Pediatr Res. 2014;76(2):190–6. https://doi.org/10.1038/1-pr.2014.68.
17. Duncan DR, Mitchell PD, Larson K, Rosen RL. Presenting signs and symptoms do not predict aspiration risk in children. J Pediatr. 2018;201:141–6. https://doi.org/10.1016/j.jpeds.2018.05.030.
18. Velayutham P, Irace AL, Kawai K, et al. Silent aspiration: who is at risk? Laryngoscope. 2018;128(8):1952–7. https://doi.org/10.1002/lary.27070.
19. Brodsky MB, Suiter DM, González-Fernández M, et al. Screening accuracy for aspiration using bedside water swallow tests: a systematic review and meta-analysis. Chest. 2016;150(1):148–63. https://doi.org/10.1016/j.chest.2016.03.059.
20. Irace AL, Dombrowski ND, Kawai K, et al. Aspiration in children with unilateral vocal fold paralysis. Laryngoscope. 2019;129(3):569–73. https://doi.org/10.1002/lary.27410.
21. Irace AL, Dombrowski ND, Kawai K, et al. Evaluation of aspiration in infants with laryngomalacia and recurrent respiratory and feeding difficulties. JAMA Otolaryngol Head Neck Surg. 2019;145(2):146–51. https://doi.org/10.1001/jamaoto.2018.3642.
22. Kieran SM, Katz E, Rosen R, Khatwa U, Martin T, Rahbar R. The lipid-laden macrophage index as a marker of aspiration in patients with type I and II laryngeal clefts. Int J Pediatr Otorhinolaryngol. 2010;74(7):743–6. https://doi.org/10.1016/j.ijporl.2010.03.028.
23. Fox MR, Bredenoord AJ. Oesophageal high-resolution manometry: moving from research into clinical practice. Gut. 2008;57:405–23.
24. Srinivasan R, Vela MF, Katz PO, et al. Esophageal function testing using multichannel intraluminal impedance. Am J Physiol Gastrointest Liver Physiol. 2001;280:G457–62.
25. Fass J, Silny J, Braun J, et al. Measuring esophageal motility with a new intraluminal impedance device. First clinical results in reflux patients. Scand J Gastroenterol. 1994;29:693–702.
26. Ghosh SK, Pandolfino JE, Zhang Q, et al. Quantifying esophageal peristalsis with high-resolution manometry: a study of asymptomatic volunteers. Am J Physiol Gastrointest Liver Physiol. 2006;290(5):G988–97. [PubMed: 16410365]
27. Ghosh SK, Pandolfino JE, Rice J, et al. Impaired deglutitive EGJ relaxation in clinical esophageal manometry: a quantitative analysis of 400 patients and 75 controls. Am J Physiol Gastrointest Liver Physiol. 2007;293(4):G878–85. [PubMed: 1769012]
28. Pandolfino JE, Ghosh SK, Rice J, et al. Classifying esophageal motility by pressure topography characteristics: a study of 400 patients and 75 controls. Am J Gastroenterol. 2008;103(1):27–37. [PubMed: 17900331]
29. Borowitz KC, Borowitz SM. Feeding problems in infants and children: assessment and etiology. Pediatr Clin N Am. 2018;65(1):59–72. https://doi.org/10.1016/j.pcl.2017.08.021.
30. Duncan DR, Larson K, Rosen RL. Clinical aspects of thickeners for pediatric gastroesophageal reflux and oropharyngeal dysphagia. Curr Gastroenterol Rep. 2019;21(7):30. https://doi.org/10.1007/s11894-019-0697-2.

31. Duncan DR, Amirault J, Johnston N, Mitchell P, Larson K, Rosen RL. Gastroesophageal reflux burden, even in children that aspirate, does not increase pediatric hospitalization. J Pediatr Gastroenterol Nutr. 2016;63(2):210–7. https://doi.org/10.1097/MPG.0000000000001092.
32. Casazza GC, Graham ME, Asfour F, O'Gorman M, Skirko J, Meier JD. Aspiration in the otherwise healthy infant—is there a natural course for improvement? [published online March 5, 2019]. Laryngoscope. 2019;130:514–20. https://doi.org/10.1002/lary.27888.
33. Walsh J, McKenna Benoit M. Ankyloglossia and other oral ties. Otolaryngol Clin N Am. 2019;52(5):795–811. https://doi.org/10.1016/j.otc.2019.06.008.
34. Simons JP, Greenberg LL, Mehta DK, Fabio A, Maguire RC, Mandell DL. Laryngomalacia and swallowing function in children. Laryngoscope. 2016;126(2):478–84. https://doi.org/10.1002/lary.25440.
35. Scott BL, Lam D, MacArthur C. Laryngomalacia and swallow dysfunction. [published online May 23, 2019]. Ear Nose Throat J. 2019;98(10):613–6. https://doi.org/10.1177/0145561319847459.
36. Johnston DR, Watters K, Ferrari LR, Rahbar R. Laryngeal cleft: evaluation and management. Int J Pediatr Otorhinolaryngol. 2014;78(6):905–11. https://doi.org/10.1016/j.ijporl.2014.03.015.

Cervical Lymphadenopathy in Children 29

Mehmet Kantar and Eda Ataseven

29.1 Introduction

Cervical lymphadenopathy is one of the most common complaints for hospital referral in children. In many cases, children have benign cervical lymph node enlargements as an immune response to viral or bacterial infections, or vaccines. Less common reasons are pathological conditions such as suppurative lymphadenitis, granulomatous lymphadenitis, malignancies, Langerhans cell histiocytosis, Rosai-Dorfman disease, and Castleman's disease that require further investigation. Besides acute suppurative lymphadenitis, children may undergo surgical excision to determine possible pathology. In a systematic review of pediatric cervical lymphadenopathy, nonspecific benign etiology is present in 67.8% while Epstein-Barr virus in 8.86%, malignancy 4.69%, and granulomatous disease 4.06% [1].

In this section, frequent causes of lymphadenopathy in children are summarized.

29.2 Reactive Lymph Node Enlargements

Lymph nodes are immune surveillance points of the immune system. Afferent lymphatics bring antigen-loaded dendritic cells to the lymph node, and they present their antigens to T cells in the paracortical areas of the lymph node. Then, T cells begin to differentiate and proliferate. T cells stimulate B cells, and then they become plasma cells to secrete antibodies. Later, CD4+ and CD8+ effector cells and antibody reach the inflammation-infection site via effect lymphatics and blood circulation.

M. Kantar (✉) · E. Ataseven
Division of Pediatric Hematology-Oncology, Department of Pediatrics, Ege University School of Medicine, Izmir, Turkey
e-mail: mehmet.kantar@ege.edu.tr

H. Yüksel et al. (eds.), *Pediatric Airway Diseases*, Comprehensive ENT, https://doi.org/10.1007/978-3-031-74853-0_29

This lymphoproliferation (functional hyperplasia) and stromal growth result in lymph node enlargement (1–3 cm). After inflammation and infection resolve, cell count returns to normal, but stromal shrinkage takes weeks. Therefore, reactive enlarged lymph nodes regress and disappear slowly. These lymph nodes are palpated as soft, nontender, and elastic in consistency. Antibiotic use in this situation is unnecessary because this is a normal immune reaction.

29.3 Vaccines

Immune cells in the lymph nodes proliferate when exposed to the vaccine antigens. Cervical as well as axillary lymphadenopathy are reported after measles, influenza, BCG, HPV, meningococci, and Covid-19 vaccines [2, 3]. Recently in Covid-19 vaccination, lymphadenopathy seems to be a reaction common to most vaccines rather than specifically to those of COVID-19. Hence, the mechanism in which lymphadenopathy occurs may be similar in all vaccine types [2].

29.4 Acute Suppurative Lymphadenitis

Suppurative lymphadenitis, secondary to a bacterial infection, is the major cause of cervical lymphadenopathy in the pediatric population. Acute bacterial lymphadenitis predominantly affects healthy preschool-aged children and infants [4]. Acute inflammatory reactions are typically the outcome of pyogenic microorganisms involving lymph nodes [5]. Most cases of acute bacterial lymphadenitis are due to Staphylococcus aureus or Streptococcus pyogenes. However, group B streptococcal lymphadenitis may present in infants. Anaerobic bacteria can occur, especially, in older children with periodontal diseases.

The diagnosis of acute bacterial lymphadenitis depends on the physical examination and the patient's medical history. Patients typically present with a history of fever, sore throat, or cough, and physical findings of pharyngitis, tonsillitis, and acute otitis media. The timing of onset will be days to a week, with fever and an enlarging neck swelling. On physical examination, lymph nodes may be firm and tender with overlying erythema, and the neck range of motion may be limited [6].

Fluctuance develops in 25% of patients with acute bacterial lymphadenitis as a sign of abscess formation. When differentiating between viral and bacterial lymphadenitis, it is essential to remember that viral lymphadenitis self-resolves. If the patient does not begin to show resolution of infection within 4–7 days, the clinician should become concerned about either primary bacterial lymphadenitis or viral lymphadenitis infected with bacteria.

The treatment for acute bacterial cervical lymphadenitis starts with appropriate antibiotics. Patients can be given oral medications such as amoxicillin/clavulanate, cephalosporins, clindamycin, or macrolides that cover the most frequent infections. In order to begin parenteral antibiotic therapy, patients with severe symptoms may need to be admitted to the hospital. The usual regimen begins with clindamycin or ampicillin/sulbactam [7]. If large fluctuant or persistent cervical lymphadenitis does not respond to antibiotic treatment within 2–3 days, the clinician should consider the possibility of abscess formation. Ultrasonography is useful for detecting abscess formation. If the lymphadenitis is highly suspicious for abscess formation and is present in an anatomical area requiring more detailed information, a computed tomographic (CT) scan or magnetic resonance image (MRI) will give more detailed information.

An abscess smaller than 1 cm may not require surgical drainage. Clinicians may consider a trial of 24–48 h of intravenous antibiotics before incision and drainage for abscesses less than 1.5–2 cm if the child is clinically stable. If the location of the abscess is anatomically tricky, or if the abscess is small but persistent, image-guided needle aspiration with or without drain placement may be appropriate. Cultures should be taken to help direct the antibiotic regimen.

29.5 Infectious Mononucleosis Due to EBV

Infectious mononucleosis due to EBV infection is frequent in the pediatric age group. Main symptoms are fever (98.3%), tonsillitis (100%), tonsillar white exudate (83.6%), cervical lymphadenopathy (98.3%), hepatomegaly (37.7%), splenomegaly (42.6%), eyelid edema (41.0%), and nasal obstruction (49.2%) [8]. Among the laboratory findings, leukocytosis with lymphocytosis and monocytosis are common as well as elevations in the levels of alanine aminotransferase, aspartate aminotransferase, and lactic dehydrogenase in the blood.

29.6 Granulomatous Lymphadenitis

The granulomatous lymphadenitis is a group of disorders that are rarely seen in children. Among them, the caseating granulomatous lymphadenitis is the result of mycobacterial infections [1]. The noncaseating granulomatous lesions are seen in cat-scratch disease, toxoplasmosis, toxocariasis, brucellosis, Kikuchi-Fujimoto disease, Kimura disease, and sarcoidosis.

29.6.1 Mycobacterial Infection

Mycobacterial infections, mainly due to Mycobacterium tuberculosis and Mycobacterium avium are the major causes of cervical granulomatous lymphadenopathy in children [9, 10]. These lymph nodes grow chronically with a purplish overlying skin color, and firm to palpation. Abscess and fistula formations are expected in clinical courses.

29.6.2 BCG Vaccine

BCG vaccine can cause lymphadenitis in 4–5 cases of 100,000 vaccine administrations [11]. The location is usually the axillary area, but supraclavicular and cervical lymph nodes can also be affected.

29.6.3 Cat-Scratch Disease

Cat-scratch disease (CSD) is characterized by regional lymphadenitis with fever caused by Bartonella henselae, a gram-negative bacillus. Cat-scratch disease follows the inoculation of Bartonella henselae through broken skin or mucous membranes and is usually transmitted by the scratch or bite of a cat [12]. A skin papule typically develops at the site of inoculation, followed by regional adenopathy 5 days to 2 months later. The cervical, axillary, or supraclavicular lymphadenopathy locations are the most frequently affected. The involved lymph nodes are initially mobile, elastic, and tender, with a typical size from 1 to 5 cm. In about 10–15% of the cases, the adenopathy evolves in a suppurative phase, lasting for months [13]. In most cases, the diagnosis is clinical and supported by a history of exposure to a cat. Serological tests can be used to confirm the diagnosis.

Cat-scratch disease is usually self-limited. In most cases, nodal enlargement resolves spontaneously after 1–3 months. In some patients, the lymph nodes may be painful and have a protracted course with the formation of abscesses and fistulas. Several studies have highlighted the need for antibiotic therapy or multiple drainages in these cases [14]. The first line of antibiotic treatment is azithromycin; however, clarithromycin, ciprofloxacin, or trimethoprim/sulfamethoxazole may be considered.

29.6.4 Sarcoidosis

Among all the causes of lymphadenopathy, sarcoidosis is reported in 0.37% as an underlying disease [1]. In pediatric sarcoidosis, there are two clinical forms reported. Children younger than 5 years of age have a triad of rash, uveitis, and arthritis. But older children have a multisystem disease that involves LAP, pulmonary involvement with fever, fatigue, and weight loss. In a pediatric series of sarcoidosis with 48 cases, peripheral lymphadenopathy is reported at 40% and hilar LAP at 71% [15]. In another large series of pediatric sarcoidosis, the percentage of peripheral LAP is 30%, hilar adenopathy 40%, and hepatosplenomegaly 30% [16]. According to the radiological findings of sarcoidosis described by Hofmann et al., chest radiographs were found normal (stage 0) in 39%; 34% had isolated bilateral hilar lymphadenopathy (stage I), 10% had bilateral hilar adenopathy with pulmonary infiltrates (stage II), and 15% had parenchymal infiltrates without hilar adenopathy (stage III) [15].

29.6.5 Kikuchi-Fujimoto Disease

Children with Kikuchi-Fujimoto disease may have enlarged cervical lymph nodes, fever, symptoms of upper respiratory tract infection, and less frequently chills, night sweats, arthralgia, rash, and weight loss. Lymph nodes are usually painful and tender; splenomegaly or hepatomegaly have sometimes been described [17].

29.7 Malignancies

Neck region may be the primary site of lymphomas, either Hodgkin's (HL) or non-Hodgkin's lymphoma (NHL), and granulocytic sarcoma, or secondary metastasis from nasopharyngeal and oropharyngeal tumors such as carcinoma, NHLs, neuroblastoma, rhabdomyosarcoma or thyroid tumors. Clinically, 70% of the HL begins in the cervical lymph nodes in children. Mediastinal involvement accompanies cervical lymph node enlargement in many cases. In NHLs, head and neck tissues may be the primary sites such as cervical lymph nodes, tonsils, nasopharyngeal area, nasal cavity, sinuses, and scalp. In acute lymphoblastic leukemia, generalized LAP is more frequent than it is in acute myeloid leukemia. Granulocytic sarcoma (chloroma) cases may primarily begin in the cervical lymph nodes without accompanying acute myeloid leukemia. Cervical lymph nodes may also be involved in histiocytosis, thyroid carcinoma, nasopharyngeal carcinoma, rhabdomyosarcoma, neuroblastoma, malignant rhabdoid tumors, osteogenic sarcoma, and Ewing family tumors of the region. In malignancies, lymph nodes are enlarged, fixed, firmed, and conglomerated without pain in palpation.

29.8 Diagnosis

All children with cervical lymphadenopathy should be evaluated clinically first. History, patient symptoms, and findings of physical examination are necessary to make the diagnosis in many cases. Laboratory (peripheral blood smear, cell count, biochemistry, serological tests) and radiological tests (especially ultrasonography) are helpful for diagnosis and differential diagnosis. In case of pathological lymphadenopathy with systemic B symptoms (fever >1 week, night sweats, weight loss >10% of body weight), palpable supraclavicular nodes, generalized lymphadenopathy, fixed, painless, matted, nontender lymph nodes, abnormal chest X-ray with mediastinal mass or adenopathy, and dyspnea, lymph node biopsy is taken to make a definitive diagnosis [16]. However, sometimes a biopsy is unnecessary. Malignancy is not found frequent among the excised lymph nodes. In a surgical analysis, biopsy yielded 48% of reactive lymph nodes, 25% tuberculosis, 11.6% neoplasm, 11.5% granulomatous lesions, 2.5% miscellaneous infections, and 1.5% normal [18].

References

1. Deosthali A, Donches K, Del Vecchio M, et al. Etiologies of pediatric cervical lymphadenopathy: a systematic review of 2687 subjects. Glob Pediatr Health. 2019;6:1–7.
2. Bshesh K, Khan W, Vattoth AL, et al. Lymphadenopathy post-COVID-19 vaccination with increased FDG uptake may be falsely attributed to oncological disorders: a systematic review. J Med Virol. 2022;94(5):1833–45.
3. Belsky JA, Carroll WR, Xu G. Side effects with a focus on lymphadenopathy following COVID-19 vaccination in pediatric and AYA oncology patients. J Pediatr Hematol Oncol. 2023;45(2):88–90. https://doi.org/10.1097/MPH.0000000000002621.

4. Howard-Jones AR, Al Abdali K, Britton PN. Acute bacterial lymphadenitis in children: a retrospective, cross-sectional study. Eur J Pediatr. 2023;82(5):2325–33. https://doi.org/10.1007/s00431-023-04861-0.
5. Kwon M, Seo JH, Cho KJ, et al. Suggested protocol for managing acute suppurative cervical lymphadenitis in children to reduce unnecessary surgical interventions. Ann Otol Rhinol Laryngal. 2016;125(12):953–8. https://doi.org/10.1177/0003489416665194.
6. Gosche JR, Vick L. Acute, subacute, and chronic cervical lymphadenitis in children. Semin Pediatr Surg. 2006;15(2):99–106. https://doi.org/10.1053/j.sempedsurg.2006.02.007.
7. Weinstock MS, Pattel NA, Smith NP. Pediatric cervical lymphadenopathy. Pediatr Rev. 2018;39(9):433–43. https://doi.org/10.1542/pir.2017-0249.
8. Wu Y, Ma S, Zhang L, et al. Clinical manifestations and laboratory results of 61 children with infectious mononucleosis. J Int Med Res. 2020;48(10):1–8. https://doi.org/10.1177/0300060520924550.
9. Haverkamp MH, Arend SM, Lindeboom JA, et al. Nontuberculous mycobacterial infection in children: a 2-year prospective surveillance study in The Netherlands. Clin Infect Dis. 2004;39(4):450–6. https://doi.org/10.1086/422319.
10. Durmuş SY, Tanır G, Kaman A. Tuberculous lymphadenitis in children. J Pediatr Inf. 2021;15(3):e139–45. https://doi.org/10.5578/ced.20219716.
11. Szczuka I. Adverse events following immunization with BCG vaccine in Poland 1994–2000. Przegl Epidemiol. 2002;56:205–16.
12. Pecora F, Abate L, Scavone S, et al. Management of infectious lymphadenitis in children. Children. 2021;8(10):860. https://doi.org/10.3390/children8100860.
13. Ridder-Schröter R, Marx A, Beer M, et al. Abscess-forming lymphadenopathy and osteomyelitis in children with Bartonella henselae infection. J Med Microbial. 2008;57(4):519–24.
14. Stevens DL, Bisno AL, Chambers HL, et al. Practice guidelines for the diagnosis and management of skin and soft-tissue infections. Clin Infect Dis. 2005;41:1373–406.
15. Hoffmann AL, Milman N, Byg KE. Childhood sarcoidosis in Denmark 1979-1994: incidence, clinical features and laboratory results at presentation in 48 children. Acta Pediatr. 2004;93(1):30–6.
16. Gedalia A, Khan TA, Avinash KS, et al. Childhood sarcoidosis: Louisiana experience. Clin Rheumatol. 2016;35:1879–84.
17. Lelii M, Senatore L, Amodeo I, et al. Kikuchi—Fujimoto disease in children: two case reports and a review of the literature. Ital J Pediatr. 2018;44:83. https://doi.org/10.1186/s13052-018-0522-9.
18. Moore SW, Schneider JW, Schaaf HS. Diagnostic aspects of cervical lymphadenopathy in children in the developing world: a study of 1,877 surgical specimens. Pediatr Surg Int. 2003;19:240–4.

Chronic Cough in Children: Upper Respiratory Tract Related Etiologies

30

Tugba Ramasli Gursoy and Laura Gochicoa-Rangel

30.1 Introduction

Cough is a forced expiratory mechanism against the glottis and protective reflex with both voluntary and involuntary control elements, necessary for the clearance of inhaled particles and mucus from airways [1]. Cough is the most common complaint in respiratory system diseases and is an irritating complaint when it is intense and prolonged [2, 3]. The presence of a persistent cough in pediatric patients has the potential to negatively impact their overall well-being, resulting in diminished quality of life, increased frequency of medical consultations, and perhaps inappropriate utilization of medications. In addition, cough can be a sign of a serious underlying disease [4]. A cough that persists for more than 4 weeks in children aged 14 years and younger is defined as a chronic cough [3]. In both adults and children aged 14 years and above, the duration of a cough over 8 weeks is classified as a chronic cough [4]. The causes of chronic cough in children are given in Table 30.1. The most common causes of upper respiratory tract related etiologies of chronic cough in children are discussed in this section.

T. Ramasli Gursoy (✉)
Department of Pediatric Pulmonology, Van Training and Research Hospital, Health Sciences University, Van, Turkey

L. Gochicoa-Rangel
Department of Respiratory Physiology, National Institute of Respiratory Diseases "Ismael Cosío Villegas", Mexico City, Mexico

H. Yüksel et al. (eds.), *Pediatric Airway Diseases*, Comprehensive ENT,
https://doi.org/10.1007/978-3-031-74853-0_30

Table 30.1 Causes of chronic cough in children

Pulmonary causes	
Asthma	Congenital lung disease
Aspiration due to swallowing dysfunction, GERD, or TEF	Tracheobronchomalacia
Cystic fibrosis	Vascular anomalies
Immunodeficiency (primary or secondary)	Environmental pollutants (tobacco smoke, vaping, air pollution)
Primary ciliary dyskinesia	**Extrapulmonary causes**
Post infection	Cardiac diseases
Protracted bacterial bronchitis	Upper respiratory tract diseases
Bronchiectasis	Ear disease
Retained inhaled foreign body	Psychogenic cough
Interstitial lung disease	Drugs (ACE inhibitors)

GERD gastroesophageal reflux disease, *TEF* tracheoesophageal fistula, *ACE* angiotensin-converting enzyme

30.2 Upper Airway Cough Syndrome

The pathogenesis of Upper Airway Cough Syndrome (UACS) is hypothesized to result from postnasal drip, wherein nasal secretions run into the nasopharynx. This condition can be associated with allergic, chronic nonallergic, or vasomotor rhinitis or rhinosinusitis. The initiation of the cough reflex is largely triggered by the activation of cough receptors situated in the mucous membranes of the larynx. This response is particularly prominent when there is a buildup of secretions in the upper respiratory tract [5]. The exact mechanism by which UACS contributes to chronic cough remains uncertain [6]. However, numerous studies have consistently demonstrated that UACS, particularly when accompanied by postnasal drip, is a common underlying factor in cases of subacute and chronic cough. The reported prevalence of UACS-associated cough varies considerably, ranging from 9% to 82% across different studies [6, 7]. The significant variation in prevalence can be primarily attributed to the slow integration of the term into clinical practice and disparities in treatment approaches across different countries. There is a prevailing agreement among experts that UACS is commonly acknowledged as either the major or secondary most prevalent cause of chronic cough in non-smokers, on a global level. UACS is frequently associated with comorbidities that can lead to the manifestation of a chronic cough [5–7]. According to Irwin et al., cough is associated with three or more etiologies (such as gastroesophageal reflux disease (GERD), drugs, asthma) in up to 42% of patients [6]. The term "postnasal drip syndrome" was commonly employed until 2006, at which point the American College of Chest Physicians (ACCP) recommended substituting it with the acronym UACS [8]. While it was previously believed that purulent nasal secretions were solely responsible for causing persistent cough, numerous studies have demonstrated that there are various underlying causes, such as inflammation and irritation of upper airway tissues, that can lead to coughing, including cases involving postnasal drip. The divergence of opinions within the academic community led the ACCP to revise the nomenclature, resulting in the adoption of the term UACS. There remains ongoing discourse regarding the appropriate terminology to delineate the experience of postnasal drip in relation to coughing [5, 8]. The reason why the European Respiratory Society (ERS) does not define UACS is that postnasal drip cannot fully explain the cough and some patients with postnasal drip do not cough. UACS and postnasal drip syndrome are classified as "rhinitis/rhinosinusitis" or upper respiratory tract diseases causing cough according to ERS [3, 5].

Initially, it is imperative to obtain a comprehensive anamnesis regarding the initiation, duration, and nature (intermittent or persistent) of the disease in children being evaluated for UACS. Additionally, it is important to inquire about symptoms such as rhinorrhea, nasal congestion, any history of allergies, sensitivity to seasonal or daily variations, as well as the severity of associated cough and headache. Characteristic features of the examination for UACS include nasal discharge and congestion, postnasal drip that can lead to symptoms of throat discharge, wheezing, and snoring, as well as a cobblestone appearance resulting from lymphoid hypertrophy in the oropharynx [5, 8].

The prioritization of therapy for UACS should be focused on addressing the underlying medical conditions that are commonly linked with it, such as GERD, uncontrolled asthma, or bronchiectasis. Nevertheless, when a specific reason cannot be determined, it is advisable to commence empirical treatment [9]. The treatments of UACS and most common underlying medical conditions are given in Table 30.2. When symptoms of rhinitis or chronic rhinosinusitis (CRS) persist despite initial empirical therapy, secondary UACS may necessitate further therapeutic approaches. Decongestants, which are believed to restrict the secretion of inflammatory cytokines, are advised for use. Patients diagnosed with allergic rhinitis (AR) are advised to utilize next-generation antihistamines; however, those with non-allergic rhinitis (NAR) or CRS should be administered first-generation antihistamines for treatment. There is a suggestion that the anticholinergic action exhibited by first generation antihistamines has a notable impact on patients with NAR and CRS in comparison to individuals with AR. In cases when antihistamines and decongestants are ineffective in managing UACS related to non-allergic rhinitis, it is advisable to explore other therapy modalities. The treatment for vasomotor rhinitis accompanied with cough typically involves the administration of antihistamines and decongestants, as

Table 30.2 The treatments of upper airway cough syndrome and most common underlying medical conditions

Allergic rhinitis	Next-generation antihistamines, decongestant, nasal steroid
Non-allergic rhinitis	First generation antihistamines, decongestant, ipratropium bromide nasal spray (alternative treatment)
Chronic rhinosinusitis	Nasal saline, nasal corticosteroids, antibiotics, endoscopic sinus surgery in selected cases
Post viral cough	First generation antihistamines, decongestants, montelukast
Gastroesophageal reflux disease	Dietary recommendations, proton pump inhibitors, antacids, histamine receptor antagonists, surgery in selected cases

these medications include anticholinergic properties, particularly in the case of first-generation antihistamines. The utilization of ipratropium bromide nasal spray may be considered in situations when contraindications are present or when alternative treatment options are deemed necessary. First generation antihistamines and decongestants may also provide relief for post viral cough resulting from a viral upper respiratory tract illness. Additionally, studies have demonstrated the potential benefits of Montelukast in the treatment of post viral cough. The management of symptoms associated with chronic rhinosinusitis often involves the use of nasal saline, topical nasal corticosteroids, and antibiotics. In certain instances where conventional medical interventions are ineffective, the necessity for endoscopic sinus surgery may arise [10]. Insufficient data exist to establish a definitive dosage or duration for the administration of non-sedating or sedative H1-histamine receptor antagonist treatment. Two distinct studies have examined the improvement in cough score at different time intervals, indicating that there is currently no universally accepted standard period for medical therapy. In a study involving a cohort of 20 patients presenting with AR, characterized by cough and rhinoconjunctivitis, the patients underwent a 4-week treatment regimen involving the administration of loratadine, with the evaluation of cough frequency and severity as the primary outcome measures. At the conclusion of the trial period, a notable enhancement in both measures was seen in comparison to the placebo group [11]. A cohort of individuals presenting with a persistent cough and concurrent eosinophilic bronchitis, commonly referred to as atopic cough, was studied. A noteworthy reduction in cough symptoms was observed after 1 week of treatment with non-sedating antihistamines [12]. It is postulated that the development of UACS may be attributed to many variables, including postnasal drip, persistent inflammation of the airway, and heightened sensitivity of the sensory nerves. Further research is required to distinguish the effects of distinct factors within, including thermal, mechanical, or chemical stimuli, on the development of chronic cough [5, 13]. The use of targeted therapy directed at particular receptors, such as transient receptor potential vanilloid 1 (TRPV1), has the potential to enhance symptom relief in individuals who exhibit resistance to conventional antihistamine and decongestant treatments [13].

30.3 Chronic Rhinosinusitis

Chronic rhinosinusitis is characterized by the presence of two or more symptoms, including purulent rhinorrhea, nasal obstruction, cough or face pressure/pain, persisting for a minimum duration of 3 months. Additionally, the condition is diagnosed based on the observation of mucosal edema, purulent discharge, or nasal polyps by endoscopic examination, and/or the identification of ostiomeatal complex or sinus edema using computer tomography (CT) scan imaging [14, 15]. The etiology of CRS in pediatric patients remains incompletely understood. Acute rhinosinusitis is predominantly caused by infection, but CRS encompasses a range of disorders that can be influenced by concomitant medical illnesses, infection, and environmental factors.

The influencing factors exhibit variation across different age groups, wherein adenoiditis emerges as a relatively significant trigger among younger children, while allergic rhinitis assumes greater importance among older children [16]. Furthermore, the presence of cystic fibrosis, primary ciliary dyskinesia, asthma, and GERD augments the prevalence of CRS. Young children have the potential to experience a range of 3–8 viral upper respiratory tract infections annually. The prevalence of acute bacterial rhinosinusitis as a complication of upper respiratory tract infections is estimated to range from 0.5% to 5%. Additionally, a subset of these cases may further proceed into CRS [17]. CRS is influenced by several environmental variables, such as exposure to smoking, industrial pollutants, and the commencement of formal education. The blockage of the ostiomeatal complex is caused by multifactorial inflammation of the sinus mucosa, whereas the impedance of the sinus ostia is a result of edema. This edema contributes to the reduction in secretions, a decrease in ciliary function, and the development of persistent bacterial infection [17, 18].

The utilization of nasal endoscopy allows for the direct observation of the nasal cavity, making it an optimal method for diagnosing CRS. Doing nasal endoscopy in children might pose difficulties, recommendations suggest that it should be considered as the first step in diagnosing CRS [14, 15]. According to the recommendations of guidelines, CT is the preferred first imaging modality for assessing chronic rhinosinusitis. CT is considered to be an optimal imaging modality due to its ability to assist with surgical navigation and its high sensitivity in detecting mucosal inflammation [15, 19]. Magnetic resonance imaging (MRI) is recommended in cases when there is suspicion of intracranial or intraorbital problems associated with sinusitis, since it offers superior vision of soft tissue, as per the established standards. According to the guidelines, the use of plain radiographs is not suggested due to their limited connection with CRS [14, 15]. A study which evaluated 6-year results of maxillary sinus punctures of children with CRS detected that the predominant bacterial species present were alpha-hemolytic Streptococcus, Haemophilus influenza, Streptococcus pneumonia, coagulase-negative Staphylococcus, Staphylococcus aureus, and anaerobic bacteria [20]. Guidelines advocate for the acquisition of cultures exclusively in cases when patients have exhibited no response to empiric therapy within a 72-h timeframe, possess notable comorbidities, or suffer from a serious sickness. Maxillary sinus aspiration is recommended as the first choice because of the high probability of microorganism isolation in culture. However, the invasiveness of the operation and the requirement for anesthesia have limitations on their applicability within the children [15].

The utilization of saline irrigations has been shown to enhance the elimination of pathogens in the nasal passage and reduce the presence of inflammatory mediators. The use of saline irrigation is supported by recommendations for the treatment of CRS due to its relative efficacy and low risk. Saline irrigation can be used as a stand-alone treatment or as an additional therapy in the management of children (especially under 6 years old) with CRS [14, 15].

The usage of nasal steroids is prevalent due to the prevailing notion that steroids possess the capacity to effectively diminish inflammation [21]. Although there is a scarcity of research specifically targeting the pediatric population, current recommendations advocate for the use of daily topical steroid spray as the primary therapeutic approach for children patients diagnosed with CRS, regardless of the presence or absence of nasal polyposis [14, 15].

In light of the established advantages associated with nasal saline irrigations, some researchers postulate that intranasal antibiotic irrigations might potentially offer the therapeutic effectiveness of antibiotics while circumventing the systemic adverse effects commonly associated with oral or intravenous administration of antibiotics [22, 23]. An examination of the existing literature pertaining to adult and pediatric populations reveals that the utilization of antibiotic nasal irrigations may be particularly advantageous when employed subsequent to endoscopic sinus surgery in the management of refractory CRS [23]. Nevertheless, due to the scarcity of information encompassing aspects such as medicine dosage and the potential for ototoxicity, it is challenging to provide definitive recommendations for pediatric patients [14].

The existing body of evidence regarding the efficacy of oral antibiotics for CRS is limited. Given the scarcity of data, the selection of antibiotics is frequently determined by treatment protocols for acute rhinosinusitis. The recommendations advocate amoxicillin for the first choice. Amoxicillin/clavulanate and cephalosporins can serve as viable options in cases when there is a perceived risk of encountering beta-lactamase generating bacteria [15]. The use of clindamycin is warranted in cases when anaerobic bacteria are detected. According to the guidelines set out by the Infectious Disease Society of America (IDSA), the preferred choice of medication is amoxicillin/clavulanate rather than amoxicillin due to the prevailing prevalence of beta-lactamase generating bacteria [24]. Consideration may be given to dual treatment with a third-generation cephalosporin and either clindamycin or levofloxacin in those who have documented allergies to penicillin [25]. The optimal length of antibiotic therapy remains undetermined due to the little information available in the existing literature. The guidelines recommend a prolonged course of treatment [14, 15].

There is a limited body of research examining the advantages of intravenous (IV) antibiotics in the pediatric chronic CRS population. While there is evidence showing therapeutic advantages, it is challenging to determine the effectiveness of IV antibiotics in isolation due to the presence of simultaneous surgical procedures and the absence of a comparison group [26, 27]. Based on the existing constraints in available data, the recommendations do not endorse the utilization of IV antibiotics as a standard practice for chronic rhinosinusitis [15]. Nevertheless, it is recommended to administer IV antibiotics in cases when there is suspicion of an intraorbital or intracranial complications arising from rhinosinusitis [14, 15].

Surgery may play a valuable role in cases whose symptoms do not improve adequately with medical treatment. Adenoidectomy is considered the primary surgical intervention for CRS. In certain instances, it is possible to integrate antral irrigation of the maxillary sinuses or balloon dilatation as complementary procedures. Endoscopic sinus surgery is a viable option for children who have had treatment failure and are afflicted with nasal polyps. The presence of foreign bodies is a rare reason for the indication of endoscopic sinus surgery. If outpatient treatment is not possible and severe sinusitis occurs, extensive examination and lengthy surgical dissection may be considered as a way to effectively drain the nasal cavities [15, 18, 28].

30.4 Gastroesophageal Reflux and Laryngopharyngeal Reflux

Gastroesophageal reflux is a physiological occurrence observed in around 40–65% of infants [29]. The occurrence of reflux often reaches its highest point between the ages of 1 and 4 months, and it tends to subside naturally by the time the child reaches 12 months of age [30]. Although reflux is a common phenomenon in infants, it becomes pathologic GERD when accompanied by additional symptoms such as recurrent regurgitation, dystonic neck posturing and back arching, cough, apnea, bradycardia episodes, and/or failure to thrive. In such cases, further investigation and intervention are necessary [31].

The challenge of establishing a connection between cough and GERD in children mostly stems from the complexities associated in diagnosing GERD. The etiology of cough is predicated upon the stimulation of vagal nerve fibers located within the esophagus, which triggers the cough reflex. Vagal stimulation subsequently elicits a parasympathetic response, resulting in the manifestation of cough and/or bronchospasm [32].

In more severe cases of GERD, passage of refluxed fluid into the larynx may result in microaspiration followed by tracheobronchitis and pneumonia. In addition, GERD can cause persistent cough even in the absence of esophagitis, that is, in the form of laryngopharyngeal reflux [33].

The identification of GERD and laryngopharyngeal reflux can be established by a comprehensive assessment of the patient's medical history and a thorough physical examination. Nevertheless, further diagnostic testing is necessary for individuals experiencing complications related to GERD. The diagnostic procedures that can be employed include barium contrast and fluoroscopic imaging of the upper gastrointestinal tract, pH meter analysis, esophageal manometry, endoscopic biopsies, and scintigraphy. Nevertheless, current recommendations do not endorse the routine utilization of these investigations for the diagnosis of GERD, except if there is a suspicion of anatomical irregularity or the presence of particular warning symptoms [31, 33].

In the management of GERD, patients are typically advised to adhere to certain dietary recommendations. These recommendations involve avoiding the consumption of a high-fat diet and, if applicable, making efforts to reduce excess body weight. Additionally, it is recommended to refrain from eating before 2 h of sleep and to abstain from consuming substances such as caffeine, carbonated beverages, alcohol, and citrus goods. It is advisable to request patients to abstain from smoking and raise the head of the bed. Proton pump inhibitors have traditionally served as the primary empirical therapy for coughs associated with GERD [34]. In the context of nonacidic reflux, drugs that function by creating a protective layer or physical barrier to prevent reflux could be used as an additional or perhaps alternative therapy approach. The etiology of GERD has been associated with gastroesophageal dysmotility, which involves anomalies in delayed gastric emptying as well as diminished pressure or improper temporary relaxation of the lower esophageal sphincter. A number of prokinetic medicines have the ability to enhance gastrointestinal motility, making them potentially valuable additions to antireflux treatment [35, 36]. The utilization of surgical interventions plays a significant role in the treatment of patients who do not respond well to conventional treatments [35].

30.5 Otogenic Cough

The phenomenon known as the ear-cough reflex was initially documented by Arnold in the year 1832, and subsequently recorded by Itard in 1842. The prevalence of this condition ranges from 1.7% to 4.2% [37]. The nerve known as Arnold's nerve originates from the jugular ganglion of the vagus nerve, and it exits through the tympanomastoid fissure. Its typical function is providing innervation to the skin of the posterior and inferior meatus. Nevertheless, the reflex of ear-cough may be induced with the stimulation of the anterior wall in approximately one-third of instances, and it is observed bilaterally in approximately two-thirds of cases. The activation of the Arnold's nerve can also result in non-respiratory manifestations, including vomiting and syncope [37, 38]. The prevailing factors contributing to this phenomenon typically involve the presence of foreign objects and impacted cerumen within the ear canal. The diagnosis is frequently made incidentally when there are no accompanying ear symptoms, as the otoscope is not regularly employed during the evaluation of a patient presenting with a persistent cough [39].

30.6 Laryngeal Clefts

Laryngeal clefts are congenital anomalies that have a relatively low prevalence and are distinguished by an atypical connection between the respiratory tract and the digestive tract. Based on the Benjamin-Inglis categorization method, there exist four distinct categories of laryngeal clefts [40]. Type 1 laryngeal cleft refers to a specific anomaly characterized by a deficiency in the interarytenoid mucosa or musculature, which does not extend beyond the voice cords. Type 1 laryngeal cleft typically manifests as persistent cough, recurring episodes of pneumonia, and difficulties with eating [41]. Type 1 laryngeal cleft has been found to have possible associations with comorbidities such as laryngomalacia, trachea-esophageal fistula, GERD, and diseases including Trisomy 21 [42]. The identification of type 1 laryngeal cleft might provide challenges in the diagnostic process, mostly because of the diverse array of non-specific symptoms exhibited by the affected individuals. The precise identification of a medical problem may experience a delay due to the potential for symptoms to be mistakenly associated with alternative disorders, such as asthma, allergies, or

GERD. Direct laryngoscopy is often regarded as the preferred diagnostic method for identifying type 1 laryngeal cleft. The management of Type 1 laryngeal cleft can be approached through conservative or surgical methods. The conservative approach to treatment encompasses the feeding and swallowing therapy. The surgical intervention involves the administration of different drugs into the interarytenoid area or the mending of the cleft using endoscopic suturing. The customization of management choices should be based on the severity of the patient's symptoms [43, 44].

30.7 Conclusion

The presence of a chronic cough is frequently observed in several illnesses, often exhibiting overlapping characteristics that transcend the boundaries of multiple medical specialties. The comprehensive evaluation of individuals experiencing persistent coughing necessitates a multidisciplinary strategy and effective collaboration among specialists in the fields of pulmonology, gastroenterology, and otolaryngology. UACS, CRS, and GERD are prevalent causes of chronic nonproductive cough observed in pediatric medical settings. A considerable number of these patients are not widely recognized for their challenging nature in terms of both diagnosis and treatment. However, employing a methodical and comprehensive approach within a multidisciplinary context has the potential to provide favorable outcomes in diagnosing and treating the majority of patients.

References

1. Song WJ, Chang YS, Faruqi S, et al. The global epidemiology of chronic cough in adults: a systematic review and meta-analysis. Eur Respir J. 2015;45:1479–81.
2. Munyard P, Bush A. How much coughing is normal? Arch Dis Child. 1996;74(6):531–4.
3. Morice AH, Millqvist E, Bieksiene K, et al. ERS guidelines on the diagnosis and treatment of chronic cough in adults and children. Eur Respir J. 55(1)1901136. 2020;55:1901136.
4. Chang AB, Robertson CF, Van Asperen PP, et al. A multicenter study on chronic cough in children: burden and etiologies based on a standardized management pathway. Chest. 2012;142(4):943–5.
5. Donaldson AM. Upper airway cough syndrome. Otolaryngol Clin N Am. 2023;56(1):147–55. https://doi.org/10.1016/j.otc.2022.09.011.
6. Irwin RS, French CL, Chang AB, et al. CHEST expert cough panel*. Classification of cough as a symptom in adults and management algorithms: CHEST guideline and expert panel report. Chest. 2018;153(1):196–209.
7. Dąbrowska M, Arcimowicz M, Grabczak EM, et al. Chronic cough related to the upper airway cough syndrome: one entity but not always the same. Eur Arch Otorrinolaringol. 2020;277(10):2753–9.
8. Pratter MR. Chronic upper airway cough syndrome secondary to rhinosinus diseases (previously referred to as postnasal drip syndrome): ACCP evidence based clinical practice guidelines. Chest. 2006;129(1 Suppl):63S–71S.
9. Lee JH, Lee JW, An J, et al. Efficacy of non-sedating H1-receptor antihistamines in adults and adolescents with chronic cough: a systematic review. World Allergy Organ J. 2021;14(8):100568.

10. Orlandi RR, Kingdom TT, Smith TL, et al. International consensus statement on allergy and rhinology: rhinosinusitis 2021. Int Forum Allergy Rhinol. 2021;11(3):213–739.
11. Ciprandi G, Buscaglia S, Catrullo A, et al. Loratadine in the treatment of cough associated with allergic rhinoconjunctivitis. Ann Allergy Asthma Immunol. 1995;75(2):115–20.
12. Shioya T, Satake M, Kagaya M, et al. Antitussive effects of the H1-receptor antagonist epinastine in patients with atopic cough (eosinophilic bronchitis). Arzneimittelforschung. 2004;54(4):207–12.
13. Lucanska M, Hajtman A, Calkovsky V, et al. Upper airway cough syndrome in pathogenesis of chronic cough. Physiol Res. 2020;69(Suppl 1):S35–42.
14. Brietzke SE, Shin JJ, Choi S, et al. Clinical consensus statement: pediatric chronic rhinosinusitis. Otolaryngol Head Neck Surg. 2014;151(4):542–53.
15. Fokkens WJ, Lund VJ, Mullol J, et al. EPOS 2012: European position paper on rhinosinusitis and nasal polyps 2012. A summary for otorhinolaryngologists. Rhinology. 2012;50(1):1–12.
16. Rizzi MD, Kazahaya K. Pediatric chronic rhinosinusitis. Curr Opin Otolaryngol Head Neck Surg. 2014;22(1):27–33.
17. Hamilos DL. Pediatric chronic rhinosinusitis. Am J Rhinol Allergy. 2015;29(6):414–20.
18. Chandy Z, Ference E, Lee JT. Clinical guidelines on chronic rhinosinusitis in children. Curr Allergy Asthma Rep. 2019;19(2):14.
19. Bhattacharyya N, Jones DT, Hill M, et al. The diagnostic accuracy of computed tomography in pediatric chronic rhinosinusitis. Arch Otolaryngol Neck Surg. 2004;130(9):1029.
20. Hsin CH, Su MC, Tsao CH, et al. Bacteriology and antimicrobial susceptibility of pediatric chronic rhinosinusitis: a 6-year result of maxillary sinus punctures. Am J Otolaryngol Head Neck Med Surg. 2010;31(3):145–9.
21. Chong LY, Head K, Hopkins C, et al. Intranasal steroids versus placebo or no intervention for chronic rhinosinusitis. Cochrane Database Syst Rev. 2016;4:CD011996.
22. Wei JL, Sykes KJ, Johnson P, et al. Safety and efficacy of once-daily nasal irrigation for the treatment of pediatric chronic rhinosinusitis. Laryngoscope. 2011;121(9):1989–2000.
23. Lee JT, Chiu AG. Topical anti-infective sinonasal irrigations: update and literature review. Am J Rhinol Allergy. 2014;28:29–38.
24. Chow AW, Benninger MS, Brook I, et al. IDSA clinical practice guideline for acute bacterial rhinosinusitis in children and adults. Clin Infect Dis. 2012;54(8):e72–e112.
25. Committee on Infectious Diseases C on ID, Jackson MA. Diseases the C on I. The use of systemic fluoroquinolones. Pediatrics. 2006;118(3):1287–92.
26. Don DM, Yellon RF, Casselbrant ML, et al. Efficacy of a stepwise protocol that includes intravenous antibiotic therapy for the management of chronic sinusitis in children and adolescents. Arch Otolaryngol Head Neck Surg. 2001;127(9):1093–8.
27. Adappa ND, Coticchia JM. Management of refractory chronic rhinosinusitis in children. Am J Otolaryngol. 2006;27(6):384–9.
28. Cardella A, Preti A, Gera R, et al. Endoscopic sinus surgery for foreign body extraction in an adult patient. Clin Case Rep. 2021;9(7):e04200.
29. Goldsobel AB, Chipps BE. Cough in the pediatric population. J Pediatr. 2010;156(3):352–8.
30. Chow PY, Ng DK. Chronic cough in children. Singapore Med J. 2004;45(10):462–8.
31. Kennedy AA, Anne S, Hart CK. Otolaryngologic management of chronic cough in school-aged children: a review. JAMA Otolaryngol Head Neck Surg. 2020;146(11):1059–64.
32. Irwin RS, Madison JM, Fraire AE. The cough reflex and its relation to gastroesophageal reflux. Am J Med. 2000;108:73–8.
33. Rosen R, Vandenplas Y, Singendonk M, et al. Pediatric gastroesophageal reflux clinical practice guidelines: joint recommendations of the North American Society for Pediatric Gastroenterology, Hepatology, and Nutrition and the European Society for Pediatric Gastroenterology, Hepatology, and Nutrition. J Pediatr Gastroenterol Nutr. 2018;66(3):516–54.
34. Irwin RS. Chronic cough due to gastroesophageal reflux disease: ACCP evidence-based clinical practice guidelines. Chest. 2006;129(1 Suppl):80S–94S.
35. Sylvester DC, Karkos PD, Vaughan C, et al. Chronic cough, reflux, postnasal drip syndrome, and the otolaryngologist. Int J Otolaryngol. 2012;2012:564852.

36. Ang D, Blondeau K, Sifrim D, et al. The spectrum of motor function abnormalities in gastroesophageal reflux disease and Barrett's esophagus. Digestion. 2009;79(3):158–68.
37. Jegoux F, Legent F, Beauvillain de Montreuil C. Chronic cough and ear wax. Lancet. 2002;360(9333):618.
38. Masson V, Kier C, Chandran L. Cough conundrums: a guide to chronic cough in the pediatric patient. Pediatr Rev. 2022;43(12):691–703.
39. Weinberger M. Chronic cough and causes in children. J Clin Med. 2023;12(12):3947.
40. Bush A, Abel RM, Chitty LS, et al. Congenital lung disease. In: Wilmott RW, Deterding RR, Li A, Ratjen F, Sly P, Zar H, Bush A, editors. Kendig's disorders of the respiratory tract in children. Philadelphia, PA: Elsevier; 2019. p. 289–337.
41. Fracchia MS, Diercks G, Cook A, et al. The diagnostic role of triple endoscopy in pediatric patients with chronic cough. Int J Pediatr Otorhinolaryngol. 2019;116:58–61.
42. Reddy P, Byun YJ, Downs J, et al. Presentation and management of type 1 laryngeal clefts: a systematic review and meta-analysis. Int J Pediatr Otorhinolaryngol. 2020;138:110370.
43. Van der Doef HP, Yntema JB, van den Hoogen FJ, et al. Clinical aspects of type 1 posterior laryngeal clefts: literature review and a report of 31 patients. Laryngoscope. 2007;117(5):859–63.
44. Mukerji SS, Yenduri NJS, Chiou E, et al. A multi-disciplinary approach to chronic cough in children. Laryngoscope Investig Otolaryngol. 2022;7(2):409–16.

Upper Respiratory Tract Comorbidities in Children with Wheezing

31

Şule Büyük Yaytokgil and Ersoy Civelek

31.1 Introduction

Multimorbidity is a common problem in patients with chronic diseases such as asthma/recurrent wheezing and may cause poor quality of life and management of diseases, and increased health care utilizations [1, 2]. Multimorbidity is more common especially in patients with difficulty treated and/or severe asthma [3]. Treating the multimorbidities may minimize future asthma exacerbations [1] and improve the asthma treatment.

Upper respiratory co-morbidities are common and important in diagnosis and management of children with recurrent wheezing/asthma, because they may confuse with wheezing and cause unnecessary treatments, or they may sometimes contribute to poor disease control by aggravating symptoms [4]. Therefore, recognizing and treating upper respiratory comorbidities in asthma/recurrent wheezing may improve their outomes [4, 5].

This chapter is an overview of the prevalence, clinical features, diagnosis, and management of the upper respiratory co-morbidities (chronic-rhinosinusitis, nasal polyposis, allergic rhinitis, vocal cord dysfunction, and obstructive sleep apnea syndrome) in children with recurrent wheezing/asthma.

Ş. Büyük Yaytokgil
Department of Pediatrics, Division of Pediatric Allergy and Immunology, Ankara Research and Training Hospital, Ankara, Turkey

E. Civelek (✉)
Department of Pediatrics, Division of Pediatric Allergy and Immunology, Private Hospital Memorial Ankara, Ankara, Turkey

H. Yüksel et al. (eds.), *Pediatric Airway Diseases*, Comprehensive ENT,
https://doi.org/10.1007/978-3-031-74853-0_31

31.2 Pathogenesis of the Upper and Lower Respiratory Diseases Comorbidities

Respiratory systems are divided into two sections: upper and lower. Diseases related with both sections may affect each other [6] and was defined as a one way or united way [7–10], because they share many anatomical and histological properties [6–8] and some mechanisms were suggested [8–11] (Table 31.1).

The first mechanism is the protective function of nose for avoiding bronchoconstriction. The nose is the entrance of air and the place where the air warms, filters, and humidifies [10], but if the nose impaired, the bronchoconstriction may occur [12]. Also, nasal breathing was reported as protected against the onset of exercise-induced asthma, whereas oral breathing is more likely to exacerbate symptoms. During the oral breathing, cold and dry air reach the lung directly and provocate bronchoconstriction [13]. Therefore, in any nasal pathology, the nasal breathing is interrupted and the nasal shielding function is cessated and consequently bronchial disorders may be triggered [10].

The second suggested mechanism is the similarity in histology [8]. Both nose and bronchi consist of a pseudostratified respiratory epithelium, and their mucosae have ciliary epithelium on the basement membrane, lamina propria, glands, and goblet cells under the basement membrane [11]. Epithelium is the first defense mechanisms for microorganisms; therefore, if any defect occurred in the epithelium, the barrier function could be lost, consequently microorganisms can penetrate the epithelium and then provocate inflammation [11]. İmpairment of the epithelium functioning is one of the contributive factors for the development of airway diseases [6, 10].

Also, there are some common immunopathology in the inflammation of the upper and lower airways, because mast cells, T lymphocytes, and eosinophils might infiltrate both airways; and may cause the symptoms [9]. Inflammation in the upper respiratory mucosa with specific allergens or microorganisms may trigger inflammation in the lower respiratory mucosa by drainage of inflammatory mediators [6, 10, 14, 15]. This mechanism, which is called as postnasal drainages of the inflammation [6, 14], is the third mechanism.

The fourth mechanism is the inflammation caused by the same triggers. One study described allergic rhinitis (AR), rhinosinusitis, and asthma as "one way and one disease" and indicated that same triggers cause inflammation in both the nose and the lungs [7]. These common triggers are allergens, pathogens, and environ-

Table 31.1 Possible mechanisms for upper respiratory comorbidities of the patients with asthma/wheezing

1. Function of nose
2. Similar epithelium and mucosal membrane
3. Postnasal drainages of the inflammations
4. İnflammation with similar agent (such as virus/bacteria/antigen)
5. Type 2 inflammation
6. Neural reflex (similar innervation)

mental factors. Previously, atopic march was considered to consist of two steps, first atopic dermatitis and then respiratory allergies, e.g., AR and asthma—as a similar tract disease [7]. However, recently a study showed that there is no specific or typical sequence of symptoms development that characterizes this atopic march, indeed the classic sequence of eczema, wheeze, and rhinitis were relatively rare (around 2–4%) by the final time [16] and increased gradually from infancy to age 4–5 years, with little change thereafter. On the other hand, some viruses affect both upper and lower respiratory systems and they may cause rhinitis, sinusitis, bronchiolitis, and pneumonia. Tobacco smoke exposure is one of the common environmental factors which also affect both upper and lower respiratory tract [17]. Also, some drugs such as aspirin and betablockers may trigger both asthma and AR symptoms [7].

The fifth mechanism is the Th2 type inflammation which may cause chronic airway diseases such as asthma, AR, and chronic sinusitis [6, 18]. Presence of the Th2-type inflammatory process dominated by eosinophils at one site of the airways may cause to release cytokines (including IL-4, IL-5, IL-13) into the blood stream which can stimulate the bone marrow and as a result of this can cause the increasing of systemic eosinophilic inflammation [6, 14]. Persistent type 2 inflammation continuously damages the epithelium and cause to exacerbate the clinical symptoms [18]. In patients with asthma, the coexistence of other type 2 inflammatory diseases produced greater decline in lung function and more symptoms [18].

"Neural reflex" is another mechanism reported that may provide communication between the nose and bronchi, because the nose and bronchi share the same adrenergic and vagal innervation [9, 19]. The nasobronchial reflex, consists of broncho constriction and increase in pulmonary resistance following the exposure of the nose to cold air or irritants [19]. Also, it was previously reported that nasal challenges induced to the bronchoconstriction and also bronchial provocations can cause the nasal reactions [14].

On the other hand, CST1 (cystatin SN gene) was detected to be higher in patients with AR and asthma than patients with AR alone; therefore, CST1 may be a biomarker for airway allergic diseases [20].

All of these mechanisms show that inflammation of the upper airway can lead to abnormal changes in the mucosa of the lower airway [14, 20]. Knowing the similarities and interactions of upper and lower airway may facilitate the managements of the respiratory diseases with coexistence of each other.

31.3 Epidemiology of Upper Respiratory Comorbidities of Asthma

Asthma is a chronic respiratory disease characterized with chronic airway inflammation [1]. The main goal of asthma therapy is achieved to the minimal or no symptoms of disease, normal sleep and activities, and optimal pulmonary function [1]. In order to achieve these goals, knowing and eliminating asthma comorbidities is important.

Mirabellia et al., reported that 87.8% of the children with asthma had other comorbidities, whereas 65% of the children without asthma had comorbidities [5]. One study reported that 21% of the patients with asthma have one to two coexisting conditions, 30% have three to four coexisting conditions, and 45% have more than five coexisting conditions [21]. Prevalence of comorbidities varies according to different studies and countries [22]. The study on asthmatic children showed that respiratory allergies were the most common detecting comorbidity (up to 30.5%) [5]. A recent study reported that only 13% of the children with asthma did not have any comorbidity, while 37% of asthmatic children had respiratory comorbidities (rhinitis or sinusitis or snoring), and 40% had both respiratory and extra-respiratory comorbidities [23]. AR were the most common respiratory comorbidities of asthma [22]. AR was detected in 64% of the asthmatic patients, and asthma was detected in 20% of AR patients. Also, 24% of the patients with chronic rhinosinusitis (CRS) was reported to have asthma and 8% of the asthmatic patients have CRS [24]. Allergic sinusitis was reported in 20% of the asthmatic children [22]. Global Initiative for Asthma (GINA) advices to evaluate the nasal involvements in asthma patients [1].

Comorbidities increase the risk of exacerbations, rates of hospitalizations, visits of emergency department (ED), and visits of unscheduled doctor ambulatory care [25]. Healthcare expenditures and hospital readmissions are directly related to the number of chronic conditions [21]. Previous studies reported that asthmatic children with respiratory comorbidities had more exacerbations, and lower sleep quality [23]. AR and sinusitis are associated with more severe symptoms, poorly controlled asthma, more exacerbations, and more sleep disturbances [26]. The frequency of asthma attack and emergency department visits were reported more in children with comorbidities compared to those without comorbidities [5].

31.4 Risk Factors for Multimorbidity/Comorbidity in Asthma

Detecting the risk factors for comorbidities of asthma may facilitate the development of preventive strategies to decrease comorbidies and its cost. There have been several studies that investigated the risk factors for developing comorbidities in patients with asthma [18, 23, 27, 28].

The EuroPrevall-iFAAM birth cohort study reported that independent to IgE sensitization, coexistence of allergic comorbidities like rhinitis and eczema were detected to be more frequent in asthmatic children than general population [27]. And Asthma comorbidities may occur as a result of both genetic and environmental factors [20, 23]. But the presence of type 2 inflammations may also increase the coexistence with other chronic airway diseases such as chronic sinusitis, AR, etc. [18].

Maternal history of asthma, breastfeeding, early mold exposure, and current environmental tobacco smokes exposure were reported as the significant risk factors for asthma-respiratory comorbidities in children [23]. Higher body mass index (BMI) was detected in asthmatic patients with respiratory comorbidities than asthmatic patients with extra-respiratory comorbidities [23]. Age may be another risk factor for asthma comorbidity, as the coexistence of CRS and asthma increased by age was reported in a small study [28].

Presence of allergy in the family, cesarean, and early-age onset-symptoms were reported as other risks for multimorbidity of allergic diseases including asthma, AR, and eczema [27]. The risk of gender is conflicted. In one study, female gender was reported as a protective factor [27]. In contrast, female was associated with increased risk of AR and sinusitis comorbidities in asthmatic patients [26]. But in another study, gender was not determined as a risk factor for comorbidities [22]. While in another study, comorbidities in asthmatic patients were more prevalent in males before puberty, and in females after puberty [29].

Also, some countries or regions had more asthma comorbidities. For example, nasal polyposis as comorbidities of asthma was less common in China compared to Europe [30]. Maybe, because in Chinese patients, nasal polyposis was less related to Th2-typed inflammation [30].

Immunological diseases such as antibody deficiency is one of the main contributors for inflammation in both upper and lower airways [31], which may increase the risk of asthma comorbidity. Some other comorbidities may increase the frequency of upper respiratory comorbidities of asthma such as hypertrophy of tonsils and adenoids [15, 32].

31.5 Upper Respiratory Comorbidities of Wheezing/Asthma

Upper respiratory comorbidities are common in patients with asthma and GINA recommend to evaluate for nasal involvements [1]. Some upper respiratory diseases such as AR and CRS may be an important risk factor for new onset asthma [9]. Bronchial hyperactivity was detected in patients with AR without asthma, forced expiratory flow at 25% and 75% (FEF 25–75) was suggested as an early marker of bronchial involvement in patients with allergic rhinitis who had only nasal symptoms [9]. Co-existence of upper respiratory comorbidities such as AR and sinusitis may increase asthma symptoms [26]. Presence of upper respiratory comorbidities increase the costs and outcomes of asthma, mimic or aggravate symptoms of asthma, decrease both adherence or effectiveness of treatments, and decrease the quality of life [4]. The upper respiratory co-morbidities of wheezy children are vocal cord dysfunction, obstructive sleep apnea syndrome (OSAS), CRS, nasal polyposis, and AR.

31.5.1 Vocal Cord Disfunction (VCD)

Vocal cord disfunction (VCD) is characterized with inappropriate movement of the vocal cords and triggered by some factors such as exercise, psychological stress, local irritation (reflux) [33]. The prevalence of the VCD in the pediatric population has not been adequately estimated [34] .VCD and asthma often coexisted with each other [33]. In a retrospective study ($n = 292$), Traister et al., reported that 32.6% of VCD patients had concomitant asthma [35].

Dyspnea, wheezing, stridor, chest pain or tightness, and throat discomfort are the most common symptoms of VCD, and they may occur both at rest and during exercised [34, 36]. Cough and wheezing are also the most important symptoms of asthma, so extensive differential diagnosis is necessary [37]. Short-acting beta-2 agonists (SABA) are not enough to control the symptoms of VCD and intermittent inspiratory symptoms occur [33]; therefore, these are important clues for differentiation of VCD from asthma. There are some other differences between characteristics of asthma and VCD. Such as the respiratory phases of symptoms; VCD occurs during inspiratory phases [34]. Also, the duration time of onset of symptoms during exercises may be different [38]. Exertional dyspnea occurs and peaks during exercise in patients with VCD, whereas it usually peaks 5–20 min after the end of exercise in patients with asthma. But if both of them coexist in the same patient, time overlap can be seen [38].

31.5.2 Obstructive Sleep Apnea Syndrome (OSAS)

OSAS was seen in 1–3% of children [15], but in asthmatic children, the prevalence of OSAS rises to 35–66% [39, 40]. A study reported that 47.3% of subjects with asthma alone and 55.9% of patients with asthma and AR had OSAS [41]. Several studies reported that OSAS and asthma were both confusing and contributed factors for each other [15, 32, 39, 40]. There were many bidirectional connections between OSAS and asthma, including incidence, risk factors, pathophysiology, and treatment [15, 32, 40].

A randomized sample survey of 1234 children aged 6–14 years in Belgium revealed a two fold increase in OSAS symptoms among children with wheezing [42]. Also, coexistence of OSAS was more frequently detected in children with uncontrolled/poorly controlled asthma than in those with controlled asthma [32, 39]. Asthma and OSAS bidirectionally increase the severity of each other [40], also, they shared multiple etiological risk factors [32], such as hypertrophy of tonsils, adenoids, and obesity [15]. The prevalence of OSAS was higher in asthmatic children with AR than asthmatic children without AR [32]. Prevalence of attention deficit hyperactivity disease was higher in asthmatic children with OSA than without OSAS [32, 41]. OSAS was reported as an independent risk factor for uncontrolled asthma in children [39]. Therefore, screening for OSAS should be performed routinely in all patients with severe, poorly controlled asthma [4]. Treating of OSAS can ameliorate the severity of asthma [15]. So, the coexisting of OSAS should be screened in patients with poorly controlled and/or severe asthma [4].

31.5.3 Allergic or Non-Allergic Rhinitis

Mucosal membranes irritations and inflammations of nose is defined as rhinitis [1]. According to the presence of allergic sensitizations, rhinitis may be classified as allergic or non-allergic rhinitis [1].

AR might promote, trigger, maintain, and worsen the asthma by several pathophysiologic mechanisms, such as the vagal reflex (rhinobronchial reflex), the continuous passage of allergic inflammation from the nose to bronchi, the systemic release of mediators and cytokines, the irritant mechanism sustained by the postnasal drip, and the oral respiration caused by nasal obstruction, which promotes bronchial hyperreactivity (BHR) as dry and cold air penetrates into the bronchi [9].

AR frequently coexist with asthmatic patients [26], even most common comorbidities of asthma [22]. AR frequently occurs before the development of asthma in children [11]. Also, AR may increase the risk of developing asthma [9]. AR may cause worsening of asthma. Asthmatic patients with a combination of lower baseline lung function and allergic rhinitis (this indicates that more severe asthma) were reported that more affected from the presence of AR [26].

Prevalences: AR is one of the most common comorbidities of asthma. Estimated prevalence of AR is 10–40% in pediatric populations [43]. Most patients with asthma, either allergic or non-allergic, have concurrent rhinitis. It is considered that 10.5–43% of patients with AR have asthma, and 40–90% of patients with asthma have rhinitis [11, 12, 37, 44]. Also, 76.2% of the children with asthma, had AR [45]. Settipane et al. reported that the risk of asthma in patients with AR are more at 3 times compared with those without AR [46]. Also, another study indicated that AR patients have eight-fold more risk of having asthma compared to patients without AR [9]. And underdiagnosis of AR in patients with asthma was more common [12].

According to Allergic Rhinitis and its Impact on Asthma (ARIA), especially patients with severe persistent rhinitis are prone to having asthma comorbidities [47]. AR comorbidities in children with asthma can cause more hospitalization and ED visits or underdiagnosed of asthma and associated with higher cost than children with asthma alone [44, 48]. In contrast to this, asthmatic participants with AR had similar exacerbation rates compared to those without AR in both the Safety of Inactivated Influenza Vaccine in Asthma in Adults and Children (SIIVA) and Low Dose Theophylline as Add-on Treatment in Asthma (LODO) cohorts [26]. Ohta et al. reported that asthma control was significantly worse in patients with a physician's diagnosis of rhinitis by comparison with those without rhinitis [44].

On the other hand, some physicians indicate that AR may be an early stage of the asthma [49]. Bronchial hyperactivity without clinical symptoms of asthma were detected in most of the patients with AR, this may predict the future development of asthma [9].

Also, Leukotriene receptor antagonists (LTRAs) may reduce the inflammation of both the nasal and bronchial mucosae, thereby improving the total symptoms score of both AR and asthma symptoms [10]. In real-life, in case of rhinitis and asthma multimorbidity, which are also affected by environmental exposures, it is recommended to give digitalize and person-focused integrated treatments [50]. Immunotherapy also decreases the risk of asthma development [51] and can reduce both nasal and bronchial symptoms [10].

31.5.4 Chronic Rhinosinusitis and Nasal Polyposis

İnflammation of nasal and paranasal sinus mucosae is called sinusitis and/or rhinosinusitis. According to durations of symptoms and inflammations, rhinosinusitis is classified as acute or chronic. Persistence of the symptoms of acute rhinosinusitis for greater than 3 months despite standard medical management, including antibiotics, steroids, saline nasal rinses, and nasal sprays is diagnosed as chronic rhinosinusitis (CRS) in children. And CRS is classified according to phenotypes with nasal polyposis (NP) and without nasal polyposis [52, 53].

CRS is one of the most frequent upper respiratory tract comorbidities of asthma [10] and associated with increasing risk of asthma exacerbations [3]. According to clinical evidences, CRS affects both occurrence and course of the asthma [6]. Also, CRS was defined as one of the markers of the severe asthma [4]. There were various inflammatory mechanisms defined, which affect the phenotypes of CRS [54]. For example, the nasal polyp phenotype with high IL-5 was detected as strongly increased the asthma prevalence [54]. Also, they reported that inflammatory phenotypes might have been an importance for comorbid asthma development [54]. In LODO cohort, sinüsitis was associated with increasing exacerbations in asthmatic patients [26].

Presence of the AR and/or CRS was associated with poorer asthma control, more exacerbations and ED visits and more difficulty in controlling the symptoms [55]. Patients with asthma with NP showed greater decline in post-bronchodilator forced expiratory volume in the first second (FEV1) per year [56].

In United states, CRS was diagnosed approximately in 2% of children per year [53]. CRS is associated with asthma, the prevalence of asthma was 5–12% in the general population and 4% in pediatric population; whereas it goes up to 25% in patients with CRS [57–59]. Tosca et al. reported rhinosinusitis in 44% of 128 asthmatic children evaluated by nasal endoscopy [60]. In another study, which investigated the CRS patients according to cluster analysis, the rate of asthma comorbidity was ranging from 7% to 71% between the CRS cluster [54]. And another study reported that 68% of the patients with asthma revealed sinus diseases which were detected by sinus computer tomography (CT). Also, they detected several mucosal thickenings which was associated with higher eosinophil levels in blood and sputum. And they reported that patients with more severe sinus disease showed a statistical trend toward lower values of mean FEV1 than others [61].

NP are benign edematous masses in the nasal cavities, paranasal cavities, or both. Nasal obstruction, rhinorrhea, postnasal drip, and loss of smell are the main symptoms of NP. And the estimated prevalence of NP is approximately 2–4% [62, 63]. The presence of NP with CRS was strongly correlated with asthma comorbidity [54]. NP were diagnosed in 7% of asthma patients, and it were more frequently seen in non-atopic asthma and late-onset asthma [6]. CRS frequently coexists with more severe asthma, especially with NP [28, 54, 62, 63]. Due to the close relations between RS and asthma, especially children and adolescents with poorly controlled asthma should be investigated for occult or manifest RS [6].

As a result of the remodeling of nasal and paranasal sinuses mucosa, NP may ocur [58]. Presence of NP affects the severity of asthma; asthma was more severe in CRS with NP (CRSwNP) than CRS without nasal polyps. But CRSwNP was associated with the late-onset, non-atopic severe asthma phenotype, so age was important for the occurence of nasal polyps [64]. Intolerance to aspirin (ASA) may also be seen in patients with CRS and may provoke asthma and rhinitis symptoms; and this was called “Non-steroidal anti-inflammatory drugs exacerbated respiratory disease” (NERD) [4].

CRS with type 2 (Th2) endotypes are more resistant to therapies compared to CRS with type 1 and 3 endotypes [58]. But biological agents are available now and they target type 2 inflammation [47]. In the very near future, personalized medicine, which is based on molecular biomarkers for the endotype or subendotype activated in an individual patient, may be used for CRS patients [58].

Nasal congestion, impaired drainage of mucus at the ostiomeatal complex, stagnation of secretions, decreased ventilation, mucosal inflammation, and decreased mucociliary transport; all of them facilitate bacterial infection [62]. Also, inflammatory discharge is dripped in to the lower airways from the nasal sinuses [11]. So, European guideline suggests that antral irrigation should be considered in addition to an adenoidectomy in children with severe asthma [57].

In asthmatic patients, endoscopic sinus surgery has been reported to improve multiple clinical asthma parameters with improved overall asthma control, reduced frequency of asthma attacks, and number of hospitalizations, as well as decreased use of oral and inhaled corticosteroids [57]. Endoscopic sinus surgery is recommended especially in older children with CRS and especially in case of failure to adenoidectomy [58].

Endoscopic sinus surgery for CRS can reduce the yearly incidence of new asthma diagnoses; those patients whose surgery is late may develop higher rates of asthma than those whose surgery is at an earlier timepoint [57].

After treatments of CRS, 79% of the poorly controlled asthmatic patients put off bronchodilator therapy and 67% of them respiratory functional tests got back to normal range [65].

Local or systemic corticosteroids, functional endoscopic sinus surgery can be used for NP. And the presence of nasal polyps in severe asthma may help with the choice of the biological therapy [1]. Because anti-IgE therapy improves both the nasal polyps scores and asthma scores compared to basal scores [66]. Also, omalizumab improved the severity of symptoms and so quality of life scores in patients with nasal polyps and comorbid asthma; the characteristics of these patients is being under Th2 type inflammations [66]. Treatment of CRS with nasal corticosteroids for 24 weeks was reported to not improve the asthma control, in their placebo control trial which investigated the effects of nasal mometasone on asthma outcome. So, treating sinonasal diseases in asthma should be determined by the need to treat sinonasal disease rather than to improve asthma control [67].

31.6 Conclusion

Multimorbidity is common in patients with difficult treated and/or severe asthma [3]. Especially, upper airway comorbidities are frequently coexistent with asthma as a result of their similar patho-physiological mechanism, immunological predisposition, chronic airway mucosal inflammation, and similar triggers [11]. Upper respiratory comorbidities are associated with poor symptoms control and increasing exacerbations [4]. Also, these comorbidities increase rates of hospitalizations, visits of ED, and visits of unscheduled doctor ambulatory care; so, this poses a significant burden on individuals with asthma and the health care system. Therefore, diagnosis and management of comorbidities are very important.

Both diagnosis and management of comorbidities should require multidisciplinary approach [4]. Because asthmatic children with multiple comorbidities are taken care from different health providers, so their managements may have became fragmented and less effective. In this perspective, comorbid disease may cause risk for bad adherence to asthma treatment [31].

Allergic multimorbidities affect quality of life of both patients and families, so treatments of asthma comorbidities may increase the quality of life [11]. Treating the upper airway (nasal) disease reduce the bronchial hyperactivities and improve the asthma symptoms [8]. Also, for decreasing the upper airway comorbidities, early preventive strategies should be developed [18].

References

1. 2023 GINA Report, Global Strategy for Asthma Management and Prevention. https://ginasthma.org/2023-gina-main-report/.
2. Wilson KC, Gould MK, Krishnan JA, et al. An Official American Thoracic Society Workshop Report. A framework for addressing multimorbidity in clinical practice guidelines for pulmonary disease, critical illness, and sleep disorders. Ann Am Thorac Soc. 2016;13:12–21.
3. Denlinger LC, Phillips BR, Ramratnam S, et al. Inflammatory and comorbid features of patients with severe asthma and frequent exacerbations. Am J Respir Crit Care Med. 2017;195:302–13.
4. Porsbjerg C, Menzies-Gow A. Co-morbidities in severe asthma: clinical impact and management. Respirology. 2017;22(4):651–61.
5. Mirabellia MC, Hsu J, Gowerb WA. Comorbidities of asthma in U.S. children. Respir Med. 2016;116:34–40.
6. Poddighea D, Brambillab I, Licarib A, et al. Pediatric rhinosinusitis and asthma. Respir Med. 2018;141:94–9.
7. Caimmi D, Marseglia A, Pieri G, et al. Nose and lungs: oneway, one disease. Ital J Pediatr. 2012;38:60.
8. Licari A, Castagnoli R, Denicolo CF, et al. The nose and the lung: united airway disease? Front Pediatr. 2017;5:44.
9. Ciprandi G, Cirillo I. The lower airway pathology of rhinitis. J Allergy Clin Immunol. 2006;118(5):1105–9.
10. Ciprandi G, Caimmi D, Giudice MMD, et al. Recent developments in united airways disease. Allergy Asthma Immunol Res. 2012;4(4):171–7.
11. Licari A, Caimmi S, Bosa L, et al. Rhinosinusitis and asthma: a very long engagement. Int J Immunopathol Pharmacol. 2014;27(4):499–508.
12. Vujnovic SD, Domuz A. Epidemiological aspects of rhinitis and asthma: comorbidity or united airway disease. INTECH. 2016; https://doi.org/10.5772/intechopen.76773.
13. Hallani M, Wheatley JR, Amis RC. Enforced mouth breathing decreases lung function in mild asthmatics. Respirology. 2008;13(4):553–8.
14. Braunstahl GJ, Kleinjan A, Overbeek SE, et al. Segmental bronchial provocation induces nasal inflammation in allergic rhinitis patients. Am J Respir Crit Care Med. 2000;161(6):2051–7.
15. Kheirandish-Gozal L, Dayyat EA, Eid NS, et al. Obstructive sleep apnea in poorly controlled asthmatic children: effect of adenotonsillectomy. Pediatr Pulmonol. 2011;46:913–8.
16. Haider S, Fontanella S, Ullah A, STELAR/UNICORN Investigators, et al. Evolution of eczema, wheeze and rhinitis from infancy to early adulthood: four birth cohort studies. Am J Respir Crit Care. 2022;206(8):950–60.

17. Gibbs K, Collaco JM, McGrath-Morrow SA. Impact of tobacco smoke and nicotine exposure on lung development. Chest. 2016;149(2):552–61.
18. Maspero J, Adir Y, Al-Ahmad M, et al. Type 2 inflammation in asthma and other airway diseases. ERJ Open Res. 2022;8:00576–2021.
19. Leonardi S, Vitaliti G, Marseglia GL, et al. Function of the airway epithelium in asthma. J Biol Regul Homeost Agents. 2012;26:S41–8.
20. Wang M, Gong L, Luo Y, et al. Transcriptomic analysis of asthma and allergic rhinitis reveals CST1 as a biomarker of unified airways. Front Immunol. 2023;14:1048195.
21. Chronic conditions among Medicare beneficiaries. Chart book. 2012th ed. Baltimore, MD: Centers for Medicare and Medicaid Services; 2012.
22. Kumar P, Singh G, Goyal JP, et al. Association of common comorbidities with asthma in children: a cross-sectional study. Sudan J Paediatr. 2019;19(2):88–92.
23. Fasola S, Ferrante G, Cilluffo G, et al. Asthma comorbidities: frequency, risk factors, and associated burden in children and adolescents. Children. 2022;9(7):1001.
24. Eriksson J, Ekerljung L, Ronmark E, et al. Rhinitis phenotypes corelates with different sympromes and risk factor patterns of asthma. Respir Med. 2011;105:1611–21.
25. Gershon AS, Wang C, Guan J, et al. Burden of comorbidity in individuals with asthma. Thorax. 2010;66:612–8.
26. Dixon AE, Kaminsky DA, Holbrook JT, et al. Allergic rhinitis and sinusitis in asthma: differential effects on symptoms and pulmonary function. Chest. 2006;130:429–35.
27. Sigurdardottir ST, Jonasson K, Clausen M, et al. Prevalence and early-life risk factors of school-age allergic multimorbidity: the EuroPrevall-iFAAM birth cohort. Allergy. 2021;76:2855–65.
28. Won H-K, Kim Y-C, Kang M-G, et al. Age-related prevalence of chronic rhinosinusitis and nasal polyps and their relationships with asthma onset. Ann Allergy Asthma Immunol. 2018;120(4):389–94.
29. Keller T, Hohmann C, Standl M, et al. The sex-shift in single disease and multimorbid asthma and rhinitis during puberty—a study by MeDALL. Allergy. 2018;73(3):602–14.
30. Wang X, Zhang N, Bo M, et al. Diversity of TH cytokine profiles in patients with chronic rhinosinusitis: a multicenter study in Europe, Asia, and Oceania. J Allergy Clin Immunol. 2016;138:1344–53.
31. Berger M, Geng B, Cameron DW, et al. Primary immune deficiency diseases as unrecognized causes of chronic respiratory disease. Respir Med. 2017;132:181–8.
32. Nguyen-Ngoc-Quynh L, Nguyen-Thi-Thanh M, Nguyen-Thi-Phuong M, et al. Clinical-functional characteristics of children with asthma and obstructive sleep apnea overlap associated with attention deficit hyperactivity disorder: a cross-sectional study. Front Neurol. 2023;13:1097202.
33. Ullman N, Mirra V. Asthma differential diagnosis and comorbidities. Front Pediatr. 2018;3(6):276.
34. Fretzayas A, Moustaki M, Loukou I. Differentiating vocal cord dysfunction from asthma. J Asthma Allergy. 2017;10:277–83.
35. Traister R, Fajt ML, Whitman-Purves E, et al. A retrospective analysis comparing subjects with isolated and co-existent vocal cord dysfunction and asthma. J Allergy Clin Immunol. 2013;131:AB63.
36. Wenzel M. Gasping for a diagnosis: pediatric vocal cord dysfunction. J Pediatr Health Care. 2019;33(1):5–13.
37. Weinberger M, Abu-Hasan M. Pseudo-asthma: when cough, wheezing, and dyspnea are not asthma. Pediatrics. 2007;120:855–64.
38. Staikunienè J, Vaitkus S, Marija L, et al. Association of chronic rhinosinusitis with nasal polyps and asthma: clinical and radiological features, allergy and inflammation markers. Medicina (Kaunas). 2008;44:257–65.
39. Ginis T, Akcan FA, Capanoglu M, et al. The frequency of sleep-disordered breathing in children with asthma and its effects on asthma control. J Asthma. 2017;54:403–10.

40. Nguyen-Hoang Y, Nguyen-Thi-Dieu T, Duong-Quy S. Study of the clinical and functional characteristics of asthmatic children with obstructive sleep apnea. J Asthma Allergy. 2017;10:285–92.
41. Braido F, Baiardini I, Lacedonia D, on behalf of the Italian Society of Respiratory Medicine (SIMeR). Sleep apnea risk in subjects with asthma with or without comorbid rhinitis. Respir Care. 2014;59(12):1851–6.
42. Desager KN, Nelen V, Weyler JJ, et al. Sleep disturbance and daytime symptoms in wheezing school-aged children. J Sleep Res. 2005;14(1):77–82.
43. Meltzer EO, Blaiss MS, Derebery MJ, et al. Burden of allergic rhinitis: results from the pediatric allergies in America survey. J Allergy Clin Immunol. 2009;124:43–70.
44. Ohta K, Bousquet PJ, Aizawa H, et al. Prevalence and impact of rhinitis in asthma. SACRA, a cross-sectional nation-wide study in Japan. Allergy. 2011;66:1287–95.
45. de Groot EP, Nijkamp A, Duiverman EJ, et al. Allergic rhinitis is associated with poor asthma control in children with asthma. Thorax. 2012;67(7):582–7.
46. Settipane RJ, Hagy GW, Settipane GA. Long-term risk factors for developing asthma and allergy rhinitis: a 23-year follow-up study of college students. Allergy Proc. 1994;15:21–5.
47. Bousquet J, Khaltaev N, Cruz AA, et al. Allergic rhinitis and its impact on asthma (ARIA) 2008 update (in collaboration with World Health Organization, GA(2)LEN and AllerGen). Allergy. 2008;63(86):8–160.
48. Bousqet J, Hellings PW, Agache I, et al. ARIA 2016: care pathways implementing emerging technologies for predictive medicine in rhinitis and asthma across the life cycle. Clin Transl Allergy. 2016;6:47.
49. Compalati E, Ridolo E, Passalacqua G, et al. The link between allergic rinitis and asthma: the united airways disease. Expert Rev Clin Immunol. 2010;6:413–23.
50. Yorgancıoğlu AA, Gemicioğlu B, Cingi C, et al. 2019 ARIA Care pathways for allergic rhinitis-Turkey. Turk Thorac J. 2020;21(2):122–33.
51. Schmitt J, Wüstenberg E, Küster D, et al. The moderating role of allergy immunotherapy in asthma progression: results of a population-based cohort study. Allergy. 2020;75(3):596–602.
52. Heath J, Hartzell L, Putt C, et al. Chronic rhinosinusitis in children: pathophysiology, evaluation, and medical management. Curr Allergy Asthma Rep. 2018;18:37.
53. Ramadan HH, Chaiban R, Makary C. Pediatric rhinosinusitis. Pediatr Clin N Am. 2022;69(2):275–86.
54. Tomassen P, Vandeplas G, Van Zele T, et al. Inflammatory endotypes of chronic rhinosinusitis based on cluster analysis of biomarkers. J Allergy Clin Immunol. 2016;137:1449–56.
55. Valovirta E, Pawankar R. Survey on the impact of comorbid allergic rhinitis in patients with asthma. BMC Pulm Med. 2006;6:S3.
56. Coumou H, Westerhof GA, de Nijs SB, et al. Predictors of accelerated decline in lung function in adult-onset asthma. Eur Respir J. 2018;51:1701785.
57. Dykewitcz MS, Wallace DW, Amrol DJ, et al. Rhinitis 2020: a practice parameter update. J Allergy Clin Immunol. 2020;146(4):721–67.
58. Fokkens W, Lund V, Hopkins C. European position paper on rhinosinusitis and nasal polyps 2020. Rhinology. 2020;58(Suppl S29):1–464.
59. Carr TF, Koterba AP, Chandra R, et al. Characterization of specific antibody deficiency in adults with medically refractory chronic rhinosinusitis. Am J Rhinol Allergy. 2011;25:241–4.
60. Tosca MA, Riccio AM, Marseglia GL, et al. Nasal endoscopy in asthmatic children: assessment of rhinosinusitis and adenoiditis incidence, correlations with cytology and microbiology. Clin Exp Allergy. 2001;31:609–15.
61. Mehta V, Campeau NG, Kita H, Hagan JB. Blood and sputum eosinophil levels in asthma and their relationship to sinus computed tomographic findings. Mayo Clin Proc. 2008;83(6):671–8.
62. Fokkens WJ, Lund VJ, Mulloy J, et al. European position paper on rhinosinusitis and nasal polyps 2012. Rhinol Suppl. 2012;23:3.
63. Fokkens W, Lund V, Mullol J. European position paper on rhinosinusitis and nasal polyps 2007. Rhinol Suppl. 2007;20:1–136.

64. Wu W, Bleecker E, Moore W, et al. Unsupervised phenotyping of severe asthma research program participants using expanded lung data. J Allergy Clin Immunol. 2015;133:1280–8.
65. Rachelefsky GS, Katz RM, Siegel SC. Chronic sinus disease with associated reactive airway disease in children. Pediatrics. 1984;73(4):526–9.
66. Gevaert P, Calus L, Van Zele T, et al. Omalizumab is effective in allergic and nonallergic patients with nasal polyps and asthma. J Allergy Clin Immunol. 2013;131:110–6.e1.
67. American Lung Association–Asthma Clinical Research Centers' Writing Committee, Dixon AE, Castro M, Cohen RI, et al. Efficacy of nasal mometasone for the treatment of chronic sinonasal disease in patients with inadequately controlled asthma. J Allergy Clin Immunol. 2015;135(3):701–9.

Hemoptysis in Children: ENT-Related Etiologies

32

Muge Ozcelik Korkmaz, Cemal Cingi, and Kamil Janeczek

32.1 Introduction

Spitting up blood from the lungs or bronchial tubes due to pulmonary or bronchial bleeding is known as hemoptysis. Based on the amount of blood lost, hemoptysis is categorized as either non-massive or massive; however, there is no consensus on what constitutes a "massive" hemoptysis. A daily blood loss of less than 200 mL is not considered substantial in this article. Both the pulmonary and bronchial arteries supply blood to the lungs. Hemostasis from the bronchi, which is under systemic pressure, is often more profuse than that from the lungs, which are under low pressure [1]. When making a diagnosis, the volume of blood loss is less helpful than when it comes to guiding treatment [2].

Hemoptysis is the term used to describe the coughing up of blood from the lungs. Hemoptysis can be mimicked by expectorating blood from the upper respiratory system, nasopharynx, or upper digestive tract [3].

M. O. Korkmaz
Department of Otorhinolaryngology, Medar Hospital, Sakarya, Türkiye

C. Cingi (✉)
Medical Faculty, Department of Otorhinolaryngology, Eskisehir Osmangazi University, Eskisehir, Turkey

K. Janeczek
Department of Pulmonary Diseases and Children Rheumatology, Medical University of Lublin, Lublin, Poland
e-mail: kamil.janeczek@umlub.pl

H. Yüksel et al. (eds.), *Pediatric Airway Diseases*, Comprehensive ENT,
https://doi.org/10.1007/978-3-031-74853-0_32

32.2 Severity of Hemoptysis

The severity of hemoptysis is not universally agreed upon. Although an estimate of the amount of hemoptysis is helpful, other patient features and clinical judgment [4, 5] are more critical in determining the best course of treatment.

Hemoptysis will be classified according to the following scale (out of 6) for this review:

- ***Scant***: Less than 5 mL (such as blood streaks) is considered "scant."
- ***Mild to moderate***: No signs of hemodynamic instability or compromised gas exchange; mild to moderate (5–200 mL within 24 h).
- ***Massive***: In the case of life-threatening or catastrophic bleeding, the amount lost must be greater than around 200 mL in less than 24 h, and there must be signs of hemodynamic instability (tachycardia, hypotension), aberrant gas exchange, difficulties keeping a patent airway, and highly rapid bleeding.

One of the most prevalent causes of hemoptysis in children is cystic fibrosis (CF), and the volume estimates given above are based in part on a consensus guideline produced for individuals with CF [6]. There is no universal threshold for what constitutes life-threatening or massive hemoptysis in adults. We use a threshold of around 200 mL, slightly lower than the threshold proposed by the CF consensus guideline (240 mL). Massive hemoptysis in younger children lacks volume estimates. Regardless, these cutoffs are approximations at best and should be considered only one part of a comprehensive clinical evaluation. It is important to remember that hemoptysis volume estimations are frequently inaccurate, do not take patient size into account, and have a limited correlation with the source of hemoptysis and clinical outcomes [3].

If feasible, firsthand observation of the bloody sputum and in-depth questioning of the patient and caretakers is necessary to evaluate its volume and appearance. Hemodynamic stability, estimated blood volume loss, and rate of bleeding are all included in the global clinical evaluation to determine the severity (minimal, severe, or fatal).

32.2.1 Non-massive Hemoptysis

Patient therapy for hemoptysis should focus on three main areas: stopping the bleeding, preventing aspiration, and treating the underlying cause. In the event of a medical emergency, the first step is always to check the "ABCs" (airway, breathing, and circulation) [2].

Acute, moderate hemoptysis due to bronchitis is the most prevalent presenting symptom. It is possible to treat low-risk individuals with normal chest radiographs as outpatients with strict supervision and suitable oral medications. An outpatient assessment by a pulmonologist should be undertaken if hemoptysis continues or is otherwise unexplained [2].

If a chest x-ray reveals an atypical mass, a bronchoscopic evaluation can be performed as an outpatient. To rule out neoplasm, outpatient fiberoptic bronchoscopy may also be necessary for patients with a normal chest radiograph and risk factors for lung cancer or recurrent hemoptysis. A high-resolution CT scan is warranted when sputum and bronchoscopy fail to reveal pathology despite a clinical suspicion of malignancy. A high-resolution CT scan is also justified when a chest X-ray indicates peripheral or other parenchymal illness [2].

32.2.2 Massive Hemoptysis

Massive hemoptysis fatality rates vary according to the severity and cause of the bleeding. Massive hemoptysis, defined as more than 1000 mL of blood lost in 24 h, is associated with an 80% fatality rate [7]. These individuals need immediate attention and a pulmonologist's opinion. Hemostasis of catastrophic or life-threatening proportions requires close medical attention. Because asphyxiation, not bleeding to death, is the leading cause of mortality, it is crucial to keep the airway open. Resuscitation measures such as providing more oxygen and fluids are essential. Since immediate surgical intervention may be required [2], getting help from a cardiothoracic surgeon is recommended.

32.3 Differential Diagnosis of Hemoptysis

Source other than the lower respiratory tract
• Upper airway (nasopharyngeal) bleeding
• Gastrointestinal bleeding [2]
Tracheobronchial source
• Neoplasm (bronchogenic carcinoma, endobronchial metastatic tumor, Kaposi's sarcoma, bronchial carcinoid)
• Bronchitis (acute or chronic)
• Bronchiectasis
• Broncholithiasis
• Airway trauma
• Foreign body [2]
Pulmonary parenchymal source
• Lung abscess
• Pneumonia
• Tuberculosis
• Mycetoma ("fungus ball")
• Goodpasture's syndrome
• Idiopathic pulmonary hemosiderosis
• Wegener's granulomatosis
• Lupus pneumonitis
• Long contusion [2]
Primary vascular source

• Arteriovenous malformation.
• Pulmonary embolism.
• Elevated pulmonary venous pressure (especially mitral stenosis).
• Pulmonary artery rupture secondary to balloon-tip pulmonary artery catheter manipulation [2]
Miscellaneous and rare causes
• Pulmonary endometriosis
• Systemic coagulopathy or use of anticoagulants or thrombolytic agents [2]

32.4 Diagnostic Evaluation

Critical blood tests (complete blood count and coagulation profile) and a chest radiograph are the initial stages in the assessment for most children presenting with hemoptysis. The results of the history and physical are used to make further diagnoses [3].

32.4.1 History

If the etiology of the hemoptysis is unclear, a complete medical history should be obtained when the patient has stabilized. The following six findings may help in determining the etiology of hemoptysis:

32.4.1.1 Infection Warning Signs

- Tracheobronchitis, pneumonia, and bronchiectasis are frequently diagnosed when blood is present in mucopurulent sputum.
- Pneumonia is suspected when there is a fever, chills, and purulent, bloody sputum.
- Anaerobic lung abscess is suspected when sputum has a putrid odor.

32.4.1.2 Choking

Even if the choking event happened days or weeks before the hemoptysis, a foreign body in the trachea or airway should be considered.

32.4.1.3 Exposures

These risk factors have been linked to hemoptysis:

- Illegal narcotics, especially cocaine, and similar inhalants.
- Nicotine or cannabis smoking can cause pneumonia-like lung symptoms [8].
- Phenytoin, retinoic acid, amiodarone, propylthiouracil, and penicillamine are all linked to an increased risk of alveolar hemorrhage.
- Medications that lower platelet counts or otherwise interfere with normal platelet function.
- Breathing in nitrogen dioxide fumes from broken ice resurfacing and ventilation equipment at a hockey rink.

- Travel and exposure—Find out whether they have ever visited or lived where TB is common or have had any recent contact with homeless people, inmates, institutions, or migrant workers. Inquire about any trips to regions known to harbor endemic mycoses or comparable exposures (such as participation in archaeological digs or spelunking) [3].

32.4.1.4 Underlying Medical Problems

Symptoms or diagnoses that point to a more serious medical issue are considered "underlying medical problems" [3].

- Trauma.
- Easy bruising, menorrhagia, or a history of bleeding that suggests a problem (such as von Willebrand disease).
- Degenerative lung or heart disease.
- Bronchiectasis is sometimes linked to systemic symptoms of collagen vascular diseases or vasculitis syndromes.
- Hematuria, which may be indicative of pulmonary-renal syndrome.

32.4.2 Physical Examination

Hemoptysis may be diagnosed based on several clues gleaned from a thorough physical examination, some of which are included in this section.

- Chest or neck bruises (a sign of trauma).
- Crepitus indicates obstruction of the airway.
- Hemangioma or telangiectasia (both of which point to arteriovenous malformations).
- Clubbed fingers (which may indicate chronic obstructive pulmonary illness, pulmonary arteriovenous malformations, or congenital heart defects).
- A lost tooth can be inhaled, especially if the kid is sleeping. It can cause bleeding in the oral cavity or nasopharynx, elevating the possibility of foreign body aspiration.
- Infectious conditions, foreign body aspiration, and localized airway, or parenchymal hemorrhage can all lead to aberrant breath sounds.

32.4.3 Laboratory Evaluation

Patients experiencing hemoptysis of at least moderate severity (5 mL blood) and unclear etiology should see a pediatric pulmonologist. These people should have routine testing for [3] conditions:

Undiagnosed hemoptysis in children [3]:

- A complete blood count.

- Coagulation tests must be performed to rule out von Willebrand disease (plasma von Willebrand factor antigen, von Willebrand factor activity, and factor VIII activity).
- Sputum should be cultured for bacteria, fungi, and viruses, and acid-fast bacilli should be stained if possible.
- Screening for hematuria using urinalysis.

32.4.4 Imaging

Radiographs of the chest taken traditionally should include at least two different angles. Parenchymal and alveolar opacities may be seen on radiographs if there has been a hemorrhage, and these opacities may be widespread or localized to one area of the lungs. Similar symptoms may present themselves in cases of nonpulmonary blood aspiration.

Some of the characteristics that point to a particular cause of bleeding are [3]:

Hyperinflation, volume loss, or localized pneumonia are all symptoms of endobronchial blockage that a foreign body may cause if it is radiopaque.

- Cavitations (which may indicate TB, a fungal infection, or granulomatosis with polyangiitis).
- Bronchiectasis—until the condition is well advanced, plain radiography has limited sensitivity for identifying bronchiectasis. A "tram-track" look has been associated with severe bronchiectasis.

Radiographs may seem normal in as much as one-third of infants with hemoptysis [9, 10].

Patients with moderate or severe hemoptysis for whom a focused history, physical, and chest radiograph have failed to yield an explanation should undergo additional evaluation using computed tomography (CT) of the chest with contrast by multidetector CT angiography [3].

The CT angiography procedure should be tailored to view the bronchial arteries since they are the most common sites of pulmonary bleeding. This method should be enough if you are checking for pulmonary embolism in the pulmonary arterial circulation [11]. Alveolar hemorrhage often presents as "ground-glass" opacities in the perivascular regions, and CT angiography will also allow evaluation of the airways and lung parenchyma. The CT scan has the potential to detect airway and vascular abnormalities.

Pulmonary arteriography should be investigated if a significant suspicion of vascular abnormalities remains despite a negative CT scan. Bronchial arteriography may help pinpoint the source of bleeding and make bronchial artery embolization (BAE) [12] more effective in cases of significant hemoptysis.

32.5 Hemoptysis: 32.5% of Cases had an ENT Cause

32.5.1 Respiratory Illness

Sixty to seventy percent of instances of hemoptysis may be attributed to infection. Infection produces inflammation and edema of the superficial mucosa, which can result in the rupture of the superficial blood vessels. Bronchitis was the leading cause of hemoptysis in a retrospective analysis [13] of inpatient and outpatient cases in the United States, followed by pneumonia (10%) and TB (8%). Most cases of hemoptysis are caused by infection with bacteria like Staphylococcus aureus or Pseudomonas aeruginosa or fungi like Aspergillus species. Severe hemoptysis can also be caused by viruses like influenza [14]. Patients with human immunodeficiency virus (HIV) infection are more likely to develop pulmonary Kaposi's sarcoma [2, 15], one of numerous illnesses that can cause hemoptysis.

In children without pulmonary, cardiac, hematologic, or neoplastic illness, infection is the leading cause of hemoptysis.

Infections, including TB, aspergilloma, and acute endemic mycoses, are common causes of hemoptysis. Hemoptysis is not prevalent in children with these infections since cavitary illness is rare in this age group [16, 17].

In addition, hemoptysis can be caused by a pulmonary infection with a common community-acquired bacterium, such as Staphylococcus, Streptococcus, Klebsiella, or Pseudomonas [18, 19]. Significant bleeding can be a symptom of the influenza virus, especially the H1N1 strain of the disease [20–22]. Evidence suggests that the immunothrombosis pathophysiology of pneumonia caused by coronavirus disease 2019 (COVID-19) can lead to alveolar bleeding [23, 24].

Finally, any acute respiratory illness that induces vigorous coughing might result in mild hemoptysis (blood-streaked sputum) due to mechanical stress on the airway. Hemoptysis of this sort typically resolves on its own [3].

32.5.2 Aspiration of a Non-native Body

Children under three are at the most risk for foreign body aspiration. Most children aspirate do not have symptoms associated with the incident until days or weeks later, when they may appear with wheezing (typically monophonic and occasionally unilateral), persistent cough, pneumonia, or hemoptysis [25]. A history of choking strongly suggests foreign body aspiration. However, the patient may not remember the episode when they present [3].

32.5.3 Trauma

Suctioning past the tracheal entrance of the tube can cause mucosal damage to the central airways and bloody sputum in children who have an endotracheal tube or tracheostomy. Very minimal bleeding occurs; this is not considered clinically significant. Humidification, soft suction catheters, and controlled suction lengths can help protect the mucosa from further injury and possibly even stop bleeding. Children who require a tracheostomy for an extended period may also experience granulation tissue formation, resulting in mild hemoptysis [3].

Bronchoscopy results may include mucosal abrasions or granulation tissue in around 10% of these children, indicating that the bleeding is more extensive than initially thought.

It is incredibly uncommon for significant hemoptysis to develop as a result of an airway tube eroding into a big vessel in the mediastinum or tracheal wall; nonetheless, some case reports describe presentations with bouts of non-massive "sentinel" bleeding [26–28]. Patients who have undergone a tracheostomy should have any signs of profuse bleeding assessed immediately by a surgical expert, usually using fiberoptic endoscopy [3].

Adult studies show that bleeding during transbronchial biopsies occurs in 0.26–5.0% of instances and is seldom significant in these people.

32.5.4 Hemoptysis Mimics

Hemoptysis is the term used to describe the expectoration of blood from the lungs. True hemoptysis [3] might be confused with bleeding from the upper respiratory tract, the oropharynx or nasopharynx, or the upper digestive tract (for example, from esophageal varices related to cirrhosis).

Children who produce injuries that seem like pulmonary bleeding on themselves have been described as having "factitious hemoptysis" [29]. A patient who appears with hemoptysis, odd symptoms, and a negative assessment [30] should be evaluated for Munchausen syndrome (or Munchausen syndrome via proxy).

References

1. Cahill BC, Ingbar DH. Massive hemoptysis. Assessment and management. Clin Chest Med. 1994;15:147–67.
2. Bidwell JL, Pachner RW. Hemoptysis: diagnosis and management. Am Fam Physician. 2005;72(7):1253–60.
3. Stillwell PC, Kupfer O. Hemoptysis in children. In: Mallory GB, Hoppin AG, editors. . UpToDate. Last updated: Feb 13, 2023.
4. Vece TJ, de Guzman MM, Langston C, Fan LL. Diffuse alveolar hemorrhage in children. In: Wilmott RW, Deterding R, Li A, Ratjen F, Sly P, editors. Kendig's disorders of the respiratory tract in children. 9th ed. Philadelphia, PA: Elsevier; 2018. p. 893.
5. Davidson K, Shojaee S. Managing massive hemoptysis. Chest. 2020;157:77.
6. Flume PA, Mogayzel PJ Jr, Robinson KA, et al. Cystic fibrosis pulmonary guidelines: pulmonary complications: hemoptysis and pneumothorax. Am J Respir Crit Care Med. 2010;182:298.
7. Jean-Baptiste E. Clinical assessment and management of massive hemoptysis. Crit Care Med. 2000;28:1642–7.
8. Reynolds C, Staples H. Hemoptysis in an adolescent with EVALI. Pediatr Pulmonol. 2022;57:2875.

9. Pianosi P, Al-sadoon H. Hemoptysis in children. Pediatr Rev. 1996;17:344.
10. Lichtenberger JP 3rd, Digumarthy SR, Abbott GF, et al. Diffuse pulmonary hemorrhage: clues to the diagnosis. Curr Probl Diagn Radiol. 2014;43:128.
11. Marquis KM, Raptis CA, Rajput MZ, et al. CT for evaluation of hemoptysis. Radiographics. 2021;41:742.
12. Noë GD, Jaffé SM, Molan MP. CT and CT angiography in massive haemoptysis with emphasis on pre-embolization assessment. Clin Radiol. 2011;66:869.
13. Reisz G, Stevens D, Boutwell C, Nair V. The causes of hemoptysis revisited. A review of the etiologies of hemoptysis between 1986 and 1995. Mo Med. 1997;94:633–5.
14. Bond D, Vyas H. Viral pneumonia and hemoptysis. Crit Care Med. 2001;29:2040–1.
15. Nelson JE, Forman M. Hemoptysis in HIV-infected patients. Chest. 1996;110:737–43.
16. Shaffer JP, Barson W, Luquette M, et al. Massive hemoptysis as the presenting manifestation in a child with histoplasmosis. Pediatr Pulmonol. 1997;24:57.
17. Morris SK, Giroux RJP, Consunji-Araneta R, et al. Epidemiology, clinical features and outcomes of incident tuberculosis in children in Canada in 2013-2016: results of a national surveillance study. Arch Dis Child. 2021;106:1165.
18. Chiel L, Welsh S, Andren K, et al. Pediatric hemoptysis without bronchiectasis or cardiac disease: etiology, recurrence, and mortality. J Pediatr. 2019;214:66.
19. Carteaux G, Contou D, Voiriot G, et al. Severe hemoptysis associated with bacterial pulmonary infection: clinical features, significance of parenchymal necrosis, and outcome. Lung. 2018;196:33.
20. Haura L, Warachit B, Makkoch J, Poovorawan Y. Hemoptysis in children with pandemic influenza H1N1 2009 infection. Southeast Asian J Trop Med Public Health. 2009;40:1259.
21. Del Bianco R, Santos MS, Ribeiro MC, et al. Clinical aspects of influenza A (H1N1) in HIV-infected individuals in São Paulo during the pandemic of 2009. Braz J Infect Dis. 2011;15:170.
22. Gilbert CR, Vipul K, Baram M. Novel H1N1 influenza A viral infection complicated by alveolar hemorrhage. Respir Care. 2010;55:623.
23. Potus F, Mai V, Lebret M, et al. Novel insights on the pulmonary vascular consequences of COVID-19. Am J Physiol Lung Cell Mol Physiol. 2020;319:L277.
24. Fireizen Y, Shahriary C, Imperial ME, et al. Pediatric P-ANCA vasculitis following COVID-19. Pediatr Pulmonol. 2021;56:3422.
25. Foltran F, Ballali S, Rodriguez H, et al. Inhaled foreign bodies in children: a global perspective on their epidemiological, clinical, and preventive aspects. Pediatr Pulmonol. 2013;48:344.
26. Ghai B, Makkar JK, Bakshi J, et al. Survival of a child without sequelae after tracheoarterial fistula. Paediatr Anaesth. 2007;17:588.
27. Ideno S, Shinto A, Matsuoka T, et al. Two cases of emergency extracorporeal membrane oxygenation support in children suffering from Tracheo-innominate artery fistula. Masui. 2016;65:146.
28. Jesus LE, Silva EWGMD, Balieiro M, et al. Post-tracheostomy tracheoinnominate fistula: endovascular treatment. Rev Paul Pediatr. 2021;40:e2020229.
29. Sood M, Clarke JR, Murphy MS. Covert biting of the buccal mucosa masquerading as haematemesis or haemoptysis in children. Acta Paediatr. 1999;88:1038.
30. Bjornson CL, Kirk VG. Munchausen's syndrome presenting as hemoptysis in a 12-year-old girl. Can Respir J. 2001;8:439.

Part IV

Pediatric Pulmonology Disease Specific Upper Respiratory Tract Involvement

Airway Inflammation: United Airway in Children

33

Mahir Serbes, Renato Cutrera, and Derya Altıntaş

33.1 Introduction

United airway disease (UAD) in children describes the shared epidemiologic, pathophysiologic, and clinical evidence that revealed the strong relationship among the most frequent and chronic inflammatory diseases of the upper and lower airways including allergic rhinitis (AR), chronic rhinosinusitis (CRS), and asthma (Table 33.1) [2, 4]. This concept proposes that these diseases are manifestations of a single unified airway inflammatory process and inflammation in one part of the airway will likely stimulate a similar reaction throughout the rest of the airway. Due to recent scientific improvements in the knowledge of mechanisms for chronic inflammation of both upper and lower airways, the concept of a single disease has been replaced by syndromes encompassing complex biological networks of distinct and interrelating inflammatory pathways (endotypes) with variable clinical presentations (phenotypes) [3].

The aim of this section was to provide a better understanding of the common pathophysiologic mechanisms of airway inflammation supporting the link between the so-called UAD in children.

M. Serbes · D. Altıntaş (✉)
Department of Pediatric Immunology and Allergy, Cukurova University, School of Medicine, Adana, Turkey

R. Cutrera
Department of Pediatric Medicine, IRCCS Bambino Gesù Children's Hospital, Rome, Italy

H. Yüksel et al. (eds.), *Pediatric Airway Diseases*, Comprehensive ENT, https://doi.org/10.1007/978-3-031-74853-0_33

Table 33.1 Evidence and mechanisms of the nose and lung interaction supporting UAD

Histological evidence[a]	Epidemiologic evidence	Pathophysiologic evidence	Clinical evidence
– The mucosa of the upper and lower airways is similar, with pseudostratified epithelium with columnar, ciliated cells located on a basement membrane. In the submucosa, there are vessels, mucus glands, fibroblasts, and some inflammatory cells [1] – Both act as transport systems moving air in and out of the lungs – Both provide defense against inhaled foreign substances	– The prevalence of AR appears to be at least triple the prevalence of asthma, and 19–38% of patients with AR have concomitant asthma, and 30–80% of asthmatics have AR [2, 3] – About 20% of patients with CRS manifest asthma, a prevalence of approximately 2–3 times greater than that of the general population. CRSwNP is more commonly associated with lower tract respiratory disorders, such as asthma and nonspecific bronchial hyper-reactivity [2] – Comorbid rhinitis/ rhinosinusitis worsens asthma outcomes [3, 4] – Colonization with S aureus and the presence of specific IgE to S. aureus enterotoxins (SAEs) were significantly higher in those patients who had both CRSwNP and asthma (66.7% and 53.8%, respectively) [5]	– The communication between the upper and lower airways is suggested to be via a bone marrow-derived systemic inflammatory response [6] – The presence of epithelial basement membrane thickening, the typical hallmark of the lower airway remodeling, not only in asthmatic patients but also in atopic patients without asthma and patients with AR [7] – In non-allergic asthma, it has been highlighted the importance of the presence of IgE in the bronchial mucosa, as in the nasal mucosa in local allergic rhinitis [8] – In a 2010 cross-sectional study, it was found that sputum eosinophilia was associated with a 52 times increase in the odds of nasal eosinophilia – Specific antibodies to SAEs can induce basophil degranulation and mast cell activation, providing another possible mechanism by which S aureus could contribute to chronic type 2 inflammation [3, 4]	– The treatment of AR can improve asthma symptoms [2] – Leukotriene receptor antagonists are known to be useful for long-term management of asthma patients complicated by AR [8] – The recombinant, humanized, monoclonal anti-IgE antibody omalizumab improved nasal and bronchial symptoms and reduced unscheduled visits due to asthma [8] – Allergen immunotherapy is effective for treating both rhinitis and asthma [8]

CRSwNP chronic rhinosinusitis with nasal polyps

[a] The absence of smooth muscles in the upper airways and the lack of extensive subepithelial capillaries, arterial systems, and venous cavernous sinusoids in the lower airways are the histological differences between upper and lower airways

33.2 Pathophysiologic Mechanisms Underlying the Relationship Between Rhinitis/Rhinosinusitis and Asthma

Local Mechanisms (1, 2, 3): Over the years, several local and systemic mechanisms explaining the interaction between the upper and lower airways have been proposed [1, 2, 4, 6]. These are summarized in Fig. 33.1. ***Mouth Breathing (1):*** In individuals with rhinitis/rhinosinusitis, the nose may be obstructed, and mouth breathing is favored, thereby eliminating this vital upper airway defense mechanism. This abnormal breathing (excluding the passage of air through the sinus system and the loss of function of inflamed/infected sinuses) compromises air warming, humidification, and purification from pollutants and irritants, allowing physical and chemical agents to have an impact on the lower airways [2, 6]. In addition, the impairment of air filtering in the presence of sinus disease may increase allergen load reaching the bronchi in allergic patients. Baraldi et al. have proposed a novel and intriguing pathogenetic hypothesis that nitric oxide, which is thought to have a modulating effect on bronchial tone and is an important host-defense molecule, is decreased during sinusitis, and that decreased physiologic autoinhalation may play a role in increasing bronchial reactivity and susceptibility to infection [2, 6]. ***Aspiration of Nasal Contents (2):*** The concept that inflammatory secretions from the upper airway of patients with rhinitis or rhinosinusitis are aspirated into the lower airway with negative consequences has traditionally been regarded as one of the primary mechanisms underlying lower airway symptoms. The few available studies, however, have not conclusively supported this hypothesis [2, 9]. ***Neural Reflexes (3):*** The presence and significance of a sinonasal-bronchial reflex, characterized by bronchoconstriction triggered by the activation of a trigeminal afferent-vagal efferent neural pathway, remains a topic of debate in human studies, despite being extensively documented in animal models [6, 9]. Rolla et al. demonstrated that damage to the pharyngeal mucosa in patients with CRS (likely mediated by the drainage of inflammatory mediators and cells and/or infected material) increased the sub-mucosal nerve's exposure to irritants, thereby activating the reflex arc [10].

Systemic (Immunological) Mechanisms (4): A large body of evidence suggests that allergic inflammation developing in the respiratory mucosa (due to allergen and/or other irritant agent exposure) may result in systemic inflammatory events and that the nose and bronchi are linked through the systemic circulation. The inflammatory process in the airways is strengthened and spread beyond its initial site by the release of immune cells and mediators from the bone marrow and other lymphoid organs. Despite the potential variability in the underlying causes, it is widely believed that the primary factor responsible for immune-mediated inflammatory mechanisms in both the upper and lower airways is the presence of widespread eosinophilic infiltration of the inflamed mucosa, which is attributed to a prevalent Th2 immune response [3, 4, 6] (Fig. 33.1).

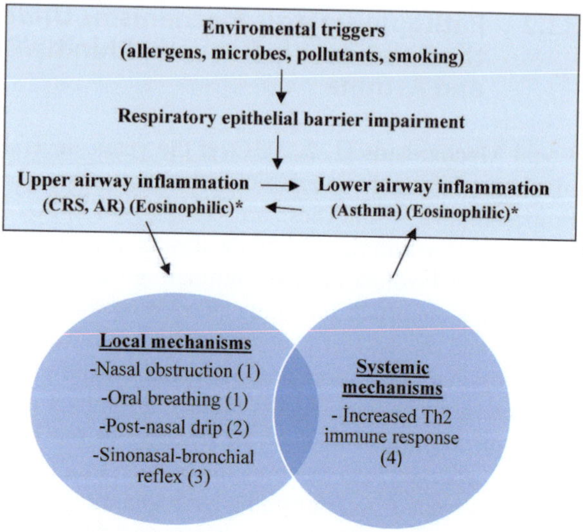

Fig. 33.1 Overview of the complex interplay between immunological (systemic) and local mechanisms (post-nasal drip, neural reflexes, mouth breathing) in patients with asthma and rhinosinusitis, according to the United Airway Disease theory (*: prevalent inflammation endotype)

33.3 Phenoendotypes of United Airway Disease Based on Inflammation

The archetype of UAD is allergic asthma-allergic rhinitis, but emerging evidence suggests that UAD is a heterogeneous condition with multiple phenotypes (observable clinical characteristics) and endotypes (pathobiological mechanisms). To improve outcomes in the classification and management of UAD, currently known phenoendotypes of UAD are proposed, in which pathophysiological mechanisms and biomarkers related to disease are identified and targeted for treatment (Table 33.2) [8, 11].

Table 33.2 Phenoendotypes of united airway disease (UAD) based on airway inflammation type

Inflammation type	Endotype	Clinical phenotype: Lower airway	Clinical phenotype: Upper airway	Assessment method/ biomarker[a]
Eosinophilic, Th2-high type	Th2, IL-4, IL-5, IL-13	CRSwNP	Eosinophilic asthma	Blood periostin, high FENO, sputum, and blood eosinophilia
Allergic, systemic	IgE-mediated	Allergic rhinitis	Allergic asthma	Blood total IgE and specific IgE, skin prick tests
Allergic, local	IgE-mediated	Local allergic rhinitis	Intrinsic asthma	Local nasal and bronchial mucosa-specific IgE
Non-allergic eosinophilic	IL-25, IL-33, TSLP, group 2 innate lymphoid cells (ILC2)	Non-allergic rhinitis with eosinophilia	Adult-onset eosinophilic asthma	Blood periostin, high FENO, sputum, and blood eosinophilia
Neutrophilic, Th2-low type	Th1, Th17, IL-17	CRsNP, Infectious rhinitis	Neutrophilic asthma, COPD	Blood IL-8 and IL-17, sputum neutrophilia

CRSwNP chronic rhinosinusitis with nasal polyps, *CRSsNP* chronic rhinosinusitis without nasal polyps, *FENO* fractional exhaled nitric oxide, *TSLP* thymic stromal lymphopoietin, *COPD* chronic obstructive pulmonary disease

[a] Serum normal periostin level is 10 $ng \cdot mL^{-1}$; a higher level identifies an inflammatory status. Blood and sputum eosinophil count of >2% or >300 cells/uL identifies airway eosinophilia (blood eosinophil count <150 cells/uL indicates low likelihood of airway eosinophilia), sputum neutrophil count ≥65% or >500 cells/10^4 mL identifies airway neutrophilia (cut-off <40% indicates low likelihood of airway neutrophilia). A FENO value <25 ppb (<20 ppb in children) is considered normal, while levels >50 ppb (>35 ppb in children) are indicative of eosinophilic inflammation. Elevated serum total IgE levels (IgE >30 and <1500 IU/mL) and positive specific IgE to at least one aeroallergen identify allergic inflammation in children (age ≥6 years) [8, 11, 12]

33.4 Pathways of Airway Inflammation in United Airway Disease

The role of airway inflammation in the development of UAD is significant and is frequently triggered by the activation of the airway epithelium due to various environmental factors such as microbes (including respiratory viruses and bacteria), pollutants, and allergens. It is a dynamic trait that changes over time and is influenced by factors such as treatment, infection, environmental exposures, and disease progression [12, 13]. The identification of the pathways of airway inflammation, which encompass intricate, interconnected, and overlapping cascades regulated by various proinflammatory cytokines, has yielded crucial and transformative knowledge regarding the specific endophenotypes of UAD [1, 11, 12]. To date, airway inflammation in the upper and lower airways is classified into 2 specific molecular pathways called *Th2-high type (eosinophilic)* and *Th2-low type (neutrophilic)*.

Th2-high inflammation is caused by both the adaptive and innate immune systems and contributes to the pathophysiology of several chronic upper and lower airway diseases, including asthma, COPD, CRSwNP, and allergic rhinitis [11, 14]. Th2 cells and group 2 innate lymphoid cells (ILC2) drive type 2 inflammation by producing type 2 cytokines such as interleukin (IL)-4, IL-5, and IL-13, as well as other inflammatory mediators [11, 14]. In the pathophysiology of type 2 inflammatory airway diseases, type 2 cytokines play a variety of roles. IL-5 is essential for the differentiation, maturation, mobilization, and survival of IL-5R+ eosinophil progenitors in the bone marrow. Furthermore, IL-5 promotes the development of other type 2 cells, which include mast cells and basophils [15]. Both IL-4 and IL-13 are involved in B-cell class switching and IgE production, which results in basophil and mast cell degranulation and the release of proinflammatory mediators, as well as barrier disruption and tissue remodeling [7, 11, 16]. Goblet-cell hyperplasia, mucus production, smooth muscle contractility, and hyperplasia are all impacted by IL-13 [11, 16]. Additionally, the development of mucus plugs as a result of mucus production is linked to IL-13-mediated damage to the epithelial barriers [17]. The trafficking of eosinophils to tissues is mediated by IL-4, IL-13, and IL-5 [11, 14–16]. Clinical symptoms of these common pathophysiological effects, which are caused by type 2 inflammation, include nasal polyps, loss of smell, nasal obstruction in allergic rhinitis and CRSwNP [18, 19], impaired lung function, wheezing, shortness of breath, chest tightness, and coughing in asthma [20]. Interleukin-5- and interleukin-13-producing group 2 innate lymphoid cells (ILC2s) have been identified as a novel subset of lymphocytes. These cells possess the ability to induce eosinophilic inflammation independently of adaptive immunity, including Th2 cells, B cells, and IgE antibodies. ILC2s are stimulated by cytokines IL-25, IL-33, and thymic stromal lymphopoietin (TSLP) that are derived from epithelial cells. These cytokines are released by epithelial cells in response to damage caused by various stimuli such as microbiota and pollutants [11, 14–16]. The corresponding phenoendotype in upper airways has been termed non-allergic rhinitis with eosinophilia syndrome (NARES) while termed non-allergic eosinophilic asthma in the lower airways in UAD (Table 33.2).

Th2-low inflammation is mainly characterized by neutrophils in nasal and bronchial mucosa [5, 21, 22]. Infections or chronic irritation, such as air pollution, can cause neutrophilic inflammation. This causes innate immune system dysregulation and activation of the IL-17 pathway, as well as neutrophil recruitment to the nasal and bronchial mucosa, which is known to be mediated by IL-8 [21, 22]. Furthermore, it has been observed that the type 1 immune response, metabolic and epigenetic factors, as well as the activation of the epithelial-mesenchymal trophic unit, can contribute to significant remodeling processes in the absence of inflammation. These factors have been recognized as influential elements in modulating neutrophilic inflammation [22, 23].

33.5 The Role of Airway Epithelium in United Airway Disease

This knowledge has been augmented by the realization of the significance of airway epithelium in inflammatory processes. The airway epithelium serves as a protective barrier and environmental sensor to triggers (allergens, pollutants, smoking, etc.) and is the first line of defense against insults inhaled. By stimulating innate and adaptive immune reactions, it promotes immunity. After epithelial damage or immune cell activation, it quickly activates epithelial cells to produce "upstream" alarmin epithelial cytokines, including IL-25, IL-33, and thymic stromal lymphopoietin (TSLP). These cytokines—TSLP in particular—provide master regulation of Th2 inflammation by guiding T-cell maturation along the Th2 cell pathway and triggering the production of downstream Th2 cytokines like IL-4, IL-5, and IL-13. Through Th1 and Th17, TSLP also contributes to inflammation that is Th2-low (neutrophilic). Remodeling of the airways also begins with the airway epithelium. The direct effects of TSLP on fibroblasts may aid in the remodeling of the airways [24, 25].

33.6 Conclusion

Complex, interactive, and redundant cascades of proinflammatory cytokines, including Th2-high, eosinophilic and Th2-low, neutrophilic inflammation, mediate airway inflammation in UAD. Consider united airway disease (UAD) in the differential diagnosis for patients presenting with both upper and lower airway inflammatory diseases. The research and efforts to better understand the pathophysiology, identify clinically useful diagnostic markers, and characterize inflammatory endotypes will result in more effective targeted therapeutics for individuals presenting with UAD.

References

1. Bachert C, Luong AU, Gevaert P, et al. The unified airway hypothesis: evidence from specific intervention with anti-IL-5 biologic therapy. J Allergy Clin Immunol Pract. 2023;11(9):2630–41. S2213-2198(23)00547-0. https://doi.org/10.1016/j.jaip.2023.05.011.
2. de Benedictis FM, Bush A. Janus looks both ways: how do the upper and lower airways interact? Paediatr Respir Rev. 2020;34:59–66. https://doi.org/10.1016/j.prrv.2019.06.004.
3. Ahmad JG, Marino MJ, Luong AU. Unified airway disease: future directions. Otolaryngol Clin North Am. 2023;56(1):181–95. https://doi.org/10.1016/j.otc.2022.09.014.
4. Poddighe D, Brambilla I, Licari A, Marseglia GL. Pediatric rhinosinusitis and asthma. Respir Med. 2018;141:94–9. https://doi.org/10.1016/j.rmed.2018.06.016.
5. De Greve G, Hellings PW, Fokkens WJ, Pugin B, Steelant B, Seys SF. Endotype-driven treatment in chronic upper airway diseases. Clin Transl Allergy. 2017;7:22. https://doi.org/10.1186/s13601-017-0157-8.
6. Kanda A, Kobayashi Y, Asako M, Tomoda K, Kawauchi H, Iwai H. Regulation of interaction between the upper and lower airways in United Airway disease. Med Sci (Basel). 2019;7(2):27. https://doi.org/10.3390/medsci7020027.
7. Samitas K, Carter A, Kariyawasam HH, Xanthou G. Upper and lower airway remodelling mechanisms in asthma, allergic rhinitis and chronic rhinosinusitis: the one airway concept revisited. Allergy. 2018;73(5):993–1002. https://doi.org/10.1111/all.13373.
8. Yii ACA, Tay TR, Choo XN, Koh MSY, Tee AKH, Wang DY. Precision medicine in united airways disease: a "treatable traits" approach. Allergy. 2018;73(10):1964–78. https://doi.org/10.1111/all.13496.

9. Lluncor M, Barranco P, Amaya ED, et al. Relationship between upper airway diseases, exhaled nitric oxide, and bronchial hyperresponsiveness to methacholine. J Asthma. 2019;56(1):53–60. https://doi.org/10.1080/02770903.2018.1429465.
10. Rolla G, Colagrande P, Scappaticci E, et al. Damage of the pharyngeal mucosa and hyperresponsiveness of airway in sinusitis. J Allergy Clin Immunol. 1997;100(1):52–7. https://doi.org/10.1016/s0091-6749(97)70194-5.
11. Maspero J, Adir Y, Al-Ahmad M, et al. Type 2 inflammation in asthma and other airway diseases. ERJ Open Res. 2022;8(3):00576–2021. https://doi.org/10.1183/23120541.00576-2021.
12. De Filippo M, Votto M, Licari A, et al. Novel therapeutic approaches targeting endotypes of severe airway disease. Expert Rev Respir Med. 2021;15(10):1303–16. https://doi.org/10.1080/17476348.2021.1937132.
13. Ricciardolo FLM, Guida G, Bertolini F, Di Stefano A, Carriero V. Phenotype overlap in the natural history of asthma. Eur Respir Rev. 2023;32(168):220201. https://doi.org/10.1183/16000617.0201-2022.
14. Busse WW, Viswanathan R. What has been learned by cytokine targeting of asthma? J Allergy Clin Immunol. 2022;150(2):235–49. https://doi.org/10.1016/j.jaci.2022.06.010.
15. Kuruvilla ME, Lee FE, Lee GB. Understanding asthma phenotypes, endotypes, and mechanisms of disease. Clin Rev Allergy Immunol. 2019;56(2):219–33. https://doi.org/10.1007/s12016-018-8712-1.
16. Akdis CA, Arkwright PD, Brüggen MC, et al. Type 2 immunity in the skin and lungs. Allergy. 2020;75(7):1582–605. https://doi.org/10.1111/all.14318.
17. Dunican EM, Elicker BM, Gierada DS, et al. Mucus plugs in patients with asthma linked to eosinophilia and airflow obstruction. J Clin Invest. 2018;128(3):997–1009. https://doi.org/10.1172/JCI95693.
18. Takabayashi T, Schleimer RP. Formation of nasal polyps: the roles of innate type 2 inflammation and deposition of fibrin. J Allergy Clin Immunol. 2020;145(3):740–50. https://doi.org/10.1016/j.jaci.2020.01.027.
19. Wise SK, Damask C, Roland LT, et al. International consensus statement on allergy and rhinology: allergic rhinitis—2023. Int Forum Allergy Rhinol. 2023;13(4):293–859. https://doi.org/10.1002/alr.23090.
20. Manti S, Licari A, Leonardi S, Marseglia GL. Management of asthma exacerbations in the paediatric population: a systematic review. Eur Respir Rev. 2021;30(161):200367. https://doi.org/10.1183/16000617.0367-2020.
21. Robinson D, Humbert M, Buhl R, et al. Revisiting type 2-high and type 2-low airway inflammation in asthma: current knowledge and therapeutic implications. Clin Exp Allergy. 2017;47(2):161–75. https://doi.org/10.1111/cea.12880.
22. Hammad H, Lambrecht BN. The basic immunology of asthma [published correction appears in Cell. 2021 Apr 29;184(9):2521-2522]. Cell. 2021;184(6):1469–85. https://doi.org/10.1016/j.cell.2021.02.016.
23. Fang L, Sun Q, Roth M. Immunologic and non-immunologic mechanisms leading to airway remodeling in asthma. Int J Mol Sci. 2020;21(3):757. https://doi.org/10.3390/ijms21030757.
24. Jakwerth CA, Ordovas-Montanes J, Blank S, Schmidt-Weber CB, Zissler UM. Role of respiratory epithelial cells in allergic diseases. Cells. 2022;11(9):1387. https://doi.org/10.3390/cells11091387.
25. Frey A, Lunding LP, Ehlers JC, Weckmann M, Zissler UM, Wegmann M. More than just a barrier: the immune functions of the airway epithelium in asthma pathogenesis. Front Immunol. 2020;11:761. https://doi.org/10.3389/fimmu.2020.00761.

Pediatric Allergic Rhinitis: Otolaryngology Perspective

34

Mert Cemal Gökgöz, Cemal Cingi, and Gabriela Kopacheva-Barsova

34.1 Introduction

Pediatric nasal obstruction is among the most common reasons for referral to pediatric otolaryngologists [1]. During the neonatal period and infancy, congenital causes are the most common causes of nasal obstruction, while in the pediatric age group in advanced ages, allergic, inflammatory, and infectious rhinitis come to the fore as the primary causes [1]. Allergic causes are not considered in the foreground in nasal congestion in the first 2 years of age, mainly since there is insufficient time for allergen exposure [2]. The presence of at least two of the complaints of nasal congestion, rhinorrhea, sneezing, and itching accompanying the inflammation of the nasal epithelium is sufficient for diagnosing rhinitis [3, 4]. Similar complaints may also occur in the presence of adenoid hypertrophy, acute and chronic sinusitis, deviation of the septum, or nasal polyp, which are other causes of nasal obstruction [5]. Allergic rhinitis is the most common chronic disease of childhood and hurts the quality of life regarding physical, social, and psychological well-being [6]. Allergic rhinitis leads to impaired sleep, daytime sleepiness, concentration impairment, and impaired cognitive functions, decreasing school success and impairing the quality of life for the child and the family. Allergic rhinitis is frequently caused by IgE-mediated early and late-phase hypersensitivity response to inhalant allergens [6].

M. C. Gökgöz
Department of Otorhinolaryngology, Manisa City Hospital, Manisa, Turkey

C. Cingi (✉)
Medical Faculty, Department of Otorhinolaryngology, Eskisehir Osmangazi University, Eskisehir, Turkey

G. Kopacheva-Barsova
Faculty of Medicine, Department of Otorhinolaryngology, Cyril and Methodius University of Skopje, Skopje, Republic of North Macedonia

H. Yüksel et al. (eds.), *Pediatric Airway Diseases*, Comprehensive ENT,
https://doi.org/10.1007/978-3-031-74853-0_34

Animal sources such as house dust, mites, pollen, cats and dogs, molds, and food allergies, which are increasingly common, can be stated as these allergens [7].

34.2 Epidemiology

34.2.1 Prevalence

In recent years, there has been an increase in the majority of allergic rhinitis, asthma, and atopic dermatitis. Environmental factors and lifestyle changes, diet changes, increased hygiene hypothesis, increased exposure to indoor antigens, and environmental toxins can be expressed as the reason for this increase [8]. In a study conducted in developed countries, the prevalence of allergic rhinitis has reached up to 50% [9]. Although the prevalence is higher in high-income countries, symptom scores reach higher levels in low- and middle-income countries [10]. Based on the study conducted by The International Study of Asthma and Allergies in Childhood in 98 countries and nearly 1.2 million children, the prevalence of allergic rhinitis is 8.5% in the 6–7 age group, while it rises to 14.6% in the 13–14 age group [11]. Regarding the prevalence of comorbid diseases, 20% of patients with asthma have allergic rhinitis, while 40% of patients diagnosed with allergic rhinitis have asthma [4].

34.2.2 Risk factors

Risk factors include family history, being male, being the first child in the family, maternal and paternal smoking, systemic antibiotic use at an early age, especially indoor allergen exposure, increased hygiene status, having a serum IgE level of >100 IU/mL before 6 years of age and the presence of allergen-specific IgE [8, 12]. In addition to that, exposure to farm animals, air pollution, and high-intensity sports in adolescence can be added to the risk factors [13]. The same risk factors often apply to asthma and atopic dermatitis.

34.3 Etiology and Pathogenesis

34.3.1 Classical Pathway

Allergen-specific IgE antibodies, formed due to previous allergen exposure, lead to the release of inflammatory mediators by binding to mast cells located in the respiratory mucosa and basophils in the circulation. Histamine, leukotrienes, and prostaglandins released by mast cells cause clinical findings by secreting platelet-activating factors and bradykinin. Moreover, the release of eosinophilic mediators increases inflammation. While the early phase occurs 15–30 min following allergen exposure, the late response peaks after 6–12 h.

34.3.2 Nasal Pathway

The nasal mucosa is the first line of defense against respiratory bacteria, viruses, and allergens. It achieves this line of protection through the immune response to the deteriorations in the mucosal integrity; in this way, it initiates protective inflammatory processes. The allergic immune reaction begins sensitizing when an allergen substance is encountered without an immune clinical response. At this stage, dendritic cells in the nasal mucosa present the allergen to CD+ T cells. Subsequently, CD+ T cells transform into allergen-specific type 2 T helper cells. B cells are transformed into allergen-specific IgE-producing plasma cells upon B cell activation. Circulating IgE binds with high affinity to its receptors located on mast cells and basophils. This process ends with allergen-specific T helper cells and B cells forming memory against this allergen.

In the pathophysiology of allergic rhinitis, respiratory allergens disrupt epithelial integrity through protease enzyme activity, stimulate previously sensitive receptors, and result in an allergen-specific response. The immune response is initiated by releasing IL (Interleukin)-33, thymic stromal lymphopoietin (TSLP), or IL-25 [14]. These, in turn, cause the release of IL-5, IL-13, and IL-4 cytokines, which provide IgE-mediated immune response and mucosal inflammation. It is considered that pollutants, irritants, and infectious agents (*Staphylococcus aureus* or viruses) could impact this pathway [15]. *S. aureus* is responsible for producing enterotoxins with superantigenic properties and is a frequently observed bacterium in the respiratory tract. Immune response to superantigens can be seen in both B and T cells. In the presence of *S. aureus* in the nasal cavity in patients with allergic rhinitis, allergic symptoms may be felt more severely with superantigens [16].

34.4 Diagnosis, Physical Examination, and Diagnostic Tests

34.4.1 Diagnosis and History

Patient history, physical examination, and allergy tests are primary in diagnosing allergic rhinitis. In the diagnosis of allergic rhinitis, as in every disease, the account to be taken from the patient in the pediatric age group and their parent is crucial in making the correct diagnosis and for patient management. There are issues to be considered in the history and physical examination when diagnosing rhinitis, determining its type, differentiating accompanying pathologies, and other diagnoses [17, 18].

Before the physical examination, the physician should also shed light on the points related to rhinitis, which might be overlooked by the parent, by asking various queries. The patient's age, since when the disease has been present, its frequency, duration, and seasonal characteristics, whether it continues throughout the year, the presence of exacerbations, whether there is a condition that causes the symptoms to occur, the impact of environmental factors originating from home or school, the presence of symptoms accompanying nasal symptoms, daily activities, school performance, sleep patterns, whether it affects the patient's and his parent's quality of life, and the presence of family history should be questioned. If any, the patient's previous allergy tests, diagnostic tests, imaging tests, the company of medications or other treatments received, and the history of surgery should be questioned [19] (Table 34.1).

34.4.2 Physical Examination

In the physical examination to be performed by an otolaryngologist, particularly, detection and differentiation of the accompanying diseases are of great importance. During the inspection, "allergic salute- transverse external crease," "Dennie-Morgan lines," allergic shiners (dark eye shadows, reflecting venous pooling in the lid vessels.), and frequent throat clearing movements, which are indicators of postnasal discharge, can be noticed. Another critical point to be evaluated during the inspection is the open-mouth breathing pattern due to chronic nasal obstruction, elongated facial appearance (adenoid facies), and accompanying dental malocclusion problems. A complete ear, nose, oropharynx, oral cavity, and neck examination should be performed in the physical examination. In the ear examination, dullness or retraction of the tympanic membrane, air-fluid levels as a result of Eustachian dysfunction due to allergic rhinitis, presence of serous otitis, and accompanying hearing loss should be evaluated via audiometric tests and tympanometry. In the nasal examination, the presence and consistency of nasal discharge in anterior rhinoscopy, septum pathologies, hypertrophies of the inferior turbinate and middle turbinate, pallor or a pale bluish hue accompanied by mucosal edema, the presence of nasal polyps or foreign bodies, crusting, and perforation can be evaluated. Albeit anterior rhinoscopy is a simple procedure to perform, patient and parent compliance is significant for nasal endoscopy. It is more challenging to apply in children younger than 2 years old. The process can be performed via rigid or flexible 2.7–4 mm endoscopes. Local anesthetic and

Table 34.1 Clinical symptoms and relation with age groups in pediatric ages

	Age groups		
Clinical symptoms	Pre-school	School	Adolescent
Rhinorrhea (watery, discolored)	x	X	X
Pruritis/itching (allergic salute, allergic crease, itchy mouth and throat)	x	X	X
Sneezing	x	X	X
Nasal congestion	x	X	X
Cough (with/without asthma)	>2 years	X	X
Eustachian dysfunction (due to nasal congestion)	x	X	
Sleep problems (due to nasal obstruction)	>2 years	x	X
Rhinosinusitis related symptoms (Nasal congestion, purulent nasal discharge, cough, facial pain and pressure, mucosal edema, polyp)		x	X
Prolonged respiratory tract infections	>2 years	x	X
Irritability, poor school performance		x	x

decongestant sprays can be used before the procedure. Endoscopic examination is crucial for the evaluation of the posterior nose and nasopharynx. Assessment of the patency of both nasal passages, the condition of the mucosa, adenoid hypertrophy, and ostium of the Eustachian Tube, and the detection of small polyps and foreign bodies that cannot be seen with anterior rhinoscopy help detect malignancies. In the oropharynx and oral cavity examination, dental malocclusion or high-arched palate associated with chronic mouth breathing, cobblestoning of the oropharyngeal wall, and pharyngeal postnasal discharge should be examined. Although viral upper respiratory tract infections exhibit similar symptoms with allergic rhinitis, they can be differentiated by the short duration of symptoms and accompanying symptoms such as fever and myalgia. Allergic conjunctivitis, watery eye discharge, and swelling in the conjunctiva are present in 50–70% of allergic rhinitis patients and are the most prominent symptom that differentiates allergic rhinitis from other forms of rhinitis [20] (Fig. 34.1).

34.4.3 Diagnostic Tests

Allergy tests are generally conducted in patients who cannot be controlled despite using antihistamines and intranasal corticosteroids for an adequate time and appropriate dose as empirical treatment, in patients with an unclear diagnosis of allergic rhinitis, and in cases where it is essential to detect the specific antigen for immuno therapy. IgE-specific allergic tests are divided into two main categories: skin and blood tests. Measurement of total Ig-E does not provide any benefit for the diagnosis of allergic rhinitis. Skin tests are considered more sensitive than blood

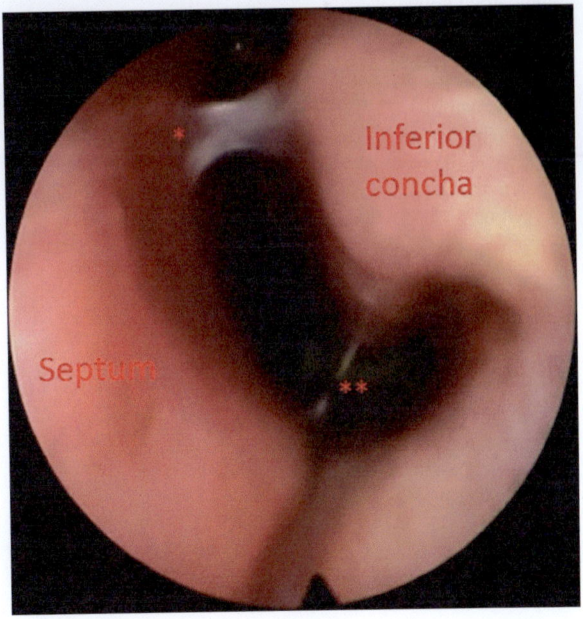

Fig. 34.1 Left nasal passage view of a 6-year-old patient with allergic rhinitis. Inferior turbinate is observed in hypertrophic and pale appearance. *: serous discharge due to allergic rhinitis, **: purulent discharge due to acute sinusitis accompanying allergic rhinitis

tests, allowing us to observe the reaction against the antigen directly. It is performed by measuring the swelling on the skin caused by the histamine released due to the rapid interaction of the antigen with IgE antibodies through mast cells. It is cheaper than blood tests but carries the risk of systemic allergic response (anaphylaxis). It can be performed at any age and has been considered sensitive-specific over 80%. Results are evaluated within 15–20 min after the application. The medication usage histories of the patients should be questioned before the allergy test (Fig. 34.2).

Blood tests are implemented by measuring the IgE-specific antigen in the patient's serum. It is specifically preferred in patients with skin-related problems, in the presence of dermatographism and severe eczema, and when the interpretation of skin tests becomes challenging. Its advantages include being unaffected by the history of medication use, no need to discontinue antihistamine therapy, and not having the risk of anaphylaxis. In the absence of contraindications, the choice of skin or blood testing can be left to the patient [21].

34.4.4 Nasal Cytology

The nasal mucosa comprises pseudostratified ciliated columnar epithelium containing mucinous cells responsible for mucus secretion. Nasal cytology is based on the principle of identification of normal and pathological cells of the nasal mucosa by

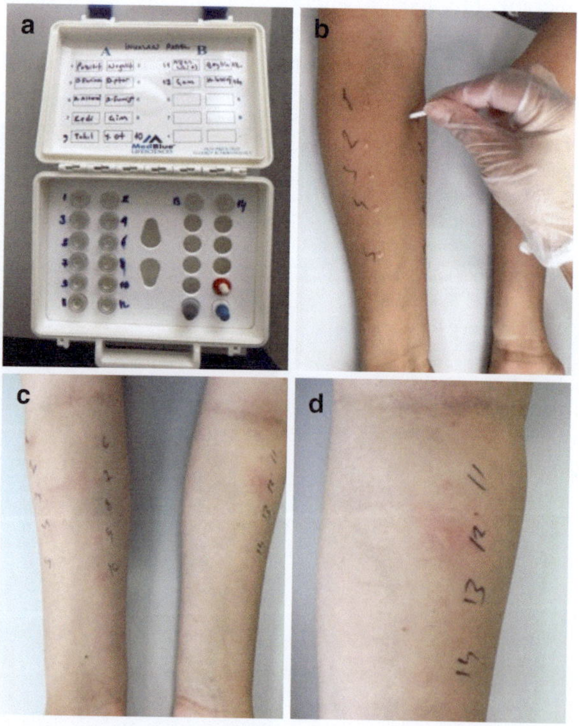

Fig. 34.2 (**a**) Inhalant panel skin prick test in which 14 different allergens are tested (grass pollen, grain pollen, weed pollen, cat, olive, etc.). (**b**) It is applied to both forearms. (**c**) Results are evaluated within 15–20 min after the application. (**d**) 6 mm level of positivity against allergen item 12 (olive)

examining the nasal cell types and morphology of the samples taken by various means (nasal lavage, micro-suction aspiration, brushing, scraping, swap, or biopsy) under the microscope [22]. It is an easy-to-apply, non-invasive, reproducible test that can be implemented without age limitations. This procedure enables the detection of normal nasal mucosal cells and inflammatory cells such as lymphocytes, neutrophils, eosinophils, and mast cells. Depending on the dominant cell type, it can help differentiate viral infections, allergic rhinitis, non-allergic rhinitis, and NARES. In allergic rhinitis, intense infiltration of eosinophils and mast cells is detected, particularly in the symptomatic period. In conditions such as house dust mite allergy that do not cause severe symptoms and last all year, cytology with minimal inflammation in which neutrophils are more dominant is observed [23].

34.4.5 Imaging

Patient history, physical examination, and allergy tests lead to allergic rhinitis diagnosis. Although there is no radiological finding that will help in the diagnosis of allergic rhinitis primarily, it can be performed in the presence of nasal polyps, chronic rhinosinusitis, and suspected malignancy accompanying allergic findings. While CT should be preferred in evaluating bone structures, orbit should be selected to assess soft tissues and tumoral structures, and MRI should be chosen to examine the skull base and intracranial extension [24].

34.5 Differential Diagnosis in Otolaryngology Perspective

34.5.1 Adenoid Hypertrophy

It can be confused with the symptoms of allergic rhinitis since it causes difficulty breathing through the nose, sleeping with the mouth open due to nasal congestion, predisposition to otitis media, and sleep disorders. Manifestations related to adenoid hypertrophy, like allergic rhinitis, often begin after the 2 years of age. Mediators released due to the inflammatory process in tonsil and adenoid tissue are effective in clinical manifestations. Allergic rhinitis is associated with adenotonsillar hypertrophy and Obstructive Sleep Apnea (OSA). The incidence of allergic rhinitis has been reported to be nearly 40% in pediatric patients who have been followed up via tonsillar hypertrophy and adenoid hypertrophy. In addition to the adenoid size, allergy also occurs due to nasal congestion caused by inflammation of the nasal mucosa. In physical examination, nasal mucosa may be observed as edematous due to nasal clearance deterioration, inflammation in anterior rhinoscopy, and occlusion due to secretion. Endoscopic examination may reveal adenoid hypertrophy, which narrows the nasopharynx and choana and closes the Eustachian tube ostium. In treating adenoid hypertrophy, intranasal corticosteroid therapy and follow-up with nasal irrigation may be recommended depending on the severity of the symptoms. OSA level, the level of obstruction caused by adenoid hypertrophy, serous otitis media, and hearing loss, are effective in the surgical decision. Reducing OSA symptoms, particularly with intranasal corticosteroids, supports the allergic background [25, 26] (Fig. 34.3).

34.5.2 Nasal Septal Deviation

It may lead to obstruction, especially more prominently on one side in the pediatric age group. It is accompanied by nasal congestion only, one of the signs of allergic rhinitis. Regarding the timing of surgery, although some studies suggest that it would not cause nasal and facial developmental disorders if performed after the age of 6, there are also studies stating that surgery can be performed from the neonatal period. There is no definite age limit for surgery yet [27]. Absolute indications include septal hematoma, septal abscess, dermoid cyst, cleft lip with the nasal component, and severe deformity secondary to nasal fracture. In contrast, the relative indication has been identified to be septum deviation causing significant nasal airway obstruction [28].

34.5.3 Chronic Rhinosinusitis

Inflammatory involvement of the sinus and nasal mucosa is defined as rhinosinusitis. Suppose nasal congestion, purulent nasal discharge, cough, facial pain and pressure, nasal polyps, and mucosal edema symptoms persist for more than 3 months despite standard treatment (antibiotics, oral or intranasal corticosteroids, nasal sprays, and nasal saline irrigation) in the pediatric age group, then

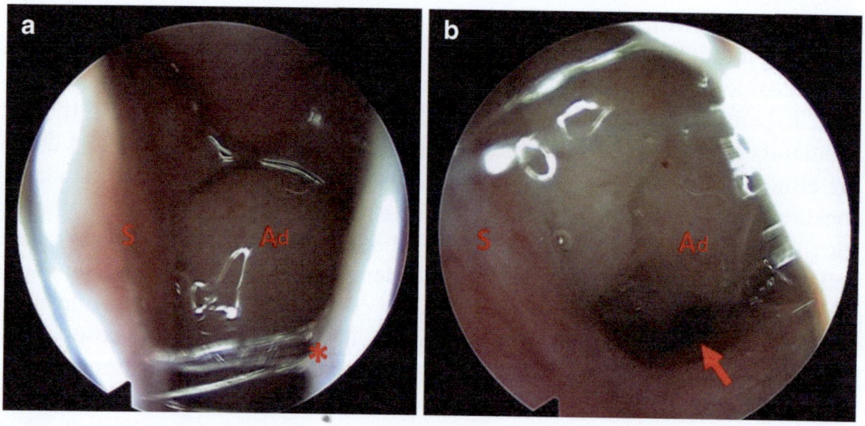

Fig. 34.3 Left nasal passage view of a 4-year-old patient with adenoid hypertrophy. (**a**) Adenoid hypertrophy obstructing the nasal passage and serous discharge. (**b**) Minimal gap in choanae due to adenoid hypertrophy. (S: Septum, Ad: Adenoid hypertrophy, *: Serous discharge, red arrow: Choanal cavity)

it is considered as chronic rhinosinusitis [29]. Mucosal inflammation, edema, impaired mucociliary clearance, and obstruction of sinus drainage due to allergic rhinitis play a significant role in the etiology of rhinosinusitis [30]. It has also been suggested that patients with allergic rhinitis are predisposed to developing rhinosinusitis and that the deterioration in sinus functions is more severe [31].

34.5.4 Turbinate Hypertrophy

It leads to allergic rhinitis-like symptoms by showing manifestations of nasal congestion and discharge, mouth breathing, and obstructive sleep apnea. In children, the effect of inferior turbinate hypertrophy is not clearly understood since adenoid hypertrophy is the most common cause of nasal obstruction. Generally, a conservative approach is followed in the pediatric age group. Patients with continuing nasal obstruction after adenoidectomy should be considered a surgical indication [32]. Studies reveal that turbinate hypertrophy surgery provides an additional benefit in addition to adenoidectomy in patients who do not respond adequately to medical treatment [33]. Surgical options include turbinectomy, cauterization or radiofrequency, and submucous micro debridement [34, 35].

34.5.5 Nasal Foreign Body

Patients typically present with unilateral discharge and obstruction. Foul-smelling unilateral discharge occurs depending on the foreign body's duration in the nasal passage. Nasal flow may be accompanied by nasal congestion, sneezing, and headache. Following anterior rhinoscopy evaluation, nasal endoscopy should be performed depending on the patient's compliance. Radiological imaging may be requested in cases where the foreign body cannot be seen, but its clinical utility is limited as most foreign bodies are radiolucent. If a foreign body is detected, it is used with a nasal speculum or endoscope-guided probe, curette, and alligator forceps removal [36].

34.5.6 Other Clinical Conditions

Although nasal polyps are rare in the pediatric age group, cystic fibrosis or ciliary dyskinesia should be considered in the etiology. In the presence of unilateral polyps, encephalocele should be considered. Nasal tumors lead to complaints of nasal discharge/nose bleeding and progression to adjacent structures, though rarely. Due to pharyngonasal reflux, symptoms such as chronic sinusitis and fluid accumulation in the ear due to Eustachian dysfunction, which can also be seen in allergic rhinitis, can be observed (Table 34.2).

Table 34.2 Differential diagnosis of allergic rhinitis in children

Differential diagnosis	Symptoms	Diagnostic tests
Adenoid hypertrophy	Difficulty in breathing through the nose, mouth breathing due to nasal congestion, predisposition to otitis media, and sleep disorders	Lateral nasopharynx X-ray graphy, endoscopic examination
Nasal septal deviation	Nasal obstruction, especially more prominently on one side, and nasal congestion	Anterior rhinoscopy, endoscopic examination
Chronic rhinosinusitis	Nasal congestion, purulent nasal discharge, cough, facial pain and pressure, mucosal edema, polyp	Anterior rhinoscopy, endoscopic examination, paranasal CT, MRI
Turbinate hypertrophy	Nasal congestion and discharge, mouth breathing, and sleep disorders	Anterior rhinoscopy, endoscopic examination
Nasal foreign body	Unilateral discharge and nasal obstruction, foul-smelling discharge	Anterior rhinoscopy, endoscopic examination, radiological tests
Cystic fibrosis/ ciliary dyskinesia	Bilateral nasal polyps, decreased mucociliary clearance	Sweat chloride test, genetic tests
Encephalocele	Unilateral nasal polyp	Endoscopic examination, paranasal, brain CT, MRI
Nasal tumors	Nasal discharge, epistaxis, progression to adjacent structures	Endoscopic examination, paranasal CT, MRI

34.6 Prevention from an Otolaryngology Perspective

34.6.1 Saline Irrigation (Douching)

Nasal irrigation has been determined to be beneficial in relieving the symptoms of allergic rhinitis in the pediatric age group [37, 38]. In addition to its mechanical cleaning effect, it is considered helpful for mucociliary clearance and removing allergens with inflammatory mediators such as histamine, prostaglandin, and leukotrienes. Nasal irrigation can be used in drops, spray, and via a pump. It is subdivided into isotonic (0.9%), hypertonic (1.5–3%), and seawater-containing types. For high-volume rinsing, pumps with a volume of 300 mL are utilized in pediatric forms. It has been suggested that adding nasal irrigation to the treatment and using intranasal corticosteroids decrease patient symptoms compared to using intranasal steroids (INS) alone and reducing the dose of INS [39]. A study on the compliance and tolerance of nasal irrigation in the pediatric age group revealed that 86% could tolerate the treatment, and 84% of the parents thought that nasal symptoms were reduced by irrigation [40]. In the same study, 21% of parents in the under-5 age group felt that their children could tolerate nasal irrigation, whereas the tolerance rate of children was 86%. When combined with nasal steroids, the benefit increases compared to INS alone [41, 42]. In addition to the signs of allergic rhinitis, it also relieves the symptoms and symptoms associated with asthma [43]. Nasal irrigation solutions should be considered an alternative that is easy to use at home, inexpensive, and has few adverse effects (Fig. 34.4). (a) The nasal irrigation bottle, used for

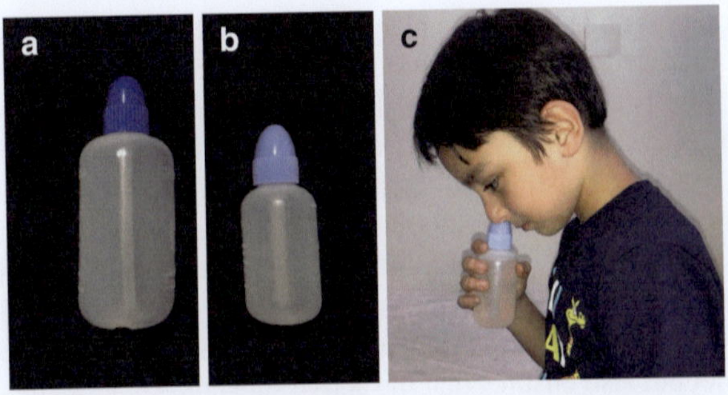

Fig. 34.4 (**a**) The nasal irrigation bottle, used for 12 years and older patients, provides high pressure washing with approximately 200 mL of water. (**b**) The nasal irrigation bottle, used for 4- to 12-years-old pediatric patients, provides high pressure washing with approximately 80–100 mL of water. (**c**) Shows how to use a nasal irrigation of a 6-year-old patient in standing position

12 years and older patients, provides high-pressure washing with approximately 200 mL of water. (b) The nasal irrigation bottle for 4- to 12-year-old pediatric patients provides high-pressure washing with about 80–100 mL of water. (c) Shows how to use nasal irrigation in the standing position of a 6-year-old child.

34.7 Treatment

34.7.1 Oral Antihistamines

Histamine is the primary mediator responsible for the symptoms of allergic rhinitis. H1 antihistamines are often used in allergic rhinitis in oral or nasal forms. They are effective for nasal flow, sneezing, itching, and congestion. As a mechanism of action, they inhibit the proinflammatory effects of histamine by blocking the histamine H1 receptor [44]. Its development starts in 1–3 h. First-generation antihistamines are not preferred as they cross the blood–brain barrier and lead to sedation, drowsiness, decreased school performance, and increased appetite. Nowadays, second generation H1 antihistamines (desloratadine, loratadine, cetirizine, levocetirizine), which have less sedating properties, and antihistamines with minimal sedation effects such as fexofenadine and bilastine have begun to be preferred [45]. New-generation antihistamines show high selectivity to H1 receptors and limitedly cross the blood–brain barrier owing to their lipophilic effect. Thanks to their cost-effectiveness and ease of use once a day, which enhances compliance with treatment, oral antihistamines are preferred, particularly in patients with mild allergic rhinitis.

34.7.2 Intranasal Steroids

Intranasal corticosteroids are the first-choice treatment modality for all stages of allergic rhinitis, from mild to persistent and severe forms [46]. It is used effectively on nasal flow, sneezing, congestion, and itching symptoms [47], in addition to reducing intranasal symptoms and relieving ocular symptoms [21]. It is in the first place regarding treatment effectiveness, albeit the onset of the duration of action is late among other allergic rhinitis treatment options. The time taken for the desired effect's beginning is 6–48 h. They are effective for nasal flow, sneezing, itching, and congestion. In addition to its anti-inflammatory effect, it reduces the release of mediators and cytokines and reduces eosinophilic, basophilic, and mononuclear cells in nasal secretions.

Moreover, INS reduces antigen-induced hyperresponsiveness [48]. Patients should be trained for the use of intranasal sprays and drops. This training not only prevents the feeling of pain in the nose and nose bleeding that may occur due to the misuse of the jet but also ensures that the active substance reaches the desired ostiomeatal complex and over the turbinates [6]. It does not result in growth retardation due to low systemic bioavailability. Fluticasone furoate, Mometasone furoate, and Fluticasone propionate are preferred in the pediatric age group as they have the most insufficient systemic bioavailability [6, 48–50]. It is also effective on ocular symptoms secondary to reducing the naso-ocular reflex [51] (Fig. 34.5).

34.7.3 Leukotriene Inhibitors

Montelukast is a selective antagonist of LTR type 1 and inhibits the proinflammatory effects of cysteinyl-leukotrienes. It has been reported that its impact is lower than antihistamines and INS [52]. Besides oral antihistamines and INS, its use helps reduce allergic rhinitis and asthma symptoms. Some studies have demonstrated that Montelukast is beneficial in combination therapy, particularly in the presence of asthma and allergic rhinitis, rather than first-line therapy [53]. It can cause mild upper respiratory tract infection, pharyngitis, headache, nausea, and vomiting as adverse effects. Still, it has been reported to occur with a frequency similar to placebo and identical drug groups [54].

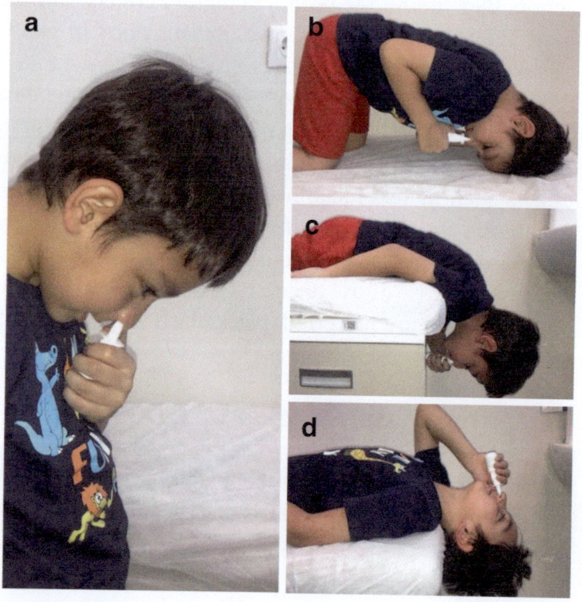

Fig. 34.5 (**a**) Shows how to use a nasal spray in a standing position using the left hand for the right nostril, and (**b–d**) Show how nasal drops should be used to reach the osteomeatal complex. (adopted from Scadding et al. [6])

34.7.4 Oral Antihistamines-Leukotriene Receptor Antagonists Combination

Studies demonstrate that this combination provides benefits compared to oral antihistamines alone and leukotriene receptor antagonists alone [55]. It is beneficial in treating persistent Allergic rhinitis (AR) in accompanying asthma and in treating grass pollen allergic rhinitis in improving lung symptoms, reducing nasal congestion, and increasing the quality of life [56]. Compared with INS, the effect of the combination on nasal symptoms was lower than with INS alone [57]. This combination of treatments should be used to assess which symptoms are predominant, specifically in the pediatric patient group [56].

34.7.5 Oral Steroids

Oral steroids should not be used except in very severe and acute conditions since they are not superior in avoiding systemic side effects and efficacy compared to intranasal steroids in the pediatric age group. It can only be used as a very short-term, low-dose, short-rescue therapy in addition to INS in patients with severe symptoms. On the other hand, depot steroid injections are not recommended since the risk outweighs the benefit [58].

34.7.6 Intranasal Antihistamines

As locally acting intranasal antihistamines, azelastine and olopatadine (there are 2 FDA-approved preparations) are used, and their effect starts in 30 min–3 h [59, 60]. For intranasal antihistamines, the age of use is 6 years and over in the pediatric group, while oral antihistamines can be used at 1 year and above. Regarding the use of olopatadine and azelastine, one puff is recommended twice a day between the ages of 6–11, while two breaths are recommended twice a day at 12 and over [61]. Some studies have revealed that intranasal antihistamines have lower systemic effects than oral antihistamines and are more effective on nasal symptoms, particularly in nasal congestion [62]. Nasal irritation, burning, accompanying pain, epistaxis, bitter taste in the mouth, mild drowsiness, and headache are everyday adverse events of nasal antihistamines.

34.7.7 Immunotherapy (Sublingual-Subcutaneous)

Allergen-specific immunotherapy is the administration of controlled repetitive doses of therapy aimed at increasing immune tolerance to the allergen in IgE-mediated AR patient groups diagnosed via medical history and allergy tests. It is the sole treatment modality with the potential to prevent AR. Merely 5% of patients can reach immunotherapy. Two types of immunotherapies are used clinically, 75% of patients receive subcutaneous therapy (SCIT), and 25% receive sublingual immunotherapy (SLIT) [63]. Immunotherapy was determined to be more effective in the pediatric age group compared to adults [64]. Although there is no specific time for the treatment period, it often takes 3–5 years. In studies demonstrating efficacy after treatment, efficacy has been shown to continue for 10 years for SCIT and 8 years for SLIT following cessation of therapy [65, 66]. Studies show that SCIT and SLIT reduce nasal symptoms more than medication use [67, 68].

Regarding the side effects, local redness and itching at the injection site can reach 58% for SCIT and 97% for SLIT in some studies. In contrast, serious adverse effects such as urticaria, wheezing, and anaphylaxis have been detected at 0.9% for SCIT and 0.056% for SLIT. It has been reported that the incidence of death due to SCIT is 1 in 2.5 million injections, whereas no death occurred due to SLIT [69]. Immunotherapy should not be performed in the presence of uncontrolled asthma, and to avoid adverse effects or unexpected effects, the first dose of the therapy should be administered under the control of a physician in the healthcare facility instead of at home, and it would be appropriate to wait 30 min after the shot, to detect the adverse effects that may occur immediately.

34.7.8 New Treatment Options: Omalizumab and Dupilumab

Omalizumab is an IgE-specific monoclonal antibody. It inhibits allergy steps by binding free-circulating allergen-specific IgEs [70]. Omalizumab can be used in children older than 6, in patients with uncontrolled, moderate–severe, and severe asthma, with increased IgE level and skin test positivity [71]. It is administered as a subcutaneous injection for 2–4 weeks. It is thought to reduce asthma exacerbations and the need for inhaled steroid usage. Many studies have demonstrated its efficacy and safety [72, 73]. Dupilumab is a humanized Ig-G4-specific monoclonal antibody developed against interleukin 4 receptor alpha. It blocks the communication of IL-4 and IL-13, suppressing the pro-allergic immune response induced by T helper two conversion [74]. It can be used in patients with moderate-to-severe and severe asthma that cannot be controlled by treatment in the presence of eosinophilic phenotype and oral corticosteroid-dependent asthma. It has been approved for use in adolescents aged 12 and over. As a subcutaneous injection, 300 mg injections are applied to two separate sites in patients over 60 kg, or 200 mg is administered at two different locations in patients weighing less than 60 kg and is repeated as a dose every 2 weeks. Comprehensive studies in the pediatric population are needed for its long-term efficacy and safety profile [75].

34.8 Conclusion

Pediatric nasal obstruction is among the most common reasons for referral to pediatric otolaryngologists. The presence of at least two of the complaints of nasal congestion, rhinorrhea, sneezing, and itching accompanying the inflammation of the nasal epithelium is sufficient for diagnosing rhinitis. Patient history, physical examination, and allergy tests are primary in diagnosing allergic rhinitis. Intranasal corticosteroids and oral antihistamines are the first-choice treatment modality for all stages of allergic rhinitis, from mild to persistent and severe forms. Regarding otolaryngology, adenoid hypertrophy, nasal septum deviation, turbinate hypertrophy, chronic sinusitis, nasal foreign bodies, cystic fibrosis/ciliary dyskinesia, and nasal tumors should be considered in the differential diagnosis in the pediatric age group. Treatment options should be determined individually according to the age and symptoms of the patients.

References

1. Smith MM, Ishman SL. Pediatric nasal obstruction. Otolaryngol Clin North Am. 2018;51(5):971–85.
2. Kulig M, Klettke U, Wahn V, et al. Development of seasonal allergic rhinitis during the first 7 years of life. J Allergy Clin Immunol. 2000;106:832–9.
3. Dykewicz MS, Wallace DV, Amrol DJ, Baroody FM, Bernstein JA, Craig TJ, et al. Rhinitis 2020: a practice parameter update. J Allergy Clin Immunol. 2020;146(4):721–67.
4. Brożek JL, Bousquet J, Agache I, Agarwal A, Bachert C, Bosnic-Anticevich S, et al. Allergic rhinitis and its impact on asthma (ARIA) guidelines-2016 revision. J Allergy Clin Immunol. 2017;140(4):950–8.
5. Roberts G, Xatzipsalti M, Borrego LM, Custovic A, Halken S, Hellings PW, et al. Paediatric rhinitis: position paper of the European Academy of Allergy and Clinical Immunology. Allergy. 2013;68(9):1102–16.
6. Scadding GK. Optimal management of allergic rhinitis. Arch Dis Child. 2015;100(6):576–82.
7. Bjorksten B, Clayton T, Ellwood P, et al. Worldwide time trends for symptoms of rhinitis and conjunctivitis: phase III of the international study of asthma and allergies in childhood. Pediatr Allergy Immunol. 2008;19:110–24.
8. Cingi C, Bayar Muluk N, Scadding GK. Will every child have allergic rhinitis soon? Int J Pediatr Otorhinolaryngol. 2019;118:53–8.
9. Bousquet PJ, Leynaert B, Neukirch F, Sunyer J, Janson CM, Anto J, Jarvis D, Burney P. Geographical distribution of atopic rhinitis in the European Community respiratory health survey I. Allergy. 2008;63(10):1301–9.
10. Aït-Khaled N, Pearce N, Anderson HR, Ellwood P, Montefort S, Shah J, ISAAC Phase Three Study Group. Global map of the prevalence of symptoms of rhinoconjunctivitis in children: the International Study of Asthma and Allergies in Childhood (ISAAC) phase three. Allergy. 2009;64(1):123–48.
11. Mallol J, Crane J, von Mutius E, Odhiambo J, Keil U, Stewart A, ISAAC Phase Three Study Group. The International Study of Asthma and Allergies in Childhood (ISAAC) phase three: a global synthesis. Allergol Immunopathol (Madr). 2013;41(2):73–85.
12. Wallace DV, Dykewicz MS, Bernstein DI, Blessing-Moore J, Cox L, Khan DA, et al.; Joint Task Force on Practice; American Academy of Allergy; Asthma & Immunology; American College of Allergy; Asthma and Immunology; Joint Council of Allergy, Asthma and Immunology. The diagnosis and management of rhinitis: an updated practice parameter. J Allergy Clin Immunol. 2008;122(2 Suppl):S1–84.
13. Asher MI, Stewart AW, Mallol J, Montefort S, Lai CK, Aït-Khaled N, Odhiambo J, ISAAC Phase One Study Group. Which population level environmental factors are associated with asthma, rhinoconjunctivitis and eczema? Review of the ecological analyses of ISAAC phase one. Respir Res. 2010;11(1):8.
14. Broide DH. Allergic rhinitis: pathophysiology. Allergy Asthma Proc. 2010;31(5):370–4.
15. Bousquet J, Anto JM, Bachert C, Baiardini I, Bosnic-Anticevich S, Walter Canonica G, Melén E, Palomares O, Scadding GK, Togias A, Toppila-Salmi S. Allergic rhinitis. Nat Rev Dis Primers. 2020;6(1):95.

16. Muluk NB, Altın F, Cingi C. Role of superantigens in allergic inflammation: their relationship to allergic rhinitis, chronic rhinosinusitis, asthma, and atopic dermatitis. Am J Rhinol Allergy. 2018;32(6):502–17.
17. Scadding G, Hellings P, Alobid I, Bachert C, Fokkens W, van Wijk RG, Gevaert P, Guilemany J, Kalogjera L, Lund V, et al. Diagnostic tools in rhinology EAACI position paper. Clin Transl Allergy. 2011;10:1–2.
18. Hellings PW, Scadding G, Alobid I, Bachert C, Fokkens WJ, Gerth van Wijk R, et al. Executive summary of European task force document on diagnostic tools in rhinology. Rhinology. 2012;50(4):339–52.
19. Doulaptsi M, Aoi N, Kawauchi H, Milioni A, Karatzanis A, Prokopakis E. Differentiating rhinitis in the paediatric population by giving focus on medical history and clinical examination. Med Sci (Basel). 2019;7(3):38.
20. Bertelsen RJ, Carlsen KC, Carlsen KH. Rhinitis in children: co-morbidities and phenotypes. Pediatr Allergy Immunol. 2010;21(4 Pt 1):612.
21. Seidman MD, Gurgel RK, Lin SY, Schwartz SR, Baroody FM, Bonner JR, et al.; Guideline Otolaryngology Development Group. AAO-HNSF. Clinical practice guideline: allergic rhinitis. Otolaryngol Head Neck Surg. 2015;152(1 Suppl):S1–43.
22. Heffler E, Landi M, Caruso C, Fichera S, Gani F, Guida G, Liuzzo MT, Pistorio MP, Pizzimenti S, Riccio AM, Seccia V, Ferrando M, Malvezzi L, Passalacqua G, Gelardi M. Nasal cytology: methodology with application to clinical practice and research. Clin Exp Allergy. 2018;48(9):1092–106.
23. Gelardi M, Iannuzzi L, Quaranta N, Landi M, Passalacqua G. NASAL cytology: practical aspects and clinical relevance. Clin Exp Allergy. 2016;46(6):785–92.
24. American College of Radiology (ACR) appropriateness criteria. Sinonasal disease. 2012. http://www.acr.org/~/media/ACR/Documents/AppCriteria/Diagnostic/SinonasalDisease.pdf. Accessed 4 Mar 2014.
25. Modrzynski M, Zawisza E. An analysis of the incidence of adenoid hypertrophy in allergic children. Int J Pediatr Otorhinolaryngol. 2007;71:713–9.
26. Sakarya EU, Bayar Muluk N, Sakalar EG, Senturk M, Aricigil M, Bafaqeeh SA, Cingi C. Use of intranasal corticosteroids in adenotonsillar hypertrophy. J Laryngol Otol. 2017;131(5):384–90.
27. Cristophel JJ, Gross CW. Pediatric septoplasty. Otolaryngol Clin North Am. 2009;42:287–94.
28. Lawrence R. Pediatric septoplasy: a review of the literature. Int J Pediatr Otorhinolaryngol. 2012;76(8):1078–81.
29. Brietzke SE, Shin JJ, Choi S, Lee JT, Parikh SR, Pena M, et al. Clinical consensus statement: pediatric chronic rhinosinusitis. Otolaryngol Head Neck Surg. 2014;151(4):542–53.
30. Vlastos I, Athanasopoulos I, Mastronikolis NS, et al. Impaired mucociliary clearance in allergic rhinitis patients is related to a predisposition to rhinosinusitis. Ear Nose Throat J. 2009;88(4):E17–9.
31. Leo G, Incorvaia C, Cazzavillan A, Consonni D, Zuccotti GV. Could seasonal allergy be a risk factor for acute rhinosinusitis in children? J Laryngol Otol. 2018;132(2):150–3.
32. Komshian SR, Cohen MB, Brook C, Levi JR. Inferior turbinate hypertrophy: a review of the evolution of management in children. Am J Rhinol Allergy. 2019;33(2):212–9.
33. Cheng P-W, Fang K-M, Su H-W, Huang T-W. Improved objective outcomes and quality of life after adenotonsillectomy with inferior turbinate reduction in pediatric obstructive sleep apnea with inferior turbinate hypertrophy. Laryngoscope. 2012;122(12):2850–4.
34. Manzi B, Sykes KJ, Wei JL. Sinonasal quality of life in children after outfracture of inferior turbinates and submucous inferior turbinoplasty for chronic nasal congestion. JAMA Otolaryngol Head Neck Surg. 2017;143(5):452–7.
35. Bitar MA, Kanaan AA, Sinno S. Efficacy and safety of inferior turbinates coblation in children. J Laryngol Otol. 2014;128(Suppl 2):S48–54.
36. Baranowski K, Al Aaraj MS, Sinha V. Nasal foreign body. In: StatPearls [Internet]. Treasure Island: StatPearls Publishing; 2021. PMID: 29083647.
37. Satdhabudha A, Poachanukoon O. Efficacy of buffered hypertonic saline nasal irrigation in children with symptomatic allergic rhinitis: a randomized double-blind study. Int J Pediatr Otorhinolaryngol. 2012;76:583–8.

38. Hermelingmeier KE, Weber RK, Hellmich M, Heubach CP, Mosges R. Nasal irrigation as an adjunctive treatment in allergic rhinitis: a systematic review and meta-analysis. Am J Rhinol Allergy. 2012;26:e119–25.
39. Chen JR, Jin L, Li XY. The effectiveness of nasal saline irrigation (seawater) in treatment of allergic rhinitis in children. Int J Pediatr Otorhinolaryngol. 2014;78(7):1115–8.
40. Jeffe JS, Bhushan B, Schroeder JW Jr. Nasal saline irrigation in children: a study of compliance and tolerance. Int J Pediatr Otorhinolaryngol. 2012;76(3):409–13.
41. Li H, Sha Q, Zuo K, et al. Nasal saline irrigation facilitates control of allergic rhinitis by topical steroid in children. ORL J Otorhinolaryngol Relat Spec. 2009;71:50–5.
42. Madison S, Brown EA, Franklin R, Wickersham EA, McCarthy LH. Clinical question: nasal saline or intranasal corticosteroids to treat allergic rhinitis in children. J Okla State Med Assoc. 2016;109(4–5):152–3.
43. Jung M, Lee JY, Ryu G, Lee KE, Hong SD, Choi J, Kim S, Ahn K, Dhong HJ, Chung SK, Kim J, Kim HY. Beneficial effect of nasal saline irrigation in children with allergic rhinitis and asthma: a randomized clinical trial. Asian Pac J Allergy Immunol. 2020;38(4):251–7.
44. Kawauchi H, Yanai K, Wang DY, Itahashi K, Okubo K. Antihistamines for allergic rhinitis treatment from the viewpoint of nonsedative properties. Int J Mol Sci. 2019;20:213.
45. Yorgancıoğlu AA, Gemicioğlu B, Cingi C, et al. 2019 ARIA Care pathways for allergic rhinitis-Turkey. Turk Thorac J. 2020;21(2):122–33.
46. Rodrigo GJ, Neffen H. Efficacy of fluticasone furoate nasal spray vs. placebo for the treatment of ocular and nasal symptoms of allergic rhinitis: a systematic review. Clin Exp Allergy. 2011;41:160–70.
47. Rachelefsky G, Farrar JR. A control model to evaluate pharmacotherapy for allergic rhinitis in children. JAMA Pediatr. 2013;167(4):380–6.
48. Bachert C, Bousquet J, Hellings P. Rapid onset of action and reduced nasal hyperreactivity: new targets in allergic rhinitis management. Clin Transl Allergy. 2018;8:25.
49. Mener DJ, Shargorodsky J, Varadhan R, Lin SY. Topical intranasal corticosteroids and growth velocity in children: a meta-analysis. Int Forum Allergy Rhinol. 2015;5:95–103.
50. Meltzer EO, Tripathy I, Maspero JF, et al. Safety and tolerability of fluticasone furoate nasal spray once daily in paediatric patients aged 6-11 years with allergic rhinitis: subanalysis of three randomized, double-blind, placebo-controlled, multicentre studies. Clin Drug Investig. 2009;29:79–86.
51. Baroody FM, Shenaq D, DeTineo M, Wang J, Naclerio RM. Fluticasone furoate nasal spray reduces the nasal-ocular reflex: a mechanism for the efficacy of topical steroids in controlling allergic eye symptoms. J Allergy Clin Immunol. 2009;123:1342–8.
52. Nayak A, Langdon RB. Montelukast in the treatment of allergic rhinitis: an evidence-based review. Drugs. 2007;67:887–901.
53. Papadopoulos NG, Philip G, Giezek H, et al. The efficacy of montelukast during the allergy season in pediatric patients with persistent asthma and seasonal aeroallergen sensitivity. J Asthma. 2009;46:413–20.
54. Bisgaard H, Skoner D, Boza ML, Tozzi CA, Newcomb K, Reiss TF, et al. Safety and tolerability of montelukast in placebo-controlled pediatric studies and their open-label extensions. Pediatr Pulmonol. 2009;44:568–79.
55. Cingi C, Gunhan K, Gage-White L, et al. Efficacy of leukotriene antagonists as concomitant therapy in allergic rhinitis. Laryngoscope. 2010;120:1718–23.
56. Yilmaz O, Altintas D, Rondon C, Cingi C, Oghan F. Effectiveness of montelukast in pediatric patients with allergic rhinitis. Int J Pediatr Otorhinolaryngol. 2013;77(12):1922–4.
57. Esteitie R, deTineo M, Naclerio RM, et al. Effect of the addition of montelukast to fluticasone proprionate for the treatment of perennial allergic rhinitis. Ann Allergy Asthma Immunol. 2010;105:155–61.
58. Roberts G, Xatzipsalti M, Borrego LM, et al. Paediatric rhinitis: position paper of the European Academy of Allergy and Clinical Immunology. Allergy. 2013;68:1102–16.
59. Patel P, D'Andrea C, Sacks HJ. Onset of action of azelastine nasal spray compared with mometasone nasal spray and placebo in subjects with seasonal allergic rhinitis evaluated in an environmental exposure chamber. Am J Rhinol. 2007;21:499–503.

60. Horak F, Zieglmayer UP, Zieglmayer R, et al. Azelastine nasal spray and Desloratadine tablets in pollen-induced seasonal allergic rhinitis: a pharmacodynamic study of onset of action and efficacy. Curr Med Res Opin. 2006;22:151–7.
61. Nickels AS, Dimov V, Wolf R. Pharmacokinetic evaluation of Oloptadine for the treatment of allergic rhinitis and conjunctivitis. Expert Opin Drug Metab Toxicol. 2011;7:1593–9.
62. Kaliner MA, Berger WE, Ratner PH, et al. The efficacy of intranasal antihistamines in the treatment of allergic rhinitis. Ann Allergy Asthma Immunol. 2011;106:S6–S11.
63. Bufe A, Roberts G. Specific immunotherapy in children. Clin Exp Allergy. 2011;41:1256–62.
64. Radulovic S, Calderon MA, Wilson D, et al. Sublingual immunotherapy for allergic rhinitis. Cochrane Database Syst Rev. 2010;(12):CD002893.
65. Jacobsen L, Niggemann B, Dreborg S, et al.; The PAT Investigator Group. Specific immunotherapy has long-term preventive effect of seasonal and perennial asthma: 10-year follow-up on the PAT study. Allergy. 2007;62(8):943–948.
66. Marogna M, Spadolini I, Massolo A, et al. Long-lasting effects of sublingual immunotherapy according to its duration: a 15 year prospective study. J Allergy Clin Immunol. 2010;126:969–75.
67. Erekosima N, Suarez-Cuervo C, Ramanathan M, et al. Effectiveness of subcutaneous immunotherapy for allergic rhinoconjunctivitis and asthma: a systematic review. Laryngoscope. 2014;124(3):616–27.
68. Hankin C, Cox L, Lang D, et al. Allergen immunotherapy and health care cost benefits for children with allergic rhinitis: a large-scale, retrospective, matched cohort study. Ann Allergy Asthma Immunol. 2010;104:79–85.
69. Bernstein DL, Wanner M, Borish L, et al.; Immunotherapy Committee, American Academy of Allergy, Asthma and Immunology. Twelve-year survey of fatal reactions to allergen injections and skin testing: 1990-2001. J Allergy Clin Immunol. 2004;113:1129–1136.
70. Pajno GB, Castagnoli R, Arasi S, Licari A, Caminiti L, Marseglia GL. Pediatric use of omalizumab for allergic asthma. Expert Opin Biol Ther. 2020;20(7):695–703.
71. Chung KF, Wenzel SE, Brozek JL, et al. International ERS/ATS guidelines on definition, evaluation and treatment of severe asthma. Eur Respir J. 2014;43(2):343–73.
72. Normansell R, Walker S, Milan SJ, et al. Omalizumab for asthma in adults and children. Cochrane Database Syst Rev. 2014;1:CD003559.
73. Corren J, Kavati A, Ortiz B, Colby JA, Ruiz K, Maiese BA, Cadarette SM, Panettieri RA Jr. Efficacy and safety of omalizumab in children and adolescents with moderate-to-severe asthma: a systematic literature review. Allergy Asthma Proc. 2017;38(4):250–63.
74. Harb H, Chatila TA. Mechanisms of Dupilumab. Clin Exp Allergy. 2020;50(1):5–14.
75. Licari A, Castagnoli R, Marseglia A, Olivero F, Votto M, Ciprandi G, Marseglia GL. Dupilumab to treat type 2 inflammatory diseases in children and adolescents. Paediatr Drugs. 2020;22(3):295–310.

35 Allergic Rhinitis: Pediatric Pulmonologist Perspective

Ahmet Turkeli and Batuhan Berk Demir

35.1 Introduction

Lung diseases in children are a leading cause of morbidity and mortality worldwide. Some of these include asthma, cystic fibrosis, neuromuscular disorders, pulmonary hypertension, interstitial and diffuse lung diseases, sleep disorders, aerodigestive disorders, opportunistic and complicated pneumonia, apnea, acute and chronic respiratory failure, primary ciliary dyskinesia, and undiagnosed genetic childhood respiratory diseases.

Allergic rhinitis (AR) is a chronic inflammatory disease of the nasal mucosa induced by environmental allergen exposure and the immunoglobulin E (IgE) response [1, 2]. AR can be intermittent or persistent, based on the duration of symptoms, and mild, moderate, or severe, based on the severity of symptoms [3]. Environmental factors that induce AR are pollen, dust mites, mold fungi, and animal dander [4]. Typical symptoms include nasal discharge, sneezing, nasal irritation, and nasal congestion [2]. Also observed are extranasal symptoms including watery eyes, redness, swelling, irritation in the eyes, itching on the palate, and itching in the ears [2, 3]. The underlying inflammatory process and/or dysfunction of the nasal mucosa [3] are responsible for these symptoms. AR can also negatively influence patients' quality of life, cause sleep disturbances, and result in poor work or school performance [3, 5].

A. Turkeli (✉)
Division of Pediatric Immunology and Allergy, Department of Pediatrics, Kutahya Health Science University Medical Faculty, Kutahya, Turkey

B. B. Demir
Department of Pediatrics, Kutahya Health Science University Medical Faculty, Kutahya, Turkey

H. Yüksel et al. (eds.), *Pediatric Airway Diseases*, Comprehensive ENT,
https://doi.org/10.1007/978-3-031-74853-0_35

Common in pediatric patients, allergic rhinitis can have significant consequences for respiratory functions. A pediatric pulmonologist must assess the effects of allergic rhinitis on the respiratory system and overall respiratory health.

35.2 Allergic Rhinitis and Asthma

The airway consists of a unified structure that extends from the nostril to the small peripheral airways [6]. Unified airway disease (UAD) refers the common epidemiological and pathophysiological relationship among chronic inflammatory diseases of the upper and lower respiratory tracts, including AR, chronic rhinosinusitis (CRS), and asthma [7–9].

Asthma is a chronic inflammatory disease of the airways characterized by structural changes and the involvement of numerous cells and cellular components, including mast cells, eosinophils, T cells, macrophages, and epithelial cells. Asthma patients exhibit wheezing, sputum production, varying degrees of ventilation limitation, and airway hypersensitivity to environmental bronchospasmogenic stimuli [10].

At the beginning of the 1990s, asthma and rhinitis were viewed as separate maladies associated with IgE sensitivity. In the European Community Respiratory Health Survey (ECRHS), rhinitis was recognized as an independent risk factor for asthma in both allergic and non-allergic patients [11].

Upper and lower airways are interconnected anatomically, histologically, and immunologically, forming a unified airway system in which inflammation in one part of the airways effects the other [7]. Numerous studies conducted in accordance with the "one airway, one disease" theory have shown that the comorbidity of rhinitis and asthma conveys a single disease pattern in the airways. AR and asthma share the same etiological factors, inflammatory cell profile, location in the respiratory system, and treatment similarities [12]. Various international guidelines, including Allergic Rhinitis and Its Impact on Asthma (ARIA), the International Consensus Statement on Allergy and Rhinology: Allergic Rhinosinusitis and Rhinosinusitis, and the European Position Paper on Rhinosinusitis and Nasal Polyps (EPOS), investigate the interaction between the upper and lower airways [7].

35.2.1 Epidemiological Relationship

Reportedly, the prevalence of AR ranges from 5 to 50% worldwide [4]. According to studies, the prevalence of AR in children may be higher than in adults, with 80% of patients experiencing symptoms before the age of 20, and in some countries, 40% of patients developing symptoms before the age of 6 [13]. In patients with rhinitis, the risk of developing asthma is three times higher than in those without rhinitis, regardless of the presence of atopy [8, 14]. There is substantial evidence that AR in childhood or adolescence is a risk factor for subsequent asthma development [10, 15, 16]. 80–90% of asthma patients have rhinitis, and 20–40% of rhinitis patients have asthma [14, 17].

Untreated or inadequately treated rhinitis can triple the risk of asthma attacks, and bronchial hyperreactivity is common among rhinitis patients [12]. It has been shown that infants with increased airway sensitivity to histamine are four times more likely to develop asthma [18]. In non-asthmatic but symptomatic patients with AR, the methacholine bronchial provocation test revealed high rates of positivity [19, 20].

The coexistence of AR and asthma poses a significant risk for deterioration in asthma control and asthma exacerbations [6]. Those who suffer from both rhinitis and asthma tend to have more severe conditions [14, 15]. Large population-based studies have demonstrated a correlation between the two diseases' severity [10, 14]. In children with asthma and AR, more frequent visits to the emergency room and admissions indicate inferior disease control, more frequent exacerbations, and increased hospitalizations. This circumstance results in increased healthcare utilization and asthma costs among asthmatic children with AR [8, 21]. In a study of approximately 30,000 asthmatic patients conducted in Japan, it was discovered that patients with concomitant AR were more likely to have uncontrolled asthma as defined by the GINA guidelines than patients without AR [22]. In contrast, Ponte and colleagues [23] demonstrated that moderate to severe rhinitis is associated with inadequately controlled asthma.

Allergens are potent inducers of AR and asthma. Indoor allergens, such as house dust mites, are linked to asthma, whereas outdoor allergens, such as pollen, are more often linked to AR [24].

35.2.2 Relationship Between the Upper and Lower Respiratory Tracts from a Pathophysiological Standpoint

The passageway that runs from the nose and paranasal sinuses to the bronchi is deemed a functional unit according to the unified airway model [10, 14]. Chronic inflammation is observed in the nasal mucosa and bronchial mucosa, the two most significant regions of this unified airway. While the nasal and bronchial mucosa share similar characteristics, such as pseudostratified epithelium and the presence of both ciliated and columnar cells on the basement membrane, they exhibit significant differences at the submucosal level. In contrast to the nasal mucosa, which is dominated by vascular structures, the bronchial airways are dominated by muscle structures encircling the airways [7, 25]. Vasodilation and edema result from inflammation of the nasal mucosa, whereas inflammation of the bronchial mucosa causes smooth muscle contraction [14].

Although there is mounting evidence that AR may influence the clinical course of asthma, the mechanisms connecting upper and lower airway dysfunction remain poorly understood. Various hypotheses, including both direct and indirect effects, have been proposed to explain the pathophysiological connection between the upper and lower respiratory tracts, specifically, an altered respiratory pattern, pulmonary aspiration of nasal contents, the nasal-bronchial reflex, and the uptake of inflammatory mediators into the systemic circulation [7, 20].

Due to its anatomical location, the nostril warms, filters, and moistens the air that is inhaled. In fact, exercise-induced bronchospasm is caused by the chilling and drying of the airways caused by forced mouth breathing during vigorous exercise. In addition, numerous submucosal glands in the nostril are capable of sterilizing the air via the release of antibacterial enzymes. Since nasal congestion in AR forces the patient to breathe through the mouth, nasal function may be completely or partially impaired. Mouth breathing allows allergens and frigid air to enter the bronchial airways directly, causing hypersensitivity in the airways [7, 26, 27].

35.2.3 Effects Systemic of Nasal Inflammation on the Lower Respiratory System

Regardless of the tissue in which the allergic reaction occurs, it triggers not only a local immune response but also a systemic response by allowing the inflammatory reaction to spread to other organs via the circulatory system. Even in the absence of clinical asthma, patients with AR exhibit not only a local inflammatory response effecting the nasal airway, but also a more widespread inflammation in the airways [14]. In patients with seasonal AR but without asthma, for instance, nasal allergen tests not only induce bronchial airway sensitization but also increase eosinophil counts in sputum samples [28]. When segmental bronchial provocation is performed on AR patients without asthma, it induces nasal inflammation and an increase in peripheral blood eosinophils [29]. It has been shown that eosinophilic inflammation occurs in the nasal mucosa of asthmatics in response to bronchial allergen provocation [26]. This occurs in the bronchial mucosa of patients with allergic rhinitis. The release of eosinophils, basophils, and their progenitor cells from the bone marrow [7] is likely caused by the absorption of inflammatory mediators (e.g., IL-5 and eotaxin) from sites of inflammation into the systemic circulation. Before and 24 h after nasal allergen testing, bronchial and nasal biopsies were performed on AR patients, and an increase in the number of eosinophils was observed in the nasal and bronchial epithelium at the end of 24 h [30].

The nasobronchial reflex is another mechanism that may explain bronchial hyperreactivity in AR patients. Bronchoconstriction is mediated by vagal, trigeminal, and afferent receptor pathways. Nose, trachea, pharynx, and respiratory tract contain receptors that are sensitive to mechanical and chemical variables. The neural signals then travel to the central nervous system and activate the efferent vagus nerve, resulting in hyperreactivity of the bronchial smooth muscle. Exposure of the nasal mucosa to cold and dry air, for instance, may induce sudden bronchoconstriction in asthmatic patients [6, 15, 31].

Impaired Mucosal Function: It has been demonstrated that allergic inflammation of the respiratory mucosa disrupts the barrier function of the epithelium. This disruption in epithelial integrity may result in increased allergen absorption and IgE synthesis, affecting the lower respiratory tract as a consequence. Alternately, impaired nasal mucosa may be more susceptible to viruses, resulting in an increase in allergic susceptibility and an increase in asthma incidence [25, 32].

35.2.4 Immunopathology

Recent research has demonstrated that the immunological mechanisms underlying AR and atopic asthma are identical. Both the upper and lower respiratory tract tissues contain structural (epithelial cells, mast cells, and dendritic cells) and infiltrative (eosinophils, Th2 cells) cell types. In allergic airway diseases, airway inflammation is characterized by Th2 cells (Th2 cells, type 2 B cells, IL-4-producing natural killer T cells (NKT cells), basophils, eosinophils, mast cells, ILC2, IL4, IL5, IL13, IL-25, IL-31, and IL-33). In addition to the adaptive immune response, the upper and lower respiratory tracts share similarities with the innate immune system, such as epithelial barrier function and innate immune cells (ILCs) [7, 9, 33]. Airway epithelial cells swiftly secrete the cytokines IL-25, IL-33, and thymic stromal lymphopoietin (TSLP) when exposed to environmental antigens, viruses, and allergens. These so-called alarmins directly activate ILC2s, which produce the prototypical type 2 cytokines IL-5 and IL-13 [7]. It is common to observe nasal inflammation in asthma patients without rhinitis symptoms and bronchial inflammation in rhinitis patients without asthma symptoms. Even in individuals with no history of bronchial hyperreactivity, nasal allergen provocation can swiftly induce significant pulmonary allergic inflammation and impaired respiratory function in patients with AR. In addition, segmental bronchial provocation may result in nasal symptoms and inflammation in patients with AR [34].

35.2.5 Effect of Rhinitis Therapy on Asthma

The most efficacious pharmacotherapy agent for AR is intranasal corticosteroids (INC). They have powerful effects on symptoms, nasal physiology, and inflammation of the upper airway mucosa. In a case-control study in which patients with both AR and asthma were treated with INC, it was found that those patients had significantly reduced risks of asthma-related emergency department visits and hospitalization [35]. Compared to placebo, a meta-analysis revealed that INC improved PFT, BHR, asthma symptom scores, asthma quality-of-life scores, and rescue medication use in patients who were not receiving adequate asthma treatment. When INC was administered to asthmatic patients receiving inhaled corticosteroids, no significant change in asthma outcomes was observed [36]. These studies demonstrate the significance of recognizing the connection between rhinitis and asthma, both in terms of reducing somatic symptoms and healthcare costs.

Contradictory effects of antihistamine medications on asthma. It is unclear whether the beneficial effects of antihistamines in asthma are due to direct effects on the physiology of the lower airways or to the alleviation of rhinitis. Antihistamines are not included in the management of asthma according to the 2022 Global Initiative for Asthma guidelines, but it is crucial to remember that asthma treatment is not "one size fits all" [37].

35.2.6 Diagnostic and Therapeutic Strategies

Patients with rhinitis and/or asthma should undergo a thorough examination and evaluation of both the upper and lower respiratory tracts [10, 27]. Symptoms, including itching, sneezing, nasal discharge, nasal obstruction, and odor, are the primary basis for a clinical suspicion of AR. These symptoms begin within minutes of allergen exposure and last for approximately 2 h. Late symptoms include nasal congestion, loss of scent, hyperreactivity of the nose, and postnasal mucus discharge [27]. Other associated symptoms (such as snoring, poor sleep quality, and ear congestion), shortness of breath with exercise, protracted cough after viral infections, and nocturnal coughs should also be investigated and taken into account when selecting a treatment [10, 38]. Evaluation of the clinical history should include an investigation of the impact of rhinitis on daily life, school performance, and sleep, as well as a comprehensive family history of allergic or immunological diseases [38].

A physical examination should also include anthropometric measurements and evaluation of the skin, ear, nose, oral cavity, and neck, with special attention devoted to signs of atopy [10, 39]. Dennie Morgan lines (is a fold or line in the skin below the lower eyelid), nasal bridging, allergic salute, conjunctivitis, and allergic shiner are typical atopy symptoms [10, 27]. An essential overview is provided by anterior rhinoscopy, or at least nasal examination, which can be performed with an otoscopc. Secretions (typically aqueous in AR, change in color in non-allergic rhinitis (NAR), or infectious rhinitis), crusts, foreign bodies, septum deviation, septum perforation, polyps, and mucosal edema are frequently observed. The use of nasal endoscopy is not required [10, 27].

In children and adolescents, allergic rhinitis is the most prevalent form of chronic rhinitis; chronic non-allergic rhinitis, or CRS, is less common [40].

To diagnose A. rhinitis and asthma, allergy skin tests (SPT) or in vitro measurements of specific IgE using the inhalant allergen panel are required. The SPT is the primary in vivo test recommended by international guidelines and is considered the most sensitive and specific test for identifying atopy [41]. This information is essential for distinguishing allergic rhinitis from non-allergic disease or other diseases such as CRS and devising an appropriate environmental control program.

Imaging is not required, but CT scanning of the nasal sinuses is recommended when sinusitis is suspected [27].

35.2.7 Non-pharmaceutical Treatment Method

It has been demonstrated that avoiding the allergen to which a person is sensitive can help control rhinitis and asthma in IgE-mediated sensitized individuals. All patients with atopy should do this. Within 3 months, the desired clinical improvement will be observed. Therefore, the effectiveness of non-pharmacological treatments is directly proportional to the duration of allergen exposure [10, 12].

35.2.8 Pharmaceutical Medication Policy

It has been demonstrated that rhinitis treatment improves asthma control. INCs are frequently the first-line treatment for AR in patients with persistent symptoms, particularly when nasal congestion is present. In addition to being an effective treatment for moderate to severe rhinitis, INC has also been demonstrated to reduce airway hyperresponsiveness (AHR) and ease asthma symptoms [10].

Oral H1 antihistamines are the most effective medications for alleviating sneezing, itching, and runny noses, while having minimal effects on nasal congestion. This is why they are frequently unified with oral decongestants like pseudoephedrine. Second-generation antihistamines effectively reduce allergy symptoms without causing sleep disturbances or adverse events [37, 42].

Montelukast has been shown to reduce all symptoms of rhinitis, including nasal congestion and allergic rhinoconjunctivitis (AR), and has been widely used in the treatment of asthma, but therapeutic consideration is limited by a Food and Drug Administration (FDA) boxed warning for potential serious neuropsychiatric side effects, such as suicidal ideation and night terrors [42].

The biologic agents omalizumab, mepolizumab, dupilumab, benralizumab, and reslizumab are examples. Although not licensed for rheumatoid arthritis (RA), patients who receive these agents for an unapproved indication may experience symptomatic improvement [42].

35.2.9 Immunotherapy Against Allergens

Allergen immunotherapy (AIT) is the only treatment modality that can alter the trajectory of allergic diseases. There are currently two primary administration routes for AIT: subcutaneous (SCIT) and sublingual (SLIT) [43]. AIT has the potential to prevent the onset of asthma, particularly in children and adolescents with AR and grass/pollen allergies [44]. A systematic review confirmed that AIT is efficacious in preventing the onset of asthma in monosensitized children when administered for at least 3 years [43]. In addition, AIT reduces the risk of new allergen sensitization in these patients, although the evidence is limited [44]. Immunotherapy is known to be effective as both a treatment and preventative measure for allergic asthma patients [45].

Compared to an open control group, 3 years of SCIT treatment in children with seasonal allergic rhinitis reduced the development of asthma symptoms and improved bronchial reactivity. SCIT should be a strong recommendation for all children with moderate to severe allergic rhinitis [46], given that it induces long-lasting alterations in AR and reduces the risk of asthma.

35.3 Allergic Rhinitis and Sleep Disorder

Disorders of sleep are prevalent in both infants and adults. Nasal congestion is the most common and bothersome symptom of rhinitis and is considered one of the primary causes of sleep disturbance in affected individuals. The severity of the disease is directly proportional to the severity of the sleep disorder. Nasal obstruction is an independent risk factor for obstructive sleep apnea (OSA) and frequently causes microarousals and fragmented sleep. Rhinitis by itself is linked to moderate OSA [27]. A systematic review of articles published within the last quarter-century revealed a statistically significant association between allergic rhinitis in infants and sleep-disordered breathing, such as snoring and OSA [47]. AR has been identified as a risk factor for nocturnal sleep-related dysfunctions including insomnia, nocturnal urination, disrupted sleep, OSA, and snoring. In addition, antiretroviral therapy has been found to increase the risk of diurnal sleep-related dysfunctions [48].

The disruption of children's nighttime sleep results in daytime fatigue and sleepiness and is frequently associated with altered immune function, anxiety, attention deficit problems, memory deficits, behavioral issues, irritability, depression, growth retardation, hormone imbalance, hypertension, poor academic performance, and increased accident rates. It is linked to substance abuse and an increased risk of cardiovascular and metabolic disorders. As a consequence, it has a negative impact on the quality of life and health-related quality [49].

Treatments that reduce nasal congestion may also improve sleep and daytime drowsiness, thereby enhancing quality of life. In addition, treatments that reduce inflammation and frequently also reduce congestion may have a beneficial effect by lowering levels of inflammatory mediators [49].

35.4 Allergic Rhinitis and Bronchiectasia

Our understanding of atopy and AR in bronchiectasis patients is limited. In a study analyzing the electronic health records of patients with bronchiectasis, the rate of AR was found to be significantly higher than in patients without bronchiectasis [50]. In an adult study, the prevalence of AR in patients with bronchiectasis was reported to be 31.7% [51]. In adult bronchiectasis patients with AR, dyspnea and the number of emergency department visits in the previous year were found to be greater than in patients without AR [51]. It was discovered that allergic rhinitis is an independent risk factor for the presence of CRS in bronchiectasis patients [52]. Multiple allergen sensitization was more prevalent in bronchiectasis than in a cohort with allergic rhinitis used as a comparison. Sensitization was associated with poor clinical outcomes, such as decreased pulmonary function and disease severity [53]. In patients with bronchiectasis, untreated and undetected AR can increase physical disability, morbidity, and healthcare utilization.

35.5 Rhinitis and Cystic Fibrosis

It is known that allergic bronchopulmonary aspergillosis (ABPA) and drug allergies are prevalent in cystic fibrosis, but the literature examining the allergy profile and possible mechanisms in CF is limited [54]. The estimated prevalence of AR in patients with CF is 48%; this rate is higher than in patients with bronchiectasis other than CF [55]. The prevalence of AR was found to be higher in a cohort of children with cystic fibrosis. Children with cystic fibrosis have impaired mucosal clearance, allowing allergens to persist in the upper airway. This, along with inflammatory changes in the airway epithelium, may produce a highly conducive environment for sensitization. AR appears prior to ABPA; if reproducible on a larger scale, this may indicate that A. fumigatus-associated allergy first manifests in the upper respiratory tract as AR prior to contributing to the pathogenesis of lower respiratory allergy (ABPA).

35.6 Conclusion

Comprehending the potential impact of allergic rhinitis on respiratory health is crucial to provide appropriate treatments and to avoid long-term complications. Common comorbidities among adolescents with AR include asthma, CRS, bronchiectasis, cystic fibrosis, and OSA. Early and effective management may reduce the risk of developing asthma in adulthood. As part of a holistic approach to care, these comorbid conditions should be taken into account during diagnosis and treatment, and the child's respiratory health should be optimized. The child's overall health and respiratory function can be enhanced by addressing the impact of AR on respiratory health, customizing treatment plans, and monitoring comorbid conditions.

References

1. Oermann CM, Lahiri T, Peterson-Carmichael SL, et al. The history of workforce concerns in pediatric pulmonary medicine. Pediatr Pulmonol. 2023;58(3):683–9.
2. Lisik D, Ermis SSÖ, Ioannidou A, et al. Siblings and risk of allergic rhinitis: a systematic review and meta-analysis. Pediatr Allergy Immunol. 2023;34(7):e13991.
3. D'Amato G, Murrieta-Aguttes M, D'Amato M, et al. Pollen respiratory allergy: is it really seasonal? World Allergy Organ J. 2023;16(7):100799.
4. Wise SK, Damask C, Roland LTC, et al. International consensus statement on allergy and rhinology: allergic rhinitis—2023. Int Forum Allergy Rhinol. 2023;13(4):293–859.
5. Bousquet J, Schünemann HJ, Togias A, et al. Next-generation allergic rhinitis and its impact on asthma (ARIA) guidelines for allergic rhinitis based on grading of recommendations assessment, development and evaluation (GRADE) and real-world evidence. J Allergy Clin Immunol. 2020;145(1):70–80.e3.
6. Bieber T. The united airway disease. In: Aksi CA, Hellings PW, Agache I, editors. The EAACI global atlas of allergic rhinitis and chronic rhinosinusitis. Zurich: European Academy of Allergy and Clinical Immunology; 2015.

7. Fokkens W, Reitsma S. Unified airway disease: a contemporary review and introduction. Otolaryngol Clin North Am. 2022;56(1):1–10.
8. Tiotiu A, Novakova P, Baiardini I, et al. Manifesto on united airways diseases (UAD): an Interasma (global asthma association—GAA) document. J Asthma. 2022;59(4):639–54.
9. Ahmad JG, Marino MJ, Luong AU. Unified airway disease: future directions. Otolaryngol Clin North Am. 2022;56(1):181–95.
10. Georgopoulos R, Krouse JH, Toskala E. Why otolaryngologists and asthma are a good match: the allergic rhinitis-asthma connection. Otolaryngol Clin North Am. 2014;47(1):1–12.
11. Bousquet J, Melén E, Haahtela T, et al. Rhinitis associated with asthma is distinct from rhinitis alone: the ARIA-MeDALL hypothesis. Allergy. 2023;78(5):1169–203.
12. Paiva Ferreira LKD, Paiva Ferreira LAM, et al. Combined allergic rhinitis and asthma syndrome (CARAS). Int Immunopharmacol. 2019;74:105718.
13. Licari A, Ciprandi G, Marseglia A, et al. Current recommendations and emerging options for the treatment of allergic rhinitis. Expert Rev Clin Immunol. 2014;10(10):1337–47.
14. Shtraks JP, Toskala E. Manifestations of inhalant allergies beyond the nose. Otolaryngol Clin North Am. 2017;50(6):1051–64.
15. Feng CH, Miller MD, Simon RA. The united allergic airway: connections between allergic rhinitis, asthma, and chronic sinusitis. Am J Rhinol Allergy. 2012;26(3):187–90.
16. Tohidinik HR, Mallah N, Takkouche B. History of allergic rhinitis and risk of asthma; a systematic review and meta-analysis. World Allergy Organ J. 2019;12(10):100069.
17. Brar T, Marino MJ, Lal D. Unified airway disease: genetics and epigenetics. Otolaryngol Clin North Am. 2023;56(1):23–38.
18. Choi SH, Yoo Y, Yu J, et al. Bronchial hyperresponsiveness in young children with allergic rhinitis and its risk factors. Allergy. 2007;62:1051 6.
19. Kirmaz C, Degirmenci PB, Tunali D, et al. Lower respiratory tract complications during nasal provocation: nonspecific stimulant or specific allergen? Ann Allergy Asthma Immunol. 2007;98(6):524–32.
20. Ciprandi G, Cirillo I, Tosca MA, et al. Bronchial hyperreactivity and spirometric impairment in patients with seasonal allergic rhinitis. Respir Med. 2004;98(9):826–31.
21. Kang HY, Park CS, Bang HR, et al. Effect of allergic rhinitis on the use and cost of health services by children with asthma. Yonsei Med J. 2008;49(4):521–9.
22. Ohta K, Bousquet PJ, Aizawa H, et al. Prevalence and impact of rhinitis in asthma. SACRA, a cross-sectional nation-wide study in Japan. Allergy. 2011;66(10):1287–95.
23. Ponte EV, Franco R, Nascimento HF, et al. Lack of control of severe asthma is associated with co-existence of moderate-to-severe rhinitis. Allergy. 2008;63:564–9.
24. Li J, Huang Y, Lin X, Zhao D, et al.; China Alliance of Research on Respiratory Allergic Disease (CARRAD). Influence of degree of specific allergic sensitivity on severity of rhinitis and asthma in Chinese allergic patients. Respir Res. 2011;12(1):95.
25. Yuksel H, Turkeli A. Airway epithelial barrier dysfunction in the pathogenesis and prognosis of respiratory tract diseases in childhood and adulthood. Tissue Barriers. 2017;5(4):e1367458.
26. Inal A, Kendirli SG, Yilmaz M, et al. Indices of lower airway inflammation in children monosensitized to house dust mite after nasal allergen challenge. Allergy. 2008;63(10):1345–51.
27. Tenero L, Vaia R, Ferrante G, et al. Diagnosis and management of allergic rhinitis in asthmatic children. J Asthma Allergy. 2023;16:45–57.
28. Bonay M, Neukirch C, Grandsaigne M, et al. Changes in airway inflammation following nasal allergic challenge in patients with seasonal rhinitis. Allergy. 2006;61:111–8.
29. Braunstahl GJ, Kleinjan A, Overbeek SE, et al. Segmental bronchial provocation induces nasal inflammation in allergic rhinitis patients. Am J Respir Crit Care Med. 2000;161:2051–7.
30. Braunstahl GJ, Overbeek SE, Kleinjan A, et al. Nasal allergen provocation induces adhesion molecule expression and tissue eosinophilia in upper and lower airways. J Allergy Clin Immunol. 2001;107:469–76.
31. Cingi C, Muluk NB, Cobanoglu B, et al. Nasobronchial interaction. World J Clin Cases. 2015;3(6):499–503.
32. Kucuksezer UC, Ozdemir C, Yazici D, et al. The epithelial barrier theory: development and exacerbation of allergic and other chronic inflammatory diseases. Asia Pac Allergy. 2023;13(1):28–39.

33. Maspero J, Adir Y, Al-Ahmad M, et al. Type 2 inflammation in asthma and other airway diseases. ERJ Open Res. 2022;8(3):00576–2021.
34. Caimmi D, Marseglia A, Pieri G, et al. Nose and lungs: one way, one disease. Ital J Pediatr. 2012;38:60.
35. Corren J, Manning BE, Thompson SF, et al. Rhinitis therapy and the prevention of hospital care for asthma: a case-control study. J Allergy Clin Immunol. 2003;113(3):415–9.
36. Lohia S, Schlosser RJ, Soler ZM. Impact of intranasal corticosteroids on asthma outcomes in allergic rhinitis: a meta-analysis. Allergy. 2013;68:569–79.
37. Linton S, Hossenbaccus L, Ellis AK. Evidence-based use of antihistamines for treatment of allergic conditions. Ann Allergy Asthma Immunol. 2023;131(4):412–20. S1081-1206(23)00524-0.
38. Doulaptsi M, Aoi N, Kawauchi H, et al. Differentiating rhinitis in the paediatric population by giving focus on medical history and clinical examination. Med Sci. 2019;7(3):38–52.
39. Roberts G, Xatzipsalti M, Borrego LM, et al. Paediatric rhinitis: position paper of the European Academy of Allergy and Clinical Immunology. Allergy. 2013;68(9):1102–16.
40. Huang Y, Zhang Y, Zhang L. Prevalence of allergic and nonallergic rhinitis in a rural area of northern China based on sensitization to specific aeroallergens. Allergy Asthma Clin Immunol. 2018;14:77.
41. Testera-Montes A, Jurado R, Salas M, et al. Diagnostic tools in allergic rhinitis. Front Allergy. 2021;2:721851.
42. Wise SK, Damask C, Greenhawt M, et al. A synopsis of guidance for allergic rhinitis diagnosis and management from ICAR 2023. J Allergy Clin Immunol Pract. 2023;11(3):773–96.
43. Farraia M, Paciência I, Castro Mendes F, et al. Allergen immunotherapy for asthma prevention: a systematic review and meta-analysis of randomized and non-randomized controlled studies. Allergy. 2022;77(6):1719–35.
44. Halken S, Larenas-Linnemann D, Roberts G, et al. EAACI guidelines on allergen immunotherapy: prevention of allergy. Pediatr Allergy Immunol. 2017;28:728–45.
45. Alamri RA, Aljabri GH, Tahlawi R, et al. Immunotherapy in the treatment of allergic rhinitis in children. Cureus. 2022;14(12):e32464.
46. Jutel M, Brüggenjürgen B, Richter H, et al. Real-world evidence of subcutaneous allergoid immunotherapy in house dust mite-induced allergic rhinitis and asthma. Allergy. 2020;75(8):2050–8.
47. Lin SY, Melvin TAN, Boss EF, et al. The association between allergic rhinitis and sleep-disordered breathing in children: a systematic review. Int Forum Allergy Rhinol. 2013;3(6):504–9.
48. Liu J, Zhang X, Zhao Y, et al. The association between allergic rhinitis and sleep: a systematic review and meta-analysis of observational studies. PLoS One. 2020;15:e0228533.
49. D'Elia C, Gozal D, Bruni O, et al. Allergic rhinitis and sleep disorders in children—coexistence and reciprocal interactions. J Pediatr (Rio J). 2021;98(5):444–54.
50. Mäntylä J, Kauppi P, Toppila-Salmi S. Chronic rhinosinusitis is associated with non-cystic fibrosis bronchiectasis: a new clinical implication? J Allergy Clin Immunol. 2022;150(3):592–3.
51. Niksarlıoğlu EY, Işık R, Uysal MA. Prevalence of atopy and allergic rhinitis in patients with adult non-cystic fibrosis bronchiectasis. Turk J Med Sci. 2019;49(2):551–7.
52. Somani SN, Kwah JH, Yeh C, et al. Prevalence and characterization of chronic rhinosinusitis in patients with non-cystic fibrosis bronchiectasis at a tertiary care center in the United States. Int Forum Allergy Rhinol. 2019;9(12):1424–9.
53. Mac Aogáin M, Tiew PY, Lim AYH, et al. Distinct "immunoallertypes" of disease and high frequencies of sensitization in non-cystic fibrosis bronchiectasis. Am J Respir Crit Care Med. 2019;199(7):842–53.
54. Elborn J. Cystic fibrosis. Lancet. 2016;388(10059):2519–31.
55. Zemke AC, Nouraie SM, Moore J, et al. Clinical predictors of cystic fibrosis chronic rhinosinusitis severity. Int Forum Allergy Rhinol. 2019;9(7):759–65.

36 Allergic Rhinitis: Clinical and Therapeutic Aspects in Asthma

Adem Yaşar, Erol A. Gaillard, and Ozge Yilmaz

36.1 Epidemiology of Coexistence of Allergic Rhinitis and Asthma

Allergic rhinitis (AR) is a common disease with symptoms such as nasal discharge congestion, and sneezing, accompanied by ocular symptoms and postnasal discharge [1]. It affects more than 400 million people of all ages, particularly children, and is significantly associated with impairment of health-related quality of life [2, 3]. Asthma is a significant burden for a population of over 300 million people worldwide and is characterized by variable, recurrent, reversible airflow obstruction, and bronchial hyperresponsiveness [4, 5]. Symptomatic patients may experience wheezing, shortness of breath, coughing, chest tightness, and pain [4]. Allergic rhinitis is usually diagnosed before asthma, and patients with AR are three times more likely to develop asthma [6]. In approximately 10–40% of patients, AR is accompanied by asthma, while in 60–80% of patients with asthma, it is accompanied by allergic rhinitis [7, 8]. Burgess et al. reported a sevenfold increase in asthma risk in patients with AR in pre-puberty and a fourfold increase in asthma risk in adolescence [9]. The frequency of asthma comorbidity was determined to be higher in patients with moderate-to-severe and persistent AR than in patients with mild AR [10]. Allergic rhinitis severity was found to be positively correlated with asthma severity, and patients with moderate-to-severe AR had a 3.8-fold higher rate of emergency department visits for asthma attacks compared to patients without AR [11]. In a study evaluating the effect of the severity of allergic rhinitis on asthma control,

A. Yaşar (✉) · O. Yilmaz
Department of Pediatric Allergy, Manisa Celal Bayar University, School of Medicine, Manisa, Turkey

E. A. Gaillard
Department of Respiratory Sciences, University of Leicester, Leicester NIHR Biomedical Research Centre (Respiratory Theme), Leicester, UK

H. Yüksel et al. (eds.), *Pediatric Airway Diseases*, Comprehensive ENT,
https://doi.org/10.1007/978-3-031-74853-0_36

uncontrolled asthma was reported in 9.2% of pediatric patients without AR, 15.3% of those with mild-to-moderate AR, and 29.2% of those with severe AR [12]. Health-related quality-of-life scales conducted in patients with allergic rhinitis have shown that quality of life deteriorates due to the disease; similarly, it has been proven in studies that asthma-related quality of life deteriorates in patients with asthma [13, 14]. In health-related quality-of-life studies in which both diseases were evaluated together, it was reported that AR patients with comorbid asthma had lower quality-of-life levels and worse symptom control than those with AR alone, using a combined quality-of-life scale for AR and asthma [3]..

36.2 Pathogenesis of Coexistence of Allergic Rhinitis and Asthma

The common characteristic in the pathogenesis of allergic rhinitis and asthma is chronic inflammation in different parts of the airways, and these two diseases should be considered together [15, 16]. Moreover, the upper and lower airways have structurally similar anatomical, functional, and immunologic features. As both diseases have similar risk factors and pathogenetic features, this association is called "one airway diseases" [15]. It is suggested that the pathophysiological events that cause allergic rhinitis may similarly cause asthma [17, 18].

Increased bronchial reactivity to methacholine was observed in approximately 23% of patients with allergic rhinitis, and more bronchial hyperreactivity was found in patients with perennial allergic rhinitis than in patients with seasonal AR [15–17, 19]. Studies have found that the level of fractionated nitric oxide (FeNO) found in patients with AR is highly correlated with the degree of bronchial hyperreactivity [18, 20]. Therefore, increased FeNO in patients with AR may be a useful indicator for assessing the risk of developing asthma [19, 21]. Furthermore, nasal mucosal inflammation can be found in asthmatic patients even in the absence of AR symptoms, whereas eosinophilic inflammation and mild basement membrane thickening in the lungs can be found in patients with AR without asthma symptoms [15, 16]. The lymphoid flow of the upper and lower respiratory tracts is located in a common pool and responds to foreign stimuli (allergens, microorganisms, etc.) through similar effector cells [7].

A study evaluating the molecular mechanisms between asthma, AR, and eczema reports that a number of protein structures and cellular mechanisms are common to atopic diseases [22]. Furthermore, a number of protein structures have been identified in the pathophysiology of asthma and AR formation, which play a crucial role in the mutual interaction [7]. The studies have found 35 proteins common to both AR and asthma, and some of these protein structures have been found to belong to the HLA-DRB and HLA-DQ families, which are involved in T-cell activation, development, and IgE response [7]. Eight common genes (CLC, EMR4P, IL5RA, FRRS1, HRH4, SLC29A1, SIGLEC8, and IL1RL1) hypothesized to be involved in the multimorbidity link between AR and asthma have been identified [23]. The solute carrier family 14 member 1 (SLCA14A1) gene, which is a significant marker in acute asthma attacks, the synuclein alpha (SNCA) gene, which plays a role in air pollution-induced asthma and is an oxidative stress gene, and the asthma-associated tensin 1 (TNS1) gene were found to be upregulated in AR asthma association, and the regulatory miRNA has-miR93-5p was found to be downregulated [24]. In one study investigating epigenetic changes in patients with allergic rhinitis and asthma, more than 10 miRNA types were identified, particularly those related to inflammatory processes regulated by miRNAs [25]. A significant association was found between single nucleotide polymorphisms in the protein tyrosine phosphatase non-receptor (PTPN22) gene and the cytotoxic T-lymphocyte-associated antigen 4 (CTLA-4) gene in patients with AR accompanied by asthma, which may be a susceptibility factor for AR and asthma [26]. Common pathways observed in the genesis of both diseases would help explain the subclinical inflammation of the lower respiratory tract detected in some cases of AR [27].

Allergen sensitization is a significant risk factor in the development of all atopic diseases [28]. Repeated inhaled allergen exposure may lead to asthma in patients with AR [29]. Some studies have reported that mite allergy is a risk factor for the development of asthma in patients with AR, while another study reported that mite sensitization is not a risk factor [30, 31]. This inconsistency between the studies was attributed to the differences in the geographical regions and climatics where the studies were conducted [7].

Harmful chemicals in tobacco smoke cause cilia loss, mucus gland hypertrophy, inflammation, and epithelial changes in the upper respiratory tract [32]. Consistent with the association between smoking and/or exposure to tobacco smoke at home and AR, tobacco exposure has also been shown to alter markers of allergic inflammation such as total IgE, skin prick test positivity, and blood eosinophilia [33]. Also, there are different types of bacteria, viruses, and fungi in the respiratory tract of healthy people, just like in the gastrointestinal tract [34]. Microbial colonization of the respiratory tract can vary depending on exposures in the living environment (e.g., tobacco smoke), and bacterial dysbiosis can occur with prolonged exposure [35]. Tobacco smoke increases mucus production in the airways, impairs mucociliary clearance, and may affect the microbiota in the respiratory tract by disrupting favorable microenvironmental conditions by causing low-grade inflammation [36]. Smoking is known to be a significant risk factor for asthma and asthma attacks in children. In patients with AR and no asthma, the risk of developing asthma was found to be higher in the smoking group than in the non-smoking group (OR 2.98) [37]. Tobacco exposure is a risk factor for both asthma and AR, as well as for their co-occurrence [37].

36.3 Coexistence of Allergic Rhinitis and Asthma in the Context of Therapeutic Approach

The systemic inflammatory nature of both AR and asthma prompts common approaches to treatment. Environmental control measures and avoidance of allergens as well as pharmacologic treatments and immunotherapy form the mainstay of treatment for AR asthma [38].

Appropriate treatment of allergic rhinitis improves control of concomitant asthma [38]. In a study including AR and asthmatic subjects, the rate of asthma-related hospitalization and emergency department admission was 1.3% in the AR-treated group, whereas the rate of hospitalization and emergency department admission was 6.6% in asthmatic subjects with untreated AR [39]. A 6-week double-blind randomized trial involving subjects with seasonal AR and mild-to-moderate asthma compared treatment with 5 mg loratadine and 120 mg pseudoephedrine twice daily with placebo. Nasal symptoms, asthma symptoms, pulmonary function, and quality of life were significantly improved in the treatment compared to the placebo group [40, 41]. In another study, it was reported that antihistaminic agents may have beneficial effects on asthma symptoms and may improve the quality of life in patients with AR and comorbid asthma [42]. It was reported that leukotriene receptor antagonists (LRTI) may be effective when used in patients with AR and asthma, especially in patients older than 6 years, and LRTI improved nasal and bronchial symptoms by reducing beta-agonist use in patients with seasonal AR and asthma comorbidity [38, 43, 44].

In patients with both AR and asthma, it was reported that intranasal corticosteroid treatment significantly reduces asthma symptom score, disease severity, and the need for rescue medication. Intranasal corticosteroid treatment also prevented exercise-associated asthma and bronchial hyperreactivity associated with seasonal pollen intake, and improved lung function [41, 45].

Allergen immunotherapy has been used to treat allergic rhinitis and asthma [46, 47]. Allergen immunotherapy for allergic rhinitis can prevent new allergen sensitization and asthma development [48]. Studies have shown that the risk of asthma was reduced by 2.68 times during the 5-year follow-up of immunotherapy patients [49, 50]. A Cochrane analysis showed positive effects of immunotherapy on asthma symptoms and bronchial hyperreactivity in patients with allergic rhinitis [51]. Meta-analyses and systematic reviews evaluating the efficacy of immunotherapy in preventing new allergic sensitization and/or onset of asthma in atopic patients reported the efficacy of immunotherapy [52, 53]. In a meta-analysis evaluating the safety, clinical, and cost-effectiveness of immunotherapy, it was concluded that the risk of developing asthma in patients with AR treated with immunotherapy was reduced in the short term, but there was no conclusive evidence in the long term [54].

Biologic agents are medications that have recently become available for the treatment of atopic diseases. Omalizumab is a recombinant, humanized, monoclonal antibody against IgE. Anti-IgE therapy omalizumab has been reported to be effective in preventing asthma exacerbations, improving symptoms of both asthma and rhinitis, and improving the quality of life [41]. In a randomized, double-blind, placebo-controlled clinical trial, improvements in polyp size, nasal obstruction, anterior rhinorrhea, anosmia, wheezing, and dyspnea were observed with the use of omalizumab [55, 56]. Another biologic agent, dupilumab, is an anti-interleukin (IL)-4 receptor-α and anti-IL-13 antibody and may be a treatment option for patients with both severe allergic asthma and allergic rhinitis [57]. In patients with uncontrolled persistent asthma who received 300 mg of dupilumab every 2 weeks, AR-related nasal symptoms were significantly improved [58]. Mepolizumab is a humanized monoclonal antibody targeting IL-5 and is used as adjunctive therapy in patients with eosinophilic asthma. A post hoc meta-analysis of four-phase IIb/III clinical trials investigating the effect of mepolizumab concluded that mepolizumab may be helpful in targeted therapy and reducing the burden of disease in individuals with severe eosinophilic asthma and comorbid disease [59].

Research is ongoing on new therapies alongside existing therapeutic agents [5]. Allergic rhinitis and asthma are common respiratory diseases that cause socioeconomic and health-related deterioration in quality of life. Allergic rhinitis is significant for the development of asthma and asthma symptom control. Due to the heterogeneous distribution of diseases, it is important to have a precise and personalized treatment plan. Over time, elucidation of the pathological mechanisms that cause diseases will lead to improvements in treatment modalities. With appropriate AR treatment, asthma morbidity can be significantly reduced. Likewise, diagnosis and appropriate treatment of allergic rhinitis in patients with asthma reduces the morbidity that may develop due to asthma and improves the quality of life.

References

1. Okubo K, Kurono Y, Ichimura K, Enomoto T, Okamoto Y, Kawauchi H, Suzaki H, Fujieda S, Masuyama K. Japanese guidelines for allergic rhinitis 2020. Allergol Int. 2020;69:331–45.
2. Brożek JL, Bousquet J, Agache I, et al. Allergic rhinitis and its impact on asthma (ARIA) guidelines-2016 revision. J Allergy Clin Immunol. 2017;140:950–8.
3. Moitra S, Simoni M, Baldacci S, et al. Symptom control and health-related quality of life in allergic rhinitis with and without comorbid asthma: a multicentre European study. Clin Transl Allergy. 2023;13:e12209.
4. Harrison D, Reibman J. World trade center-related asthma: clinical care essentials. Arch Environ Occup Health. 2023;78(4):206–11.
5. Massoth L, Anderson C, McKinney KA. Asthma and chronic rhinosinusitis: diagnosis and medical management. Med Sci. 2019;7:53.
6. Khan DA. Allergic rhinitis and asthma: epidemiology and common pathophysiology. Allergy Asthma Proc. 2014;35:357–61.
7. Morjaria JB, Caruso M, Emma R, Russo C, Polosa R. Treatment of allergic rhinitis as a strategy for preventing asthma. Curr Allergy Asthma Rep. 2018;18:23.
8. Wise SK, Lin SY, Toskala E, et al. International consensus statement on allergy and rhinology: allergic rhinitis. Int Forum Allergy Rhinol. 2018;8:108–352.
9. Burgess JA, Walters EH, Byrnes GB, Matheson MC, Jenkins MA, Wharton CL, Johns DP, Abramson MJ, Hopper JL, Dharmage SC. Childhood allergic rhinitis predicts asthma incidence and persistence to middle age: a longitudinal study. J Allergy Clin Immunol. 2007;120:863–9.
10. Bousquet J, Annesi-Maesano I, Carat F, Léger D, Rugina M, Pribil C, El Hasnaoui A, Chanal I. Characteristics of intermittent and persistent allergic rhinitis: DREAMS study group. Clin Exp Allergy. 2005;35:728–32.
11. Ponte EV, Franco R, Nascimento HF, Souza-Machado A, Cunha S, Barreto ML, Naspitz C, Cruz ÁA. Lack of control of severe asthma is associated with co-existence of moderate-to-severe rhinitis. Allergy. 2008;63:564–9.
12. Sasaki M, Yoshida K, Adachi Y, Furukawa M, Itazawa T, Odajima H, Saito H, Akasawa A. Factors associated with asthma control in children: findings from a national web-based survey. Pediatr Allergy Immunol. 2014;25:804–9.
13. Ozoh OB, Aderibigbe SA, Ayuk AC, Dede SK, Egbagbe E, Babashani M. Health-related quality of life in asthma measured by the World Health Organization brief questionnaire (WHO-

BREF) and the effect of concomitant allergic rhinitis-a population-based study. Clin Respir J. 2023;1:10.

14. Ödling M, Andersson N, Janson C, Melén E, Bergström A, Kull I. Health-related quality of life decreases in young people with asthma during the transition from adolescence to young adulthood: a birth cohort study. BMC Pulm Med. 2023;23:34.
15. Paiva Ferreira LKD, Paiva Ferreira LAM, Monteiro TM, Bezerra GC, Bernardo LR, Piuvezam MR. Combined allergic rhinitis and asthma syndrome (CARAS). Int Immunopharmacol. 2019;74:105718.
16. Riccioni G, Della Vecchia R, Castronuovo M, Di Pietro V, Spoltore R, De Benedictis M, Di Iorio A, Di Gioacchino M, Guagnano MT. Bronchial hyperresponsiveness in adults with seasonal and perennial rhinitis: is there a link for asthma and rhinitis? Int J Immunopathol Pharmacol. 2002;15:69–73.
17. Bousquet J, Anto JM, Wickman M, et al. Are allergic multimorbidities and IgE polysensitization associated with the persistence or re-occurrence of foetal type 2 signalling? The MeDALL hypothesis. Allergy. 2015;70:1062–78.
18. Liu AH, Babineau DC, Krouse RZ, et al. Pathways through which asthma risk factors contribute to asthma severity in inner-city children. J Allergy Clin Immunol. 2016;138:1042–50.
19. Ciprandi G, Ricciardolo FLM, Schiavetti I, Cirillo I. Allergic rhinitis phenotypes based on bronchial hyperreactivity to methacholine. Am J Rhinol Allergy. 2014;28:e214–8.
20. Ciprandi G, Tosca MA, Capasso M. Exhaled nitric oxide in children with allergic rhinitis and/or asthma: a relationship with bronchial hyperreactivity. J Asthma. 2010;47:1142–7.
21. Cirillo I, Ricciardolo FLM, Medusei G, Signori A, Ciprandi G. Exhaled nitric oxide may predict bronchial hyperreactivity in patients with allergic rhinitis. Int Arch Allergy Immunol. 2013;160:322–8.
22. Aguilar D, Pinart M, Koppelman GH, et al. Computational analysis of multimorbidity between asthma, eczema and rhinitis. PLoS One. 2017;12:e0179125.
23. Lemonnier N, Melén E, Jiang Y, et al. A novel whole blood gene expression signature for asthma, dermatitis, and rhinitis multimorbidity in children and adolescents. Allergy. 2020;75:3248–60.
24. Mao Z, Shi Y, Cao Q, Chen Y, Sun Y, Liu Z, Zhang Q, Huang M. Transcriptional regulation on the gene expression signature in combined allergic rhinitis and asthma syndrome. Epigenomics. 2018;10:119–31.
25. Panganiban RP, Wang Y, Howrylak J, Chinchilli VM, Craig TJ, August A, Ishmael FT. Circulating microRNAs as biomarkers in patients with allergic rhinitis and asthma. J Allergy Clin Immunol. 2016;137:1423–32.
26. Ke X, Song S, Wang X, Shen Y, Kang H, Hong S. Associations of single nucleotide polymorphisms of PTPN22 and Ctla4 genes with the risk of allergic rhinitis in a Chinese Han population. Hum Immunol. 2017;78:227–31.
27. Canonica GW, Compalati E. Minimal persistent inflammation in allergic rhinitis: implications for current treatment strategies. Clin Exp Immunol. 2009;158:260.
28. Salo PM, Arbes SJ, Jaramillo R, et al. Prevalence of allergic sensitization in the United States: results from the National Health and Nutrition Examination Survey (NHANES) 2005-2006. J Allergy Clin Immunol. 2014;134:350–9.
29. Halken S, Larenas-Linnemann D, Roberts G, et al. EAACI guidelines on allergen immunotherapy: prevention of allergy. Pediatr Allergy Immunol. 2017;28:728–45.
30. Meng Q, Liu X, Li P, He L, Xie J, Gao X, Wu X, Su F, Liang Y. The influence of house dust mite sublingual immunotherapy on the TSLP-OX40L signaling pathway in patients with allergic rhinitis. Int Forum Allergy Rhinol. 2016;6:862–70.
31. Polosa R, Al-Delaimy WK, Russo C, Piccillo G, Sarvà M. Greater risk of incident asthma cases in adults with allergic rhinitis and effect of allergen immunotherapy: a retrospective cohort study. Respir Res. 2005;6:153.
32. Testa D, Di Bari M, Nunziata M, De Cristofaro G, Massaro G, Marcuccio G, Motta G. Allergic rhinitis and asthma assessment of risk factors in pediatric patients: a systematic review. Int J Pediatr Otorhinolaryngol. 2020;129:109759.

33. Baldacci S, Omenaas E, Oryszczyn MP. Allergy markers in respiratory epidemiology. Eur Respir J. 2001;17:773–90.
34. Sbihi H, Boutin RCT, Cutler C, Suen M, Finlay BB, Turvey SE. Thinking bigger: how early-life environmental exposures shape the gut microbiome and influence the development of asthma and allergic disease. Allergy. 2019;74:2103–15.
35. Marsland BJ, Gollwitzer ES. Host-microorganism interactions in lung diseases. Nat Rev Immunol. 2014;14:827–35.
36. Eguiluz-Gracia I, Mathioudakis AG, Bartel S, et al. The need for clean air: the way air pollution and climate change affect allergic rhinitis and asthma. Allergy. 2020;75:2170–84.
37. Polosa R, Knoke JD, Russo C, Piccillo G, Caponnetto P, Sarvà M, Proietti L, Al-Delaimy WK. Cigarette smoking is associated with a greater risk of incident asthma in allergic rhinitis. J Allergy Clin Immunol. 2008;121:1428–34.
38. Bousquet J, Khaltaev N, Cruz AA, et al. Allergic rhinitis and its impact on asthma (ARIA) 2008 update (in collaboration with the World Health Organization, GA(2)LEN and AllerGen). Allergy. 2008;63(Suppl 86):8–160.
39. Crystal-Peters J, Neslusan C, Crown WH, Torres A. Treating allergic rhinitis in patients with comorbid asthma: the risk of asthma-related hospitalizations and emergency department visits. J Allergy Clin Immunol. 2002;109:57–62.
40. Corren J, Harris AG, Aaronson D, et al. Efficacy and safety of loratadine plus pseudoephedrine in patients with seasonal allergic rhinitis and mild asthma. J Allergy Clin Immunol. 1997;100:781–8.
41. Tiotiu A, Plavec D, Novakova S, Mihaicuta S, Novakova P, Labor M, Bikov A. Current opinions for the management of asthma associated with ear, nose and throat comorbidities. Eur Respir Rev. 2018;27:180056.
42. Bachert C, Maspero J. Efficacy of second-generation antihistamines in patients with allergic rhinitis and comorbid asthma. J Asthma. 2011;48:965–73.
43. Philip G, Nayak AS, Berger WE, Leynadier F, Vrijens F, Dass SB, Reiss TF. The effect of montelukast on rhinitis symptoms in patients with asthma and seasonal allergic rhinitis. Curr Med Res Opin. 2004;20:1549–58.
44. Busse WW, Casale TB, Dykewicz MS, Meltzer EO, Bird SR, Hustad CM, Grant E, Zeldin RK, Edelman JM. Efficacy of montelukast during the allergy season in patients with chronic asthma and seasonal aeroallergen sensitivity. Ann Allergy Asthma Immunol. 2006;96:60–8.
45. Lohia S, Schlosser RJ, Soler ZM. Impact of intranasal corticosteroids on asthma outcomes in allergic rhinitis: a meta-analysis. Allergy. 2013;68:569–79.
46. Demoly P, Emminger W, Rehm D, Backer V, Tommerup L, Kleine-Tebbe J. Effective treatment of house dust mite-induced allergic rhinitis with 2 doses of the SQ HDM SLIT-tablet: results from a randomized, double-blind, placebo-controlled phase III trial. J Allergy Clin Immunol. 2016;137:444–451.e8.
47. Virchow JC, Backer V, Kuna P, Prieto L, Nolte H, Villesen HH, Ljørring C, Riis B, De Blay F. Efficacy of a house dust mite sublingual allergen immunotherapy tablet in adults with allergic asthma: a randomized clinical trial. JAMA. 2016;315:1715–25.
48. Valovirta E, Petersen TH, Piotrowska T, et al. Results from the 5-year SQ grass sublingual immunotherapy tablet asthma prevention (GAP) trial in children with grass pollen allergy. J Allergy Clin Immunol. 2018;141(2):529–538.e13.
49. Möller C, Dreborg S, Ferdousi HA, et al. Pollen immunotherapy reduces the development of asthma in children with seasonal rhinoconjunctivitis (the PAT-study). J Allergy Clin Immunol. 2002;109:251–6.
50. Niggemann B, Jacobsen L, Dreborg S, et al. Five-year follow-up on the PAT study: specific immunotherapy and long-term prevention of asthma in children. Allergy. 2006;61:855–9.
51. Abramson MJ, Puy RM, Weiner JM. Injection allergen immunotherapy for asthma. Cochrane Database Syst Rev. 2010;(8):CD001186.
52. Dhami S, Nurmatov U, Arasi S, et al. Allergen immunotherapy for allergic rhinoconjunctivitis: a systematic review and meta-analysis. Allergy. 2017;72:1597–631.

53. Di Bona D, Plaia A, Leto-Barone MS, La Piana S, Macchia L, Di Lorenzo G. Efficacy of allergen immunotherapy in reducing the likelihood of developing new allergen sensitizations: a systematic review. Allergy. 2017;72:691–704.
54. Kristiansen M, Dhami S, Netuveli G, et al. Allergen immunotherapy for the prevention of allergy: a systematic review and meta-analysis. Pediatr Allergy Immunol. 2017;28:18–29.
55. Avdeeva K, Fokkens W. Precision medicine in chronic rhinosinusitis with nasal polyps. Curr Allergy Asthma Rep. 2018;18:25.
56. Gevaert P, Calus L, Van Zele T, et al. Omalizumab is effective in allergic and nonallergic patients with nasal polyps and asthma. J Allergy Clin Immunol. 2013;1311:110–6.e1.
57. Busse WW, Maspero JF, Lu Y, et al. Efficacy of dupilumab on clinical outcomes in patients with asthma and perennial allergic rhinitis. Ann Allergy Asthma Immunol. 2020;125:565–576.e1.
58. Weinstein SF, Katial R, Jayawardena S, et al. Efficacy and safety of dupilumab in perennial allergic rhinitis and comorbid asthma. J Allergy Clin Immunol. 2018;142:171–177.e1.
59. Gibson PG, Prazma CM, Chupp GL, Bradford ES, Forshag M, Mallett SA, Yancey SW, Smith SG, Bel EH. Mepolizumab improves clinical outcomes in patients with severe asthma and comorbid conditions. Respir Res. 2021;22:171.

Meeting Organ for ENT and Pediatric Pulmonology: Adenoids

37

Çiğdem Firat Koca, Cemal Cingi, and Sergei Karpischenko

37.1 Introduction

The adenoid tissue is a lymphoid aggregate on the posterior and superior nasopharyngeal area [1]. The nasopharynx region is located at the posterior continuing of nasal openings, where the inferior turbinate and the septum terminate. The soft palate divides the oropharynx and nasopharynx. The Mucoperiosteum of the upper clivus creates the structure of the nasopharyngeal roof. The mucosa, the prevertebral fascia, the superior pharyngeal constrictor, and the longus capitis muscles comprise the nasopharynx's posterior side. The rear nasopharyngeal wall stands mid to clivus, the anterior side of the foramen magnum, and the atlas. The orifice of the Eustachian tube exists in the lateral nasopharyngeal wall. The Rosenmüller fossa (pharyngeal recess) is situated at the joint of lateral and posterior nasopharyngeal walls [2].

Adenoids are components of Waldeyer's ring. Waldeyer's ring, with its lymphoid nature, is formed by superiorly pharyngeal tonsils (adenoids), laterally two palatine tonsils, inferiorly from the lingual tonsils, and located at the base of the tongue [3]. Adenoid tissue development begins in the third month of fetal life. Lymphocytes infiltrate the glandular primordial situated in the posterior nasopharynx. Sagittal masses that create pharyngeal crypts appear in the fifth month. The surface of this formation is covered by pseudostratified ciliated columnar

Ç. F. Koca
Medical Faculty, Department of Otorhynolaryngology, Malatya Turgut Özal University, Malatya, Turkey

C. Cingi (✉)
Medical Faculty, Department of Otorhinolaryngology, Eskisehir Osmangazi University, Eskişehir, Turkey

S. Karpischenko
Department of Otorhinolaryngology, The First Pavlov State Medical University of Saint Petersburg, Saint Petersburg, Russia

H. Yüksel et al. (eds.), *Pediatric Airway Diseases*, Comprehensive ENT,
https://doi.org/10.1007/978-3-031-74853-0_37

epithelium, and the development of adenoids is completed in the seventh month of fetal development [4]. The ascending pharyngeal artery, pharyngeal division of the maxillary artery, and the cervical ascending arteries originating from the thyrocervical trunk provide blood supply to the adenoid tissue. Venous drainage is maintained via the pterygoid and pharyngeal to the internal jugular and facial veins. Adenoid tissue is innervated with glossopharyngeal and branches of the vagus and has no afferent lymphatics. Efferent lymphatic drainage is to the retropharyngeal and upper cervical lymph nodes [4].

This chapter aimed to address adenoid and adenoid-related diseases and their treatment modalities.

37.2 Adenoid Hypertrophy

Adenoid hypertrophy is a frequent problem among pediatrics. When adenoid hypertrophy exceeds a certain level, fills the nasopharyngeal space, and extends the choana, it can cause upper-airway obstruction [1]. Adenoid tissue is small in the neonatal period. It begins to grow in the first years of life, reaches its maximum size by age 5, and regresses after age 8 [5]. Chronic nasal obstruction due to adenoid hypertrophy may cause symptoms include the following: hyponasality of voice, obstructive sleep apnea (OSA), daytime sleepiness, behavioral and mouth breathing, snoring, attention problems, growth retardation, rhinorrhea, failure to thrive, enuresis, and craniofacial issues. Severe obstructive sleep apnea may cause cor pulmonale with right heart failure [6].

37.3 Adenoid Hypertrophy and Craniofacial Development

The upper-airway obstruction due to enlarged adenoids may cause maxillofacial dysfunctions [4]. The face shape that occurs due to chronic nasal obstruction due to adenoid hypertrophy is the adenoid face. Adenoid face can be described as having a short upper lip, a posterior positioned hyoid bone, a constricted upper dental arch, a posterior position of mandibular incisors, an elongated anterior face, a constricted or "V"-formed maxillary arc, a high mandibular plane angle, and a posterior positioned mandible [7]. Intraoral examination shows constricted maxillary and elevated palatal arcs and dental malocclusion [8].

Nasal obstruction may cause mouth breathing. Therefore, incisors face wetness and get cold due to the vaporization. The mean results in pain, which initiates the tongue-pushing reflex to maintain optimal temperature for the incisors. Prolonged breathing in the open-mouth position due to chronic obstruction induces the tongue-pushing reflex and anterior displacement of the tongue, and this chronic situation may result in anterior open bite deformity [9]. Koca et al. detected a statistically significant elevation in the anterior face height and identified the posterior replacement of the mandible due to the hypertrophied adenoids. They also underlined the importance of early intervention to the nasal obstruction in pediatrics to maintain healthy dentofacial development [10]. Timing of adenoidectomy is critical to support the normal craniofacial development [7]. Average mandibular growth has been clarified after the adenoidectomy procedure with improved nasal breathing [8].

37.4 Adenoid Hypertrophy and Pediatric Sleep Breathing Disorders

Childhood OSA can be described as partial or complete obstruction of the upper airway during sleep. Some associated symptoms are sleep disorders, hypercapnia, hypoxemia, daytime sleepiness, snoring, enuresis, mouth breathing, and behavioral and neurocognitive difficulties. Enlarged adenoids alone, or with tonsil enlargement, are the most common predisposition factors for pediatric OSA due to nasopharyngeal and oropharyngeal obstruction. Adenoid tissue is a member of the Waldeyer ring that completes its rapid growth between the ages of 2 and 8. Although no direct relationship has been found between the thickness of adenoids and OSAS, the OSAS clinic, considered an upper-airway motor or tonus disorder, causes dynamic airway stenosis during sleep together with adenoid hypertrophy. Sleep disruption, fragmentation, hypoxia, and hypercapnia are some mechanisms accused of neurocognitive and behavioral dysfunctions in pediatric sleep-disordered breathing (SDB). Pediatric SDB may cause cardiac dysfunctions, blood pressure dysregulation, and growth retardation [11].

Intermittent hypoxia during sleep may influence the neurochemical structure of the brain and growth hormone secretion. Cardiovascular pathologies are associated with increased intrathoracic pressure, excessive free circulating inflammatory mediators, and increased insulin resistance. Pediatric OSA has been observed most frequently between the ages of 2 and 6 due to the largest size of adenoids. Adenoid hypertrophy may cause obstructive problems, including nasal obstruction that causes chronic mouth breathing, rhinorrhea, and dysphagia. Hypertrophy of adenoids due to an acute upper-respiratory system infection may lead to snoring and nighttime breathing problems; this clinical period may end when the condition improves, but this may be the onset of a challenging chronic upper-respiratory system obstruction [11]. Adenoid hypertrophy may cause neurocognitive changes, including headache, daytime sleepiness, poor school performance, and learning difficulties [5]. The mechanism of the neurobehavioral problems observed due to sleep interruption is unclear. The possible tool is that sleep disruption and chronic hypoxia may lead to functional impairments due to the alterations in the prefrontal cortex. Low lingual visual capacity and poor school performance support that pediatrics having hypertrophied adenoid tissue have difficulties with their prefrontal cortex. An essential academic improvement has been detected following adenoidectomy [12, 13]. Koca et al. observed lower academic performance in the children with hypertrophied adenoid tissue compared with the control group [10].

Sleep apnea requires a detailed examination by an ENT doctor and a sleep medicine physician. It is critical to underline that OSA in children has different clinical features from adults, as it is presented with more corrupted nocturnal sleep than excessive daytime sleepiness and prominent behavioral disorders, including hyperactivity, enuresis nocturna, poor school performance, and psychiatric problems. Polysomnography (PSG) is an accurate evaluation instrument that clarifies the obstructive events and facilitates the classification of the severity of OSA. Enlargement of adenotonsillar tissue blocks the upper airway, and surgical intervention overcomes obstructive symptoms. Surgical procedure forms the first treatment modality in OSA due to adenotonsillar hypertrophy [14]. Adenoidectomy is a standard surgical procedure carried out alone or combined with tonsillectomy for pediatric patients with OSA. A clinical study reported adenoidectomy's success in OSA treatment as 80% [4, 15, 16].

37.5 Diagnosis of Adenoid Hypertrophy

The nasopharynx is an anatomical location that is difficult to examine, with one end extending from the base of the skull and the other to the soft palate. A small dental mirror and a headlamp may help analyze the nasopharynx. A fiberoptic nasopharyngoscope is another alternative visualization method to maintain a perfect sight of the nasopharyngeal area [17]. Posterior rhinoscopy and nasopharyngeal radiological scans form the methods for evaluating adenoidal tissue. Flexible fiberoptic nasal endoscopy is a popular, well-established, and commonly used procedure in otolaryngological practice, as it provides a perfect visualization and facilitates a correct diagnosis to be performed. Nasal flexible fiberoptic endoscopy is a safe method for examining the nasopharyngeal region in children [18, 19]. Endoscopy provides a direct visualization of nasal cavities and nasopharynx. Several techniques for grading enlarged adenoids have been published in the literature [18, 20]. The grading system described by Parikh et al. (2006) has been most accepted for examining the extension of adenoids over the posterior choanae; grade 1 for adenoids with no contiguity with adjacent textures, grade 2 adenoids close contiguity with the torus tuberous; grade 3 adenoids contiguity with the vomer and finally grade 4 adenoids have close contiguity with the soft palate [21]. Lateral radiological examination of the nasopharyngeal region has been carried out in pediatrics for many years to determine the size of adenoid tissue. Paradise et al. reported that the radiograph was in good accordance with the size of adenoids removed intraoperatively. Radiographs are objective and noninvasive instruments for assessing the adenoidal size [22]. It is not easy to perform this imaging modality for infants, and radiation exposure is a disadvantage of the procedure that should not be neglected [23].

37.6 Surgical Indications for Adenoidectomy

1. Four or more attacks of recurrent purulent rhinorrhea in the previous 12-month period in a child younger than 12.
2. Resistant complaints of adenoiditis despite antibiotic therapy (two courses of therapy) (one antibiotic treatment period should be at least 14 days and with a beta-lactamase agent).

3. It prolonged sleep-related problems due to nasal blockage for at least 3 months.
4. Hyponasality while speaking.
5. Serous otitis media persisting for longer than 3 months period.
6. Dental malocclusion or orofacial developmental problems diagnosed by an orthodontist.
7. Cor pulmonale, right ventricular hypertrophy, and pulmonary hypertension due to upper-airway blockage.
8. Serous otitis media in the ages of 4 or older [24].

37.7 Preoperative Evaluation

Bleeding is the major complication of the adenoidectomy procedure. Bleeding diathesis of the medical and family history of the patient should be questioned in detail. In suspicion of bleeding diathesis, a detailed hematologic evaluation is required. A thorough otorhinolaryngological examination is essential in the presence of cleft palate, submucous cleft palate, and velopharyngeal functions. Detection of bifid uvula should be reminded of the possibility of a submucous cleft palate. The atlantoaxial subluxation can be observed in pediatrics with Down syndrome. Before surgery in children with Down syndrome, the C1–2 joint should be examined with cervical radiographs. Surgery can be performed in a neutral position in case of any pathology.

37.8 Contraindications

The presence of bleeding diathesis creates a definite contraindication for adenoidectomy. The existence of a cleft palate may lead to postoperative velopharyngeal failure. A cleft palate is a contraindication for adenoidectomy due to the possibility of postoperative velopharyngeal failure. Surgery should be avoided during poliomyelitis epidemics.

37.9 Complications

37.9.1 Bleeding

If the coagulation functions are standard in the patient, excessive bleeding is not expected during the operation. Fibrosis due to recurring infections and active infections may cause bleeding. Adenoidectomy procedures can be carried out alone or in combination with tonsillectomy. Bleeding prevalence has been reported between 0.1 and 58% after tonsillectomy and adenoidectomy. Bleeding in the postoperative period is divided into early and late. Early period bleedings occur in the first 24 hours after surgery. The most severe bleedings arise due to insufficient hemostasis during the first hour after surgery and are often noticed in the recovery room afterward.

First, the location of the bleeding should be determined. If the bleeding is severe and the patient's cooperation is difficult, intubation under general anesthesia should be carried out to achieve appropriate hemostasis. Posterior packing can be placed to control excessive bleeding. The posterior packing can be removed after 24–48 h. A blood transfusion may be required if the bleeding is severe, especially in children. The most common cause of late-period bleedings, which occur in postoperative 5–7 days, is infection. Late-period bleedings are treated in the same way.

37.9.2 Hypernasality

Severe hypernasality incidence due to adenoidectomy and tonsillectomy has been reported between 1/1500 and 1/10,000. Preoperative cleft palate or submucosal cleft existence and velopharyngeal dysfunctions should alert the surgeon not to perform adenoidectomy. The patient is followed up for 3 months postoperatively. Speech therapy should be started unless the compensation develops. Surgical intervention may be required in severe hypernasality. Bipolar cautery is recommended for hemostasis intraoperative rather than unipolar cautery due to the harmful effect of unipolar cautery on the nerves.

37.9.3 Surgical Traumas

The mouth opener can traumatize the tongue, lips, teeth, and temporomandibular joint. Teeth can be detached, and the patient can aspirate these broken teeth. The uvula, soft palate, and pharyngeal mucosa may be damaged. Burns may occur due to cautery or laser devices used in the surgery.

37.9.4 Torticollis

Superior pharyngeal constrictor muscle may be traumatized while adenoid tissue is curetted over the vertebrae in the posterior nasopharynx. Traumatization of the muscle may cause neck spasms, pain, and rarely torticollis. Grisel syndrome should be suspected if neck movement limitation is accompanied by neck pain. Grisel's syndrome can be described, as the nontraumatic subluxation or dislocation of the atlantoaxial joint or the C1 and C2 vertebrae. Warm compress, anti-inflammatory medication can be useful for resolving the spasm. Surgical treatment is rarely required.

37.9.5 Otitis Media

Otitis media may occur after adenoidectomy surgery. Patients having otalgia following adenoidectomy should be evaluated by otoscopy.

37.9.6 Psychological Trauma

Surgical intervention may cause psychological trauma, particularly in pediatrics younger than 5. Sleep problems, behavioral disorders, and depression may be observed in the postoperative period. Postoperative pain, young age, and previous psychological problems can trigger postoperative behavioral disorders [25].

37.9.7 Nasopharyngeal Stenosis

An uncommon complication may be seen after a long period following the adenoidectomy procedure due to excessive mucosal destruction and infections [26]. Its treatment is surgery.

37.9.8 Recurrence

Although it is rare, recurrence may be observed after adenoidectomies. The recurrence rate has been reported as 0.55% [27]. If adenoidectomy is performed young, adenoid tissue can grow again during the child's growth period.

37.10 Postoperative Care

After patients are discharged and sent home, close observation by their parents should be recommended at home. Heavy physical activities are prohibited for 1–2 weeks after surgery. Children can continue school a week later. A cold or warm liquid diet is applied, particularly in the first few days [4].

37.11 Surgery

Adenoidectomy is a frequent surgery carried out by otolaryngologists. The most frequent indications are obstructive pathologies, including OSA, nasal obstruction, recurrent OM, and otitis media with effusion. The classical transoral adenoidectomy method is performed with an adenoid curette or an adenectomy, usually under general anesthesia. The surgery is always carried out without viewing the nasopharyngeal region. Classical transoral adenoidectomy may fail to achieve sufficient removal of adenoids in one-third of cases, particularly when the existence of an intranasal, superior, or peritubaric extension [28–33]. Complete removal of the whole hypertrophied adenoids is the main aim of this procedure and suppresses the recurrences. Digital control of the curetted area intraoperatively helps the surgeon determine whether there is any rest tissue. Angle mirrors or endoscopic evaluation are superior to directly visualizing the region [34]. With the endoscopic evaluation,

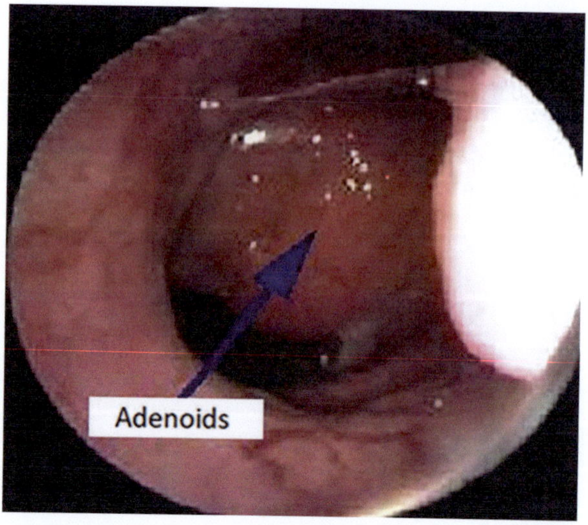

Fig. 37.1 Endoscopic image of adenoids

the removal of peritubaric and perichoanal adenoidal tissues can be achieved, and the boundaries and depth of the resection can be controlled [35] (Fig. 37.1).

37.12 Adenoids and Related Diseases

37.12.1 Adenoiditis

Adenoiditis can be described as the inflammation of the adenoidal tissue due to infections, allergies, or stomach acid irritation. Adenoiditis is often not alone and is found as part of more complicated clinical situations, including adenotonsillitis, pharyngitis, rhinosinusitis, and laryngopharyngeal reflux [36].

Purulent, runny nose, postnasal discharge, fever, and cough should suggest the diagnosis of adenoiditis. Cervical lymphadenopathy, sinusitis, and otitis media can also accompany adenoiditis. Over four repetitions of this clinical situation annually can be defined as recurrent adenoiditis [4, 37]. If these symptoms persist despite the appropriate treatment without any improvement, this clinical situation is called chronic adenoiditis [4]. Numerous microorganisms may cause inflammation in the adenoidal tissue. Upper-respiratory tract infections due to viral agents frequently initiate the adenoiditis process and facilitate bacterial infections and proliferation in the adenoidal tissue. *Haemophilus influenza*, *Streptococcus pyogenes*, *Streptococcus pneumonia*, and *Staphylococcus aureus* are the most frequent bacterial agents detected from adenoid tissue [38]. Chronic irritation due to gastroesophageal reflux may be a factor in adenoiditis and enlargement of adenoid tissue, especially in infants and pediatric patients [39]. The precise incidence and prevalence ratio for adenoiditis remains unclear. If there is only a viral upper-respiratory tract infection, the doctor can follow up without antibiotics, as many viral infections are self-limiting and improve within 5–7 days. If complaints persist or a bacterial infection is considered, the first-step treatment is appropriate antibiotics. Amoxicillin is the first choice. Cefdinir or cefuroxime may be a second alternative if there is insufficient response to amoxicillin treatment. In the case of penicillin allergy, azithromycin or clarithromycin may be alternative agents. The treatment period should be 10 days to suppress relapse rates and antibiotic resistance [36]. Amoxicillin-clavunate combination is a good alternative for treating beta-lactamase-forming agents [40]. Nasal steroid sprays, oral steroids, and oral antihistamines create the treatment for adenoiditis that occurs due to allergic conditions. Reflux treatment should be given if adenoiditis is considered to develop due to reflux [39]. Differential diagnosis should be made in adenoiditis with sinusitis, rhinosinusitis, pharyngitis, tonsillitis, nasal polyposis, seasonal allergies, and laryngopharyngeal reflux [36].

Adenoidectomy is recommended for recurrent or chronic adenoiditis that persists despite appropriate antimicrobial treatments [6, 41].

37.12.2 Adenoids and Ear Diseases

The nasopharynx creates the most superior part of the pharynx, restricted by the skull base superiorly, by the soft palate inferiorly, by the nasal cavity anteriorly, by posterior pharyngeal wall posteriorly, the medial pterygoid plates and superior pharyngeal constrictor muscle laterally. The nasopharynx creates a connection between the nasal cavity and the oropharynx. Eustachian tube (ET) orifices and adenoidal tissue exist in the nasopharyngeal region [42–44]. The relationship between adenoids and ET dysfunctions has been the issue of many studies in the literature. Different studies have determined that the adenoids contain excessively more mast cells in cases with ET impairments and otitis media (OM) with effusion [45]. Bacteria creating biofilm have been obtained from adenoidal tissues of pediatric patients with repetitive acute OM and resistant OM with flow. The more common localization of bacterial biofilms is around the ET ostium, which shows that adenoid tissue is a reservoir for bacteria and adenoiditis and can lead to otitis, rhinosinusitis, or similar upper-respiratory infections.

Additionally, adenoid hypertrophy can obstruct the ET mechanically, and this mechanical blockage leads to more difficult middle ear diseases [35]. Adenoid hypertrophy may block the nasopharyngeal space and occlude the ET. This blockage disrupts the ventilation of the middle ear and the mastoid system [46]. Adenoidectomy may provide recovery in children with recurrent otitis media but is not suggested as a first-step treatment unless recommended for upper-airway obstruction [47].

37.12.3 Adenoids and Rhinosinusitis

Chronic rhinosinusitis (CRS) can be described as nasal inflammation, and the paranasal sinuses presented by two or more symptoms for at least 12 weeks without cessation including nasal blockage, nasal congestion or discharge, facial pain or pressure, and cough [48, 49]. The diagnosis depends on an endoscopic examination and computed tomography (CT) scan. Although CRS is a frequent disease, the definite incidence in children is unknown [49]. Nasal congestion, cough, rhinorrhea, and postnasal drip create the most frequent symptoms of CRS [50, 51]. Tatli et al. reported that 66% of children with chronic cough symptoms had CT scan pathologies in the paranasal sinuses [52]. The diagnosis of CRS in pediatrics is difficult due to the similar symptomatology to viral upper-respiratory tract infections, adenoiditis/adenoid hypertrophy and allergic rhinitis. At this point of distinction, families may not always be able to give a clear anamnesis, and it is difficult to perform an endoscopy on a young child [49]. The adenoid tissue is closely associated with the paranasal sinuses. Adenoidectomy is sufficient in treating complaints in some children with CRS [49]. According to the analysis of a study in the literature, it was considered that enlarged adenoids have similar bacteriology with the middle meatus of children with chronic or recurrent sinusitis [53]. In children with severe sinusitis reflected on radiological imaging, it has been shown that there is a direct correlation between the incidence of bacterial isolation from the adenoid tissue and the size of the adenoids [54, 55]. This result suggests that adenoiditis may cause nasal discharge, and the effect of the adenoids on CRS may be related to their bacterial reservoir rather than their size [49]. The diagnosis of CRS in pediatrics is based on clinical symptoms. Although physical examination and clinical history are helpful in diagnosis, they cannot distinguish CRS from adenoiditis, especially in smaller pediatrics. Paranasal CT is the most frequently used radiological modality in diagnosing CRS. Direct radiography is more diagnostic than CT. Adenoidectomy, combined with a maxillary sinus wash procedure following functional endoscopic sinus surgery, is the most preferred surgical procedure in CRS cases that have no improvement despite optimal medical therapy [49]. Ramadan and Tiu reported that children smaller than 7 years of age with asthma had a lower improvement rate and required additional endoscopic sinus surgery procedures [56]. Maxillary antral irrigation is commonly carried out in addition to adenoidectomy. Ramada et al. reported 60 pediatrics who experienced adenoidectomy due to CRS and observed that children who experienced adenoidectomy solely had a 61% success range at 12 months. On the other hand, patients who had adenoidectomy combined with a sinus wash had an 88% success ratio [57]. Paranasal sinus CT scan studies showed that 18–45% of children with CRS have radiographic pathologies [58, 59]. The Lund-Mackay scoring system was described to determine CRS-dependent CT findings. A study showed a mean Lund-Mackay score of 2.8 in a pediatric group without complaints of rhinosinusitis. Lund-Mackay scores of 2 or fewer create a perfect negative predictive value. On the other hand, scores of 5 or bigger have an ideal positive predictive value for CRS [49, 60, 61] (Fig. 37.2).

37.12.4 Adenoids and Allergic Rhinitis

Adenoids are members of upper-respiratory tract-associated lymphoid tissues and create the organism's first step of immune protective barrier and are critical structures in both mucosal and systemic adaptive immunity mechanisms. They play

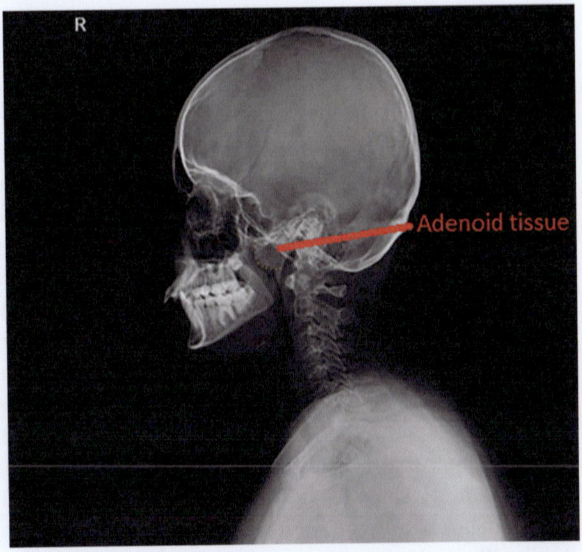

Fig. 37.2 Lateral radiographic image of adenoid tissue

crucial functions in mediating local and regional immune mechanisms, as they meet antigens [35]. Various factors may cause adenoid hypertrophy, but it is frequently suggested that passive smoking and allergic diseases induce repetitive respiratory inflammation in children via decreased IFN-gamma-generating CD8+ T lymphocytes. Additionally, adenoid tissue is an essential location of allergic inflammation due to the production of total and specific IgEs by adenoid mast cells [62].

Adenoids are formed by lymphoepithelial tissue and consist of lymphocytes, epithelial cells, macrophages, and dendritic cells. The localization and rule of effector T cells is critical for maintaining an efficient immune reaction. In particular, CD8+ T lymphocytes may be used in two main ways: cytolysis and synthesis of chemokines, cytokines, and microbicidal particles. When the synthesis of IFN-gamma by Th1 adenoidal lymphocytes is decreased, patients become more vulnerable to infectious viral diseases, facilitating the proliferation of pathogenic bacteria in adenoids [63]. Secretory IgA is the primary antibody in adenoids and plays a critical role in mucosal immunity, connecting to bacteria and preventing bacterial replication in the epithelium. According to the results of some studies, it was reported that IgA synthesis is seriously lower than in the adenoidal tissue of children diagnosed with OM with effusion [64]. Toll-like receptors (TLRs) mediate the active relation between innate and adaptive immunity mechanisms and mechanical factors, including ciliary movement. Recurrent respiratory infections and exposure to cigarette smoke may decrease the number of TLRs [65]. The over-expression of TLR7 in pediatrics with OM with effusion may indicate the significant task of these proteins in the immunological and antimicrobial reaction [66]. De Amici et al. analyzed the potential effects of various serum mediators that may be indicators of adenoidal hypertrophy in pediatrics. Primarily, increased serum levels of myeloperoxidase, which is an indicator of neutrophil activation, is determined in pediatrics with repetitive lower respiratory disease; high serum levels of eosinophilic cationic protein, a classical indicator of eosinophil over functions, are observed in children with repetitive upper-respiratory diseases; an increased levels of CD163 glycoprotein, a characteristic indicator of monocyte/macrophage activation, may demonstrate the enlargement of adenoidal hypertrophy [67]. These negative results may devastate the protective structures of the nose, facilitating the development of resistant adenotonsillar and respiratory diseases, including pharyngitis, rhinitis, otitis, laryngitis, sinusitis, pneumonia bronchitis, and allergic conditions. The relationship between adenoidal diseases and allergy is still unclear. Some papers in the literature declared a potential location of allergic pediatrics, as detected by myriad brightly fluorescent IgE mast cells, by the local production of total and specific IgE, and by the evident eosinophilic inflammatory process, classical in atopic cases. IgA receptors' synthesis on eosinophils is high in allergic cases, and infected adenoid tissue may have a different cell content from healthy adenoids. Although allergic rhinitis is accepted as an important predisposing factor for adenoid hypertrophy, it is infrequent in the ages when the frequency of adenoid hypertrophy is high. The clinical complaints of both diseases are similar. Possibly, only one of the diseases can be diagnosed. Allergic rhinitis and hypertrophied adenoids may cause nasal obstructive symptoms [35]. Ameli et al. reported that large-sized adenoid tissue can be related to the absence of allergic conditions, whereas large turbinates may have a relationship with small adenoidal tissue [68]. In pediatrics with allergic rhinitis associated with hypersensitivity to dust mites, adenoid hypertrophy develops excessively more frequently than in children with other allergic problems (asthma/atopic dermatitis) or no allergies. Meeting a sensitizing agent may be the leading cause of adenoidal hypertrophy in pediatrics with allergic rhinitis, and an appropriate treatment for allergic rhinitis could decrease the ratio of adenoid hypertrophy in atopic children [35]. A relationship has been found between childhood exposure to cigarette smoke and many childhood respiratory diseases. IFN-gamma synthesis by CD8+ T cells is inaccurate in these pediatric patients, creating susceptibility to recurrent respiratory infections [69]. Passive cigarette smoking elevates the level of proinflammatory molecules, decreases the Th1/Th2 ratio, and activates numerous structural changes in the respiratory nasal mucosa that effect negatively its ciliary functions [70]. Cytotoxic effects may occur due to the high concentration of nitric oxide. Smoking activates the production of heat shock proteins. These proteins are produced in tissues as a response to stressor factors. Smoking achieves its destructive effects in adenoid tissue via reagent oxygen and nitrogen products. Heat shock protein 70 has been accused of adenoidal hypertrophy in pediatrics exposed to smoking [71]. Koca et al. detected an increased smoking ratio in parents of children with adenoids compared with the control group [10].

37.12.5 Adenoids and Asthma

Di Matiro et al. reported that enlarged adenoids may affect expiratory nasal flow [72]. Obturation can be described as decreased airflow in the respiratory tract. This entity causes a reduction of maximum flow values and air volumes in the unit of time during forced expiration in proportion to vital capacity. Obturation is a decline in the

Tiffaneau index (FEV1%/VC). This index is an essential marker of obturation. Niedzielska et al. found an improvement in the Tiffaneau index in their patients after adenoidectomy (VC: vital capacity) (FEV1: Forced expiratory volume during the first second of expiration) [73]. Madrzynski and Zawisza analyzed the incidence of adenoidal hypertrophy in pediatrics with allergic rhinitis, and they pointed out that allergic situations such as allergic rhinitis, atopic dermatitis, and bronchial asthma enhanced the adenoidal tissue enlargement risk [74]. Kavukcu et al. suggested the evaluation of spirometric results for adenoid surgery. They observed the improvement of airway obstruction problems in their patients after the adenoid procedure. According to the study results, the authors declared that PEF, FVC, FEV1/PEF, and FEV1/FVC values recovered after adenoidectomy [75]. Aykan et al. suggested that pulmonary function tests may determine patients with mild degrees of adenoid hypertrophy to assess whether they are candidates for surgery (FEV1: Forced expiratory volume during the first second of expiration, PVC: forced vital capacity) [76].

Additionally, adenoid hypertrophy has been observed in cases with allergic rhinitis and asthma. According to one study, 52% of patients with only adenoid hypertrophy had signs of lower respiratory tract obstruction detected in pulmonary function tests [77].

References

1. Duan H, Xia L, He W, et al. Accuracy of lateral cephalogram for diagnosis of adenoid hypertrophy and posterior upper-airway obstruction: a meta-analysis. Int J Pediatr Otorhinolaryngol. 2019;119:1–9.
2. Stamm AC, Pignatari SSN, Balsalobre L. Chapter 175. Transnasal endoscopic-assisted surgery of the anterior skull base. In: Flint PW, Haughey BH, Lund V, et al., editors. Cummings otolaryngology: head & neck surgery. 6th ed. Philadelphia: Elsevier Saunders; 2015.
3. Casselbrant ML. What is wrong in chronic adenoiditis/tonsillitis anatomical considerations. Int J Pediatr Otorhinolaryngol. 1999;49:133–5.
4. Kara CO. Chapter 6. Tonsil-adenoid and pharynx infections. In: Koc C, editor. Ear nose throat diseases and head and neck surgery. 2nd ed. Ankara: Guneş Medicine Bookstores; 2013.
5. Guilleminault C, Stoohs R. Chronic snoring and obstructive sleep apnea syndrome in children. Lung. 1990;168(Suppl):912–9.
6. Wine TM, Yellon RF. Chapter 71. Infectious and inflammatory disease of the oral cavity, oropharynx, and nasopharynx. In: Wackym PA, Snow JB, editors. Ballenger's otorhinolaryngology head and neck surgery. 18th ed. Shelton: People's Medical Publishing House; 2016.
7. Arsalah R, Waheed H, Fatima J. Cephalometric assessment of patients with adenoidal faces. J Pak Med Assoc. 2009;59:747–52.
8. Peltomaki T. The effect of mode of breathing on craniofacial growth. Eur J Orthod. 2007;29:426–9.
9. Mizrahi E. A review of anterior open bite. Br J Orthod. 1978;5:21–7.
10. Koca CF, Erdem T, Bayındır T. The effect of adenoid hypertrophy on maxillofacial development: an objective photographic analysis. J Otolaryngol Head Neck Surg. 2016;45(1):48.
11. Goldstein NA. Chapter 184. Evaluation and management of pediatric obstructive sleep apnea. In: Flint PW, Haughey BH, Lund V, et al., editors. Cummings otolaryngology: head & neck surgery. 6th ed. Philadelphia: Elsevier Saunders; 2015.
12. Gottlieb DJ, Chase C, Vezina RM, Heeren TC, Corwin MJ, Auerbcah SH, et al. Sleep- disordered breathing symptoms are associated with poorer cognitive function in 5-year-old children. J Pediatr. 2004;145:458–64.

13. Rhodes SK, Shimoda KC, Wald LR, O'Neil PM, Oexmann MJ, Collop NA. Neurocognitive deficits in morbidly obese children with obstructive sleep apnea. J Pediatr. 1995;127:741–4.
14. Kumari S, Bagla J, Singla A. Pediatric obstructive sleep apnea: a review of approach to management. Indian Sleep Med. 2019;14(2):32–7.
15. Joshua B, Bahar G, Sulkes J, et al. Adenoidectomy: long-term follow-up. Otolaryngol Head Neck Surg. 2006;135:576–80.
16. Ishman SL, Kimple AJ. Chapter 72. Pediatric sleep disordered breathing. In: Wackym PA, Snow JB, editors. Ballenger's otorhinolaryngology head and neck surgery. 18th ed. Shelton: People's Medical Publishing House; 2016.
17. King EF, Couch ME. Chapter 4. History, physical examination, and the preoperative evaluation. In: Flint PW, Haughey BH, Lund V, et al., editors. Cummings otolaryngology: head & neck surgery. 6th ed. Philadelphia: Elsevier Saunders; 2015.
18. Cassano P, Gelardi M, Cassano M, Fiorella ML, Fiorella R. Adenoid tissue rhinopharyngeal obstruction grading based on fiberendoscopic findings: a novel approach to therapeutic management. Int J Pediatr Otorhinolaryngol. 2003;67:1303–9.
19. Chien CY, Chen AM, Hwang CF, Su CY. The clinical significance of adenoid-choanae area ratio in children with adenoid hypertrophy. Int J Pediatr Otorhinolaryngol. 2005;69:235–9.
20. Josephson GD, Duckworth L, Hossain J. Proposed definitive grading system tool for the assessment of adenoid hyperplasia. Laryngoscope. 2011;121:187–93.
21. Parikh SR, Coronel M, Lee JJ, Brown SM. Validation of a new grading system for endoscopic examination of adenoid hypertrophy. Otolaryngol Head Neck Surg. 2006;135:684–7.
22. Paradise JL, Bernard BS, Colborn DK, Janosky JE. Assessment of adenoidal obstruction in children: clinical signs versus roentgenographic findings. Pediatrics. 1998;101:979–86.
23. Cho JH, Lee DH, Lee NS, Won YS, Yoon HR, Suh BD. Size assessment of adenoid and nasopharyngeal airway by acoustic rhinometry in children. J Laryngol Otol. 1999;113:899–905.
24. Schupper AJ, Nation J, Pransky S. Adenoidectomy in children: what is the evidence and what is its role? Curr Otorhinolaryngol Rep. 2018;6(1):64–73.
25. Fortier MA, Del Rosario AM, Rosenbaum A, Kain ZN. Beyond pain: predictors of postoperative maladaptive behavior change in children. Paediatr Anaesth. 2010;20:445–53.
26. Koç C, Kocaman F, Aygenç E, Özdem C, Çekiç A. The use of preoperative lidocaine to prevent stridor and laryngospasm after tonsillectomy and adenoidectomy. Otolaryngol Head Neck Surg. 1998;118:880–2.
27. Simonsen AR, Duncavage A, Becker SS. A review of malpractice cases after tonsillectomy and adenoidectomy. Int J Pediatr Otorhinolaryngol. 2010;74:977–9.
28. Pagella F, Matti E, Colombo A, Giourgos G, Mira E. How we do it: a combined method of traditional curette and power-assisted endoscopic adenoidectomy. Acta Otolaryngol. 1996;129:556–9.
29. Buchinsky FJ, Lowry MA, Isaacson G. Do adenoids regrow after excision? Otolaryngol Head Neck Surg. 2000;123:576–81.
30. Stanislaw P Jr, Koltai PJ, Feustel PJ. Comparison of powerassisted adenoidectomy vs adenoid curette adenoidectomy. Arch Otolaryngol Head Neck Surg. 2000;126:845–9.
31. Elluru RG, Johnson L, Myer CM. Electrocautery adenoidectomy compared with curettage and power-assisted methods. Laryngoscope. 2002;112:23–5.
32. Havas T, Lowinger D. Obstructive adenoid tissue: an indication for powered-shaver adenoidectomy. Arch Otolaryngol Head Neck Surg. 2002;128:789–91.
33. Murray N, Fitzpatrick P, Guarisco JL. Powered partial adenoidectomy. Arch Otolaryngol Head Neck Surg. 2002;128:792–6.
34. Ezzat WF. Role of endoscopic nasal examination in reduction of nasopharyngeal adenoid recurrence rates. Int J Pediatr Otorhinolaryngol. 2010;74:404–6.
35. Brambilla I, Pusateri A, Pagella F, Caimmi D, Caimmi S, Licari A, et al. Adenoids in children: advances in immunology, diagnosis, and surgery. Clin Anat. 2014;27(3):346–52.
36. Bowers I, Shermetaro C. Adenoiditis. In: StatPearls [Internet]. Treasure Island: StatPearls Publishing; 2021.

37. Brodsky L. Tonsil adenoid disorders. In: Gates GA, editor. Current therapy in otolaryngology-head and neck surgery. St. Louis: Mosby; 1998. p. 414–7.
38. Shin KS, Cho SH, Kim KR, Tae K, Lee SH, Park CW, Jeong JH. The role of adenoids in pediatric rhinosinusitis. Int J Pediatr Otorhinolaryngol. 2008;72(11):1643–50.
39. Niu X, Wu ZH, Xiao XY, Chen X. The relationship between adenoid hypertrophy and gastroesophageal reflux disease: a meta-analysis. Medicine (Baltimore). 2018;97(41):e12540.
40. American Academy of Pediatrics; Subcommittee on Management of Sinusitis and Committee on Quality Improvement. Clinical practice guideline: management of sinusitis. Pediatrics. 2001;108(3):798–808.
41. Rosenfeld RM. Pilot study of outcomes in pediatric rhinosinusitis. Arch Otolaryngol Head Neck Surg. 1995;121(7):729–36.
42. Chong VF, Ong CK. Nasopharyngeal carcinoma. Eur J Radiol. 2008;66(3):437–47.
43. Mukherji SK, Castillo M. Normal cross-sectional anatomy of the nasopharynx, oropharynx, and oral cavity. Neuroimaging Clin N Am. 1998;8(1):211–8.
44. Mankowski NL, Bordoni B. Anatomy, head and neck, nasopharynx. In: StatPearls [Internet]. Treasure Island: StatPearls Publishing; 2021.
45. Bylander-Groth A, Stenström C. Eustachian tube function and otitis media in children. Ear Nose Throat J. 1998;77:762–4, 766, 768–769.
46. Bluestone CD. Eustachian tube function: physiology, pathophysiology, and role of allergy in pathogenesis of otitis media. J Allergy Clin Immunol. 1983;72(3):242–51.
47. Casselbrant ML, Mandel EM, Marchisio P. Chapter 16. Acute otitis media and middle-ear effusions. In: Wackym PA, Snow JB, editors. Ballenger's otorhinolaryngology head and neck surgery. 18th ed. Shelton: People's Medical Publishing House; 2016.
48. Fokkens WJ, Lund VJ, Mullol J, et al. The European position paper on rhinosinusitis and nasal polyps 2012. Rhinology. 2012;23:1–298.
49. Baroody FM. Chapter 196. Pediatric chronic rhinosinusitis. In: Flint PW, Haughey BH, Lund V, et al., editors. Cummings otolaryngology: head & neck surgery. 6th ed. Philadelphia: Elsevier Saunders; 2015.
50. Rachelefsky GS, Goldberg M, Katz RM, et al. Sinus disease in children with respiratory allergy. J Allergy Clin Immunol. 1978;61:310–4.
51. Rachelefsky GS, Shapiro GG. Diseases of paranasal sinuses in children. In: Bierman W, Pearlman D, editors. Management of upper respiratory tract disease. Philadelphia: WB Saunders; 1980.
52. Tatli MM, San I, Karaoglanoglu M. Paranasal sinus computed tomographic findings of children with chronic cough. Int J Pediatr Otorhinolaryngol. 2001;60(3):213–7.
53. Elwany S, El-Dine AN, El-Medany A, et al. Relationship between bacteriology of the adenoid core and middle meatus in children with sinusitis. J Laryngol Otol. 2011;125(3):279–81.
54. Shin KS, Cho SH, Kim KR, et al. The role of adenoids in pediatric rhinosinusitis. Int J Pediatr Otorhinolaryngol. 2008;72:1643–50.
55. Bercin AS, Ural A, Kutluhan A, et al. Relationship between sinusitis and adenoid size in pediatric age group. Ann Otol Rhinol Laryngol. 2007;116(7):550–3.
56. Ramadan HH, Tiu J. Failures of adenoidectomy for chronic rhinosinusitis in children: for whom and when do they fail? Laryngoscope. 2007;117(60):1080–3.
57. Ramadan HH, Cost JL. Outcome of adenoidectomy versus adenoidectomy with maxillary sinus wash for chronic rhinosinusitis in children. Laryngoscope. 2008;118(5):871–3.
58. Glasier CM, Ascher DP, Williams KD. Incidental paranasal sinus abnormalities on CT of children: clinical correlation. Am J Neuroradiol. 1986;7(5):861–4.
59. Diament MJ, Senac MO Jr, Gilsanz V, et al. Prevalence of incidental paranasal sinuses opacification in pediatric patients: a CT study. J Comput Assist Tomogr. 1987;11(3):426–31.
60. Hill M, Bhattacharyya N, Hall TR, et al. Incidental paranasal sinus imaging abnormalities and the normal Lund score in children. Otolaryngol Head Neck Surg. 2004;130:171–5.
61. Bhattacharyya N, Jones DT, Hill M, et al. The diagnostic accuracy of computed tomography in pediatric chronic rhinosinusitis. Arch Otolaryngol Head Neck Surg. 2004;130:1029–32.

62. Marseglia GL, Caimmi D, Pagella F, Matti E, Labo E, Licari A. Adenoids during childhood: the facts. Int J Immunopathol Pharmacol. 2011;24(4 Suppl):1–5.
63. Avanzini AM, Castellazzi AM, Marconi M, Valsecchi C, Marseglia A, Ciprandi G. Children with recurrent otitis show defective IFN-gamma producing cells in adenoids. Pediatr Allergy Immunol. 2008;19:523–6.
64. Wang B, Tang X, Xu J, Yao H. Differential expression of immunoglobulin A in the adenoids of children with and without exudative otitis media. Int J Pediatr Otorhinolaryngol. 2012;76:728–30.
65. Ricci A, Avanzini MA, Scaramuzza C, Castellazzi AM, Marconi M, Marseglia GL. Toll-like receptor 2-positive and Toll-like receptor 4-positive cells in adenoids of children exposed to passive smoking. J Allergy Clin Immunol. 2005;115:631–2.
66. Granath A, Uddman R, Cardell LO. Increased TLR7 expression in the adenoids among children with otitis media with effusion. Acta Otolaryngol. 2010;130:57–61.
67. De Amici M, Ciprandi G, Marseglia A, Licari A, Matti E, Caputo M. Adenoid hypetrophy: definition of some risk factors. J Biol Regul Homeost Agents. 2012;26(1 Suppl):S1–7.
68. Ameli F, Brocchetti F, Tosca MA, Signori A, Ciprandi G. Adenoidal hypertrophy and allergic rhinitis: is there an inverse relationship? Am J Rhinol Allergy. 2013;27:e5–10.
69. Marseglia GL, Avanzini MA, Caimmi S, Caimmi D, Marseglia A, Valsecchi C, et al. Passive exposure to smoke results in defective IFN-gamma production by adenoids in children with recurrent respiratory infections. J Interferon Cytokine Res. 2009;29:427–32.
70. Elwany S, Ibrahim AA, Mandour Z, Talaat I. Effect of passive smoking on the ultrastructure of the nasal mucosa in children. Laryngoscope. 2012;122:965–9.
71. Aycicek A, Dilek H, Sargın R, Sahin O, Kenar F, Derekoy SO. Heat shock protein 70 and inducible nitric oxide synthase expression in adenoid tissue of children exposed to passive smoke. Türkiye Klinikleri J Med Sci. 2009;29:1528–34.
72. Di Martino E, Mlynski G, Mlynski B. Effect of adenoid hyperplasia on nasal airflow. Laryngorhinootologie. 1998;77(5):272–4.
73. Niedzielska G, Kotowski M, Niedzielski A. Assessment of pulmonary function and nasal flow in children with adenoid hypertrophy. Int J Pediatr Otorhinolaryngol. 2008;72(3):333–5.
74. Modrzynski M, Zawisza E. An analysis of the incidence of adenoid hypertrophy in allergic children. Int J Pediatr Otorhinolaryngol. 2007;71:713–9.
75. Kavukcu S, Coskun S, Cevik N, Kuscu B, Akkoclu A. The importance of pulmonary function tests in adenotonsillectomy indications. Indian J Pediatr. 1993;60:249–55.
76. Aykan M, Aydın S, Öktem S, Demir MG, Tutar E. Effect of adenoid hypertrophy and pulmonary function tests in children with mild asthma. Kulak Burun Bogaz Ihtis Derg. 2016;26(5):253–7.
77. Maurizi M, Paludetti G, Todisco T, Dottorini M, Grassi V. Pulmonary function studies in adenoid hypertrophy. Int J Pediatr Otorhinolaryngol. 1980;2:243–50.

Meeting Organ for ENT and Pediatric Pulmonology: Tonsils

38

Duygu Demirbaş Keskin, Ayşe Seçil Kayalı Dinç, and Andrew A. Winkler

38.1 Introduction

Tonsils are lymphoid tissue structures positioned close to the entrance of the digestive and respiratory tracts and play a key role in our immune system. Together, the lingual tonsil at the posterior third of the tongue, the paired palatine tonsils laterally, the nasopharyngeal tonsil (adenoid) posterosuperior, and the paired tubal tonsils at the pharyngeal openings of the Eustachian tubes form a ring of lymphoid tissue called Waldeyer's ring [1–5]. They are crucial in preventing infection and act as the first defense against ingested or inhaled pathogens [2].

38.2 Anatomy

38.2.1 Palatine Tonsils (Faucial Tonsils)

The palatine tonsils are the most significant lymphoid tissue aggregation in Waldeyer's ring, first described by German anatomist Heinrich Wilhelm Gottfried von Waldeyer-Hartz [2, 5] and generally referred to as "the tonsils."

D. D. Keskin (✉)
Department of Otorhynolaryngology, Acıbadem Zekeriyakoy Medical Center, Department of Medical education PhD.c., Acıbadem MAA University Institute of Health Sciences, İstanbul, Turkey

A. S. K. Dinç
Department of Otorhynolaryngology, Ankara Bilkent City Hospital, Ankara, Turkey

A. A. Winkler
Department of Otolaryngology, University of Colorado School of Medicine, Aurora, CO, USA

H. Yüksel et al. (eds.), *Pediatric Airway Diseases*, Comprehensive ENT,
https://doi.org/10.1007/978-3-031-74853-0_38

They are found in the tonsillar fossa of the lateral oropharyngeal wall, between the palatoglossal arch (anterior) and the palatopharyngeal arch (posterior). The medial surface is the free mucosal part of the tonsil facing the oropharynx. The epithelium of the tonsil is the stratified squamous, nonkeratinized epithelium, which contains blind tubules from the epithelium on the surface of the tonsil and extends deep into this tissue, leading into tonsillar crypts [1]. About 10–30 branching and anastomosing crypts increase the tonsils' surface area for interactions between antigens and the nodular lymphoid tissue [1, 5, 6]. They increase the surface area of the tonsil up to 300 cm^2 [2, 6, 7]. The tonsil is surrounded by a capsule of loose connective tissue and is separated from the superior pharyngeal constrictor fascia on the deep surface of the tonsil [1, 3]. The surface epithelia are underlined by a band of thick connective tissue containing many vessels, nerves, and lymphatics [1].

The arterial blood supplies of the tonsils are the anterior tonsillar artery, from dorsal lingual branches of the lingual artery, the posterior tonsillar artery, and the ascending palatine branch of the facial. Ascending pharyngeal arteries, a superior tonsillar artery from a more significant palatine branch of maxillary artery, and inferior tonsillar artery (main artery) from facial artery [1, 3, 4]. The venous drainage is via the tonsillar vein (drains into the facial vein), and paratonsillar veins, which drain into the pharyngeal plexus and then internal jugular vein [1, 3, 4]. The palatine tonsils receive innervation from the maxillary nerve and glossopharyngeal nerve. The lymphatic drainage of the palatine tonsils through to the jugulodigastric and upper deep cervical lymph nodes located behind the angle of the mandible [1, 3, 4].

38.2.2 Lingual Tonsil

The lingual tonsil comprises numerous lymphoid nodules within the posterior third of the tongue. A stratified nonkeratinized squamous epithelium covers the lingual tonsil. The lingual artery's dorsal and the lingual vein's dorsal lingual branches perform the vascular supply. Innervation is from the glossopharyngeal nerve. Lymphatic fluid from the lingual tonsil drains into the jugulodigastric and deep cervical lymph nodes [1, 3, 4].

38.2.3 Adenoids (Pharyngeal Tonsil)

The pharyngeal tonsil, also known as the adenoid, is composed of lymphoid tissue within the mucosa of the roof of the nasopharynx. The pharyngeal tonsil is lined by pseudostratified ciliated columnar epithelium (respiratory epithelium) that is plicated to form numerous surface folds. The arterial supply of the adenoids is from the basisphenoid artery, the ascending pharyngeal artery, the ascending palatine artery, the pharyngeal branch of the maxillary artery, the tonsillar branch of the facial artery, and the artery of the pterygoid canal. Venous drainage is to the pharyngeal plexus, which communicates with the pterygoid plexus and drains into the internal jugular and facial veins. The nerve supply is from the pharyngeal plexus. The efferent lymphatic drainage of the adenoids is to the retropharyngeal and pharyngomaxillary space lymph nodes [1, 3, 4].

38.2.4 Tubal Tonsils

The tubal tonsils are the small aggregates of lymphoid tissue around the Eustachian tube's opening in the nasopharynx's lateral wall. They form the lateral aspect of Waldeyer's ring. The epithelial covering of the tubal tonsils is ciliated pseudostratified epithelium with no crypts. Arterial supply is from the ascending pharyngeal artery, and venous drainage is to the pharyngeal plexus. Innervation is via the maxillary and glossopharyngeal nerves. The retropharyngeal and the deep cervical lymph nodes drain the tubal tonsils [1, 3, 4].

38.3 Embryology of the Tonsils

Tonsils are derived from the second pharyngeal pouch. Tonsilla palatina begins to develop in the 14th gestational week and is characterized by the development of invaginations of the epithelium in the underlying mesenchymal cells and the infiltration of the stroma by lymphoid cells [8, 9]. About the 16th gestational week, epithelial crypts develop into connective tissue and are infiltrated with T lymphocytes [8, 9]. A progressive development of complex epithelial invagination (tubules and crypts) occurs with the parallel development of lymphocytic tissue. Primary follicles contain precursors of dendritic reticulum cells and lymphoid cells that belong to the B-cell line and are considered the first B-cell regions in fetal lymphoid tissue [8, 9]. In embryonic life, no germinal center is observed in the lymphatic follicles of the tonsil [9]. Present at birth, the tonsils tend to reach their full size between the sixth and eighth years of life. Between the 4th and 12th year of life, tonsils and adenoids are found to be the most immunologically active and begin to involute/atrophy shortly after the first decade, directly proportional to the bacterial load and the number of B and T cells [1, 3, 10].

38.4 Immunology of the Tonsils

Tonsils are lymphoid tissue structures positioned close to the entrance of the digestive and respiratory tracts and play a key role in our immune system as part of secondary lymphoid organs [2]. The mucosal-associated lymphoid tissues (MALT) are considered a special type of secondary lymphoid organ concerned with immunity at mucosal surfaces of the aerodigestive tract [7, 11]. The MALT includes Peyer's patches, appendix, and tonsils as nasopharynx-associated lymphoid tissue (NALT), known as Waldeyer's ring [2, 6, 7, 11].

Tonsils are designed to carry foreign bodies from the outside to lymphoid cells. This contrasts with the lymph nodes, which depend on antigenic administration via the lymphatic pathway [1]. In the tonsils, immune-reactive lymphoid cells are found in four separate areas: the reticular cell epithelium, the extrafollicular area, the mantle zone of the lymphoid follicle, and the germinal center of the lymphoid follicle [1]. The germinal center and the mantle zone define the lymphoid follicle.

Mature B lymphocytes make up the mantle zone surrounding the germ center. It is surrounded by T cells in the extrafollicular area [2, 12, 13].

The reticulated crypt epithelium, also known as lymphoepithelium [2], plays a vital role in beginning immune responses in the palatine tonsils when antigens are inhaled or ingested [1, 2]. The antigen is transported by specialized membranous (M) cells at the base of the reticulated crypt epithelium [7, 10–12]. After detecting an antigen, M cells activate T and B cells in the tonsils, triggering an immunological response [1–3]. B lymphocytes and T helper cells (CD4+) make up the majority of lymphoid cells detected in the spaces of the reticulated crypt epithelium of the human palatine tonsil. Approximately 50–90% of the intraepithelial lymphocytes are B cells. Antigens enter the extrafollicular area of lymphoid follicles after passing through the crypt epithelium. T cells (mainly of the CD4+ helper phenotype), interdigitating dendritic cells (IDC), macrophages, and specialized venules known as high endothelial venules (HEV) are found in the extrafollicular region. HEV is necessary to enter T and B cells from the blood into the tonsils. Activated T cells produce and release biologically active protein cytokines. T helper lymphocytes (CD4) stimulate B cells and facilitate their transformation into plasma cells (producing antibodies), and T cytotoxic lymphocytes (CD8) kill antigen-containing cells by direct contact and by release of cytokines. B memory cells develop and are maintained at the germinal center for repeated antigen exposure, whereas antibody-producing plasma cells migrate from the germinal zone to the mantle zone. The palatine tonsils produce a variety of Ig isotypes (IgD, IgM, IgG, and IgA) [2, 7, 12, 13].

IgA is an antibody that functions as a mucosal antiseptic' and plays a vital role in mucus immune activity [1, 3, 11, 12]. The J-chain is required for the epithelial transport of Ig polymers and is produced by Ig-producing cells. The presence of the J-chain in the IgA polymer is needed in a stable complex. IgA binds to pathogens and other molecules, either blocking or rendering them harmless, allowing them to be absorbed, transported as an immunological complex, and dealt with by the reticuloendothelial system. J-chain is also found in IgM, allowing it to be secreted in the same way as IgA. In patients with selective IgA deficiency, secretory IgA (sIgA) is lacking but may be replaced by secretory IgM, which is also protective. Immunoregulatory compensation occurs in other IgA-deficient patients, resulting in many IgD-producing cells in the respiratory mucosa. Because this cannot function as a secretory antibody, these people are prone to repeated respiratory tract infections. Tonsillectomy specimens show an increase in IgD-bearing cells [2, 7, 11].

The number of lymphocytes in children's tonsils is higher than in adults' tonsils, and the number of helper and cytotoxic T lymphocytes is higher in sick tonsils. Also, the persistent antigenic stimulation from infected tonsils causes increased levels of immunoglobulins throughout the pretonsillectomy period [2, 11].

38.5 Etiology and Pathogenesis

Normal flora in the upper respiratory tract is established from birth. After birth, the tonsils are one of the first organs to accept external antigenic stimuli with respiration and digestion. The pathophysiology of disease in the tonsils is likely multifactorial [4]. Multiple organisms, including aerobic and anaerobic bacteria, viruses, fungi, and parasites, can infect tonsils; some are part of the normal oral pharyngeal flora, while others are external pathogens [1, 4, 14].

The mostly found aerobic bacteria in tonsils and adenoids are Streptococci (groups A, B, C, G), *Hemophilus influenza*, *Streptococcus pneumoniae*, *Branhamella cattarhalis*, *Staphylococcus aureus*, Mycobacterium sp., and Neisseria sp. [4]. As anaerobic, we may list *Bacteroides* sp., *Actinomycosis* sp., *Peptococcus* sp., and *Peptostreptococcus* sp. [4].

38.5.1 Viral Tonsillitis

The most prevalent viral causes are rhinovirus, respiratory syncytial virus, adenovirus, and coronavirus, which all cause the common cold. These are typically low-virulent, mild, and self-limiting infections that do not require special treatment and rarely cause complications. The majority of patients have a fever and erythematous pharyngeal mucosa. Although the tonsils may be swollen, no associated exudate usually exists [1]. Tonsilitis can be caused by various viruses, including Epstein-Barr (which causes mononucleosis), CMV, herpesvirus, hepatitis A, rubella, and HIV [1, 13, 15]. Coxsackievirus, herpesvirus, and Epstein-Barr virus may affect the tonsils and produce symptoms of exudative and nonexudative tonsils [1, 13, 15–17].

High fever, general malaise, large, palatal petechia, swollen, dirty-gray tonsils, posterior cervical lymphadenopathy, hepatosplenomegaly, and exhaustion are all symptoms of mononucleosis caused by EBV [1, 13, 15, 16]. The diagnosis of Epstein-Barr virus can be confirmed by laboratory testing in conjunction with physical exam findings. A differential blood count indicating lymphocytosis (50% lymphocytes with 10% atypical cells) supports a diagnosis, as are heterophil antibody titers [1, 15, 16]. The disease may still be present if the heterophil antibody agglutination test is negative. Only 60% of individuals with infectious mononucleosis have a positive result during the first 2 weeks of illness onset; 90% have a positive impact one month later [1]. Patients should avoid contact sports during their sickness due to the link between hepatosplenomegaly and mononucleosis syndrome, since they risk splenic rupture [13]. Symptomatic treatment is used to treat this condition. When given to mononucleosis patients, amoxicillin-related drugs have been reported to trigger an immune-mediated rash. Antibiotics should not be used in patients diagnosed with EBV tonsillitis or suspected of having it [1, 13]. Upper airway obstruction from severely enlarged tonsils can be life-threatening and should be managed promptly with the insertion of a nasopharyngeal airway and short-term high-dose steroid therapy. Tonsillectomy or tracheotomy may be indicated if the obstruction is severe and these methods do not relieve it [1, 13].

Small vesicles with erythematous bases form ulcers and extend over the anterior pillar tonsils, palate, and posterior pharynx in Herpangina caused by coxsackievirus [1, 13]. It could be a part of the hand, foot, and mouth syndrome, with blisters on the palms and soles. Hydration, antipyretics, and analgesics are commonly supportive treatments [1, 13, 17].

38.5.2 Bacterial Tonsillitis

GABHS (group A beta-hemolytic Streptococcus) is the most common cause of bacterial infections, though *Staphylococcus aureus*, *Streptococcus pneumoniae*, and *Haemophilus influenzae* have all been cultured. Symptoms of acute bacterial tonsillitis include throat soreness, swollen erythematous or exudative tonsils, stinking breath, and painful cervical lymph nodes. It might be difficult to distinguish between bacterial and viral causes of tonsillitis and pharyngitis. At the same time, supportive care treats viral infections, pain management, and antibiotics (amoxicillin or macrolides). They are used to treat ordinary, moderate bacterial tonsillitis [1, 4, 13]. The most prevalent bacterial cause of acute tonsillitis is Group A B-hemolytic streptococcus. Because this organism is a known precursor of acute rheumatic fever and glomerulonephritis, which develops due to an autoimmune response, it is a severe infectious condition [1, 4, 13, 17]. As a result, most authorities advise that microbiologic testing be used to confirm or rule out a diagnosis of group A-hemolytic streptococcal (GABHS) tonsillitis. Selective use of throat cultures is a time-honored medical practice, the usefulness of which is somewhat limited by the delay in obtaining results [1, 4, 17]. The use of throat cultures is a long-honored medical practice, but its utility is restricted by the time it takes to get results [1, 4, 17]. The 18- to 36-h wait for positive cultures may cause the patient extra suffering and lengthen the clinical course [1, 4, 17]. The development of rapid strep detection tests for detecting the group A streptococcal antigen has represented a helpful advance. Rapid streptococcus antigen tests are very specific but less sensitive than a throat culture [1, 18]. This test is particular (ranging from 88 to 100%). However, it is not exposed (61–95%) [14]. The quick strep test is the most accurate and cost-effective way to diagnose acute GABHS infection. A standard throat culture is performed in individuals with a negative immediate strep test result and a strong suspicion of streptococcal tonsillitis [1, 4, 13, 17, 18].

Other bacteria, such as Streptococci of Group C and G, *Haemophilus influenzae*, *Nocardia*, *Corynebacteria*, and *Neisseria gonorrhoeae*, must be evaluated more seldom. Vincent's angina is caused by the bacterial symbiosis of *Fusobacterium nucleatum* and *Borrelia vincentii*, characterized by a generally unilateral, ulcerating tonsillitis with halitosis. Patients complain of a high headache, fever, sore throat, cervical lymphadenopathy, and a membrane on the tonsil that, when removed, reveals an ulcer that is restricted to the surrounding tissue and resolves in 7–10 days. Treatment usually involves debridement, antiseptic mouthwashes such as chlorhexidine, pain control, and antibiotics, including clindamycin, penicillin, or erythromycin [1, 13, 17].

Diphtheria tonsillitis has decreased dramatically since the introduction of diphtheria toxin immunization. This organism produces a thick pharyngeal membrane and early exudative pharyngotonsillitis. When this membrane is removed, it causes bleeding. After that, the infection might spread to the throat, palate, tonsils, and larynx [1, 13]. Airway obstruction can occur when laryngeal inflammation is accompanied by an exudative, necrotic gray pharyngeal membrane [1, 13].

The organisms of C. diphtheriae also release a fatal exotoxin that can damage cells in distant organs. Myocarditis and neurologic sequelae resembling features of poliomyelitis may result [1, 13]. Fluorescent antibody studies are used to identify the organism. Gram staining can detect the presence of Klebs-Löffler bacillus in the membrane. Because diphtheria is a life-threatening condition, antitoxin must be administered within 48 h of the onset of symptoms. Airway obstruction should be managed with tracheotomy. Penicillin should be given in high dosages [1, 13].

One of the most common sexually transmitted bacterial infections is gonorrhea. While oral-genital infections are most commonly transferred through sexual contact, transmission from mother to fetus during pregnancy might result in systemic or ophthalmic diseases. As a result, N. gonorrhoeae and C. trachomatis are uncommonly found in pediatric patients [13]. Unfortunately, because the physical findings in the pharynx are not specific enough to reveal the etiology, the diagnosis is frequently made clinically, depending on the patient's history and risk factors. Mild pharyngeal pain and dysphagia are among the pharyngeal symptoms. Despite the start of empiric antibiotic treatment, pharyngeal culture explicitly aimed at identifying gonorrhea is frequently conducted. Notably, *C. trachomatis*, a gram-negative intracellular bacterium, is known to be capable of causing a similar pharyngeal infection and often coexists with pharyngeal gonorrhea in patients. Despite signs of systemic disease, chlamydial conditions are rarely found in pharyngeal culture, unlike gonorrhea. As a result, both *N. gonorrhoeae* and *C. trachomatis* should be treated. Intramuscular ceftriaxone in combination with azithromycin or doxycycline is the preferred treatment [1, 13, 19].

Oral pharyngeal lesions have been linked to *Treponema pallidum* infections in both the primary and later stages of syphilis. Oral chancres are common in primary syphilis, while grayish superficial mucous membrane patches with an erythematous border are standard in secondary syphilis. A dark-field microscope inspection of the lesions and a serological test are used to confirm the diagnosis [1, 19].

38.5.3 Candida

Although thrush is frequent in newborns, *Candida albicans* infection of the pharynx is uncommon in healthy children and adults. Candidiasis can cause severe pharyngitis, especially in immunocompromised patients or those treated with antimicrobial drugs. The lesions are patchy white "in color," and when the exudate is removed, a shallow reddish ulcer is revealed. The usual yeast forms in stained smears and cultures are used to confirm the diagnosis. In resistant cases, Nystatin or fluconazole are used to treat the infection [1, 19].

38.6 Complications of Tonsillitis

The complications of tonsillitis can be divided into suppurative and nonsuppurative difficulties [1].

38.6.1 Suppurative Complications

38.6.1.1 Peritonsillar Abscess (Quincy Tonsil)

Peritonsillar abscess is the most common complication of acute tonsillitis. It is a purulent fluid in the space surrounding the tonsils between the tonsillar capsule and the superior constrictor muscle [3]. Patients with recurrent tonsillitis or chronic tonsillitis that has not been appropriately treated are more likely to develop peritonsillar abscess [1, 15, 20]. Patients usually present with unilateral pain that causes odynophagia, ipsilateral otalgia, and classic "hot potato" or muffled voice [1, 3]. The odynophagia may be so acute that the patient cannot swallow, resulting in dehydration. Oropharyngeal asymmetry can be demonstrated clinically by moving the affected side's tonsil toward the median [1, 20, 21]. Trismus is frequently present due to irritation of the pterygoid musculature by the pus and inflammation [1]. Peritonsillar abscess cultures typically reveal a polymicrobial infection, both aerobic and anaerobic. In recent studies, *Fusobacterium necrophorum*, also responsible for Lemierre's syndrome, is a prominent and prevalent pathogen in peritonsillar abscesses [22]. In some circumstances, a single needle aspirate or a series of needle aspirates may be sufficient to resolve abscess formation.

In some cases, broader drainage may be required to clear the infection. If there has been a previous history of tonsillitis, a Quinsy tonsillectomy may be highly beneficial in circumstances where incision and drainage cannot be performed without general anesthesia. Although tonsillectomy is not required for all peritonsillar abscesses, it is the preferred treatment for recurrent infection [1, 15, 20, 21, 23]. Intratonsillar abscesses are usually found in association with peritonsillar abscesses [20, 22, 23]. Peritonsillar abscess complications are relatively uncommon. Parapharyngeal and retropharyngeal abscesses, upper airway obstruction [13], Lemierre's syndrome [24, 25], mediastinitis [26], and other abnormal conditions are among them.

38.6.1.2 Parapharyngeal and Retropharyngeal Space Abscess

Parapharyngeal abscess is located between the superior constrictor muscle and the deep cervical fascia [1, 20]. A patient with a parapharyngeal space infection typically has fever, leukocytosis, and pain. Tonsil displacement is found in the anterior-medial direction. A CT scan with contrast enhancement should be conducted if this is suspected to be a parapharyngeal abscess. Aggressive antibiotic medication, fluid replacement, and close observation should all be used to treat lateral pharyngeal space infections [1, 20]. The resolution of these infections frequently necessitates surgical intervention. Intraoral methods should be utilized to treat peritonsillar abscesses; they should not be utilized to treat lateral pharyngeal space abscesses due to insufficient exposure in the event of heavy bleeding [1, 15, 20].

In pediatric populations, retropharyngeal abscesses represent the predominant deep neck infections after peritonsillar infections. Infection arises from the lymph nodes that drain the upper airway and oropharynx. The abscess infectious process may progress down the carotid sheath and into the mediastinum. Infections of the retropharyngeal space are most frequent in children under the age of two. Irritability, fever, dysphagia, airway obstruction, unilateral pain, torticollis, and cervical lymphadenopathy are common symptoms in children with retropharyngeal infections. A CT scan is an excellent way to determine the size and extent of an abscess invasion [1, 15, 21, 23]. A transoral approach is recommended for incision and drainage of retropharyngeal space abscesses. An external approach should be performed if the abscess extends inferiorly below the hyoid bone (as revealed on the CT scan) [1].

Lemierre's Syndrome
Lemierre syndrome commonly presents as sepsis following a sore throat with associated thrombosis of the internal jugular vein and septic emboli. It is most often linked to *Fusobacterium necrophorum*, although it has also been linked to Staphylococcal and Streptococcal infections. It most commonly affects healthy teenagers and young adults. At the onset of the disease, patients present with nonspecific symptoms such as exudative tonsillitis, high fever, oropharyngeal ulcers, cervical lymphadenopathy, and pharyngeal hyperemia. Internal jugular vein thrombophlebitis, which commonly manifests as pain and unilateral swelling around the angle of the jaw and along the sternocleidomastoid muscle and is sometimes associated with trismus, is caused by the second stage of the infection, which involves invasion of the anterior compartment. Invasion of the posterior compartment, on the other hand, can cause Horner syndrome or cranial nerve X–XII palsies [27]. The third stage is the metastatic stage, in which septic emboli can induce characteristic clinical signs and symptoms depending on the location of the embolism. The most prevalent location of metastatic dissemination is the lungs, where embolic illness causes symptoms similar to an aseptic pulmonary embolism [25, 27]. Accurate diagnosis necessitates a high level of clinical suspicion. Early CT/US imaging and polymerase chain reaction–based serological screening are recommended to reduce diagnostic delays. The effective treatment of Lemierre syndrome requires a combination of early diagnosis and aggressive antimicrobial therapy. Despite being a rare clinical entity today, Lemierre syndrome is nevertheless a condition with significant morbidity and death [24, 25, 27].

38.6.2 Nonsuppurative Complications

38.6.2.1 Acute Rheumatic Fever

Rheumatic fever (RF) is an inflammatory, immunological condition caused by group A *Streptococcus* infection. Patients aged 5–18 years old are the most typically affected. While rare in the developed world, the incidence is high in developing nations. RF usually appears 2–3 weeks after a rheumatogenic streptococcus throat infection, but it can present as early as 1 week and as late as 5 weeks. Multiple organ systems are affected, and the presentation can have different degrees of severity. A diagnosis of acute rheumatic fever cannot be made using a specific laboratory test. It is a clinical diagnosis based on the Jones criteria (table) and supported by clinical immunology and microbiology lab data [1, 14, 15, 25]. For diagnosis of ARF, according to Jones Criteria, two major or one significant and two minor manifestations must be present, plus evidence of antecedent group A streptococcus infection. Chorea and carditis do not require evidence of antecedent group A streptococcus infection [14].

Cardiac manifestations such as pericarditis, myocarditis, and endocarditis are common. Carditis affects approximately half of all patients and is frequently associated with valvular disease, particularly the mitral valve. Arthralgia, arthritis, skin lesions, and central nervous system involvement (chorea) may be seen. Arthritis in the major joints is frequently migratory, asymmetrical, and painful. Involuntary movements of the limbs and facial muscles and speech and gait problems characterize Sydenham chorea. Patients may present with a rash called erythema marginatum and subcutaneous nodules [1, 15, 25].

Elevated streptococcal antibody titers or demonstration of bacteria in the throat are required to diagnose acute rheumatic fever. The ASO test may be administered first. Anti-DNAse B, antistreptokinase, or antihyaluronidase tests may be obtained if the titer is not increased. To monitor disease activity, the preferred tests are C-reactive protein and erythrocyte sedimentation rate to inflammatory activity [1, 14, 15].

The use of antimicrobial medicincs has reduced the incidence of rheumatic fever. A single dose of penicillin, 1.2 million units intramuscularly for individuals weighing more than 27 kg and 600,000 units for those weighing less than 27 kg, is suggested. Penicillin V is the preferred oral antibiotic, which should be taken twice to thrice daily [1, 14, 15, 25]. For those allergic to penicillin, erythromycin (20–40 mg/kg/day for 10 days) is a good option. Patients allergic to penicillin who do not have acute hypersensitivity to beta-lactam antibiotics may benefit from first- or second-generation cephalosporins [1, 14]. Azithromycin and clarithromycin, two newer macrolides, show fewer side effects in the stomach than erythromycin and have similar sensitivity patterns to group A streptococcus. The inflammatory process involving numerous organ systems should be targeted for symptomatic treatment of rheumatic fever. Because it has a higher risk of morbidity, the duration and kind of therapy are determined mainly by the existence and severity of carditis during the initial attack. The routine use of corticosteroids is not recommended. They should only be used in the case of severe carditis, where they appear to help reduce mortality during an acute episode. The drug of choice is prednisone, given at 1–2 mg/kg/day for 2–3 weeks. Rest for at least 4 weeks is recommended. Arthritis caused by acute rheumatic fever responds well to salicylates, with significant clinical improvement. Treatment should last at least 2 weeks and up to 6 weeks to avoid rebound.

Sydenham's chorea (SC) is not a self-limited or benign disease. SC mainly affects children between 5 and 15 years old and appears to predominate in girls. After Group A B-hemolytic streptococcal pharyngitis, the condition usually takes 6–8 weeks to manifest. It does not happen as a result of a skin disease. Family investigations in both SC and RF patients have indicated a significant incidence of a favorable family history. The main feature of SC is the involuntary movements. These might be general or unilateral, with the most commonly affected areas of the extremities and face. The signs occur at rest, may start gradually or abruptly, and are exacerbated by stress. They disappear during sleep, however. Depression, anxiety, personality changes, emotional lability, OCD, tics, and attention deficit disorder are some psychological and psychiatric symptoms of patients with SC. Cases of disability and social isolation have been reported. It has been suggested that haloperidol be used to treat chorea. However, sodium valproate has also been proven helpful. In this situation, there is no evidence that steroids or nonsteroidal anti-inflammatory medicines are beneficial [1, 14].

38.6.2.2 Poststreptococcal Glomerulonephritis

Post-streptococcal glomerulonephritis (PSGN) is an immune-mediated disorder following infection with Group A streptococcus. PSGN usually appears 1–2 weeks after a streptococcal throat infection or 6 weeks after a streptococcal skin infection (impetigo) in children. PSGN clinical symptoms are more prevalent in males than females, with a 2:1 ratio. Patients present with hypertension, edema, abnormalities on urine sediment, elevated inflammatory markers, hypoproteinemia, and low complement levels. The situation is secondary to the presence of a common antigen of the glomerulus with the streptococcus. Approximately 50% of children with PSGN are asymptomatic and are discovered accidentally during routine urine analysis.

In most cases, PSGN is a self-limiting disease that only requires symptomatic treatment. During the acute phase of the disease, supportive treatment aims to control the complications of volume overload, such as hypertension and edema. There is no indication that antibiotic medication modifies the natural history of glomerulonephritis, and penicillin management may not reduce the attack rate. A tonsillectomy may be required to eradicate the cause of infection [1, 25].

38.6.2.3 Scarlet Fever

Scarlet fever is related to the production of endotoxins by the group A streptococcal bacteria. An erythematous rash, acute lymphadenopathy with a painful throat, vomiting, headache, fever, erythematous tonsils, pharynx, tachycardia, and a yellow exudate across the tonsils, pharynx, and nasopharynx are the most common symptoms of scarlet fever. A strawberry tongue with a rash and large glossal papillae is a good diagnostic sign. Diagnosis of scarlet fever is made by culture and positive result of the Dick test, which is an intradermal injection of dilute streptococcal toxin. The rash is not harmful, but it is a sign of group A streptococcus infection, which can cause suppurative and non-suppurative problems. To avoid severe problems, it is necessary to treat the acute infection. Penicillin is the first-line therapy of choice [1, 15, 17].

38.6.2.4 Pediatric Autoimmune Neuropsychiatric Disorder Associated with Streptococcal Infection (PANDAS)

Anxiety disorders, obsessive-compulsive characteristics, and pathologic compulsive tics associated with streptococcal tonsillitis and pharyngitis are increasingly being recognized as a single entity. The symptoms start within weeks after the pharyngeal or tonsillar infection, and it is limited to the pediatric group by definition [13]. Antibasal ganglia antibodies (ABGA) were detected in 95–100% of Sydenham Corea (SC) patients and 64–94% of PANDAS patients [28]. Streptococcal infections may trigger an autoimmune response to the basal ganglia through a molecular mimicry mechanism [13, 28, 29]. A tonsillectomy is an option for treatment [13].

Tonsillectomy has been proposed as a treatment for PANDAS, but the evidence is limited, and the condition is poorly understood. A recent comprehensive study showed no recommendations for or against tonsillectomy as a treatment for PANDAS [30, 31].

38.6.2.5 Periodic Fever, Aphthous Stomatitis, Pharyngitis, and Adenopathy Syndrome (PFAPA)

PFAPA syndrome (periodic fever, aphthous stomatitis, pharyngitis, and cervical adenitis) is a recurrent febrile condition primarily affecting children aged 2–6, with a minor male predisposition. The sudden onset of fever, pharyngitis, tender cervical lymphadenopathy, or aphthous ulcers characterizes it [13, 32, 33]. Clinical criteria are used to make a diagnosis. Despite research that shows a hereditary origin, the genetic origins, and etiology of PFAPA syndrome remain unknown. The cornerstone of treatment is corticosteroids. However, tonsillectomy has also been shown to induce remission and/or minimize the severity of episodes [32, 33]. Although there have been isolated reports of sporadic cases in adults, they become less common after age 10 [13].

38.6.2.6 Palmoplantar Pustulosis (PPP)

Palmoplantar pustulosis (PPP) is defined by the recurrence of sterile pustules on the palms and soles, accompanied by scaly and erythematous skin that might fissure [34, 35]. PPP patients have an intraepidermal aggregation of neutrophils in the upper dermis and a mixed perivascular, diffuse infiltrate with inflammatory cells. Molecular investigations of PPP reveal that CD4-positive T cells in the tonsils and peripheral blood detect streptococcal antigens and exhibit increased levels of immunological markers such as beta-1integrin and CCR6 in PPP patients. Immune complexes, antikeratin antibodies, and inflammatory cytokines (IL-6, IFN-, and TNF-) were found to be elevated in PPP patients, and changes in these levels following tonsillectomy were found to be closely connected with the prevalence of skin lesions [34, 36]. As a result, tonsillectomy appears to decrease the number of autoreactive cells. Tonsillectomy has effectively improved PPP skin lesions in several studies [34–36].

38.6.2.7 IgA Nephropathy

The most frequent type of glomerulonephritis in the world is IgA nephropathy. Progress takes 10–20 years and can lead to end-stage renal failure. It is caused by immunoglobulin A (IgA) protein deposits inside the kidney's filters (glomeruli) [36, 37]. Upper respiratory infections, such as tonsillitis, frequently manifest with macroscopic hematuria in IgAN patients. There is a link between tonsillar immunity and pathophysiology, according to clinical data. Tonsillar immunity is a type of mucosal immunity in which antigen-presenting cells, such as macrophages, form the starting point for B cells and plasma cells to make antibodies, including IgA, when exposed to pathogens (e.g., bacteria and their constituents) [38]. Hotta et al. were the first to propose that for IgAN patients, a tonsillectomy combined with steroid pulse therapy will reduce hematuria/proteinuria and increase remission rates [36–39].

38.7 Clinical Manifestation

The most prevalent upper respiratory tract disorders are recurrent acute tonsillitis (RT) and obstructive diseases induced by tonsillar hyperplasia (TH). Although the severity of frailty varies, many patients suffer from chronic and recurrent medical conditions that have an impact on their physical and mental health, as well as their educational performance and healthcare costs [40].

38.7.1 Infection

Acute tonsillitis is a clinical diagnosis. It can be challenging to distinguish between bacterial and viral causes, but it is necessary to avoid antibiotic overuse. To differentiate between viral and bacterial tonsillitis, data such as the patient's history, clinical symptoms, and laboratory data are required [17, 41]. In 70–95% of patients, viral infection causes acute tonsillitis [41]. Epstein-Barr virus (EBV), rhinovirus, enterovirus, influenza, and adenovirus are viral infections that frequently cause acute tonsillitis [1, 13]. The most prevalent bacterial etiology is Group A beta-hemolytic streptococcus (GABHS) [1, 4, 13, 17]. Different pathogen spectrums are detected depending on age [17, 41]. Streptococcal pharyngitis affects people of all ages, though it is most frequent in children and teenagers—the infection peaks between the ages of 3 and 14. Although the disease is more common in the winter and early spring, it can strike any time of year. The incubation period is between 2 and 5 days [41]. Both aerobic and anaerobic microorganisms can cause bacterial tonsillitis.

Histologically, a necrotic crypt epithelium, leukocytes within the crypts (empyema), and numerous bacterial colonies are all signs of acute bacterial tonsillitis. Chronic inflammation, on the other hand, is defined by larger and activated germinal centers, as well as a significant rise in IgG production. Crypts are dilated and frequently include debris, bacteria, and calcification (tonsillithiasis).

38.7.2 Obstruction

In the pediatric population, obstructive sleep apnea is the most common reason for tonsillectomy [1]. Sleep apnea syndrome (SAS) is a common disorder characterized by snoring and partial or intermittent obstruction of the upper airway during sleep. It is estimated to occur in 1–3% of children with a peak age of 2–5 years. Common symptoms include chronic snoring, difficulty breathing during sleep, restlessness, and witnessed apnea. The most prevalent related condition in otherwise healthy children is adenotonsillar hypertrophy, but cranial-facial deformities, neuromuscular disorders, and obesity are risk factors. Excessive daytime sleepiness, growth failure, school failure, behavioral issues, cor pulmonale, and even death can be significant neurobehavioral and cardiorespiratory consequences of severe OSAS. Diagnosis is based on data from the history, physical exam, and laboratory studies that confirm the presence and severity of the upper airway obstruction.

The diagnostic tool of choice has been polysomnography. The severity of the symptoms, as well as the underlying anatomic and physiologic abnormalities, determine treatment options. Because adenotonsillar hypertrophy is generally present in children with OSAS, most cases can be treated surgically [1, 42–45].

Snoring should be monitored in all children and adolescents. If polysomnography is unavailable, alternative diagnostic testing or referral to a specialist for a complete assessment should be considered in children/adolescents with snoring and symptoms/signs of OSAS. Patients with adenotonsillar hypertrophy should receive adenotonsillectomy as a first-line treatment. If adenotonsillectomy is not performed or if OSAS persists after surgery, continuous positive airway pressure is indicated as a therapy. In patients who are overweight or obese, weight loss is shown in addition to other treatments. Intranasal corticosteroids are an option for children with minor OSAS who are not candidates for adenotonsillectomy or who have minor OSAS after surgery [45].

38.7.3 Neoplasia

Tumors in the oropharynx are most commonly found in the anterior tonsillar pillar and the tonsil. Lesions on the anterior tonsillar most widely manifest as regions of leukoplakia or erythroplakia and are often asymptomatic. Exophytic or ulcerative lesions, predominantly in the tonsillar fossa, are more common. Tonsil lesions are at a significant risk of spreading to regional lymph nodes due to lymphatic drainage. They may also be the unobvious primary site when carcinoma appears in the lymph nodes with no known place of origin in the pharynx. Lymphoma, Hodgkin's disease, and tonsil cancer have been the most prevalent lesions [19]. Asymmetric tonsil enlargement is uncommon and may indicate the necessity for tonsillectomy to confirm the diagnosis [1, 4, 15, 19]. Patients with concomitant symptoms suggestive of a malignant process, such as adenopathy over 3 cm, dysphagia, night sweats, and fevers, may consider tonsillectomy for tonsil asymmetry [46].

38.8 Diagnosis

38.8.1 Symptoms and Signs

The most prevalent upper respiratory tract disorders are recurrent acute tonsillitis (RT) and obstructive infections caused by tonsillar hyperplasia (TH) [40]. Children who have tonsillar diseases present variably. Fever, tonsillar exudates, sore throat, odynophagia, halitosis, and sensitive anterior cervical chain lymphadenopathy are common symptoms of infection [1, 13, 25, 47]. Patients may also have dysphagia secondary to tonsillar swelling. A complete history and physical exam should be performed first, and the results can be used to calculate a Centor Score or McIsaac score (modified Centor score) [17, 48]. According to national and international guidelines, the McIsaac Score for clinical assessment of the possibility of GABHS tonsillitis is still recommended as the preferred clinical screening technique. According to McIsaac, the modified Centor score is correct for age and may thus be utilized in both adults and children [17, 48]. Both methods were created to determine the likelihood that streptococcal bacteria and guiding treatment cause pharyngitis. A rapid test or culture should only be considered if the patient scores 3 or above (Centor or McIsaac). This is not recommended for people with a score of 2 or less unless they have a persistent illness or a unilateral finding [17, 48].

38.8.2 Physical Examination

There have been no standard recommendations for the clinical assessment of the tonsils. To prevent gagging, a tongue depressor is softly placed on the anterior two-thirds of the tongue in front of the circumvallate papillae [4]. The palatine tonsils can often be seen in a pediatric child by steadily depressing the posterior oral tongue using a tongue depressor. Conversely, involution may make the palatine tonsil less visible in the adult patient [4, 13].

Brodsky and colleagues developed a tonsillar hypertrophy assessment scale [4].

38.8.3 Laboratory

Acute tonsillitis is a clinical diagnosis. Acute tonsillitis will be diagnosed clinically. To distinguish between viral and bacterial tonsillitis, information such as the patient's history, clinical symptoms, and test data are required [17].

GABHS can be detected using throat culture alone or with rapid antigen testing. It is vital to remember that while rapid antigen testing is specific (88–100%), it is not sensitive (61–95%); false negatives are possible. Clinicians should consider acquiring pharyngeal swabs for gonorrhea, chlamydia, and HIV in the appropriate clinical situation. When the Ebstein-Barr virus is suspected, a mononucleosis spot test may be considered [25].

The sampling technique is essential for the diagnostic quality of the pharyngeal swab [49]. The tongue should be forced down, and the swab should be wiped across both tonsils and the posterior pharyngeal wall in a rotating motion. The intraoral mucosa and saliva should not be touched [49]. If the rapid test findings are negative and there is a strong suspicion of bacterial pharyngeal infection, a microbiological culture should be used to identify the bacteria [17, 48, 49]. Mostly, microbiological culture is less expensive than rapid test procedures. However, one disadvantage of culturing is the time required until the test result is available [17]. Multiplex PCR can offer molecular genetic confirmation of viral (tonsillitis) infections. Rapid tests or multiplex PCR for virus identification are nearly always unimportant in the clinical routine for different viruses (e.g., adenoviruses) due to the lack of therapeutic significance [25].

The human antibody production against such streptococcal antigens is measured by antistreptolysin O titer (ASLO titer) values. An acute b-hemolytic streptococcal infection could trigger the development of antibodies. The ASLO titer and all other currently known human antibody titers against b-hemolytic streptococci (e.g., anti-hyaluronidase, and anti-DNase B) do not provide valid diagnostic criteria for the diagnostics. An increased antibody response to streptococci (e.g., an increased ASL titer) does not indicate protection from acute streptococcal infections, nor does it imply an increased risk of acute streptococcal disease, nor does it indicate an increased risk of purulent or immunogenic streptococcal secondary illness [17, 50].

38.8.4 Imagining

A lateral neck film can occasionally help identify the tonsils' inferior extension; however, this modality cannot precisely evaluate the tonsils' relative airway size [4, 51].

A more thorough examination may be required in complicated infections, such as those involving patients with unstable vital signs, toxic appearance, difficulties swallowing, inability to accept oral intake, or trismus. CT imaging of the neck with intravenous contrast can rule out dangerous conditions such as abscess, Lemierre disease, and epiglottitis [25]. Imaging with head and neck magnetic resonance imaging (MRI) or computed tomography (CT) is appropriate if abscessing is suspected beyond the peritonsillar region. A CT scan can confirm the diagnosis of peritonsillar abscess with a sensitivity of up to 100% and a specificity of up to 75%, and it can also identify additional abscessing and is nearly always available and cost-effective. Because MRI enables higher soft tissue resolution and visualization of vessels without exposing patients to radiation, it is highly suggested for children [17, 51].

38.8.5 Polysomnography

According to the American Academy of Pediatrics, the gold standard tool for diagnosing OSAS in children is overnight, attended, in-laboratory polysomnography [45, 52]. Video recording, electro-encephalogram; electrooculogram, submental and leg electromyogram, oronasal airflow; abdominal and chest wall movements; pulse oximetry, and end-tidal or transcutaneous partial pressure of carbon dioxide (PCO_2) should all be recorded during polysomnography (PSG) [1, 4, 45, 51, 52]. Despite its high cost and scheduling challenges, PSG is still the gold standard for objectively correlating ventilatory problems with sleep-disordered breathing (SBD). Other evaluation procedures, such as audiotaping, videotaping, and home PSG, have generated promising findings but need more research [46]. Abbreviated PSG (i.e., nocturnal oximetry or nap PSG) has been demonstrated to have a high positive predictive value and a low negative predictive value, indicating that patients with negative results may require further testing [46]. When polysomnography is unavailable, nocturnal pulse oximetry is a low-cost, easy-to-use diagnostic method for detecting OSAS in children with SDB symptoms. Oximetry results can facilitate treatment decisions and help predict immediate major respiratory complications postadenotonsillectomy [52].

PSG avoids unnecessary or ineffective surgery in children with primarily nonobstructive events or central apnea [43]. Before performing tonsillectomy, the clinician should refer children with sleep-disordered breathing (SDB) for PSG if they exhibit any of the following: obesity, Down syndrome, craniofacial abnormalities, neuromuscular disorders, sickle cell disease, or mucopolysaccharidoses [43]. When the need for surgery is uncertain or when there is a discrepancy between tonsillar size on physical examination and the reported severity of SDB, the doctor should advocate for PSG before tonsillectomy for SDB in children without any of the comorbidities described earlier [43]. Provide a baseline PSG for comparison after surgery. Persistent SDB or OSA, despite surgery, is more common in high-risk patients than in otherwise healthy children [43].

38.9 Treatments

38.9.1 Medical Treatment

An acute episode of tonsillitis, with or without a documented GABHS infection, usually has a self-limiting clinical course. Because viral etiologies are so common, supportive care, such as analgesics and hydration, is the basis of treatment for acute tonsillitis; patients rarely require hospitalization. NSAIDs, for example, can help with symptom relief [4].

Antibiotics are frequently used in treating patients at high risk of bacterial pharyngitis based on Centor or McIsaac criteria and antigen testing or throat culture. Patients with streptococcal pharyngotonsillitis should be treated with an antibiotic in the proper dosage for the duration required to eradicate GABHS from the pharynx once diagnosed. Inadequate administration of antibiotic therapy may result in bacterial resistance. Penicillin and amoxicillin are recommended as first-line antibiotics for those not allergic to them.

In patients allergic to penicillin, treatment for streptococcal pharyngotonsillitis should include (except for cross-reactions) a first-generation/second-generation cephalosporin for 10 days (5–6 days for a third generation) clarithromycin for 10 days, or azithromycin for 5 days, erythromycin for 5 days recommended for patients with demonstrated IgE-mediated allergy to beta-lactam. In most cases, treatment of the carrier state is not necessary [13, 15, 17, 18, 53]. Most patients, particularly adolescents and adults, are symptom-free within 48 h of receiving appropriate treatment. Except in patients with risk factors (such as a history of ARF), there is no need to do a pharyngeal swab following antibiotic medication [17]. Antibiotic-treated patients are no longer contagious after at least 24 h. It can reduce purulent complications. Immunogenic secondary diseases such as acute rheumatic fever (ARF) or acute post-streptococcal glomerulonephritis (APSGN) are potentially avoided [17]. Increased antibacterial resistance, GI distress, diarrhea, *Clostridium difficile* infection, and cost are among the risks associated with antibiotic use [17].

38.9.2 Surgery

Recurrent throat infections and obstructive sleep-disordered breathing (SDB), which can significantly impact a child's health and quality of life, are two of the most common reasons for surgery [30]. With the decline of infection as a reason for surgery in children, the prevalence of obstructive sleep-disordered breathing (oSDB) as a primary reason for surgery has risen, particularly in children under three [30, 54, 55]. Although tonsillectomy has advantages, it can also have complications, such as throat pain, postoperative nausea and vomiting, dehydration, delayed nutrition, speech problems (e.g., velopharyngeal incompetence), bleeding, and death [30, 56].

The criteria for surgical management decision-making are outlined by the American Academy of Otolaryngology, Head, and Neck Surgery and updated 2011 guidelines in 2019 for tonsillectomy [30].

1. Clinicians should recommend watchful waiting for recurrent throat infections if there have been <7 episodes in the past year, <5 episodes per year in the past 2 years, or 3 episodes per year in the past 3 years.
2. Clinicians may recommend tonsillectomy for recurrent throat infection with a frequency of at least 7 episodes in the past year, at least 5 episodes per year for 2 years, or at least 3 episodes per year for 3 years with documentation in the medical record for each episode of sore throat and >1 of the following: temperature >38.3 °C (101 °F), cervical adenopathy, tonsillar exudate, or positive test for group A beta-hemolytic streptococcus.
3. Clinicians should evaluate children with recurrent throat infections who do not fulfill the criteria for tonsillectomy, have multiple antibiotic allergies/intolerance, PFAPA, or have a history of more than one peritonsillar abscess.
4. Children with obstructive sleep-disordered breathing (SDB), should be referred for polysomnography (PSG) if they are <2 years old or have any of the following: obesity, Down syndrome, craniofacial abnormalities, neuromuscular problems, sickle cell disease, or mucopolysaccharidoses.
5. Tonsillectomy should be recommended for children who have obstructive sleep apnea (OSA), as evidenced by overnight polysomnography (PSG).
6. Children undergoing tonsillectomy should not be given or prescribed perioperative antibiotics.
7. For pain relief following tonsillectomy, doctors should prescribe ibuprofen, acetaminophen, or both. After tonsillectomy in children under 12, clinicians must not provide or prescribe codeine or any drug-containing codeine.
8. If children <3 years old or have severe obstructive sleep apnea (OSA; apnea-hypopnea index [AHI] >10 obstructive events/hour, oxygen saturation <80%, or both), clinicians should arrange for overnight hospital monitoring after tonsillectomy.
9. Children undergoing tonsillectomy should receive a single intraoperative dose of intravenous dexamethasone. They reduced postoperative nausea and vomiting (PONV) up to 24 h after tonsillectomy, shorter time to first oral intake, and less

pain, as evaluated by lower pain scores and longer latency times to painkiller administration.

Chronic tonsillitis, febrile seizures, muffled ("hot potato") speech, halitosis, malocclusion of teeth, tonsillar hypertrophy, cryptic tonsils, and chronic pharyngeal carriage of GABHS are among the poorly validated indications for tonsillectomy that have not been assessed in any controlled trials or case series. When considering tonsillectomy for one of these conditions, there is a significant role for shared decision-making with caregivers, with individualized decisions considering the severity of the illness and quality of life [30].

38.9.2.1 Tonsillotomy (Partial Tonsillectomy, Intracapsular Tonsillectomy)

Tonsillotomy is the partial intracapsular removal of tonsil tissue instead of tonsillectomy, which is the complete extracapsular removal. Tonsillotomy, partial tonsillectomy, tonsil ablation, intra-capsular tonsillectomy, radiofrequency-induced thermotherapy (RFITT) of the tonsils, and subtotal tonsillectomy are some of the terms used in the literature to describe the partial removal of tonsils. Tonsillotomy has been performed with several surgical devices, including CO_2-Laser, diathermy, radiofrequency, microdebrider, coblation, bipolar, and cold-steel tonsillectomy. Tonsillotomy is usually done under general anesthesia. However, it can also be done with local anesthesia. Tonsillotomy is mainly used in pediatric obstructive sleep apnoea syndrome (pOSAS) children and is performed under general anesthesia [57].

38.9.2.2 Tonsillectomy

The surgical removal of the palatine tonsils, known as a tonsillectomy, is one of the most common surgical procedures in the head and neck area. Tonsillectomy is a surgical operation that completely removes the tonsil, including its capsule, by dissecting the peritonsillar space between the tonsil capsule and the muscle wall, with or without adenoidectomy [30].

Tonsillotomy has shown to be as successful as tonsillectomy in treating tonsillar hypertrophy. Conversely, tonsillotomy reduces the risk of subsequent bleeding by 79%, reduces the severity of postoperative pain, and allows earlier return to regular diet and exercise [1, 57–61]. After tonsillectomy, postoperative hemorrhages were more common; tonsillotomy may lower the risk of bleeding that necessitates a hospital visit (tonsillotomy: 2/1000; tonsillectomy: 14/1000) [57, 58]. Furthermore, the changing trends from tonsillectomy to tonsillotomy reduced the need for and expense of healthcare services. Only 1.5% of patients required resurgery following tonsillotomy [59, 61].

There was no difference in postoperative discomfort and bleeding in the tonsillotomy between the microdebrider and the coblator. No substantial infection was observed despite the possibility of tonsillar remaining following tonsillotomy. Regarding sleep disturbance and quality of life, there is no benefit to utilizing tonsillotomy versus tonsillectomy [60, 61].

38.9.3 Complications of Tonsil Surgery

One of the most common operations performed by otolaryngologists is tonsillectomy. The number of complications associated with tonsillectomy has decreased dramatically due to meticulous surgical techniques and technological advances in modern anesthesiology [1].

38.9.3.1 Intraoperative Complications

Within the first 24 h, primary complications develop intraoperatively or soon after tonsillectomy. Complications from anesthesia are a significant worry. Intraoperative complications include atlantoaxial subluxation, temporomandibular joint dislocation, loose teeth dislodging, accidental extubation, or kinking of the endotracheal tube. To reduce the danger of laryngospasm and aspiration after extubation, secretions, or blood in the hypopharynx must be suctioned. One of the most severe complications of tonsillectomy is bleeding, which can happen at any time during the perioperative period. Intraoperative bleeding may be related to an underlying coagulopathy or possibly to major arterial damage in severe cases. With the use of electrocautery, intraoperative bleeding is substantially less common. Detecting underlying coagulation problems through history and physical findings, as well as preoperative screening in carefully selected individuals, can help avoid severe intraoperative blood loss. Suction cautery or ligation, or even the implantation of a pack in the tonsillar fossa and over-suturing of the tonsillar pillars to give continual compression of the fossa, are all options for controlling significant intraoperative hemorrhage. Ligating larger arteries through an open-neck exploration may be necessary in severe cases. However, this should be an extremely uncommon step [1, 56].

38.9.3.2 Postoperative Early Complications (<24 h)

Most patients have nausea, vomiting, oropharyngeal pain, or referred otalgia in the early postoperatively period. Dehydration can arise due to poorly controlled pain, intractable nausea, and vomiting, which is frequently caused by the use of narcotic painkillers. One of the most severe complications of tonsillectomy is bleeding, which can happen at any time during the perioperative period. Pulmonary edema may occur. After a long-standing upper airway obstruction, the removal of the tonsils and an increase in intrathoracic pressure can rapidly increase pulmonary hydrostatic pressure, resulting in fluid transudation into the pulmonary interstitium. Patients with a long history of obstructive sleep apnea, as demonstrated by polysomnography and cor pulmonale, should be closely monitored with pulse oximetry in a monitored setting following surgery. Patients with prolonged hypercapnia may require planned mechanical breathing after surgery until their Pco_2 levels return to normal [1, 56].

38.9.3.3 Postoperative Late Complications (>24 h–2 weeks)

Pharyngitis can occur in dehydrated patients and necessitates the use of systemic antibiotics. Atelectasis or aspiration of loose teeth, blood, or tissue can cause lung infections. The most common manifestation of postoperative bleeding is delayed hemorrhage, which occurs between days 5 and 10 after surgery due to premature eschar separation, which causes retraction of small surface arteries and the creation of an overlaying clot. If the surgeon is unsure whether active bleeding is occurring, the lump should be suctioned to allow for a more thorough examination. Blood clots can hide bleeding veins and, as a result of fibrinolysis, can inhibit proper coagulation. Patients with a blood clot in the tonsillar fossa and a delayed hemorrhage who are not actively bleeding should be admitted for at least overnight observation. It is necessary to get a coagulation profile and a hematocrit measurement [1, 56].

38.9.3.4 Postoperative Long-Term Complications (>weeks)

Eagle syndrome (ossification of the stylohyoid ligament) is a rare condition with a poorly known pathophysiologic basis for its symptoms. Patients with face pain or dysphagia may present months or years following tonsillectomy [56].

38.9.4 Immunological Effects of Tonsil Surgery

Due to the limited availability of sequential studies, these have yet to be thoroughly investigated, the fact that any immunological deficiency could have existed prior to surgery should be taken into consideration. However, there is evidence of a reduction in the number of activated B cells and a decrease in secretory IgA and other immunoglobulins, but only to the lower end of the normal range [1, 11]. The number of lymphocytes in children's tonsils is higher than in adults' tonsils, and the number of helper and cytotoxic T lymphocytes is higher in sick tonsils. Also, the persistent antigenic stimulation from infected tonsils causes increased levels of immunoglobulins throughout the pretonsillectomy interval. It was found that following tonsillectomy, the immune response was decreased and that the greater levels of immunoglobulin in the preoperative period were related to bacterial activation of lymphocytes [62].

Tonsillar lymphocytes can become so overstimulated by antigenic stimulation that they lose their ability to respond to other antigens. When this immunologic impairment develops, the tonsil can no longer provide adequate local protection or reinforce the upper respiratory tract's secretory immune system. As a result, removing recurrently sick tonsils has a therapeutic benefit [30]. Some studies, however, found minimal changes in Ig concentrations in the serum and surrounding tissues after tonsillectomy. Nonetheless, no research has shown that tonsillectomy has a significant clinical influence on the immune system [30].

After tonsillectomy and adenoidectomy, children who had previously been immunized orally with live poliovirus vaccine saw their titers decline three- to fourfold. Attempts to vaccinate seronegative children who had tonsillectomy and adenoidectomy resulted in delayed and reduced nasopharyngeal secretory immune responses, as evaluated by poliovirus IgA antibodies [1, 11].

38.10 Conclusion

Understanding the anatomy, embryology, and physiology of tonsils is crucial for diagnosing and treating diseases of this area. The physician must be familiar with and capable of analyzing a variety of infections that can be found. Once pharyngitis and tonsillar diseases have been diagnosed, the physician must know the treatment choices and potential complications. The critical component of proper tonsillar disease treatment is a complete history and physical examination. Tonsillectomy has been done using a variety of methods. The surgeon must be familiar with all of the surgical options available. Whatever procedure is used, it is critical to use meticulous surgical skills and to be mindful of potential complications. The surgeon must not only be able to deal with probable difficulties but also know how to avoid them.

References

1. Shirley WP, Wiatrak BJ, Woolley AL. Pharyngitis and adenotonsillar disease. In: Cummings CW, editor. Otolaryngology—Head and neck surgery. 5th ed. Philadelphia: Mosby, Inc.; 2010. p. 2782–811.
2. Perry M, Whyte A. Immunology of the tonsils. Immunol Today. 1998;19(9):414–21. https://doi.org/10.1016/s0167-5699(98)01307-3.
3. Meegalla N, Downs BW. Anatomy, head and neck, palatine tonsil (Faucial tonsils). In: StatPearls. StatPearls Publishing; 2020.
4. Brodsky L, Poje C. Tonsillitis, tonsillectomy, and adenoidectomy. In: Bailey BJ, Johnson JT, Newlands SD, editors. Head and neck surgery—otolaryngology. 4th ed. Philadelphia: Lippincott Williams & Wilkins; 2006. p. 1183–95.
5. Regauer S. Chapter 6. Nasopharynx and Waldeyer's ring. In: Cardesa A, Slootweg PJ, editors. Pathology of the head & neck. New York: Springer; 2006. p. 183–9.
6. Açar G. Surgical anatomy of the tonsils. In: Sridharan G, editor. Oral and maxillofacial surgery. IntechOpen; 2020. https://doi.org/10.5772/intechopen.93038. https://www.intechopen.com/books/oral-and-maxillofacial-surgery/surgical-anatomy-of-the-tonsils.
7. Nave H, Gebert A, Pabst R. Morphology and immunology of the human palatine tonsil. Anat Embryol. 2001;204(5):367–73. https://doi.org/10.1007/s004290100210.
8. von Gaudecker B, Müller-Hermelink HK. The development of the human tonsilla palatina. Cell Tissue Res. 1982;224(3):579–600. https://doi.org/10.1007/BF00213754.
9. Noussios G, Xanthopoulos J, Zaraboukas T, Vital V, Konstantinidis I. Morphological study of development and functional activity of palatine tonsils in embryonic age. Acta Otorhinolaryngol Ital. 2003;23(2):98–101.
10. Siegel G, Linse R, Macheleidt S. Factors of tonsillar involution: age-dependent changes in B-cell activation and Langerhans' cell density. Arch Otorhinolaryngol. 1982;236(3):261–9. https://doi.org/10.1007/BF00454218.
11. Scadding GK. Immunology of the tonsil: a review. J R Soc Med. 1990;83(2):104–7. https://doi.org/10.1177/014107689008300216.
12. Brandtzaeg P, Baekkevold ES, Farstad IN, Jahnsen FL, Johansen FE, Nilsen EM, Yamanaka T. Regional specialization in the mucosal immune system: what happens in the microcompartments? Immunol Today. 1999;20(3):141–51. https://doi.org/10.1016/s0167-5699(98)01413-3.
13. Sidell D, Shapiro NL. Acute tonsillitis. Infect Disord Drug Targets. 2012;12(4):271–6. https://doi.org/10.2174/187152612801319230.
14. Rullan E, Sigal LH. Rheumatic fever. Curr Rheumatol Rep. 2001;3(5):445–52. https://doi.org/10.1007/s11926-996-0016-4.

15. Guidelines for the diagnosis of rheumatic fever. Jones criteria, 1992 update. Special Writing Group of the Committee on Rheumatic Fever, Endocarditis, and Kawasaki Disease of the Council on Cardiovascular Disease in the Young of the American Heart Association. JAMA.1992;268(15):2069–2073.
16. Kobayashi R, Takeuchi H, Sasaki M, Hasegawa M, Hirai K. Detection of Epstein-Barr virus infection in the epithelial cells and lymphocytes of non-neoplastic tonsils by in situ hybridization and in situ PCR. Arch Virol. 1998;143(4):803–13. https://doi.org/10.1007/s007050050332.
17. Windfuhr JP, Toepfner N, Steffen G, Waldfahrer F, Berner R. Clinical practice guideline: tonsillitis I. Diagnostics and nonsurgical management. Eur Arch Otorhinolaryngol. 2016;273(4):973–87. https://doi.org/10.1007/s00405-015-3872-6.
18. Di Muzio F, Barucco M, Guerriero F. Diagnosis and treatment of acute pharyngitis/tonsillitis: a preliminary observational study in general medicine. Eur Rev Med Pharmacol Sci. 2016;20(23):4950–4.
19. Weinstein L. Diseases of the tonsils and adenoids in adults. Ann Otol Rhinol Laryngol. 1975;84(2 Pt2 Suppl 19):34–6. https://doi.org/10.1177/00034894750840S208.
20. Tagliareni JM, Clarkson EI. Tonsillitis, peritonsillar and lateral pharyngeal abscesses. Oral Maxillofac Surg Clin North Am. 2012;24(2):197, viii. https://doi.org/10.1016/j.coms.2012.01.014.
21. Johnson BC, Alvi A. Cost-effective workup for tonsillitis. Testing, treatment, and potential complications. Postgrad Med. 2003;113(3):115–21. https://doi.org/10.3810/pgm.2003.03.1391.
22. Klug TE. Peritonsillar abscess: clinical aspects of microbiology, risk factors, and the association with parapharyngeal abscess. Dan Med J. 2017;64(3):B5333.
23. Childs EW, Baugh RF, Diaz JA. Tonsillar abscess. J Natl Med Assoc. 1991;83(4):333–6.
24. Karkos PD, Asrani S, Karkos CD, Leong SC, Theochari EG, Alexopoulou TD, Assimakopoulos AD. Lemierre's syndrome: a systematic review. Laryngoscope. 2009;119(8):1552–9. https://doi.org/10.1002/lary.20542.
25. Anderson J, Paterek E. Tonsillitis. In: StatPearls. StatPearls Publishing; 2020.
26. Bell Z, Menezes AA, Primrose WJ, et al. Mediastinitis: a life-threatening complication of acute tonsillitis. J Laryngol Otol. 2005;119:743–5.
27. Ridgway JM, Parikh DA, Wright R, Holden P, Armstrong W, Camilon F, Wong BJ. Lemierre syndrome: a pediatric case series and review of literature. Am J Otolaryngol. 2010;31(1):38–45. https://doi.org/10.1016/j.amjoto.2008.09.006.
28. Church AJ, Dale RC, Giovannoni G. Anti-basal ganglia antibodies: a possible diagnostic utility in idiopathic movement disorders? Arch Dis Child. 2004;89(7):611–4. https://doi.org/10.1136/adc.2003.031880.
29. Sanchez-Carpintero R, Albesa SA, Crespo N, Villoslada P, Narbona J. A preliminary study of the frequency of anti-basal ganglia antibodies and streptococcal infection in attention deficit/hyperactivity disorder. J Neurol. 2009;256(7):1103–8. https://doi.org/10.1007/s00415-009-5076-8.
30. Guideline.
31. Pavone P, Rapisarda V, Serra A, Nicita F, Spalice A, Parano E, Rizzo R, Maiolino L, Di Mauro P, Vitaliti G, Coco A, Falsaperla R, Trifiletti RR, Cocuzza S. Pediatric autoimmune neuropsychiatric disorder associated with group a streptococcal infection: the role of surgical treatment. Int J Immunopathol Pharmacol. 2014;27(3):371–8. https://doi.org/10.1177/039463201402700307.
32. Cochard M, Clet J, Le L, Pillet P, Onrubia X, Guéron T, Faouzi M, Hofer M. PFAPA syndrome is not a sporadic disease. Rheumatology (Oxford). 2010;49(10):1984–7. https://doi.org/10.1093/rheumatology/keq187.
33. Adachi M, Watanabe A, Nishiyama A, Oyazato Y, Kamioka I, Murase M, Ishida A, Sakai H, Nishikomori R, Heike T. Familial cases of periodic fever with aphthous stomatitis, pharyngitis, and cervical adenitis syndrome. J Pediatr. 2011;158(1):155–9. https://doi.org/10.1016/j.jpeds.2010.09.054.
34. Harabuchi Y, Takahara M. Pathogenic role of palatine tonsils in palmoplantar pustulosis: a review. J Dermatol. 2019;46(11):931–9. https://doi.org/10.1111/1346-8138.15100.

35. Wu W, Debbaneh M, Moslehi H, Koo J, Liao W. Tonsillectomy as a treatment for psoriasis: a review. J Dermatolog Treat. 2014;25(6):482–6. https://doi.org/10.3109/09546634.2013.848258.
36. Yamashita K, Ichimiya S, Kamekura R, Nagaya T, Jitsukawa S, Matsumiya H, Takano K, Himi T. Studies of tonsils in basic and clinical perspectives: from the past to the future. Adv Otorhinolaryngol. 2016;77:119–24. https://doi.org/10.1159/000441902.
37. Ito S, Misaki T, Naka S, Wato K, Nagasawa Y, Nomura R, Otsugu M, Matsumoto-Nakano M, Nakano K, Kumagai H, Oshima N. Specific strains of Streptococcus mutans, a pathogen of dental caries, in the tonsils, are associated with IgA nephropathy. Sci Rep. 2019;9(1):20130. https://doi.org/10.1038/s41598-019-56679-2.
38. Béné MC, Hurault de Ligny B, Kessler M, Foliguet B, Faure GC. Tonsils in IgA nephropathy. Contrib Nephrol. 1993;104:153–61. https://doi.org/10.1159/000422408.
39. Hotta O, Miyazaki M, Furuta T, Tomioka S, Chiba S, Horigome I, Abe K, Taguma Y. Tonsillectomy and steroid pulse therapy significantly impact on clinical remission in patients with IgA nephropathy. Am J Kidney Dis. 2001;38(4):736–43. https://doi.org/10.1053/ajkd.2001.27690.
40. Silva J, Almeida E, Sousa JC, Reis L, Sousa JB, Etchebehere RM. Tonsillar hyperplasia and recurrent acute tonsillitis in children: immunohistochemical evaluation of the lymphatic tissue. Int J Pediatr Otorhinolaryngol. 2019;121:15–9. https://doi.org/10.1016/j.ijporl.2019.02.032.
41. Chiappini E, Regoli M, Bonsignori F, Sollai S, Parretti A, Galli L, de Martino M. Analysis of different recommendations from international guidelines for the management of acute pharyngitis in adults and children. Clin Ther. 2011;33(1):48–58. https://doi.org/10.1016/j.clinthera.2011.02.001.
42. Deutsch ES, Isaacson GC. Tonsils and adenoids: an update. Pediatr Rev. 1995;16(1):17–21. https://doi.org/10.1542/pir.16-1-17.
43. Roland PS, Rosenfeld RM, Brooks LJ, Friedman NR, Jones J, Kim TW, Kuhar S, Mitchell RB, Seidman MD, Sheldon SH, Jones S, Robertson P, American Academy of Otolaryngology—Head and Neck Surgery Foundation. Clinical practice guideline: polysomnography for sleep-disordered breathing prior to tonsillectomy in children. Otolaryngol Head Neck Surg. 2011;145(1 Suppl):S1–S15. https://doi.org/10.1177/0194599811409837.
44. Mitchell RB, Pereira KD, Friedman NR. Sleep-disordered breathing in children: survey of current practice. Laryngoscope. 2006;116(6):956–8. https://doi.org/10.1097/01.MLG.0000216413.22408.FD.
45. Marcus CL, Brooks LJ, Draper KA, Gozal D, Halbower AC, Jones J, Schechter MS, Sheldon SH, Spruyt K, Ward SD, Lehmann C, Shiffman RN, American Academy of Pediatrics. Diagnosis and management of childhood obstructive sleep apnea syndrome. Pediatrics. 2012;130(3):576–84. https://doi.org/10.1542/peds.2012-1671. Epub 2012 Aug 27. PMID: 22926173.
46. Darrow DH, Siemens C. Indications for tonsillectomy and adenoidectomy. Laryngoscope. 2002;112(8 Pt 2 Suppl 100):6–10. https://doi.org/10.1002/lary.5541121404.
47. Ferguson M, Aydin M, Mickel J. Halitosis and the tonsils: a review of management. Otolaryngol Head Neck Surg. 2014;151(4):567–74. https://doi.org/10.1177/0194599814544881.
48. McIsaac WJ, Kellner JD, Aufricht P, Vanjaka A, Low DE. Empirical validation of guidelines for the management of pharyngitis in children and adults. JAMA. 2004;291(13):1587–95. https://doi.org/10.1001/jama.291.13.1587.
49. Kurtz B, Kurtz M, Roe M, Todd J. Importance of inoculum size and sampling effect in rapid antigen detection for diagnosis of Streptococcus pyogenes pharyngitis. J Clin Microbiol. 2000;38(1):279–81.
50. Johnson DR, Kurlan R, Leckman J, Kaplan EL. The human immune response to streptococcal extracellular antigens: clinical, diagnostic, and potential pathogenetic implications. Clin Infect Dis. 2010;50(4):481–90. https://doi.org/10.1086/650167.
51. Gross CW, Harrison SE. Tonsils and adenoids. Pediatr Rev. 2000;21(3):75–8. https://doi.org/10.1542/pir.21-3-75.

52. Kaditis A, Kheirandish-Gozal L, Gozal D. Pediatric OSAS: oximetry can provide answers when polysomnography is not available. Sleep Med Rev. 2016;27:96–105. https://doi.org/10.1016/j.smrv.2015.05.008.
53. Pichichero ME, Casey JR. Bacterial eradication rates with shortened courses of 2nd- and 3rd-generation cephalosporins versus 10 days of penicillin for treatment of group A streptococcal tonsillopharyngitis in adults. Diagn Microbiol Infect Dis. 2007;59(2):127–30. https://doi.org/10.1016/j.diagmicrobio.2007.04.010.
54. Parker NP, Walner DL. Trends in the indications for pediatric tonsillectomy or adenotonsillectomy. Int J Pediatr Otorhinolaryngol. 2011;75(2):282–5. https://doi.org/10.1016/j.ijporl.2010.11.019.
55. Erickson BK, Larson DR, St Sauver JL, Meverden RA, Orvidas LJ. Changes in incidence and indications of tonsillectomy and adenotonsillectomy, 1970-2005. Otolaryngol Head Neck Surg. 2009;140(6):894–901. https://doi.org/10.1016/j.otohns.2009.01.044.
56. Johnson LB, Elluru RG, Myer CM 3rd. Complications of adenotonsillectomy. Laryngoscope. 2002;112(8 Pt 2 Suppl 100):35–6. https://doi.org/10.1002/lary.5541121413.
57. Wong Chung J, van Benthem P, Blom HM. Tonsillotomy versus tonsillectomy in adults suffering from tonsil-related afflictions: a systematic review. Acta Otolaryngol. 2018;138(5):492–501. https://doi.org/10.1080/00016489.2017.1412500.
58. Zhang LY, Zhong L, David M, Cervin A. Tonsillectomy or tonsillotomy? A systematic review for paediatric sleep-disordered breathing. Int J Pediatr Otorhinolaryngol. 2017;103:41–50. https://doi.org/10.1016/j.ijporl.2017.10.008.
59. Sakki A, Mäkinen LK, Roine RP, Nokso-Koivisto J. Changing trends in pediatric tonsil surgery. Int J Pediatr Otorhinolaryngol. 2019;118:84–9. https://doi.org/10.1016/j.ijporl.2018.12.028.
60. Kim JS, Kwon SH, Lee EJ, Yoon YJ. Can intracapsular tonsillectomy be an alternative to classical tonsillectomy? A meta-analysis. Otolaryngol Head Neck Surg. 2017;157(2):178–89. https://doi.org/10.1177/0194599817700374.
61. Acevedo JL, Shah RK, Brietzke SE. Systematic review of complications of tonsillotomy versus tonsillectomy. Otolaryngol Head Neck Surg. 2012;146(6):871–9. https://doi.org/10.1177/0194599812439017.
62. Kaygusuz I, Alpay HC, Gödekmerdan A, Karlidag T, Keles E, Yalcin S, Demir N. Evaluation of long-term impacts of tonsillectomy on immune functions of children: a follow-up study. Int J Pediatr Otorhinolaryngol. 2009;73(3):445–9. https://doi.org/10.1016/j.ijporl.2008.11.014.

Overview of Pediatric Rhinosinusitis

39

Oben Yıldırım and Yusuf Dundar

39.1 Introduction

The nasal cavity and paranasal sinuses are lined with the same mucosa and are affected by the same factors because they are continuous with each other. For this reason, the term rhinosinusitis is used rather than rhinitis or sinusitis.

Inflammation of the sinus and nasal mucosa characterizes rhinosinusitis, a frequent condition. Acute rhinosinusitis lasts less than a month, subacute lasts between 1 and 3 months, and chronicities lasts more than 3 months [1].

Adult guidelines recommend considering a diagnosis of acute rhinosinusitis when one or more of the following symptoms are present: facial pain, facial pressure, facial congestion, hyposmia or anosmia, nasal congestion, nasal discharge, purulence or discolored postnasal discharge, and fever. Similar recommendations have been made for kids with acute sinusitis [2]. The preceding symptoms of acute rhinosinusitis persisting for more than 3 months despite routine medical care (antibiotics, steroids, saline nasal rinses, and nasal sprays) are diagnostic criteria for children's chronic rhinosinusitis (CRS). At least two of the following symptoms are required for a diagnosis of CRS, as outlined in the most recent clinical consensus statement [3]: nasal obstruction, purulent rhinorrhea, cough, facial pressure or pain, purulent drainage, endoscopic or CT scan findings consistent with the diagnosis, mucosal edema, or nasal polyposis.

O. Yıldırım (✉)
Private ENT Clinic, İzmir, Turkey

Y. Dundar
Department of Otolaryngology—Head and Neck Surgery, Texas Tech University, Health Sciences Center, Lubbock, TX, USA

H. Yüksel et al. (eds.), *Pediatric Airway Diseases*, Comprehensive ENT,
https://doi.org/10.1007/978-3-031-74853-0_39

39.2 Embryology and Anatomy

It is necessary to have a good grasp of the anatomy and development of the paranasal sinus to understand the effect of rhinosinusitis in children, interpret radiological examinations, plan surgical intervention if necessary, and avoid complications during surgical interventions. Since structures such as turbinates, uncinate process, infundibulum, and hiatus semilunaris are developed during the newborn period, there is no significant change in the form of the osteomeatal complex after birth. Maxillary sinuses appear in the ethmoid section of the lateral nasal wall in the third month of fetal life. The development of this cell progresses slowly throughout fetal life, and at birth, the dimensions of the maxillary sinus are approximately 10 × 4 × 3 mm, and it is located medial to the orbit. They show two periods of rapid development in the first 3 years of life and between the ages of 7 and 12. They change little after the age of 12. The anterior and middle ethmoid sinuses appear as protrusions on the lateral nasal wall in the third month of gestation. Posterior ethmoid cells are 4–5 in the upper meatus. It occurs in months. The front and the posterior ethmoids are complete in number at birth but small in size, and there is plenty of connective tissue. The ethmoid sinuses continue to develop after birth and reach adult size between the ages of 8–12. Frontal sinuses are formed by the progression of anterior ethmoid cells towards the frontal bone. They are not apparent at birth. They begin to expand at age 4, and their development continues until age 20. The sphenoid sinuses emerge from the posterior nasal capsule by pocketing in the fourth month of gestation. The sphenoid sinus is filled with red marrow and is not ventilated, but its ostium may be present [4, 5]. They start growing from age 3 and reach adulthood between 7 and 12.

39.3 Etiopathogenesis

Mucus-producing goblet cells and pseudostratified ciliated columnar epithelium line the sinuses, air-filled pockets within the facial bones. The presence of cilia in the sinuses aids in the removal of secretions. The osteomeatal complex (OMC) is the passageway that links most sinuses to the middle meatus. This includes the frontal, anterior ethmoidal, and maxillary sinuses. Sinusitis in children frequently begins with obstruction of the OMC because the resulting negative pressure in the sinuses encourages mucus production and retention, which can then progress to infections [6].

In children, CRS can be triggered by various risk factors.

Children with frequent URTIs have a relatively immature immune system compared to adults. They are more likely to be affected by allergic rhinitis, adenoid hypertrophy, and bacterial colonization in the nasopharynx. Gastroesophageal reflux is also common in children with rhinosinusitis. Foreign body, cystic fibrosis, and immotile cilia syndromes may also lead to rhinosinusitis.

CRS may also be caused, at least in part, by enlarged adenoids, according to many studies [7–11]. In one research, children with CRS were shown to have more oversized adenoids compared to children with obstructive sleep apnea. It has been hypothesized that enlarged adenoids might impede the sinonasal airways and serve as a breeding ground for bacteria [12, 13]. These findings bolstered the utility of adenoidectomy as an early therapeutic option for children with CRS [14, 15].

The high prevalence of viral infections in kids is clearly to blame.

Inflammation caused by viral infections and allergic rhinitis causes mucosal destruction and impairs ciliary function, leading to secretion stasis and condition of the relevant sinus. Children generally average 3–8 viral infections each year, which subjects them to an increased risk of developing acute bacterial sinusitis [16]. The frequency of rhinosinusitis also increases in autumn and winter, when viral upper respiratory tract infections increase [17].

There needs to be more consensus on whether or not allergic sensitization plays a significant role in the onset of CRS, both in children and in adults. Some research has shown a link, whereas others have found no link [3]. Allergic rhinitis was revealed to be the most prevalent comorbidity among a large group of 4044 pediatric patients with CRS [18]. The hypothesis of an "allergic dose-response" leading to CRS was disproved in another research by the same group, which found that patients with allergic rhinitis who developed later CRS did not have more severe allergic rhinitis [19]. Current research suggests that allergy sensitization may play a role in the onset of CRS, particularly in older children [3, 20]. Considering the OMC's part in CRS development, it becomes apparent that IgE-mediated mast cell degranulation can cause nasal mucosal edema and that the presence of eosinophils in the noses of people with allergic rhinitis might impair mucociliary clearance [21–23]. Therefore, the authors believe all children with CRS should have allergy sensitivities evaluated.

In addition, some anatomical problems also play a role in etiology. These include turbinate bullosa, paradoxical middle turbinate presence, hypoplastic sinuses, infraorbital (Haller) cells, and nasal septum deviation.

Diseases such as cleft palate-lip, Down syndrome, and choanal atresia also increase the frequency of rhinosinusitis.

The foreign body in the nose is a common problem in children. It is manifested by unilateral, foul-smelling discharge and may obstruct the sinus ostium, resulting in rhinosinusitis.

Local predisposing factors may include allergic rhinitis, upper respiratory infections, anatomic abnormalities such as a deviated septum, concha bullosa, enlarged adenoids, nasal polyps, and tumors [1].

Systemic predisposing factors may be listed as immune deficiency, such as IgA deficiency, pan hypo-gammaglobulinemia, IgG subclass deficiency, and HIV, cystic fibrosis, and ciliary disorders [1].

Gastroesophageal reflux (GER) is another influential factor in the development of otitis and rhinosinusitis. It should be considered in children with chronic nasal discharge and congestion, hoarseness, and stridor who do not show adequate improvement despite optimal medical or surgical treatment. Endoscopic examination is essential in these patients. Diagnosis can be made by 24-h pH monitoring.

CRS can occur in children due to disorders that hinder ciliary motility. The most prevalent disease seen in these patients is cystic fibrosis (CF), which has been linked to CRS with nasal polyps (NP). Virtually, all people with CF will develop CRS at some point [24–28]. However, CF's total contribution to the prevalence of CRS is modest [1, 29] due to the disease's rarity. In the setting of poor weight growth, respiratory illness, and gastrointestinal abnormalities, doctors treating children with polyps and sinus disease should have a high index of suspicion for CF.

Primary ciliary dyskinesia (PCD), also known as Kartagener's syndrome, is a condition that causes defective mucociliary clearance. PCD, an autosomal recessive disorder, causes inefficient and disorganized ciliary movement. Frequent sinus and ear infections, infertility in 50% of males diagnosed, and heterotaxy or situs ambiguus in 12% of those diagnosed are all related to this condition [30]. Older children diagnosed with PCD had acute and CRS at the time of diagnosis between 11 and 71% of the time [31–33].

39.4 Microbiology

The number of studies investigating pediatric rhinosinusitis microbiology could be much higher because it is difficult to reach the paranasal sinuses in children and obtain aspirate from the sinus contents for culture. Although viruses cannot be overproduced in cultures obtained from sinus aspirates, they facilitate bacterial infections by disrupting the mucosal structure and ciliary function. The causative bacteria in acute sinusitis are the same as those in the etiology of otitis media: Streptococcus pneumoniae, Moraxella catarrhalis, and Haemophilus influenza. Anaerobic bacteria also play a role in infection. In chronic rhinosinusitis, the causative bacteria are similar, but staphylococci and alpha-hemolytic streptococci are more common among aerobes, and streptococci, peptostreptococci, and Bacteroides strains are more common among anaerobes. In patients with cystic fibrosis, pseudomonas aeruginosa, Haemophilus influenza, and alpha-hemolytic streptococci are frequently encountered as causative agents. Fungal sinusitis is more common in patients with immunodeficiency.

39.5 Symptoms and Signs

Multiple indicators are used to diagnose acute bacterial rhinosinusitis in a child. A severe onset of symptoms such as fever or purulent nasal discharge lasting more than three consecutive days associated with facial tenderness or headache [34] or recurrence of symptoms after initial improvement: fever, worsening cough, or worsening or new purulent rhinorrhea. Pathogens such as Streptococcus pneumonia, Influenza A virus, and Moraxella catarrhalis are frequently associated with ABRS. In children, ABRS can develop from 5 to 10% of viral upper respiratory tract infections [3, 35], and many cases of ABRS lead to chronic rhinosinusitis. Since viral rhinosinusitis shares many of ABRS's clinical and radiological hallmarks, distinguishing between the two can be challenging.

According to the IDSA recommendations, the following clinical presentations qualify as indicators of ABRS:

1. Upper respiratory infection (URI) symptoms that have persisted for more than 10 days;
2. High-grade fever (>39 °C), face discomfort, or purulent nasal discharge that has been present for longer than 3–4 days;
3. "Double-sickening" occurs when symptoms, such as a fresh beginning of fever, headache, or rise in nasal discharge, appear 3 days after a normal viral URI that lasted 5–6 days and were initially recovering.

The relationship between the cause of cough and rhinosinusitis is not very clear. The first hypothesis on this subject is that nasal secretions cause airway irritation. The second hypothesis is that a reflex arc thought to exist between the paranasal sinuses and bronchi causes cough [36].

Headache and fever are the most prominent symptoms of acute rhinosinusitis.

Nasal congestion is evident in chronic rhinosinusitis. Mouth breathing, bad breath, postnasal discharge, and accompanying ear problems (such as serous otitis media) may occur.

39.6 Medical and Surgical Management of Pediatric Rhinosinusitis

Acute and chronic rhinosinusitis are often treated with medical therapy. Most people get well only from receiving medical care. The typical course of treatment for acute sinusitis is 10–14 days. If symptoms are not improving, it may be time to switch antibiotics or commit to a longer course of therapy. Treatment for chronic rhinosinusitis often takes 3–4 weeks.

Reducing inflammation, enhancing drainage, and eliminating infections are the first medical aims in treating juvenile CRS [20]. Antibiotics, nasal irrigation, topical and possible oral steroids, and allergen immunotherapy in the right setting are all necessary to achieve this goal.

When medication treatment fails, procedures such as balloon sinuplasty, adenoidectomy, endoscopic sinus surgery, open surgical methods, and turbinate reduction may be performed [35]. Sinonasal aeration and drainage are improved, and potential bacterial reservoirs are eliminated with these treatments [18].

39.6.1 Medical Treatment

The use of antibiotics is crucial to the healing process. If you have a common infection, your doctor may recommend an antibiotic as a precaution. Streptococcus pneumonia, Hemophilus influenzae, Moraxella catarrhalis, and beta-hemolytic Streptococcus pyogenes are some of the most prevalent bacterial infections in children [37–39]. When conventional antibiotics fail to work, it may be time to switch to a more targeted approach based on a patient's culture [37].

Patients with penicillin allergies have other options, including clindamycin, azithromycin, clarithromycin, and erythromycin. However, amoxicillin at a high dosage (90 mg/kg) is an effective first-line oral drug for empiric treatment in pediatric CRS [37].

Adding clavulanic acid to amoxicillin gives an advantage over amoxicillin alone since the number of cases caused by Haemophilus influenza is likely growing, and the rate of B-lactamase generation by this organism is probably increasing.

Although cephalosporins like cefpodoxime, cefdinir, and cefuroxime are less effective against S pneumonia than amoxicillin-clavulanate, they are still viable alternatives.

Cefixime (or cefdinir) and linezolid may be used as an alternative to parenteral antimicrobial medicines in children who do not respond to amoxicillin-clavulanate or second or third-generation cephalosporins. Patients allergic to or intolerant to beta-lactam antibiotics can take doxycycline or a respiratory fluoroquinolone (levofloxacin or moxifloxacin).

Children with sinusitis who comply with treatment with an effective antimicrobial medication show a quick response to treatment. Symptoms (such as fever, cough, and discharge) often subside after 48 h. Clinical reevaluation is necessary [32] if symptoms increase within 72 h or do not improve within 3–5 days. A second-line antibiotic should be provided if the diagnosis is not modified. Sinus aspiration is another option that can help pinpoint the offending microorganism.

The duration of antimicrobial treatment has yet to be examined extensively. In most cases, 10 days of medication is sufficient for children who quickly respond to the commencement of antimicrobial treatment. Treatment should continue until the patient is symptom-free, an extra 7 days for those who respond more slowly [38].

Nasal saline irrigation is a standard treatment for CRS [3, 40] because it is efficient, safe, and well-tolerated. In children with CRS, saline irrigation of the nasal passages is a viable therapy option. Because sinus rinses clear the nasal and sinus mucosa of debris and mucus, using topical steroids in conjunction with them can be adequate. Overall, this treatment has been shown to lessen the need for sinus operations and boost the health and happiness of people with CRS [41].

Treatment of pediatric CRS might include intranasal steroids alone or in conjunction with other therapies. They are routinely part of the first round of medical treatment [42]. When intranasal steroid sprays are used with oral antibiotics in pediatric CRS, symptoms, such as cough and postnasal drainage, are alleviated, and mucosal inflammation is reduced [14, 29, 43].

Oral steroids have been debated as a viable therapeutic option for CRS, with some researchers finding that they benefit individuals who will soon undergo surgery [42]. When polyps are removed surgically (also called a medical polypectomy), oral steroids are often prescribed for use after surgery to reduce the high risk of recurrence [20, 29].

Because of the severe risks of long-term use, especially in children, oral steroids should be administered cautiously and only when necessary.

It is essential to teach children diagnosed with allergies to avoid their allergens. Patients with well-described environmental allergies may also benefit from allergen immunotherapy (IT). While there is evidence for the effectiveness of immunotherapy in treating allergic rhinitis, this is not the case for people with CRS.

39.6.2 Surgical Treatment

However, surgery may be necessary in cases of complications, medical therapy failure, or when anatomic anomalies are detected in people with CRS [35].

Sinus surgeries to treat sinusitis may be broken down into indirect and direct categories. Indirect sinus operations are procedures outside the sinuses that aim to improve sinus function. Septorhinoplasty and adenoidectomy are examples of indirect procedures. Interventions involving the sinuses are included in direct sinus surgery.

Children of any size who suffer from CRS benefit from having their adenoids removed since they serve as a bacterial reservoir [44, 45]. While adenoidectomy is a successful first surgical therapy for children under 6, its effectiveness declines between 6 and 12. However, the panel could not agree on a course of action for pediatric patients aged 13 and up [3]. Treatment of PCRS with tonsillectomy alone (without adenoidectomy) is unsuccessful [3].

Antral lavage was used for diagnosis and treatment and was popular in the 1970s. Its diagnostic use is limited to the maxillary sinus. It is not a very suitable approach in children due to the small size of the maxillary sinus, the necessity of general anesthesia, and the lack of intervention for the disease in the ethmoid sinuses. Its effect on chronic rhinosinusitis has not been proven [36].

Since the effect of antral lavage was short-lived, permanent antrostomy or opening a nasal antral window at the lower meatus was used as an alternative surgical treatment in patients requiring continuous antral lavage. However, inferior meatal antrostomy (nasal antral window) is an abandoned technique today because it generally tends to close on its own, cannot be opened large enough in children, and ciliary activity is directed towards the natural ostium and secretions is not directed towards the newly opened window.

It is recommended that the Caldwell-Luc technique not be used in young children unless necessary due to the risk of damaging permanent teeth and affecting tooth development.

With the development of technology and surgical instruments, the popularity of functional endoscopic sinus surgery (FESS) in treating pediatric rhinosinusitis has increased. FESS is a surgery with a high risk of complications in pediatric patients due to the small size of the nasal cavity, the proximity of the lateral nasal wall to the orbit, and the short distance to the anterior cranial fossa. However, today, effective results can be achieved by using appropriate techniques. Since the sinuses and faces in children are in the process of growth, a conservative approach should be taken as much as possible. Chronic sinusitis in children most commonly affects the anterior ethmoids and maxillary sinuses. For this reason, in most cases, a limited surgery involving only the ethmoid and maxillary sinuses is sufficient. Approximately less than 10% of children with chronic rhinosinusitis require opening of the sphenoid sinus [46]. However, in cases of massive polyposis in patients with cystic fibrosis, wide sphenoethmoidectomy may be required.

39.7 Complications

Sinusitis complications
Orbital
Preseptal cellulitis
Orbital cellulite
Subperiastal abscess
Orbital abscess
Cavernous sinus thrombosis
Intracranial
Meningitis and encephalitis
Epidural abscess
Subdural abscess
Brain abscess

39.7.1 Orbital Complications

Orbital complications generally develop after acute sinusitis. The infection spreads to the adjacent orbit and cranial cavity.

Limited preseptal inflammation seen in the eyelid in rhinosinusitis is a benign event. When the inflammation extends beyond the septum, which is the continuation of the orbital periosteum forward into the eyelid tissues, the condition becomes severe and requires urgent treatment. Openings in the lamina paprisea and valveless orbital veins predispose to this spread of inflammation and ultimately orbital complications.

The classification made by Chandler et al. regarding orbital complications is the most accepted.

1. Preseptal cellulitis: There is inflammatory edema and venous drainage obstruction in the eyelids (preseptal region). There is no loss of vision or restriction of eye movements.
2. Orbital cellulitis: Diffuse edema of adipose tissue in the orbit and orbital cellulitis secondary to bacterial infection or inflammation. There is no abscess formation yet.
3. Subperiosteal abscess is the formation of an abscess between the orbital periosteum and the bony orbital wall. The resulting abscess pushes the eyeball. The resulting proptosis may cause impairment in eye movements and visual acuity.

4. Orbital abscess: There is an abscess limited to the orbit. Advanced proptosis is observed. There is complete ophthalmoplegia. It results in approximately 10–15% vision loss.
5. Cavernous sinus thrombosis: Infection of the paranasal sinuses or orbit can spread to the cavernous sinus due to the absence of valves in the orbital veins. Even if diagnosed early, it can progress rapidly to vision loss, meningitis, and even death.

If the infection originates from the sinuses, possible factors are S. pneumoniae, H. influenza, M. catarrhalis, and S. pyogenes, which also cause acute sinusitis. Staphylococcus aureus is more common in chronic infections and older children.

Treatment of these complications requires collaboration of more than one branch. Medical treatment begins with IV antibiotics that cross the blood-brain barrier to prevent intracranial infection. Fever, visual acuity, and eye movements should be monitored closely. If there is no improvement within 24–48 h and the clinic worsens, CT should be performed to detect possible abscess. If an abscess is seen, it is drained.

Progressive vision loss is a condition that requires rapid diagnosis and treatment. Vision loss may be secondary to direct optic nerve compression or neuritis. When the abscess is drained in time, vision loss returns.

Urgent CT and contrast-enhanced MRI are indicated if cavernous sinus thrombosis or intracranial complications are suspected. If the cavernous sinus is thrombosed, a decrease in contrast enhancement is seen on that side on CT. In this case, exophthalmos, chemosis, ophthalmoplegia, vision loss, and pain occur in the opposite eye of the patient with a toxic appearance, previously having complaints in one eye. This situation is explained by the infection passing to the opposite side through the intercavernous sinus. Involvement of the third, fourth, fifth (ophthalmic and maxillary branches), and sixth cranial nerves may be seen. It is the most severe form of orbital complications. It is a complication with a risk of mortality. Aggressive IV antibiotic therapy should be designed to cover gram-positive cocci and gram-negative bacilli.

In addition to the Chandler classification, there are additional problems that may develop during the course of orbital complications.

Mucocele formation is considered among the complications of chronic sinusitis. Cysts of the paranasal sinuses according to their pathogenesis: It is divided into three types: retention cyst, mucocele, and antral pseudocyst, and the most common among them is retention cysts. Sinus mucoceles, unlike other mucoceles, are surrounded by epithelium and have thick, well-developed cyst epithelium. Although they are benign, when they reach large sizes, they can cause bone destruction by putting pressure on the surrounding bone tissue. This feature is the most important difference between them and retention cysts. If not infected, clear watery fluid containing mucoid material may be aspirated.

Carotid artery occlusion is a serious complication that may develop after cavernous sinus thrombosis.

Skull osteomyelitis is a rapidly spreading, life-threatening condition. It may occur mostly after frontal sinusitis. Subperiosteal abscess accompanied by osteomyelitis that develops after frontal sinusitis is defined as Pott's puffy tumor. In young patients, it may occur through septic thrombophlebitis or valveless communicating veins of Breschet.

39.7.2 Intracranial Complications

Intracranial complications occur due to the progression of pathogenic organisms through bone openings and diploic veins. Intracranial complications include meningitis, epidural, subdural abscess, and acute and chronic brain abscess.

The most common intracranial complication is meningitis. It is characterized by headache and neck stiffness. The patient appears toxic and has a fever. Cranial nerve paralysis may occur. The patient may experience long-term sensorineural hearing loss and mild mental status disorders.

In epidural abscess, osteitis on the posterior wall of the frontal sinus infection causes spreading to the epidural distance. The patient has a persistent dull headache, suddenly rising fever, and normal CSF findings. An undetected epidural abscess can tear the dura and cause subdural empyema. Frontal sinus infection may cause osteitis in the anterior wall, and if it spreads from there, it may cause pus accumulation under the frontal periosteum. This is called Pott's puffy tumor.

Infection may be carried back through diploic veins and cause septic thrombophlebitis. As a result, sagittal sinus thrombosis may occur. This clinical condition is often found together with other complications.

Subdural abscess results from the migration of infection into the subdural space. The patient appears toxic, mental status is impaired, and there are signs of meningeal irritation, optic neuritis, and papilledema. CSF is cloudy, and leukocytes are present. Focal neurological findings may be seen.

Acute brain abscess occurs due to retrograde septic embolism. The abscess does not cause signs of meningeal irritation unless it opens into the ventricular system. Subacute and chronic brain abscess creates a less toxic condition for the patient than acute brain abscess. Headache, nausea, vomiting, and mild fever may occur. Focal neurological findings and seizures may be observed.

Intracranial abscess factors are similar to the pathogens of ear infections and acute sinusitis (S. pneumoniae, H. influenza, and M. catarrhalis). In addition to chronic sinusitis, S. aureus and alpha-hemolytic streptococci should not be forgotten. The antibiotics must pass the blood-brain barrier and are effective against the most frequently isolated microorganisms.

The guidebook called "The Pocket Book of Pediatric Antimicrobial Therapy" recommends that a combination of methicillin (150–200 mg/kg/day IV every 6 h, in total) and aminoglycoside or cefotaxime (a total dose every 6 h) until the agent is isolated. It recommends a combination of 150–200 mg/kg/day IV) and metronidazole (30 mg/kg/day IV every 8 h). The duration of treatment is determined according to the patient's condition. Medical treatment is essential in the process leading to abscess formation. However, it may only sometimes be enough on its own. Surgical treatment depends on the location and extent of the pathology. The location of the pathology determines the type of intracranial approach.

References

1. Badr DT, Gaffin JM, Phipatanakul W. Pediatric rhinosinusitis. Curr Treat Options Allergy. 2016;3(3):268–81. https://doi.org/10.1007/s40521-016-0096-y.
2. Brook I. Acute sinusitis in children. Pediatr Clin North Am. 2013;60(2):409–24. https://doi.org/10.1016/j.pcl.2012.12.002.
3. Brietzke SE, Shin JJ, Choi S, Lee JT, Parikh SR, Pena M, et al. Clinical consensus statement: pediatric chronic rhinosinusitis. Otolaryngol Head Neck Surg. 2014;151(4):542–53. https://doi.org/10.1177/0194599814549302.
4. Scuderi AJ, Harnsberger HR, Boyer RS. Pneumatization of paranasal sinuses: normal features of importance to the accurate interpretation of CT scans and MR images. Am J Radiol. 1993;160:1101–4.
5. Wolf G, Anderhuber W, Kuhn F. Development of the paranasal sinuses in children: implications for paranasal sinus surgery. Ann Otol Rhinol Laryngol. 1993;102:705–11.
6. Shahid SK. Rhinosinusitis in children. ISRN Otolaryngol. 2012;2012:851831. https://doi.org/10.5402/2012/851831.
7. Lee D, Rosenfeld RM. Adenoid bacteriology and sinonasal symptoms in children. Otolaryngol Head Neck Surg. 1997;116(3):301–7. https://doi.org/10.1016/S0194-59989770264-X.
8. Paul D. Sinus infection and adenotonsillitis in pediatric patients. Laryngoscope. 1981;91(6):997–1000.
9. Ramadan HH. Revision endoscopic sinus surgery in children: surgical causes of failure. Laryngoscope. 2009;119(6):1214–7. https://doi.org/10.1002/lary.20230.
10. Rosenfeld RM. Pilot study of outcomes in pediatric rhinosinusitis. Arch Otolaryngol Head Neck Surg. 1995;121(7):729–36.
11. Talaat AM, Bahgat YS, el-Ghazzawy E, Elwany S. Nasopharyngeal bacterial flora before and after adenoidectomy. J Laryngol Otol. 1989;103(4):372–4.
12. Soler ZM, Rosenbloom JS, Skarada D, Gutman M, Hoy MJ, Nguyen SA. Prospective, multicenter evaluation of balloon sinus dilation for treatment of pediatric chronic rhinosinusitis. Int Forum Allergy Rhinol. 2017;7(3):221–9. https://doi.org/10.1002/alr.21889.
13. Zuliani G, Carron M, Gurrola J, Coleman C, Haupert M, Berk R, et al. Identification of adenoid biofilms in chronic rhinosinusitis. Int J Pediatr Otorhinolaryngol. 2006;70(9):1613–7. https://doi.org/10.1016/j.ijporl.2006.05.002.
14. Brietzke SE, Brigger MT. Adenoidectomy outcomes in pediatric rhinosinusitis: a meta-analysis. Int J Pediatr Otorhinolaryngol. 2008;72(10):1541–5. https://doi.org/10.1016/j.ijporl.2008.07.008.
15. Vandenberg SJ, Heatley DG. Efficacy of adenoidectomy in relieving symptoms of chronic sinusitis in children. Arch Otolaryngol Head Neck Surg. 1997;123(7):675–8.
16. Hamilos DL. Pediatric chronic rhinosinusitis. Am J Rhinol Allergy. 2015;29(6):414–20. https://doi.org/10.2500/ajra.2015.29.4238.
17. Heath J, Hartzell L, Putt C, Kennedy JL. Chronic rhinosinusitis in children: pathophysiology, evaluation and medical management. Curr Allergy Asthma Rep. 2018;18:37. https://doi.org/10.1007/s11882-018-0792-8.
18. Sedaghat AR, Phipatanakul W, Cunningham MJ. Prevalence of and associations with allergic rhinitis in children with chronic rhinosinusitis. Int J Pediatr Otorhinolaryngol. 2014;78(2):343–7. https://doi.org/10.1016/j.ijporl.2013.12.006.
19. Sedaghat AR, Phipatanakul W, Cunningham MJ. Atopy and the development of chronic rhinosinusitis in children with allergic rhinitis. J Allergy Clin Immunol Pract. 2013;6(1):689–91.e2.

20. Halderman AA, Tully LJ. The role of allergy in chronic rhinosinusitis. Otolaryngol Clin North Am. 2017;50(6):1077–90. https://doi.org/10.1016/j.otc.2017.08.003.
21. Baroody FM, Mucha SM, Detineo M, Naclerio RM. Nasal challenge with allergen leads to maxillary sinus inflammation. J Allergy Clin Immunol. 2008;121(5):1126–32.e7. https://doi.org/10.1016/j.jaci.2008.02.010.
22. Kennedy JL, Borish L. Chronic sinusitis pathophysiology: the role of allergy. Am J Rhinol Allergy. 2013;27(5):367–71. https://doi.org/10.2500/ajra.2013.27.3906.
23. Melen I, Ivarsson A, Schrewelius C. Ostial function in allergic rhinitis. Acta Otolaryngol Suppl. 1992;492:82–5.
24. Cepero R, Smith RJ, Catlin FI, Bressler KL, Furuta GT, Shandera KC. Cystic fibrosis—an otolaryngologic perspective. Otolaryngol Head Neck Surg. 1987;97(4):356–60. https://doi.org/10.1177/019459988709700403.
25. Kerrebijn JD, Poublon RM, Overbeek SE. Nasal and paranasal disease in adult cystic fibrosis patients. Eur Respir J. 1992;5(10):1239–42.
26. Oomen KP, April MM. Sinonasal manifestations in cystic fibrosis. Int J Otolaryngol. 2012;2012:789572. https://doi.org/10.1155/2012/789572.
27. Steinke JW, Payne SC, Chen PG, Negri J, Stelow EB, Borish L. Etiology of nasal polyps in cystic fibrosis: not a unimodal disease. Ann Otol Rhinol Laryngol. 2012;121(9):579–86. https://doi.org/10.1177/000348941212100904.
28. Tandon R, Derkay C. Contemporary management of rhinosinusitis and cystic fibrosis. Curr Opin Otolaryngol Head Neck Surg. 2003;11(1):41–4.
29. Magit A. Pediatric rhinosinusitis. Otolaryngol Clin North Am. 2014;47(5):733–46. https://doi.org/10.1016/j.otc.2014.06.003.
30. Fretzayas A, MoustakiM. Clinical spectrum of primary ciliary dyskinesia in childhood. World J Clin Pediatr. 2016;5(1):57–62. https://doi.org/10.5409/wjcp.v5.i1.57.
31. Coren ME, Meeks M, Morrison I, Buchdahl RM, Bush A. Primary ciliary dyskinesia: age at diagnosis and symptom history. Acta Paediatr. 2002;91(6):667–9.
32. Hosie PH, Fitzgerald DA, Jaffe A, Birman CS, Rutland J, Morgan LC. Presentation of primary ciliary dyskinesia in children: 30 years' experience. J Paediatr Child Health. 2015;51(7):722–6. https://doi.org/10.1111/jpc.12791.
33. Sommer JU, Schafer K, Omran H, Olbrich H, Wallmeier J, Blum A, et al. ENT manifestations in patients with primary ciliary dyskinesia: prevalence and significance of otorhinolaryngologic co-morbidities. Eur Arch Otorrinolaringol. 2011;268(3):383–8. https://doi.org/10.1007/s00405-010-1341-9.
34. Chow AW, Benninger MS, Brook I, Brozek JL, Goldstein EJ, Hicks LA, et al. IDSA clinical practice guideline for acute bacterial rhinosinusitis in children and adults. Clin Infect Dis. 2012;54(8):e72–e112. https://doi.org/10.1093/cid/cir1043. [PubMed: 22438350] [Large evidence based guidelines and recommendations for acute bacterial rhinosinusitis.]
35. Wald ER, Applegate KE, Bordley C, Darrow DH, Glode MP, Marcy SM, et al. Clinical practice guideline for the diagnosis and management of acute bacterial sinusitis in children aged 1 to 18 years. Pediatrics. 2013;132(1):e262–80. https://doi.org/10.1542/peds.2013-1071. [PubMed: 23796742]
36. Cummings CW, Frederickson JM, Harker LA, Krause CJ, Richardson MA, Schuller DE. Otolaryngology—Head and neck surgery. St Louis: Mosby Yearbook Inc.; 1998.
37. Brook I. The role of antibiotics in pediatric chronic rhinosinusitis. Laryngoscope Investig Otolaryngol. 2017;2(3):104–8. https://doi.org/10.1002/lio2.67.
38. DeMuri G, Wald ER. Acute bacterial sinusitis in children. Pediatr Rev. 2013;34(10):429–37; quiz 37. https://doi.org/10.1542/pir.34-10-429.
39. Marom T, Alvarez-Fernandez PE, Jennings K, Patel JA, McCormick DP, Chonmaitree T. Acute bacterial sinusitis complicating viral upper respiratory tract infection in young children. Pediatr Infect Dis J. 2014;33(8):803–8. https://doi.org/10.1097/INF.0000000000000278.
40. Beswick DM, Ramadan H, Baroody FM, Hwang PH. Practice patterns in pediatric chronic rhinosinusitis: a survey of the American Rhinologic Society. Am J Rhinol Allergy. 2016;30(6):418–23. https://doi.org/10.2500/ajra.2016.30.4373.

41. Steinke JW, Payne SC, Tessier ME, Borish LO, Han JK, Borish LC. Pilot study of budesonide inhalant suspension irrigations for chronic eosinophilic sinusitis. J Allergy Clin Immunol. 2009;124(6):1352–4 e7. https://doi.org/10.1016/j.jaci.2009.09.018.
42. Beswick DM, Messner AH, Hwang PH. Pediatric chronic rhinosinusitis management in rhinologists and pediatric otolaryngologists. Ann Otol Rhinol Laryngol. 2017;126(9):634–9. https://doi.org/10.1177/0003489417719717.
43. Rose AS, Thorp BD, Zanation AM, Ebert CS Jr. Chronic rhinosinusitis in children. Pediatr Clin North Am. 2013;60(4):979–91. https://doi.org/10.1016/j.pcl.2013.04.001.
44. Anfuso A, Ramadan H, Terrell A, Demirdag Y, Walton C, Skoner DP, et al. Sinus and adenoid inflammation in children with chronic rhinosinusitis and asthma. Ann Allergy Asthma Immunol. 2015;114(2):103–10. https://doi.org/10.1016/j.anai.2014.10.024.
45. Neff L, Adil EA. What is the role of the adenoid in pediatric chronic rhinosinusitis? Laryngoscope. 2015;125(6):1282–3. https://doi.org/10.1002/lary.25090. [PubMed: 25523938].
46. Sinüs hastalıkları s.255–9 Kennedy, Bolger, Zinnreich 2003 Nobel Tıp Kitapevi.

Pediatric Rhinosinusitis and Comorbid Asthma

40

Beste Ozsezen and Hossein Sadeghi

40.1 Introduction

Pediatric rhinosinusitis is characterized by the inflammation of the nose and the paranasal sinuses accompanied by at least two symptoms such as nasal obstruction, nasal congestion, or nasal discharge. Facial pain, facial pressure, and cough can accompany these symptoms [1, 2]. Rhinosinusitis must be suspected in children who have these symptoms persisting more than 7–10 days without any improvement. It affects 5–12% of the population [3]. However, these symptoms may be present in upper respiratory tract infections caused by viral pathogens which resolve within 7–10 days [2, 4]. Additional support for rhinosinusitis includes endoscopic findings of nasal polyps, mucosal obstruction in the middle meatus, and mucosal changes of ostiomeatal complex or sinuses on computed tomography [5].

The separating factor for acute and chronic rhinosinusitis is the duration of the symptoms. Acute rhinosinusitis lasts <12 weeks where the symptoms occur suddenly. Viruses are the main cause of acute upper airway infections. However, in some children underlying allergic status like allergic rhinitis may aggravate the clinical condition. In chronic rhinosinusitis, symptoms carry on for at least 12 weeks. According to nasal endoscopic and CT findings, the two major phenotypes of CRS are CRS with nasal polyposis (CRSwNP) and CRSsine nasal polyposis (CRSsNP) [5]. CRSsNP is twice as common compared to CRSwNP in pediatric population.

B. Ozsezen (✉)
Department of Pediatric Pulmonology, Dokuz Eylul University, İzmir, Turkey

H. Sadeghi
Sue & John L. Weinberg Cystic Fibrosis Center, New York, NY, USA

Division of Pediatric Pulmonology and Sleep Medicine, Columbia University Irving Medical Center, New York, NY, USA
e-mail: hs762@cumc.columbia.edu

H. Yüksel et al. (eds.), *Pediatric Airway Diseases*, Comprehensive ENT,
https://doi.org/10.1007/978-3-031-74853-0_40

Even though less prevalent, CRSwNP is more frequent in patients with asthma which share the same T helper 2 immune response.

Asthma is characterized by chronic inflammation of the airways showing variable airflow limitation and bronchial hyperresponsiveness. The chronic inflammation leads to airway remodeling [6]. Nocturnal cough, shortness of breath, and wheezing are the most frequent symptoms. Older children may complain of chest tightness, whereas in younger children may have recurrent chest pain [7]. Symptoms are triggered by inhalant allergens, respiratory infections, and exposure to cold air or physical activity.

According to the underlying biological mechanisms, there are two types of asthma: eosinophilic (type 2) or non-eosinophilic (non-type 2) endotype [8, 9]. Type 2 asthma endotype is characterized by the existence of Th2 cytokines associated with airway and peripheral blood eosinophilia. The two mechanisms that play a role in airway inflammation in type 2 asthma are allergic eosinophilic airway inflammation and non-allergic eosinophilic airway inflammation. In allergic eosinophilic inflammation (atopic asthma), IgE-mediated mast cell degranulation takes place, whereas in non-allergic eosinophilic inflammation (non-atopic asthma) innate immune cells, basophils, group 2 innate lymphocyte cells (ILC2), and eosinophils are present without allergen-specific IgE [10].

The allergic eosinophilic inflammation cascade is as follows: dendritic cells located in the airway epithelium recognized the allergen. The allergen is presented to naive T cells via dendritic cells in the secondary lymphoid organ. Naive T cells that recognize the antigen transform into Th2 cells or follicular T cells. Follicular T cells stimulate antigen-specific B cells to synthesize IgE. Allergen-specific IgE binds to high-affinity FcEpsilonRI receptors on the mast cell surface. As a result of cross-linking of IgE and antigens on the mast cell surface, inflammatory mediators are released from mast cells. After re-contact with the antigen, Th2 cells move to the area of inflammation and produce Th2 cytokines. IL-5 and IL-9 cause tissue eosinophilia and mast cell hyperplasia, while IL-13 is responsible for mucus production from goblet cells and airway hyperresponsiveness [10].

However, in the nonallergic eosinophilic inflammation cascade allergens with protease activity (e.g., house dust mite) disrupt barrier integrity in epithelial cells and stimulate the release of damage-related cytokines. IL-33 and TSLP (thymic stromal lymphopoietin) released from epithelial cells stimulate basophils and ILC2 cells, causing the release of Th2 cytokines. IL-33 and basophil-derived IL-4, on the other hand, stimulate ILC2 cells synergistically, increasing the release of chemoattractants such as CCL11, and causing aggregation of eosinophils in the lung. IL-5 and IL-13 released from activated ILC2 cause eosinophilia and mucus production. IL-33, on the other hand, causes the activation of Treg cells by stimulating the release of IL-2 from activated mast cells. The IL-33-ICL2-IL-5/IL-13 axis is a crucial path in protease-induced airway inflammation. Innate immunity cells have a part in Th2-mediated inflammation by stimulating Th2 cytokines directly or indirectly [10–12].

40.2 Comorbidities of CRS

Presence of comorbidities like adenoid hypertrophy, allergic rhinitis, gastroesophageal reflux, and asthma may cause negative clinical consequences and week disease control in patients who have CRS. Adenoid tissue may behave as a bacterial reservoir [13, 14]. Studies show that there is an atopic predilection in patients with CRS and is related with the severity of sinus disease. All these findings highlight the causal relationship between CRS and AR and that AR is a comorbidity of CRS [15, 16]. On the other hand, among the comorbidities of asthma, CRS is the most frequent one. Besides disease control, the outcome is worse in patients with asthma and comorbid CRS [17, 18].

40.3 Epidemiology and Prevalence

CRSwNP accounts for roughly 20% of CRS patients [19]. The prevalence ranges between 1 and 10% for CRSsNP and 4% for CRSwNP for the general population [20]. On the contrary, 40–67% of CRSwNP patients have asthma [21, 22]. The incidence of CRS is also higher in asthmatic patients compared to non-asthmatic patients. Jarvis et al. showed a strong association between asthma and CRS in their screening of 52,000 patients aged 18–75 years [23]. This association was stronger in patients who have both CRS and allergic rhinitis. Matsuno et al. [1] showed a CRS prevalence of 36.7% in patients with asthma. Abnormal sinus CT findings were present in 66.3% of the asthma patients and more frequent in patients with moderate-to-severe asthma compared to those with mild asthma [24]. The CRS prevalence was 35–45% in asthma patients, and mucosal thickening was significantly more pronounced in the sinuses compared to the control group according to the study by Crater et al. [25]. In the European Unbiased Biomarkers for the Prediction of Respiratory Disease Outcomes (UBIOPRED), cohort of 25% of the adult patient with severe asthma had nasal polyps [18]. The limited number of pediatric studies showed similar results [18, 26–28]. Fuller et al. [26] stated that 27% of severe asthma patients had abnormal sinus findings. Later on, Tosco et al. showed that among persistent asthma patients almost half had rhinosinusitis detected by nasal endoscopy [27]. Marseglia et al. performed nasal endoscopy in 294 pediatric patients and showed that 7.5% had sinus abnormalities whom had poorly controlled asthma [28]. In addition, patients with CRS have severe asthma, uncontrolled asthma, and more frequent asthma attacks. Interestingly, the methacholine challenge test was positive in many patients with CRS who did not have any asthma symptoms [29]. Parson et al. demonstrated a reduction in asthma symptoms by 96%, as well as asthma exacerbations and outpatient visits after the surgical treatment for CRS [30].

40.4 The United Airway Disease

Many children have complaints involving both upper and lower airways. The "united airway disease" term is used the define the link between upper and lower airways. The upper and lower airways have many anatomical, pathophysiological, and therapeutic similarities [31, 32].

Although the common mechanism in the development of allergic rhinitis and asthma has been demonstrated, the relationship between asthma and CRS has not yet been clearly determined [33]. There are many studies examining the relationship between CRS and asthma. In the Galen study, in which 52,000 adult patients were evaluated by questionnaire, a higher rate of CRS was present in patients with asthma compared to the normal population [23]. In a large retrospective study, it was stated that patients with newly diagnosed CRS had a higher probability of previous asthma diagnosis [34].

In patients who have asthma, abnormal sinus findings were detected by sinus X-ray in 47% of the patients and this rate was found to be significantly higher than patients who were only diagnosed with rhinitis [35]. On the other hand, patients with severe mucosal changes on computed tomography who had sinus surgery were more likely to have a wheezing episode in any period of time compared to patients with mild-moderate mucosal changes [36]. Lately, Lee et al. implied that patients with radiologically confirmed sinus disease had significantly lower FEV1/FVC ratio and higher bronchial hyperreactivity than subjects without sinusitis finding these patients. Besides FEV1/FVC ratio was lower in patients with extensive sinusitis compared to patients with limited disease [37].

40.5 Anatomical Similarities

The nose and the bronchi are histologically lined with pseudostratified respiratory epithelium with columnar ciliated cells. Along the respiratory tree, the basement membrane and ciliary epithelium with glands and goblet cells are present [2, 31]. An intact upper airway is necessary to protect the respiratory tract from harmful external agents. İmpaired nasal breathing caused by rhinosinusitis impairs air warming, humidification, and purification from pollutants and irritants; it triggers bronchial disorders caused by the inhalation of cold, dry air, and possible irritants. In addition, the conductive airways prevent the passage of particles with a diameter of 5–10 microns into the lower airways. This ensures that the distal airways are protected from possible toxic substances. Besides, in allergic patients with CRS, the mouth breathing leads to impairment of air filtering which may increase the concentration of aeroallergens reaching the bronchial system.

40.6 Pathogenesis of Upper and Lower Airway Inflammation in CRS and Asthma

Regardless of the underlying etiological factor, it is known that the most prominent pathological finding in CRS is eosinophilic infiltration in the inflamed tissue, and this finding is found at a similar rate in allergic and non-allergic patients [4]. The pathological findings may be related to the predominant Th2 immune response and similar cytokine pattern with increased production of IL-4 and TNF-alfa independent from the Ig-E mediated period. In patients with CRSwNP, eosinophils are the main cells responsible for tissue damage in the sinus mucosa.

An altered epithelial innate immunity and Th2 response is present in this group of patients [38, 39]. These underlying risk factors facilitates the settlement of bacteria into the sinus cavity. *Staphylococcus aureus* stimulates the adaptive immune system by super antigenic stimulation via its exotoxins. In addition, it causes eosinophilic inflammation by creating a biofilm layer and increasing eosinophilic cationic protein and IL-5 levels [40, 41].

The allergic and non-allergic eosinophilic inflammation stimulates the bone marrow which produces inflammatory cells and mediators acting in respiratory airways. For this reason, the coexistence of CRS and asthma occurs with the interaction of many different mechanisms that act both in the respiratory system and outside the respiratory system [4]. Novel evidence supports that systemic immune arises through immune cells and mediators released from bone marrow and other lymphoid organs and this response strengthens inflammation in the airways and carries its effect beyond. Although local factors such as nasal-pharyngeal bronchial reflexes, post-nasal discharge and inhalation of polluted cold air may exacerbate inflammation in the upper and lower airways, they are not the main determinants of inflammation [4].

Other than the classical 2 major phenotypes based on the presence of nasal polyposis, CRS can similarly be classified as type 2 and non-type 2 endotypes. While 80% of CRSwNP patients have type 2 endotype, type 1 and type 3 inflammation are in the foreground in CRSsNP and are regulated by cytokines such as IL-6, IL-8, IL-17, and TNF-alpha [42–44].

CRSwNP and asthma have the similar type 2 immunopathology and epithelial barrier dysfunction [45]. T helper type 2 (Th2), type 2 innate lymphoid cells (ILC2), innate like lymphocytes (ILL), and effectors cells such as mast cells, basophils, and eosinophils regulate the production of type 2 cytokines (IL-4, IL-5, IL-13) [46–48]. The remodeling of the airways is the straightforward reaction of inflammation and repair cycle [1].

IL-5, IL-13 generating ILC2 is elevated in sputum and nasal mucosa of patients who have type 2 asthma and CRSwNP, respectively. However, there are some pathological differences between type 2 and non-type2 phenotypes and between asthma and CRSwNP or CRSsNP [1]. For example, in CRSwNP and CRSsNP, the remodeling is caused by increased collagen deposition [49, 50]. Besides even though type 2 inflammation with increased eosinophils and IL-4, IL-5, IL-13 are the hallmark of the disease, remodeling is also present in CRS patients where neutrophils are evident. These findings suggest that eosinophils are not fundamental remodeling formation [51].

In summary, in asthma, chronic eosinophilic type 2 inflammation leading to airway remodeling, whereas in allergic rhinitis, no remodeling occurs even though type 2 inflammation is present. Patients who have CRSwNP the present remodeling caused by type 2 inflammation which leads to nasal polyp development is characterized by pseudocyst formation, stromal edema, and collagen deposition. Finally, patients who have CRSsNP where type 1 and 3 neutrophilic inflammation is prominent remodeling consists of basal membrane thickening, fibrosis, and goblet cell hyperplasia [1].

40.7 Treatment

The first-line treatment is medical treatment by long-term oral antibiotics (3–6 weeks) in CRS aiming the most frequent microorganisms (*Streptococcus pneumoniae, Moraxella catarrhalis, Hemophilus influenza*, beta-hemolytic *Streptococcus pyogenes*). Amoxicillin, amoxicillin-clavulanate, or third- or fourth-generation cephalosporins can be initiated. Clindamycin may be chosen if the patient has penicillin allergy [52]. Nasal saline and intranasal corticosteroids are added to oral antibiotic therapy. The effectiveness of nasal saline has also been demonstrated by the Cochrane review. Intranasal corticosteroids which act via the eosinophilic pathway in alliance with nasal saline irrigation is the backbone treatment for CRSwNP and CRSsNP [53]. The resistance to standardized therapies is uncommon, called as difficult to treat rhinosinusitis, and usually seen in patients with CRSwNP who present type 2 endotype [2].

Surgery is applied in patients who are unresponsive to medical therapy. Considering that similar bacteria are detected in cultures taken from adenoid tissue and sinuses, unlike adults, adenoidectomy only can be an adequate treatment choice in patients with CRS [54, 55]. Risk factors like asthma and young age (<7 years) should be sought in patients who require functional endoscopic sinus surgery despite adenoidectomy [56]. Balloon sinuplasty is an alternative surgical technique. However, adenoidectomy alone is the most cost-effective first procedure for pediatric CRS [57]. The recurrence ratio following the sinus surgery is up to 80%, which is greater in patients who have CRSwNP, elevated eosinophil counts, IL-5, and IgE in nasal tissue [58]. These findings suggest that surgery must be combined with medical therapy.

The effect of upper airway pathologies on the severity and control of asthma has been shown in many studies. Early detection of upper airway pathologies is crucial, especially in patients who have severe asthma. For this reason, nasal endoscopy and imaging are recommended in these patients [59–61]. In patients with asthma, rhinosinusitis treatment improves asthma symptoms, respiratory function, and airway hyperreactivity. In addition, recovery in asthma symptoms quality of life scores was observed after endoscopic sinus surgery in patients with CRS resistant to medical treatment and comorbid asthma [62].

Some patients who have type 2 immune-mediated, severe, and recurring CRSwNP and comorbid asthma are unresponsive to standardized treatment modalities. These group of patients are candidates for biological therapies [63]. Monoclonal antibodies against IgE (omalizumab), IL-5 (mepolizumab), and IL-4 or IL-13 (dupilumab) improved nasal symptoms and polyp size in patients with CRSwNP [64, 65]. Presently, omalizumab, mepolizumab, and dupilumab is approved for use in children between 6 and 11 years.

40.8 Conclusion

CRS and asthma are meticulously connected with one another. They are both characterized by eosinophilic inflammation. Eosinophilic inflammation is more severe in patients with CRS and comorbid asthma.

Contrarily, the probability of detecting CRS is higher in severe asthma patients. It is necessary to detect upper airway pathologies in patients with asthma in the early period, especially to detect patients at risk of severe disease.

High index of suspicion and early attention and treatment of both CRS and asthma are required for successful clinical management of CRS and asthma.

References

1. Matucci A, Bormioli S, Nencini F, et al. Asthma and chronic rhinosinusitis: how similar are they in pathogenesis and treatment responses? Int J Mol Sci. 2021;22(7):3340. https://doi.org/10.3390/ijms22073340.
2. Licari A, Brambilla I, Castagnoli R, et al. Rhinosinusitis and asthma in children. Sinusitis. 2018;3:3. https://doi.org/10.3390/sinusitis3020003.
3. Fokkens WJ, Lund VJ, Mullol J, et al. European position paper on rhinosinusitis and nasal polyps 2012. Rhinol Suppl. 2012;23:1–299.
4. Poddighe D, Brambilla I, Licari A, et al. Pediatric rhinosinusitis and asthma. Respir Med. 2018;141:94–9. https://doi.org/10.1016/j.rmed.2018.06.016.
5. Alobid I. Chronic rhinosinusitis and nasal polyps: the role of generic and specific questionnaires on assessing its impact on patient's quality of life. Allergy. 2008;63(10):1267–79.
6. Gandhi NA, Bennett BL, Graham NMH, et al. Targeting key proximal drivers of type 2 inflammation in disease. Nat Rev Drug Discov. 2016;15:35–50.
7. Liu AH, Covar RA, Spahn JD, Leung DYM. Childhood asthma; 2011. issn:978-1-4377-0755-7. https://doi.org/10.1016/B978-1-4377-0755-7.00138-X
8. Wenzel SE, Schwartz LB, Langmack EL, et al. Evidence that severe asthma can be divided pathologically into two inflammatory subtypes with distinct physiologic and clinical characteristics. Am J Respir Crit Care Med. 1999;160:1001–8.
9. Carr TF, Zeki AA, Kraft M. Eosinophilic and non eosinophilic asthma. Am J Respir Crit Care Med. 2018;197:22–37.
10. Russell RJ, Brightling C. Pathogenesis of asthma: implications for precision medicine. Clin Sci. 2017;131:1723–35.
11. Kubo M. Innate and adaptive type 2 immunity in lung allergic inflammation. Immunol Rev. 2017;278:162–72.
12. Bel EH, Brinke AT. New anti-eosinophil drugs for asthma and COPD. Chest. 2017;152:1276–82.
13. Prokopakis EP, Kalogjera L, Karatzanis AD. Pediatric severe chronic upper airway disease (P-SCUAD). Curr Allergy Asthma Rep. 2015;15:68.
14. Karatzanis A, Kalogjera L, Scadding G, et al. Severe chronic upper airway disease (SCUAD) in children. Definition issues and requirements. Int J Pediatr Otorhinolaryngol. 2015;79:965–8.
15. Brambilla I, Pusateri A, Pagella F, et al. Adenoids in children: advances in immunology, diagnosis, and surgery. Clin Anat. 2014;27:346–52.
16. Georgalas C, Vlastos I, Picavet V, et al. Is chronic rhinosinusitis related to allergic rhinitis in adults and children? Applying epidemiological guidelines for causation. Allergy. 2014;69:828–33.
17. Ten Brinke A, Sterk PJ, Masclee AA, et al. Risk factors of frequent exacerbations in difficult-to-treat asthma. Eur Respir J. 2005;26:812–8.

18. Shaw DE, Sousa AR, Fowler SJ, et al. Clinical and inflammatory characteristics of the European U-BIOPRED adult severe asthma cohort. Eur Respir J. 2015;46:1308–21.
19. Benjamin MR, Stevens WW, Li N, et al. Clinical characteristics of patients with chronic rhinosinusitis without nasal polyps in an academic setting. J Allergy Clin Immunol Pract. 2019;7(3):1010–6. https://doi.org/10.1016/j.jaip.2018.10.014.
20. Global Initiative for Asthma. Global strategy for asthma management and prevention. 2023. https://ginasthma.org/2023-gina-main-report/. Accessed 23 Aug 2023.
21. Mullol J, Azar A, Buchheit KM, et al. Chronic rhinosinusitis with nasal polyps: quality of life in the biologics era. J Allergy Clin Immunol Pract. 2022;10(6):1434–1453.e9. https://doi.org/10.1016/j.jaip.2022.03.002.
22. Laidlaw TM, Mullol J, Woessner KM, et al. Chronic rhinosinusitis with nasal polyps and asthma. J Allergy Clin Immunol Pract. 2021;9:1133–41.
23. Jarvis D, Newson R, Lotvall J, et al. Asthma in adults and its association with chronic rhinosinusitis: the GA2LEN survey in Europe. Allergy. 2012;67:91–8.
24. Matsuno O, Ono E, Takenaka R, et al. Asthma and sinusitis: association and implication. Int Arch Allergy Immunol. 2008;147(1):52–8.
25. Crater SE, Peters EJ, Phillips CD, et al. Prospective analysis of CT of the sinuses in acute asthma. AJR Am J Roentgenol. 1999;173(1):127–31.
26. Fuller CG, Schoettler JJ, Gilsanz V, et al. Sinusitis in status asthmaticus. Clin Pediatr. 1994;33(12):712–9. https://doi.org/10.1177/000992289403301202.
27. Tosca MA, Cosentino C, Pallestrini E, et al. Improvement of clinical and immunopathologic parameters in asthmatic children treated for concomitant chronic rhinosinusitis. Ann Allergy Asthma Immunol. 2003;91(1):71–8.
28. Marseglia GL, Caimmi S, Marseglia A, et al. Occult sinusitis may be a key feature for non-controlled asthma in children. J Biol Regul Homeost Agents. 2012;26(1 Suppl):S125–31.
29. Dixon AE, Kaminsky DA, Holbrook JT, et al. Allergic rhinitis and sinusitis in asthma: differential effects on symptoms and pulmonary function. Chest. 2006;130:429–35.
30. Parsons DS, Phillips SE. Functional endoscopic surgery in children: a retrospective analysis of results. Laryngoscope. 1993;103(8):899–903.
31. Licari A, Castagnoli R, Denicolò CF, et al. The nose and the lung: united airway disease? Front Pediatr. 2017;5:44.
32. Hellings PW, Prokopakis EP. Global airway disease beyond allergy. Curr Allergy Asthma Rep. 2010;10:143–9.
33. Tint D, Kubala S, Toskala E. Risk factors and comorbidities in chronic rhinosinusitis. Curr Allergy Asthma Rep. 2016;16:16. https://doi.org/10.1007/s11882-015-0589-y.
34. Tan BK, Chandra RK, Pollak J, et al. Incidence and associated premorbid diagnoses of patients with chronic rhinosinusitis. J Allergy Clin Immunol. 2013;131(5):1350–60.
35. Schwartz HJ, Thompson JS, Sher TH, et al. Occult sinus abnormalities in the asthmatic patient. Arch Intern Med. 1987;147(12):2194–6.
36. Newman LJ, Platts-Mills TA, Phillips CD, et al. Chronic sinusitis. Relationship of computed tomographic findings to allergy, asthma, and eosinophilia. JAMA. 1994;271(5):363–7.
37. Lee SY, Yoon SH, Song WJ, et al. Influence of chronic sinusitis and nasal polyp on the lower airway of subjects without lower airway diseases. Allergy Asthma Immunol Res. 2014;6(4):310–5.
38. Frieri M. Asthma linked with rhinosinusitis: an extensive review. Allergy Rhinol (Providence). 2014;5(1):41–9.
39. Hamilos DL. Pediatric chronic rhinosinusitis. Am J Rhinol Allergy. 2015;29(6):414–20.
40. Foreman A, Boase S, Psaltis A, Wormald PJ, et al. Role of bacterial and fungal biofilms in chronic rhinosinusitis. Curr Allergy Asthma Rep. 2012;12(2):127–35.
41. Madeo J, Frieri M. Bacterial biofilms and chronic rhinosinusitis. Allergy Asthma Proc. 2013;34(4):335–41.
42. Delemarre T, Holtappels G, De Ruyck Zhang N, et al. Type 2 inflammation in chronic rhinosinusitis without nasal polyps: another relevant endotype. J Allergy Clin Immunol. 2020;146:337–43.

43. Cho SH, Kim DW, Gevaert P. Chronic rhinosinusitis without nasal polyps. J Allergy Clin Immunol Pract. 2016;4:575–82.
44. Tomassen P, Vandeplas G, Van Zele T, et al. Inflammatory endotypes of chronic rhinosinusitis based on cluster analysis of biomarkers. J Allergy Clin Immunol. 2016;137:1449–56.
45. Schleich F, Brusselle G, Louis R, et al. Heterogeneity of phenotypes in severe asthmatics. The Belgian severe asthma registry (BSAR). Respir Med. 2014;108(12):1723–32. https://doi.org/10.1016/j.rmed.2014.10.007.
46. Maggi L, Montaini G, Mazzoni A, et al. Human circulating group 2 innate lymphoid cells can express CD154 and promote IgE production. J Allergy Clin Immunol. 2017;139:964–76.
47. Koh Y-I, Shim J-U. Association between sputum natural killer T cells and eosinophilic airway inflammation in human asthma. Int Arch Allergy Immunol. 2010;153:239–48.
48. Acharya KR, Ackerman SJ. Eosinophil granule proteins: form and function. J Biol Chem. 2014;289:17406–15.
49. De Borja CF, Picado C, Martinez-Anton A, et al. Differential expression of remodeling markers by tissue structure in nasal polyposis. Am J Rhinol Allergy. 2013;27:e69–74.
50. Wang L-F, Chien C-Y, Chiang F-Y, et al. Corelationship between matrix metalloproteinase 2 and 9 expression and severity of chronic rhinosinusitis with nasal polyposis. Am J Rhinol Allergy. 2012;26:e1–4.
51. Li X, Meng J, Qiao X, et al. Expression of TGF, matrix metalloproteinases, and tissue inhibitors in Chinese chronic rhinosinusitis. J Allergy Clin Immunol. 2010;125:1061–8.
52. Quantilla LAM. Curr Treat Options Pediatr. 2018;4(4):413–24. https://doi.org/10.1007/s40746-018-0142-z.
53. Fokkens WJ, Lund VJ, Hopkins C, et al. European position paper on rhinosinusitis and nasal polyps 2020. Rhinology. 2020;58:1–464.
54. Elwany S, El-Dine AN, El-Medany A, et al. Relationship between bacteriology of the adenoid core and middle meatus in children with sinusitis. J Laryngol Otol. 2011;125(3):279–81. [PubMed: 21144114].
55. Zuliani G, Carron M, Gurrola J, et al. Identification of adenoid biofilms in chronic rhinosinusitis. Int J Pediatr Otorhinolaryngol. 2006;70(9):1613–7. [PubMed: 16781783].
56. Brietzke SE, Brigger MT. Adenoidectomy outcomes in pediatric rhinosinusitis: a meta analysis. Int J Pediatr Otorhinolaryngol. 2008;72(10):1541–5. [PubMed: 18723228].
57. House LK, Lewis AF, Ashmead MG. A cost-effectiveness analysis of the up-front use of balloon catheter dilation in the treatment of pediatric chronic rhinosinusitis. Am J Otolaryngol. 2018;39(4):418–22. [PubMed: 29706456].
58. Van Zele T, Holtappels G, Gevaert P, et al. Differences in initial immunoprofiles between recurrent and nonrecurrent chronic rhinosinusitis with nasal polyps. Am J Rhinol Allergy. 2014;28:192–8.
59. Amelink M, de Groot JC, de Nijs SB, et al. Severe adult-onset asthma: a distinct phenotype. J Allergy Clin Immunol. 2013;132:336–41.
60. Phillips KM, Hoehle LP, Bergmark RW, et al. Chronic rhinosinusitis severity is associated with need for asthma-related systemic corticosteroids. Rhinology. 2017;55:211–7.
61. Chung KF, Wenzel SE, Brozek JL, et al. International ERS/ATS guidelines on definition, evaluation and treatment of severe asthma. Eur Respir J. 2014;43:343–73.
62. Schlosser RJ, Smith TL, Mace J, et al. Asthma quality of life and control after sinus surgery in patients with chronic rhinosinusitis. Allergy. 2017;72:483–91.
63. Bachert C, Gevaert P, Hellings P. Biotherapeutics in chronic rhinosinusitis with and without nasal polyps. J Allergy Clin Immunol Pract. 2017;5:1512–6.
64. Gevaert P, Omachi TA, Corren J, et al. Efficacy and safety of omalizumab in nasal polyposis: 2 randomized phase 3 trials. J Allergy Clin Immunol. 2020;146:595–605.
65. Bachert C, Sousa AR, Lund VJ, et al. Reduced need for surgery in severe nasal polyposis with mepolizumab: randomized trial. J Allergy Clin Immunol. 2017;140:1024–1031.e1014.

41 Pediatric Otitis Media and Comorbid Asthma

Dilber Ademhan Tural, Şule Selin Akyan Soydaş, and Refiloe Masekela

41.1 Pediatric Otitis Media

Otitis media (OM) is a term for infection or inflammation accompanied by effusion of the middle ear. It is divided into two main categories such as acute otitis media (AOM) and otitis media with effusion (OME) [1]. OM peaks during the first 2 years of life. It is particularly prevalent in children under 5, with cumulative incidence exceeding 80% by age three [2–4]. OM is one of the most common reasons for physician visits and the use of antibiotics and should be in the differential diagnosis of fever in childhood [5]. OM is also the most common cause of acquired hearing loss in children [1]. The recurrence, severity, and persistence of middle ear effusion are strongly related to the earlier in life a child experiences the first episode of OM [2].

Acute otitis media (AOM) is one of the most common infectious diseases in early childhood [1]. It is estimated that more than 50% of children have had at least one episode of AOM in their first year of life [1–4]. AOM is one of the most common reasons for antibiotic prescription in children under 3 years of age [5–7]. The symptoms can be obscure, especially in infants, and difficulties on the tympanic membrane and middle ear area visualization may result in under- and overdiagnosis of AOM [1, 2].

Otitis media with effusion (OME) is caused by the nonpurulent fluid accumulation in the middle ear area without signs of acute infection [1]. OME affected more than 60% of children under the age of 2. The prevalence is increasing in children with craniofacial abnormalities and comorbidities [1–4]. The attacks mostly resolve spontaneously within 3 months, but approximately 40% of children have recurrent

D. Ademhan Tural (✉) · Ş. S. A. Soydaş
Department of Pediatric Pulmonology, Ankara Bilkent City Hospital, Ankara, Turkey

R. Masekela
Department of Pediatric Pulmonology, University of KwaZulu Natal, Durban, South Africa
e-mail: masekelar@ukzn.ac.za

H. Yüksel et al. (eds.), *Pediatric Airway Diseases*, Comprehensive ENT, https://doi.org/10.1007/978-3-031-74853-0_41

Table 41.1 Effective factors in the epidemiology of otitis media

Host-related factors	Environmental factors
Age	Socioeconomic status
Gender	Breast milk-formula feeding
Race	Exposure to other children
Genetic background	Exposure to the tobacco smoke
Craniofacial anomalies	Season
Allergy and immunocompetence	Pacifier use

OME. Recurrent and persistent OME may result in hearing loss, speech delay, and behavioral disturbances [1, 8, 9].

41.2 Epidemiology

Several factors affect the occurrence of OM. These can be divided into two main categories, including host-related and environmental factors, summarized in Table 41.1.

41.3 Host-Related Factors

41.3.1 Age

The prevalence of OM is higher in infants and younger children [1, 2]. The highest rate of OM is seen in the first 20 months of life, and the prevalence progressively declines after the second year of life [10]. OM is also relatively common in early school-age years. The first OM episode has been reported to be seen at a rate of up to 85% in the first year of age and up to 99% by the second year of age [1–3, 10]. The immaturity of the immune system and the structure and dysfunction of the Eustachian tube are the most likely reasons for the higher prevalence of OM in infants and young children [1, 10]. The onset age of OM is an essential predictor of developing recurrent and chronic OM; earlier age increases these risks [9, 10].

41.3.2 Gender

The incidence and persistence of OM have been reported to be higher in boys, but some studies have shown no gender-related difference [7, 11].

41.3.3 Race

OM is particularly common and severe in Native American, Inuit, and indigenous Australian children. There are inconsistencies in the results of the studies that compare the occurrence of OM in Caucasian and black children [11].

41.3.4 Genetic Background

The occurrence of OM is much greater among monozygotic than among dizygotic twins. Twin and genome studies suggest that OM has a heritable component [12, 13].

41.3.5 Craniofacial Anomalies

OM is universal among infants with unrepaired palatal cleft and is also very prevalent in children with cleft lip, submucous cleft palate, and other craniofacial anomalies [1, 14]. These congenital anomalies cause Eustachian tube dysfunction, thus predisposing children to the recurrence of middle ear disease [1, 2]. Repair of the palate reduces the incidence of OM, but many children require multiple tube insertions. An ear examination and placement of ear tubes are recommended at the time of cleft palate repair [14].

41.3.6 Allergy and Immunocompetence

The role of asthma, allergic rhinitis, and atopic diseases as primary etiologic agents in OM is uncertain. However, it is possible that OM is aggravated and persistency increased by the allergy [14–16]. Defective or immature immunologic responses may contribute to the occurrence and persistency of OM in children [1, 2]. The decrease in the incidence of OM with age may be related to the maturation of immunity with age [1].

41.4 Environmental Factors

41.4.1 Socioeconomic Status

The frequency of OM increases with low socioeconomic conditions due to crowding, poor hygiene and nutritional status, limited access to medical care, and prescribed medications [14, 17].

41.4.2 Breast Milk-Formula Feeding

Breast milk feeding has been found protective against OM, especially in the first 6 months of life [18].

41.4.3 Exposure to Other Children

Exposure to other children is an important identifiable risk factor for developing OM [1, 14, 17]. Children having older siblings have more OM in the first 2 years of life than firstborn children. Children in daycare have an increased incidence of OM and tympanostomy tube insertion than children cared for at home [17, 19].

41.4.4 Exposure to Tobacco Smoke

Studies that have used measures of nicotine metabolites have consistently identified a significant linkage between exposure to tobacco smoke and OM [20, 21]. Tobacco smoke exposure is a preventable risk factor for OM occurrences [1, 14, 20].

41.4.5 Season

Occurrences of OM reach the highest rates during the fall and winter when upper respiratory tract infection incidence is also highest. These findings reflect the significant association of OM with viral respiratory illnesses [1, 14, 22].

41.4.6 Pacifier Use

Pacifier use increased the incidence of OM and recurrence of OM by up to 30%, although the exact role and contribution of pacifier use are still unclear [14, 23].

41.4.7 Pathophysiology and Pathogenesis

Otitis media is a multifactorial disease. Host and environmental factors affect the progression of the disease. Pathogenesis begins with early bacterial colonization of the nasopharynx. Continuous exposure to infective agents may eventually cause severe chronic ear disease. Mechanisms and causal pathways for otitis media are summarized in Fig. 41.1 (Fig. 41.1 adapted from the study of Schilder et al. [1]).

41.4.8 Eustachian Tube Dysfunction

The Eustachian tube protects the middle ear against the influx of bacterial and viral pathogens, equalizes the middle ear pressure, and drains secretions from the middle ear [1]. The tube has three main functions such as ventilation, protection, and clearance of the middle ear. Impairment of these functions results in an increased risk of OM.

The Eustachian tube is shorter, wider, and more horizontal in infants and young children. These anatomical differences impair the protection and cleaning functions of the tube and increase the risk of OM [24]. The angle and length of the Eustachian tube increase with growth, and the tube gets the adult configuration at the end of the first decade of life. These anatomical changes might reduce the risk of OM with age, even in children at high risk of OM [1, 24].

Tubal obstruction, caused mainly by hypertrophied adenoid tissue and inflammatory edema of the tubal mucosa by a viral infection, interrupts the ventilation and initiates an inflammatory response that includes secretory metaplasia, compromise of the mucociliary transport system, and effusion of liquid into the tympanic cavity [24].

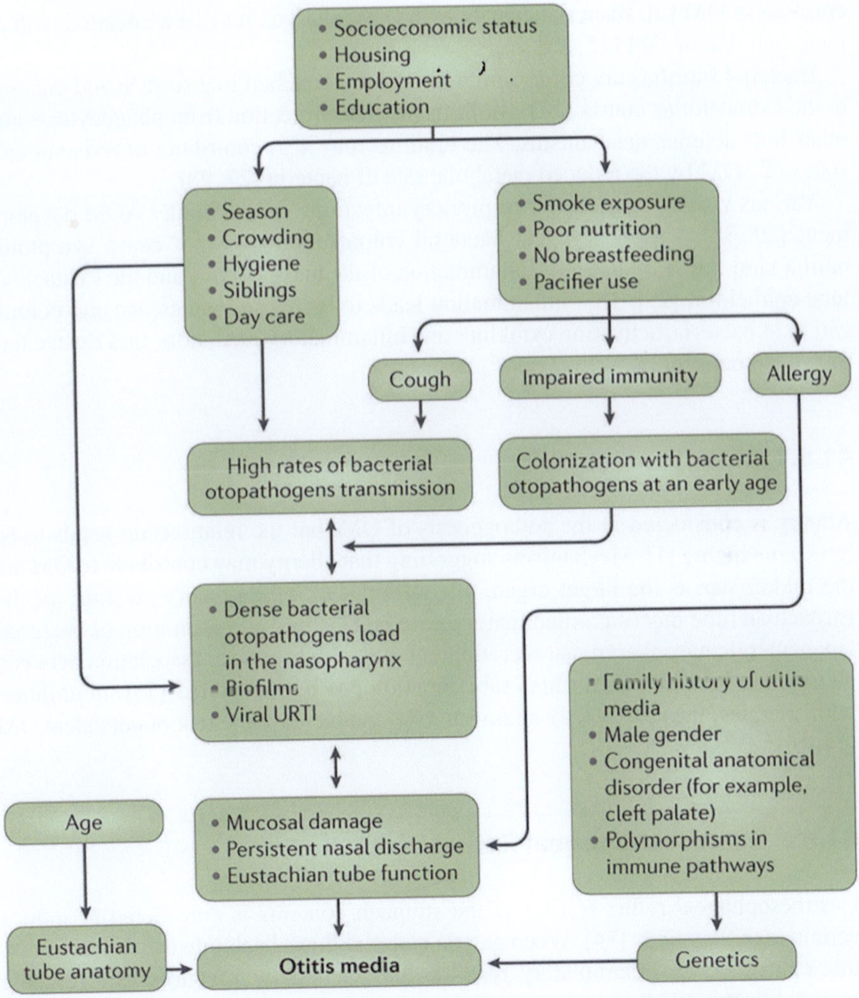

Fig. 41.1 Mechanisms and causal pathways for otitis media. The diagram shows that host and environmental factors put children at risk for otitis media through various mechanisms

In children with craniofacial abnormalities, the main factor underlying the chronic middle-ear inflammation appears to be impairment of the Eustachian tube functions [1, 14, 24].

41.5 Bacterial and Viral Infection

Streptococcus pneumoniae, nontypeable *Haemophilus influenzae*, and *Moraxella catarrhalis* are the most common bacterial pathogens in OM [25]. These pathogens also cause bacterial colonization in the middle ear. Early colonization of the nasopharynx with bacterial pathogens considerably increases the risk of subsequent episodes of OM [2]. Bacterial density in the nasopharynx may be associated with an increased risk of OM [25, 26].

Bacterial biofilms are colonization of bacteria attached to a surface and encased in the extracellular matrix [27]. Biofilms provide protection from phagocytosis and other host defense mechanisms. The biofilms may also contribute to resistant episodes of AOM by the reduced metabolic rate of bacteria [27, 28].

Various viruses cause upper respiratory infections, which induce AOM development [29, 30]. Nasopharyngeal bacterial colonization does not cause symptoms until a viral infection initiates inflammation of the nasopharynx and the Eustachian tube epithelium [29]. This inflammation leads to increasing adherence and colonization of bacteria, activating cytokines and inflammatory mediators, and Eustachian tube dysfunction [31, 32].

41.5.1 Allergy

Allergy is considered in the pathogenesis of OM, but the relationship needs to be more convincing [1]. Mechanisms suggesting that allergy may contribute to OM are the middle ear as the target organ, allergy-induced inflammatory swelling of the Eustachian tube mucosa, inflammatory nose congestion, and aspiration of bacteria-laden allergic nasopharyngeal secretion into the middle ear. An association between allergy and impaired Eustachian tube function has been reported [33]. In children with allergies, the allergy may aggravate OM and increase the risk of persistent OM [14–16].

41.6 Gastroesophageal Reflux Disease

Gastroesophageal reflux (GER) of the stomach contents is considered to induce certain manifestations [34]. When gastric material flows back into the nasopharynx, this can cause an inflammatory reaction and secondary infection. The refluxed material in the middle ear cavity causes inflammation of the Eustachian tube and middle ear mucosa. This inflammation results in impaired mucociliary clearance and ventilatory function of the Eustachian tube, resulting in chronic otitis media [34–36].

A recent metaanalysis suggested a significant association between OME and GER disease [37].

41.6.1 Diagnosis

AOM diagnosis is based on otoscopic findings of inflammation with symptoms and can be further assessed using a symptom severity scale [2].

OME is diagnosed by pneumatic otoscopy, with acoustic reflectometry and tympanometry as valuable adjunct measures [2].

According to the 2013 American Academy of Pediatrics guidelines suggestions, the diagnosis of AOM should be made in children presenting with [2] new-onset otorrhea not caused by otitis externa or moderate to severe bulging of the tympanic membrane, ear pain that started in the last 48 h and mild bulging of the tympanic membrane or intense tympanic membrane erythema.

41.6.2 Symptoms

Symptoms of AOM are variable, especially in infants and young children, even though there may be no symptoms. Systemic symptoms (nausea, irritability, sleep disturbance, and loss of appetite) and upper respiratory tract infection symptoms also can be seen [1, 2]. The Acute Otitis Media Severity of Symptom (AOM-SOS) scale is a parent-reported measure of AOM severity. It is used to rate severity and follows the course of the disease and outcomes [38].

Ear pain: Ear pain (otalgia) is the most consistent symptom of AOM. In young children, evidence of ear pain may be manifested by irritability or a change in sleeping or appetite and holding or tugging at the ear.

Fever: It is one of the most common symptoms of AOM. Fever may occasionally be the only sign of AOM.

Otorrhea: Rupture of the TM with purulent otorrhea is uncommon (Fig. 41.2).

41.6.3 Otoscopy

Bulging of the tympanic membrane, visualized by otoscopy, is a key diagnostic feature of AOM. The clinician can assess and record the tympanic membrane's color, opacity, position, and integrity by performing an otoscopy [1, 2, 39] (Fig. 41.2).

Pneumatic otoscopy is the primary diagnostic method for OME with high diagnostic accuracy. In pneumatic otoscopy, impaired tympanic membrane motility is highly predictive of OME [2, 40].

41.6.4 Tympanometry

Tympanometry is an objective, simple, and rapid measure of middle ear mobility and function [41]. The tympanometry assesses tympanic membrane compliance with a graph, showing how energy admitted to the ear canal is reflected in an internal microphone while the canal pressure varies from negative to positive.

41.6.5 Acoustic Reflectometry

Acoustic reflectometry measures how much sound is reflected off the tympanic membrane. Higher reflectivity levels indicate a greater probability of effusion. It evaluates only the effusion, not the middle ear function [42].

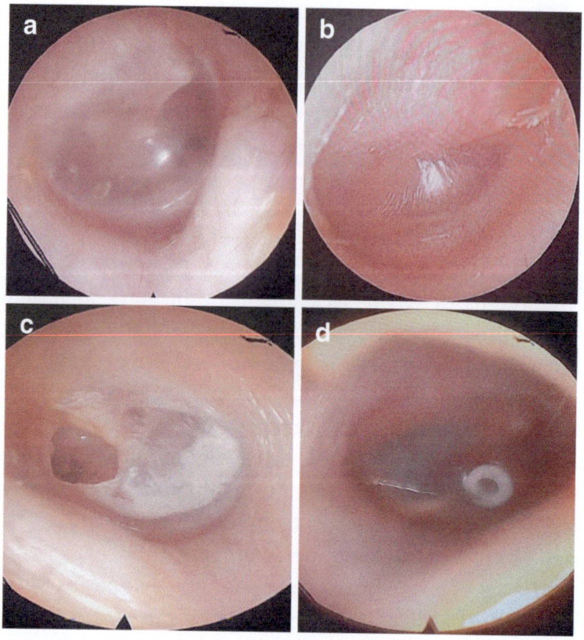

Fig. 41.2 Otoscopic findings. (**a**) Normal tympanic membrane. (**b**) Red and bulging tympanic membrane indicative of acute otitis media. (**c**) Perforated tympanic membrane. (**d**) Presence of a ventilation tube in the tympanic membrane

41.6.6 Management

41.6.6.1 Acute Otitis Media

Acetaminophen and paracetamol are recommended to relieve ear pain, fever, and irritability [1, 2].

Topical and oral decongestants, antihistamines, and corticosteroids have not been proven effective in resolving symptoms of AOM [1, 2].

Antibiotics should be routinely prescribed for infants under 6 months old (even with suspicion of AOM), children older than 6 months with severe signs and symptoms, and children younger than 2 years with bilateral AOM [2].

Watchful waiting or delayed antibiotic prescription is recommended for unilateral or bilateral OM in children older than 2 years with mild symptoms [2]. Watchful waiting includes careful monitoring by caregivers of the course of illness with advice to return if symptoms persist or the child's condition worsens [1, 2].

First-line antibiotic treatment includes 10 days of amoxicillin (80–90 mg/kg/day in divided doses) with or without clavulanic acid. In patients with penicillin allergy, cefdinir, cefuroxime, or clarithromycin can be chosen as first-line treatment [2].

41.6.6.2 Otitis Media with Effusion

Antibiotics, decongestants, and nasal steroids are not recommended in treating OME [2].

Children with OME who are not at particular risk for speech, language, or learning problems are recommended to follow-up every 3-month period [2, 40].

Ventilation tubes (tympanostomy tubes) are an appropriate option for children with bilateral OME for 3 months or longer with documented hearing difficulties. Children with recurrent AOM with evidence of middle ear effusion at the assessment time are also appropriate for the ventilation tubes.

Children with chronic OME who did not receive tubes should be reevaluated every 3–6 months until the effusion is no longer present or complications are detected [2, 40].

Adenoidectomy as a standalone operation or addition to ventilation tube insertion is most beneficial in children with OME ≥4 years of age [43].

41.7 Asthma

Asthma is a chronic respiratory condition characterized by recurring episodes of airflow obstruction, inflammation, and hyperresponsiveness of the airway [44]. Around 14% of children worldwide have a diagnosis of asthma, making it the most common chronic respiratory disease of childhood, making it a substantial public health concern [44].

41.7.1 Pathophysiology and Pathogenesis

The primary underlying pathology involves chronic inflammation of the airways. The airway lining becomes inflamed in response to various triggers, leading to swelling and increased mucus production [44]. The contraction of the muscles surrounding the airways also contributes to the narrowing passage of the airflow [44, 45].

Pediatric asthma is a multifactorial condition influenced by genetic, environmental, and immunological factors [46]. Asthma risk factors are personal or family history of atopy (eczema, allergic rhinitis, or nasal polyposis), family history of asthma, exposure to tobacco smoke, preterm birth, low birth weight, obesity, mold and dampness, and air pollution [45, 46].

Asthma may be triggered by a wide range of factors, including allergens (pollens, dust mites, animal dander, mold spores, and cockroach droppings), viral respiratory tract infections, irritants (exposure to tobacco smoke, air pollution), exercise, GERD, obesity, certain medications (beta-blockers, aspirin), atopic conditions (eczema, allergic rhinitis), and psychosocial factors (stress, anxiety, and depression) [46–48].

41.7.2 Diagnosis

There is no gold-standard test that accurately diagnoses asthma. Diagnosis should be made based on characteristic symptom patterns, evidence of variability in airflow limitation, and treatment response [46]. Therefore, diagnosis involves assessing physical examination, medical history, and spirometry [46]. The classic symptoms of asthma, including wheezing, shortness of breath, coughing, and chest tightness, are the results of these processes. Severe symptoms and life-threatening attacks may occur in some children [49]. Subsequently, identifying asthma phenotypes, such as allergic, eosinophilic, or viral-triggered, informs targeted treatment plans [45].

41.7.3 Management

The asthma management aims to achieve optimal control of symptoms and prevent exacerbations [45, 50]. A personalized action plan should be performed for the management. This plan includes daily medication and steps to take during worsening symptoms or emergencies [45, 50].

If triggers are defined, avoiding them is essential [48].

Short-acting bronchodilators (salbutamol albuterol) are used for rapid relief of symptoms [50].

Inhaled corticosteroids are the most effective medications for reducing inflammation and preventing symptoms. They are long-term control medications that can combine with long-acting beta-agonists (formoterol, salmeterol) [50].

Leukotriene modifiers and immunomodulators are also long-term disease control medication options [45, 50].

41.8 Otitis Media and Comorbid Asthma

Otitis media and asthma are among the most common childhood diseases. The relationship between these two diseases is controversial and still debated. Many studies proposed an association between otitis media and asthma [51, 52].

Early-life OM was found to be positively associated with school-age asthma [51, 53–55]. Recurrence of OM might increase the risk of asthma [52, 54, 55]. The risk of occurrence and recurrence of OM was found to be higher in asthmatic children than in healthy controls in a recent study [52]. OM could be a predictive factor for asthma in children [52].

41.8.1 Possible Mechanism and Pathogenesis

Multiple pathophysiologies might be involved in the relationship between asthma and otitis media in children. Eustachian tube dysfunction and airway inflammation might impact the relationship between repeated otitis media and asthma in children [52].

41.8.2 Eustachian Tube Dysfunction

In asthmatic children, the inflammation and mucosal swelling of the airway, including the Eustachian tube, could narrow the Eustachian tube, increasing susceptibility to otitis media [56, 57].

Lower airway inflammation in asthma occurs due to T helper type 1 and T helper type 2 (Th2) immune responses according to asthma types [45, 46].

This airway inflammation may induce the inflammation of the Eustachian tube mucosa, interrupting the ventilation of the middle ear. Moreover, recurrent wheezing and airway secretions in asthma patients could physically obstruct the Eustachian tube [56, 57]. This obstruction initiates an inflammatory response that results in impaired mucociliary clearance and accumulation effusion into the tympanic cavity [24, 57].

The middle ear connects to the airway via the Eustachian tube. Especially in young children, the Eustachian tube immaturity could be more involved in the potential for the development of asthma in children with otitis media. The occurrence or recurrence of otitis media might increase the risk of asthma [51–57].

41.8.3 Infections and Inflammation

Asthma induces airway inflammation and may lead to viral and bacterial infection susceptibility, causing otitis media [45, 52]. A skewed Th2 immune response and eosinophilia could elevate the risk of eosinophilic otitis media in asthmatic children. Eosinophilic otitis media has middle ear effusion rich in eosinophils and is prevalent among asthma patients [58]. The Th2 immune response and eosinophilia extending to the middle ear might be one of the links between otitis media and asthma.

Asthma causes chronic inflammation of the airways and impaired mucociliary clearance, making the host more susceptible to pathogens [45, 46, 50]. This chronic inflammation results in increased mucus production, epithelium disruption, and modification in innate or adaptive immune responses [59].

On the other hand, middle ear inflammation in otitis media may be a risk for asthma due to the sharing airway. Many studies reported that airway respiratory infections in early childhood have increased the risk of asthma [59–62]. Recurrent airway infections in childhood could compromise airway immunity and change the airway microbiome, thereby increasing the risk of asthma [63, 64].

Opportunistic viral or bacterial infection might contribute to the reciprocal relationship between otitis media and asthma in children [52].

41.9 Conclusion

Many studies proposed an association between otitis media and asthma. Clinicians should consider the possibility of asthma in children presenting with recurrent or chronic otitis media. Conversely, children with asthma should be monitored for signs and complications of otitis media. Asthma in children with otitis media may complicate the clinical picture. Children with both conditions might experience more severe symptoms during ear infections, as the underlying inflammation from asthma can exacerbate the discomfort associated with otitis media.

A comprehensive understanding of this relationship is essential for healthcare providers to effectively manage these conditions, ensuring the best possible outcomes for their young patients' health and quality of life. Future research should focus on elucidating the precise mechanisms driving their interaction.

References

1. Schilder AG, Chonmaitree T, Cripps AW, et al. Otitis media. Nat Rev Dis Primers. 2016;2(1):16063. https://doi.org/10.1038/nrdp.2016.63.
2. Lieberthal AS, Carroll AE, Chonmaitree T, et al. The diagnosis and management of acute otitis media. Pediatrics. 2014;133(2):346. https://doi.org/10.1542/peds.2012-3488.
3. Teele DW, Klein JO, Rosner B. Epidemiology of otitis media during the first seven years of life in children in greater Boston: a prospective, cohort study. J Infect Dis. 1989;160(1):83–94. https://doi.org/10.1093/infdis/160.1.83.
4. Kaur R, Morris M, Pichichero ME. Epidemiology of acute otitis media in the postpneumococcal conjugate vaccine era. Pediatrics. 2017;140(3):e20170181. https://doi.org/10.1542/peds.2017-0181.
5. Thompson PL, Gilbert RE, Long PF, Saxena S, Sharland M, Wong IC. Has UK guidance affected general practitioner antibiotic prescribing for otitis media in children? J Public Health (Oxf). 2008;30(4):479–86. https://doi.org/10.1093/pubmed/fdn072.
6. Coker TR, Chan LS, Newberry SJ, et al. Diagnosis, microbial epidemiology, and antibiotic treatment of acute otitis media in children: a systematic review. JAMA. 2010;304(19):2161–9. https://doi.org/10.1001/jama.2010.1651.
7. Leibovitz E. Acute otitis media in pediatric medicine: current issues in epidemiology, diagnosis, and management. Paediatr Drugs. 2003;5:1–12.
8. Aarhus L, Tambs K, Kvestad E, Engdahl B. Childhood otitis media: a cohort study with 30-year follow-up of hearing (the HUNT study). Ear Hear. 2015;36(3):302–8. https://doi.org/10.1097/AUD.0000000000000118.
9. Blanc F, Ayache D, Calmels MN, et al. Management of otitis media with effusion in children. Société française d'ORL et de chirurgie cervico-faciale clinical practice guidelines. Eur Ann Otorhinolaryngol Head Neck Dis. 2018;135(4):269–73. https://doi.org/10.1016/j.anorl.2018.04.008.
10. Bluestone CD, Klein JO. Otitis media in infants and children. PMPH-USA; 2007.
11. Casselbrant ML, Mandel EM. Diagnosis and management of otitis media. In: Pereira K, Mitchell R, editors. Pediatric otolaryngology for the clinician. Totowa: Humana Press; 2009. https://doi.org/10.1007/978-1-60327-127-1_7.
12. Daly KA, Brown WM, Segade F, et al. Chronic and recurrent otitis media: a genome scan for susceptibility loci. Am J Hum Genet. 2004;75(6):988–97. https://doi.org/10.1086/426061.
13. Casselbrant ML, Mandel EM, Fall PA, et al. The heritability of otitis media: a twin and triplet study. JAMA. 1999;282(22):2125–30. https://doi.org/10.1001/jama.282.22.2125.
14. Otteson T. Otitis media and tympanostomy tubes. Pediatr Clin North Am. 2022;69(2):203–19. https://doi.org/10.1016/j.pcl.2022.01.001.
15. Kwon C, Lee HY, Kim MG, Boo SH, Yeo SG. Allergic diseases in children with otitis media with effusion. Int J Pediatr Otorhinolaryngol. 2013;77(2):158–61. https://doi.org/10.1016/j.ijporl.2012.09.039.
16. Luong A, Roland PS. The link between allergic rhinitis and chronic otitis media with effusion in atopic patients. Otolaryngol Clin North Am. 2008;41(2):311–vi. https://doi.org/10.1016/j.otc.2007.11.004.
17. Smith DF, Boss EF. Racial/ethnic and socioeconomic disparities in the prevalence and treatment of otitis media in children in the United States. Laryngoscope. 2010;120(11):2306–12. https://doi.org/10.1002/lary.21090.

18. Bowatte G, Tham R, Allen KJ, et al. Breastfeeding and childhood acute otitis media: a systematic review and meta-analysis. Acta Paediatr. 2015;104(467):85–95. https://doi.org/10.1111/apa.13151.
19. Fiellau-Nikolajsen M. Tympanometry in 3-year-old children. Type of care as an epidemiological factor in secretory otitis media and tubal dysfunction in unselected populations of 3-year-old children. ORL J Otorhinolaryngol Relat Spec. 1979;41(4):193–205. https://doi.org/10.1159/000275459.
20. Tarhun YM. The effect of passive smoking on the etiology of serous otitis media in children. Am J Otolaryngol. 2020;41(3):102398. https://doi.org/10.1016/j.amjoto.2020.102398.
21. Erdivanli OC, Coskun ZO, Kazikdas KC, Demirci M. Prevalence of otitis media with effusion among primary school children in eastern Black Sea, in Turkey and the effect of smoking in the development of otitis media with effusion. Indian J Otolaryngol Head Neck Surg. 2012;64(1):17–21. https://doi.org/10.1007/s12070-011-0131-z.
22. Heikkinen T, Thint M, Chonmaitree T. Prevalence of various respiratory viruses in the middle ear during acute otitis media. N Engl J Med. 1999;340(4):260–4. https://doi.org/10.1056/NEJM199901283400402.
23. Niemelä M, Pihakari O, Pokka T, Uhari M. Pacifier as a risk factor for acute otitis media: a randomized, controlled trial of parental counseling. Pediatrics. 2000;106(3):483–8. https://doi.org/10.1542/peds.106.3.483.
24. Bluestone CD, Tunkel DE, Grundfast KM. Pediatric otolaryngology. Pediatr Clin North Am. 2003;50(2):xiii–xiv. https://doi.org/10.1016/S0031-3955(03)00035-X.
25. Watson K, Carville K, Bowman J, et al. Upper respiratory tract bacterial carriage in aboriginal and non-aboriginal children in a semi-arid area of Western Australia. Pediatr Infect Dis J. 2006;25(9):782–90. https://doi.org/10.1097/01.inf.0000232705.49634.68.
26. Smith-Vaughan H, Byun R, Nadkarni M, et al. Measuring nasal bacterial load and its association with otitis media. BMC Ear Nose Throat Disord. 2006;6:10. https://doi.org/10.1186/1472-6815-6-10.
27. García-Cobos S, Moscoso M, Pumarola F, et al. Frequent carriage of resistance mechanisms to β-lactams and biofilm formation in Haemophilus influenzae causing treatment failure and recurrent otitis media in young children. J Antimicrob Chemother. 2014;69(9):2394–9. https://doi.org/10.1093/jac/dku158.
28. Hall-Stoodley L, Hu FZ, Gieseke A, et al. Direct detection of bacterial biofilms on the middle-ear mucosa of children with chronic otitis media. JAMA. 2006;296(2):202–11. https://doi.org/10.1001/jama.296.2.202.
29. Nokso-Koivisto J, Marom T, Chonmaitree T. Importance of viruses in acute otitis media. Curr Opin Pediatr. 2015;27(1):110–5. https://doi.org/10.1097/MOP.0000000000000184.
30. Chonmaitree T. Viral upper respiratory tract infection and otitis media complication in young children. Clin Infect Dis. 2008;46:815–23. https://doi.org/10.1086/528685.
31. Patel JA, Nair S, Revai K, Grady J, Chonmaitree T. Nasopharyngeal acute phase cytokines in viral upper respiratory infection: impact on acute otitis media in children. Pediatr Infect Dis J. 2009;28(11):1002–7. https://doi.org/10.1097/INF.0b013e3181aa5b13.
32. Bakaletz LO. Immunopathogenesis of polymicrobial otitis media. J Leukoc Biol. 2010;87(2):213–22. https://doi.org/10.1189/jlb.0709518.
33. Hurst DS, Denne CM. The relation of allergy to Eustachian tube dysfunction and the subsequent need for insertion of pressure equalization tubes. Ear Nose Throat J. 2020;99(1_suppl):39S–47S. https://doi.org/10.1177/0145561320918805.
34. Miura MS, Mascaro M, Rosenfeld RM. Association between otitis media and gastroesophageal reflux: a systematic review. Otolaryngol Head Neck Surg. 2012;146(3):345–52. https://doi.org/10.1177/0194599811430809.
35. White DR, Heavner SB, Hardy SM, Prazma J. Gastroesophageal reflux and eustachian tube dysfunction in an animal model. Laryngoscope. 2002;112(6):955–61. https://doi.org/10.1097/00005537-200206000-00004.

36. Poelmans J, Tack J, Feenstra L. Prospective study on the incidence of chronic ear complaints related to gastroesophageal reflux and on the outcome of antireflux therapy. Ann Otol Rhinol Laryngol. 2002;111(10):933–8. https://doi.org/10.1177/000348940211101013.
37. Wu ZH, Tang Y, Niu X, Sun HY, Chen X. The relationship between otitis media with effusion and gastroesophageal reflux disease: a meta-analysis. Otol Neurotol. 2021;42(3):e245–53. https://doi.org/10.1097/MAO.0000000000002945.
38. Shaikh N, Hoberman A, Paradise JL, et al. Responsiveness and construct validity of a symptom scale for acute otitis media. Pediatr Infect Dis J. 2009;28(1):9–12. https://doi.org/10.1097/INF.0b013e318185a3a0.
39. Shaikh N. Otoscopic signs of otitis media. Pediatr Infect Dis J. 2011;30:822–6. https://doi.org/10.1097/INF.0b013e31822e6637.
40. Rosenfeld RM, Shin JJ, Schwartz SR, et al. Clinical practice guideline: otitis media with effusion (update). Otolaryngol Head Neck Surg. 2016;154(1 Suppl):S1–S41. https://doi.org/10.1177/0194599815623467.
41. Onusko E. Tympanometry. Am Fam Physician. 2004;70(9):1713–20.
42. Erkkola-Anttinen N, Laine MK, Tähtinen PA, Ruohola A. Parental role in the diagnostics of otitis media: can layman parents use spectral gradient acoustic reflectometry reliably? Int J Pediatr Otorhinolaryngol. 2015;79(9):1516–21. https://doi.org/10.1016/j.ijporl.2015.06.040.
43. Boonacker CW. Adenoidectomy with or without grommets for children with otitis media: an individual patient data meta-analysis. Health Technol Assess. 2014;18:1–118. https://doi.org/10.3310/hta18050.
44. Zar HJ, Ferkol TW. The global burden of respiratory disease-impact on child health. Pediatr Pulmonol. 2014;49:430–4. https://doi.org/10.1002/ppul.23030.
45. Martin J, Townshend J, Brodlie M. Diagnosis and management of asthma in children. BMJ Paediatr Open. 2022;6(1):e001277. https://doi.org/10.1136/bmjpo-2021-001277.
46. Tarasidis GS, Wilson KF. Diagnosis of asthma: clinical assessment. Int Forum Allergy Rhinol. 2015;5(Suppl 1):S23–6. https://doi.org/10.1002/alr.21518.
47. Win PH, Hussain I. Asthma triggers: what really matters? Clin Asthma. 2008:149–156.
48. Gautier C, Charpin D. Environmental triggers and avoidance in the management of asthma. J Asthma Allergy. 2017;10:47–56. https://doi.org/10.2147/JAA.S121276.
49. FitzGerald JM, Barnes PJ, Chipps BE, et al. The burden of exacerbations in mild asthma: a systematic review. ERJ Open Res. 2020;6:00359–2019. https://doi.org/10.1183/23120541.00359-2019.
50. Bush A, Pavord ID. The Lancet Asthma Commission: treating children in primary care. Prescriber. 2018;29:28–32. https://doi.org/10.1002/psb.1719.
51. MacIntyre EA, Heinrich J. Otitis media in infancy and the development of asthma and atopic disease. Curr Allergy Asthma Rep. 2012;12(6):547–50. https://doi.org/10.1007/s11882-012-0308-x.
52. Kim SY, Kim HR, Min C, Choi HG. Bidirectional association between asthma and otitis media in children. Allergy Asthma Clin Immunol. 2021;17(1):7. https://doi.org/10.1186/s13223-020-00500-7.
53. Eldeirawi K, Persky VW. History of ear infections and prevalence of asthma in a national sample of children aged 2 to 11 years: the third National Health and Nutrition Examination Survey, 1988 to 1994. Chest. 2004;125(5):1685–92. https://doi.org/10.1378/chest.125.5.1685.
54. Nafstad P, Magnus P, Jaakkola JJ. Early respiratory infections and childhood asthma. Pediatrics. 2000;106:E38. https://doi.org/10.1542/peds.106.3.e38.
55. Nafstad P, Brunekreef B, Skrondal A, Nystad W. Early respiratory infections, asthma, and allergy: 10-year follow-up of the Oslo Birth Cohort. Pediatrics. 2005;116(2):e255–62. https://doi.org/10.1542/peds.2004-2785.
56. Juszczak HM, Loftus PA. Role of allergy in Eustachian tube dysfunction. Curr Allergy Asthma Rep. 2020;20(10):54. https://doi.org/10.1007/s11882-020-00951-3.
57. Cunsolo E, Marchioni D, Leo G, Incorvaia C, Presutti L. Functional anatomy of the Eustachian tube. Int J Immunopathol Pharmacol. 2010;23(1 Suppl):4–7.

58. Seo Y, Nonaka M, Tagaya E, Tamaoki J, Yoshihara T. Eosinophilic otitis media is associated with asthma severity and smoking history. ORL J Otorhinolaryngol Relat Spec. 2015;77(1):1–9. https://doi.org/10.1159/000370122.
59. Hartert TV. Are persons with asthma at increased risk of pneumococcal infections, and can we prevent them? J Allergy Clin Immunol. 2008;122(4):724–5. https://doi.org/10.1016/j.jaci.2008.09.008.
60. Toivonen L, Forsström V, Waris M, Peltola V. Acute respiratory infections in early childhood and risk of asthma at age 7 years. J Allergy Clin Immunol. 2019;143(1):407–410.e6. https://doi.org/10.1016/j.jaci.2018.08.025.
61. van Meel ER, den Dekker HT, Elbert NJ, et al. A population-based prospective cohort study examining the influence of early-life respiratory tract infections on school-age lung function and asthma. Thorax. 2018;73(2):167–73. https://doi.org/10.1136/thoraxjnl-2017-210149.
62. Bønnelykke K, Vissing NH, Sevelsted A, Johnston SL, Bisgaard H. Association between respiratory infections in early life and later asthma is independent of virus type. J Allergy Clin Immunol. 2015;136(1):81–86.e4. https://doi.org/10.1016/j.jaci.2015.02.024.
63. Feldman AS, He Y, Moore ML, Hershenson MB, Hartert TV. Toward primary prevention of asthma. Reviewing the evidence for early-life respiratory viral infections as modifiable risk factors to prevent childhood asthma. Am J Respir Crit Care Med. 2015;191(1):34–44. https://doi.org/10.1164/rccm.201405-0901PP.
64. Teo SM, Mok D, Pham K, et al. The infant nasopharyngeal microbiome impacts severity of lower respiratory infection and risk of asthma development. Cell Host Microbe. 2015;17(5):704–15. https://doi.org/10.1016/j.chom.2015.03.008.

Pneumonia in Children and Comorbid Rhinosinusitis

42

Gökçen Kartal Öztürk, Zorika Zivkovic, and Demet Can

42.1 Pneumonia in Children

Pneumonia is usually defined as acute inflammation of the lung parenchyma. Although hospital-acquired pneumonia and immunocompromised pneumonia are defined, in the childhood age group, community-acquired pneumonia (CAP) is the most common subtype. The definition of CAP varies among the different guidelines but is usually used for pneumonia caused by an infection acquired outside the hospital in a previously healthy child [1–4].

42.1.1 Epidemiology

CAP is the major infectious disease cause of death in children worldwide, with the deaths of 740,180 children younger than 5 years of age in 2019. It is responsible for 22% of all deaths in children aged 1–5 years and constitutes an important preventable health problem, especially in low- and middle-income countries [5].

The incidence of pneumonia varies regionally depending on vaccination status and diagnostic criteria. In a worldwide burden of childhood pneumonia series, the incidence of episodes per child aged 0–4 years was reported for the American,

G. K. Öztürk (✉)
Department of Pediatrics Pulmonology, Ege University, Faculty of Medicine, Izmir, Turkey

Z. Zivkovic
Faculty of Pharmacy in Novi Sad, University Business Academy, Novi Sad, Serbia

Medical Center "Dr Dragisa Misovic", Children's Hospital for Lung Diseases and Tuberculosis, Belgrade, Serbia

D. Can
Department of Pediatric Pulmonology and Pediatric Allergy, University of Health Sciences Turkey, İzmir Faculty of Medicine, Dr. Behçet Uz Children's Hospital, İzmir, Turkey

H. Yüksel et al. (eds.), *Pediatric Airway Diseases*, Comprehensive ENT,
https://doi.org/10.1007/978-3-031-74853-0_42

European, and global regions as 0.08 (0.04–0.18), 0.19 (0.10–0.44), and 0.03 (0.02–0.04), respectively. The regions of Southeast Asia [0.26 (0.13–0.61)] and Africa [0.27 (0.14–0.63)] had the highest incidence [6].

Despite the mortality rate that decreases with the years, 80% of deaths from pneumonia occur in the first 2 years of age. The majority of deaths were in sub-Saharan African regions [6, 7]. With the improvement in diagnostic tests, antimicrobial treatments, and preventive immunization strategies, childhood pneumonia mortality rates decreased in all age groups. However, CAP is still the most common cause of pediatric emergency department visits and hospitalization in developed countries. In a multicenter study in the United States (US), the annual incidence of hospital admissions due to pneumonia was 15.7/10,000 children [8].

42.1.2 Risk Factors

Various risk factors can affect both the frequency and severity of pneumonia. In a meta-analysis of risk factors for severe pneumonia in children under 5 years of age, seven definite risk factors (low birth weight, lack of breastfeeding, undernutrition, indoor air pollution, crowding, incomplete immunization, and HIV infection) were determined. Moreover, lack of maternal education, parental smoking, male sex, preterm births, vitamin D deficiency, anemia, and zinc deficiency were detected as likely risk factors. Daycare, birth interval (<24 months), birth order (>3 pregnancies), previous history of acute lower respiratory infections, and vitamin A deficiency were identified as possible risk factors [9].

42.1.3 Etiology

Pneumonia can be caused by different pathogens most prominently viruses and bacteria; however, determining the etiology is often difficult in children because invasive diagnostic samples are not preferred in most centers.

According to age groups and immunization status, different pathogens may come to the fore in etiology (Table 42.1). Viruses are more foremost in children under 2 years of age, and bacterial pathogens cause in older children. Despite a decrease in incidence with vaccination policies against *Streptococcus pneumoniae* and *Haemophilus influenzae*, they continue to be the most common bacterial pathogens in childhood pneumonia. In a multicenter prospective population-based surveillance study in the US, bacterial pathogens were detected in 15% of hospitalized children with CAP. Compared to previous etiological studies, the decreased incidence of bacterial pathogens in this study was suggested, reflects the vaccination with pneumococcal conjugate vaccine (PCV) and *Haemophilus influenzae* type B (HiB) [8]. There are many serotypes of pneumococci, and they have been associated with CAP in different regions. The 13-valent pneumococcal vaccine is effective against many important serotypes. In a study determining the etiology of CAP under 5 years of age in China between 2001 and 2015, the most frequently detected

Table 42.1 According to age groups most common causative pathogens in children with CAP [1, 2]

Age	
Newborns	Enteric Gram-negative bacteria Group B Streptococcus
İnfant	Viruses *Streptococcus pneumoniae* *Haemophilus influenzae* *Moraxella catarrhalis* *Staphylococcus aureus* *Chlamydia trachomatis* *Bordetella pertussis*
<5 years children	Viruses *Streptococcus pneumoniae* *Haemophilus influenzae* *Moraxella catarrhalis* *Staphylococcus aureus* Group A streptococcus *Chlamydia pneumonia* *Mycoplasma pneumonia*
>5 years children	Viruses *Chlamydia pneumonia* *Mycoplasma pneumonia* *Streptococcus pneumoniae* *Haemophilus influenzae*

bacterial pathogens were *Klebsiella pneumoniae* (5.4%), *Streptococcus pneumoniae* (5.2%), *Escherichia coli* (5.2%), *Staphylococcus aureus* (3.9%), *Haemophilus influenza* (3.6%), and *Haemophilus parainfluenzae* (3.3%) [10].

In recent years, *Staphylococcus aureus* was noted in the increased frequency of the etiology of complicated pneumonia in hospitalized children [11]. The prevalence of community-acquired methicillin-resistant *Staphylococcus aureus* pneumonia has increased in the past decade and has commonly been associated with hospitalized complicated pneumonia and severe disease [11, 12].

Chlamydia pneumonia and *Mycoplasma pneumonia* infections occur more often in CAP with school-age children [1, 2]. In a meta-analysis of the prevalence of atypical pathogens in CAP, the prevalence of *M. pneumoniae* (peak at 6 years of age) was 10.1% (7.1–13.1%) and *C. pneumoniae* was 3.5% (2.2–4.9%) [13]. Viral and bacterial pathogen coinfections and two or more viruses were documented in approximately 30% of CAP [14].

Respiratory syncytial virus and *Rhinovirus* are the most common viral pathogens in CAP. Other viruses such as adenoviruses, influenza A and B, parainfluenza, bocavirus, human metapneumovirus, and coronaviruses are detected in about 10% of CAP. In a meta-analysis representing 152,209 children with CAP, it was reported that one or more respiratory viruses were detected in 50% of CAP, and nonsignificant variation in the prevalence of CAP was found by the country's national income, under 5 years mortality rate, and World Health Organization (WHO) regions [15].

Mycobacterium tuberculosis is increasingly detected in childhood pneumonia and is a cause of morbidity and mortality in high-endemic areas. Children with comorbid disease (asthma, neurological and cardiological diseases, immunodeficiency, and congenital lung diseases, etc.) have a higher incidence of pneumonia and various etiologic pathogens (Gram-negative bacilli, nontypeable *H. influenzae*, cytomegalovirus, etc.) may be causative pathogens in this group.

42.1.4 Clinical Features and Diagnosis

The clinical manifestation of pneumonia varies depending on age, etiologic pathogens, and disease severity and may occasionally be unclear, especially in infants. Common signs and symptoms are fever, cough, tachypnea, retractions, breathlessness, and chest pain. Other nonspecific symptoms, such as low-grade fever, abdominal pain, vomiting, malaise, myalgia, or headache occur especially in pneumonia caused by viruses or atypical pathogens. Rales, crackles, decreased breath sounds in consolidation areas, and bronchial breath sounds may be present in lung auscultation. The normal auscultation findings do not rule out pneumonia [16]. The presence of hypoxia positively correlates with the severity of pneumonia and is one of the most beneficial findings in the diagnosis of pneumonia [1].

The WHO recommends using tachypnea and retractions to diagnose pneumonia in children younger than 5 years. While children with tachypnea were classified as "pneumonia," children who had retractions with or without tachypnea were classified as "severe pneumonia." Children with danger signs and symptoms (lethargy, respiratory distress, apnea, dehydration, toxic appearance, seizures, and cyanosis, etc.) were classified as "severe pneumonia or very severe disease" [5]. Definitions for mild, moderate, and severe pneumonia vary in the literature, further complicating the validation of the development of standardized severity criteria.

These signs and symptoms are nonspecific and are not sufficient to diagnose pneumonia. In a systematic review of 23 prospective cohort studies (13,833 children), fever (temperature >37.5 °C) and tachypnea (respiratory rate >40 breaths/min) were not associated strongly with pneumonia. The presence of moderate hypoxemia (oxygen saturation ≤96%) and increased work of breathing (grunting, flaring, and retractions) were the most associated signs with pneumonia. No single symptom and auscultation findings were found associated with pneumonia diagnosis [17].

42.1.5 Laboratory Tests

Laboratory tests [white blood cell counts, absolute neutrophil count, C-reactive protein (CRP), and erythrocyte sedimentation rate (ESR)] are not useful for diagnosing pneumonia and determining the etiology, and should not be performed routinely [2]. The increase in these parameters is more suggestive of bacterial pathogens and may also be present in coinfection. Procalcitonin (PCT) may be the most effective test for determining bacterial CAP, evaluating the disease severity, and guiding the treatment [18, 19].

42.1.6 Imaging Techniques

In the guidelines, chest radiography is not routinely recommended for diagnosing pneumonia in outpatients. It should be slated for hospitalized patients and children with suspected inadequate treatment and pneumonia complications. Although radiographic findings may be normal in the early stages of the disease, consolidation and parenchymal infiltrates are observed. Alveolar infiltrates are more suggestive of CAP caused by bacterial pathogens, while interstitial infiltrations suggest viral or atypical pathogens [1, 2, 20] (Fig. 42.1). In a study to evaluate the association between consolidation and bacterial etiology of CAP, consolidation was observed in 74% of typical bacterial CAP, 58% in atypical bacterial CAP, and 54% in viral CAP. Positive and negative predictive value of consolidation for bacterial CAP were found at 12% and 96%, respectively [21].

Chest X-ray is insufficient to differentiate between viral and bacterial pathogens in CAP. Lateral X-rays are not routinely performed in diagnosing CAP because of further radiation and lack of superiority compared to anterior-posterior X-rays. In recent years, because of bedside use and no radiation exposure, lung ultrasound has been used for the diagnosis and follow-up of pneumonia [22]. In a meta-analysis to evaluate the accuracy of lung ultrasound compared to X-ray for the diagnosis of CAP, while specificity was similar to lung ultrasound and X-ray (95.3% and 98.2%), ultrasound had a significantly higher sensitivity (95.5–86.8%) [23]. Computed tomography (CT) is not a first-line imaging tool for diagnosis and may be considered when complications are suspected and there is difficulty in differentiating pneumonia from other diseases.

42.1.7 Microbiological Tests

Microbiological investigations for the etiology of CAP are difficult in children and are not routinely recommended in nonsevere patients due to low-grade sensitivity and high cost. Detection of the etiological pathogens can be made by microbiological demonstration of the pathogens (sputum, blood, lung tissue, aspiration, and pleural fluid cultures) and immunological and serological tests.

Gram staining and culture can be performed from sputum samples in older children and adolescents, while throat and nasopharyngeal aspirates and induced sputum sampling in younger children. Because many potential pathogenic microorganisms colonize the upper respiratory tract flora, the results should be considered when evaluating the tests. Blood culture is used for bacterial pathogens. The positivity rate is below 10% but increases up to 30% in the parapneumonic effusion. Therefore, the CAP guidelines recommend its use only in hospitalized patients. If

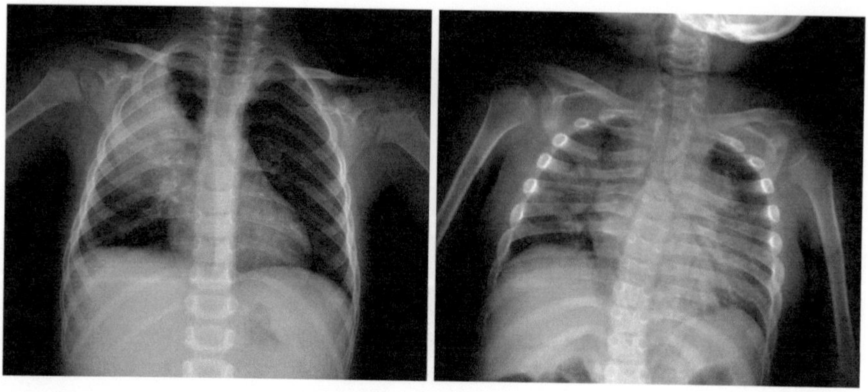

Fig. 42.1 Right upper lobe consolidation in a child with bacterial pneumonia (left image) and bilateral interstitial infiltrates and patchy atelectasis with adenovirus pneumonia (right image)

indicated, bronchoalveolar lavage (BAL) and pleural fluid cultures have higher positivity rates and provide more information about etiology in CAP [1–3, 24, 25].

The pneumococcal urinary antigen test is not useful in children with CAP due to high false-positive rates [26]. Rapid molecular diagnostic techniques [polymerase chain reaction (PCR)] can be performed on either viruses or bacterial pathogens in many diagnostic samples such as blood, sputum, nasopharyngeal secretions, BAL, and pleural fluids. Because of reasons such as conflicting results, low sensitivity and specificity, and the presence of colonization, the results should be interpreted with caution in children. Serologic testing for *M. pneumoniae* and *C. pneumoniae* requires a comparison of two samples at acute phase and convalescence, so is not usually useful for management [27].

42.1.8 Management

After a child is diagnosed with pneumonia, primarily must decide whether hospitalization is required. Children with nonsevere CAP can be managed at home. These children should be reexamined within 48 h after treatment started. If there is no significant improvement, children must be reviewed for diagnosis, treatment effectiveness, and presence of complications (pleural effusion, necrotizing pneumonia, and lung abscess) [1, 2, 28].

There are no validated pneumonia scoring systems in pediatric populations. Many guidelines have suggested definitions of severity and criteria for indications of hospitalization according to the clinical findings and appearance of the children (Table 42.2). In a systematic review of factors associated with pneumonia severity in children, age <3–6 months, altered mental status, hypoxemia, dyspnea, multilobar infiltrates, and moderate/large pleural effusions were found the most predictive factors of pneumonia severity in children [29]. A multicenter, prospective cohort study has developed a prediction model for severe outcomes. The most important

Table 42.2 Hospitalization criteria for a child with CAP [1, 2, 28]

Respiratory distress
Tachypnea[a]
Retractions
Nasal flaring
Grunting
Cyanosis
SO_2 <90–92%
Dyspnea, apnea
Vomiting, not feeding
Dehydration
Capillary refill time ≥2 min
Shock
Malnutrition
Etiological pathogens (MRSA, co-infections)
Comorbidities (e.g., chronic lung disease of prematurity, chronic respiratory conditions, congenital heart disease, and immunodeficiency)

[a]Adjusted with age

predictors in hospitalized children with CAP were age extremes, vital signs, chest indrawing, and radiographic infiltrate patterns [30].

Before starting treatment, patients are classified as mild-moderate and severe pneumonia according to the severity of the disease. Severe pneumonia is considered if at least one of the following criteria was present: SpO_2 <90% (in ambient air), impaired consciousness (tendency to sleep, lethargy, confusion, and unresponsiveness to painful stimulant), apnea, 2nd or 3rd stage intensive care or mechanical ventilation support requirement, excessive dehydration, and development of atelectasis or effusion [31].

General management for pneumonia includes antipyretics and, if needed, hydration, oxygen supplementation, and ventilation support. Studies have not recommended chest physiotherapy, mucolytic, and antitussive treatments due to no beneficial effects and no reliable conclusions [1, 32, 33].

Treatment decisions in children with CAP are made according to age, clinical, laboratory, and radiological findings, regional and seasonal prevalence of microorganisms, risk factors, disease severity, and antibiotic resistance. In outpatient treatments, antimicrobial therapy is not routinely recommended for <5-year-old children with CAP due to viral pathogens being responsible for the vast majority of diseases. Antibiotic treatment should be started for all children diagnosed with CAP when bacterial pathogens are considered or bacterial and viral pathogens cannot be reliably distinguished [2]. Various guidelines recommend that amoxicillin be used as first-line treatment in outpatient for previously healthy and appropriately vaccinated children with pneumonia caused by bacterial pathogens. Macrolides are also recommended as a first-line treatment if the child is allergic to penicillin or *M. pneumonia* and *C. pneumonia* are suspected pathogens in school-aged children and adolescents [34]. In outpatient treatments, the duration of antibiotic use is recommended 7–10 days. Studies have shown that a short-course (3 days) antibiotic treatment is as effective as a long-course (5 days) with rates of clinical cure, treatment failure, and relapse for non-severe pneumonia at <5 years of age [35]. In a retrospective cohort study from 2010 to 2016, short-course (5–9 days) and long-course (10–14 days) antibiotic therapy in outpatient children with CAP (n = 121,846) were compared. The most frequently prescribed antibiotic duration was 10 days (82.8% of prescriptions). There was no significant difference in the rates of hospitalization, new antibiotic prescriptions, and acute care visits between both groups [36]. The SAFER (Short-Course Antimicrobial Therapy for Pediatric Respiratory Infections) 2-center, parallel-group, randomized clinical trial study has shown that short-course (5 days) antibiotic therapy appeared to be comparable to standard-course for the treatment of previously healthy children with not hospitalized CAP [37]. Short (5 days)- and standard-course (10 days) outpatient antibiotic therapy in children with CAP were compared in a randomized, double-blind, placebo-controlled SCOUT-CAP clinical trial. The short-course therapy resulted in a similar clinical response and antibiotic-associated adverse effects while reducing antibiotic exposure and resistance [38].

In inpatient treatment, various guidelines recommend intravenous penicillin/ampicillin, amoxicillin-clavulanate, cefuroxime, and cefotaxime/ceftriaxone for severe pneumonia. The prevalence of penicillin and macrolide resistance is increasing and varies according to countries and regions. Avoiding unnecessary antibiotic use, choosing specific narrow-spectrum antibiotics, and using the appropriate duration of antimicrobial treatment are necessary to prevent antibiotic resistance. Macrolides are added to the treatment if *M. pneumonia* and *C. pneumonia* are suspected or no improvement or resolution of symptoms after 48 h. Vancomycin or clindamycin should be added if clinical, laboratory, or imaging findings are consistent with *S. aureus* infection. Antiviral therapy should be administered to children with severe CAP during the influenza season [1–3, 28, 39]. There are no data from randomized controlled trials and observational studies evaluating the optimal duration of treatment for inpatient treatment. Treatment periods of 10–14 days are generally recommended depending on the severity of the disease and recovery time. There are no randomized controlled trials with short- and long-course intravenous therapy for severe pneumonia in hospitalized children aged 2–59 months [40]. Oral therapy should be considered if there is clear evidence of improvement in a patient receiving intravenous antibiotic therapy such as increased activity and appetite, absence of fever for 12–24 h, and SO_2 >90–92% in room air.

In the evaluation 48–72 h after the start of treatment, if fever persists and there is no clinical response, it should be investigated whether the treatment failure, the presence of a resistant microorganism, the development of complications (pleural effusion, empyema, pneumatocele, necrotizing pneumonia, abscess, etc.) or immunosuppression or concomitant disease.

42.1.9 Prevention

Despite widespread vaccination policies, CAP still constitutes one of the most important preventable infections in childhood. Education, nutrition, the importance of breast milk, hand washing, improvement of crowded living conditions, prevention of smoking, and vaccination are the primary policies for preventing pneumonia. Annual vaccination with inactivated influenza vaccine is recommended in all children older than 6 months, especially in high-risk groups. Also, prophylaxis with a specific monoclonal antibody for RSV is effective for preventing pneumonia in infants at high risk of RSV disease.

The vaccination with pneumococcal conjugate vaccine and HiB has recently become widespread; however, many children are still not vaccinated especially in low-income countries. Both 10-valent (PCV-10) and 13-valent (PCV-13) pneumococcal conjugate vaccines in >150 countries' pediatric immunization programs decreased the incidence of pneumonia and hospitalizations due to severe disease. The most resistant pneumococcus strains are serogroups 23F, 6A, 6B, 9V, 19A, 19F, and 14, and all are included in the PCV-13. In a meta-analysis comparing the effects of different types of PCVs on the frequency of hospitalization at <2 years of age, 20 studies were included. Pneumococcal conjugate vaccines 10 or 13 had independent associations in reducing the frequency of hospitalizations compared to no vaccine or PCV-7 [41].

42.2 Comorbid Rhinosinusitis

42.2.1 Rhinosinusitis

Rhinosinusitis is defined as an inflammation of the sinus and nasal mucosa. Upper respiratory tract infections (URTI) are common in children and may be presented with acute rhinosinusitis. The vast majority of rhinosinusitis spontaneously resolves nevertheless, approximately 5–10% of viral URTIs may be complicated by secondary bacterial rhinosinusitis. It may cause health problems and negatively affect the daily function and quality of life of children [42–45].

Rhinosinusitis is classified according to the duration of symptoms; acute (<1 month), subacute (1–3 months), or chronic (>3 months) [42]. Lasting up to 1-month rhinosinusitis is called acute rhinosinusitis, and can be caused by infections (viral, bacteria, or fungi), environmental irritants, and allergies. Acute rhinosinusitis is usually seen in children aged 1–5 years. The mucociliary clearance impairment and blockage of sinus drainage are the pathophysiological mechanisms responsible for rhinosinusitis. The addition of bacterial microorganisms to these mechanisms causes acute bacterial rhinosinusitis (ABR) [46].

Acute bacterial rhinosinusitis is diagnosed in children with any of the clinical presentations:

1. Persistent symptoms and signs (cough, nasal obstruction, or discharge) lasting >10 days without any clinical improvement.
2. Severe symptoms such as fever, purulent nasal discharge, or facial pain from the onset of the disease.
3. Recurrence after initial improvement, or worsening symptoms and signs (new onset fever, increased nasal discharge, or severe headache).

Postnasal drip, malaise, sinus tenderness or pain, sore throat, halitosis, facial congestion, and pressure can occur in patients. However, signs and symptoms may be uncertain in children. The incidence of ABR in children is exactly unknown. The common causes of bacterial microorganisms are *Streptococcus pneumoniae*, *Haemophilus influenzae*, and *Moraxella catarrhalis*. In one-third of the patients, more than one microorganism may be responsible for the disease. When ARB is diagnosed in children, 10–14 days of empirical antibiotic therapy is recommended [46, 47]. Some of acute bacterial rhinosinusitis may progress to chronic rhinosinusitis (CRS), but there is no definite information about this rate in children.

CRS in children is diagnosed with the persistence of two or more symptoms (purulent rhinorrhea, nasal obstruction, facial pressure/pain, or cough) corresponding with endoscopic (mucosal edema, purulent drainage, or nasal polyps) and/or CT findings (ostiomeatal complex or sinus edema) at least three months despite standard medical treatment [48]. Despite these, due to presenting with nonspecific symptoms, the diagnosis of CRS is difficult in children. In a study evaluating clinical diagnosis of CRS in children as confirmed by nasal fibroendoscopy, rhinorrhea was found as the strongest predictor of CRS. In the multivariate logistic regression for CRS symptoms (halitosis, cough, facial pain, rhinorrhea, and nasal obstruction), the probability of CRS was 77–91% with three symptoms, was over 93% with four symptoms and was 100% with all five symptoms [49].

The prevalence of CRS in children is around 5–15%, between the ages of 5 and 15 years children are the most affected by the disease. CRS can lead to complaints such as limitations in daily activities, concentration problems, and impairment of sleep quality by impairing the quality of life in children [50, 51]. In a multicenter study in the US between 2005 and 2012, CRS accounted for 5.6 million acute care visits (range, 3.7–7.5 million) per annum patients with 0–20 years of age. Among all visits, CRS was diagnosed in 2.1% and was significantly more prevalent than acute rhinosinusitis (relative risk, 3.40; 95% CI, 2.70–4.10; $P < 0.0001$) [52].

The pathogenesis of CRS is multifactorial and characterized by mainly inflammatory processes accompanying various contributing factors such as genetic, environmental (smoke exposure, industrial pollution), allergens, irritants, and comorbid predisposing diseases including allergic rhinitis, asthma, cystic fibrosis (CF), primary ciliary dyskinesia, immunodeficiency, and eosinophilic granulomatosis with polyangiitis (EGPA) [42, 51, 53]. In response to the contributing factors, inflammation with eosinophils, neutrophils, lymphocytes, cytokines, and chemokines are shown in CRS. While type 2 eosinophilic inflammation contributes to the development of nasal polyposis in patients with CRS, type 1 and type 3 inflammation dominated by neutrophils are seen in CRS without nasal polyps. Inflammation and infection trigger each other, causing the progression of the pathological process [54].

The management of CRS contains medical treatment for bacterial infections and inflammation reduction. To determine the underlying etiology and associated comorbidities, a detailed evaluation should be performed. Surgical approaches are considered in patients with inadequate response to medical treatments [55].

42.2.2 Pneumonia Comorbid Rhinosinusitis

The relationship between the upper and lower airways suggests that the upper and lower airways are a single functional unit. The relationship between CRS and lower airway diseases supports this idea. Despite this association, few studies have evaluated pneumonia and rhinosinusitis, and these studies were conducted in adult patients [56–58]. In a retrospective study, the sinusitis frequency was found 84% in patients with pneumonia. These findings have suggested that sinusitis may be an important causative factor for pneumonia [57]. In another study to examine the relationship between CRS and CAP, an association has been shown between sphenoid rhinosinusitis and CAP [odds ratio 19.76, 95% CI 8.78–44.47] [58]. Also, a longitudinal follow-up study using a national health screening cohort showed the association between CRS and pneumonia, and this association was seen only in the younger age, female sex, and CRS without nasal polyps subgroups [56]. The presence of impaired mucociliary function in CRS, associated primary respiratory tract pathogens that play a role in both rhinosinusitis and pneumonia, and the increase in cytokines causes inflammation in the lungs induced by CRS are possible mechanisms, underlying the relationship between CRS and pneumonia [56]. However, both diseases may be simply different manifestations of common pathophysiology.

Comorbid rhinosinusitis may occur due to viral upper respiratory tract infections, active and passive smoking, noxious inhalants and air pollution (ozone, chlorine, sulfur dioxide), indoor dampness and mold exposure, predisposing diseases, and chronic aspiration [gastro-oesophageal reflux (GER), incoordinate swallowing]. Studies have shown that esophageal reflux occurs in 63% of children with CRS, and most children with GER demonstrated improvement in sinus disease after treatment of GER. Gastroesophageal reflux disease (GERD) is suggested to relate to comorbid rhinosinusitis in some pediatric patients, but its association with respiratory diseases is conflicting [53–55, 59]. Additionally, in the presence of pneumonia comorbid rhinosinusitis, diseases that cause recurrent respiratory infections or complaints (allergic rhinitis, CF, primary ciliary dyskinesia, primary immunodeficiency, asthma, EGPA, sickle cell anemia, etc.) should be investigated.

42.2.3 Allergic Rhinitis

Allergic inflammation causes nasal congestion and impairs mucociliary function. Although this is seen as a risk factor for the development of CRS, the contribution of allergic rhinitis (AR) to CRS in children is controversial. The epidemiology of AR in children with CRS has not been as fully characterized as other comorbidities. Approximately 17–52% of CRS is associated with nonallergic rhinitis [51, 53]. In a study that evaluated comorbidities in children with CRS, allergic rhinitis was found the most common comorbidity in this population [60]. Although few studies have shown an association between AR and CRS, other studies suggest that allergy is not a significant factor in developing CRS [48]. Allergic rhinitis is known to cause recurrent rhinosinusitis. There is a tendency for lower respiratory tract infections in atopic children. CRS and pneumonia coexistence are observed in children with allergic rhinitis.

42.2.4 Cystic Fibrosis

CF is an autosomal recessive disease caused by various mutations in the CF transmembrane conductance regulator gene. The disease is characterized by sinopulmonary diseases such as recurrent sinusitis, nasal polyps, and pulmonary infections. Due to defective CFTR protein, mucous obstructions of the sinus ostia cause rhinosinusitis and nasal polyposis. While the prevalence of CRS in CF patients is nearly 100%, the prevalence of nasal polyposis is more variable and increases with age. *P. aeruginosa* and *S. aureus* are the most common microorganisms which affect the paranasal sinuses. The management of CRS in CF consists of local and/or systemic antiinflammatory medications and antibiotics. Approximately 20–25% of patients require sinus surgery due to failed medical treatment [61, 62].

42.2.5 Primary Ciliary Dyskinesia

Primary ciliary dyskinesia (PCD) is a disease characterized by impaired mucociliary clearance. Patients have persistent rhinosinusitis, recurrent otitis media, and respiratory infections [63]. CRS is found in all patients and causes impaired quality of life in patients. Bacterial sinusitis has been reported in 88% of PCD patients with CRS [64]. Kartagener's syndrome is a triad of rhinosinusitis, bronchiectasis, and situs inversus totalis in 50% of patients with PCD.

42.2.6 Immunodeficiency

CRS is a common disease in immunodeficiency, especially primary immunodeficiency. Antibodies deficiency leads to the development of recurrent otitis media, rhinosinusitis, and lower respiratory tract infections with insufficiency of protecting mucosal surfaces in the respiratory airway. The prevalence of CRS has been evaluated in children with specific immunodeficiencies in many studies and has confirmed that the disease is common. Also, the prevalence of immunodeficiency has been evaluated in CRS [65–68]. In a meta-analysis, a prevalence of pooled IgG, IgA, and IgM deficiencies was found in 13% of patients with recurrent CRS and 23% of patients with difficult-to-treat CRS [66]. Responsible bacterial microorganisms (*M. catarrhalis*, *S. pneumoniae*, *S. aureus*, and *H. influenzae*) are similar in CRS and immunodeficiency. To evaluate, immunodeficiency is recommended when a patient is poorly responsive to therapies of CRS [69].

42.2.7 Asthma

Studies show that about 40% of children with CRS have asthma and the presence of CRS is associated with worse outcomes in children with asthma [53, 70]. Both diseases are highly heterogeneous with contributing factors, structural and inflammatory pathophysiology, and are also linked through the underlying T2 inflammation. In CRS, as in asthma, remodeling processes such as goblet cell hyperplasia, epithelial barrier abnormalities, and polyp formation can be observed. For this reason, asthma symptoms can be improved by medical management of CRS [71, 72]. Chronic sinusitis and asthma are shown to be risk factors in children with recurrent CAP [73].

42.2.8 Eosinophilic Granulomatosis with Polyangiitis

Eosinophilic granulomatosis with polyangiitis (EGPA) is a small-vessel vasculitis characterized by necrotizing vasculitis and eosinophil-rich granulomatous inflammation. The vast majority of patients with EGPA are affected by asthma accompanied by CRS with nasal polyps. Apart from this, eosinophilia, eosinophilic tissue infiltrates, and clinical manifestations due to vasculitis can be seen in patients [74]. In a review comparison of the clinical characteristics of children with adult patients, asthma and rhinosinusitis were frequent in all patients [75]. Patients with accompanying rhinosinusitis are associated with a more severe course of asthma [76].

42.2.9 Sickle Cell Anemia

Sickle cell disease (SCD) is the most common hereditary blood disorder and has chronic respiratory complications including an increased risk of invasive bacterial diseases such as *S. pneumoniae*, *Neisseria meningitidis*, and *H. influenzae* type B, and noninvasive diseases like otitis media and rhinosinusitis due to splenic dysfunction. Pneumonia and acute chest syndrome are the primary causes of hospitalization and mortality in children with SCD [77, 78].

References

1. Harris M, Clark J, Coote N, et al. British Thoracic Society guidelines for the management of community-acquired pneumonia in children: update 2011. Thorax. 2011;66(Suppl 2):ii1–23. https://doi.org/10.1136/thoraxjnl-2011-200598.
2. Bradley JS, Byington CL, Shah SS, et al. The management of community-acquired pneumonia in infants and children older than 3 months of age: clinical practice guidelines by the Pediatric Infectious Diseases Society and the Infectious Diseases Society of America. Clin Infect Dis. 2011;53(7):e25–76. https://doi.org/10.1093/cid/cir531.
3. Andrés-Martín A, Escribano Montaner A, Figuerola Mulet J, et al. Consensus document on community-acquired pneumonia in children. SENP-SEPAR-SEIP. Arch Bronconeumol (Engl Ed). 2020;56(11):725–41. https://doi.org/10.1016/j.arbres.2020.03.025.

4. Katz SE, Williams DJ. Pediatric community-acquired pneumonia in the United States: changing epidemiology, diagnostic and therapeutic challenges, and areas for future research. Infect Dis Clin N Am. 2018;32(1):47–63. https://doi.org/10.1016/j.idc.2017.11.002.
5. World Health Organization. Pneumonia. https://www.who.int/news-room/fact-sheets/detail/pneumonia.
6. Walker CLF, Rudan I, Liu L, et al. Global burden of childhood pneumonia and diarrhoea. Lancet. 2013;381(9875):1405–16. https://doi.org/10.1016/s0140-6736(13)60222-6.
7. Liu L, Oza S, Hogan D, et al. Global, regional, and national causes of under-5 mortality in 2000–2015: an updated systematic analysis with implications for the Sustainable Development Goals. Lancet. 2016;388(10063):3027–35. https://doi.org/10.1016/s0140-6736(16)31593-8.
8. Jain S, Williams DJ, Arnold SR, et al. Community-acquired pneumonia requiring hospitalization among U.S. children. N Engl J Med. 2015;372(9):835–45. https://doi.org/10.1056/NEJMoa1405870.
9. Jackson S, Mathews KH, Pulanic D, et al. Risk factors for severe acute lower respiratory infections in children: a systematic review and meta-analysis. Croat Med J. 2013;54(2):110–21. https://doi.org/10.3325/cmj.2013.54.110.
10. Ning G, Wang X, Wu D, et al. The etiology of community-acquired pneumonia among children under 5 years of age in mainland China, 2001–2015: a systematic review. Hum Vaccines Immunother. 2017;13(11):2742–50. https://doi.org/10.1080/21645515.2017.1371381.
11. Ensinck G, Lazarte G, Ernst A, et al. Community-acquired methicillin-resistant *Staphylococcus aureus* pneumonia in a children's hospital. Our 10-year experience. Arch Argent Pediatr. 2021;119(1):11–7. https://doi.org/10.5546/aap.2021.eng.11.
12. Carrillo-Marquez MA, Hulten KG, Hammerman W, Lamberth L, Mason EO, Kaplan SL. *Staphylococcus aureus* pneumonia in children in the era of community-acquired methicillin-resistance at Texas Children's Hospital. Pediatr Infect Dis J. 2011;30(7):545–50. https://doi.org/10.1097/INF.0b013e31821618be.
13. Marchello C, Dale AP, Thai TN, Han DS, Ebell MH. Prevalence of atypical pathogens in patients with cough and community-acquired pneumonia: a meta-analysis. Ann Fam Med. 2016;14(6):552–66. https://doi.org/10.1370/afm.1993.
14. García-García ML, Calvo C, Pozo F, Villadangos PA, Pérez-Breña P, Casas I. Spectrum of respiratory viruses in children with community-acquired pneumonia. Pediatr Infect Dis J. 2012;31(8):808–13. https://doi.org/10.1097/INF.0b013e3182568c67.
15. Pratt MTG, Abdalla T, Richmond PC, et al. Prevalence of respiratory viruses in community-acquired pneumonia in children: a systematic review and meta-analysis. Lancet Child Adolesc Health. 2022;6(8):555–70. https://doi.org/10.1016/s2352-4642(22)00092-x.
16. Gereige RS, Laufer PM. Pneumonia. Pediatr Rev. 2013;34(10):438–56.; quiz 455–6. https://doi.org/10.1542/pir.34-10-438.
17. Shah SN, Bachur RG, Simel DL, Neuman MI. Does this child have pneumonia? The rational clinical examination systematic review. Jama. 2017;318(5):462–71. https://doi.org/10.1001/jama.2017.9039.
18. Florin TA, Ambroggio L, Brokamp C, et al. Biomarkers and disease severity in children with community-acquired pneumonia. Pediatrics. 2020;145(6):e20193728. https://doi.org/10.1542/peds.2019-3728.
19. Principi N, Esposito S. Biomarkers in pediatric community-acquired pneumonia. Int J Mol Sci. 2017;18(2):447. https://doi.org/10.3390/ijms18020447.
20. Andronikou S, Lambert E, Halton J, et al. Guidelines for the use of chest radiographs in community-acquired pneumonia in children and adolescents. Pediatr Radiol. 2017;47(11):1405–11. https://doi.org/10.1007/s00247-017-3944-4.
21. Arnold SR, Jain S, Dansie D, et al. Association of radiology findings with etiology of community acquired pneumonia among children. J Pediatr. 2023;261:113333. https://doi.org/10.1016/j.jpeds.2023.01.010.
22. Stadler JAM, Andronikou S, Zar HJ. Lung ultrasound for the diagnosis of community-acquired pneumonia in children. Pediatr Radiol. 2017;47(11):1412–9. https://doi.org/10.1007/s00247-017-3910-1.

23. Balk DS, Lee C, Schafer J, et al. Lung ultrasound compared to chest X-ray for diagnosis of pediatric pneumonia: a meta-analysis. Pediatr Pulmonol. 2018;53(8):1130–9. https://doi.org/10.1002/ppul.24020.
24. Shah SS, Dugan MH, Bell LM, et al. Blood cultures in the emergency department evaluation of childhood pneumonia. Pediatr Infect Dis J. 2011;30(6):475–9. https://doi.org/10.1097/INF.0b013e31820a5adb.
25. Cevey-Macherel M, Galetto-Lacour A, Gervaix A, et al. Etiology of community-acquired pneumonia in hospitalized children based on WHO clinical guidelines. Eur J Pediatr. 2009;168(12):1429–36. https://doi.org/10.1007/s00431-009-0943-y.
26. Charkaluk ML, Kalach N, Mvogo H, et al. Assessment of a rapid urinary antigen detection by an immunochromatographic test for diagnosis of pneumococcal infection in children. Diagn Microbiol Infect Dis. 2006;55(2):89–94. https://doi.org/10.1016/j.diagmicrobio.2005.10.013.
27. Chang HY, Chang LY, Shao PL, et al. Comparison of real-time polymerase chain reaction and serological tests for the confirmation of *Mycoplasma pneumoniae* infection in children with clinical diagnosis of atypical pneumonia. J Microbiol Immunol Infect. 2014;47(2):137–44. https://doi.org/10.1016/j.jmii.2013.03.015.
28. Esposito S, Cohen R, Domingo JD, et al. Antibiotic therapy for pediatric community-acquired pneumonia: do we know when, what and for how long to treat? Pediatr Infect Dis J. 2012;31(6):e78–85. https://doi.org/10.1097/INF.0b013e318255dc5b.
29. Dean P, Florin TA. Factors associated with pneumonia severity in children: a systematic review. J Pediatric Infect Dis Soc. 2018;7(4):323–34. https://doi.org/10.1093/jpids/piy046.
30. Williams DJ, Zhu Y, Grijalva CG, et al. Predicting severe pneumonia outcomes in children. Pediatrics. 2016;138(4):e20161019. https://doi.org/10.1542/peds.2016-1019.
31. Erdem SB, Can D, Girit S, et al. Does atopy affect the course of viral pneumonia? Allergol Immunopathol (Madr). 2018;46(2):119–26. https://doi.org/10.1016/j.aller.2017.04.003.
32. Chang CC, Cheng AC, Chang AB. Over-the-counter (OTC) medications to reduce cough as an adjunct to antibiotics for acute pneumonia in children and adults. Cochrane Database Syst Rev. 2012;2:Cd006088. https://doi.org/10.1002/14651858.CD006088.pub3.
33. Chaves GS, Freitas DA, Santino TA, Nogueira PAM, Fregonezi GA, Mendonça KM. Chest physiotherapy for pneumonia in children. Cochrane Database Syst Rev. 2019;1(1):Cd010277. https://doi.org/10.1002/14651858.CD010277.pub3.
34. Mathur S, Fuchs A, Bielicki J, Van Den Anker J, Sharland M. Antibiotic use for community-acquired pneumonia in neonates and children: WHO evidence review. Paediatr Int Child Health. 2018;38(sup1):S66–s75. https://doi.org/10.1080/20469047.2017.1409455.
35. Haider BA, Saeed MA, Bhutta ZA. Short-course versus long-course antibiotic therapy for non-severe community-acquired pneumonia in children aged 2 months to 59 months. Cochrane Database Syst Rev. 2008;2):Cd005976. https://doi.org/10.1002/14651858.CD005976.pub2.
36. Shapiro DJ, Hall M, Lipsett SC, et al. Short-versus prolonged-duration antibiotics for outpatient pneumonia in children. J Pediatr. 2021;234:205–211.e1. https://doi.org/10.1016/j.jpeds.2021.03.017.
37. Pernica JM, Harman S, Kam AJ, et al. Short-course antimicrobial therapy for pediatric community-acquired pneumonia: the SAFER randomized clinical trial. JAMA Pediatr. 2021;175(5):475–82. https://doi.org/10.1001/jamapediatrics.2020.6735.
38. Williams DJ, Creech CB, Walter EB, et al. Short- vs standard-course outpatient antibiotic therapy for community-acquired pneumonia in children: the SCOUT-CAP randomized clinical trial. JAMA Pediatr. 2022;176(3):253–61. https://doi.org/10.1001/jamapediatrics.2021.5547.
39. Le Saux N, Robinson JL. Uncomplicated pneumonia in healthy Canadian children and youth: practice points for management. Paediatr Child Health. 2015;20(8):441–50. https://doi.org/10.1093/pch/20.8.441.
40. Lassi ZS, Imdad A, Bhutta ZA. Short-course versus long-course intravenous therapy with the same antibiotic for severe community-acquired pneumonia in children aged two months to 59 months. Cochrane Database Syst Rev. 2017;10(10):Cd008032. https://doi.org/10.1002/14651858.CD008032.pub3.

41. Zhu X, Li X. Pneumococcal vaccine effect on hospitalisation rates of pneumonia in children: a meta-analysis. Int J Clin Pract. 2021;75(11):e14739. https://doi.org/10.1111/ijcp.14739.
42. Badr DT, Gaffin JM, Phipatanakul W. Pediatric rhinosinusitis. Curr Treat Options Allergy. 2016;3(3):268–81. https://doi.org/10.1007/s40521-016-0096-y.
43. Wald ER, Applegate KE, Bordley C, et al. Clinical practice guideline for the diagnosis and management of acute bacterial sinusitis in children aged 1–18 years. Pediatrics. 2013;132(1):e262–80. https://doi.org/10.1542/peds.2013-1071.
44. Tan R, Spector S. Pediatric sinusitis. Curr Allergy Asthma Rep. 2007;7(6):421–6. https://doi.org/10.1007/s11882-007-0064-5.
45. DeMuri G, Wald ER. Acute bacterial sinusitis in children. Pediatr Rev. 2013;34(10):429–37.; quiz 437. https://doi.org/10.1542/pir.34-10-429.
46. Brook I. Acute sinusitis in children. Pediatr Clin N Am. 2013;60(2):409–24. https://doi.org/10.1016/j.pcl.2012.12.002.
47. Chow AW, Benninger MS, Brook I, et al. IDSA clinical practice guideline for acute bacterial rhinosinusitis in children and adults. Clin Infect Dis. 2012;54(8):e72–e112. https://doi.org/10.1093/cid/cir1043.
48. Brietzke SE, Shin JJ, Choi S, et al. Clinical consensus statement: pediatric chronic rhinosinusitis. Otolaryngol Head Neck Surg. 2014;151(4):542–53. https://doi.org/10.1177/0194599814549302.
49. Leo G, Incorvaia C, Cazzavillan A, Consonni D. May chronic rhinosinusitis in children be diagnosed by clinical symptoms? Int J Pediatr Otorhinolaryngol. 2015;79(6):825–8. https://doi.org/10.1016/j.ijporl.2015.03.011.
50. Fokkens WJ, Lund VJ, Mullol J, et al. European position paper on rhinosinusitis and nasal polyps 2012. Rhinology. 2012;50(Suppl 23):1–298.
51. Snidvongs K, Sangubol M, Poachanukoon O. Pediatric versus adult chronic rhinosinusitis. Curr Allergy Asthma Rep. 2020;20(8):29. https://doi.org/10.1007/s11882-020-00924-6.
52. Gilani S, Shin JJ. The burden and visit prevalence of pediatric chronic rhinosinusitis. Otolaryngol Head Neck Surg. 2017;157(6):1048–52. https://doi.org/10.1177/0194599817721177.
53. Silviu-Dan F. Pediatric chronic rhinosinusitis. Pediatr Ann. 2014;43(8):e201–9. https://doi.org/10.3928/00904481-20140723-10.
54. Delemarre T, Holtappels G, De Ruyck N, et al. Type 2 inflammation in chronic rhinosinusitis without nasal polyps: another relevant endotype. J Allergy Clin Immunol. 2020;146(2):337–343.e6. https://doi.org/10.1016/j.jaci.2020.04.040.
55. Isaacson G. Surgical treatment of pediatric rhinosinusitis. Minerva Pediatr. 2015;67(4):357–68.
56. Wee JH, Min C, Jung HJ, Park MW, Park B, Choi HG. Association between chronic rhinosinusitis and pneumonia: a longitudinal follow-up study using a national health screening cohort. Sci Rep. 2022;12(1):5498. https://doi.org/10.1038/s41598-022-09552-8.
57. Ozbay B, Arslan H. Frequency of sinusitis in the patients with pneumonia. Clin Imaging. 2002;26(2):92–4. https://doi.org/10.1016/s0899-7071(01)00377-1.
58. McQuitty R, Bui R, Chaaban MR. Retrospective study: association of chronic sphenoid rhinosinusitis with community acquired pneumonia. Am J Rhinol Allergy. 2019;33(6):751–6. https://doi.org/10.1177/1945892419865651.
59. Phipps CD, Wood WE, Gibson WS, Cochran WJ. Gastroesophageal reflux contributing to chronic sinus disease in children: a prospective analysis. Arch Otolaryngol Head Neck Surg. 2000;126(7):831–6. https://doi.org/10.1001/archotol.126.7.831.
60. Sedaghat AR, Phipatanakul W, Cunningham MJ. Prevalence of and associations with allergic rhinitis in children with chronic rhinosinusitis. Int J Pediatr Otorhinolaryngol. 2014;78(2):343–7. https://doi.org/10.1016/j.ijporl.2013.12.006.
61. Dickinson KM, Collaco JM. Cystic fibrosis. Pediatr Rev. 2021;42(2):55–67. https://doi.org/10.1542/pir.2019-0212.
62. Oomen KP, April MM. Sinonasal manifestations in cystic fibrosis. Int J Otolaryngol. 2012;2012:789572. https://doi.org/10.1155/2012/789572.
63. Horani A, Ferkol TW. Understanding primary ciliary dyskinesia and other ciliopathies. J Pediatr. 2021;230:15–22.e1. https://doi.org/10.1016/j.jpeds.2020.11.040.

64. Lucas JS, Alanin MC, Collins S, et al. Clinical care of children with primary ciliary dyskinesia. Expert Rev Respir Med. 2017;11(10):779–90. https://doi.org/10.1080/17476348.2017.1360770.
65. Karadeniz EB, Aliyeva C, Aydemir S, et al. Chronic rhinosinusitis in patients with primary immunodeficiency. Int Arch Allergy Immunol. 2023;184(3):302–10. https://doi.org/10.1159/000527265.
66. Schwitzguébel AJ, Jandus P, Lacroix JS, Seebach JD, Harr T. Immunoglobulin deficiency in patients with chronic rhinosinusitis: systematic review of the literature and meta-analysis. J Allergy Clin Immunol. 2015;136(6):1523–31. https://doi.org/10.1016/j.jaci.2015.07.016.
67. Huwyler C, Lin SY, Liang J. Primary immunodeficiency and rhinosinusitis. Immunol Allergy Clin N Am. 2020;40(2):233–49. https://doi.org/10.1016/j.iac.2019.12.003.
68. Bernatowska E, Mikołuć B, Krzeski A, Piatosa B, Gromek I. Chronic rhinosinusitis in primary antibody immunodeficient patients. Int J Pediatr Otorhinolaryngol. 2006;70(9):1587–92. https://doi.org/10.1016/j.ijporl.2006.04.013.
69. Chiarella SE, Grammer LC. Immune deficiency in chronic rhinosinusitis: screening and treatment. Expert Rev Clin Immunol. 2017;13(2):117–23. https://doi.org/10.1080/1744666x.2016.1216790.
70. Matucci A, Bormioli S, Nencini F, et al. Asthma and chronic rhinosinusitis: how similar are they in pathogenesis and treatment responses? Int J Mol Sci. 2021;22(7):3340. https://doi.org/10.3390/ijms22073340.
71. Striz I, Golebski K, Strizova Z, et al. New insights into the pathophysiology and therapeutic targets of asthma and comorbid chronic rhinosinusitis with or without nasal polyposis. Clin Sci (Lond). 2023;137(9):727–53. https://doi.org/10.1042/cs20190281.
72. Frieri M. Asthma linked with rhinosinusitis: an extensive review. Allergy Rhinol (Providence). 2014;5(1):41–9. https://doi.org/10.2500/ar.2014.5.0083.
73. Patria F, Longhi B, Tagliabue C, et al. Clinical profile of recurrent community-acquired pneumonia in children. BMC Pulm Med. 2013;13:60. https://doi.org/10.1186/1471-2466-13-60.
74. Emmi G, Bettiol A, Gelain E, et al. Evidence-based guideline for the diagnosis and management of eosinophilic granulomatosis with polyangiitis. Nat Rev Rheumatol. 2023;19(6):378–93. https://doi.org/10.1038/s41584-023-00958-w.
75. Zwerina J, Eger G, Englbrecht M, Manger B, Schett G. Churg-Strauss syndrome in childhood: a systematic literature review and clinical comparison with adult patients. Semin Arthritis Rheum. 2009;39(2):108–15. https://doi.org/10.1016/j.semarthrit.2008.05.004.
76. Berti A, Cornec D, Casal Moura M, et al. Eosinophilic granulomatosis with polyangiitis: clinical predictors of long-term asthma severity. Chest. 2020;157(5):1086–99. https://doi.org/10.1016/j.chest.2019.11.045.
77. Arigliani M, Gupta A. Management of chronic respiratory complications in children and adolescents with sickle cell disease. Eur Respir Rev. 2020;29(157):200054. https://doi.org/10.1183/16000617.0054-2020.
78. Oligbu G, Fallaha M, Pay L, Ladhani S. Risk of invasive pneumococcal disease in children with sickle cell disease in the era of conjugate vaccines: a systematic review of the literature. Br J Haematol. 2019;185(4):743–51. https://doi.org/10.1111/bjh.15846.

Sleep-Related Breathing Disorder: Upper Respiratory Tract-Related Etiologies

43

Birce Sunman and Uğur Özçelik

43.1 Sleep-Related Breathing Disorder: Upper Respiratory Tract-Related Etiologies

43.1.1 Introduction

Sleep-related breathing disorders (SRBDs), also referred to as sleep-disordered breathing, are characterized by atypical respiratory patterns occurring during sleep. SRBDs are common in the pediatric population and consist of a spectrum of disorders, varying in severity from habitual snoring to obstructive sleep apnea (OSA) syndrome [1]. The prevalence in children has been documented to be 5.1–13.3%, with the highest incidence between the ages of 2 and 8 years [2]. Based on the third version of the International Classification of Sleep Disorders (ICSD-3), SRBDs are divided into four groups such as sleep-related hypoxemia disorder, sleep-related hypoventilation, OSA, and central sleep apnea [3].

OSA is the most prevalent type of SRBDs in all ages and is defined by episodes of partial (also known as hypopnea) or complete (referred to as apnea) obstructions in the upper respiratory tract with an associated decrease in oxygen saturation or arousal from sleep [4]. The American Academy of Pediatrics (AAP) Subcommittee on Pediatric Sleep estimates that OSA affects between 1.2 and 5.7% of children [5].

B. Sunman
Department of Pediatric Pulmonology, Hacettepe University Faculty of Medicine, Ihsan Dogramaci Children's Hospital, Ankara, Turkey

U. Özçelik (✉)
Department of Pediatric Pulmonology, Hacettepe University Faculty of Medicine, Ihsan Dogramaci Children's Hospital, Ankara, Turkey

Department of Pediatric Pulmonology, School of Medicine, Hacettepe University, Ihsan Dogramaci Children's Hospital, Ankara, Turkey
e-mail: uozcelik@hacettepe.edu.tr

H. Yüksel et al. (eds.), *Pediatric Airway Diseases*, Comprehensive ENT,
https://doi.org/10.1007/978-3-031-74853-0_43

Children with OSA have a complex etiology for upper airway obstruction which includes anatomical obstruction, abnormal neuromotor tone, and disorders in ventilatory drive [6].

43.1.2 Pathophysiology of Upper Airway Obstruction in Obstructive Sleep Apnea

The upper airway is comprised of several anatomical structures, namely, the nose, paranasal sinuses, nasopharynx, oropharynx, and larynx. The nasal cavity serves as the initial point of entrance and contributes to approximately 50% of the overall resistance encountered in the upper respiratory tract [7]. Although the contribution of anatomical stenosis is obvious, it is becoming increasingly apparent that there is a problem beyond this basic structural obstruction of the airway. The pathogenesis of OSA is still controversial, as the neural regulation of the upper respiratory tract remains to be elucidated.

The upper airways should be collapsible to function properly during breathing, especially during sleep. Neuromuscular tone in the pharynx rises to keep the upper airway from collapsing when we are awake. However, during sleep, this mechanism decreases, paving the way for upper airway obstruction [8]. The tasks of protection of the airway and preservation of its patency are fulfilled by the central respiratory drive and upper airway reflexes [9]. In healthy children, airway patency is maintained during sleep by an increase in upper airway neuromotor tone caused by increased central respiratory stimulation.

Upper airway obstruction during sleep results in decreased oxygen saturation and causes interrupted sleep and impaired sleep quality. Hypoxemia, hypercapnia, and pharyngeal subatmospheric pressure generated during episodes of apnea activate the upper airway dilator muscles. Obstructive apnea ends as a result of the reopening of the airway following activation of the upper airway dilator muscles [6].

Two main factors that result in OSA are decrement in intrinsic upper airway diameter and increment in collapsibility of the upper airway. A decrease in ventilatory drive or any lesion in the reflex pathway may lead to a more collapsible upper airway [10]. Prior research has established that upper airway mucosal sensory receptors also regulate upper airway tone, contributing to the termination of apnea. It has been shown in these studies that upper airway anesthesia administration results in apnea and hypopnea during sleep even in healthy people. These findings suggest that the disruption of the sensory function of the mucosa in the upper airway could participate in the pathogenesis of the upper airway collapse during sleep [11]. Table 43.1 displays the most commonly encountered anatomical abnormalities that contribute to increased airway resistance and neuromuscular abnormalities which prevent the proper functioning of the dilator muscles.

Table 43.1 Disorders affecting upper airway size resulting in obstructive sleep apnea in children

Craniofacial anomalies
Down syndrome
Beckwith–Wiedemann syndrome
Mucopolysaccharidoses
Treacher-Collins syndrome
Robin sequence
Goldenhar syndrome
Neurologic disorders
Cerebral palsy
Arnold–Chiari malformation
Poliomyelitis
Other disorders
Obesity
Prader–Willi
Congenital hypothyroidism
Subglottic stenosis
Allergic rhinitis

43.1.3 Anatomical Obstruction Leading to Upper Airway Narrowing in Obstructive Sleep Apnea

Altered anatomical structures surrounding the airway affect the size and shape of the respiratory passage and may contribute to upper airway narrowing, increasing the risk for OSA in children. Soft tissues, especially the tonsils and adenoids, narrow the upper airway [8]. Adenotonsillar hypertrophy is considered the primary predisposing factor for OSA in children. It is most commonly observed in children aged 2–8 years [12]. In the majority of cases, the obstructive clinical symptoms of OSA can be attributed to enlarged tonsils, adenoids, or both (Fig. 43.1). In addition, the role of inflammation in the pathogenesis of adenotonsillar hypertrophy and OSA was studied. Improvement was observed after treatment with antiinflammatory agents (such as nasal steroids and antileukotrienes), although adenotonsillectomy remains the gold standard treatment. This suggests a multidisciplinary approach to treatment [13].

In addition to the tonsils and adenoid, the tongue constitutes one of the biggest anatomical components that comprise the anterior boundary of the oropharyngeal airway. The position and size of the airway can be influenced by the positioning and dimensions of the tongue. Macroglossia is a substantial contributor to upper airway narrowing and is usually seen in combination with specific disorders, such as Down syndrome, as well as a variety of metabolic and storage disorders, such as mucopolysaccharidosis and Beckwith–Wiedemann syndrome. Furthermore, backwards positioning of the tongue, known as glossoptosis, can lead to airway obstruction. Glossoptosis is frequently observed in individuals diagnosed with Robin sequence and Down syndrome [8].

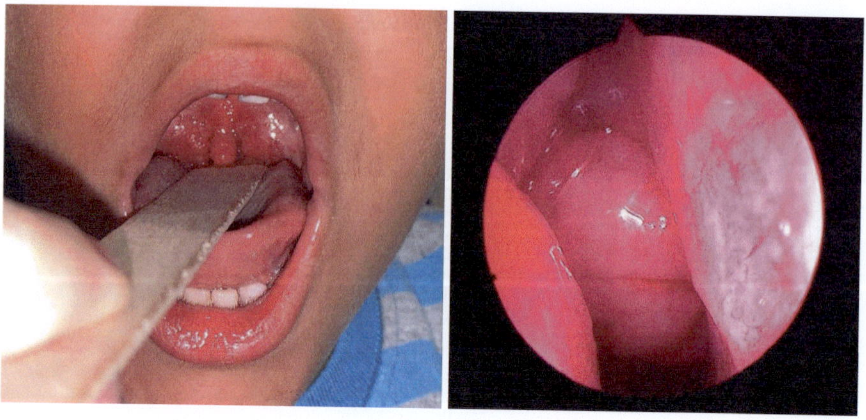

Fig. 43.1 Adenotonsillar hypertrophy. (**a**) A child with grade III tonsils. (**b**) Adenoid hypertrophy in a child narrowing the passage by 60%

Other anatomical factors participating in the development of OSA are craniofacial anomalies such as obstruction at the nasal level, an enlarged tongue, retrognathia, a high-arched palate, short or posteriorly placed mandible and midface hypoplasia [6]. Midface hypoplasia is characterized by a somewhat slower growth of the nasal, maxillary, and zygomatic bones in the cheek compared to other facial structures. Underdevelopment of the maxilla results in a reduction in the nasopharyngeal airway space, leading to OSA. Midface hypoplasia can arise as a result of genetic abnormalities, epigenetic factors, or traumatic events occurring during early developmental stages [14].

There are two groups of craniofacial anomalies: syndromic craniofacial anomalies (Crouzon, Apert, Pfeiffer, Treacher-Collins syndrome, Goldenhar syndrome, and DiGeorge syndrome) and nonsyndromic craniofacial anomalies (micrognathia, skeletal retrusion, malocclusion, macroglossia, high-arch palate, cleft lip/palate, and Pierre Robin sequence) [15]. Children with Pierre Robin anomaly or Treacher Collins syndrome experience nasal obstruction along with oral pharyngeal obstruction associated with OSA [16]. Children with Beckwith–Wiedemann syndrome, achondroplasia, Chiari malformation, trisomy 21, and mucopolysaccharidoses also have anatomical characteristics that contribute to OSA [12]. Various factors such as adenoid and tonsillar hypertrophy, midfacial and mandibular hypoplasia, laryngotracheal abnormalities, glossoptosis, and obesity may contribute to the airway narrowing in children with Down syndrome [13].

Obesity is an independent risk factor for OSA in the pediatric population. Multiple mechanisms, such as narrowing of the upper airway by local fat infiltration, are described as causes of OSA in obese children [17]. The excessive accumulation of adipose tissue surrounding the airway in these children increases airway resistance and obstruction [8]. Su et al. found that overweight or obese children have a higher risk of developing OSA compared with children of normal weight. Weight loss is one of the main treatment methods for obesity-related OSA in children and adolescents [18].

Additionally, allergic rhinitis is thought to have a variety of potential sleep-related effects and raises the likelihood of developing OSA due to two main factors. First, symptoms of allergic rhinitis, particularly rhinorrhea and congestion, can contribute to increased nasal resistance. Second, decreased pharyngeal diameter from mouth breathing shifts the mandible inferiorly, resulting in a narrow upper airway. Furthermore, previous studies have provided evidence indicating that the presence of additional inflammatory mediators, such as histamine, which is found at elevated levels in individuals with allergic rhinitis, can have a detrimental impact on the quality of sleep [19].

43.1.4 Neuromotor Factors Resulting in Increased Upper Airway Collapsibility

Besides the upper airway anatomic obstruction being the main causative factor in OSA, other contributing factors are believed to influence the development of OSA. One notable observation is that individuals diagnosed with OSA do not have airway obstruction in wakefulness state, as their upper airway dilator muscles exhibit increased tone during this period. In addition, surgical interventions targeting upper airway obstruction exhibit suboptimal outcomes as the results are not as satisfactory as expected and they often fail to achieve the desired improvement in the apnea hypopnea index (AHI). Additional evidence for the contribution of other factors besides anatomical obstruction was shown in the study by Guilleminault et al. In this study, resolution of OSA after tonsillectomy in children was subsequently followed by recurrence in adolescence. Moreover, OSA was not observed in other children with adenotonsillar hypertrophy [20]. These findings suggest that in some children with OSA upper airway collapse occurs as a result of the narrowing of the anatomical tract due to excessive soft tissue such as pharyngeal tissues and palatine tonsils [21]. However, in others, distinct underlying causes leading to defective neuromuscular control to maintain airway patency may be the reason [22].

The upper airway situated superior to the cartilaginous part is a collapsible muscular tube that possesses the ability to undergo compression, hence aiding in the processes of speech and swallowing. It contains over 30 pairs of muscles. Studies using upper airway dilating muscle denervation have demonstrated that the collapsibility of the upper airway is increased in instances where there is a reduction in the functioning of the upper airway muscles. On the other hand, muscular stimulation in the upper airway reduces collapsibility. Neuromotor control of this region is essential for maintaining airway patency and is regulated during sleep by central ventilatory drive, which is triggered by hypercapnia and pharyngeal subatmospheric pressure. In response to an increased central ventilatory drive, alteration of the upper airway dilatory muscles from a hypotonic to an activated state occurs to open the obstruction [23]. Prior studies have demonstrated that the activation of the upper airway in response to subatmospheric pressure does not occur immediately, but rather manifests after around three respiratory cycles. Consequently, the increased collapsibility of the upper airways in children with OSA is due to decreased neuromotor responses of the upper airway muscles to respiratory stimuli. To clarify, individuals diagnosed with OSA exhibit a notable absence of upper airway neuromotor reactions to hypercapnia and negative pressure while asleep, which distinguishes them from healthy pediatric populations [24].

As in diseases like cerebral palsy, neuromuscular disorders, and myelomeningocele, altered neurological reflexes of the upper airway muscles are common factors, leading to increased upper airway collapsibility [10].

Moreover, a range of central nervous system illnesses can lead to a decrease in muscle tone in the pharynx, which increases the likelihood of experiencing sleep-related breathing problems and obstruction of the airway. Frequent etiologies encompass elevated intracranial pressure, brain stem compression or dysplasia, specifically recurrent laryngeal nerve palsy, Arnold–Chiari malformations, and cranial nerve palsies.

43.1.5 Recognition and Management of Upper Airway Obstruction in Obstructive Sleep Apnea

The defining characteristic of upper airway blockage is the reduction or absence of airflow despite ongoing respiratory exertion. Silentness characterizes complete upper airway obstruction, whereas snoring (in the case of supralaryngeal obstruction) or inspiratory stridor (in the case of perilaryngeal obstruction) accompanies partial obstruction. Continuous inspiratory efforts against a partially or completely closed airway results in considerable negative intrathoracic pressure fluctuations, which are typically accompanied by a paradoxical movement of the anterior ribs, as well as decreased chest wall movement and distortion. There are numerous techniques to assess the upper airway obstruction. One of them is drug-induced sleep endoscopy (DISE) which identifies the anatomical segment responsible for obstructing the upper airway during drug induced sedation that mimics natural sleep. However, DISE cannot give information about whole sleep phases in a night, especially about rapid eye movement (REM) sleep phase in which respiratory events frequently occurs. Obstruction can also be diagnosed during polysomnography in the sleep laboratory by comparing measures of breathing effort (chest wall motion) with those of ventilation (oronasal airflow) [25].

There exists a range of both surgical and nonsurgical therapy modalities for pediatric OSA. Several therapeutic options are available for addressing the condition, including adenotonsillectomy, lingual tonsillectomy, continuous positive airway pressure (CPAP), supraglottoplasty, rapid maxillary expansion, antiinflammatory therapies, oral appliance therapy, and supplementary oxygen. Additional surgical techniques include midline posterior glossectomy, adenotonsillotomy (as an alternative to adenotonsillectomy), mandibular distraction for tongue base obstruction resulting from retrognathia, bariatric surgery interventions for individuals with morbid obesity, midface advancement procedures, and the insertion of tracheostomy tubes [6].

The primary treatment approach for pediatric patients with OSA syndrome, if there are no contraindications to surgical intervention, continues to be adenotonsillectomy [26]. For children with residual OSA after adenotonsillectomy or those in whom surgery is contraindicated, CPAP is frequently highly efficacious and well tolerated. In patients who cannot tolerate CPAP, young children with persistent OSA following adenotonsillectomy, and newborns with OSA, some tests are performed to see whether any obstructive lesions can be surgically corrected.

In a retrospective study conducted in 2018, it was shown that maxillomandibular advancement (MMA) surgery is considered the preferred treatment for children with syndromic craniofacial anomalies. This mechanism facilitates the expansion of the nasopharynx, oropharynx, and hypopharynx through the anterior movement of the soft palate and tongue, as well as the constriction of the lateral pharyngeal walls [27]. In order to widen the palate and flatten the palatal arch, rapid maxillary expansion is also used, which involves the use of orthodontic appliances. A recent meta-analysis has demonstrated a notable enhancement in the AHI when utilizing rapid maxillary expansion in pediatric patients [28]. A further therapeutic modality entails the utilization of oral appliance therapy, which encompasses the application of a detachable mandibular positioning device during periods of sleep to advance the mandible and facilitate the expansion of the airway. Although there has been much research conducted on these devices in adults, the available literature on their efficacy in children is limited to a single study, which reported a minimum 50% reduction in AHI [29].

References

1. Blumer S, Eli I, Kaminsky-Kurtz S, Shreiber-Fridman Y, Dolev E, Emodi-Perlman A. Sleep-related breathing disorders in children-red flags in pediatric care. J Clin Med. 2022;11(19):5570. https://doi.org/10.3390/jcm11195570.
2. Guo Y, Pan Z, Gao F, et al. Characteristics and risk factors of children with sleep-disordered breathing in Wuxi, China. BMC Pediatr. 2020;20(1):310. https://doi.org/10.1186/s12887-020-02207-5.
3. Sateia MJ. International classification of sleep disorders-third edition: highlights and modifications. Chest. 2014;146(5):1387–94. https://doi.org/10.1378/chest.14-0970.
4. Slowik JM, Sankari A, Collen JF. Obstructive sleep apnea. StatPearls; 2023.
5. Gipson K, Lu M, Kinane TB. Sleep-disordered breathing in children. Pediatr Rev. 2019;40(1):3–13. https://doi.org/10.1542/pir.2018-0142.
6. Brockbank JC. Update on pathophysiology and treatment of childhood obstructive sleep apnea syndrome. Paediatr Respir Rev. 2017;24:21–3. https://doi.org/10.1016/j.prrv.2017.06.003.
7. Wilhelm CP, deShazo RD, Tamanna S, Ullah MI, Skipworth LB. The nose, upper airway, and obstructive sleep apnea. Ann Allergy Asthma Immunol. 2015;115(2):96–102. https://doi.org/10.1016/j.anai.2015.06.011.
8. Arens R, Marcus CL. Pathophysiology of upper airway obstruction: a developmental perspective. Sleep. 2004;27(5):997–1019. https://doi.org/10.1093/sleep/27.5.997.
9. Nishino T. Physiological and pathophysiological implications of upper airway reflexes in humans. Jpn J Physiol. 2000;50(1):3–14. https://doi.org/10.2170/jjphysiol.50.3.
10. Grime C, Tan HL. Sleep disordered breathing in children. Indian J Pediatr. 2015;82(10):945–55. https://doi.org/10.1007/s12098-015-1857-5.

11. Tapia IE, Bandla P, Traylor J, Karamessinis L, Huang J, Marcus CL. Upper airway sensory function in children with obstructive sleep apnea syndrome. Sleep. 2010;33(7):968–72. https://doi.org/10.1093/sleep/33.7.968.
12. Solano-Perez E, Coso C, Castillo-Garcia M, et al. Diagnosis and treatment of sleep apnea in children: a future perspective is needed. Biomedicines. 2023;11(6):1708. https://doi.org/10.3390/biomedicines11061708.
13. Gulotta G, Iannella G, Vicini C, et al. Risk factors for obstructive sleep apnea syndrome in children: state of the art. Int J Environ Res Public Health. 2019;16(18):3235. https://doi.org/10.3390/ijerph16183235.
14. Marulanda J, Eimar H, McKee MD, et al. Matrix Gla protein deficiency impairs nasal septum growth, causing midface hypoplasia. J Biol Chem. 2017;292(27):11400–12. https://doi.org/10.1074/jbc.M116.769802.
15. Pongchangyoo J, Hantragool S, Rojvachiranonda N, Niyomkarn W. Sleep-disordered breathing in children with craniofacial anomalies. J Craniofac Surg. 2023;34(7):1962–5. https://doi.org/10.1097/SCS.0000000000009470.
16. Crysdale WS, Djupesland P. Nasal obstruction in children with craniofacial malformations. Int J Pediatr Otorhinolaryngol. 1999;49(Suppl 1):S63–7. https://doi.org/10.1016/s0165-5876(99)00135-4.
17. Sanchez T, Rojas C, Casals M, et al. Prevalence and risk factors for sleep-disordered breathing in chilean school children. Rev Child Pediatr. 2018;89(6):718–25. https://doi.org/10.4067/S0370-41062018005000902.
18. Su MS, Zhang HL, Cai XH, et al. Obesity in children with different risk factors for obstructive sleep apnea: a community-based study. Eur J Pediatr. 2016;175(2):211–20. https://doi.org/10.1007/s00431-015-2613-6.
19. Chirakalwasan N, Ruxrungtham K. The linkage of allergic rhinitis and obstructive sleep apnea. Asian Pac J Allergy Immunol. 2014;32(4):276–86.
20. Guilleminault C, Partinen M, Praud JP, Quera-Salva MA, Powell N, Riley R. Morphometric facial changes and obstructive sleep apnea in adolescents. J Pediatr. 1989;114(6):997–9. https://doi.org/10.1016/s0022-3476(89)80447-0.
21. Marcus CL. Pathophysiology of childhood obstructive sleep apnea: current concepts. Respir Physiol. 2000;119(2–3):143–54. https://doi.org/10.1016/s0034-5687(99)00109-7.
22. Duan X, Li M, Liu F, et al. Sensorimotor nerve lesion of upper airway in patients with obstructive sleep apnea. Respir Physiol Neurobiol. 2021;293:103720. https://doi.org/10.1016/j.resp.2021.103720.
23. Marcus CL, Katz ES, Lutz J, Black CA, Galster P, Carson KA. Upper airway dynamic responses in children with the obstructive sleep apnea syndrome. Pediatr Res. 2005;57(1):99–107. https://doi.org/10.1203/01.PDR.0000147565.74947.14.
24. Marcus CL, Fernandes Do Prado LB, Lutz J, et al. Developmental changes in upper airway dynamics. J Appl Physiol (1985). 2004;97(1):98–108. https://doi.org/10.1152/japplphysiol.00462.2003.
25. Hillman DR, Platt PR, Eastwood PR. The upper airway during anaesthesia. Br J Anaesth. 2003;91(1):31–9. https://doi.org/10.1093/bja/aeg126.
26. Marcus CL, Brooks LJ, Draper KA, et al. Diagnosis and management of childhood obstructive sleep apnea syndrome. Pediatrics. 2012;130(3):e714–55. https://doi.org/10.1542/peds.2012-1672.
27. Saxby C, Stephenson KA, Steele K, Ifeacho S, Wyatt ME, Samuels M. The effect of midface advancement surgery on obstructive sleep apnoea in syndromic craniosynostosis. J Craniofac Surg. 2018;29(1):92–5. https://doi.org/10.1097/SCS.0000000000004105.
28. Camacho M, Chang ET, Song SA, et al. Rapid maxillary expansion for pediatric obstructive sleep apnea: a systematic review and meta-analysis. Laryngoscope. 2017;127(7):1712–9. https://doi.org/10.1002/lary.26352.
29. Villa MP, Bernkopf E, Pagani J, Broia V, Montesano M, Ronchetti R. Randomized controlled study of an oral jaw-positioning appliance for the treatment of obstructive sleep apnea in children with malocclusion. Am J Respir Crit Care Med. 2002;165(1):123–7. https://doi.org/10.1164/ajrccm.165.1.2011031.

44 Upper Respiratory Tract Involvement in Cystic Fibrosis: Genetics and Developmental Basis

Azer Kilic Baskan, Ayse Ayzit Kilinc Sakallı, and Bruce K. Rubin

44.1 Characteristics of Sinonasal Disease in CF

Sinonasal disease is the prevailing otolaryngological manifestation of cystic fibrosis (CF) [1]. This arises due to poor mucociliary clearance (MCC) and defective bacterial immune responses. In addition, the hypoxic environment in the sinuses leads to chronic bacterial colonization [2]. Sinonasal disease commonly presents as chronic rhinosinusitis (CRS) [3]. CRS has been reported in pediatric and adult patients with CF at varying rates ranging from 40 to 60% in different studies [4, 5]. The most common symptoms reported are nasal congestion, obstruction, and rhinorrhea. Additional symptoms include headache, facial pain, olfactory dysfunction, and mouth breathing [6]. The criteria most frequently used for CRS are derived from The EAACI position paper on Rhinosinusitis and Nasal Polyps and are presented as follows [7].

(A) Inflammation of the nose and the paranasal sinuses with two or more symptoms for more than 12 weeks:
   1. nasal obstruction,
   2. congestion,
   3. rhinorrhea,
   4. nasal discharge,
   5. facial pain/pressure,
   6. reduction in olfaction

A. K. Baskan · A. A. K. Sakallı (✉)
Department of Pediatric Pulmonology, Istanbul University-Cerrahpasa, Cerrahpasa Faculty of Medicine, Istanbul, Turkey

B. K. Rubin
Pediatrics and Biomedical Engineering, Virginia Commonwealth University School of Medicine, Richmond, VA, USA

H. Yüksel et al. (eds.), *Pediatric Airway Diseases*, Comprehensive ENT,
https://doi.org/10.1007/978-3-031-74853-0_44

(B) With at least one of the following findings:
1. nasal polyps,
2. mucopurulent discharge (yellow-green sticky secretions of infected mucus),
3. mucosal edema/changes,
4. radiological findings of disease on a computer tomography (CT) scan

Computed tomography (CT) or nasal endoscopy examination can diagnose CF sinonasal disease. Nasal endoscopy detects nasal polyps and allows sinus cultures to be taken.

Endoscopic evaluation may also reveal the presence of mucopurulent material in the anterior nasal cavity, cobblestone formation in the posterior pharynx, and adenoid enlargement. Concha obstruction, nasal polyposis, and anomalies of the lateral nasal wall are frequently seen in patients with CF [8]. Sinus CT scanning helps determine the extent of CRS and other sinonasal abnormalities. Studies have shown that CF patients typically have pansinusitis rather than inflammation limited to specific sinuses. CT findings usually present as hypoplastic sinuses, pseudo-mucocele, opacification, and osteitis. Hypoplastic sinuses are mainly caused by growth restriction caused by severe chronic infections or improper embryogenesis due to genetic mutation [9]. CRS may also be present in patients without sinus CT abnormalities [1, 3]. It is recommended that imaging indications be limited to preoperative planning purposes only in pediatric patients to limit radiation exposure. Although endoscopic examination or CT can detect sinonasal abnormalities, many people with CF do not report significant symptoms as the disease progresses [10]. This may be explained by the chronicity of symptoms [11].

Nasal polyps may accompany CRS. However, 90–100% of CF patients have pulmonary and sinonasal involvement, despite the disease having a diverse phenotypic presentation [10]. In a study of children with cystic fibrosis, Yung et al. reported that 57% of children between the ages of 5 and 18 years had nasal polyps [6]. In contrast to nasal polyps in the non-CF population, nasal polyp formation in CF is primarily associated with an inflammatory response characterized by neutrophilic activity and predominance of T1 and T17 inflammatory mediators such as IL-1β, IL-8, IL-17, and myeloperoxidase [12]. Several studies have shown that children with CF, significant nasal polyps, or recurrent polyposis are more likely to have milder lung disease than their peers of the same age. Rubin et al. suggest polyps may be an overabundant manifestation of the epithelial repair process [13]. The process of inflammation and remodeling promotes the formation of nasal polyps and contributes to the age-related increase in prevalence.

Diverse pathogenic organisms predominate in the sinonasal cavity, causing cycles of infection and inflammation [14]. The temporal relationship between acute exacerbation of pulmonary disease and sinonasal symptoms suggests bacterial infection from the upper respiratory tract to the lower respiratory tract. The sinonasal cavity may be a reservoir for bacteria that infect the lungs [15, 16]. Furthermore, the observation that nasal symptoms appear before lower respiratory tract (LRT) symptoms means that the nasal cavity is likely the primary site of viral entry. The main linking factor between CRS and pulmonary exacerbations is thought to be postnasal drip, which carries pathogens into the LRT [3]. Similar pathogen profiles in lung and sinonasal cultures (e.g., *Pseudomonas aeruginosa* and *Staphylococcus aureus*) also support this [17, 18]. Studies have shown a correlation between sinonasal cultures and lower airway cultures obtained from patients undergoing lung transplantation for CF [19].

44.1.1 Effects on the Senses of Taste and Smell

Persons with CF may have olfactory and taste disorders. Loss of smell may occur due to sinonasal disease, a common condition in most CF patients. The etiology of olfactory disturbances in CF is poorly understood. However, it has been suggested that this may be due to peripheral olfactory dysfunction associated with sensorineural or central components. One study of CF patients found that almost 2/3 had impaired olfactory function. In addition to reducing quality of life, this increases the risk of malnutrition [20, 21].

The presence of taste abnormalities in people with CF is controversial. Because CF suffers from salt loss due to the malfunction of CFTR, studies have prioritized investigating salt taste sensitivity [22, 23], but it has been found that taste sensation is not primarily affected [24].

Another noteworthy issue in CF is the association of taste receptor defects with airway disease. Some isoforms of Tat family two receptors (T2Rs), necessary for the perception of bitter taste on the tongue, are found in limited numbers in bronchial and nasal cilia (i.e., T2Rs 4, 14, 16, and 38). These are G protein-coupled receptors. *P. aeruginosa* metabolites trigger these receptors in the nasal area and induce nitric oxide formation. This triggers the activation of protein kinase G and phosphorylation of proteins associated with cilia function. NO can also neutralize infectious agents through its effect on the cell wall and DNA. Defective alleles of one of the isoforms, T2R38 (alanine–valine–isoleucine/AVI variant), have been associated with resistant CRS in individuals without CF. A correlation between the T2R38 genotype and variability in sinonasal quality of life and severity of CRS was observed in CF patients homozygous for phe.508.del. There is a suggestion that individuals AVI-homozygous for T2R38 may have increased susceptibility to Gram-negative upper respiratory tract infection and CRS [25].

44.2 Ear Disease in CF

Unlike sinonasal disease, acute otitis media (AOM) is uncommon in patients with CF. Many studies have suggested that the prevalence of AOM in CF varies between 3 and 43% [26–29]. A study conducted in 2021 indicated that middle ear involvement should not be ignored in patients with cystic fibrosis (CF), as moderate ear abnormalities were detected in CF at rates similar to the general population [30]. Kaffenberger et al. also conducted a study evaluating the association of CFTR mutations with the risk of AOM and showed that more severe classes of CFTR mutation

(Classes I–III) not only have more severe clinical phenotypes compared to mild classes but may also have unexpected additional complications such as middle ear disease [31]. This is important because this study shows an increased risk of moderate ear disease in individuals with severe CFTR mutations. On the other hand, despite the extraordinarily high prevalence of sinus problems, there is little evidence to suggest that middle ear disease is becoming more common.

44.3 Effect of Upper Airway Disease on Quality of LIFE (QoL)

CRS negatively impacts QoL. The CF Questionnaire-Revised (CFQ-R) is a tool often used to evaluate the QoL of CF patients. However, it does not assess the effects of sinonasal dysfunction [32]. The most extensively used questionnaire to evaluate rhinologic dysfunction is the Sino-Nasal Outcome Test-22 (SNOT-22) [32]. The Sinus and Nasal Quality of Life

Questionnaire (SN-5) is a scale used to assess sinonasal disease in children aged 2–12 years.

However, there are insufficient data regarding the use of SNOT-22 and SN-5 in children with CF [33]. In a study conducted by Thamboo et al. using the SNOT-22 questionnaire on children with cystic fibrosis aged 6–18 years, a correlation was discovered between questionnaire scores exceeding 11 and the presence of nasal polyps [33]. In addition, some studies have demonstrated a possible correlation between compromised sinus quality of life, impaired lung health, and decreased disease-specific QoL in individuals with CF [34].

44.4 Treatment

Conservative treatment is preferred for CF-related CRS. Nasal saline irrigation, topical and systemic antibiotics, and macrolide antibiotics as immunomodulators treat CRS associated with CF [35].

1. *Dornase alfa*: Dornase alfa is a mucolytic drug that degrades extracellular polymeric deoxyribonucleic acid (DNA). It reduces mucus stickiness, thus facilitating the clearance of mucus. Administered by a nebulizer at a dose of 2.5 mg once daily, dornase alfa has been suggested to improve sinonasal symptoms [35–37] and SNOT-20 scores [36, 38] and decrease the need for surgery [39].
2. *Nasal saline irrigations*: Nasal lavage is used to help clear secretions. A multidisciplinary council specifically recommends sinonasal irrigation with isotonic saline (0.9% saline solution) for the treatment of CRS associated with CF [40]. There is insufficient information on sinonasal lavage with hypertonic saline (3–7% saline solutions). Care should be taken when using hypertonic solutions, which may cause ciliostasis and mucosal irritation. Both treatments (0.9% saline solution and 6.0% NaCl) have similar effects on SNOT-20 scores [41].

3. *Corticosteroids*: Corticosteroids are potent immunosuppressants that effectively treat CRS by suppressing the T2 inflammatory response. They can be administered orally or topically. Topical application increases the drug's local effect and prevents systemic side effects. Topical corticosteroids have been used to reduce nasal polyp formation due to their anti-inflammatory properties [42, 43]. Suppression of inflammation provides regression of edema and drainage of secretions from the sinuses [35]. Its antiinflammatory properties are effective in allergy-related rhinosinusitis [42], but there is no recommendation for using nasal steroids in CF rhinosinusitis [1]. Neutrophils are the predominant inflammatory cells in the pathogenesis of CF disease, and this type of inflammation is not responsive to therapy with corticosteroids. Data suggest that chronic low-dose macrolide therapy is more effective in ameliorating nasal polyps associated with neutrophilic inflammation.
4. *Antibiotics*: Colistin and tobramycin are the two topical antibiotics that are most frequently used [35]. Using inhaled antibiotics in CF upper respiratory tract disease has been shown to reduce chronic sinonasal infection, mainly of *P. aeruginosa* and *S. aureus,* and improve symptoms [44]. Using topical antibiotics in the postoperative period delays the recurrence of CF sinus exacerbations for up to two years following surgery [45]. The benefits of topical antibiotic therapy include minimizing the risk of systemic absorption and side effects and achieving therapeutically effective drug concentrations in the nose, but perhaps not in the sinuses. It has been reported that nebulization of tobramycin (80 mg/2 mL) once daily for 28 days reduces bacterial load in secretions, and adding 20 mg of tobramycin to 50 mL of nasal saline irrigation once a day decreases the frequency of exacerbations in persons with CF and improves sinus MRI scans [45, 46]. CF patients with CRS undergoing endoscopic sinus surgery may benefit from 2 weeks of postoperative broad-spectrum intravenous antibiotics, daily colistimethate sodium and nasal saline lavage for at least 6 months, and topical nasal mometasone furoate for at least 6 months [47].
5. *Ibuprofen*: Information on the effect of ibuprofen use in CF is limited. Although ibuprofen treatment reduces nasal polyp formation in some patients, these effects are short-lived [48]. This effect may be attributable to ibuprofen's ability to inhibit cyclooxygenase enzymes and prevent neutrophil activation and migration [49]. Ibuprofen may also regulate microtubule function in nasal epithelial cells [50].
6. *Macrolides*: Most studies investigating the potential benefit of macrolides in treating CF have focused on the effects of macrolide administration on chronic lung disease [51, 52]. The comparable pathophysiological mechanism contributing to chronic lung disease suggests these drugs may benefit CF-related CRS [53]. Macrolides, a class of antibiotics with immunomodulatory properties, are believed to have therapeutic potential for treating nasal polyps-related CRS [54]. Macrolides also promote tissue repair by inhibiting neutrophil chemotaxis and recruitment, mucus production, and airway transport. Administration of clarithromycin for 2–3 months in non-CF patients with nasal polyps decreased the size of the polyps and CXCL8 in nasal lavage [55]. In a randomized controlled

trial, 64 subjects with non-CF CRS were given either low-dose roxithromycin or a placebo for 3 months. The macrolide group had significant improvements in the sinonasal outcome test-20 score, nasal endoscopy findings, saccharin transit time, and CXCL8 levels ($p < 0.05$) [56].

7. *Endoscopic sinus surgery*: The endoscopic surgical treatment option is not typically considered for CRS associated with CF. Patient selection for sinus surgery in the CF population is very important. Sinus surgery may be indicated in CF in the following situations [13, 57]:
   (a) Persistent nasal congestion that remains unresolved despite medical interventions
   (b) Presence of an anatomical obstruction as evidenced by nasal endoscopy or CT imaging
   (c) Substantial impairment in quality of life resulting from symptomatic manifestations.

CT scans cannot be used as a criterion for sinus surgery as results poorly correlate with clinical symptoms. CT scanning should only be used to evaluate anatomy and assess the extent of disease [58].

Functional endoscopic sinus surgery (FESS) is regarded as the prevailing surgical approach for CRS, particularly in cases of CRS with nasal polyposis. In a broad sense, it is advisable to contemplate FESS as a possible option for patients CF who have sinonasal symptoms that do not improve with medical management, especially in association with anatomic abnormalities [59]. In children with CF, there are often anatomical variations in the development and pneumatization of the sinuses, and these increase the possibility of encountering difficulties during surgery. Sinus surgery is generally well tolerated in CF, and the incidence of complications in CF patients is comparable to that in the general population [60]. However, sinus surgery is palliative and does not change the pathogenic pathways and mucosa contributing to CRS.

In some children with CRS and nasal polyposis, polypectomy may be an alternative to FEES. However, patients with CF have a high recurrence rate after polypectomy, and symptomatic improvement is only temporary [61].

44.4.1 Effect of Highly Effective Modulator Therapy (HEMT) on Upper Airway Disease in CF

HEMT has been a life-changing therapy for CF patients, resulting in fewer respiratory symptoms, pulmonary exacerbations, and improved lung function and quality of life. The effects of CFTR-modulator therapy have been demonstrated in CF-CRS [62]. It has been reported that ivacaftor treatment used in CF patients with G551D mutation improved sinonasal symptoms and radiologic findings [63–65] and positively affected QoL, psychological, and sleep domains assessed by the SNOT-22 questionnaire [66]. The combination of ivacaftor and lumacaftor has not been reported to have any apparent positive effect on CRS, nor has the use of tezacaftor/ivacaftor improved sinonasal symptoms. However, a longitudinal paranasal sinus

MRI imaging study showed that lumacaftor/ivacaftor treatment improved paranasal sinus abnormalities in children with CF starting at school age while preventing the increase in paranasal sinus abnormalities in preschool-aged children [67]. Triple therapy with ivacaftor and the correctors tezacaftor and elexacaftor (ETI—the most effective combination for patients with the phe.508.del mutation) results in dramatic improvements in pulmonary function, QoL, body mass index, and frequency of exacerbations. For this reason, it has been termed "highly effective CFTR-modulatory therapy" or HEMT [68, 69]. ETI treatment significantly improves CFTR function in the nasal epithelium [70]. ETI therapy decreases CRS and respiratory symptoms in CF. The observed advantages were more notable among patients who began ETI treatment early [71–74]. ETI significantly decreased sinus CT opacification and sinonasal QoL. Improvements in QoL began in the first month of treatment and continued throughout a 6-month study period [74]. Radiologic imaging demonstrates fewer paranasal sinus abnormalities in adults after the initiation of HEMT [74, 75]. In another study, sinonasal symptoms improved rapidly and permanently for at least 180 days with ETI treatment, and objective evaluations of the disease, including endoscopic and CT findings, also improved [76]. In a study conducted in CF patients while receiving CFTR modulator therapy, it was thought that the improvement in imaging findings on CT was closely related to improved SNOT-22 and that CT could be an objective indicator of sinonasal disease in the follow-up of patients receiving HEMT [77]. The administration of ETI over a period of 6 months does not appear to improve olfaction [78, 79].

References

1. Krajewska J, Zub K, Slowikowski A, et al. Chronic rhinosinusitis in cystic fibrosis: a review of therapeutic options. Eur Arch Oto-Rhino-Laryngol. 2022;279:1–24.
2. Chaaban MR, Kejner A, Rowe SM, et al. Cystic fibrosis chronic rhinosinusitis: a comprehensive review. Am J Rhinol Allergy. 2013;27(5):387–95.
3. Kang SH, Dalcin PDTR, Piltcher OB, et al. Chronic rhinosinusitis and nasal polyposis in cystic fibrosis: update on diagnosis and treatment. J Bras Pneumol. 2015;41(1):65–76.
4. Gentile VG, Isaacson G. Patterns of sinusitis in cystic fibrosis. Laryngoscope. 1996;106:1005–9.
5. Casserly P, Harrison M, O'Connell O, et al. Nasal endoscopy and paranasal sinus computerized tomography (CT) findings in an Irish cystic fibrosis adult patient group. Eur Arch Otorhinolaryngol. 2015;272:3353–9.
6. Yung MW, Gould J, Upton GJG. Nasal polyposis in children with cystic fibrosis: a long-term follow-up study. Ann Otol Rhinol Laryngol. 2002;111(12):1081–6.
7. Fokkens W, Lund VJ, Mullol J, et al. European position paper on rhinosinusitis and nasal polyps 2012. A summary for otorhinolaryngologists. Rhinology. 2012;50:1–12.
8. Spielman DB, Beswick DM, Kimple AJ, et al. The management of cystic fibrosis chronic rhinosinusitis: an evidenced-based review with recommendations. Int Forum Allergy Rhinol. 2022;12(9):1148–83.
9. Kang SH, Piltcher OB, de Dalcin PT. Sinonasal alterations in computed tomography scans in cystic fibrosis: a literature review of observational studies. Int Forum Allergy Rhinol. 2014;4(3):223–31.
10. Oomen KP, April MM. Sinonasal manifestations in cystic fibrosis. Int J Otolaryngol. 2012;2012:789572.

11. Kikuchi Y, Okabe S, Tamura G, et al. Chemosensitivity and perception of dyspnea in patient with a history of near-fatal asthma. N Engl J Med. 1994;330(19):1329–34.
12. Derycke L, Eyerich S, van Crombruggen K, et al. Mixed T helper cell signatures in chronic rhinosinusitis with and without polyps. PLoS One. 2014;9(6):e97581.
13. Robertson JM, Friedman EM, Rubin BK. Nazal and sinüs disease in cystic fibrosis. Paediatr Respir Rev. 2008;9:213–9.
14. Whiteson KL, Bailey B, Bergkessel M, et al. The upper respiratory tract as a microbial source for pulmonary infections in cystic fibrosis. Parallels from island biogeography. Am J Respir Crit Care Med. 2014;189:1309–15.
15. Nelson J, Karempelis P, Dunitz J, et al. Pulmonary aspiration of sinus secretions in patients with cystic fibrosis. Int Forum of Allergy Rhinol. 2018;8:385–8.
16. Zemke Anna C, Mehdi NS, John M, et al. Clinical predictors of cystic fibrosis chronic rhinosinusitis severity. Int Forum Allergy Rhinol. 2019;9(7):759–65.
17. Mainz JG, Naehrlich L, Schien M, et al. Concordant genotype of upper and lower airways *P. aeruginosa* and *S. aureus* isolates in cystic fibrosis. Thorax. 2009;64(6):535–40.
18. Lavin J, Bhushan B, Schroeder JW Jr. Correlation between respiratory and sinus cultures in children with cystic fibrosis. Int J Pediatr Otorhinolaryngol. 2013;77:686–9.
19. Choi KJ, Cheng TZ, Honeybrook AL, et al. Correlation between sinus and lung cultures in lung transplant patients with cystic fibrosis. Int Forum Allergy Rhinol. 2018;8(3):389–93.
20. Lindig J, Steger C, Beiersdorf N. Smell in cystic fibrosis. Eur Arch Otorhinolaryngol. 2013;270:915–21.
21. Mueller CA, Quint C, Gulesserian T, et al. Olfactory function in children with cystic fibrosis. Acta Paediatr. 2007;96:145–9.
22. Lullo MA, Lacotucci P, Comegna M. Cystic fibrosis: the sense of smell. Am J Rhinol Allergy. 2020;34(1):35–42.
23. Henkin RI, Powell GF. Increased sensitivity of taste and smell in cystic fibrosis. Science. 1962;138:1107–8.
24. Laing DG, Armstrong JE, Aitken M, et al. Chemosensory function and food preferences of children with cystic fibrosis. Pediatr Pulmonol. 2010;45:807–15.
25. Lee RJ, Cohen NA. Role of the bitter taste receptor T2R38 in upper respiratory infection and chronic rhinosinusitis. Curr Opin Allergy Clin Immunol. 2015;15(1):14–20.
26. Cipolli M, Canciani M, Cavazzani M, Uras P, Zampieri P, Mastella G. Ear disease is not a common complication in cystic fibrosis. Eur J Pediatr. 1993;152(3):265–6.
27. Bak-Pedersen K, Larsen PK. Inflammatory middle ear diseases in patients with cystic fibrosis. Acta Otolaryngol Suppl. 1979;360:138–40.
28. Forcucci RA, Stark EW. Hearing loss, speech-language, and cystic fibrosis. Arch Otolaryngol. 1972;96(4):361–4.
29. Haddad J, Gonzalez C, Kurland G, Orenstein DM, Casselbrant ML. Ear disease in children with cystic fibrosis. Arch Otolaryngol Head Neck Surg. 1994;120:491–3.
30. McCoy JL, Kaffenberger TM, Yang TS, et al. Otitis media prone children with cystic fibrosis: a new normal. Am J Otolaryngol. 2021;42(5):103137.
31. Kaffenberger TM, Eichar BW, McCoy JL, et al. Cystic fibrosis mutation classes in pediatric otitis media—Fickle or faulty? Am J Otolaryngol. 2021;42(6):103067.
32. Virgin FW. Clinical chronic rhinosinusitis outcomes in pediatric patients with cystic fibrosis. Laryngosc Investig Otolaryngol. 2017;2(5):276–80.
33. Thamboo A, Santos RCD, Naidoo L, et al. Use of the SNOT-22 and UPSIT to appropriately select pediatric patients with cystic fibrosis who should be referred to an otolaryngologist. JAMA Otolaryngol Neck Surg. 2014;140(10):934.
34. Safi C, DiMango E, Keating C, et al. Sinonasal quality-of-life declines in cystic fibrosis patients with pulmonary exacerbations. Int Forum Allergy Rhinol. 2020;10(2):194–8.
35. Karanth TK, Karanth VKLKL, Ward BK, et al. Medical interventions for chronic rhinosinusitis in cystic fibrosis. Cochrane Database Syst Rev. 2022;4(4):CD012979.
36. Mainz JG, Schien C, Schiller I, et al. Sinonasal inhalation of dornase alfa administered by vibrating aerosol to cystic fibrosis patients: a double-blind placebo-controlled cross-over trial. J Cyst Fibros. 2014;13(4):461–70.

37. Cimmino M, Nardone M, Cavaliere M, et al. Dornase alfa as postoperative therapy in cystic fibrosis sinonasal disease. Arch Otolaryngol Neck Surg. 2005;131(12):1097.
38. Mainz JG, Schiller I, Ritschel C, et al. Sinonasal inhalation of dornase alfa in CF: a double-blind placebo-controlled cross-over pilot trial. Auris Nasus Larynx. 2011;38(2):220–7.
39. Raynor EM, Butler A, Guill M, Bent JP. Nasally inhaled dornase alfa in the postoperative management of chronic sinusitis due to cystic fibrosis. Arch Otolaryngol Neck Surg. 2000;126(5):581.
40. Jayawardena ADL, Fracchia MS, Bartley BL, et al. Working towards consensus in the management of pediatric chronic rhinosinusitis in cystic fibrosis. Int J Pediatr Otorhinolaryngol. 2020;135:110047.
41. Mainz JG, Schumacher U, Schädlich K, et al. Sino nasal inhalation of isotonic versus hypertonic saline (6.0%) in CF patients with chronic rhinosinusitis—results of a multicenter, prospective, randomized, double-blind, controlled trial. J Cyst Fibros. 2016;15(6):e57–66.
42. Costantini D, Di Cicco M, Giunta A, et al. Nasal polyposis in cystic fibrosis treated by beclomethasone dipropionate. Acta Universitatis Carolinae Medica. 1990;36(1–4):220–1.
43. Hadfield PJ, Rowe-Jones JM, Mackay IS. A prospective treatment trial of nasal polyps in adults with cystic fibrosis. Rhinology. 2000;38(2):63–5.
44. Mainz JG, Koitschev A. Pathogenesis and management of nasal polyposis in cystic fibrosis. Curr Allergy Asthma Rep. 2012;12(2):163–74.
45. Davidson TM, Murphy C, Mitchell M, et al. Management of chronic sinusitis in cystic fibrosis. Laryngoscope. 1995;105(4):354–8.
46. Mainz JG, Schaedlich K, Schien C, et al. Sinonasal inhalation of tobramycin vibrating aerosol in cystic fibrosis patients with upper airway *Pseudomonas aeruginosa* colonization: results of a randomized, double-blind, placebo-controlled pilot study. Drug Des Dev Ther. 2014;8:209.
47. Aanaes K, von Buchwald C, Hjuler T, et al. The effect of sinus surgery with intensive follow up on pathogenic sinus bacteria in patients with cystic fibrosis. Am J Rhinol Allergy. 2013;27(1):e1–4.
48. Lindstrom DR, Conley SF, Splaingard ML, et al. Ibuprofen therapy and nasal polyposis in cystic fibrosis patients. J Otolaryngol. 2007;36(05):309.
49. Crosby DL, Adappa ND. What is the optimal management of chronic rhinosinusitis in cystic fibrosis? Curr Opin Otolaryngol Head Neck Surg. 2014;22(1):42–6.
50. Rymut SM, Kampman CM, Corey DA, et al. Ibuprofen regulation of microtubule dynamics in cystic fibrosis epithelial cells. Am J Physiol Cell Mol Physiol. 2016;311(2):317–27.
51. Zimmermann P, Ziesenitz VC, Curtis N, et al. The immunomodulatory effects of macrolides—a systematic review of the underlying mechanisms. Front Immunol. 2018;13(9):302.
52. Southern KW, Barker PM, Solis-Moya A, Patel L. Macrolide antibiotics for cystic fibrosis. Cochrane Database Syst Rev. 2012;11(11):CD002203.
53. Shimizu T, Suzaki H. Past, present and future of macrolide therapy for chronic rhinosinusitis in Japan. Auris Nasus Larynx. 2016;43(2):131–6.
54. Oakley GM, Harvey RJ, Lund VJ. The role of macrolides in chronic rhinosinusitis (CRSsNP and CRSwNP). Curr Allergy Asthma Rep. 2017;17(5):30.
55. Yamada T, Fujieda S, Mori S, et al. Macrolide treatment decreased the size of nasal polyps and IL-8 levels in nasal lavage. Am J Rhinol. 2000;14:143–8.
56. Wallwork B, Coman W, Mackay-Sim A, et al. A double-blind, randomized, placebo-controlled trial of macrolide in the treatment of chronic rhinosinusitis. Laryngoscope. 2006;116:189–93.
57. Brook CD, Maxfield AZ, Ahmed H, et al. Factors influencing the need for endoscopic sinus surgery in adult patients with cystic fibrosis. Am J Rhinol Allergy. 2017;31:44–7.
58. Carter JM, Johnson BT, Patel A, et al. Lund-Mackay staging system in cystic fibrosis: a prognostic factor for revision surgery? Ochsner J. 2014;14(2):184–7.
59. Keck T, Rozsasi A. Medium-term symptom outcomes after paranasal sinus surgery in children and young adults with cystic fibrosis. Laryngoscope. 2007;117(3):475–9.
60. Van Peteghem A, Clement PAR. Influence of extensive functional endoscopic sinus surgery (FESS) on facial growth in children with cystic fibrosis. Int J Pediatr Otorhinolaryngol. 2006;70(8):1407–13.

61. Virgin FW, Huang L, Roberson DW, et al. Inter-hospital variation in the frequency of sinus surgery in children with cystic fibrosis. Pediatr Pulmonol. 2015;50(3):231–5.
62. Bode SFN, Rapp H, Lienert N. Effects of CFTR-modulator triple therapy on sinonasal symptoms in children and adults with cystic fibrosis. Eur Arch Oto-Rhino-Laryngol. 2023;280:3271–7.
63. Hayes D Jr, McCoy KS, Sheikh SI. Improvement of sinus disease in cystic fibrosis with ivacaftor therapy. Am J Respir Crit Care Med. 2014;190(4):468.
64. Sheikh SI, Long FR, McCoy KS, et al. Ivacaftor improves appearance of sinus disease on computerized tomography in cystic fibrosis patients with G551D mutation. Clin Otolaryngol. 2015;40(1):16–21.
65. Vreede CL, Berkhout MC, Sprij AJ, et al. Ivacaftor and sinonasal pathology in a cystic fibrosis patient with genotype deltaF508/S1215N. J Cyst Fibros. 2015;14(3):412–3.
66. McCormick J, Cho DY, Lampkin B, et al. Ivacaftor improves rhinologic, psychologic, and sleep-related quality of life in G551D cystic fibrosis patients. Int Forum Allergy Rhinol. 2019;9(3):292–7.
67. Wucherpfennig L, Wuennemann F, Eichinger M, et al. Long-term effects of lumacaftor/ivacaftor on paranasal sinus abnormalities in children with cystic fibrosis detected with magnetic resonance imaging. Front Pharmacol. 2022;10(14):1161891.
68. Keating D, Marigowda G, Burr L, et al. VX-445-tezacaftor–ivacaftor in patients with cystic fibrosis and one or two Phe508del alleles. N Engl J Med. 2018;379(17):1612–20.
69. Middleton PG, Mall MA, Drevinek P, et al. Elexacaftor–tezacaftor–ivacaftor for cystic fibrosis with a single Phe508del allele. N Engl J Med. 2019;381(19):1809–19.
70. Graeber SY, Vitzthum C, Pallenberg ST, et al. Effects of elexacaftor/tezacaftor/ivacaftor therapy on CFTR function in patients with cystic fibrosis and one or two F508del alleles. Am J Respir Crit Care Med. 2022;205(5):540–9.
71. DiMango E, Overdevest J, Keating C, et al. Effect of highly effective modulator treatment on sinonasal symptoms in cystic fibrosis. J Cyst Fibros. 2021;20(3):460–3.
72. Douglas JE, Civantos AM, Locke TB. Impact of novel CFTR modulator on sinonasal quality of life in adult patients with cystic fibrosis. Int Forum Allergy Rhinol. 2021;11(2):201–3.
73. Shakir S, Echevarria C, Doe S, et al. Elexacaftor–tezacaftor–ivacaftor improve gastro-oesophageal reflux and sinonasal symptoms in advanced cystic fibrosis. J Cyst Fibros. 2022;21(5):807–10.
74. Beswick DM, Humphries SM, Balkissoon CD, et al. Impact of cystic fibrosis transmembrane conductance regulator therapy on chronic rhinosinusitis and health status: deep learning CT analysis and patient-reported outcomes. Ann Am Thorac Soc. 2022;19(1):12–9.
75. Wucherpfennig L, Triphan SMF, Wege S, et al. Magnetic resonance imaging detects improvements of pulmonary and paranasal sinus abnormalities in response to elexacaftor/tezacaftor/ivacaftor therapy in adults with cystic fibrosis. J Cyst Fibros. 2022;21(6):1053–60.
76. Stapleton AL, Kimple AJ, Goralski JL, et al. Elexacaftor–tezacaftor–ivacaftor improves sinonasal outcomes in cystic fibrosis. J Cyst Fibros. 2022;21(5):792–9.
77. Tagliati C, Pantano S, Lanni G, et al. Sinus disease grading on computed tomography before and after modulating therapy in adult patients with cystic fibrosis. J Belg Soc Radiol. 2022;106(1):57.
78. Bacon DR, Stapleton AL, Goralaski JL, et al. Olfaction before and after initiation of elexacaftor–tezacaftor–ivacaftor in a cystic fibrosis cohort. Int Forum Allergy Rhinol. 2021;12(2):223–6.
79. Beswick DM, Humphries SM, Balkissoon CD, et al. Olfactory dysfunction in cystic fibrosis: impact of CFTR modulator therapy. J Cyst Fibros. 2021;21(2):e141147.

45 Upper Respiratory Tract Involvement in Cystic Fibrosis: Clinics and Diagnosis

Pelin Asfuroğlu and Larry C. Lands

45.1 Introduction

Cystic fibrosis (CF) is an autosomal recessive genetic disease caused by mutations in the cystic fibrosis transmembrane conductivity regulator (*CFTR*) gene, encoding the CFTR protein, an apical cell membrane ion channel. Mutations in *CFTR* result in viscous mucus that impairs mucociliary clearance in both the upper and lower airways.

Upper respiratory tract involvement, such as sinonasal diseases, nasal polyps, and otic diseases, is common in CF. Anosmia, headache, facial pain, nasal congestion, chronic congestion, runny nose, abnormal hearing or hearing loss, dizziness, and vertigo can be seen as symptoms of upper respiratory tract involvement in CF. These symptoms can also affect children's quality of life. Since upper respiratory tract involvement is common in CF, these children need to be followed regularly.

P. Asfuroğlu (✉)
Pediatric Pulmonology Clinic, Gaziantep Cengiz Gökçek Gynecology and Pediatrics Hospital, Gaziantep, Turkey

L. C. Lands
Department of Pediatric Respiratory Medicine and Pediatric Cystic Fibrosis Clinic, McGill University Health Centre, Montreal Children's Hospital, Montreal, QC, Canada
e-mail: larry.lands@mcgill.ca

H. Yüksel et al. (eds.), *Pediatric Airway Diseases*, Comprehensive ENT,
https://doi.org/10.1007/978-3-031-74853-0_45

45.2 Upper Respiratory Tract Involvement in Cystic Fibrosis: Clinics and Diagnosis

45.2.1 What Is CF, Includıng Genes and Pathophysiology of CFTR Dysfunction

Cystic fibrosis (CF) is the most common autosomal recessive disease caused by mutations in the cystic fibrosis transmembrane conductance regulator (*CFTR*) gene, which encodes the CFTR protein, in the Caucasian population [1]. The CFTR protein is the main regulator of fluid and electrolyte homeostasis of the mucosal surface. The structural and functional defect in the CFTR protein causes increased viscosity of secretions in the pulmonary, gastrointestinal, and reproductive systems. The viscous mucus leads to inflammation, infections, malnutrition, and multiorgan dysfunction [2]. CFTR mutations are classified based on how they reduce CFTR protein synthesis, function or stability [1]. The absence of CFTR protein is seen in class I mutations, the limited trafficking of CFTR to the apical cell membrane is seen in class II mutations, defective regulation of CFTR gating and disruption of channel opening are seen in class III mutations, impaired conductivity of the CFTR channel is seen in class IV mutations, reduced amounts of normal CFTR protein with alternative splicing mutations is seen in class V mutations, unstable and prematurely destroyed CFTR protein is seen in class VI mutations, and the absence of mRNA transcription required for protein synthesis and inability to produce CFTR protein are seen in class VII mutations [1, 3, 4]. Note that certain mutations can affect several aspects related to functional CFTR abundance at the cell surface. The most common variant worldwide is c.1521_1523delCTT (delF508), class II mutation [3, 4]. Class 1, 2, 3, and 7 mutations are clinically severe and the disease has a more severe course. Class 4 and 5 mutations show a milder, late-onset clinical course [5–7].

45.2.2 Sinonasal Disease in CF

Thickened secretions with impaired mucociliary clearance as a result of defective CFTR function affect both the upper airways and lower airways [8]. Nasal and sinus disease may be presenting or persisting symptoms of CF, and are quite common [9].

45.2.2.1 Sinus Disease in CF

Anosmia, headache, facial pain, nasal congestion, chronic congestion, and runny nose are symptoms associated with sinus disease in CF [10]. Sinusitis can severely affect quality of life by causing nasal congestion, obstructive sleep apnea, and developmental growth delay [10].

Histologically, chronic neutrophil inflammatory cells can be seen predominantly in CF [11]. Although it may be lymphocytic in the early stages, it later turns into chronic neutrophilic inflammation [9, 11].

The details of bone and soft tissue anatomy can be provided by sinus computed tomography (CT). Characteristic sinonasal CT anomalies in CF are findings such as bulging/displacement of the lateral nasal wall and demineralization of the uncinate process [9]. In a study on sinus imaging, it was determined that the decision of treatment was based on clinical status rather than imaging findings, and it was concluded that it would be valuable to make a multidisciplinary imaging decision in all patients with CF [12]. It was reported that those with class 1–3 mutations had worse sinus hypoplasia, opacification, associated maxillary sinus osteitis, smaller frontal and sphenoid sinuses on CT scan than those with class 4 and 5 mutations, and it was concluded that the genotype affected the severity of the sinus disease in CF [13]. Sinus CT scans are not a useful criterion for deciding medical or surgical management of sinus disease in CF [9]. Bacterial density and endoscopic evaluation may be more useful in the treatment decision [9]. It is important to determine when sinus CT imaging is truly required to affect therapeutic decisions in children with CF [12].

Lung transplantation is an effective treatment option for CF patients with end-stage pulmonary disease [14]. In a study of sinus disease in CF patients who underwent lung transplantation, it was shown that sinus disease is common in transplant recipients [15].

Patient-reported specific questionnaires such as Sinonasal Quality of Life Survey (SN-5) and SinoNasal Outcome Test (SNOT-22) are available to assess quality of life in those with sinonasal disease [16, 17]. These questionnaires are predictive tools for diagnosis, outcome of an intervention and treatment preferences [18]. For patients aged 5 years and below, SN-5 can be used, and for patients above 5 years of age, SNOT-22 can be used. SN-5 contains of 5 items and the maximum score is 7 [16, 19]. SNOT-22 contains of 6 levels and includes 22 items (increasing scores from 0 to 5), and the final score is obtained by summing the scores of the items (0: best, 110: worst quality of life) [17]. SN-5 and SNOT-22 have higher scores in the presence of more sinonasal symptoms [16].

45.2.2.2 Nasal Polyposis in CF

The prevalence of nasal polyposis in CF varies; however, prevalence increases with age [9, 20]. The frequency of detection by nasal endoscopy has increased to approximately 57% [9]. Although the pathogenesis of nasal polyposis is unclear, the most relevant factor is predicted to be chronic inflammation [21]. Another prediction is that enlarged mucus glands cause occlusion of capillaries and disruption of blood flow, resulting in local edema and stroma prolapse, resulting in polyps [22]. The histopathology of CF-related polyps is different from atopy-related polyps [22, 23]. In CF-related polyps, a thin basal membrane, neutrophil infiltration and mucus glands with predominantly acid mucin are seen, but no eosinophil infiltration and hyalinization of the submucosa [22, 23]. In contrast, atopy-related polyps demonstrate thick basal membrane, eosinophil infiltration, and neutral mucin in the mucous glands [22, 23]. Nasal obstruction is the most important complaint of patients with nasal polyps [22]. Runny nose, facial pain, and decreased or loss of smell may be other complaints [13]. In CF with nasal polyps, the lateral wall of the bone may be eroded or even completely destroyed [22]. Physical examination such as broadening of nasal bridge, hypertelorism, and mouth breathing in CF can provide evidence of a nasal polyp [22]. Endoscopic examination reveals mucopurulent discharge from the middle meatus, along with edema and mucosal obstruction in that area [13]. CT scans show mucosal changes within the ostiomeatal complex or sinuses [13].

45.2.2.3 Highly Effective CFTR Modulator Therapy in Sinonasal Disease

CFTR modulators, which improve the function of the CFTR protein by various mechanisms, have been used more widely recently [8]. Modulators work to increase the transport of CFTR to the apical surface of epithelial cells and increase channel opening. Modulators with different mechanisms were combined to increase CFTR function [8]. Studies have found beneficial effects of ivacaftor on symptoms of chronic rhinosinusitis [8, 24]. In another study with a small CF patient group, sinus disease was evaluated with imaging before and after the initiation of ivacaftor, and it was reported that ivacaftor also improved imaging [25]. Other studies investigating the effects of elexacaftor/tezacaftor/ivacaftor treatment on sinonasal disease in CF patients also observed improvement in sinonasal symptoms and SNOT-22 [8, 26, 27]. In a recent study in adults with CF, although there was no difference in SNOT-22 scores in modulator users compared to nonusers, significantly lower CT scores and a lower colonization rate in upper respiratory tract cultures were found [28].

45.2.3 Microbiology and Its Relation to Lower Airways Microbiology

The upper and lower respiratory tracts have different microbiota, and their homeostasis is regulated by the immune system of host [29]. Bacterial colonization in the upper respiratory tract is known to be a common source of bacterial migration to the lung. However, not all migrating bacteria may reproduce in the lower respiratory tract [29].

Studies on the colonization of the upper respiratory tract before or together with the lower respiratory tract in CF indicate that the nasal cavity may function as a bacterial reservoir and that pathogens may migrate from upper to lower respiratory tract [30]. Bacterial colonization with *Pseudomonas aeruginosa* (PsA), *Achromobacteria xylosoxidans*, *Burkholderia cepacia*, methicillin-sensitive, and methicillin-resistant *Staphylococcus aureus* (MSSA, MRSA) can be associated with poor transplant outcomes [14]. Studies show that the microorganisms detected in the sinuses correlate with those detected in the transplanted lungs in CF. In a study conducted with cultures from the sinuses and lungs before and after lung transplantation, it was shown that the detection of PsA, MRSA, and Burkholderia in the sinuses before lung transplantation was associated with the detection of the same pathogens in the lungs after lung transplantation [14]. This was thought to be due to the high microorganism load in the sinuses of CF patients [14]. Although there are studies showing that posttransplant sinus surgeries and some treatment protocols can reduce lower respiratory tract infection and colonization in CF patients with lung transplantation, studies on this subject are insufficient [14].

Another study in CF showed that *P. aeruginosa* settled in the transplanted lung tissue after lung transplantation, and it was thought to adapted to the non-CF donor lung originating from the sinuses [31].

45.2.4 Otic Disease in CF

Previously, the CF was accepted as "protective" against otitis media [32]. This was explained by the hypothesis that frequent and long-term antibiotics used for respiratory and sinonasal infections lead to changes in the mucosa of the middle ear and therefore lead to a lower incidence otitis media [33]. Although the prevalence of otitis media in CF has been variable in the literature, it shows an increasing tendency in recent years. In a recent study, the highest otitis media prevalence was 52.6% and tube placement occurred in 9%; however, no predictive factors specific to otitis media in CF was found [34]. Aminoglycosides, frequently used to treat lung infections in CF, can have a toxic effect on the inner ear structures [35]. Aminoglycoside-related vestibulotoxicity occurs as a result of damage to hair cells in the vestibular system and may cause vestibular symptoms such as dizziness and vertigo [35, 36]. Aminoglycoside-related ototoxicity occurs as a result of degeneration of cochlear hair cells in the basal turn, which are necessary for high-frequency sounds, secondary to the production of reactive oxygen samples [35, 36]. Although the American Academy of Audiology does not specify a specific screening method, it recommends screening per week or once every 2 weeks during aminoglycoside treatment and a few months after treatment [37]. Although methods such as standard pure-tone audiometry, high frequency pure-tone audiometry, otoacoustic emissions, distortion product otoacoustic emissions, and automated auditory brainstem response can be used for hearing assessment, no single routinely recommended method for screening has been defined [37]. Some studies also recommend hearing screening in CF patients who are not exposed to aminoglyoses [37]. The European Cystic Fibrosis Society (ECFS) 2018 guideline recommends that CF centers should perform evaluation for aminoglycoside-related ototoxicity by audiology tests for patients with complaints or as a part of a routine evaluation [38].

In conclusion, upper respiratory tract involvement is common in CF. In children with CF, the sinuses may serve as reservoirs for lower respiratory tract microorganisms. Imaging for upper respiratory tract involvement during follow-up may result in abnormal findings even in asymptomatic children. Modulatory treatments, which have been shown to be highly effective in CF, have also been shown to improve upper respiratory tract symptoms. It should not be forgotten that upper respiratory tract involvement, which can also affect the quality of life of children, is common in CF and children with CF should be followed up in terms of upper respiratory tract involvement even if they are asymptomatic.

References

1. De Boeck K. Cystic fibrosis in the year 2020: a disease with a new face. Acta Paediatr. 2020;109:893–9. https://doi.org/10.1111/apa.15155. Epub 2020 Jan 22.
2. Bierlaagh MC, Muilwijk D, Beekman JM, et al. A new era for people with cystic fibrosis. Eur J Pediatr. 2021;180:2731–9. https://doi.org/10.1007/s00431-021-04168-y. Epub 2021 Jul 2.
3. Lopes-Pacheco M. CFTR modulators: shedding light on precision medicine for cystic fibrosis. Front Pharmacol. 2016;7:275. https://doi.org/10.3389/fphar.2016.00275.
4. Dabrowski M, Bukowy-Bieryllo Z, Zietkiewicz E. Advances in therapeutic use of a drug-stimulated translational read through of premature termination codons. Mol Med. 2018;24:25. https://doi.org/10.1186/s10020-018-0024-7.
5. The CFTR mutations database. http://www.umd.be/CFTR/W_CFTR/gene.html. Accessed 19 July 2023.
6. Singh VK, Schwarzenberg SJ. Pancreatic insufficiency in cystic fibrosis. J Cyst Fibros. 2017;16(Suppl 2):S70–8. https://doi.org/10.1016/j.jcf.2017.06.011.
7. Marson FAL, Bertuzzo CS, Ribeiro JD. Classification of CFTR mutation classes. Lancet Respir Med. 2016;4:e37–8. https://doi.org/10.1016/S2213-2600(16)30188-6. Epub 2016 Jul 1.
8. Spielman DB, Beswick DM, Kimple AJ, et al. The management of cystic fibrosis chronic rhinosinusitis: an evidenced-based review with recommendations. Int Forum Allergy Rhinol. 2022;12:1148–83. https://doi.org/10.1002/alr.22953. Epub 2022 Jan 10.
9. Robertson JM, Friedman EM, Rubin BK. Nasal and sinus disease in cystic fibrosis. Paediatr Respir Rev. 2008;9:213–9. https://doi.org/10.1016/j.prrv.2008.04.003. Epub 2008 Jul 31.
10. Le C, McCrary HC, Chang E. Cystic fibrosis sinusitis. Adv Otorhinolaryngol. 2016;79:29–37. https://doi.org/10.1159/000444959. Epub 2016 Jul 28.
11. Mainz JG, Koitschev A. Pathogenesis and management of nasal polyposis in cystic fibrosis. Curr Allergy Asthma Rep. 2012;12:163–74. https://doi.org/10.1007/s11882-012-0250-y.
12. Gergin O, Kawai K, MacDougall RD, et al. Sinus computed tomography imaging in pediatric cystic fibrosis: added value? Otolaryngol Head Neck Surg. 2016;155:160–5. https://doi.org/10.1177/0194599816634671. Epub 2016 Mar 1.
13. Berkhout MC, van Rooden CJ, Rijntjes E, et al. Sinonasal manifestations of cystic fibrosis: a correlation between genotype and phenotype? J Cyst Fibros. 2014;13:442–8. https://doi.org/10.1016/j.jcf.2013.10.011. Epub 2013 Nov 5.
14. Choi KJ, Cheng TZ, Honeybrook AL, et al. Correlation between sinus and lung cultures in lung transplant patients with cystic fibrosis. Int Forum Allergy Rhinol. 2018;8:389–93. https://doi.org/10.1002/alr.22067. Epub 2017 Dec 14.
15. Morlacchi LC, Greer M, Tudorache I, et al. The burden of sinus disease in cystic fibrosis lung transplant recipients. Transpl Infect Dis. 2018;20:e12924. https://doi.org/10.1111/tid.12924. Epub 2018 Jun 28.
16. Weinstock MS, Shaffer AD, Stapleton AL. Predictors of sinonasal disease onset, progression, and severity in pediatric cystic fibrosis patients. Am J Otolaryngol. 2021;42(5):103016. https://doi.org/10.1016/j.amjoto.2021.103016. Epub 2021 Mar 31.
17. Hancı D, Altun H, Şahin E, et al. Turkish translation, cross-cultural adaptation and validation of the SinoNasal Outcome Test (SNOT)-22. ENT Updates. 2015;5:51–7.
18. Liu M, Liu J, Weitzel EK, et al. The predictive utility of the 22-item sino-nasal outcome test (SNOT-22): a scoping review. Int Forum Allergy Rhinol. 2022;12:83–102. https://doi.org/10.1002/alr.22888. Epub 2021 Sep 28.
19. Kay DJ, Rosenfeld RM. Quality of life for children with persistent sinonasal symptoms. Otolaryngol Head Neck Surg. 2003;128:17–26. https://doi.org/10.1067/mhn.2003.41.
20. Steinke JW, Payne SC, Chen PG, et al. Etiology of nasal polyps in cystic fibrosis: not a unimodal disease. Ann Otol Rhinol Laryngol. 2012;121:579–86. https://doi.org/10.1177/000348941212100904.

21. Tandon R, Derkay C. Contemporary management of rhinosinusitis and cystic fibrosis. Curr Opin Otolaryngol Head Neck Surg. 2003;11:41–4. https://doi.org/10.1097/00020840-200302000-00009.
22. Gysin C, Alothman GA, Papsin BC. Sinonasal disease in cystic fibrosis: clinical characteristics, diagnosis, and management. Pediatr Pulmonol. 2000;30:481–9. https://doi.org/10.1002/1099-0496(200012)30:6<481::aid-ppul8>3.0.co;2-n.
23. Illing EA, Woodworth BA. Management of the upper airway in cystic fibrosis. Curr Opin Pulm Med. 2014;20:623–31. https://doi.org/10.1097/MCP.0000000000000107.
24. Sergeev V, Chou FY, Lam GY, et al. The extrapulmonary effects of cystic fibrosis transmembrane conductance regulator modulators in cystic fibrosis. Ann Am Thorac Soc. 2020;17:147–54. https://doi.org/10.1513/AnnalsATS.201909-671CME.
25. Sheikh SI, Long FR, McCoy KS, et al. Ivacaftor improves appearance of sinus disease on computerised tomography in cystic fibrosis patients with G551D mutation. Clin Otolaryngol. 2015;40:16–21. https://doi.org/10.1111/coa.12310.
26. Beswick DM, Humphries SM, Balkissoon CD, et al. Impact of cystic fibrosis transmembrane conductance regulator therapy on chronic rhinosinusitis and health status: deep learning CT analysis and patient-reported outcomes. Ann Am Thorac Soc. 2022;19:12–9. https://doi.org/10.1513/AnnalsATS.202101-057OC.
27. Stapleton AL, Kimple AJ, Goralski JL, et al. Elexacaftor–tezacaftor–ivacaftor improves sinonasal outcomes in cystic fibrosis. J Cyst Fibros. 2022;21:792–9. https://doi.org/10.1016/j.jcf.2022.03.002.
28. Uyttebroek S, Dupont L, Jorissen M, et al. Upper airway disease in adults with cystic fibrosis in the era of CFTR modulators. Laryngoscope. 2023;133(11):2898–909. (Epub ahead of print). https://doi.org/10.1002/lary.30642.
29. Mendez R, Banerjee S, Bhattacharya SK, et al. Lung inflammation and disease: a perspective on microbial homeostasis and metabolism. IUBMB Life. 2019;71:152–65. https://doi.org/10.1002/iub.1969. Epub 2018 Nov 22.
30. Steffen LM, Pezzin LS, Sulis N, et al. Upper airway findings and markers of lung disease progression in patients with cystic fibrosis. Int Arch Otorhinolaryngol. 2020;24:e434–7. https://doi.org/10.1055/s-0039-3402434. Epub 2020 Mar 11.
31. Beaume M, Köhler T, Greub G, Swiss Transplant Cohort Study, et al. Rapid adaptation drives invasion of airway donor microbiota by Pseudomonas after lung transplantation. Sci Rep. 2017;7:40309. https://doi.org/10.1038/srep40309.
32. Haddad J Jr, Gonzalez C, Kurland G, et al. Ear disease in children with cystic fibrosis. Arch Otolaryngol Head Neck Surg. 1994;120:491–3. https://doi.org/10.1001/archotol.1994.01880290009002.
33. Taylor B, Evans JN, Hope GA, et al. Upper respiratory tract in cystic fibrosis. Ear-nose-throat survey of 50 children. Arch Dis Child. 1974;49:133–6. https://doi.org/10.1136/adc.49.2.133.
34. McCoy JL, Kaffenberger TM, Yang TS, et al. Middle ear disease in CF? It's not just about the sinuses anymore! Int J Pediatr Otorhinolaryngol. 2020;134:110032. https://doi.org/10.1016/j.ijporl.2020.110032. Epub 2020 Apr 1.
35. Pauna HF, Monsanto RC, Kurata N, et al. Changes in the inner ear structures in cystic fibrosis patients. Int J Pediatr Otorhinolaryngol. 2017;92:108–14. https://doi.org/10.1016/j.ijporl.2016.11.013. Epub 2016 Nov 16.
36. Prayle A, Watson A, Fortnum H, et al. Side effects of aminoglycosides on the kidney, ear and balance in cystic fibrosis. Thorax. 2010;65:654–8. https://doi.org/10.1136/thx.2009.131532.
37. Farzal Z, Kou YF, St John R, et al. The role of routine hearing screening in children with cystic fibrosis on aminoglycosides: a systematic review. Laryngoscope. 2016;126:228–35. https://doi.org/10.1002/lary.25409. Epub 2015 Jul 7.
38. Castellani C, Duff AJA, Bell SC, et al. ECFS best practice guidelines: the 2018 revision. J Cyst Fibros. 2018;17:153–78. https://doi.org/10.1016/j.jcf.2018.02.006. Epub 2018 Mar 3.

Upper Respiratory Tract Involvement in Cystic Fibrosis

46

Raziye Atan and Deniz Doğru Ersöz

46.1 Introduction

Upper respiratory tract involvement is a prevalent comorbidity in patients with CF, which starts from early childhood and increases with age. For this reason, the upper airways of patients should be examined and their symptoms should be evaluated regularly. Medical treatment of upper respiratory tract involvement of CF includes nasal saline irrigation, nasal steroids, dornase alfa, and systemic or local antibiotics. With advances in treatment, recent studies show that using CFTR modulators reduce chronic rhinosinusitis severity. Surgical intervention is only recommended in specific cases. Functional endoscopic sinus surgery is often the primary surgical choice, although some patients may require more comprehensive or repeated surgery. Upper airway problems should be treated in close collaboration with an otolaryngologist who has experience with CF disease. Sinus infections can trigger lower respiratory exacerbation, and nasal polyps can cause sleep disorders. In this way, they can also be the cause of systemic problems. It is therefore important to maintain treatment.

46.2 Therapeutic Continuity

High-level recommendations for the management of chronic rhinosinusitis (CRS) due to CF have not yet been in place. To date, most research on the management of CRS in persons with CF have relied on small cohorts. In addition, the majority of research made no distinction based on age. Various treatments with nasal corticosteroids, nasal saline rinses, local antibiotics, and dornase alfa are reported medical

R. Atan · D. Doğru Ersöz (✉)
Division of Pediatric Pulmonology, Hacettepe University Faculty of Medicine, Ankara, Turkey
e-mail: ddogru@hacettepe.edu.tr

H. Yüksel et al. (eds.), *Pediatric Airway Diseases*, Comprehensive ENT,
https://doi.org/10.1007/978-3-031-74853-0_46

therapies [1]. Although aggressive surgery in intractable disease has demonstrated some clinical relief, there is no clear consensus on surgical criteria or approach [2]. Endoscopic sinus surgery may benefit some patients whose sinuses serve as a reservoir for recurrent lung infections [3]. Conservative management is considered the first step in the treatment of CRS in CF patients.

Nasal irrigation aids in the elimination of bacteria-infested dried mucous crusts, debris, and viscous sinonasal secretions. The saline-induced mucolytic activity may be useful in CF patients due to the retention of substantial volumes of viscous mucus in sinonasal cavities. It also aids in the localization of topical medicines. To wash secretions, normal saline (0.9% saline solution) or hypertonic saline is recommended, and there are a number of studies that compare these treatments. Results from a multicentre, randomized, controlled trial show that both treatment arms were well tolerated and showed slight improvements in quality of life scores, with no significant difference [4].

Corticosteroids reduce nasal discharge and oedema, aid in the evacuation of sinus fluids, and cause nasal polyp shrinking. Corticosteroids are used in CF because of their antiinflammatory effects. According to a multidisciplinary group of pediatricians, otolaryngologists, and pulmonologists, intranasal steroids should be considered in the treatment of CF-related CRS [5]. However, regardless of mode of administration, prolonged use has been linked to adrenal suppression and growth failure [6]. For severe numerous recurring polyps, oral steroid regimens are occasionally used [7]. To date, there are no strong recommendations for or against short-term or long-term systemic corticosteroid use in people with CF [8].

Nasal decongestants relieve the inferior blockage caused by nasal congestion but have no direct effect on the sinuses. If decongestants are used for more than 1 week, they might cause rebound congestion, which can develop to physical dependence and drug-induced rhinitis; thus, their regular usage is discouraged [7].

Dornase alfa, a recombinant human DNase, is a mucolytic agent that decreases the viscosity of secretions in CF patients' airways by cleaving extracellular DNA, which is found in large amounts in CF patients' respiratory tracts as a result of neutrophil destruction. The use of sinonasal inhalation of dornase alfa in the treatment of CRS in CF has been demonstrated [9].

Antibiotics are important in the pharmacological treatment of rhinosinusitis in people with CF because of chronic colonization, primarily by *P. aeruginosa* and *S. aureus*. If *P. aeruginosa* is isolated from the nasal swab or sinus rinse sample, nebulized antibiotics such as colistin or tobramycin may be administered nasally using a sinus nebulizer, which creates aerosol pulses that are then delivered to the paranasal sinuses. Inhaled antibiotics enter the sinonasal mucosa more effectively than systemically delivered antibiotics, making them more efficacious than oral or intravenous treatment. Furthermore, inhaling antibiotics is safer because it eliminates the negative effects of systemic use. Long-term oral macrolide treatment is recommended for CF patients, although the ideal duration has not yet been defined [10]. In addition to their antibacterial activity, macrolides play a significant role in the modulation of chronic inflammation. Previous researches have shown that macrolides reduce IL-8 production and thus the growth of nasal polyps [11].

New therapeutic strategies to improve CFTR activity have been created for specific mutations in CF patients. CFTR modulators that target the underlying genetic defect have already shown promising results in CF therapy. There are two types of CFTR modulators and combinations of them: correctors, which increase the transfer of CFTR to the cell surface membrane, and potentiators, which improve CFTR function and transmembrane ion flux. Because CFTR modulators improve the activity of the CFTR protein, resulting in increased chloride transmembrane transport and decreased mucus viscosity, they may also interfere with the pathophysiology of CRS and hence alleviate CRS symptoms in CF patients. There are studies showing that highly effective CFTR modulator treatment improves upper airway symptoms and quality of life in CF patients [12–16]. Although MRI is not an excellent test to assess sinusitis, one study showed an improvement in the MRI findings of the sinuses with modulator therapy in patients with CF [17].

Surgery is not recommended as the first-line treatment for CF-related CRS. Most patients with CRS and nasal polyps require sinus surgery if they do not improve sufficiently with standard medical management. Specific indications for surgical intervention include failure of the initial medical therapies mentioned above, severe symptoms or inability to use topical medications due to polyposis, bony erosion or disease progression outside the sinuses. Nasal and paranasal sinus mucoceles can also be effectively treated with endoscopic sinus surgery (ESS). ESS is recommended as a first-line surgical treatment for resistant CRS. However, extended surgical procedures or combined surgical methods are required for patients who have recurrent ESS [18].

As people with CF live longer lives, further research about medical therapy, the effect of CFTR modulators on sinonasal therapies and surgical methods and their results are definitely needed [3].

References

1. Kang SH, Dalcin PT, Piltcher OB, et al. Chronic rhinosinusitis and nasal polyposis in cystic fibrosis: update on diagnosis and treatment. J Bras Pneumol. 2015;41:65–76. https://doi.org/10.1590/S1806-37132015000100009.
2. Weinstock MS, Shaffer AD, Stapleton AL. Predictors of sinonasal disease onset, progression, and severity in pediatric cystic fibrosis patients. Am J Otolaryngol. 2021;42(5):103016. https://doi.org/10.1016/j.amjoto.2021.103016.
3. Johnson BJ, Choby GW, O'Brien EK. Chronic rhinosinusitis in patients with cystic fibrosis—current management and new treatments. Laryngosc Investig Otolaryngol. 2020;5(3):368–74. https://doi.org/10.1002/lio2.401.
4. Mainz JG, Schumacher U, Schädlich K, et al. Sino nasal inhalation of isotonic versus hypertonic saline (6.0%) in CF patients with chronic rhinosinusitis—results of a multicenter, prospective, randomized, double-blind, controlled trial. J Cyst Fibros. 2016;15(6):e57–66. https://doi.org/10.1016/j.jcf.2016.05.003.
5. Jayawardena AD, Fracchia MS, Bartley BL, et al. Working towards consensus in the management of pediatric chronic rhinosinusitis in cystic fibrosis. Int J Pediatr Otorhinolaryngol. 2020;135:110047. https://doi.org/10.1016/j.ijporl.2020.110047.
6. Broersen LH, Pereira AM, Jørgensen JOL, et al. Adrenal insufficiency in corticosteroids use: systematic review and meta-analysis. J Clin Endocrinol Metab. 2015;100(6):2171–80. https://doi.org/10.1210/jc.2015-1218.

7. Fokkens WJ, Lund VJ, Hopkins C, et al. European position paper on rhinosinusitis and nasal polyps. 2020. https://helda.helsinki.fi/bitstream/handle/10138/328733/supplement_29.pdf?sequence=1. Accessed 31 Aug 2023.
8. Chinese Experts Cystic Fibrosis Consensus Committee; Chinese Alliance for Rare Lung Diseases; Chinese Alliance for Rare Diseases, Bronchiectasis-China. Chinese experts consensus statement: diagnosis and treatment of cystic fibrosis. Zhonghua Jie He He Hu Xi Za Zhi. 2023;46(4):352–72. https://doi.org/10.3760/cma.j.cn112147-20221214-00971.
9. Mainz JG, Schien C, Schiller I, et al. Sinonasal inhalation of dornase alfa administered by vibrating aerosol to cystic fibrosis patients: a double-blind placebo-controlled cross-over trial. J Cyst Fibros. 2014;13(4):461–70. https://doi.org/10.1016/j.jcf.2014.02.005.
10. Karanth TK, Karanth VKLK, Ward BK, et al. Medical interventions for chronic rhinosinusitis in cystic fibrosis. Cochrane Database Syst Rev. 2022;10(10):CD012979. https://doi.org/10.1002/14651858.CD012979.pub3.
11. Zimmermann P, Ziesenitz VC, Curtis N, et al. The immunomodulatory effects of macrolides—a systematic review of the underlying mechanisms. Front Immunol. 2018;9:302. https://doi.org/10.3389/fimmu.2018.00302.
12. Bode SF, Rapp H, Lienert N, et al. Effects of CFTR-modulator triple therapy on sinunasal symptoms in children and adults with cystic fibrosis. Eur Arch Otorhinolaryngol. 2023;280:3271–7. https://doi.org/10.1007/s00405-023-07859-4.
13. McCormick J, Cho DY, Lampkin B, et al. Ivacaftor improves rhinologic, psychologic, and sleep-related quality of life in G551D cystic fibrosis patients. Int Forum Allergy Rhinol. 2019;9(3):292–7. https://doi.org/10.1002/alr.22251.
14. DiMango E, Overdevest J, Keating C, et al. Effect of highly effective modulator treatment on sinonasal symptoms in cystic fibrosis. J Cyst Fibros. 2021;20(3):460–3. https://doi.org/10.1016/j.jcf.2020.07.002.
15. Douglas JE, Civantos AM, Locke TB, et al. Impact of novel CFTR modulator on sinonasal quality of life in adult patients with cystic fibrosis. Int Forum Allergy Rhinol. 2021;11(2):201–3. https://doi.org/10.1002/alr.22716.
16. King JA, Nichols AL, Bentley S, et al. An update on CFTR modulators as new therapies for cystic fibrosis. Paediatr Drugs. 2022;24(4):321–33. https://doi.org/10.1007/s40272-022-00509-y.
17. Wucherpfennig L, Wuennemann F, Eichinger M, et al. Longitudinal magnetic resonance imaging detects onset and progression of chronic rhinosinusitis from infancy to school age in cystic fibrosis. Ann Am Thorac Soc. 2023;20(5):687–97. https://doi.org/10.1513/AnnalsATS.202209-763OC.
18. Krajewska J, Zub K, Słowikowski A, et al. Chronic rhinosinusitis in cystic fibrosis: a review of therapeutic options. Eur Arch Otorhinolaryngol. 2022;279:1–24. https://doi.org/10.1007/s00405-021-06875-6.

Upper Respiratory Tract Involvement in Primary Ciliary Dyskinesia: Genetics and Developmental Abnormalities

47

Meltem Akgül Erdal, Nagehan Emiralioğlu Ordukaya, and Samya Nasr

47.1 Introduction

Primary ciliary dyskinesia (PCD) is a genetic disorder caused by abnormal function, and anatomy of the epithelial cilia. The abnormality in the cilia can result in nonmotile or abnormally motile cilia. The estimated incidence ranges from 1:7500 to 1:20,000 [1]. Normal beating function of cilia clears the mucus, microorganisms, and particles from the airways. Abnormal beating patterns, ultrastructural defects, and reduced number/absence of the cilia reduce mucociliary clearance of airways, resulting in chronic and recurrent upper and lower respiratory tract infections.

47.1.1 Developmental Basis of PCD

The different types of cilia that are found in different parts of the body are involved in a variety of processes such as the proper function and alignment of organs in the body [2, 3].

The importance of the ciliary function in the respiratory system was recognized with the identification of Kartgener's syndrome (KS) characterized by nodal ciliary dysfunction. The ultrastructural defect of the cilia was first identified by electron microscopy of immotile spermatozoa in brothers with KS, which showed the absence of dynein arms [4]. Disorders of nodal cilia can lead to conditions such as laterality defects during embryogenesis, infertility due to defects in the reproductive

M. A. Erdal · N. E. Ordukaya (✉)
Department of Pediatric Pulmonology, Hacettepe University Faculty of Medicine, Ihsan Dogramaci Children's Hospital, Ankara, Turkey

S. Nasr
Division of Pediatric Pulmonology, University of Michigan, Ann Arbor, MI, USA
e-mail: snasr@med.umich.edu

H. Yüksel et al. (eds.), *Pediatric Airway Diseases*, Comprehensive ENT,
https://doi.org/10.1007/978-3-031-74853-0_47

organs (sperm, vas deferens, and/or fallopian tubes), and hydrocephalus due to defects in the ependymal cilia movements in the central nervous system [5]. Motile cilia in the fallopian tubes, cerebral ependyma, nose, paranasal sinuses, Eustachian tubes in the upper airways, and trachea were later found to lack dynein arms. Patients exhibiting symptoms of chronic or recurrent rhinitis, sinusitis, bronchitis, and otitis media were found to have immotility or dismotility in their nasal/bronchial cilia examinations. The term "primary ciliary dyskinesia" has been proposed for patients with congenitally abnormal ciliary structure, and as a result, abnormal coordination of ciliary movements [6].

47.1.1.1 Cilia

The flagella of unicellular eukaryotes (9 + 2) are the ancestors for the motile cilia, found in humans. Many evidence have been shown that its structure is well conserved throughout the course of evolution to humans [5]. Cilia are thin, hair-like, and microtubule-containing projection from the cell surface. It is composed of a basal body and an axoneme. The basal bodies are a barrel-shaped cylindrical array of centrioles consisting of nine doublet microtubule filaments. The ciliary axoneme, the microtubule cytoskeleton of the cilium, is an extension of the ninefold symmetry of the centriole [7]. A cilium consists of an axoneme and basal body [8].

Motile cilia project from cells as a single cilium (monocilium) or cilia bundles of 200–300 individual cilia per cell. The axonemes of the monocilia and the multiple motile cilia have different structures. The axoneme of a single multiple cilium (9 + 2, respiratory cilium) contains a central pair of singlet microtubules surrounded by the nine doublet microtubules, and a single cilium (9 + 0, nodal cilium) has an axoneme in which the central pair of microtubules is missing [2]. Ciliary axonemes contain protein complexes consisting of outer (ODA) and inner dynein arms (IDA), central pair complex (CPC), nexin-dynein regulatory complexes (N-DRC), radial spokes (RS), microtubule internal proteins (MIPs), and their connections. Ultrastructure of a normal cilium shows a "9 + 2" microtubule pattern. This intricate structure results in multiple cilia, exhibiting a unique type of motion, characterized by a continuous, synchronized, and rhythmic beat. ODA regulates the beating frequency of the cilium, while others generate ciliary bending movements that influence the ciliary beating pattern [9, 10]. This stroke patterns of cilia guide the overlying mucus across the epithelium.

The movements of the cilia reveal different roles in the human body. A motile monocilium plays a role in embryogenesis, generating a flow of fluid that directs cell migration in the early embryo and ensures left-right symmetry and proper organ alignment [11]. Multiple cilia in the respiratory tract move in an orchestrated motion directing mucus, particles, and microorganisms along the epithelial layer and clearing the airways. The ultrastructural defects of these complexes cilia generate abnormalities in the movement pattern of the cilia, resulting in heterogeneous clinical manifestations in PCD, such as male infertility, chronic airway diseases, chronic otitis media, and situs abnormalities [12–15].

Because of the abnormal movement of the cilia in PCD, it leads to the use of the term "dyskinesia." However, the reduced number of cilia with normal movement pattern is also identified in PCD. Therefore, the term "primary respiratory ciliopathy" may be more appropriate instead of "dyskinesia" [16].

47.1.2 PCD Genetics

PCD is primarily inherited as an autosomal recessive trait, but can also be inherited as autosomal dominant or X-linked [17–20]. There are more than 50 genes that have been identified as involved in ciliary structure and function. The complex axonemal structure, consisting of hundreds of proteins, causes a wide range of genetic heterogeneity in PCD [21].

Prevalence of PCD genotype shows regional and ethnic differences [22]. DNAH5, DNAH11, DNAI1, CCDC39, and CCDC40 have been identified as the most common genes in North America and Europe [5]. A study conducted with Chinese PCD patients showed similar mutation spectrum, in addition to a higher rate of HYDIN mutation [23]. Recent studies in Japanese and Korean populations revealed different mutations (biallelic 27,748 bp deletion exons of DRC1) as the most common cause of PCD [24–27].

PCD-causing genes are associated with specific ciliary defects that can be demonstrated through the use of electron microscopy. The most common genes, DNAH5, DNAI1, and DNAI2, are only associated with defects in ODA with immotile or minimal residual motile cilia. Whereas DNAH11 shows hyperkinetic and stiff beating pattern with normal electron microscopic findings [28]. There are also other mutations such as CCDC11, DRC1, GAS8, and DNAH9 that do not show any ultrastructural defects. Some other PCD-causing genes such as LRRC6, CCDC103, and DNAAF1-2-3 related with combined ODA/IDA or IDA/CA/MTD (microtubular disorganization) defects. CCDC40 results in a microtubular disorganization (MTD), radial spokes, nexin link defects, and absence of inner dynein arms. Biallelic CCDC40 and CCDC39 mutations have ciliary movements with a reduced amplitude [29, 30]. CCNO mutation causes oligocilia, RSPH4A, RSPH1, and RSPH9 causes absence of RS apparatus of cilia [31].

The ultrastructural defects of axonemes have been associated with clinical symptoms including neonatal respiratory distress, chronic cough, chronic nasal congestion, and chronic otitis media [31]. However, the clinical features associated with specific genotypes can vary widely, and the severity of the respiratory symptoms may depend on the genetic variant. *DNAH11*, *DNAH9*, and *RSPH1* mutations are associated with mild respiratory symptoms [28, 32, 33]. Biallelic *RSPH1*, RSPH4A, and RSPH9 mutations can cause mild to severe respiratory manifestations and situs abnormalities [34, 32]. The pathologic variant of CCNO has been found to be associated with the low body mass index in children [35]. The most frequent cause of lateralization defect is DNAH5 mutation [36]. However, PKD1L1 and Pitchfork (PIFO) heterozygous mutations have also found linked to right-left asymmetry [37, 38]. Linkage between congenital cardiac defects and PCD-causing genes are contradictory [39]. The combined results of laterality defects and CHD rates in PCD suggest a wide prevalence range (3.5–25.2% of patients) in PCD with cardiovascular malformations [40, 41]. Some studies investigating genotype–phenotype correlations confirm the possibility of a genetic predisposition to CHD and/or laterality defects in PCD, as some PCD genes are not clearly associated with situs problems [39]. A recent study evaluating the ciliary ultrastructural markers have been shown a greater prevalence of absence of *RSPH1*, *RSPH4A*, *RSPH9*, and *DNAH5* expressions in patients with nasal polyps which can be seen in PCD patients [42].

In summary, PCD is a heterogeneous disorder of motile ciliary dysfunction, in which mutations have been found in a relatively large number of genes. In addition to genes encoding structural components of ciliary axonemia, mutations in genes encoding novel cytoplasmic and regulatory proteins have been discovered in recent years. Future studies are ongoing for new gene associations with PCD.

References

1. Hannah WB, Seifert BA, Truty R, Zariwala MA, Ameel K, Zhao Y, et al. The global prevalence and ethnic heterogeneity of primary ciliary dyskinesia gene variants: a genetic database analysis. Lancet Respir Med. 2022;10:459–68.
2. Fliegauf M, Benzing T, Omran H. When cilia go bad: cilia defects and ciliopathies. Nat Rev Mol Cell Biol. 2007;8:880–93.
3. Horani A, Brody SL, Ferkol TW. Picking up speed: advances in the genetics of primary ciliary dyskinesia. Pediatr Res. 2014;75:158–64.
4. Afzelius B. Electron microscopy of the sperm tail results obtained with a new fixative. J Cell Biol. 1959;5:269–78.
5. Wallmeier J, Nielsen KG, Kuehni CE, Lucas JS, Leigh MW, Zariwala MA, et al. Motile ciliopathies. Nat Rev Dis Primers. 2020;6:77.
6. Afzelius BA. Cilia-related diseases. J Pathol. 2004;204:470–7.
7. Satir P, Christensen ST. Overview of structure and function of mammalian cilia. Annu Rev Physiol. 2007;69:377–400.
8. Peabody JE, Shei R-J, Bermingham BM, Phillips SE, Turner B, Rowe SM, et al. Seeing cilia: imaging modalities for ciliary motion and clinical connections. Am J Phsyiol Lung Cell Mol Physiol. 2018;314:L909–21.
9. Gibbons BH, Gibbons I. The effect of partial extraction of dynein arms on the movement of reactivated sea-urchin sperm. J Cell Sci. 1973;13:337–57.
10. Kamiya R, Yagi T. Functional diversity of axonemal dyneins as assessed by in vitro and in vivo motility assays of Chlamydomonas mutants. Zool Sci. 2014;31:633–44.
11. Afzelius BA. A human syndrome caused by immotile cilia. Science. 1976;193:317–9.
12. Afzelius B, Eliasson R. Male and female infertility problems in the immotile-cilia syndrome. Eur J Respir Suppl. 1983;127:144–7.
13. Coren M, Meeks M, Morrison I, Buchdahl R, Bush A. Primary ciliary dyskinesia: age at diagnosis and symptom history. Acta Paediatr. 2002;91:667–9.
14. Eliasson R, Mossberg B, Camner P, Afzelius BA. The immotile-cilia syndrome: a congenital ciliary abnormality as an etiologic factor in chronic airway infections and male sterility. N Engl J Med. 1977;297:1–6.
15. Noone PG, Leigh MW, Sannuti A, Minnix SL, Carson JL, Hazucha M, et al. Primary ciliary dyskinesia: diagnostic and phenotypic features. Am J Respir Crit Care Med. 2004;169:459–67.
16. Paff T, Omran H, Nielsen KG, Haarman EG. Current and future treatments in primary ciliary dyskinesia. Int J Mol Sci. 2021;22:9834.
17. Höben IM, Hjeij R, Olbrich H, Dougherty GW, Nöthe-Menchen T, Aprea I, et al. Mutations in C11orf70 cause primary ciliary dyskinesia with randomization of left/right body asymmetry due to defects of outer and inner dynein arms. Am J Hum Genet. 2018;102:973–84.

18. Lucas JS, Davis SD, Omran H, Shoemark A. Primary ciliary dyskinesia in the genomics age. Lancet Respir Med. 2020;8:202–16.
19. Paff T, Loges NT, Aprea I, Wu K, Bakey Z, Haarman EG, et al. Mutations in PIH1D3 cause X-linked primary ciliary dyskinesia with outer and inner dynein arm defects. Am J Hum Genet. 2017;100:160–8.
20. Wallmeier J, Frank D, Shoemark A, Nöthe-Menchen T, Cindric S, Olbrich H, et al. De novo mutations in FOXJ1 result in a motile ciliopathy with hydrocephalus and randomization of left/right body asymmetry. Am J Hum Genet. 2019;105:1030–9.
21. Pazour GJ, Agrin N, Leszyk J, Witman GB. Proteomic analysis of a eukaryotic cilium. J Cell Biol. 2005;170:103–13.
22. Fassad MR, Patel MP, Shoemark A, Cullup T, Hayward J, Dixon M, et al. Clinical utility of NGS diagnosis and disease stratification in a multiethnic primary ciliary dyskinesia cohort. J Med Genet. 2020;57:322–30.
23. Peng B, Gao Y-H, Xie J-Q, He X-W, Wang C-C, Xu J-F, et al. Clinical and genetic spectrum of primary ciliary dyskinesia in Chinese patients: a systematic review. Orphanet J Rare Dis. 2022;17:283.
24. Keicho N, Hijikata M, Morimoto K, Homma S, Taguchi Y, Azuma A, et al. Primary ciliary dyskinesia caused by a large homozygous deletion including exons 1–4 of DRC1 in Japanese patients with recurrent sinopulmonary infection. Mol Genet Genomic Med. 2020;8:1033.
25. Kim MJ, Kim S, Chae SW, Lee S, Yoon JG, Kim B, et al. Prevalence and founder effect of DRC1 exon 1–4 deletion in Korean patients with primary ciliary dyskinesia. J Hum Genet. 2023;68:369–74.
26. Morimoto K, Hijikata M, Zariwala MA, Nykamp K, Inaba A, Guo TC, et al. Recurring large deletion in DRC1 (CCDC164) identified as causing primary ciliary dyskinesia in two Asian patients. Mol Genet Genomic Med. 2019;7:838.
27. Xu Y, Feng G, Yano T, Masuda S, Nagao M, Gotoh S, et al. Characteristic genetic spectrum of primary ciliary dyskinesia in Japanese patients and global ethnic heterogeneity: population-based genomic variation database analysis. J Hum Genet. 2023;68:455–61.
28. Dougherty GW, Loges NT, Klinkenbusch JA, Olbrich H, Pennekamp P, Menchen T, et al. DNAH11 localization in the proximal region of respiratory cilia defines distinct outer dynein arm complexes. Am J Respir Cell Mol Biol. 2016;55:213–24.
29. Becker-Heck A, Zohn IE, Okabe N, Pollock A, Lenhart KB, Sullivan-Brown J, et al. The coiled-coil domain containing protein CCDC40 is essential for motile cilia function and left-right axis formation. Nat Genet. 2011;43:79–84.
30. Merveille A-C, Davis EE, Becker-Heck A, Legendre M, Amirav I, Bataille G, et al. CCDC39 is required for assembly of inner dynein arms and the dynein regulatory complex and for normal ciliary motility in humans and dogs. Nat Genet. 2011;43:72–8.
31. Davis SD, Rosenfeld M, Lee H-S, Ferkol TW, Sagel SD, Dell SD, et al. Primary ciliary dyskinesia: longitudinal study of lung disease by ultrastructure defect and genotype. Am J Respir Crit Care Med. 2019;199:190–8.
32. Knowles MR, Ostrowski LE, Leigh MW, Sears PR, Davis SD, Wolf WE, et al. Mutations in RSPH1 cause primary ciliary dyskinesia with a unique clinical and ciliary phenotype. Am J Respir Crit Care Med. 2014;189:707–17.
33. Loges NT, Antony D, Maver A, Deardorff MA, Güleç EY, Gezdirici A, et al. Recessive DNAH9 loss-of-function mutations cause laterality defects and subtle respiratory ciliary-beating defects. Am J Respir Crit Care Med. 2018;103:995–1008.
34. Castleman VH, Romio L, Chodhari R, Hirst RA, de Castro SC, Parker KA, et al. Mutations in radial spoke head protein genes RSPH9 and RSPH4A cause primary ciliary dyskinesia with central-microtubular-pair abnormalities. Am J Hum Genet. 2009;84:197–209.
35. Emiralioğlu N, Taşkıran EZ, Koşukcu C, Bilgiç E, Atilla P, Kaya B, et al. Genotype and phenotype evaluation of patients with primary ciliary dyskinesia: first results from Turkey. Pediatr Pulmonol. 2020;55:383–93.
36. Nöthe-Menchen T, Wallmeier J, Pennekamp P, Höben IM, Olbrich H, Loges NT, et al. Randomization of left-right asymmetry and congenital heart defects: the role of DNAH5 in humans and mice. Circ Genom Precis Med. 2019;12:002686.

37. Delling M, DeCaen PG, Doerner JF, Febvay S, Clapham DE. Primary cilia are specialized calcium signalling organelles. Nature. 2013;504:311–4.
38. Kinzel D, Boldt K, Davis EE, Burtscher I, Trümbach D, Diplas B, et al. Pitchfork regulates primary cilia disassembly and left-right asymmetry. Dev Cell. 2010;19:66–77.
39. Antony D, Gulec Yilmaz E, Gezdirici A, Slagter L, Bakey Z, Bornaun H, et al. Spectrum of genetic variants in a cohort of 37 laterality defect cases. Front Genet. 2022;13:861236.
40. Best S, Shoemark A, Rubbo B, Patel MP, Fassad MR, Dixon M, et al. Risk factors for situs defects and congenital heart disease in primary ciliary dyskinesia. Thorax. 2019;74:203–5.
41. Harrison MJ, Shapiro AJ, Kennedy MP. Congenital heart disease and primary ciliary dyskinesia. Paediatr Respir Rev. 2016;18:25–32.
42. Zi X-X, Guan W-J, Peng Y, Tan KS, Liu J, He T-T, et al. An integrated analysis of radial spoke head and outer dynein arm protein defects and ciliogenesis abnormality in nasal polyps. Front Genet. 2019;10:1083.

Upper Respiratory Tract Involvement in Primary Ciliary Dyskinesia: Clinics and Diagnosis

48

Pelin Asfuroglu, Ophir Bar-On,
and Tugba Sismanlar Eyuboglu

48.1 Upper Respiratory Tract Involvement in Primary Ciliary Dyskinesia: Clinics and Diagnosis

Primary ciliary dyskinesia (PCD) is an autosomal recessive inherited disease that results from impaired mucociliary activity [1]. The prevalence of PCD is 1 in 10,000–20,000 live-born children [2]. Disruption in the structure or function of motile cilia causes a wide variety of symptoms in many organ systems, which could be observed from birth [1, 3].

In patients with PCD, the lungs, brain ependyma, and reproductive systems are affected, as well as the middle ear and paranasal sinuses [1, 3]. Chronic perennial productive cough, neonatal respiratory distress, hydrocephalus, nasal congestion, nasal drainage, nasal polyposis, chronic rhinosinusitis, recurrent acute and chronic purulent otitis media, conductive hearing loss, left-right laterality abnormalities (including situs inversus totalis and heterotaxy syndromes), and infertility/subfertility are clinical manifestations of PCD [3, 4]. If a child has persistent wet cough accompanied by history of neonatal respiratory distress, persistent rhinitis, chronic middle ear disease with or without hearing loss, and laterality disorder, the child should be investigated for PCD [5].

The number of diagnostic tests which are performed on people with clinical findings compatible with PCD has increased; however, the diagnosis of PCD is still difficult and no single test can diagnose every child with PCD [3, 6]. A simple

P. Asfuroglu
Pediatric Pulmonology Clinic, Gaziantep Cengiz Gökçek Gynecology and Pediatrics Hospital, Gaziantep, Turkey

O. Bar-On
Pulmonology Institute, Schneider Children's Medical Center of Israel, Petah Tikva, Israel

T. Sismanlar Eyuboglu (✉)
Department of Pediatric Pulmonology, Gazi University Faculty of Medicine, Ankara, Turkey

H. Yüksel et al. (eds.), *Pediatric Airway Diseases*, Comprehensive ENT,
https://doi.org/10.1007/978-3-031-74853-0_48

clinical diagnostic scoring tool, PICADAR (Primary Ciliary Dyskinesia A Rule), was designed to predict whether or not PCD is present for a child with a relevant clinical suspicion, including chronic daily wet cough [2]. Term gestation, neonatal chest symptoms, admission to neonatal intensive care unit, situs inversus (Fig. 48.1), congenital heart defect, chronic rhinitis, and ear symptoms are the parameters used in the PICADAR score [2]. Diagnosis of PCD usually requires a combination of investigations such as measurement of exhaled nasal nitric oxide (nNO), high-speed video microscopy analysis, high-resolution immunofluorescence analysis, and transmission electron microscopy [6]. Exhaled nNO is a useful screening tool for PCD, and demonstrates a reduced nNO level in most PCD patients [5–7]. High-speed video microscopy analysis is a method of recording the ciliary beat pattern and frequency in a sample of respiratory epithelium taken by brushing the nose or lower airways [5, 6]. Transmission electron microscopy is used to detect ciliary ultrastructure defects in the various proteins which comprise the cilia core, such as irregular microtubules, absence of inner or outer dynein arms, and radial spokes [5, 6]. High-resolution immunofluorescence analysis is used to detect presence or absence of normal ciliary proteins in the respiratory epithelium [5, 6]. Finally, genetic testing is used to confirm the diagnosis by identifying known mutations in cilia proteins [5]. All of these analyzes can confirm the diagnosis; however, they do not always rule out the diagnosis [6].

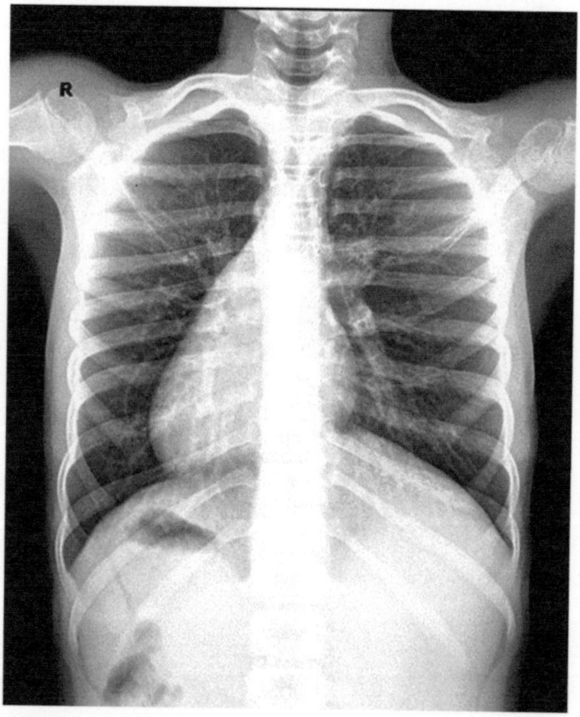

Fig. 48.1 Chest X-ray of a child with PCD with situs inversus totalis

48.2 Upper Respiratory Tract Involvement in Primary Ciliary Dyskinesia

The prevalence of ear–nose–throat (ENT) symptoms in PCD varies among patients; however, recurrent otitis media and chronic rhinosinusitis are present in most patients with PCD throughout the year, and are the most common reason for hospital admission [8].

Nasal congestion, anterior or posterior rhinorrhea, hyposmia/anosmia, and nasal polyposis are symptoms that may be seen in patients with PCD [7, 9]. There is no defined relationship between the ultrastructural abnormality of the cilia and the severity of clinical symptoms [9]. Recurrent purulent acute otitis media, otitis media with effusion, chronic otitis media, and conductive hearing loss can be seen as otological complications of PCD [7, 10].

Persistent nasal congestion is common in patients with PCD at any age, and has many different causes [6, 9]. Patients with PCD suffer from daily stuffy nose throughout the year, which is especially more prevalent in the first years of life [6]. The appearance in the nose is not specific for PCD. PCD-associated nasal disease, similar to perennial allergic rhinitis, is usually present year-round and does not show improvement between seasons or viral infections [9]. Studies show that chronic rhinorrhea complicated by anosmia is seen in 76–100% of children with PCD, and this may also cause sleep-disordered breathing [6].

Nasal polyps, which are rare in the general pediatric population, can be seen in 15–30% of children with PCD and can be unilateral or bilateral [11, 12]. Nasal polyps are usually characterized by a neutrophilic histotype because of bacterial colonization due to defective mucociliary clearance in patients with PCD [13]. In children with PCD, the incidence of nasal polyps increases with increasing age [11]. A nasal polyp should be suspected and evaluated if a child with PCD complains of nasal congestion, decreased or loss of smell [12].

Chronic rhinosinusitis, which is common in PCD, is characterized by inflammation of the nasal mucosa and paranasal sinuses [7, 9]. Chronic rhinosinusitis may develop as a result of disruption of the host defense mechanisms of the mucosa, such as epithelial damage, increased mucus production, and chronic inflammation [9, 14]. The biofilm is a source of bacteria that can cause systemic inflammation and recurrent infections [14]. In patients with chronic rhinosinusitis in PCD, the paranasal sinuses are often colonized with bacteria [15]. The most common pathogens detected in sinonasal infections in PCD are *Haemophilus influenzae*, *Streptococcus pneumoniae*, and *Pseudomonas aeruginosa* [15, 16]. In other studies, the most common pathogens detected in nasal swabs in PCD are *Staphylococcus aureus*, *Streptococcus pneumoniae*, *Haemophilus influenzae*, and *Moraxella catarrhalis*, respectively [17]. These bacteria may form a biofilm, which can cause systemic inflammation and recurrent infections [14], and obstruct antibiotic penetration.

Bilateral ethmoid sinus mucoceles can also be detected in children with PCD [7]. Sinus hypoplasia, which has recently been accepted as a specific feature of PCD, can be commonly detected in PCD [9]. Sinonasal involvement in PCD should be followed closely as it may result in aplastic or hypoplastic sinuses and exacerbate pulmonary and otological diseases [6, 7].

Adenoidal hypertrophy can also be seen in PCD [18]. As the degree of adenoid hypertrophy increases, nasal nitric oxide gradually decreases [18]. In one study, adenoid hypertrophy was detected in 20% of children with PCD [19]. In this study, the tonsil size was found to be larger than normal in all children with PCD, but in most of them, the tonsil size was evaluated as occupying less than 25% of the oropharyngeal width [19].

Most children with PCD have recurrent chronic otitis media with effusion [9]. Sequelae of chronic otologic infections such as tympanosclerosis, retraction of the eardrum, atelectasis, cholesteatoma, and keratosis obturans may also be detected in PCD [10]. In studies, cholesteatoma has been rarely reported in patients with PCD. It was thought that this might be associated with a high rate of ventilation tube insertion in PCD [7, 20].

Otitis media with effusion is the most common cause of acquired conductive hearing loss in the pediatric age group, with a prevalence of 10–30% in the 1–3 year old age group [7, 21]. In PCD, the severity of hearing loss due to otological involvement can be variable. Hearing loss may be fluctuating, and may extend into adulthood [7]. In PCD, otitis media with effusion should be closely monitored for complications that may occur as a result of hearing loss, such as speech and language delay [7]. Tympanometry and hearing tests are the most reliable way to decide on the need for treatment [9]. It is important to aim to prevent hearing loss and related disorders in cognition, speech and language development that may be caused by otological involvement in children with PCD [7].

In addition to otological disorders, vestibular pathologies such as balance impairment can also be seen in children with PCD [22, 23]. In a pilot study conducted with a small number of participants, cilia structure and/or motility were suggested to be associated with decreased saccular and utricular function in PCD, unilateral/bilateral decreased or unobtainable vestibular evoked myogenic potentials were detected in all participants [23]. In another study, children with PCD had further vestibular tests, and vestibular disorders were detected in 76% of children with PCD [22].

Children with PCD may complain of mouth breathing and snoring [24]. Upper respiratory tract involvement of PCD may cause sleep-disordered breathing by increasing the resistance of the upper airway [19]. Gas exchange abnormalities such as hypoxemia and hypercapnia resulting from airflow obstruction and air trapping may lead to sleep-disordered breathing [19]. In studies, sleep-disordered breathing was found to be high in children with PCD [19, 24–26]. In a case series study, it was determined that the obstructive apnea-hypopnea index was higher in the polysomnography of children with PCD [25]. In another questionnaire study evaluating sleep in children with PCD, it was found that sleep disorders scores were high for PCD patients [26].

In the follow-up of patients with PCD, it is also recommended to perform a detailed otoscopic examination, and report the history of ventilation tube and postoperative otorrhea [8]. According to the consensus statement from the Genetic Disorders of Mucociliary Clearance Consortium and PCD Foundation, children with PCD should undergo an initial audiology evaluation at diagnosis and visit a pediatric otolaryngologist at least once or twice a year for follow-up [27].

Studies show that the majority of patients with recurrent nasal problems undergo at least one advanced radiology examination such as X-ray or computed tomography (CT) [10]. It is recommended that children with PCD should be evaluated periodically (once or twice annually) by otolaryngologists for sinonasal diseases [8, 27]. As permitted according to the child's age, evaluation by nasal endoscopy can be used specifically to identify polyps that may exacerbate mucociliary clearance [27].

In children with sinus CT, the Lund-Mackay scoring system can be used to evaluate each sinus [28, 29]. It is an important radiological scoring tool to determine the severity of rhinosinusitis [30]. In the scoring system, 0 indicates no opacification, 1 indicates partial opacification, and 2 indicates full opacification [29]. Left and right sides are evaluated separately, and the total score is obtained; the total score ranges from 0 to 24 for each patient [29]. The modified Lund-Mackay score was developed for patients with sinus hypoplasia or aplasia [8], and it provides a more precise score by subtracting the hypoplastic or aplastic sinus from the total score calculation [8].

In conclusion, PCD is a heterogeneous disease that is occasionally difficult to diagnose, and hence is often diagnosed late. Symptoms of PCD in the upper respiratory tract are common, have an early onset, are perennial, and persist throughout life. Follow-up and management of upper respiratory tract involvement are important in terms of quality of life and prevention of sequelae. Patients with PCD who need multidisciplinary care should be routinely under the control of a pulmonologist, combined with an ENT physician, and follow-up should aim to prevent permanent sinonasal or vestibulocochlear damage.

References

1. Lucas JS, Burgess A, Mitchison HM, National PCD Service, UK, et al. Diagnosis and management of primary ciliary dyskinesia. Arch Dis Child. 2014;99:850–6. https://doi.org/10.1136/archdischild-2013-304831.
2. Behan L, Dimitrov BD, Kuehni CE, et al. PICADAR: a diagnostic predictive tool for primary ciliary dyskinesia. Eur Respir J. 2016;47:1103–12. https://doi.org/10.1183/13993003.01551-2015.
3. Horani A, Ferkol TW. Understanding primary ciliary dyskinesia and other ciliopathies. J Pediatr. 2021;230:15–22.e1. https://doi.org/10.1016/j.jpeds.2020.11.040. Epub 2020 Nov 23.
4. Fretzayas A, Moustaki M. Clinical spectrum of primary ciliary dyskinesia in childhood. World J Clin Pediatr. 2016;5:57–62. https://doi.org/10.5409/wjcp.v5.i1.57.
5. Dalrymple RA, Kenia P. European Respiratory Society guidelines for the diagnosis of primary ciliary dyskinesia: a guideline review. Arch Dis Child Educ Pract Ed. 2019;104:265–9. https://doi.org/10.1136/archdischild-2017-312902.
6. Mirra V, Werner C, Santamaria F. Primary ciliary dyskinesia: an update on clinical aspects, genetics, diagnosis, and future treatment strategies. Front Pediatr. 2017;5:135. https://doi.org/10.3389/fped.2017.00135.
7. Campbell R. Managing upper respiratory tract complications of primary ciliary dyskinesia in children. Curr Opin Allergy Clin Immunol. 2012;12:32–8. https://doi.org/10.1097/ACI.0b013e32834eccc6.
8. Alexandru M, Veil R, Rubbo B, et al. Ear and upper airway clinical outcome measures for use in primary ciliary dyskinesia research: a scoping review. Eur Respir Rev. 2023;32:220200. https://doi.org/10.1183/16000617.0200-2022.
9. Morgan LC, Birman CS. The impact of primary ciliary dyskinesia on the upper respiratory tract. Paediatr Respir Rev. 2016;18:33–8. https://doi.org/10.1016/j.prrv.2015.09.006.

10. Sommer JU, Schäfer K, Omran H, et al. ENT manifestations in patients with primary ciliary dyskinesia: prevalence and significance of otorhinolaryngologic co-morbidities. Eur Arch Otorhinolaryngol. 2011;268:383–8. https://doi.org/10.1007/s00405-010-1341-9.
11. Lam YT, Papon JF, Alexandru M, EPIC-PCD Team, Goutaki M, et al. Sinonasal disease among patients with primary ciliary dyskinesia: an international study. ERJ Open Res. 2023;9:00701–2022. https://doi.org/10.1183/23120541.00701-2022.
12. Sitzia E, Santarsiero S, Marini G, et al. Endotypes of nasal polyps in children: a multidisciplinary approach. J Pers Med. 2023;13:707. https://doi.org/10.3390/jpm13050707.
13. Brescia G, Zanotti C, Parrino D, et al. Nasal polyposis pathophysiology: endotype and phenotype open issues. Am J Otolaryngol. 2018;39:441–4. https://doi.org/10.1016/j.amjoto.2018.03.020.
14. Al-Mutairi D, Kilty SJ. Bacterial biofilms and the pathophysiology of chronic rhinosinusitis. Curr Opin Allergy Clin Immunol. 2011;11:18–23. https://doi.org/10.1097/ACI.0b013e3283423376.
15. Alanin MC. Bacteriology and treatment of infections in the upper and lower airways in patients with primary ciliary dyskinesia: addressing the paranasal sinuses. Dan Med J. 2017;64:B5361.
16. Møller ME, Alanin MC, Grønhøj C, et al. Sinus bacteriology in patients with cystic fibrosis or primary ciliary dyskinesia: a systematic review. Am J Rhinol Allergy. 2017;31:293–8. https://doi.org/10.2500/ajra.2017.31.4461.
17. Günaydın RÖ, Eroğlu E, Tellioğlu B, et al. Evaluation of otorhinolaryngological manifestations in patients with primary ciliary dyskinesia. Int J Pediatr Otorhinolaryngol. 2023;168:111520. https://doi.org/10.1016/j.ijporl.2023.111520.
18. Rybnikar T, Senkerik M, Chladek J, et al. Adenoid hypertrophy affects screening for primary ciliary dyskinesia using nasal nitric oxide. Int J Pediatr Otorhinolaryngol. 2018;115:6–9. https://doi.org/10.1016/j.ijporl.2018.09.007.
19. Oktem S, Karadag B, Erdem E, et al. Sleep disordered breathing in patients with primary ciliary dyskinesia. Pediatr Pulmonol. 2013;48:897–903. https://doi.org/10.1002/ppul.22710.
20. Prulière-Escabasse V, Coste A, Chauvin P, et al. Otologic features in children with primary ciliary dyskinesia. Arch Otolaryngol Head Neck Surg. 2010;136(11):1121–6. https://doi.org/10.1001/archoto.2010.183.
21. Yumuşakhuylu AC, Gündoğdu Y, Asya O. Approach to the ear nose and throat problems in primary ciliary dyskinesia. In: Erdem Eralp E, Karadağ BT, editors. Current approaches in primary ciliary dyskinesia. 1st ed. Ankara: Türkiye Klinikleri; 2022.
22. Zawawi F, Papsin BC, Dell S, et al. Vestibular and balance impairment is common in children with primary ciliary dyskinesia. Otol Neurotol. 2022;43(3):e355–60. https://doi.org/10.1097/MAO.0000000000003455.
23. Rimmer J, Patel M, Agarwal K, et al. Peripheral vestibular dysfunction in patients with primary ciliary dyskinesia: abnormal otoconial development? Otol Neurotol. 2015;36:662–9. https://doi.org/10.1097/MAO.0000000000000592.
24. Zawawi F, Shapiro AJ, Dell S, et al. Otolaryngology manifestations of primary ciliary dyskinesia: a multicenter study. Otolaryngol Head Neck Surg. 2022;166:540–7. https://doi.org/10.1177/01945998211019320.
25. Santamaria F, Esposito M, Montella S, et al. Sleep disordered breathing and airway disease in primary ciliary dyskinesia. Respirology. 2014;19:570–5. https://doi.org/10.1111/resp.12273.
26. Şişmanlar Eyüboğlu T, Aslan AT, Ceylan A, et al. Neurocognitive disorders and sleep in children with primary ciliary dyskinesia. Pediatr Pulmonol. 2018;53:1436–41. https://doi.org/10.1002/ppul.24133.
27. Shapiro AJ, Zariwala MA, Ferkol T, Genetic Disorders of Mucociliary Clearance Consortium, et al. Diagnosis, monitoring, and treatment of primary ciliary dyskinesia: PCD foundation consensus recommendations based on state of the art review. Pediatr Pulmonol. 2016;51:115–32. https://doi.org/10.1002/ppul.23304.
28. Plantier DB, Pilan RRM, Athanazio R, et al. Computed tomography evaluation of the paranasal sinuses in adults with primary ciliary dyskinesia. Int Arch Otorhinolaryngol. 2022;27:e130–7. https://doi.org/10.1055/s-0042-1749392.

29. Bhattacharyya N, Jones DT, Hill M, et al. The diagnostic accuracy of computed tomography in pediatric chronic rhinosinusitis. Arch Otolaryngol Head Neck Surg. 2004;130:1029–32. https://doi.org/10.1001/archotol.130.9.1029.
30. Lyu H, Guo Z, Chen C, et al. CT imaging features of paranasal sinuses in children with primary ciliary dyskinesia. Acta Otolaryngol. 2022;142:691–5. https://doi.org/10.1080/00016489.2022.2118371.

Upper Respiratory Tract Involvement in Primary Ciliary Dyskinesia: Therapeutic Continuity

49

Handan Kekeç, Lina Jankauskaite, and Ayşe Tana Aslan

49.1 Introduction

Primary ciliary dyskinesia (PCD) is a rare autosomal recessive genetic disease characterized by cilia dysfunction [1]. X-linked or autosomal dominant inheritance can be seen very rarely [2]. There are a lot of mutations identified in PCD, the existing mutations have an effect on the clinical progress and the severity of the disease [3]. Its incidence has been reported as 1/15–30,000 live births, but it is estimated to be more common because it can be overlooked in diagnosis for heterogeneous course of the disease [4, 5]. Mucociliary clearance increases as a result of absent or abnormal ciliary function [6]. In the upper airways, chronic rhinosinusitis, rhinorrhea or nasal congestion, acute otitis, recurrent otitis media with effusion, hearing impairment, and speech problems can be seen [7, 8]. Recurrent infections and bronchiectasis can be seen in the lower respiratory tract [9]. In addition, findings such as retinitis pigmentosa, congenital heart diseases, situs anomalies, accessory spleen or absence of spleen, reproductive difficulties, and deterioration in quality of life can be seen [8, 10, 11].

However, the characteristics of clinical findings can be variable according to the age. PCD findings may be presented such as unexplained respiratory distress in term infants, transient tachypnea in the newborn period, and the need for incubator care [12]. Recurrent ear and sinus infections, recurrent pneumonia, bronchiectasis, and daily wet sputum cough come to the fore in the clinical course going from childhood to adulthood [8, 13]. Situs inversus anomaly finding can be encountered in all

H. Kekeç · A. T. Aslan (✉)
Department of Pediatric Pulmonology, Ankara Gazi University Faculty of Medicine, Ankara, Turkey

L. Jankauskaite
Medical Academy, Lithuanian University of Health Sciences, Kaunas, Lithuania

H. Yüksel et al. (eds.), *Pediatric Airway Diseases*, Comprehensive ENT,
https://doi.org/10.1007/978-3-031-74853-0_49

age groups and the rate of situs anomaly can be seen less than 50% of the patient with PCD [10, 13].

The fact that PCD can affect many systems requires a multidisciplinary approach in long-term follow-up. According to the PCD foundation consensus, visits of otolaryngologist for 1–2 times a year and pulmonologist for 2–4 times a year are recommended for the follow-up of children with PCD. Audiologist examination is recommended when the first diagnosis and whenever the otolaryngologist seems it necessary. Patients with PCD should also be followed up by a reproductive specialist when the clinician considers it necessary [13, 14].

In this section, we aim to describe current treatment approaches in PCD.

49.2 Treatment Approaches in PCD

Although studies have been conducted on the lung involvement of PCD, its relationship with genetics and respiratory function capacities, studies on the effects on the upper airways, follow-up and treatment approaches are limited. Since there is no specific treatment or cure defined for PCD yet, the main goals in PCD treatment are to increase mucociliary clearance, to prevent repeated upper and lower respiratory tract infections due to mucociliary activity disorder and reduce inflammation. Approaches to this in treatment come to the fore [15–17]. Due to the mucociliary activity disorder, recurrent lung and upper airway infections, especially in patients with severe phenotype, may develop complications such as decreased lung capacity, bronchiectasis, and even have a serious clinical course that may require lung transplantation [6, 18, 19]. Therefore, it is necessary to diagnose and start treatment as early as possible [20].

49.2.1 Preventive Advice and Vaccine Prophylaxis

Growth and developmental retardation can be seen in children with PCD perhaps due to recurrent infections, malnutrition, and higher respiratory workload. In PCD patients body mass index z-scores and respiratory functions are closely related. For this reason, it should be ensured that children with PCD have a daily calorie intake appropriate for their age, and if necessary, vitamin supplements should be given to keep them in the appropriate percentiles with their peers. And they should be followed up by developmental pediatrics [21].

PCD is characterized by increased inflammation in the respiratory tract [22]. Precautions should be taken to protect against inflammation triggering agents and infections. Children with PCD should avoid active and passive smoking and should not be exposed to cigarette smoke [23].

In addition to preventive measures, azithromycin can be used as a prophylactic treatment by the clinician in children with PCD who have frequent infections, need additional antibiotic use and consequently have limitations in their daily activities and progress with intense inflammation. The immunomodulatory effect of azithromycin, a macrolide, is known. Use of azithromycin, 3 days a week for 6 months, has been shown to reduce lung exacerbations in patients with PCD in a multicenter study [24]. In another study, it was shown that the frequency of lung exacerbations decreased in the group using 10 mg/kg/day azithromycin as a long-term prophylactic. In addition, exercise intolerance was less common in this group than in the other group, and sputum volume decreased [25].

Children with PCD should receive pneumococcal and annual influenza vaccinations in addition to the routine recommended vaccination schedule.

49.2.2 Treatment of Otological Disease

In the otological involvement of PCD due to impaired cilia function and increased mucociliary clearance, middle ear structures (tympanic cavity, aditus, middle ear cavity, and mastoid air cells) and Eustachian tube are affected and cause recurrent microbial infections [26, 27]. The otologic presentation of PCD may be seen with findings such as acute otitis media (AOM), chronic otitis media (COM), effusion, tympanic membrane perforation, cholesteatoma, otorrhea, vertigo or balance impairment, hearing loss, and speech disorder secondary to this if hearing loss occurs at an early age. These findings may have a recurrent course or may be resistant to treatment in PCD [15, 27, 28]. Hearing protection treatments are one of the main points in the autological management of children with PCD [7]. It is aimed to ensure that language development is normal and to prevent complications related to the eardrum [29, 30].

The treatment management in otitis media may vary according to the age of the patient, the severity of the clinic, the feature of recurrence, whether or not there is accompanying effusion, and the presence of complications. Systemically effective antibiotics, especially high-dose amoxicillin clavulanate (90 mg/kg/day), can be used in the treatment of acute otitis media. The frequency of attacks and effusion status of the patient should be considered when deciding on the ventilation tube [31].

Otitis Media with Effusion (OME) can be defined due to the presence of liquid in the middle ear and as the absence of any sign of active infection [29]. Surgery is not required to all children with OME, in some children, effusion may be spontaneously regressed, or medical treatments such as antibiotics, nasal decongestants, lavages, and steroids can be applied [6, 29]. In OME, if surgery is required, then options will be as follows;

49.2.2.1 Myringotomy

Myringotomy is the process of opening a therapeutic incision in the tympanic membrane in order to drain the accumulated middle ear fluid or to provide air flow [30].

49.2.2.2 Grommet Insertion May Be Applied (Ventilation or Tympanostomy Tubes)

Ventilation tubes (VT) can be used to provide the flow between the middle ear and the Eustachian tube and equalizes the pressure. After tube insertion, patients should definitely go to their controls with 3–6 months period. But these tubes can be cause chronic otorrhea. In addition to the ventilation tube, adenoidectomy can also be applied to ensure ventilation of the Eustachian tube and to support the prevention of microbial colonization and adenoidectomy can be applied as an adjuvant treatment option [13, 30, 32]. If hearing loss has developed in patients, the use of hearing aids may be recommended in addition to or as an alternative to ventilation tube application [30].

49.2.3 Treatment of Sinonasal Disease

Findings such as nasal secretion, nasal polyp, nasal obstruction and discharge, decreased sense of smell, chronic rhinosinusitis (CRS), sinus aplasia/hypoplasia, sinus mucoceles, and hydrocephalus can be observed in the sinonasal involvement of PCD [7, 15, 33]. Sinonasal and otological symptoms are as common as pulmonary findings in PCD. CRS is an increased sinonasal complaint of the patients [34]. CRS can be defined as an inflammation of the paranasal sinuses lasting longer than 12 weeks and accompanying symptoms. Approximately 70% of children with PCD have CRS and 15–30% have nasal polyps [35].

Sleep disorders are also an important comorbid condition in children, with PCD and obstructive sleep apnea syndrome (OSAS) is quite common among sleep disorders. OSAS is defined as partial reduction or complete cessation of airflow during sleep. It has been shown to have negative effects on growth, cardiovascular system, behavioral and cognitive development when sleep disorders in children are not treated. In the long term, learning difficulties, poor school performance, attention deficit, hyperactivity disorder, and a decrease in general quality of life can be observed. If the patient has accompanying symptoms such as sleeping with an open mouth, snoring, and daytime sleepiness, the patient's upper airway should be evaluated endoscopically for the presence of adenotonsillar hypertrophy, nasal polyps, and CRS, especially with an upper airway obstructive course. Nasal polyps and CRS are related condition which is among the inflammatory causes of childhood obstructive sleep apnea syndrome. A home sleep study test can be done to detect OSAS. Children with OSAS benefit greatly from adenotonsillectomy. In the presence of chronic rhinosinusitis and nasal polyps, intranasal steroids and lavage can be used, and if the polyp is occlusive, polypectomy can be applied [36, 37].

In the sinonasal involvement of PCD, the treatment approach should be primarily medical treatments, if no response is obtained or if necessary, surgical treatment options can be applied. Saline lavage can be applied daily to clean the nasal cavity and increase mucociliary clearance. In the presence of nasal polyps, nasal steroid therapy can be used to shrink the polyp, reduce the inflammations and symptoms [38].

If the patient has recurrent acute and chronic sinusitis and it is unresponsive to antibiotics or if long-term antibiotic use is required, endoscopic sinus surgery (ESS) can be applied to this group of patients. The severity of the patient and CT images are evaluated together when deciding on the surgical procedure. The purpose of ESS is to ventilate the sinuses and provide airflow [35, 39, 40].

49.2.4 Treatment of Pulmonary Disease

According to the European Respiratory Society consensus of definition for pulmonary exacerbations,

- Changes in sputum character such as darkening of sputum color/increase in quantity/increase in frequency
- A feeling of an increased tightness or shortness of breath that the patient described or noticed by the patient's relatives
- Body temperature above 38 °C
- Description of symptoms such as weakness, fatigue, and exhaustion
- Planning to start antibiotics and/or needing to change the current antibiotic therapy as a result of evaluation of pulmonary findings
- Complain of increased cough
- Detection of hemoptysis and/or increase in existing hemoptysis

The presence of three or more of the above points is considered an acute exacerbation in children with PCD [41].

Lung exacerbations should be kept under control because they both affect the psychological health of the patient and important for the development of bronchiectasis [42]. It is recommended to give sputum or cough swab culture every 3 months in children with PCD. The most frequently microorganisms are often isolated such as *Haemophilus influenzae, Streptococcus pneumonia, Staphylococcus aureus, Pseudomonas aeruginosa* (PA), *Moraxella catarrhalis,* and *nontuberculous mycobacteria* in sputum culture [23, 43]. If there is an active upper airway infection or pulmonary exacerbation, the patient should be treated with appropriate antibiotics for a sufficient duration and dose according to the microorganism isolated in the cultures. If it is *Pseudomonas aeruginosa* grown in culture, eradication treatment is recommended in PCD, with long-term nebulized antibiotics just like in CF [23]. Modified Leeds criteria can be used to define the patient's PA infection status. If more than 50% of the cultures taken in the last 12 months have specific microorganisms, it is defined as a chronic infection. Defined as intermittent infection in the presence of specific microorganisms detected in 50% or less of cultures taken in the last 12 months. It is considered free infection when no growth or colonization is detected in cultures taken in the last 12 months [44, 45]. Although different centers may apply different treatment and eradication protocols in intermittent and chronic PA. In the management of PA eradication, 2–4 weeks of oral ciprofloxacin plus inhaled tobramycin/colistin for 1–3 months can be used. If the PA infection is recurrent or accompanied by acute exacerbation, intravenous carbapenem or ceftazidime may be added to the treatment. It is thought that a microbial colonization in the upper airway may also pose a risk for the lower airways [45]. This situation should be considered and the upper and lower airways should be evaluated together. Due care should be taken in the follow-up.

On the lack of sufficient data and studies on lung involvement and disease severity of PCD; in a study including 991 patients who can perform PFT by Halbeisen et al. FEV1 and FVC *z*-score values of patients were compared with data collected from healthy children and children with cystic fibrosis. It was shown that lung involvement of patients with PCD was similar affected to that of children with CF. It was observed that FEV1 and FVC values of children with PCD were lower than healthy children [46, 47]. Based on this, it should be taken into account that PCD can be seriously affect the lungs and reduce the lung capacity and should not be underestimated. In particularly, patients should regularly apply respiratory physiotherapy and the clinician should periodically monitor lung function spirometrically.

49.2.5 Physiotherapy and Physical Exercises

Increasing physical activity in addition to daily respiratory physiotherapy recommended to improve airway clearance in children with PCD contributes to a better clinical course of patients [48]. In addition to increasing lung capacity, physical activity has been shown to increase bone mineral density and reduce the rates of anxiety and depression in children [49].

49.2.6 Inhaler Treatments

49.2.6.1 Hyperosmolar Agents

The aim of inhaled hyperosmolar agents is to increase mucociliary clearance and to ensure fluidity of the mucus. For this purpose, 3–7% hypertonic saline or inhaled mannitol can be used. Although these agents are not routinely used in the treatment of PCD, they may be preferred in cases deemed appropriate by the clinician [7, 13].

49.2.6.2 DNase (Recombinant Human Dornase Alfa)

Nebulized rhDNase (PulmozymeTM) which is a part of the inhaler treatment of cystic fibrosis and acts by breaking down the DNA in the dense sticky mucus, has been shown to reduce sputum viscosity and improve lung functions in regular daily use [50]. Due to the lack of clinical experience regarding the use of rhDNase in PCD, its use cannot be recommended [6], but in a study with two case [51] it has been shown that lung functions have improved in patients with PCD. Maybe it can also be used in the treatment of PCD in only selected patients [13].

49.2.6.3 Inhale Bronchodilators and Inhale Corticosteroids

Although it has been observed that bronchodilator and inhaled corticosteroids are prescribed in PCD, routine use is not recommended in the guidelines. If the patient has a comorbid disease with a bronchodilator response, such as asthma, a response is expected. The response status of the patient should be evaluated and prescribed accordingly [52, 53].

49.2.7 Pulmonary Surgical Options and Transplant

Lobectomy or segmentectomy can be applied only in selected patients who develop severe localized bronchiectasis unresponsive to medical treatments. Not recommended to apply routinely and clinical benefit has not been proven [54, 55]. In order for lung transplantation to be performed in PCD, end-stage disease must be defined and the number of cases performed is very low [19].

References

1. Damseh N, Quercia N, Rumman N, et al. Primary ciliary dyskinesia: mechanisms and management. Appl Clin Genet. 2017;10:67–74.
2. Shapiro AJ, Kaspy K, Daniels MLA, et al. Autosomal dominant variants in FOXJ1 causing primary ciliary dyskinesia in two patients with obstructive hydrocephalus. Mol Genet Genom Med. 2021;9(7):e1726.
3. Shoemark A, Rubbo B, Legendre M, et al. Topological data analysis reveals genotype–phenotype relationships in primary ciliary dyskinesia. Eur Respir J. 2021;58(2):2002359.
4. Bush A, Chodhari R, Collins N, et al. Primary ciliary dyskinesia: current state of the art. Arch Dis Child. 2007;92(12):1136–40.
5. O'Callaghan C, Chetcuti P, Moya E. High prevalence of primary ciliary dyskinesia in a British Asian population. Arch Dis Child. 2010;95(1):51–2.
6. Paff T, Omran H, Nielsen KG. Current and future treatments in primary ciliary dyskinesia. Int J Mol Sci. 2021;22(18):9834.
7. Campbell R. Managing upper respiratory tract complications of primary ciliary dyskinesia in children. Curr Opin Allergy Clin Immunol. 2012;12(1):32–8.
8. Goutaki M, Shoemark A. Diagnosis of primary ciliary dyskinesia. Clin Chest Med. 2022;43(1):127–40.
9. Goutaki M, Meier AB, Halbeisen FS, et al. Clinical manifestations in primary ciliary dyskinesia: systematic review and meta-analysis. Eur Respir J. 2016;48(4):1081–95.
10. Mirra V, Werner C, Santamaria F. Primary ciliary dyskinesia: an update on clinical aspects, genetics, diagnosis, and future treatment strategies. Front Pediatr. 2017;5:135.
11. Emiralioğlu N, Karadağ B, Özçelik HU. Quality of life questionnaire for Turkish patients with primary ciliary dyskinesia. Turk Thorac J. 2017;18(1):19–22.
12. Ferkol T, Leigh M. Primary ciliary dyskinesia and newborn respiratory distress. Semin Perinatol. 2006;30(6):335–40.
13. Shapiro AJ, Zariwala MA, Ferkol T, Genetic Disorders of Mucociliary Clearance Consortium, et al. Diagnosis, monitoring, and treatment of primary ciliary dyskinesia: PCD foundation consensus recommendations based on state of the art review. Pediatr Pulmonol. 2016;51(2):115–32.
14. Lucas JS, Barbato A, Collins SA, et al. European Respiratory Society guidelines for the diagnosis of primary ciliary dyskinesia. Eur Respir J. 2017;49(1):1601090.
15. Zawawi F, Shapiro AJ, Dell S, et al. Otolaryngology manifestations of primary ciliary dyskinesia: a multicenter study. Otolaryngol Head Neck Surg. 2022;166(3):540–7.
16. Goutaki M, Lam YT, Alexandru M, et al. Study protocol: the ear–nose–throat (ENT) prospective international cohort of patients with primary ciliary dyskinesia (EPIC-PCD). BMJ Open. 2021;11(10):e051433.
17. Blanter M, Cockx M, Wittebols L, et al. Sputum from patients with primary ciliary dyskinesia contains high numbers of dysfunctional neutrophils and inhibits efferocytosis. Respir Res. 2022;23(1):359.
18. Davis SD, Ferkol TW, Rosenfeld M, et al. Clinical features of childhood primary ciliary dyskinesia by genotype and ultrastructural phenotype. Am J Respir Crit Care Med. 2015;191(3):316–24.

19. Marro M, Leiva-Juárez MM, D'Ovidio F. Lung transplantation for primary ciliary dyskinesia and Kartagener syndrome: a multicenter study. Transplant Int. 2023;36:10819.
20. Goutaki M, Halbeisen FS, Barbato A, et al. Late diagnosis of infants with PCD and neonatal respiratory distress. J Clin Med. 2020;9(9):2871.
21. Marino LV, Harris A, Johnstone C, et al. Characterising the nutritional status of children with primary ciliary dyskinesia. Clin Nutr (Edinburgh, Scotland). 2019;38(5):2127–35.
22. Sagel SD, Kupfer O, Wagner BD, et al. Airway inflammation in children with primary ciliary dyskinesia. Ann Am Thorac Soc. 2023;20(1):67–74.
23. Barbato A, Frischer T, Kuehni CE, et al. Primary ciliary dyskinesia: a consensus statement on diagnostic and treatment approaches in children. Eur Respir J. 2009;34(6):1264–76.
24. Kobbernagel HE, Buchvald FF, Haarman EG, et al. Efficacy and safety of azithromycin maintenance therapy in primary ciliary dyskinesia (BESTCILIA): a multicentre, double-blind, randomised, placebo-controlled phase 3 trial. Lancet Respir Med. 2020;8(5):493–505.
25. Guan Y, Zhang X, Yang H, et al. Long-term azithromycin treatment in pediatric primary ciliary dyskinesia: a retrospective study. Front Pediatr. 2022;10:905253.
26. Noone PG, Leigh MW, Sannuti A, et al. Primary ciliary dyskinesia: diagnostic and phenotypic features. Am J Respir Crit Care Med. 2004;169(4):459–67.
27. Andersen TN, Alanin MC, von Buchwald C, et al. A longitudinal evaluation of hearing and ventilation tube insertion in patients with primary ciliary dyskinesia. Int J Pediatr Otorhinolaryngol. 2016;89:164–8.
28. Prulière-Escabasse V, Coste A, Chauvin P, et al. Otologic features in children with primary ciliary dyskinesia. Arch Otolaryngol Head & Neck Surg. 2010;136(11):1121–6.
29. Lous J, Burton MJ, Felding JU, et al. Grommets (ventilation tubes) for hearing loss associated with otitis media with effusion in children. Cochrane Database Syst Rev. 2005;1:CD001801.
30. Rosenfeld RM, Tunkel DE, Schwartz SR, et al. Clinical practice guideline: tympanostomy tubes in children (update). Otolaryngol Head Neck Surg. 2022;166(1_suppl):S1–S55.
31. Otteson T. Otitis media and tympanostomy tubes. Pediatr Clin N Am. 2022;69(2):203–19.
32. Campbell RG, Birman CS, Morgan L. Management of otitis media with effusion in children with primary ciliary dyskinesia: a literature review. Int J Pediatr Otorhinolaryngol. 2009;73(12):1630–8.
33. Pappa AK, Sullivan KM, Lopez EM, et al. Sinus development and pneumatization in a primary ciliary dyskinesia cohort. Am J Rhinol Allergy. 2021;35(1):72–6.
34. Lam YT, Papon JF, Alexandru M, et al. Sinonasal disease among patients with primary ciliary dyskinesia: an international study. ERJ Open Res. 2023;9(3):00701–2022.
35. Alanin MC, Aanaes K, Høiby N, et al. Sinus surgery can improve quality of life, lung infections, and lung function in patients with primary ciliary dyskinesia. Int Forum Allergy Rhinol. 2017;7(3):240–7.
36. Li Z, Celestin J, Lockey RF. Pediatric sleep apnea syndrome: an update. J Allergy Clin Immunol. 2016;4(5):852–61.
37. Santamaria F, Esposito M, Montella S, et al. Sleep disordered breathing and airway disease in primary ciliary dyskinesia. Respirology. 2014;19(4):570–5.
38. Lucas JS, Alanin MC, Collins S, et al. Clinical care of children with primary ciliary dyskinesia. Expert Rev Respir Med. 2017;11(10):779–90.
39. Mener DJ, Lin SY, Ishman SL, et al. Treatment and outcomes of chronic rhinosinusitis in children with primary ciliary dyskinesia: where is the evidence? A qualitative systematic review. Int Forum Allergy Rhinol. 2013;3(12):986–91.
40. Parsons DS, Greene BA. A treatment for primary ciliary dyskinesia: efficacy of functional endoscopic sinus surgery. Laryngoscope. 1993;103(11 Pt 1):1269–72.
41. Lucas JS, Gahleitner F, Amorim A, et al. Pulmonary exacerbations in patients with primary ciliary dyskinesia: an expert consensus definition for use in clinical trials. ERJ Open Res. 2019;5(1):00147–2018.
42. Chang AB, Morgan LC, Duncan EL, et al. Reducing exacerbations in children and adults with primary ciliary dyskinesia using erdosteine and/or azithromycin therapy (REPEAT trial):

study protocol for a multicentre, double-blind, double-dummy, 2 × 2 partial factorial, randomised controlled trial. BMJ Open Respir Res. 2022;9(1):e001236.
43. Knowles MR, Daniels LA, Davis SD, et al. Primary ciliary dyskinesia. Recent advances in diagnostics, genetics, and characterization of clinical disease. Am J Respir Crit Care Med. 2013;188(8):913–22.
44. Alanin MC, Nielsen KG, von Buchwald C, et al. A longitudinal study of lung bacterial pathogens in patients with primary ciliary dyskinesia. Clin Microbiol Infect. 2015;21(12):1093.e1–7.
45. Crowley S, Holgersen MG, Nielsen KG. Variation in treatment strategies for the eradication of *Pseudomonas aeruginosa* in primary ciliary dyskinesia across European centers. Chronic Respir Dis. 2019;16:1479972318787919.
46. Halbeisen FS, Goutaki M, Spycher BD, et al. Lung function in patients with primary ciliary dyskinesia: an iPCD Cohort study. Eur Respir J. 2018;52(2):1801040.
47. Saglani S. Lung function in primary ciliary dyskinesia: breaking the myth that this is a mild disease. Eur Respir J. 2018;52(2):1801365.
48. Schumann M, Freitag N, Haag E, et al. Individualized physical training in the therapy of primary ciliary dyskinesia—a case report. Respir Med Case Rep. 2019;28:100925.
49. Valerio G, Giallauria F, Montella S, et al. Cardiopulmonary assessment in primary ciliary dyskinesia. Eur J Clin Investig. 2012;42(6):617–22.
50. Altaf R, Parmar M. Dornase alfa. In: StatPearls. StatPearls Publishing; 2023.
51. El-Abiad NM, Clifton S, Nasr SZ. Long-term use of nebulized human recombinant DNase1 in two siblings with primary ciliary dyskinesia. Respir Med. 2007;101(10):2224–6.
52. Dehlink E, Richardson C, Marsh G, et al. Are inhaled corticosteroids prescribed rationally in primary ciliary dyskinesia? Eur Respir J. 2018;51(3):1702221.
53. Levine H, Bar-On O, Nir V, et al. Reversible bronchial obstruction in primary ciliary dyskinesia. J Clin Med. 2022;11(22):6791.
54. Sendon CS, Cowles RA, Worhunsky DJ, et al. Pediatric unilobar resection in primary ciliary dyskinesia. Minerva Pediatr. 2022;74(5):593–9.
55. Kouis P, Goutaki M, Halbeisen FS, et al. Prevalence and course of disease after lung resection in primary ciliary dyskinesia: a cohort and nested case-control study. Respir Res. 2019;20(1):212.

Primary Immunodeficiencies: Upper Respiratory Tract Consequences

50

Zeynep Meric, Zita Chovancova, and Ayca Kiykim

50.1 Upper Respiratory Tract Infections

Acute otitis media (AOM) is very common in childhood, and up to 60% of children suffer from at least one episode of otitis media in the first 3 years of life [1]. It is defined as inflammation of the middle ear and usually occurs in one of three forms: AOM, otitis media with effusion (OME), or chronic suppurative otitis media (CSOM). AOM is usually self-limiting and is often associated with a viral upper respiratory tract infection. Complications like bacterial OM may be seen during the disease course, especially in young children. AOM is often accompanied by ear pain and fever. If not properly treated, it can lead to complications such as tympanic membrane perforation or mastoiditis [1].

OME is a well-known cause of hearing loss in children, and is defined as an accumulation of fluid in the middle ear due to negative pressure caused by altered function of the Eustachian tube. It can occur due to allergy, bacterial otitis media, or viral infection. When the fluid in the middle ear space increases, it causes conductive hearing loss [1].

CSOM is an active middle ear infection with perforation of the tympanic membrane. It manifests as otorrhea, resulting in hearing loss. The most common microorganism causing CSOM is *Pseudomonas aeruginosa*. The other microorganisms isolated from culture are coagulase-negative *Staphylococcus aerius*, *Escherichia coli*, *Proteus mirabilis*, and *Bacteroides fragilis*.

Z. Meric · A. Kiykim (✉)
Department of Pediatric Immunology and Allergy, Cerrahpasa School of Medicine, Istanbul University-Cerrahpasa, Istanbul, Turkey

Z. Chovancova
Department of Clinical Immunology and Allergology, St. Anne's University Hospital in Brno and Faculty of Medicine, Masaryk University, Brno, Czech Republic
e-mail: zita.chovancova@fnusa.cz

H. Yüksel et al. (eds.), *Pediatric Airway Diseases*, Comprehensive ENT,
https://doi.org/10.1007/978-3-031-74853-0_50

Immature anatomy of the Eustachian tube, other anatomic anomalies including cleft palate, genetic conditions with craniofacial anomalies, and also adenoid hypertrophy, daycare attendance, and parental smoking contribute to the higher rates of otitis media in children [2]. Breastfeeding for at least 4–6 months is beneficial in reducing the number and duration of all OM infections. On the other hand, an underlying immune deficiency may contribute to otitis media [3].

In 1987, Vicki and Fred Modell established the Jeffrey Modell Foundation (JMF) in memory of their son Jeffrey, who died as a result of IEI. In 1993, ten Warning Signs of IEI were proposed by this foundation with the help of immunologists to raise awareness among physicians. It is recommended that physicians should suspect IEI if more than two warning signs are present. Experiencing at least four serious ear infections in a year is one of them (Table 50.1) [4, 5]. Recurrent middle ear infections are very frequent in IEI, although may vary among different forms of IEI. In particular, if AOM is frequent, purulent, the response is poor to antibiotics, unusual organisms have been found, or occurs in association with other lung infections, failure to thrive or atopic dermatitis, we should consider IEI (Table 50.2) [2, 6].

In 2016, Pichichero first described a nomenclature for children at risk for otitis. They defined children as at risk for otitis if they had 3 episodes of AOM in 6 months or 4 episodes in 12 months. They prospectively screened children for almost any disease and confirmed almost any clinical diagnosis of AOM by middle ear fluid (MEF) culture by tympanocentesis from 6 to 36 months of age. The initial findings were that pediatricians diagnosed excessive AOM, consistent with ENT physicians. On immunologic evaluation, these patients showed a low antibody response to routine pediatric vaccines (including antibody response to *Streptococcus pneumoniae* and *Haemophilus influenzae*). In addition, antigen-specific memory B-cell

Table 50.1 Warning signs for inborn errors of immunity in children

1. More than 4 otitis in 1 year
2. More than 2 sinusitis in 1 year
3. More than 2 lower respiratory tract infections in 1 year
4. Recurrent, deep skin or organ abscesses
5. Persistent oral moniliasis or skin infections with fungus
6. More than 2 deep-seated infections (including septicemia)
7. More than 2 months on antibiotics with poor response
8. Necessitation of parenteral antibiotics for infections
9. Failure to thrive
10. Affected individuals in the family

Table 50.2 Warning signs to investigate IEI in otitis

1. Otitis progressing to mastoiditis, systemic infections or abscesses
2. Poor response to antibiotics
3. Presence of other infections
4. Recurrent, deep skin or organ abscesses
5. Recurrent otitis leading to failure to thrive and general developmental delay
6. Affected individuals in the family or consanguinity

populations exhibited mechanistic dysfunction that impaired proliferation or differentiation into plasma cells [7].

Since AOM is very common in childhood, it is very important to know which patients need a thorough immunologic evaluation. A thorough immunologic evaluation should be performed if the following warning signs are present: progression to mastoiditis; cooccurrence of abscesses or systemic infections; poor response to appropriate antibiotic treatment; or association of unusual, severe, or frequently recurring infections elsewhere [6] (Table 50.2). The presence of failure to thrive should be evaluated for IEI [8]. In addition, if a family history and/or consanguineous marriage is present, an underlying IEI should be considered [4].

Rhinosinusitis is the inflammation of the nasal cavity and sinuses. Common symptoms include purulent nasal discharge, postnasal drainage, facial or headache, nasal congestion, and anosmia [9].

Rhinosinusitis is defined as acute if it lasts <12 weeks and chronic if it lasts longer than 12 weeks. Acute rhinosinusitis (ARS) can be viral or bacterial in origin, and recurrent acute rhinosinusitis (RARS) consists of at least three acute bacterial rhinosinusitis (ABRS) within a year. Chronic rhinosinusitis (CRS) is further divided into CRS with nasal polyps (CRSwNP) and CRS without nasal polyps (CRSsNP) [9].

Acute rhinosinusitis is most commonly viral, and ABRS accounts for nearly 1.5% in the general population. Acute bacterial rhinosinusitis is predominantly caused by *Streptococcus pneumoniae*, *Moraxella catarrhalis*, and *Haemophilus influenzae* [10].

In addition to the bacterial causes mentioned above, *Staphylococcus aureus*, *Pseudomonas aeruginosa*, and others may be found in CRS patients. The preferred treatment for ABRS is antibiotics; however, overdiagnosis of ABRS may lead to inappropriate antibiotic use. The diagnosis of ABRS is likely when symptoms preceding a cold initially improve and then worsen with the appearance of fever and purulent nasal discharge. Aspiration of the maxillary sinus or a culture from the middle nasal passage by endoscopic sampling is best suited for the detection of the causative microorganism [9].

Antibiotic use is controversial at CRS and limited to acute exacerbations and patients with persistent purulent discharge. Sinus culture is strongly recommended for persistent purulent discharge [9]. Anatomic defects, foreign bodies, tumors, allergic and nonallergic rhinitis may predispose to RARS and CRS [9, 10]. In patients with RARS and CRS, the differential diagnosis should include cystic fibrosis, primary ciliary dyskinesia, and immunodeficiencies.

Primary immunodeficiencies (PIDs) include at least 485 genetic disorders classified into ten subgroups; (1) combined immunodeficiencies, (2) combined immunodeficiencies (CIDs) with associated or syndromic features, (3) predominantly antibody deficiencies, (4) diseases of immune dysregulation (ID), (5) congenital defects of phagocyte number and/or function, (6) intrinsic and innate immune defects, (7) autoinflammatory disorders, (8) complement deficiencies, (9) bone marrow failure, and (10) phenocopies of PID [11].

More than 70% of PIDs initially present with infections [12]. Recurrent upper respiratory tract infections (URTIs), including recurrent otitis and sinusitis, are among the 10 warning signs recommended by the Jeffrey Modell Foundation for early diagnosis of PIDs [5]. The incidence of URTIs can be as high as 90% [13]. Among them, antibody deficiencies (PAD) form the majority of CRS [14]. In the metaanalysis published by Schwitzguebel et al. [15], they showed that common variable immunodeficiencies (CVID) and unclassified IgG deficiencies were more common in patients with CRS (0–10% and 0–16%, respectively). When CVID, unclassified IgG, selective IgA, and selective IgM deficiencies were evaluated together, the prevalence was even higher in patients with difficult-to-treat CRS (22.8%).

50.1.1 Selective IgA Deficiency

Selective immunoglobulin A deficiency (sIgAD) is the most common primary immunodeficiency, with a frequency of 1:600, defined as a deficiency of IgA (less than 7 mg/L) in children >4 years [16, 17]. Immunoglobulin A is the major antibody in secretions covering mucosal surfaces of the respiratory, gastrointestinal, and genitourinary tracts and is an important member of the defense [18]. Although IgA deficiency is associated with a higher incidence of URTIs and OM, the majority of individuals with a diagnosis of an IgA deficiency lives without significant morbidity [19].

Due to the very mild phenotype of selective IgA deficiency, patients with recurrent or chronic otitis media with low IgA serum levels should be thoroughly investigated. These patients may have a deficient antibody response to vaccination and decreased memory B cells, leading to a diagnosis of CVID on follow-up [20]. Immunoglobulin replacement therapy is not indicated in sIgAD and may lead to hypersensitivity reactions [21, 22]. Antibiotic prophylaxis with amoxicillin on a continuous or seasonal intermittent basis may be beneficial in recurrent AOM [23].

Patients with sIgAD frequently present CRS (up to 78%), and of those with CRS, only 6.2 % meet the criteria for sIgAD [24]. The role of IgA in mucosal defense is still not well understood [25], higher levels can be found in CRS patients. It has been hypothesized that increased local IgA levels may be produced by type 2 hyperinflamed tissue [26]. Given the high prevalence of IgA deficiency and the fact that few are symptomatic, isolated IgA deficiency is still controversial in the differential diagnosis of CRS. Some authors believe that it should be associated with other IgG subclasses or specific antibody deficiencies to cause severe refractory infections [27].

50.1.2 Immunoglobulin Subclass Deficiencies

Selective IgG subclass deficiency is defined as a significant decrease (below 2 SD of the mean) in one or more IgG subgroups in the presence of normal total IgG, IgA, and IgM levels. These defects may occur singly or in combination with IgA deficiency. In one study, otitis-prone children had up to 33% low serum IgG2 levels, while other immunoglobulin levels were within the normal range [28]. IgG2 is related to the humoral response to polysaccharide antigens and thus to encapsulated bacteria in adults [29]. In recurrent AOM, the diagnostic approach may include quantification of IgG subclasses so that these children can be successfully treated with antibiotic prophylaxis and IVIG replacement [8].

The most common subgroup deficiency in children is IgG2 and is associated with upper and lower RTIs. It can be isolated or together with IgG4 subclass deficiency. In contrast, IgG3 deficiency is more prominent in adults. In a retrospective study by Vanlerberghe et al. IgG2 deficiency was found in 2% and IgG3 deficiency in 17.9% of 307 patients with CRS [30]. However, this study did not record specific antibody responses to vaccination. In another study by May et al. that also included pneumococcal antibody responses, 245 patients with refractory rhinosinusitis (CRS) were found to have 17 IgG subclass deficiencies, most of them IgG2 deficient (IgG2:10, IgG1:5). Almost half of the patients with IgG subclass deficiency were found to have a lower pneumococcal antibody response [31]. The presence of functional antibody responses should be investigated before inferring low IgG subclass levels as a direct cause of therapy-refractory CRS. Low IgG subclass levels may occasionally occur in 2–20% of healthy individuals [32]. Patients with a deficiency in functional antibody responses may benefit from IVIG.

50.1.3 Common Variable Immunodeficiency

Common Variable Immunodeficiency (CVID) is a primary antibody deficiency, often symptomatic and is very common (1:25,000–1:50,000) [33]. CVID is a disorder of B cell development and/or function that results in low serum Ig levels with reduced or absent antibody response to vaccines. The diagnosis of CVID should be based on low IgG levels, either low IgM or IgA levels and the absence of specific antibody responses in individuals over 4 years of age regarding International Consensus Document released in 2016 [34]. A similar diagnostic criteria was proposed by The European Society of Immune Deficiencies (ESID); the presence of symptoms including unexplained polyclonal lymphoproliferation, infections, affected family member or granulomatous disease with antibody deficiency and poor response to vaccination or decreased memory B cells, without severe cellular deficiency or secondary hypogammaglobulinemia to establish a diagnosis of CVID [35]. As can be seen, the disease can present with many different clinical and laboratory findings across a broad spectrum.

A long-term follow-up study of CVID patients showed that the most common clinical symptoms was recurrent infections (89.0%), predominantly RTIs, followed by immune dysregulation (42.5%) [36]. Otitis media is very common among CVID patients. In a systematic review and meta-analysis of CVID patients, a history of upper and/or lower RTIs was present in 75% of patients at the time of diagnosis (with sinusitis in 59%, and otitis in 39%) [37]. Another study showed a higher prevalence of recurrent or chronic otitis media, with a prevalence of 69% [38]. Similar results were obtained in other cohorts [39]. Mastoiditis occurred in 10% of children with CVID, indicating an uncontrolled infection. Unlike to the agammaglobulinemic patients, in CVID, secondary lymphoid tissue is present and is often hypertrophic, promoting the development of otitis media due to mechanical obstruction [8].

The treatment of choice in CVID is immunoglobulin replacement which reduces the rate of infections [21]. Besides, antibiotic prophylaxis could be beneficial in these patients. However, some patients may require drainage of the middle ear and long-term antibiotic treatment for otitis. The molecular defects that lead to CVID have yet to be discovered, but the current state of knowledge already sheds light on the mechanisms and possible targeted treatments [40].

Impaired Ig production puts patients at risk for respiratory infections, mainly from encapsulated bacteria, leading to chronic lung disease and chronic sinusitis. *Haemophilus influenza*, *Streptococcus pneumoniae*, Mycoplasma, *Pseudomonas* spp., Moraxella, *Klebsiella pneumonia* and *Staphylococcus* spp., and are common respiratory infections in CVID [41]. The most common upper respiratory viruses include human rhinoviruses (HRV), followed by adenoviruses, respiratory syncytial viruses, and seasonal coronaviruses.

Chronic rhinosinusitis is a common feature in CVID and may occur in nearly 40% of patients [42–44]. In the study published by Bondioni et al. sinus changes were found in 25 of 27 patients with CVID, with mucosal thickening being the most common change [45]. The maxillary sinus was affected in 96% of cases, and bilaterally in 41.6%. Ethmoid and frontal sinus followed in 44% and 40% of patients, respectively. Bone sclerosis was found in 7 of 25 patients, affecting the maxillary sinus (57.1%), followed by the ethmoid sinus (42.8%), frontal sinus, and sphenoid sinus (28.5%). Similarly, polyposis was found in the maxillary sinus (71.4%), ethmoid sinus (57.1%), and frontal sinus (14.2%) in 28% of patients [45]. Despite the high frequency of CRS in PIDs, Odat et al. found no significant difference in age, sex, polyp status, and allergy between patients with and without immunodeficiency [46].

Antibiotic prophylaxis and immunoglobulin replacement are the treatment options for CVID and with severe and recurrent infections. There is no consensus on the choice of prophylactic antibiotics, but beta-lactams, trimethoprim-sulfamethoxazole, and azithromycin are preferred [27].

Conventional treatment of CRS should include early initiation of antibiotics according to nasal culture and steroids (intranasal and/or systemic), and surgical intervention if necessary. Although replacement of immunoglobulins is the main therapy for respiratory infections, the benefit is less likely in the case of CRS [47]. Quinti et al. showed that only 8% of patients improved with immunoglobulin replacement therapy (IgRT) and documented an increase in the percentage of CRS patients (36–53%) despite IgRT [47]. Depending on patient characteristics, either intravenous (IVIG) or subcutaneous (SCIG) administration can be chosen, with an initial dose of 400–600 mg/kg every 3–4 weeks intravenously or 100 mg/kg/week subcutaneously with a trough level of 800 mg/dL to prevent chronic lung disease [48].

50.1.4 X-Linked and Autosomal Agammaglobulinemia

X-linked agammaglobulinemia (XLA) is an early developmental defect of B cells and is caused by a mutation in the Bruton tyrosine kinase (BTK) gene [49]. The diagnostic features of XLA include the absence of B cells and immunoglobulin levels. In the absence of BTK, immunoglobulin gene rearrangement is impaired, and B cell maturation stops at the pro-B cell level and fails to develop into mature B cells. It is characterized by lack of B cells in the circulation and the absence of organized lymph nodes with low immunoglobulin levels [50].

X-linked agammaglobulinemia is the most common cause of agammaglobulinemia with an estimated incidence of between 1:100,000 and 1:200,000. Typically, the majority of patients presents with early-onset infections, very low B cells and panhypogammaglobulinemia. In addition, autosomal recessive (μ-heavy chain gene) and autosomal dominant (LRRC8A gene and TCF3 gene) forms of agammaglobulinemia have been described [51, 52].

Recurrent or chronic otitis media is very common. In a metaanalysis, these patients were found to have AOM in up to 73% [51]. Bacterial infections usually occur in the 6th–12th month of life, when maternal serum IgG levels fall below protective levels. The absence of a humoral immune response, including secretory IgG deficiency, predisposes these patients to upper respiratory tract bacterial infections. Despite recurrent URTIs, the absence of enlarged lymph nodes and small tonsils may be indicate agammaglobulinemia [49].

In an Italian multicenter study, the authors collected data from 73 patients with XLA. Respiratory infections were the most common manifestations in 68.5% (50/73) of patients. Both lower and respiratory tracts were affected in 39 patients, and only URTIs occurred in 11 patients. Age at diagnosis was lower only in the URTI group. Chronic sinusitis was diagnosed in 15 of 73 patients based on clinical and/or computed tomographic findings. Age at diagnosis was higher in patients with CRS than in those without CRS. And interestingly, half of the patients with CRS also had chronic lung disease. The authors suggest that prolonged postnasal drip may increase the risk of developing chronic lung disease [53]. In a recent cohort from the United States, the presence of sinusitis was documented in 54.6% of patients. They also found that patients continued to have otitis and sinusitis despite adequate Ig substitution [54]. In the study by Bondioni et al. sinusal changes were detected in 88.8% of 18 patients with agammaglobulinemia [45]. Mucosal thickening was the most common finding in 93.7% of cases, followed by bone sclerosis and polyposis (31.2% and 18.7%, respectively). The maxillary sinus, ethmoid sinus, and sphenoid sinus were most commonly affected (87.5%, 56.2%, and 43.7%, respectively). Unfortunately, despite early diagnosis and adequate replacement therapy, few patients show improvement [45].

A history of invasive infections, especially with encapsulated bacteria, enteroviral meningoencephalitis, chronic diarrhea with *Giardia lamblia*, should suggest a thorough investigation [51].

Neutrophil and lymphocyte counts are usually normal, while findings of agamaglobulinemia and lack of B cells are typical. Genetic analysis should be performed to confirm the diagnosis [8].

The standard treatment includes immunoglobulin replacement therapy. Not surprisingly, however, the incidence of URTI does not really change with the administration of IgRT, since the mucosal immune response requires prompt IgA and IgM functions that cannot be replaced by current Ig therapies [53].

In the long term, these patients should be carefully monitored for CSOM, hearing loss, and other otitis complications [51].

50.1.5 Specific Antibody Deficiency

Determination of serum immunoglobulin level is the first level of assessment in suspected immunodeficiency. Specific antibody deficiency (SAD) is a condition associated with normal Ig levels but deficient antibody response to polysaccharide antigens [55]. An adequate antipneumococcal antibody response is defined as a postvaccination Ig level of ≥1.3 μg/mL or at least a fourfold increase from baseline. Such an immune response is not expected in children younger than 2 years of age because of the immaturity of the polysaccharide antigen response.

Similar to other predominantly antibody deficiencies, susceptibility to sinopulmonary infections is the hallmark of SAD. Infections with encapsulated bacteria are expected, including *Haemophilus influenza* and *Streptococcus pneumonia* [56]. In a study by Misbah et al. they examined patients with recurrent otitis media requiring tympanostomy and found a low response to antipneumococcal antibodies in 20% of patients [57]. In another study by Boyle, SAD was found in 15% of patients and was associated with allergic rhinitis [58]. SAD may also contribute to CRS. In a retrospective study by Carr, among 129 patients with CRS, SAD was found in 11.6% [55].

50.1.6 Congenital Defects of Phagocyte

Phagocytes are part of the innate immune system and not only fight invading pathogens, but are also necessary for wound healing. Monogenic defects has been described that impair phagocyte number and/or function. Increased susceptibility to severe bacterial and fungal infections is a common feature of these defects. Typical sites of infection include the skin, lymph nodes, gums, lungs, and other internal organs. Patients with phagocytic defects are also susceptible to recurrent AOM [59].

Chronic granulomatous disease (CGD) is characterized by defective nicotinamide adenine dinucleotide phosphate oxidase (NADPH) enzyme system. The formation of reactive oxygen intermediates are required for the optimal killing of bacteria and fungi. Affected patients frequently show infections with catalase-positive microorganisms such as *Klebsiella pneumoniae*, *Staphylococcus aureus*, *Burkholderia cepacia*, *Salmonella* spp., Aspergillus, Nocardia, or Candida. In addition, CGD may also lead to granuloma formation by abnormal inflammatory responses. In a large cohort of CGD patients, AOM is the first symptom in 4.6% of patients, and AOM was the most common clinical manifestation in 21.6% of patients [60]. AOM may rarely occur in CGD patients with subsequent granulomatous complications. Chang et al. reported a child with CGD who underwent radical mastoidectomy due to granulation tissue on the tympanic membrane and oto mastoiditiss [61]. Sinusitis was documented in 1.2% of patients at initial presentation and was more common in X-linked CGD than in autosomal recessive forms (24% and

18.9%, respectively) [60]. External ear and mastoid infections can progress rapidly despite antibiotics, and surgery may be required. Granuloma formation as a hallmark of CGD is most commonly observed in the gastrointestinal tract and urinary system, but granulomas can also affect the head and neck and lead to severe obstruction. In most cases, aggressive treatment with antibiotics along with surgery may be required. Severe granulomas causing obstruction may respond to steroids [62].

In case of clinical suspicion, the nitroblue tetrazolium dye reduction (NBT) test is used as screening test for CGD. Flow-cytometry-based dihydrorhodamine (DHR) assay and genetic examination are required for the definitive diagnosis of patients [63].

Conventional treatment of CGD is based on prophylactic antibiotics and antifungals. Prophylaxis with trimethoprim-sulfamethoxazole and itraconazole reduces the frequency and severity of infections. IFN-γ prophylaxis may also be beneficial. The decision to use IFN-γ prophylaxis is made on a case-by-case basis and is particularly recommended in patients with increased infections. The only curative treatment for CGD is allogeneic HSCT and can reduce both inflammatory and infectious complications [63].

Another common congenital defect of phagocytes is leukocyte adhesion deficiencies (LAD). Severe bacterial and fungal infections, granulocytosis, and cord complications (delayed detachment or omphalitis) are the most common manifestations in LAD patients. In a comprehensive review of all published cases, the most common infections in 85 cases were respiratory (39%, including LRTIs), sepsis (29%), and otitis media (27%). The most common infections in 69 cases were periodontitis (52%), otitis media (36%), and sepsis (25%). Flow cytometry and genetic evaluation can aid in diagnosis and prognosis. The curative treatment for LAD-1 is allogeneic HSCT [64].

50.1.7 Complement Deficiencies

The complement system is an important component of the innate and adaptive immune defense against infections. Activation of the complement system can be mediated via the classical, lectin, and alternative pathways. The classical complement pathway includes C1, C2, C4, C3, while the alternative pathway includes C3, factor B, factor D and properdin. Complement defects in early stages can lead to severe bacterial infections [65].

Complement deficiencies comprise 5% of PIDs and are usually associated with severe bacterial infections such as meningitis and bacteremia, especially with *Neisseria* spp. or *Streptococcus pneumoniae* [66]. AOM has been described as a clinical manifestation in factor I, C4b, C7, C1r, and C2 deficiency [2]. Recently, a family with properdin deficiency was reported in which affected members had recurrent AOM due to *Neisseria meningitidis* [67].

Recurrent sinusitis has been associated with complement defects, particularly C2 deficiency [68]. In a recent study, CRS was more common in patients with C3, C4, and mannose-binding lectin (MBL) deficiency [69]. However, no correlation was found between the type of defect and severity CRS [70].

Diagnosis is based on classical (CH50) and alternative (AP50) hemolytic activity [71].

50.1.8 Combined Immunodeficiency

Combined immunodeficiencies (CIDs) are a group of monogenic IEIs with T and B cell defects that are associated with severe infections, lymphoproliferation, autoimmunity and malignancy. Severe combined immunodeficiencies (SCID) can lead to early death if left untreated. Patients with SCID are susceptible to a broad spectrum of microorganisms and opportunistic pathogens. These children often suffer from chronic diarrhea and failure to thrive besides infections [72].

Among CIDs, there is a group of disorders associated with syndromic features. In addition to immunologic abnormalities, patients may have skeletal, neurologic, or gastrointestinal dysfunction or development [73]. Respiratory infections such as AOM are an important cause of mortality and morbidity in these diseases. In one study, AOM was observed in 57.1% of patients with hyper-IgM syndrome and in 50% of patients with ataxia-telangiectasia syndrome [74]. Hyperimmunoglobulin M syndrome (HIGM) can be caused by either T or B cell defects and is characterized by recurrent infections, decreased IgG, IgA, and IgE serum levels despite normal or increased IgM. In another cohort, AOM was observed as the second respiratory manifestation (45.1%) in these patients, similar to previously reported rates [75, 76].

Hyper-IgE (HIES) is a syndrome with severe eczema, recurrent sinopulmonary and skin infections, and extremely high IgE associated with a high incidence of AOM; some patients develop complications such as mastoiditis and external otitis like the other PID patients. Most AD-HIES patients have a history of AOM [77]. In a cohort of Iranian HIES patients, 25.5% suffered from recurrent AOM [78]. In a French national study AD-HIES, the incidence was as high as 73% [79].

Combined immunodeficiencies may be associated with hearing loss, as in adenosine deaminase deficiency (ADA). Recurrent URTIs may occur in SCID patients but may be overlooked because of the severe pulmonary and gastrointestinal manifestations [80]. Patients with Wiskott–Aldrich syndrome (WAS) usually present with eczema, recurrent infections, and thrombocytopenia. Malignancies and autoimmune diseases are also expected in severe patients. The immunodeficiency underlying WAS affects both the humoral and cellular immune systems. The impaired antibody response makes them susceptible to infections with encapsulated bacteria. Middle ear infection is very common, along with other respiratory infections. Allergic manifestations can complicate the clinical picture with allergic rhinosinusitis and asthma [62].

The propensity for recurrent RTIs with encapsulated bacteria is also a common feature in patients with ataxia and telangiectasia (AT). AT is a syndromic CID, caused by DNA repair defects. Patients present with ataxia in early childhood, which is later followed by oculocutaneous telangiectasia. Cerebellar involvement is progressive and patients become wheelchair dependent over time. T-cell defects are associated with humoral immunodeficiency. Recurrent otitis and rhinosinusitis are common in AT patients. Due to the underlying DNA repair defect, patients are prone to develop malignancies [80].

DiGeorge syndrome (DGS) or velocardiofacial syndrome is described as an association of cardiac abnormalities, hypoparathyroidism, and a variable degree of T-cell deficiency secondary to impaired development of the thymus. Other comorbidities, such as gastroesophageal reflux and rhinitis, may also predispose 22q11.2DS patients to respiratory infections. In a large cohort, recurrent or chronic otitis media with effusion was observed in 32.5% of patients with DiGeorge syndrome [81].

Panhypogammaglobulinemia, elevated IgE levels, lymphopenia, and defective lymphocyte proliferation may be seen. The absence of a thymic shadow on X-ray is the warning sign of DiGeorge syndrome or the other SCIDs.

SCID is a medical emergency and must be treated immediately. Initial treatment includes infection therapy with antimicrobials and IgG replacement. Curative therapy is HSCT and should be performed as soon as possible. Outcomes are greatly improved by early intervention [72].

50.1.9 Management

In patients who do not respond to conventional treatments for upper respiratory tract infections, immunologic testing should be performed. As a first step, a complete blood count, Ig levels, and specific antibody responses should be examined. Lymphocyte phenotyping, including T-cell enumeration, and assessment of phagocyte function using oxidative burst testing can be reviewed as needed.

AOM in children is caused by both viral and bacterial respiratory pathogens. Viral pathogens commonly associated with AOM include adenovirus (AdV), respiratory syncytial virus (RSV), parainfluenza virus (PIV), coronavirus, rhinovirus (RV), influenza virus and enterovirus. AOM is caused by interactions between a previous viral infection and colonized bacteria in the nasopharynx. The most common bacteria causing AOM are *Streptococcus pneumoniae*, *Moraxella catarrhalis*, and *Haemophilus influenzae* found in 70% of bacterial culture tests [82].

Increased susceptibility to encapsulated bacteria is the most common clinical manifestation of PID, which is characterized by a predominant defect in the antibody and complement systems. Infections with catalase-positive microorganisms, atypical mycobacteria, or fungi indicate both phagocytic defects and combined immunodeficiencies. The pathogens associated with the immunodeficiencies are listed in Table 50.3 [6, 83]. Detection of respiratory viruses and bacteria in nasopharyngeal aspirates and middle ear fluid can aid in treatment, diagnostic algorithm, and laboratory testing for underlying immunodeficiencies [83].

Treatment of AOM in patients with underlying IEI is similar to other patients but should be more aggressive. These children are more likely to develop fulminant systemic infections than local infection due to their defective immune system and may need to be started on antibiotic therapy earlier. Cultures from myringotomies

Table 50.3 Common pathogens according to the immune defects

Immunologic defect	Pathogens
Antibody deficiency	*Streptococcus pneumoniae, Haemophilus influenzae, Moraxella catarrhalis, Staphylococcus aureus, Bordetella pertussis, Pseudomonas aeruginosa,* Mycoplasma, Chlamydophila Rhinovirus, Herpes simplex virus, Cytomegalovirus
T and B cell immunodeficiencies	*Streptococcus pneumoniae, Staphylococcus aureus, Haemophilus influenzae*, and *Moraxella catarrhalis* RSV, Adenovirus, Parainfluenza 3, paramyxovirus, Cytomegalovirus *Pseudomonas aeruginosa, Pneumocystis jiroveci* Atypical mycobacteria, BCG Aspergillus, Scedosporium, Candida, Histoplasma, Cryptococcus
Phagocytic defects	Staphylococcus, Burkholderia, Pseudomonas, Serratia Aspergillus, Nocardia, Candida Atypical mycobacteria, BCG
Complement immunodeficiencies	*Neisseria* spp., *Streptococcus pneumoniae*

may be helpful in identifying the organisms and selecting the antibiotic. Consultation with an otolaryngologist may be required in case of severe complications including mastoiditis, and also for the insertion of ventilation tube [2].

A metaanalysis found that antibiotic prophylaxis in children prone to otitis media reduced the incidence of AOM episodes per year from about three to about 1.55 [84]. However, this positive effect of prophylactic antibiotics was also accompanied by antibiotic resistance and drug-related side effects. Some studies showed variable benefit of prophylactic antibiotics in preventing OM. Consequently, further studies could provide evidence on the efficacy of antibiotic prophylaxis in recurrent AOM [85].

Chronic rhinosinusitis should be treated aggressively in PIDs, including prophylactic antibiotics, culture-guided antimicrobial treatment, and IgRT if indicated. Allergic manifestations are not uncommon in PIDs and should be investigated if CRS. Endoscopic sinus surgery (ESS) may be a treatment option for recurrent CRS. Khalid et al. found similar postoperative outcomes in terms of quality of life and endoscopic improvement compared with immunocompetent patients [86].

50.2 Congenital Malformations

Congenital malformations are structural abnormalities present at birth which can affect various part of the body including upper respiratory tract. Although congenital malformations are not a defining characteristic of PIDs and are relatively rare within this context some of them are associated with PIDs due to the complex interactions between genetic factors affecting both the immune system and other developmental processes. Congenital malformations in ear, nose, and throat (ENT) region can contribute to an increased susceptibility to infections due to various factors related to the anatomy, immune function, and physiological processes of these structures [87].

The most common PIDs with congenital malformations of upper respiratory tract are DiGeorge syndrome (DGS) and CHARGE syndrome. These syndromes at two distinct genetic disorders that can both affect multiple systems in the body. Although both syndromes have a mutual clinical overlap, they are caused by different genetic mutations and have distinct sets of features [88]. DGS syndrome is caused by mutation in TBX1 gene (also known as T-box 1) located on chromosome 22q11.2. This gene plays a significant role in embryonic development and is associated with several genetic disorders. TBX1 gene encodes a transcription factor, which is a protein that helps regulate the expression of other genes during the development of various organs and tissues. Mutations, deletions, or variations in this gene are associated with a spectrum of developmental disorders, most notably DGS. CHARGE syndrome is caused by chromodomain helicase DNA-binding 7 (CHD7) gene mutations inherited in autosomal dominant manner [89]. The CHD7 gene is located on chromosome 8q12.1 and encodes a protein that functions as a chromatin remodeler. Chromatin remodeling is a process that affects how DNA is packaged within the nucleus of cells, thereby regulating gene expression and controlling the access of transcription factors to specific DNA sequences. The CHD7 protein is involved in controlling the structure and function of chromatin during embryonic development and plays a crucial role in the differentiation and development of various tissues and organs [89]. Although the interaction of CHD7 and TBX1 is not yet clear, the presence of a common embryonic pathway can explain the underlying pathogenesis of abnormal thymus development and the presence of T-cell deficiency in patients with thymic aplasia [90]. Except the DGS and CHARGE syndrome, Otofaciocervical Syndrome Type 2 (OSCF2) was recently described. Facial anomalies, hearing loss, branchial defects, skeletal anomalies, and mild mental retardation accompanies T-cell immunodeficiency due to abnormal thymic development with recurrent severe infections [91].

50.2.1 DiGeorge Syndrome (22q11.2 Deletion Syndrome)

DiGeorge Syndrome (DGS) is named after Dr. Angelo DiGeorge, who first described the disorder in the 1960s [92]. Its incidence is 1/4000 live newborns affecting both sexes [93]. DGS is a genetic disorder caused by the deletion of the 22q11.2 region on chromosome 22, which can be partial or nearly complete. The deletion, which involves a significant portion of genetic material in the 22q11.2 region, leads to a more severe and pronounced set of symptoms and features compared to partial deletions. This leads to a wide range of developmental and health issues, affecting various systems in the body. DGS is the most common of the other rare syndromes within the same chromosomal region.

This multisystem disorder is characterized by broad clinical variability where specific features and severity clinical phenotype can vary among individuals and can range from seemingly normal to significant features. Some individuals may exhibit more severe cardiac issues, while others might have more pronounced immune system dysfunction. Common features and symptoms associated with DGS include mainly cardiac anomalies, hypocalcemia, and thymic hypoplasia. Congenital heart defects including tetralogy of Fallot, aortic arch defects, truncus arteriosus, ventricular septal defect or patent ductus arteriosus occur in majority of DGS patients [94]. The parathyroid glands, which regulate calcium levels in the body, are often affected in DGS, leading to low blood calcium levels and related symptoms like muscle cramps and seizures [95]. Developmental and speech delay as well as learning deficits and differences in behavior are another common reason for ascertainment and diagnosis of DGS in childhood. On the other hand, psychiatric issues as anxiety, attention deficit, autism spectrum disorders, and schizophrenia are frequent in adult patients and it can later lead to the diagnosis of DGS [96]. Renal abnormalities, hypothyroidism, laryngo-tracheo-esophageal abnormalities, intrauterine growth retardation, vertebral abnormalities, polydactyly, scoliosis, hearing loss, microcephaly, or thrombocytopenia are less frequently seen in DGS [93].

Immune system abnormalities of DGS vary from milder immune system dysfunction due to partial thymus underdevelopment or dysfunction to profound immune deficiency, making individuals highly susceptible to severe and recurrent infections. Thymic hypoplasia results in a spectrum of T-cell deficiency, ranging from only a slight reduction in T-cell numbers without overt clinical immunodeficiency to patients suffering from a complete absence of thymic tissue associated with severe combined immunodeficiency which is life threatening if not corrected with thymic transplantation. Large survey from Europe of patients with DGS found an infection frequency of just 7% [97]. According to study of Jawad et al. 27% children with diagnosis of DGS had recurrent sinusitis, 25% had recurrent OM, 7% had recurrent bronchitis, and 4% had recurrent LRTIs [98].

In patients with thymic aplasia and missing T-cells, a suitable T-cell transfer from siblings or thymus transplantation is required [99]. Some patients with DGS may have milder antibody deficiencies [96], and immunoglobulin replacement therapy is required in more than 3% [100]. Prophylactic antibiotics are frequently used, although there are no reliable studies [96].

50.2.2 CHARGE Syndrome

CHARGE syndrome is a rare complex autosomal-dominant malformation syndrome comprised of congenital abnormalities that can affect multiple systems including central nervous system, eye, ear, nose, and mediastinal organs [101]. The estimated incidence of CHARGE syndrome ranges between 1/8500 and 1/12,000 newborns [102]. Designation "CHARGE" is an acronym for a syndrome comprised of ocular coloboma, heart defects, atresia of the choanae, retarded growth and development, genitourinary hypoplasia, and ear abnormalities [103]. Other systems may be compromised including the immune system. This genetic disorder is caused by loss-of-function mutation in the gene encoding chromodomain helicase DNA-binding 7 (CHD7), and 97% of CHD7 mutations are de novo [104]. This protein affects several signaling pathways and controls organ development. The minor and major criteria of CHARGE syndrome was first described by Blake et al. and then modified by Sanlaville et al. who emphasized the importance of coloboma, choanal atresia, and presence of abnormal semicircular canals [104, 105]. Abnormal facial features, orofacial clefts, limb anomalies, tracheoesophageal fistulas, and some degree of immune deficiency may also occur.

Coloboma and other ocular abnormalities (75–90%) and cardiac malformations (75–85%) are reported in the majority of patients [106, 107]. Genital hypoplasia (micropenis, cryptorchidism, and reduced clitoral size) is a further common feature of patients with CHARGE syndrome [108] and is thought to be secondary to hypogonadotropic hypogonadism. Although the majority of children with CHARGE syndrome have a normal birth weight and height, many of them show poor growth in late infancy [109]. Patients with CHARGE syndrome suffer from developmental delays (84%), mental retardation (64%), aggressive behaviour (48%), self-injurious behaviour (44%), and sleep disorders (45%) [110]. A meta-regression revealed significant associations between mental retardation and choanal atresia, mental retardation and inner ear anomalies, sleep disturbances and growth deficits, and sleep disturbances and gross motor difficulties [110]. ENT abnormalities are common features of CHARGE syndrome. Choanal atresia is the partial or complete blockage of the nasal passages at the back of the nasal cavity. Choanal stenosis refers to a narrowing of these passages. Both conditions can lead to breathing difficulties, feeding issues in newborns, and an increased susceptibility to upper respiratory infections. Choanal atresia was reported in 65% patients with CHARGE syndrome [109]. Airway obstruction below the choanae is present in 70% of patients, half of whom have multiple levels of obstruction. Laryngomalacia is found in 40% of patients, tracheomalacia in 20%, and subglottic stenosis in 10% [111]. Sensorineural hearing loss is also a common feature of CHARGE syndrome [112]. The hearing loss can range from mild to profound and can affect one or both ears. It may be due to structural abnormalities in the ear, such as malformation of the cochlea or the auditory nerve. Children with CHARGE syndrome are prone to recurrent ear infections, particularly otitis media. These infections can contribute to hearing loss. The patients can have also abnormalities of tympanic membrane. Patients with CHARGE syndrome can suffer from external and inner ear abnormalities. They might have malformed or absent external ears (microtia) or ear tags (preauricular tags). Malformations of the inner ear can contribute to hearing loss and vestibular (balance) issues. Malformations of the facial nerve can lead to facial weakness or asymmetry. A cleft palate, a gap or opening in the roof of the mouth, can also occur. This can lead to feeding difficulties, speech problems, and an increased risk of ear infections. The severity and combination of ENT abnormalities can vary widely among individuals with CHARGE syndrome.

While the frequency and type of immunodeficiencies in 22q11.2 deletion have been well studied, the opposite is true for CHARGE syndrome. Manifestations of immunodeficiencies occurring in CHARGE syndrome are relatively new and originate from case reports and small case series [109]. The possible contribution of immunological abnormalities to these infections has not been systematically investigated. Many children with CHARGE syndrome have recurrent suppurative ear and chest infections, probably due to anatomical anomalies of the craniofacial region and upper respiratory tract, as well as cranial nerve problems leading to dysphagia and aspiration [113]. The immunodeficiency in CHARGE syndrome is largely due to an impairment of thymus development and thus of functional T-cell production. The severity of the immunodeficiency is related to the extent of thymic underdevelopment. The very rare complete thymic aplasia leads to a severe immunodeficiency with complete or almost complete absence of T-cells and abnormal B-cell function with associated hypogammaglobulinemia requiring immune reconstitution. Partial thymic aplasia may lead to a reduction in T-cells with no clinical consequences, or to a more severe reduction in T-cells with associated impairment of B cell function, leading to recurrent infections requiring prophylactic antibiotics and/or immunoglobulin infusions. Pure B-cell or antibody defects are rarely described in CHARGE syndrome [114].

Due to the potential impact on hearing, speech, breathing, and overall quality of life, early and comprehensive evaluation by a team of medical professionals, including otolaryngologists, audiologists, immunologists and geneticists, is crucial for accurate diagnosis and appropriate management of individuals with CHARGE syndrome.

50.2.3 Autosomal Recessive Otofaciocervical Syndrome Type 2 (OTFCS2)

First cases of otofaciocervical syndrome (OTFCS) were described in 1967 [115]. The characteristics originally described included a short stature, a long face with a broad forehead, a narrow nose and lower jaw, sunken nasal roots, a high arched palate, protruding ears with large auricles and preauricular fistulae. Some family members also had lateral cervical fistulae, a long neck with drooping shoulders and collarbones and winged scapulae. They had bilateral conductive hearing loss and mild mental retardation [116]. Both autosomal dominant (OTFCS1) and autosomal recessive (OTFCS2) forms are reported. Originally described autosomal dominant OTFCS1 syndrome has been found to be due to EYA1 variants [117]. Later described OTFCS2 syndrome with associated T-cell deficiency has been found to be due to biallelic variants in PAX1 [118].

The PAX1 protein belongs to the PAX transcription factor family (paired box) and plays a role during embryogenesis in the patterning of the pharyngeal endoderm, from which the thymus, tonsils, parathyroid glands, thyroid gland and middle ear emerge [119]. Descriptions of PAX1-associated otofaciocervical syndrome (OTFCS2) remain limited as only thirteen cases from five consanguineous families have been documented to date, most of which have had a poor outcome due to associated immunodeficiency [116]. OTFCS2 is characterized by facial dysmorphism, anomalies of the auricles, hearing loss, branchial cysts or fistulas, anomalies of the shoulder girdle and mild mental retardation. PAX1 mutations with loss of function have been identified as the cause of a syndromic form of SCID that is due to impaired thymus development [120].

50.3 Adenoid Hypertrophy

The adenoid is a lymphoid tissue, and located in the posterior wall of the nasopharyngeal tip and contributes to Waldeyer's ring. It plays an important role in the first line of defense as an immune barrier in the digestive and respiratory tract [121]. Tonsillar and adenoid hypertrophy is a common manifestation of some PID groups, especially those associated with lymphoproliferation which may be oligoclonal, polyclonal, or monoclonal origin [122].

In a cohort of patients with activated phosphoinositide 3-kinase d syndrome 2 (APDS2), three (11 %) patients were found to have chronic lymphoid hyperplasia without the need for surgical intervention, seven (26 %) patients had adenoidectomy, tonsillectomy, or both, and three patients had multiple surgical resections. For example, one six-year-old patient required multiple surgical procedures, including multiple adenoidectomies and tonsillectomies, and developed postoperative pharyngeal stenosis requiring tracheostomy [123]. CD25 deficiency is also a rare CID, associated with lymphoproliferation. Caudy et al. reported on a boy diagnosed with CD25 deficiency who developed diffuse eczema, systemic lymphadenopathy, hepatosplenomegaly, enlarged tonsils and symptoms of sleep apnea requiring tonsillectomy and adenoidectomy [124].

Adenoid hypertrophy (AH) is the leading cause of upper airway obstruction and can cause mouth breathing, speech problems, and obstructive sleep apnea in children and adolescents. Nasal endoscopy is the current diagnostic tool with a comprehensive clinical evaluation in the diagnosis of AH. Adenoid-related airway obstruction is graded by an experienced otolaryngologist using various scales. Adenoidectomy is the standard treatment for moderate to severe adenoid hypertrophy, although pain, bleeding and anesthetic complications can occur. The development of respiratory, allergic, and infectious diseases in adulthood is also possible [121, 125]. Drug treatment with rapamycin has been used to treat benign lymphoproliferative disorders in some groups of PIDs, but no respiratory-specific results have been published. In the study of the selective PI3Kδ inhibitor leniolisib in patients with APDS1, no respiratory outcomes were reported either, but improvements in lymphoproliferation were reported [126].

50.4 Allergic Manifestations

Allergic manifestation in the ENT region encompasses a range of allergic conditions, affecting the upper respiratory tract, including mainly allergic rhinitis, sinusitis, and related symptoms. Atopy in the setting of immunodeficiency can be common but is often overlooked [127]. Although allergic diseases have long been observed in patients with IEI, the prevalence has not been thoroughly investigated [128]. According to a worldwide study focused on allergic manifestation in patients with IEI, it seems that allergic diseases are most commonly seen in patients with primary antibody deficiencies (PAD; 25%) and combined immunodeficiencies (CID; 20%) [128]. Furthermore, the most common occurrence of allergic diseases was in patients with selective IgA deficiency (53.6%) from PAD group and patients with HIES (43%) and WAS (38%) from CID group [128]. In patients with immune dysregulation and congenital phagocytic defects, allergy was less frequent with a frequency of 14% (0–33.8%) and 9% (0–20%), respectively [128]. According to the USIDNET dataset, which includes 2332 patients, 68.8% of IEI patients had concomitant allergic diseases, primarily bronchial asthma in 46.9%, followed by atopic dermatitis in 23.7% and allergic rhinitis in 8.2% [128]. According to data from 8450 IEI patients, allergic diseases occurred in 16.3% (10–28.8%) of patients during the course of their IEI, as follows: 3.6% (1.3–11.3%) had bronchial asthma, 3.6% (1.9–9.1%) atopic dermatitis, 3.0% (1.0–7.8%) allergic rhinitis and 1.3% (0.5–3.3%) food allergy [128]. Estimates of prevalence of allergic rhinitis vary enormously worldwide. For example, the affected population of adults is estimated to be 23–30% in Europe, 12–30% in the USA and 26% in the UK [129]. According to these data, it seems that allergic rhinitis is occuring but not dominant clinical manifestation of allergy in patients with IEI.

Increased serum concentration or number of humoral or cellular components of immune system related to type I hypersensitivity in patients with inborn errors of immunity may mean a true allergy or it may only reflect the activation of Th2 mechanisms due to different defects in the immune system pathways [130]. Misdiagnosis of inborn errors of immunity as allergy is well described and may be complicated by cooccurrence of allergy as a clinical manifestation [131]. The term "primary atopic disorders" was proposed to classify heritable genetic disorders that are associated with deregulated pathogenic allergic effector responses independent of sensitization [132]. These include genetic disorders leading to abnormal mast cell degranulation, chronic Th2 and eosinophil-mediated allergic inflammation and excessive IgE production [132]. These congenital defects of immunity manifest themselves in various types of allergies (urticaria, food allergy, asthma, and atopic dermatitis) or eosinophilia and elevated serum IgE [133]. For example elevated serum levels of IgE and eosinophilia is associated with autosomal dominant STAT3 loss of function hyper IgE syndrome (AD STAT3-HIES; Job's syndrome) and defects in STAT3 pathway, clinical manifestation of atopy (atopic dermatitis, asthma, food allergy or anaphylaxis) with Wiskott-Aldrich syndrome (WAS) and defects in DOCK8, ARPC1B, CARMIL2, CARD9, CARD11, CARD14, MALT1, and PGM3, severe atopic dermatitis and/or erythroderma or ichtyosis with Omenn's syndrome, Comel-Netherton syndrome (CNS) and JAK1 gain of function mutation, urticaria, and anaphylaxis with STAT5b gain of function mutations and other nosological entities [130].

References

1. Kaur R, Morris M, Pichichero ME. Epidemiology of acute otitis media in the postpneumococcal conjugate vaccine era. Pediatrics. 2017;140(3):e20174067.
2. Wilson NW, Hogan MB. Otitis media as a presenting complaint in childhood immunodeficiency diseases. Curr Allergy Asthma Rep. 2008;8(6):519–24.
3. Lieberthal AS, Carroll AE, Chonmaitree T, Ganiats TG, Hoberman A, Jackson MA, et al. The diagnosis and management of acute otitis media. Pediatrics. 2013;131(3):e964–e99.

4. Arkwright PD, Gennery AR. Ten warning signs of primary immunodeficiency: a new paradigm is needed for the 21st century. Ann N Y Acad Sci. 2011;1238(1):7–14.
5. Jeffrey Modell Foundation, Educational Materials. https://info4pi.org/library/educational-materials/. Accessed 21 Aug 2023.
6. Bardou ML, Pontarolli D, Grumach AS. Otitis media and inborn errors of immunity. Curr Allergy Asthma Rep. 2020;20:1–5.
7. Pichichero ME. Ten year study of the stringently defined otitis prone child in Rochester, NY. Pediatr Infect Dis J. 2016;35(9):1033.
8. Urschel S. Otitis media in children with congenital immunodeficiencies. Curr Allergy Asthma Rep. 2010;10:425–33.
9. Peters AT, Spector S, Hsu J, Hamilos DL, Baroody FM, Chandra RK, et al. Diagnosis and management of rhinosinusitis: a practice parameter update. Ann Allergy Asthma Immunol. 2014;113(4):347–85.
10. Dass K, Peters AT. Diagnosis and management of rhinosinusitis: highlights from the 2015 practice parameter. Curr Allergy Asthma Rep. 2016;16:1–7.
11. Bousfiha A, Moundir A, Tangye SG, Picard C, Jeddane L, Al-Herz W, et al. The 2022 update of IUIS phenotypical classification for human inborn errors of immunity. J Clin Immunol. 2022;42(7):1508–20.
12. Sanchez LA, Maggadottir SM, Pantell MS, Lugar P, Rundles CC, Sullivan KE, et al. Two sides of the same coin: pediatric-onset and adult-onset common variable immune deficiency. J Clin Immunol. 2017;37:592–602.
13. Aldırmaz S, Yücel E, Kıykım A, Çokuğraş H, Akçakaya N, Camcıoğlu Y. Profile of the patients who present to immunology outpatient clinics because of frequent infections. Turk Arch Pediatr. 2014;49(3):210.
14. Thalhammer J, Kindle G, Nieters A, Rusch S, Seppänen MR, Fischer A, et al. Initial presenting manifestations in 16,486 patients with inborn errors of immunity include infections and noninfectious manifestations. J Allergy Clin Immunol. 2021;148(5):1332–41.
15. Schwitzguébel AJ-P, Jandus P, Lacroix J-S, Seebach JD, Harr T. Immunoglobulin deficiency in patients with chronic rhinosinusitis: systematic review of the literature and meta-analysis. J Allergy Clin Immunol. 2015;136(6):1523–31.
16. Picard C, Al-Herz W, Bousfiha A, Casanova J-L, Chatila T, Conley ME, et al. Primary immunodeficiency diseases: an update on the classification from the International Union of Immunological Societies Expert Committee for Primary Immunodeficiency 2015. J Clin Immunol. 2015;35:696–726.
17. Pan-Hammarström Q, Hammarström L. Antibody deficiency diseases. Eur J Immunol. 2008;38(2):327–33.
18. Woof JM, Kerr MA. The function of immunoglobulin A in immunity. J Pathol. 2006;208(2):270–82.
19. Moschese V, Chini L, Graziani S, Sgrulletti M, Gallo V, Di Matteo G, et al. Follow-up and outcome of symptomatic partial or absolute IgA deficiency in children. Eur J Pediatr. 2019;178:51–60.
20. Lougaris V, Sorlini A, Monfredini C, Ingrasciotta G, Caravaggio A, Lorenzini T, et al. Clinical and laboratory features of 184 Italian pediatric patients affected with selective IgA deficiency (SIgAD): a longitudinal single-center study. J Clin Immunol. 2019;39:470–5.
21. Perez EE, Orange JS, Bonilla F, Chinen J, Chinn IK, Dorsey M, et al. Update on the use of immunoglobulin in human disease: a review of evidence. J Allergy Clin Immunol. 2017;139(3):S1–S46.
22. Carbone J. Adverse reactions and pathogen safety of intravenous immunoglobulin. Curr Drug Saf. 2007;2(1):9–18.
23. Kuruvilla M, De la Morena MT. Antibiotic prophylaxis in primary immune deficiency disorders. J Allergy Clin Immunol. 2013;1(6):573–82.
24. Sánchez Montalvo A, Gohy S, Rombaux P, Pilette C, Hox V. The role of IgA in chronic upper airway disease: friend or foe? Front Allergy. 2022;3:26.

25. Kıykım AA, Topçuoğlu N, Külekçi G, Çokuğraş H, Akçakaya N, Camcıoğlu Y. Comparison of oral microflora in selective IgA deficiency and X linked agammaglobulinemia cases with control group. Turk Arch Pediatr. 2013;48(3):204–9.
26. Sánchez-Segura A, Antonio Brieva J, Rodríguez C. Regulation of immunoglobulin secretion by plasma cells infiltrating nasal polyps. Laryngosc. 2000;110(7):1183–8.
27. Ocampo CJ, Peters AT. Antibody deficiency in chronic rhinosinusitis: epidemiology and burden of illness. Am J Rhinol Allergy. 2013;27(1):34–8.
28. Veenhoven R, Rijkers G, Schilder A, Adelmeijer J, Uiterwaal C, Kuis W, et al. Immunoglobulins in otitis-prone children. Pediatr Res. 2004;55(1):159–62.
29. Abrahamian F, Agrawal S, Gupta S. Immunological and clinical profile of adult patients with selective immunoglobulin subclass deficiency: response to intravenous immunoglobulin therapy. Clin Exp Immunol. 2010;159(3):344–50.
30. Vanlerberghe L, Joniau S, Jorissen M. The prevalence of humoral immunodeficiency in refractory rhinosinusitis: a retrospective analysis. B ENT. 2006;4:161.
31. May A, Zielen S, Von Ilberg C, Weber A. Immunoglobulin deficiency and determination of pneumococcal antibody titers in patients with therapy-refractory recurrent rhinosinusitis. Eur Arch Oto-Rhino-Laryngol. 1999;256:445–9.
32. Fried AJ, Bonilla FA. Pathogenesis, diagnosis, and management of primary antibody deficiencies and infections. Clin Microbiol Rev. 2009;22(3):396–414.
33. Cunningham-Rundles C, Maglione PJ. Common variable immunodeficiency. J Allergy Clin Immunol. 2012;129(5):1425–6. e3
34. Bonilla FA, Barlan I, Chapel H, Costa-Carvalho BT, Cunningham-Rundles C, de la Morena MT, et al. International Consensus Document (ICON): common variable immunodeficiency disorders. J Allergy Clin Immunol. 2016;4(1):38–59.
35. Seidel MG, Kindle G, Gathmann B, Quinti I, Buckland M, van Montfrans J, et al. The European Society for Immunodeficiencies (ESID) registry working definitions for the clinical diagnosis of inborn errors of immunity. J Allergy Clin Immunol. 2019;7(6):1763–70.
36. Carrabba M, Salvi M, Baselli LA, Serafino S, Zarantonello M, Trombetta E, et al. Long-term follow-up in common variable immunodeficiency: the pediatric-onset and adult-onset landscape. Front Pediatr. 2023;11:1125994.
37. Janssen LM, van der Flier M, de Vries E. Lessons learned from the clinical presentation of common variable immunodeficiency disorders: a systematic review and meta-analysis. Front Immunol. 2021;12:620709.
38. Urschel S, Kayikci L, Wintergerst U, Notheis G, Jansson A, Belohradsky BH. Common variable immunodeficiency disorders in children: delayed diagnosis despite typical clinical presentation. J Pediatr. 2009;154(6):888–94.
39. Cunningham-Rundles C, Bodian C. Common variable immunodeficiency: clinical and immunological features of 248 patients. Clin Immunol. 1999;92(1):34–48.
40. Sogkas G, Dubrowinskaja N, Schütz K, Steinbrück L, Götting J, Schwerk N, et al. Diagnostic yield and therapeutic consequences of targeted next-generation sequencing in sporadic primary immunodeficiency. Int Arch Allergy Immunol. 2022;183(3):337–49.
41. Demirdag YY, Gupta S. Update on infections in primary antibody deficiencies. Front Immunol. 2021;12:634181.
42. Stevens WW, Peters AT. Immunodeficiency in chronic sinusitis: recognition and treatment. Am J Rhinol Allergy. 2015;29(2):115–8.
43. Oksenhendler E, Gérard L, Fieschi C, Malphettes M, Mouillot G, Jaussaud R, et al. Infections in 252 patients with common variable immunodeficiency. Clin Infect Dis. 2008;46(10):1547–54.
44. Karadeniz EB, Aliyeva C, Aydemir S, Karaaslan BG, Mustu U, Ada M, et al. Chronic rhinosinusitis in patients with primary immunodeficiency. Int Arch Allergy Immunol. 2023;184(3):302–10.
45. Bondioni MP, Duse M, Plebani A, Soresina A, Notarangelo LD, Berlucchi M, et al. Pulmonary and sinusal changes in 45 patients with primary immunodeficiencies: computed tomography evaluation. J Comput Assist Tomogr. 2007;31(4):620–8.

46. Odat H, Alqudah M. Prevalence and pattern of humoral immunodeficiency in chronic refractory sinusitis. Eur Arch Oto-Rhino-Laryngol. 2016;273:3189–93.
47. Quinti I, Soresina A, Spadaro G, Martino S, Donnanno S, Agostini C, et al. Long-term follow-up and outcome of a large cohort of patients with common variable immunodeficiency. J Clin Immunol. 2007;27:308–16.
48. Ballow M. Optimizing immunoglobulin treatment for patients with primary immunodeficiency disease to prevent pneumonia and infection incidence: review of the current data. Ann Allergy Asthma Immunol. 2013;111(6):S2–5.
49. Ochs HD, Smith CE. X-linked agammaglobulinemia a clinical and molecular analysis. Medicine. 1996;75(6):287–99.
50. Maas A, Hendriks RW. Role of Bruton's tyrosine kinase in B cell development. J Immunol Res. 2001;8:171–81.
51. El-Sayed ZA, Abramova I, Aldave JC, Al-Herz W, Bezrodnik L, Boukari R, et al. X-linked agammaglobulinemia (XLA): phenotype, diagnosis, and therapeutic challenges around the world. World Allergy Organ J. 2019;12(3):100018.
52. Boisson B, Wang Y-D, Bosompem A, Ma CS, Lim A, Kochetkov T, et al. A recurrent dominant negative E47 mutation causes agammaglobulinemia and BCR-B cells. J Clin Investig. 2013;123(11):4781–5.
53. Plebani A, Soresina A, Rondelli R, Amato GM, Azzari C, Cardinale F, et al. Clinical, immunological, and molecular analysis in a large cohort of patients with X-linked agammaglobulinemia: an Italian multicenter study. Clin Immunol. 2002;104(3):221–30.
54. Hernandez-Trujillo V, Zhou C, Scalchunes C, Ochs HD, Sullivan KE, Cunningham-Rundles C, et al. A registry study of 240 patients with X-linked agammaglobulinemia living in the USA. J Clin Immunol. 2023;43:1468.
55. Carr TF, Koterba AP, Chandra R, Grammer LC, Conley DB, Harris KE, et al. Characterization of specific antibody deficiency in adults with medically refractory chronic rhinosinusitis. Am J Rhinol Allergy. 2011;25(4):241–4.
56. Bonilla FA, Bernstein IL, Khan DA, Ballas ZK, Chinen J, Frank MM, et al. Practice parameter for the diagnosis and management of primary immunodeficiency. Ann Allergy Asthma Immunol. 2005;94(5):S1–S63.
57. Misbah S, Griffiths H, Mitchell T, Freeland A, Haeney M, Chapel H. Antipolysaccharide antibodies in 450 children with otitis media. Clin Exp Immunol. 1997;109(1):67–72.
58. Boyle R, Le C, Balloch A, Tang ML. The clinical syndrome of specific antibody deficiency in children. Clin Exp Immunol. 2006;146(3):486–92.
59. Bogaert DJ, Haerynck F. Congenital defects of phagocytes. In: Cellular primary immunodeficiencies. Springer; 2021. p. 97–176.
60. Abd Elaziz D, El Hawary R, Meshaal S, Alkady R, Lotfy S, Eldash A, et al. Chronic granulomatous disease: a cohort of 173 patients—10-years single center experience from Egypt. J Clin Immunol. 2023;43(8):1799–811.
61. Chang SW, Kang HS, Song CI. Mastoidectomy in a child with chronic granulomatous disease. Br J Hosp Med. 2017;78(10):586–7.
62. Sikora AG, Lee KC. Otolaryngologic manifestations of immunodeficiency. Otolaryngol Clin N Am. 2003;36(4):647–72.
63. Arnold DE, Heimall JR. A review of chronic granulomatous disease. Adv Ther. 2017;34:2543–57.
64. Novoa EA, Kasbekar S, Thrasher AJ, Kohn DB, Sevilla J, Nguyen T, et al. Leukocyte adhesion deficiency-I: a comprehensive review of all published cases. J Allergy Clin Immunol. 2018;6(4):1418–20. e10
65. Tong HH, Li YX, Stahl GL, Thurman JM. Enhanced susceptibility to acute pneumococcal otitis media in mice deficient in complement C1qa, factor B, and factor B/C2. Infect Immun. 2010;78(3):976–83.
66. El Sissy C, Rosain J, Vieira-Martins P, Bordereau P, Gruber A, Devriese M, et al. Clinical and genetic spectrum of a large cohort with total and sub-total complement deficiencies. Front Immunol. 2019;10:1936.

67. Schejbel L, Rosenfeldt V, Marquart H, Valerius NH, Garred P. Properdin deficiency associated with recurrent otitis media and pneumonia, and identification of male carrier with Klinefelter syndrome. Clin Immunol. 2009;131(3):456–62.
68. Jönsson G, Truedsson L, Sturfelt G, Oxelius V-A, Braconier JH, Sjöholm AG. Hereditary C2 deficiency in Sweden: frequent occurrence of invasive infection, atherosclerosis, and rheumatic disease. Medicine. 2005;84(1):23–34.
69. Cui Y-H, Zhang F, Xiong Z-G, You X-J, Gao Q-X, Liu Z. Increased serum complement component 3 and mannose-binding lectin levels in adult Chinese patients with chronic rhinosinusitis. Rhinology. 2009;47(2):187.
70. Seppänen M, Suvilehto J, Lokki M-L, Notkola I-L, Järvinen A, Jarva H, et al. Immunoglobulins and complement factor C4 in adult rhinosinusitis. Clin Exp Immunol. 2006;145(2):219–27.
71. Brodszki N, Frazer-Abel A, Grumach AS, Kirschfink M, Litzman J, Perez E, et al. European society for immunodeficiencies (ESID) and European reference network on rare primary immunodeficiency, autoinflammatory and autoimmune diseases (ERN RITA) complement guideline: deficiencies, diagnosis, and management. J Clin Immunol. 2020;40:576–91.
72. Bonilla FA, Khan DA, Ballas ZK, Chinen J, Frank MM, Hsu JT, et al. Practice parameter for the diagnosis and management of primary immunodeficiency. J Allergy Clin Immunol. 2015;136(5):1186–205. e78
73. Tangye SG, Al-Herz W, Bousfiha A, Cunningham-Rundles C, Franco JL, Holland SM, et al. Human inborn errors of immunity: 2022 update on the classification from the international union of immunological societies expert committee. J Clin Immunol. 2022;42(7):1473–507.
74. Bazregari S, Azizi G, Tavakol M, Asgardoon MH, Kiaee F, Tavakolinia N, et al. Evaluation of infectious and non-infectious complications in patients with primary immunodeficiency. Cent Eur J Immunol. 2017;42(4):336–41.
75. Moazzami B, Yazdani R, Azizi G, Kiaei F, Tafakori M, Modaresi M, et al. Respiratory complications in patients with hyper IgM syndrome. J Clin Immunol. 2019;39:557–68.
76. Leven EA, Maffucci P, Ochs HD, Scholl PR, Buckley RH, Fuleihan RL, et al. Hyper IgM syndrome: a report from the USIDNET registry. J Clin Immunol. 2016;36:490–501.
77. Wu J, Hong L, Chen T-X. Clinical manifestation of hyper IgE syndrome including otitis media. Curr Allergy Asthma Rep. 2018;18:1–7.
78. Tavassoli M, Abolhassani H, Yazdani R, Ghadami M, Azizi G, Abdolrahim Poor Heravi S, et al. The first cohort of Iranian patients with hyper immunoglobulin E syndrome: a long-term follow-up and genetic analysis. Pediatr Allergy Immunol. 2019;30(4):469–78.
79. Chandesris M-O, Melki I, Natividad A, Puel A, Fieschi C, Yun L, et al. Autosomal dominant STAT3 deficiency and hyper-IgE syndrome molecular, cellular, and clinical features from a French National Survey. Medicine. 2012;91(4):e1.
80. Mohammadi F, Yadegar A, Mardani M, Ayati A, Abolhassani H, Rezaei N. Organ-based clues for diagnosis of inborn errors of immunity: a practical guide for clinicians. Immun Inflamm Dis. 2023;11(4):e833.
81. Giardino G, Radwan N, Koletsi P, Morrogh DM, Adams S, Ip W, et al. Clinical and immunological features in a cohort of patients with partial DiGeorge syndrome followed at a single center. Blood. 2019;133(24):2586–96.
82. Sawada S, Okutani F, Kobayashi T. Comprehensive detection of respiratory bacterial and viral pathogens in the middle ear fluid and nasopharynx of pediatric patients with acute otitis media. Pediatr Infect Dis J. 2019;38(12):1199–203.
83. Yamanaka N, Hotomi M, Billal DS. Clinical bacteriology and immunology in acute otitis media in children. J Infect Chemother. 2008;14(3):180–7.
84. Leach AJ, Morris PS. Antibiotics for the prevention of acute and chronic suppurative otitis media in children. Cochrane Database Syst Rev. 2006;4:CD004401.
85. Ballow M, Paris K, de la Morena M. Should antibiotic prophylaxis be routinely used in patients with antibody-mediated primary immunodeficiency? J Allergy Clin Immunol. 2018;6(2):421–6.
86. Khalid AN, Mace JC, Smith TL. Outcomes of sinus surgery in ambulatory patients with immune dysfunction. Am J Rhinol Allergy. 2010;24(3):230–3.

87. Daniel SJ. The upper airway: congenital malformations. Paediatr Respir Rev. 2006;7(Suppl 1):S260–3.
88. Uchiyama T, Kawakami S, Masuda H, Yoshida K, Niizeki H, Mochizuki E, et al. A distinct feature of T cell subpopulations in a patient with CHARGE syndrome and Omenn syndrome. J Clin Immunol. 2021;41(1):233–7.
89. Janssen N, Bergman JE, Swertz MA, Tranebjaerg L, Lodahl M, Schoots J, et al. Mutation update on the CHD7 gene involved in CHARGE syndrome. Hum Mutat. 2012;33(8):1149–60.
90. Randall V, McCue K, Roberts C, Kyriakopoulou V, Beddow S, Barrett AN, et al. Great vessel development requires biallelic expression of Chd7 and Tbx1 in pharyngeal ectoderm in mice. J Clin Invest. 2009;119(11):3301–10.
91. Paganini I, Sestini R, Capone GL, Putignano AL, Contini E, Giotti I, et al. A novel PAX1 null homozygous mutation in autosomal recessive otofaciocervical syndrome associated with severe combined immunodeficiency. Clin Genet. 2017;92(6):664–8.
92. Kirkpatrick JA, DiGeorge AM. Congenital absence of the thymus. Am J Roentgenol Radium Ther Nucl Med. 1968;103(1):32–7.
93. Cortés-Martín J, Peñuela NL, Sánchez-García JC, Montiel-Troya M, Díaz-Rodríguez L, Rodríguez-Blanque R. Deletion syndrome 22q11.2: a systematic review. Children (Basel). 2022;9(8):1168.
94. Butensky A, de Rinaldis CP, Patel S, Edman S, Bailey A, McGinn DE, et al. Cardiac evaluation of patients with 22q11.2 duplication syndrome. Am J Med Genet A. 2021;185(3):753–8.
95. Cheung EN, George SR, Costain GA, Andrade DM, Chow EW, Silversides CK, et al. Prevalence of hypocalcaemia and its associated features in 22q11.2 deletion syndrome. Clin Endocrinol (Oxf). 2014;81(2):190–6.
96. Sullivan KE. Chromosome 22q11.2 deletion syndrome and DiGeorge syndrome. Immunol Rev. 2019;287(1):186–201.
97. Ryan AK, Goodship JA, Wilson DI, Philip N, Levy A, Seidel H, et al. Spectrum of clinical features associated with interstitial chromosome 22q11 deletions: a European collaborative study. J Med Genet. 1997;34(10):798–804.
98. Jawad AF, McDonald-Mcginn DM, Zackai E, Sullivan KE. Immunologic features of chromosome 22q11.2 deletion syndrome (DiGeorge syndrome/velocardiofacial syndrome). J Pediatr. 2001;139(5):715–23.
99. Davies EG, Cheung M, Gilmour K, Maimaris J, Curry J, Furmanski A, et al. Thymus transplantation for complete DiGeorge syndrome: European experience. J Allergy Clin Immunol. 2017;140(6):1660–70.e16.
100. Patel K, Akhter J, Kobrynski L, Benjamin Gathmann MA, Davis O, Sullivan KE, et al. Immunoglobulin deficiencies: the B-lymphocyte side of DiGeorge syndrome. J Pediatr. 2012;161(5):950–3.
101. Vissers LE, van Ravenswaaij CM, Admiraal R, Hurst JA, de Vries BB, Janssen IM, et al. Mutations in a new member of the chromodomain gene family cause CHARGE syndrome. Nat Genet. 2004;36(9):955–7.
102. Aksel Kılıçarslan Ö, Ataman E, Gürsoy S, Hazan F, Randa C, Çankaya T, et al. Phenotypic spectrum of CHARGE syndrome based on clinical characteristics. Turk J Med Sci. 2018;48(5):911–5.
103. Pagon RA. Velo-cardio-facial syndrome vs. CHARGE "association". Am J Med Genet. 1987;28(3):751–8.
104. Sanlaville D, Verloes A. CHARGE syndrome: an update. Eur J Hum Genet. 2007;15(4):389–99.
105. Blake KD, Davenport SL, Hall BD, Hefner MA, Pagon RA, Williams MS, et al. CHARGE association: an update and review for the primary pediatrician. Clin Pediatr (Phila). 1998;37(3):159–73.
106. Russell-Eggitt IM, Blake KD, Taylor DS, Wyse RK. The eye in the CHARGE association. Br J Ophthalmol. 1990;74(7):421–6.
107. Blake KD, Prasad C. CHARGE syndrome. Orphanet J Rare Dis. 2006;1:34.
108. Wheeler PG, Quigley CA, Sadeghi-Nejad A, Weaver DD. Hypogonadism and CHARGE association. Am J Med Genet. 2000;94(3):228–31.

109. Hsu P, Ma A, Wilson M, Williams G, Curotta J, Munns CF, et al. CHARGE syndrome: a review. J Paediatr Child Health. 2014;50(7):504–11.
110. Thomas AT, Waite J, Williams CA, Kirk J, Oliver C, Richards C. Phenotypic characteristics and variability in CHARGE syndrome: a PRISMA compliant systematic review and meta-analysis. J Neurodev Disord. 2022;14(1):49.
111. Morgan D, Bailey M, Phelps P, Bellman S, Grace A, Wyse R. Ear–nose–throat abnormalities in the CHARGE association. Arch Otolaryngol Head Neck Surg. 1993;119(1):49–54.
112. Holcomb MA, Rumboldt Z, White DR. Cochlear nerve deficiency in children with CHARGE syndrome. Laryngoscope. 2013;123(3):793–6.
113. Wong MT, Lambeck AJ, van der Burg M, la Bastide-van GS, Hogendorf LA, van Ravenswaaij-Arts CM, et al. Immune dysfunction in children with CHARGE syndrome: a cross-sectional study. PLoS One. 2015;10(11):e0142350.
114. Mehr S, Hsu P, Campbell D. Immunodeficiency in CHARGE syndrome. Am J Med Genet C Semin Med Genet. 2017;175(4):516–23.
115. Fára M, Chlupácková V, Hrivnákova J. Familial oto-facio-cervical dysmorphia. Acta Chir Orthop Traumatol Cech. 1967;34(6):511–20.
116. Sherlaw-Sturrock C, Austin T, Baptista J, Gilmour K, Naik S. Dysmorphism and immunodeficiency—one of the differential diagnoses is PAX1 related otofaciocervical syndrome type 2. Eur J Med Genet. 2022;65(7):104523.
117. Rickard S, Parker M, van't Hoff W, Barnicoat A, Russell-Eggitt I, Winter RM, et al. Oto-facio-cervical (OFC) syndrome is a contiguous gene deletion syndrome involving EYA1: molecular analysis confirms allelism with BOR syndrome and further narrows the Duane syndrome critical region to 1 cM. Hum Genet. 2001;108(5):398–403.
118. Pohl E, Aykut A, Beleggia F, Karaca E, Durmaz B, Keupp K, et al. A hypofunctional PAX1 mutation causes autosomal recessively inherited otofaciocervical syndrome. Hum Genet. 2013;132(11):1311–20.
119. Wu W, Kong X, Jia Y, Ou W, Dai C, Li G, et al. An overview of PAX1: expression, function and regulation in development and diseases. Front Cell Dev Biol. 2022;10:1051102.
120. Yamazaki Y, Urrutia R, Franco LM, Giliani S, Zhang K, Alazami AM, et al. PAX1 is essential for development and function of the human thymus. Sci Immunol. 2020;5(44):eaax1036.
121. Pereira L, Monyror J, Almeida FT, Almeida FR, Guerra E, Flores-Mir C, et al. Prevalence of adenoid hypertrophy: a systematic review and meta-analysis. Sleep Med Rev. 2018;38:101–12.
122. Sharma S, Pilania RK, Anjani G, Sudhakar M, Arora K, Tyagi R, et al. Lymphoproliferation in inborn errors of immunity: the eye does not see what the mind does not know. Front Immunol. 2022;13:856601.
123. Elkaim E, Neven B, Bruneau J, Mitsui-Sekinaka K, Stanislas A, Heurtier L, et al. Clinical and immunologic phenotype associated with activated phosphoinositide 3-kinase δ syndrome 2: a cohort study. J Allergy Clin Immunol. 2016;138(1):210–8.
124. Caudy AA, Reddy ST, Chatila T, Atkinson JP, Verbsky JW. CD25 deficiency causes an immune dysregulation, polyendocrinopathy, enteropathy, X-linked-like syndrome, and defective IL-10 expression from CD4 lymphocytes. J Allergy Clin Immunol. 2007;119(2):482–7.
125. Byars SG, Stearns SC, Boomsma JJ. Association of long-term risk of respiratory, allergic, and infectious diseases with removal of adenoids and tonsils in childhood. JAMA Otolaryngol Head Neck Surg. 2018;144(7):594–603.
126. Condliffe AM, Chandra A. Respiratory manifestations of the activated phosphoinositide 3-kinase delta syndrome. Front Immunol. 2018;9:338.
127. Sokol K, Milner JD. The overlap between allergy and immunodeficiency. Curr Opin Pediatr. 2018;30(6):848–54.
128. El-Sayed ZA, El-Ghoneimy DH, Ortega-Martell JA, Radwan N, Aldave JC, Al-Herz W, et al. Allergic manifestations of inborn errors of immunity and their impact on the diagnosis: a worldwide study. World Allergy Organ J. 2022;15(6):100657.
129. Siddiqui ZA, Walker A, Pirwani MM, Tahiri M, Syed I. Allergic rhinitis: diagnosis and management. Br J Hosp Med (Lond). 2022;83(2):1–9.

130. Goudouris ES. Immunodeficiencies: non-infectious manifestations. J Pediatr (Rio J). 2021;97(Suppl 1):S24–33.
131. Ponsford MJ, Klocperk A, Pulvirenti F, Dalm VASH, Milota T, Cinetto F, et al. Hyper IgE in the allergy clinic—when is it primary immunodeficiency? Allergy. 2018;73(11):2122–36.
132. Lyons JJ, Milner JD. Primary atopic disorders. J Exp Med. 2018;215(4):1009–22.
133. Milner JD. Primary atopic disorders. Annu Rev Immunol. 2020;38:785–808.

Foreign Bodies in Children as A Cause of Upper and Lower Airways Infection

51

Melih Hangul, Mehmet Kose, and Hannah Blau

Foreign body aspiration (FBA) continues to be an important contributor to morbidity or mortality in children, attributable to both anatomical and developmental factors [1]. The term “choking” is commonly used to describe a situation where a foreign object in the airway causes partial or complete obstruction to the passage of air [2]. Obstruction can give rise to challenges in terms of ventilation and oxygenation, thereby leading to notable morbidity or mortality. Around 80% of incidents of pediatric FBA are observed in children below the age of three, with the highest incidence observed between the ages of 1 and 2 years [2–6]. During this developmental stage, the majority of children demonstrate the ability to achieve independent mobility, thereby enabling them to actively engage with their surroundings through oral exploration. Additionally, infants possess the requisite fine motor abilities to orally manipulate small objects. However, due to the absence of molars, their ability to effectively chew food is limited, potentially resulting in uncoordinated or underdeveloped swallowing processes [7]. There are other factors that can contribute to the occurrence of FBA in this particular age group. These factors include the availability of and access to inappropriate foods or small items, engaging in other activities while eating, and the presence of older siblings who may introduce food or objects into the mouths of infants or toddlers. Young children are also at a heightened risk of FBA due to the narrower diameter of their airway, which makes them more susceptible to obstruction [8, 9]. Frequently encountered FBA in children comprises a variety of substances, with peanuts accounting for a substantial

M. Hangul
Pediatric Pulmonology Department, Adana City Hospital, Adana, Turkey

M. Kose (✉)
Pediatric Pulmonology Department, Erciyes University of Medicine, Kayseri, Turkey
e-mail: dr.mkose@erciyes.edu.tr

H. Blau
Faculty of Medicine, Tel Aviv University, Tel Aviv, Israel

H. Yüksel et al. (eds.), *Pediatric Airway Diseases*, Comprehensive ENT,
https://doi.org/10.1007/978-3-031-74853-0_51

proportion (ranging from 36 to 55%) in Western societies. Additionally, various types of nuts, seeds (notably watermelon seeds in Middle Eastern nations), popcorn, food particles, hardware, and fragments of toys are commonly reported FBA in this population [2–6]. Infants and toddlers frequently aspirate food items, while older children tend to aspirate nonedible objects such as coins, paper clips, pins, and pen caps [10, 11]. Toy balloons, as well as other inflated objects such as gloves or condoms, have been identified as the primary items associated with fatal childhood FBA [8].

The bronchi are the primary site of aspiration for the majority of foreign bodies in children [6, 11, 12]. Foreign bodies in the larynx and trachea occur less frequently. In a comprehensive study examining over 1000 cases of foreign body aspirations in children, the locations where the foreign bodies were lodged were documented [1]. The distribution of foreign body locations was as follows: the larynx accounted for approximately 3%, the trachea and carina contributed to around 13%, the right lung comprised 60% (with 52% in the main bronchus, 6% in the lower lobe bronchus, and less than 1% in the middle lobe bronchus), the left lung constituted 23% (with 18% in the main bronchus and 5% in the lower bronchus), and both lungs together represented 2% [1, 12, 13].

When the diameter of the foreign object is bigger, there is an increased likelihood of obstruction occurring in the upper airways, specifically the larynx or trachea. Consequently, symptoms such as asphyxia become quickly apparent following inhalation. In such instances, prompt intervention with first aid techniques is imperative. In cases where the foreign object possesses a reduced diameter, there is an increased propensity for it to become lodged within the steeper segments of the bronchial tree. The most common clinical manifestations include coughing, localized wheezing, and diminished breath sounds in the affected area [14]. However, it is important to note that these symptoms are observed in less than 40% of children, indicating that the clinical findings have a low diagnostic sensitivity. Consequently, it is not possible to completely rule out FBA in asymptomatic individuals [15]. Clinical history is most important, when the incident is observed, and includes the triad of a sudden onset of choking or coughing, in a previously healthy child, with ongoing symptoms following the episode [16].

The manifestation of FBA is contingent upon several factors, including the extent of airway obstruction, the object's location, the child's age, the characteristics of the aspirated object (specifically, its size and composition), and the duration since the incident. Regrettably, delayed presentation is a prevalent occurrence, particularly when the incident was not observed. The occurrence of presentation and diagnosis within a 24-h timeframe following aspiration is observed in around 50–60% of cases, as reported in previous studies [7, 11]. It is advisable to maintain a heightened level of suspicion for FBA in order to prevent delayed diagnosis and the resulting morbidity [5].

Delayed diagnosis can result in patients presenting days or weeks after aspiration, leading to the development of symptoms caused by complications associated with the presence of FBA. These complications may include ***infection and inflammation*** of the airway. These complications occur in up to 16%, in those where diagnosis is delayed [16]. In these cases, the symptoms are typically moderate or imperceptible, and the foreign object has the potential to persist within the bronchial passages for extended durations, ranging from months to even years. The clinical symptoms, physical signs, and radiographic findings resulting from the presence of foreign bodies often lack specificity. Distinguishing this particular form of FBA from conditions such as lung infections, asthma, and congenital airway stenosis is a challenge, perhaps resulting in instances of undiagnosed or incorrectly diagnosed cases. The utilization of bronchoscopy is frequently necessary in order to identify the presence of foreign objects.

These particular instances are referred to as protracted, suspected, or occult foreign body aspiration [17]. Patients may have fever and clinical manifestations indicative of pneumonia. If the patient does not have a previous history of choking, then it is possible that FBA will not be suspected. Furthermore, patients presenting with occult FBA may improve clinically after the use of antibiotic medication. Nevertheless, the infiltrate observed on the chest radiograph typically does not disappear, and it is common for pneumonia to recur. The presence of asymptomatic or long-standing undetected FBA can lead to permanent consequences, including bronchiectasis, bronchopleural fistula, recurrent pneumonia, lung abscess, atelectasis, and potentially fatal outcomes [7, 17].

Children with lower airway FBA may present with subtle or nonspecific symptoms, and have a normal chest radiograph, which can delay the diagnosis. Radiological examinations may be used to corroborate aspiration, but not to rule it out. Therefore, they may not seek medical care until they develop dyspnea, wheezing, a chronic cough, or recurrent pneumonia [18]. Other contributors to diagnostic delay include unwitnessed aspiration, the decision by the parent/caregiver or clinician not to pursue evaluation once the acute choking episode has resolved, and the misinterpretation of symptoms as evidence supporting the diagnosis of de novo pneumonia, asthma, or asthma exacerbation, or bronchiolitis [7, 18]. According to a review of the systematic literature, the duration of occult foreign body retention ranges from 18.4 to 25.8 months [7]. A persistent foreign body in the bronchial tree causes irritation and inflammation, as well as the formation of obstructive granulation tissue. According to our observation, any delayed obstruction of the bronchus and atelectasis can damage the architecture of the lung and lead to bronchiectasis and complications such as hemoptysis, empyema, and recurrent pneumonia [19].

A 2-year-old female patient presented with a chronic cough and recurrent pneumonia. The symptoms started for the first time 6 months ago. Despite antibiotic treatment, the patient's complaints did not improve. She was referred to our chest disease clinic for further investigation and treatment. Figure 51.1 shows the chest X-ray, thorax tomography, and bronchoscopic findings of a patient with a delayed diagnosis of foreign name aspiration.

Saki et al. found that among 1015 patients who underwent bronchoscopy for suspected FBA, 73.03% presented with cough, 13.18% with cyanosis, 4.6% with dyspnea, 2.2% with wheezing, 1.73% with unresolved lung infections, 3.2% with coughing, and 0.89% with stridor, while 1.13% were asymptomatic [20]. This explains why FBA is frequently misdiagnosed. Karakoc et al. demonstrated that 32 of 654 patients who underwent bronchoscopy with an ambiguous respiratory

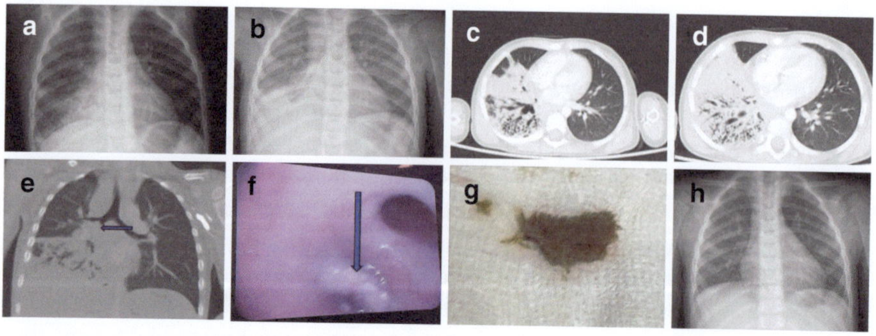

Fig. 51.1 (**a**) Chest X-ray when the patient's symptoms first started (6 months ago). (**b**) There is a chest X-ray finding that did not improve despite treatment (6 months later). (**c**, **d**) There was bronchiectatic change and consolidation area in the right middle and lower lobe. (**e**) The right intermediate bronchus was occluded. (**f**) Bronchoscopy shows that the right intermediate bronchus was occluded. (**g**) Image of the removed foreign body. (**h**) The chest radiograph 5 months after treatment

clinical picture had FBA and a prior misdiagnosis of bronchitis, pneumonia, tuberculosis, or croup [21].

In cases where the medical history lacks clarity and presents inconclusive evidence, it is imperative to exhaust all efforts in order to ascertain or eliminate the diagnosis. According to previous research [6], it has been observed that not all intrabronchial foreign entities exhibit radiopacity on chest X-rays. The prevailing observations mostly consist of radiological indicators associated with problems, including parenchyma pulmonary infiltrate, atelectasis, hyperinflation, and bronchiectasis [20].

In a study of 174 children with FBA, once again, the risk of long-term complications increased with delayed diagnosis. Bronchiectases were a major complication in 25% of those where diagnosis was delayed more than 30 days and three of these required lobectomy. Organic FBA was associated with an increased risk of persistent symptoms and bronchiectasis. Even after foreign body removal, some patients required ongoing bronchodilators, inhaled corticosteroids, airway clearance physiotherapy, and antibiotics [22].

The inclusion of FBA in the differential diagnosis of chronic or recurrent respiratory disorders is imperative, regardless of the absence of a prior choking incident. It is imperative to thoroughly assess clinical and radiological observations in order to consider the potential presence of a FBA. It is imperative to minimize any delays in the identification and treatment of FBA in order to mitigate the risk of potential consequences.

References

1. Eren S, Balci AE, Dikici B, et al. Foreign body aspiration in children: experience of 1160 cases. Ann Trop Paediatr. 2003;23:31.
2. Burton EM, Brick WG, Hall JD, et al. Tracheobronchial foreign body aspiration in children. S Med J. 1996;89:195.

3. Mu L, He P, Sun D. Inhalation of foreign bodies in Chinese children: a review of 400 cases. Laryngoscope. 1991;101:657.
4. Schmidt H, Manegold BC. Foreign body aspiration in children. Surg Endosc. 2000;14:644.
5. Altkorn R, Chen X, Milkovich S, et al. Fatal and non-fatal food injuries among children (aged 0–14 years). Int J Pediatr Otorhinolaryngol. 2008;72:1041.
6. Ciftci AO, Bingöl-Kologlu M, Senocak ME, et al. Bronchoscopy for evaluation of foreign body aspiration in children. J Pediatr Surg. 2003;38:1170.
7. Laya BF, Restrepo R, Lee EY. Practical imaging evaluation of foreign bodies in children: an update. Radiol Clin N Am. 2017;55:845.
8. Committee on Injury, Violence, and Poison Prevention. Prevention of choking among children. Pediatrics. 2010;125:601.
9. DeRowe A, Massick D, Beste DJ. Clinical characteristics of aero-digestive foreign bodies in neurologically impaired children. Int J Pediatr Otorhinolaryngol. 2002;62:243.
10. Rimell FL, Thome A Jr, Stool S, et al. Characteristics of objects that cause choking in children. JAMA. 1995;274:1763.
11. Fitzpatrick PC, Guarisco JL. Pediatric airway foreign bodies. J La State Med Soc. 1998;150:138.
12. Black RE, Johnson DG, Matlak ME. Bronchoscopic removal of aspirated foreign bodies in children. J Pediatr Surg. 1994;29:682.
13. Tan HK, Brown K, McGill T, et al. Airway foreign bodies (FB): a 10-year review. Int J Pediatr Otorhinolaryngol. 2000;56:91.
14. Sink JR, Kitsko DJ, Georg MW, Winger DG, Simons JP. Predictors of foreign body aspiration in children. Otolaryngol Head Neck Surg. 2016;155:501–7.
15. Janahi IA, Khan S, Chandra P, Al-Marri N, Saadoon A, Al-Naimi L, Al-Thani M, Greer W. A new clinical algorithm scoring for management of suspected foreign body aspiration in children. BMC Pulm Med. 2017;17:61.
16. Antón-Pacheco JL, Martín-Alelú R, López M, et al. Foreign body aspiration in children: treatment timing and related complications. Int J Pediatr Otorhinolaryngol. 2021;144:110690.
17. Liu B, Ding F, An Y, et al. Occult foreign body aspirations in pediatric patients: 20-years of experience. BMC Pulm Med. 2020;20(1):320.
18. Mu L, He P, Sun D. The causes and complications of late diagnosis of foreign body aspiration in children. Report of 210 cases. Arch Otolaryngol Head Neck Surg. 1991;117:876.
19. Razafimanjato NNM, Ralaivao RA, Ravelomihary TDN, Hunald FA, Rakotovao JLH. Pneumonectomy in a child due to belated diagnosis of foreign body aspiration: a case report. J Med Case Rep. 2021;15(1):533.
20. Saki N, Nikakhlagh S, Rahim F, Abshirini H. Foreign body aspirations in infancy: a 20-year experience 2009. Int J Med Sci. 2009;6:322–8.
21. Karakoc F, Cakir E, Ersu R, et al. Late diagnosis of foreign body aspiration in children with chronic respiratory symptoms. Int J Pediatr Otorhinolaryngol. 2007;71(2):241–6.
22. Karakoc F, Karadag B, Akbenlioglu C, et al. Foreign body aspiration: what is the outcome? Pediatr Pulmonol. 2002;34:30–6.

Part V

Infectious Diseases of the Pediatric Airway

Rhinosinusitis in Children

52

Bünyamin Kutlu, Cemal Cingi, and Glenis Scadding

52.1 Introduction

Primary care physicians and otolaryngologists frequently encounter pediatric rhinosinusitis. Even though this condition has been studied for centuries, we have recently begun to understand its entire nature, etiology, diagnosis, therapy, and complications. Acute rhinosinusitis can be successfully treated in children with short courses of antibiotic therapy following the common cold. However, intranasal corticosteroids are superior in those without severe pain and fever over 38 °C, with fewer adverse events, probably because most infections are viral rather than bacterial [1].

Chronic and recurring rhinosinusitis can be more challenging to treat, causing frustration for doctors and patients' loved ones. The doctor may also need to diagnose and treat any contributory underlying illnesses [2].

Treatment for these children entails a combination of therapy, not always antibiotics, and the management of any underlying problems until the symptoms subside and sinus physiology and mucociliary clearance return to normal. In this piece, we'll talk about how to treat pediatric rhinosinusitis medically.

B. Kutlu
Department of Otorhinplaryngology, Medicalpark Hospital, Trabzon, Türkiye

C. Cingi (✉)
Department of Otorhinolaryngology, Eskisehir Osmangazi University, Medical Faculty, Eskisehir, Turkey

G. Scadding
Consultant Allergist & Rhinologist, RNENT Hospital, University College Hospital, London, UK

H. Yüksel et al. (eds.), *Pediatric Airway Diseases*, Comprehensive ENT,
https://doi.org/10.1007/978-3-031-74853-0_52

52.2 Anatomy

Outgrowths of the nasal cavity give rise to the paranasal sinuses [1, 2]. Paranasal sinus development begins at different ages and lasts for other times in various anatomical areas. By age 12, the nasal cavities and paranasal sinuses have grown to almost adult size [3, 4].

The maxillary sinuses appear shortly after birth and develop rapidly by age four [3]. The ostia of the maxillary sinus are situated high on the medial walls. Therefore, ciliary action is required to outflow secretions into the nose.

The ethmoid sinuses are preexisting structures that consist of several small air cells, each with its passage leading into the nasal cavity [3].

By age five, the sphenoid sinuses have usually been pneumatized; by age 12, they have reached their final size [3].

The frontal sinuses do not constantly fully develop [2]. They are radiographically distinguishable from the ethmoid sinuses [4] by age 6–8 but do not finish development for another 8–10 years.

Frontal sinus agenesis affects 1–4% of adults; the remaining 80% have bilateral frontal sinuses, and the remaining 2% have unilateral frontal sinus hypoplasia [2].

52.3 Pathophysiology

The ostiomeatal complex (OMC) is present in all neonates, though not at full size. It is thought to be the critical anatomic structure in sinusitis. The uncinate process, infundibulum ethmoidalis, hiatus semilunaris, ethmoid bulla, and frontal recess comprise the ostia media and cauda, or OMC, located within the middle meatus. Changes in the anterior ethmoids hinder drainage through the OMC, leading to chronic maxillary sinusitis and, rarely, frontal sinusitis [5]. However, obstruction of the OMC has not been demonstrated to be the predominant etiology of pediatric sinusitis.

Inflammation of the mucosa can impede the normal metachronous flow of mucus toward the natural ostia of the sinuses and, ultimately, the nasopharynx. Common causes include viral URTIs, nasal allergies, and the immune response to these infections or allergens. Allergic rhinitis, structural abnormalities, gastroesophageal reflux (GER), immunological insufficiency, and problems of ciliary function are just a few of the many risk factors for developing a chronic illness [5].

Acute sinusitis has been linked to a decrease in the relative abundance of specific taxa in the nasopharyngeal microbiota, according to a prospective cohort research conducted by Santee et al. *Faecalibacterium prausnitzii* and Akkermansia species were considerably reduced in participants with a history of acute sinusitis, whereas the relative abundance of the bacterium *Moraxella nonliquefaciens* was enriched. The study comprised 47 healthy children aged 49–84 months. According to the researchers, children who acquired acute sinusitis over the study period of 1 year were likewise characterized by enrichment of *M. nonliquefaciens* [6].

52.4 Predisposing Factors

Acute bacterial rhinosinusitis (ABRS) is most commonly associated with a viral upper respiratory infection (URI) [7–9]. Children in daycare are likelier to get a viral URI [10]. The incidence of URIs was higher among children who developed ABRS (three per year vs. one per year) in a study of 237 children aged 48–96 months who were observed for a year. Sinusitis is a common complication of URIs, and respiratory syncytial virus has been found more frequently than other respiratory viruses in these cases. Separate sections are devoted to the epidemiology and clinical presentation of viral URI.

Allergic rhinitis is also a risk factor for ABRS [11–13].

Anatomic obstruction (for example, nasal septal abnormalities, craniofacial malformations, adenoidal hypertrophy, cysts of the maxillary antrum, or nasal foreign bodies, masses, or polyps) is a less prevalent risk factor for ABRS [2, 4].

Investigations for cystic fibrosis (CF) and allergy should be undertaken in children with nasal polyps [14].

52.5 Classification

52.5.1 Acute Sinusitis

- Acute sinusitis is suspected if URTI symptoms last longer than 10 days.
- A cough and runny nose during the day are the most typical manifestations.
- The following are some additional common symptoms:
  - Congestion in the nose
  - Otitis media (affecting 50–60% of patients) intermittent low-grade fever
  - Mood swings and pain in the head
- The following are some signs of a severe infection, more likely to be bacterial:
  - High fever (i.e., >39 °C)
  - Periorbital edema
  - Purulent rhinorrhea
- About 40% of those with uncomplicated sinusitis see their symptoms go away independently within 30 days [5].

Recurrent acute sinusitis occurs when the about lasts less than 30 days and is separated by symptom-free periods of at least 10 days [5].

Subacute sinusitis occurs with signs and symptoms lasting between 30 and 90 days [5].

Chronic sinusitis occurs when signs and symptoms remain for more than 90 days without resolution.

- There may be a history of acute exacerbations, with the patient never fully recovering in between.
- Coughing is more common at night [2].

52.6 Acute Bacterial Rhinosinusitis

52.6.1 Clinical Features

Acute bacterial rhinosinusitis (ABRS) in children has symptoms that overlap with those of viral upper respiratory infections (URTIs) [15]. Differentiating between simple viral URTI and ABRS depends on the clinical history, significantly the persistence and severity of symptoms [7, 16–18].

There needs to be more data connecting the microbiology of ABRS with its clinical manifestations. Children with straightforward ABRS are not typically subjected to the invasive process of sinus aspiration.

52.6.1.1 Cough

A dry or wet cough is a significant sign of ABRS. Eighteen percent [19] of the 30 children in observational research with culture-confirmed maxillary ABRS reported cough as their primary symptom.

More extended periods of illness are associated with a more severe cough [2]. While a cough is always present, many people say theirs is worse at night [16, 17]. Without other symptoms, a persistent cough at night is most likely due to postnasal drip or reactive airway disease [20].

52.6.1.2 Nasal Symptoms

ABRS nasal symptoms include nasal congestion, blockage, and discharge. Among 30 children with culture-confirmed maxillary ABRS, 23 reported nasal symptoms, with 10 reporting only nasal symptoms [18].

The consistency of the nasal discharge can vary widely. While posttussive emesis is more common, postnasal eruption can also trigger vomiting [4].

On examination, mild erythema and swelling of the nasal turbinates may be present, along with mucopurulent anterior nasal discharge. The purulent material in the posterior pharynx may originate in the drainage of the posterior ethmoids [4].

52.6.1.3 Fever

ABRS patients may also experience problems, some of which include fever. Fever was not a primary complaint among the 30 children in an observational study who had culture-confirmed maxillary ABRS [20].

The severe form of ABRS includes a temperature of 39 °C (102.2 °F) or below for at least 3 days. In cases of viral URI without complications, fever often develops in the first few days of the disease and subsides in 2 days [21].

52.6.1.4 Other Findings

Headaches and facial pain complaints are also not uniform; however, they are rare in young children [18, 22]. Migraine may occur, and irritability is common.

On examination, percussion of the upper molars, or percussion or direct pressure over the body of the frontal or maxillary sinuses [23, 24], can elicit sinus discomfort (rare in young infants). Otitis media occurs in 50% of ABRS, so the ears should be examined.

Although some children may complain of a sore throat or bad breath, these symptoms rarely prompt a visit to the doctor [4, 18].

52.6.2 Complications

Bacterial rhinosinusitis in children can have profound implications, such as orbital cellulitis and cerebral infection if left untreated. This is estimated to occur in around 5% of people admitted to the hospital with rhinosinusitis [19, 25].

52.6.3 Orbit-Related Complications

52.6.3.1 Cellulitis in the Preseptal (Periorbital) Space

One of the most prevalent side effects of ABRS is modest but serious preseptal cellulitis (inflammatory edema or sympathetic effusion). There is no proptosis or restriction of eye movement, but there is redness and swelling of the lids and periorbital area [26]. Preseptal cellulitis implies obstruction to venous flow, even if the infection is restricted to the sinuses (often the ethmoid sinuses). Presented cellulitis-complicating sinusitis is much more dangerous than uncomplicated sinusitis.

Orbital cellulitis, subperiosteal abscess, and orbital abscess [4] are all postsinusitis sequelae that can affect the orbit.

Postseptal complications of sinusitis share several diagnostic criteria and may include [24, 26–28]:

- Periorbital edema
- Eyelid edema
- Pain with blinking
- Swelling of the conjunctiva
- Proptosis
- Ophthalmoplegia (weakness of the eye muscles)
- Diplopia
- Vision loss

Imaging can assist in differentiating between subperiosteal abscess, orbital abscess, and orbital cellulitis when the above clinical symptoms suggest a postseptal consequence of ABRS [28, 29]. Computed tomography (CT) scans show subperiosteal and orbital abscesses as low-density collections. Location close to the ethmoid sinus is common. Subperiosteal abscesses may form between the periosteum and the bony sinus wall [4].

52.6.3.2 Orbital Subperiosteal Abscess

Postsinusitis complications in children often include orbital subperiosteal abscesses [29–34]. Orbital subperiosteal abscess was found in 9–23% of children with ABRS-related orbital sequelae in two single-institution, 10-year analyses [34, 35].

Subperiosteal abscesses in younger children typically develop medially in orbit [36], are surgically avoidable when slight or manifest as poorly organized phlegmons [36–38], and are colonized by a single aerobic species [38]. Older patients are more likely to need drainage for abscesses because they are more likely to include aerobic and anaerobic microorganisms [39, 40]. The risk of intracranial dissemination appears to be most significant for nonmedial abscesses in older children and superiorly situated abscesses (near the frontal sinus).

52.6.3.3 Orbital Abscess

Signs (proptosis, ophthalmoplegia) and symptoms (pain with eye movements) in patients with orbital abscesses are often more severe than in patients without them [35, 41].

Six (2%) of the 298 children who were brought to a pediatric emergency room and scanned with CT for acute periorbital (preseptal) or orbital cellulitis were found to have an orbital abscess [41]. An orbital abscess was linked to proptosis, pain with external ocular movement, and ophthalmoplegia, while 51% of patients with abscesses did not have these characteristics. On a multivariate analysis, the lack of conjunctivitis, periorbital edema, age greater than 3 years, and prior antibiotic medication were all risk factors for orbital abscess [4].

52.6.3.4 Intracranial Complications

Frontal and sphenoidal sinusitis are most likely to lead to intracranial complications, which may require surgical intervention and lead to permanent neurologic disability and rarely death. Headache is a prominent symptom in these patients [42, 43].

Findings that should prompt consideration of intracranial extension include [37, 44, 45]:

- The combination of eye swelling with persistent headache and vomiting
- Vomiting and headache that requires hospital admission, particularly in older children
- Vomiting that persists for more than 24 h
- Altered level of consciousness
- Focal neurologic deficits
- Signs of meningeal irritation (e.g., stiff neck)

Clinical manifestations specific to intracranial complications of rhinosinusitis are listed below [46–50]:

- Septic cavernous sinus thrombosis—Bilateral ptosis, proptosis, ophthalmoplegia, bilateral periorbital edema, headache, change in mental status.

- Meningitis—Fever, headache, nuchal rigidity, and change in mental status.
- Osteomyelitis of the frontal bone associated with a subperiosteal abscess (Pott puffy tumor)—Forehead or scalp swelling and tenderness, headache, photophobia, fever, vomiting, lethargy [51].
- Epidural abscess—Papilledema, focal neurologic signs, headache, lethargy, nausea, and vomiting.
- Subdural abscess—Fever, severe headache, meningeal irritation, progressive neurologic deficits, seizures, and signs of increased intracranial pressure (papilledema, vomiting) [3].
- Brain abscess—Headache, neck stiffness, changes in mental status, vomiting, focal neurologic deficits, seizures, third and sixth cranial nerve deficits, and papilledema [4].

52.6.4 Radiologic Features

CT findings that are compatible with sinus inflammation include [14, 52, 53]:

- Complete opacification
- Mucosal thickening of at least 4 mm
- Air-fluid level

However, abnormal imaging studies cannot distinguish between bacterial, viral, or other causes of sinus inflammation [16, 54]. Observational studies performed with radiographs, CT, and magnetic resonance imaging have demonstrated frequent abnormalities in the paranasal sinuses [55–58] and adults with uncomplicated viral upper respiratory infection [59].

52.7 Chronic Rhinosinusitis

Chronic rhinosinusitis (CRS) is a syndrome characterized by persistent inflammation of the mucosa of the nose and paranasal sinuses. In children, this results in the symptoms of chronic nasal congestion, purulent rhinorrhea, facial pain and pressure, and cough. The etiology and pathogenesis of this inflammation may represent an inappropriate or excessive immune response to an external stimulus inhaled through the nasal airway [60].

Pediatric CRS can be subclassified into CRS with or without nasal polyposis. In the Clinical Consensus Statement for pediatric CRS, there was a strong consensus that children who present with polyps represent a distinct patient subgroup compared to those without [4]. Patients with nasal polyposis are thought to constitute a different subtype of CRS with differing pathophysiology and optimal management. Specifically, these children carry an increased risk of underlying conditions such as cystic fibrosis, allergic fungal sinusitis, and antrochoanal polyps. An assessment of these conditions needs to be considered in their workup [60].

52.7.1 Pathophysiology of CRS

The path to developing bacterial rhinosinusitis usually begins with a viral respiratory infection with concomitant mucosal inflammation. This results in obstruction of the sinus ostia with impaired aeration of the sinuses decreased ciliary function, and stasis of secretions within the sinuses. These factors are believed to constitute the primary factors in sinus disease pathophysiology, leading to secondary infection by bacteria residing within the nose and nasopharynx [61, 62]. It has been estimated that 0.5–13% of children's upper respiratory infections (URIs) progress into bacterial rhinosinusitis [61, 63].

A multitude of factors exist that could lead to a predisposition for CRS. Anything that contributes to immune deficiency or obstruction of the sinus ostia would constitute such a factor. Extrinsic factors consist of nasal foreign bodies, including nasogastric and nasotracheal tubes. Other factors could exist that lead to a chronic inflammatory state and, therefore, cause inflamed sinonasal mucosa that then obstructs sinus flow; some examples include allergic rhinitis, allergic fungal sinusitis (a hypersensitivity reaction of the sinus mucosa to airborne fungal species in immunocompetent individuals), gastroesophageal reflux, and tobacco smoke [62, 64]. A recent systematic review noted inferior surgery outcomes for CRS among children exposed to second-hand smoke [65].

52.7.2 Microbiology

Viral upper respiratory tract infections frequently precede bacterial infections of the sinuses. The most common causal organisms of acute and subacute rhinosinusitis are *Streptococcus pneumoniae, Haemophilus influenza,* and *Moraxella catarrhalis* [66]. I*n* contrast, the most common bacteria found in CRS are alpha-hemolytic streptococci *and Staphylococcus aureus,* followed by *S. pneumoniae, H. influenza,* and *M. catarrhalis* [67]. Other common bacterial species include *Pseudomonas aeruginosa* and anaerobes [68]. *P. aeruginosa* and other aerobic Gram-negative rods are more common in sinusitis of nosocomial origin, immunocompromised individuals, or those with CF [60, 64].

The prevalence of penicillin-resistant organisms in rhinosinusitis can be significant. *S. pneumoniae* has geographic variation but is thought to have a 15–50% resistance rate to penicillin [66, 69]. Both *H. influenzae* and *M. catarrhalis* can produce β-lactamase and are resistant to penicillin and its derivatives. The prevalence of macrolide-resistant *S. pneumoniae* is 10–40% [60].

Fungi are increasingly being recognized as an etiologic factor in CRS. The most commonly involved pathogens are *Bipolaris, Curvularia, Aspergillus,* and *Dreschlera* species [60].

Biofilms and bacterial exotoxins have been implicated in the pathogenesis of CRS. Biofilms are bacteria aggregating on surfaces within an external polysaccharide, nucleic acids, and protein matrix. Biofilms provide a protected environment for pathogens and may be responsible for persistent or recurrent diseases. In CRS, biofilm formation may decrease the efficacy of antibiotics by as much as 100-fold, allowing bacteria to thrive in the nose and sinuses. Other studies have reported the presence of biofilms in adenoid tissue from patients with chronic infectious diseases of the upper airways [62]. Bacteria release exotoxins and may trigger a symptomatic immune response [60].

52.7.3 Clinical Presentation

Because the symptoms of pediatric CRS are more sluggish and nonspecific than an episode of ARS, it can be difficult to distinguish from recurrent viral upper respiratory infections, chronic allergic rhinitis, or chronic nasal congestion due to adenoid hypertrophy. Adenoid hypertrophy and adenoiditis are prominent contributors to the pathogenesis of CRS in young children and may not be possible to differentiate from CRS in this age group. As noted previously, the AAO-HNS Clinical Consensus Statement defined pediatric CRS as at least 90 continuous days of 2 or more symptoms of purulent rhinorrhea, nasal obstruction, facial pressure/pain, or cough. Chronic cough lasting more than 4 weeks, mainly if associated with rhinorrhea and nasal congestion, should prompt an evaluation for CRS. Unlike in adults, hyposmia and headache are less common in children, though there may be more significant irritability and behavioral changes. In addition, these symptoms should be accompanied by at least one objective sign from a nasal endoscopic exam (mucosal edema, purulent drainage from one or more sinuses, nasal polyposis). Abnormalities on a sinus CT can be used to back up a diagnosis of CRS, but alone cannot be diagnostic since CT sinus abnormalities are present in 45% of children due to frequent colds [60, 63].

52.7.4 Complications of CRS

Complications of CRS with or without nasal polyps are rare and less dramatic than those of ARS, such as subperiosteal abscess formation. They include bony erosion and expansion due to polyps or mucoceles, sclerosis due to chronic osteitis, and recurrent pulmonary exacerbations in the setting of asthma or cystic fibrosis. In addition, sleep has detrimental effects, leading to tiredness, poor concentration, irritability, and reduced attention/ performance in school [60].

Mucoceles are fluid-filled epithelial-lined sacs that are typically unilocular and slow-growing. They can eventually fill an entire sinus and cause expansion or erosion of the surrounding bone, particularly if an acute bacterial infection results in a pyocele. Mucoceles tend to be unilateral and occur most commonly in the fronto-ethmoid sinuses. The mass effect caused by a sizeable fronto-ethmoid mucocele can cause orbital displacement and proptosis. Fortunately, such mucoceles are rare in children and generally respond well with endoscopic marsupialization, with reported recurrence rates ranging from 0 to 13% [70, 71].

Chronic nasal polyposis can similarly exert a mass effect with thinning of bone, most often affecting the ethmoid sinuses and lamina papyracea. A condition that can often predispose to nasal polyposis in children is allergic fungal sinusitis (AFS). AFS is caused by a type I hypersensitivity to fungal pathogens, most commonly Bipolaris, Aspergillus, Alternaria, Curvularia, and Dreschslera species. It leads to a chronic eosinophilic infiltrate and inflammation of the sinus mucosa. This can often result in polyposis, unilateral sinus opacification, and expansion [72].

52.8 Diagnosis and Management of Rhinosinusitis

The diagnosis is usually made on the history, supported by endoscopic findings. Many children are catarrhal in early childhood, it is only those in whom the symptoms never abate that investigation is needed [73].

Laboratory tests can be essential in determining whether associated conditions such as allergic rhinitis, cystic fibrosis, or immunodeficiency are present. In addition, in patients with suppurative complications or a very toxic-appearing child, blood cultures may help determine treatment [5].

Computed tomography (CT) scanning is the criterion for evaluating mucosal inflammation and anatomic abnormalities in the paranasal sinuses. CT scanning provides a reliable picture of the ostiomeatal complex (OMC) in a noninvasive fashion [5]. It is rarely needed in uncomplicated CRS in children. Since an abnormal CT scan is found in many children due to frequent colds, it is not diagnostic alone and no treatment is necessary in an asymptomatic child [73].

Various procedures in patients' workups include the following [5]:

- Rigid or flexible nasal endoscopy—Provides an excellent view of OMC
- Middle meatal swab

Indications for antibiotic therapy for acute sinusitis are as follows: [5]

- Persistent acute sinusitis
- Severe acute sinusitis
- Toxic child with suspected complications

Surgical approaches include the following [5]: *surgery is very rarely necessary in children who tend to outgrow their CRS (EPOS 2020)* [74]

- Adenoidectomy
- Functional endoscopic sinus surgery
- Uncinate removal, anterior ethmoidectomy, and maxillary antrostomy
- Balloon sinuplasty

References

1. Meltzer EO, Bachert C, Staudinger H. Treating acute rhinosinusitis: comparing efficacy and safety of mometasone furoate nasal spray, amoxicillin, and placebo. J Allergy Clin Immunol. 2005;116(6):1289–95.
2. Cherry JD, Kuan EC, Shapiro NL. Rhinosinusitis. In: Cherry JD, Harrison G, Kaplan SL, et al., editors. Feigin and Cherry's textbook of pediatric infectious diseases. 8th ed. Philadelphia: Elsevier; 2018. p. 137.
3. Wolf G, Anderhuber W, Kuhn F. Development of the paranasal sinuses in children: implications for paranasal sinus surgery. Ann Otol Rhinol Laryngol. 1993;102:705.
4. Wald ER. Acute bacterial rhinosinusitis in children: clinical features and diagnosis. In: Kaplan SL, Wood RA, Isaacson GC, Blake D, editors. ; 2022.

5. Ramadan HH. Medical treatment of pediatric sinusitis clinical presentation. Meyers AD Medscape. 2022. https://emedicine.medscape.com/article/873149-clinical. Accessed 3 June 2023.
6. Santee CA, Nagalingam NA, Faruqi AA, et al. Nasopharyngeal microbiota composition of children is related to the frequency of upper respiratory infection and acute sinusitis. Microbiome. 2016;4(1):34.
7. DeMuri GP, Gern JE, Moyer SC, et al. Clinical features, virus identification, and sinusitis as a complication of upper respiratory tract illness in children ages 4–7 years. J Pediatr. 2016;171:133.
8. DeMuri GP, Eickhoff JC, Gern JC, Wald ER. Clinical and virological characteristics of acute sinusitis in children. Clin Infect Dis. 2019;69:1764.
9. Revai K, Dobbs LA, Nair S, et al. Incidence of acute otitis media and sinusitis complicating upper respiratory tract infection: the effect of age. Pediatrics. 2007;119:e1408.
10. Wald ER, Dashefsky B, Byers C, et al. Frequency and severity of infections in day care. J Pediatr. 1988;112:540.
11. Rachelefsky GS, Katz RM, Siegel SC. Chronic sinusitis in children with respiratory allergy: the role of antimicrobials. J Allergy Clin Immunol. 1982;69:382.
12. Rachelefsky GS, Katz RM, Siegel SC. Chronic sinusitis in the allergic child. Pediatr Clin N Am. 1988;35:1091.
13. Furukawa CT. The role of allergy in sinusitis in children. J Allergy Clin Immunol. 1992;90:515.
14. Peters AT, Spector S, Hsu J, et al. Diagnosis and management of rhinosinusitis: a practice parameter update. Ann Allergy Asthma Immunol. 2014;113:347.
15. Lusk RP, Stankiewicz JA. Pediatric rhinosinusitis. Otolaryngol Head Neck Surg. 1997;117:S53.
16. Chow AW, Benninger MS, Brook I, et al. IDSA clinical practice guideline for acute bacterial rhinosinusitis in children and adults. Clin Infect Dis. 2012;54:e72.
17. Wald ER, Applegate KE, Bordley C, et al. Clinical practice guideline for the diagnosis and management of acute bacterial sinusitis in children aged 1–18 years. Pediatrics. 2013;132:e262.
18. Wald ER, Milmoe GJ, Bowen A, et al. Acute maxillary sinusitis in children. N Engl J Med. 1981;304:749.
19. Brook I. Microbiology and antimicrobial treatment of orbital and intracranial complications of sinusitis in children and their management. Int J Pediatr Otorhinolaryngol. 2009;73:1183.
20. DeMuri GP, Wald ER. Clinical practice. Acute bacterial sinusitis in children. N Engl J Med. 2012;367:1128.
21. Gwaltney JM Jr, Hendley JO, Simon G, Jordan WS Jr. Rhinovirus infections in an industrial population. II. Characteristics of illness and antibody response. JAMA. 1967;202:494.
22. Kogutt MS, Swischuk LE. Diagnosis of sinusitis in infants and children. Pediatrics. 1973;52:121.
23. Williams JW Jr, Simel DL. Does this patient have sinusitis? Diagnosing acute sinusitis by history and physical examination. JAMA. 1993;270:1242.
24. Fireman P. Diagnosis of sinusitis in children: emphasis on the history and physical examination. J Allergy Clin Immunol. 1992;90:433.
25. Clayman GL, Adams GL, Paugh DR, Koopmann CF Jr. Intracranial complications of paranasal sinusitis: a combined institutional review. Laryngoscope. 1991;101:234.
26. Chandler JR, Langenbrunner DJ, Stevens ER. The pathogenesis of orbital complications in acute sinusitis. Laryngoscope. 1970;80:1414.
27. Sultész M, Csákányi Z, Majoros T, et al. Acute bacterial rhinosinusitis and its complications in our pediatric otolaryngological department between 1997 and 2006. Int J Pediatr Otorhinolaryngol. 2009;73:1507.
28. Soon VT. Pediatric subperiosteal orbital abscess secondary to acute sinusitis: a 5-year review. Am J Otolaryngol. 2011;32:62.
29. Botting AM, McIntosh D, Mahadevan M. Paediatric pre- and post-septal peri-orbital infections are different diseases. A retrospective review of 262 cases. Int J Pediatr Otorhinolaryngol. 2008;72:377.
30. Seltz LB, Smith J, Durairaj VD, et al. Microbiology and antibiotic management of orbital cellulitis. Pediatrics. 2011;127:e566.

31. Nageswaran S, Woods CR, Benjamin DK Jr, et al. Orbital cellulitis in children. Pediatr Infect Dis J. 2006;25:695.
32. Ryan JT, Preciado DA, Bauman N, et al. Management of pediatric orbital cellulitis in patients with radiographic findings of subperiosteal abscess. Otolaryngol Head Neck Surg. 2009;140:907.
33. Wong SJ, Levi J. Management of pediatric orbital cellulitis: a systematic review. Int J Pediatr Otorhinolaryngol. 2018;110:123.
34. Saltagi MZ, Rabbani CC, Patel KS, et al. Orbital complications of acute sinusitis in pediatric patients: management of Chandler III patients. Allergy Rhinol (Providence). 2022;13:21526575221097311.
35. Sobol SE, Marchand J, Tewfik TL, et al. Orbital complications of sinusitis in children. J Otolaryngol. 2002;31:131.
36. Greenberg MF, Pollard ZF. Medical treatment of pediatric subperiosteal orbital abscess secondary to sinusitis. J AAPOS. 1998;2:351.
37. Goytia VK, Giannoni CM, Edwards MS. Intraorbital and intracranial extension of sinusitis: comparative morbidity. J Pediatr. 2011;158:486.
38. Harris GJ. Subperiosteal abscess of the orbit. Age as a factor in the bacteriology and response to treatment. Ophthalmology. 1994;101:585.
39. Bergin DJ, Wright JE. Orbital cellulitis. Br J Ophthalmol. 1986;70:174.
40. Brook I, Frazier EH. Microbiology of subperiosteal orbital abscess and associated maxillary sinusitis. Laryngoscope. 1996;106:1010.
41. Rudloe TF, Harper MB, Prabhu SP, et al. Acute periorbital infections: who needs emergent imaging? Pediatrics. 2010;125:e719.
42. Clement WA, Sooby P, Doherty C, et al. Acute isolated sphenoid sinusitis in children: a case series and systematic review of the literature. Int J Pediatr Otorhinolaryngol. 2021;140:110492.
43. Milinis K, Thompson N, Atsmoni SC, Sharma SD. Sinogenic intracranial suppuration in children: systematic review and meta-analysis. Otolaryngol Head Neck Surg. 2022;167:215.
44. Hicks CW, Weber JG, Reid JR, Moodley M. Identifying and managing intracranial complications of sinusitis in children: a retrospective series. Pediatr Infect Dis J. 2011;30:222.
45. Otto WR, Paden WZ, Connors M, et al. Suppurative intracranial complications of pediatric sinusitis: a single-center experience. J Pediatr Infect Dis Soc. 2021;10:309.
46. Sable NS, Hengerer A, Powell KR. Acute frontal sinusitis with intracranial complications. Pediatr Infect Dis. 1984;3:58.
47. Wassermann D. Acute paranasal sinusitis and cavernous sinus thrombosis. Arch Otolaryngol. 1967;86:205.
48. Whitaker CW. Intracranial complications of ear, nose, and throat infections. Laryngoscope. 1971;81:1375.
49. Germiller JA, Monin DL, Sparano AM, Tom LW. Intracranial complications of sinusitis in children and adolescents and their outcomes. Arch Otolaryngol Head Neck Surg. 2006;132:969.
50. Bair-Merritt MH, Shah SS, Zaoutis TE, et al. Suppurative intracranial complications of sinusitis in previously healthy children. Pediatr Infect Dis J. 2005;24:384.
51. Bambakidis NC, Cohen AR. Intracranial complications of frontal sinusitis in children: Pott's puffy tumor revisited. Pediatr Neurosurg. 2001;35:82.
52. Diament MJ. The diagnosis of sinusitis in infants and children: X-ray, computed tomography, and magnetic resonance imaging. Diagnostic imaging of pediatric sinusitis. J Allergy Clin Immunol. 1992;90:442.
53. Jones NS. CT of the paranasal sinuses: a review of the correlation with clinical, surgical and histopathological findings. Clin Otolaryngol Allied Sci. 2002;27(1):11–7. https://doi.org/10.1046/j.0307-7772.2001.00525.x. PMID: 11903365.
54. American College of Radiology. ACR appropriateness criteria. Sinusitis—Child. 2018. https://www.acr.org/Clinical-Resources/ACR-Appropriateness-Criteria. Accessed 31 Oct 2022.
55. Diament MJ, Senac MO Jr, Gilsanz V, et al. Prevalence of incidental paranasal sinuses opacification in pediatric patients: a CT study. J Comput Assist Tomogr. 1987;11:426.

56. Kristo A, Alho OP, Luotonen J, et al. Cross-sectional survey of paranasal sinus magnetic resonance imaging findings in schoolchildren. Acta Paediatr. 2003;92:34.
57. Glasier CM, Mallory GB Jr, Steele RW. Significance of opacification of the maxillary and ethmoid sinuses in infants. J Pediatr. 1989;114:45.
58. Kovatch AL, Wald ER, Ledesma-Medina J, et al. Maxillary sinus radiographs in children with nonrespiratory complaints. Pediatrics. 1984;73:306.
59. Gwaltney JM Jr, Phillips CD, Miller RD, Riker DK. Computed tomographic study of the common cold. N Engl J Med. 1994;330:25.
60. Quintanilla-Dieck L, Lam DJ. Chronic rhinosinusitis in children. Curr Treat Options Pediatr. 2018;4(4):413–24. https://doi.org/10.1007/s40746-018-0142-z. Epub 2018 Sep 25. PMID: 33312844; PMCID: PMC7728295.
61. Magit A. Pediatric rhinosinusitis. Otolaryngol Clin N Am. 2014;47(5):733–46.
62. Rose AS, Thorp BD, Zanation AM, Ebert CS Jr. Chronic rhinosinusitis in children. Pediatr Clin N Am. 2013;60(4):979–91.
63. Brietzke SE, Shin JJ, Choi S, et al. Clinical consensus statement: pediatric chronic rhinosinusitis. Otolaryngol Head Neck Surg. 2014;151(4):542–53.
64. Zacharisen M, Casper R. Pediatric sinusitis. Immunol Allergy Clin N Am. 2005;25(2):313–32.
65. Christensen DN, Franks ZG, McCrary HC, Saleh AA, Chang EH. A systematic review of the association between cigarette smoke exposure and chronic rhinosinusitis. Otolaryngol Head Neck Surg. 2018;158(5):801–16.
66. Principi N, Esposito S. New insights into pediatric rhinosinusitis. Pediatr Allergy Immunol. 2007;18(Suppl 18):7–9.
67. Muntz HR, Lusk RP. Bacteriology of the ethmoid bullae in children with chronic sinusitis. Arch Otolaryngol Head Neck Surg. 1991;117(2):179–81.
68. Gilani S, Shin JJ. The burden and visit prevalence of pediatric chronic rhinosinusitis. Otolaryngol Head Neck Surg. 2017;157(6):1048–52.
69. Novembre E, Mori F, Pucci N, Bernardini R, Vierucci A, de Martino M. Systemic treatment of rhinosinusitis in children. Pediatr Allergy Immunol. 2007;18(Suppl 18):56–61.
70. Hill M, Bhattacharyya N, Hall TR, Lufkin R, Shapiro NL. Incidental paranasal sinus imaging abnormalities and the normal Lund score in children. Otolaryngol Head Neck Surg. 2004;130(2):171–5.
71. Kennedy DW, Josephson JS, Zinreich SJ, Mattox DE, Goldsmith MM. Endoscopic sinus surgery for mucoceles: a viable alternative. Laryngoscope. 1989;99(9):885–95.
72. Benninger MS, Marks S. The endoscopic management of sphenoid and ethmoid mucoceles with orbital and intranasal extension. Rhinology. 1995;33(3):157–61.
73. Scadding GK. The catarrhal child. Paediatr Child Health. 2015;26(1):21–5. https://doi.org/10.1016/j.paed.2015.08.002.
74. Fokkens WJ, Lund VJ, Hopkins C, Hellings PW, Kern R, Reitsma S, Toppila-Salmi S, Bernal-Sprekelsen M, Mullol J, Alobid I, Terezinha Anselmo-Lima W, Bachert C, Baroody F, von Buchwald C, Cervin A, Cohen N, Constantinidis J, De Gabory L, Desrosiers M, Diamant Z, Douglas RG, Gevaert PH, Hafner A, Harvey RJ, Joos GF, Kalogjera L, Knill A, Kocks JH, Landis BN, Limpens J, Lebeer S, Lourenco O, Meco C, Matricardi PM, O'Mahony L, Philpott CM, Ryan D, Schlosser R, Senior B, Smith TL, Teeling T, Tomazic PV, Wang DY, Wang D, Zhang L, Agius AM, Ahlstrom-Emanuelsson C, Alabri R, Albu S, Alhabash S, Aleksic A, Aloulah M, Al-Qudah M, Alsaleh S, Baban MA, Baudoin T, Balvers T, Battaglia P, Bedoya JD, Beule A, Bofares KM, Braverman I, Brozek-Madry E, Richard B, Callejas C, Carrie S, Caulley L, Chussi D, de Corso E, Coste A, El Hadi U, Elfarouk A, Eloy PH, Farrokhi S, Felisati G, Ferrari MD, Fishchuk R, Grayson W, Goncalves PM, Grdinic B, Grgic V, Hamizan AW, Heinichen JV, Husain S, Ping TI, Ivaska J, Jakimovska F, Jovancevic L, Kakande E, Kamel R, Karpischenko S, Kariyawasam HH, Kawauchi H, Kjeldsen A, Klimek L, Krzeski A, Kopacheva Barsova G, Kim SW, Lal D, Letort JJ, Lopatin A, Mahdjoubi A, Mesbahi A, Netkovski J, Nyenbue Tshipukane D, Obando-Valverde A, Okano M, Onerci M, Ong YK, Orlandi R, Otori N, Ouennoughy K, Ozkan M, Peric A, Plzak J, Prokopakis E, Prepageran N, Psaltis A, Pugin B, Raftopulos M, Rombaux P, Riechelmann H, Sahtout S, Sarafoleanu CC,

Searyoh K, Rhee CS, Shi J, Shkoukani M, Shukuryan AK, Sicak M, Smyth D, Sindvongs K, Soklic Kosak T, Stjarne P, Sutikno B, Steinsvag S, Tantilipikorn P, Thanaviratananich S, Tran T, Urbancic J, Valiulius A, Vasquez de Aparicio C, Vicheva D, Virkkula PM, Vicente G, Voegels R, Wagenmann MM, Wardani RS, Welge-Lussen A, Witterick I, Wright E, Zabolotniy D, Zsolt B, Zwetsloot CP. European position paper on rhinosinusitis and nasal polyps 2020. Rhinology. 2020;58(Suppl S29):1–464.

Adenoiditis in Children

53

Samet Aydemir, Cemal Cingi, and Luisa Maria Bellussi

53.1 Introduction

A collection of lymphoid tissue known as the tonsil, adenoid pad, or adenoids is situated on the posterior wall of the nasopharynx, just above the level of the soft palate. Waldeyer's ring, a circumferential collection of lymphoid tissue that surrounds the upper aerodigestive tract, is comprised of the adenoids, faucial tonsils, lingual tonsils, and tubal tonsils of Gerlach and was named for Heinrich Wilhelm Gottfried von Waldeyer-Hartz, a German anatomist at the turn of the twentieth century [1]. These tissues work together to form an essential aspect of the developing human immune system. IgA antibodies are produced by the immune cells of Waldeyer's ring once they come into contact with antigens presented through the oral and nasal canals. Researchers believe this "priming" of the immune system occurs throughout early childhood [2].

53.2 Adenoids

Although they are present at birth, the adenoids do not reach their full size until about seven. Most people see a significant reduction in their size throughout puberty, and some see them almost entirely disappear. Adenoiditis occurs often throughout these

S. Aydemir
Department of Otorhinolaryngology, Samsun Training and Research Hospital, Samsun, Turkey

C. Cingi (✉)
Department of Otorhinolaryngology, Eskisehir Osmangazi University, Medical Faculty, Eskisehir, Turkey

L. M. Bellussi
ENT Clinic, University of Siena, Siena, Italy

H. Yüksel et al. (eds.), *Pediatric Airway Diseases*, Comprehensive ENT, https://doi.org/10.1007/978-3-031-74853-0_53

years because of this. Infection, allergies, or irritation from stomach acid as part of laryngopharyngeal reflux (LPR) can all lead to inflammation of the adenoid tissue, a condition known as "adenoiditis." However, adenotonsillitis, pharyngitis, rhinosinusitis, and other similar infections almost always accompany adenoiditis. Many of the side effects of adenoid illness, such as eustachian tube dysfunction and recurrent acute otitis media, can be traced back to adenoid hypertrophy, which can be caused by chronic irritation. There are two types of adenoiditis such as acute and chronic [3].

The adenoids are located on the wall of the nasopharynx behind the nose. In the 16th week of pregnancy, lymphocytes infiltrate the subepithelial space. The adenoids, palatine tonsils, and lingual tonsils comprise the Waldeyer ring of lymphoid tissue in the oropharynx and nasopharynx [4].

The adenoids are initially small, but they gradually grow in size. Like the tonsils, they keep growing until a child ages seven. Symptoms associated with the adenoids, including snoring, nasal airway blockage, and blocked breathing during sleep, often emerge between 18 and 24 months. Symptoms often subside as a kid reaches school age, and by the time they reach their adolescent or teenage years, their adenoids are usually tiny enough to cause any problems [4].

Many germs and bacteria can quickly enter the nasopharynx and adenoids after a baby is born. At birth, the upper respiratory system begins to develop. Bacteria such as lactobacilli, anaerobic streptococci, actinomycosis, Fusobacterium species, and Nocardia species are all found in children as young as 6 months old. Alpha-hemolytic streptococci and enterococci, Corynebacterium species, coagulase-negative staphylococci, Neisseria species, Haemophilus species, Micrococcus species, and Stomatococcus species are all members of the normal flora of the adenoid. Diseases of the ears, nose, and sinuses (ENT) can be caused by adenoids becoming inflamed and harboring dangerous bacteria [4].

53.3 Pathophysiology

Adenoids, which can house a chronic infection, have been linked to chronic sinusitis and persistent or recurrent ear infections in the existing literature. The sickness and the child's age appear to affect the kind and number of harmful bacteria [5].

The most often cultivated bacteria are *Haemophilus influenzae*, group A beta-hemolytic Streptococcus, *Staphylococcus aureus*, *Moraxella catarrhalis*, and *Streptococcus pneumoniae*. The author has discovered antibiotic-resistant strains of the three most prevalent causes of ear infections and sinus infections in children (*H. influenzae*, *M. catarrhalis*, and *S. pneumoniae*) [4].

Studies on children over 3 years found that adenoidectomy, regardless of adenoid size, relieved symptoms of rhinosinusitis and decreased the recurrence of chronic middle ear effusions or infections [4].

53.3.1 Recurrent or Persistent Middle Ear Effusion

The causes and severity of recurrent or chronic otitis media vary with age. Middle ear diseases can be attributed to a breakdown in the immune system or eustachian tube function. The immune system and the eustachian tube function are naturally lower in infants and develop as the baby grows. As a result of this maturation, many youngsters eventually outgrow their ear infections. Children who suffer from recurrent ear infections or fluid issues often have underdeveloped eustachian tube function, a chronic adenoid infection, or eustachian tube dysfunction due to congestion from allergic rhinitis. Several studies show that after adenoidectomy, eustachian tube function is enhanced and fluid accumulation is avoided, despite the size of the adenoids [4].

The pathophysiology of the adenoids' function in generating ear infections has been the subject of conflicting investigations throughout the past two decades. The etiology of eustachian tube dysfunction was first unclear, with researchers debating whether a physical blockage or the presence of a persistent infection was to blame. Multiple publications evaluated the bacterial load in the adenoids of children with various diseases (such as chronic ear infections or difficulty breathing through the nose). Children without any head and neck pathology or infection [4] or children with adenoid hypertrophy alone and no ear infections were often used as controls for those with middle ear effusions.

Patients with recurrent otitis media had more pathogenic germs in their adenoid beds than those with chronic serous otitis media or hypertrophy, as shown by a culture [6]. When comparing patients with and without head and neck infections, Brodsky and Koch cultured more bacteria from the adenoids of patients with recurrent or chronic otitis media [7].

When comparing the adenoids of patients with otitis media and rhinosinusitis to those of patients with solely adenoid hyperplasia-producing nasal airway obstruction, Brodsky et al. observed no significant difference in the number of harmful bacteria. Adding to the mystery, Maw and Speller [8] discovered that individuals with otitis media with effusion had the same number of harmful bacteria in their adenoids and tonsils as healthy controls.

Adenoidectomy has been proven to help treat chronic persistent otitis media with effusion and probably recurrent otitis media in children older than 4 years old, and this benefit appears to be independent of adenoid size. However, the efficacy of adenoidectomy in treating recurrent otitis media or rhinosinusitis in children younger than 3 years of age has not been shown [4].

It is unknown whether bacteria that live in the adenoids irritate the lining of the eustachian tube, leading to malfunction, or whether they create a chronic low-grade infection in the middle ear area, leading to persistent fluid or recurring infections [4].

53.3.2 The Chronic Sinusitis

The adenoid appears to be a source of infection for people who suffer from chronic sinusitis. Lee and Rosenfeld (1997) [9] showed that the symptoms of chronic sinusitis in children improved after adenoidectomy regardless of the size of the adenoids. The pathogenic bacteria found in the adenoids were also cultivated from the middle meatus, close to the drainage site for the anterior sinuses [10], as demonstrated by Brodsky et al. McClay also showed [11] that antibiotic-resistant bacteria were present in the adenoid bed.

Nasal airway obstruction causes sinusitis and other sinus infections.

The physical blockage of the back of the nose by enlarged adenoids can also lead to clinical symptoms such as nasal congestion, snoring, and mouth breathing. Nasal airway obstruction can cause symptoms similar to those of chronic sinusitis, and the physical block can exacerbate sinusitis by preventing the usual passage of nasal secretions and air out of the sinuses from the back of the nose [4].

Overgrown adenoids (and tonsils) can block airflow, leading to youngsters' sleep apnea and other breathing problems. Only their size causes an obstruction—the possibility of a persistent infection in larger adenoids [4].

53.4 Etiology

A wide variety of substances and infections can cause adenoid inflammation. Acute adenoiditis typically follows a viral upper respiratory tract illness (URI). Superinfection by bacterial pathogens and subsequent tissue proliferation can occur in this condition [3].

Three types of bacteria are routinely isolated as pathogens from adenoid biopsies.

- *Haemophilus influenzae*
- *Staphylococcus aureus*
- *Streptococcus pyogenes*
- *Streptococcus pneumoniae* [12]

More frequently than not, anaerobic pathogens are part of the polymicrobial infection that causes chronic adenoiditis. Biofilm formation is a common cause of chronic adenoiditis, which may contribute to upper respiratory tract infections in children. Adenoiditis is usually connected to occurrences of pediatric rhinosinusitis [13]. Adenoiditis and the ensuing enlargement of the adenoids are thought to be triggered by allergies. The adenoid tissue comes into touch with allergens breathed through the nose, prompting the adenoid to grow to trigger an immune response and manufacture IgA [14]. Adenoiditis and adenoid hypertrophy may be caused, in part, by the chronic irritation caused by stomach acid in the context of gastroesophageal reflux disease (GERD), especially in newborns and young children [15].

53.5 Epidemiology

Since adenoiditis is typically handled in the context of a regional disease process like rhinosinusitis and adenotonsillar illness, it is difficult to determine the exact incidence and prevalence numbers for adenoiditis alone. Adenoiditis is often a condition in children since adenoid tissue atrophies throughout puberty. Parental smoking has been positively connected with this disease, although the available data do not imply a preference for gender, race, geography, or socioeconomic level [16].

Differentiating adenoiditis from bacterial sinusitis in children might be difficult. Therefore, the prevalence of adenoiditis may be estimated using data on the incidence of sinusitis in children. Six to eight viral upper respiratory infections (URIs) are reported annually among youngsters. Sinusitis and adenoiditis can develop as complications of a viral upper respiratory infection in 5–13% of cases [17].

53.6 Diagnosis and Evaluation

The usual patient with adenoiditis is a prepubescent child who has just recovered from an upper respiratory infection (URI), as adenoid tissue generally regresses around puberty. Recurrent acute otitis media, chronic nasal obstruction with mouth-breathing, chronic otitis media, sleep-disordered breathing/obstructive sleep apnea, or gastroesophageal reflux disease/lower esophageal reflux disease [3] are all possible in this patient.

Symptoms include a bad smell in the mouth, snoring, fever, breathing via the mouth, and nasal blockage. Although difficult to conduct on youngsters, an indirect mirror exam may allow the practitioner to see larger adenoids with exudates. The adenoids can be evaluated more thoroughly using a flexible nasal and laryngeal endoscopic exam. However, using one properly can be tricky and may need special training and the participation of the patient's kid and parents. If the adenoid is very big, it can sometimes be seen protruding below the soft palate's lateral border (picture). Acute or chronic adenoid growth that displaces the soft palate might harm a patient's ability to communicate clearly [18].

The condition known as adenoid facies, or long-face syndrome, can occur in young children who suffer from chronic adenoiditis and consequent adenoid enlargement. Obligate mouth breathing from a blocked nasopharynx is associated with craniofacial anomalies such as a high-arched palate and a retrognathic jaw in children with enlarged adenoids [19].

53.7 Clinical Evaluation

Acute adenoiditis is clinically diagnosed when three criteria are met.

- Concurrent acute otitis media is a possibility.

- Symptoms include fever, purulent rhinorrhea, postnasal drip, nasal blockage, throat discomfort, and bad breath.
- A laryngeal mirror or nasal endoscope can be used to check the adenoids visually.

53.8 Laboratory Testing

Testing for allergies, strep throat, and other infections

- Rapid Strep test
- Cultures
- Allergy testing [3]

Clinicians may order a quick Strep test if adenoiditis is suspected in a patient with pharyngitis. This has a dual purpose. First, it will provide a conclusive diagnosis of the patient's illness, directing the selection of antibiotics. Second, the results of any strep tests administered will be on file, which will be considered when determining whether or not an adenoidectomy and tonsillectomy are necessary. Adenoiditis is still diagnosed clinically. Therefore, if the Strep test returns negative, the doctor can assume that the symptoms are caused by anything other than Strep [3].

As direct cultures of the adenoids may be challenging in the office environment, the doctor may elect to perform throat cultures in cases of persistent infection despite antibiotic therapy to assist in identifying the causative agent and guide treatment. Complete blood count and HIV testing are other tests to consider [3].

Allergic skin tests may assist guide treatment [3] if it is suspected that seasonal or environmental allergies are to blame for the adenoiditis.

X-ray of the sinuses and the side of the neck. Computed tomography (CT) scan of the sinuses.

If a sinus infection is suspected clinically, an X-ray or CT scan of the sinuses may be performed to locate the infection. This is typically optional for everyday situations. X-rays taken from the side of the neck can help diagnose adenoid hypertrophy. If the patient has adenoid hypertrophy and snores, a sleep study can be performed to rule out obstructive sleep apnea [3].

Adenoiditis is a common symptom of upper respiratory tract infections, including rhinosinusitis and pharyngitis. Adenoiditis is generally treated like that of rhinosinusitis and pharyngitis by medical professionals [20, 21].

- Computed tomography (CT) or CT scans are not often utilized to assess the adenoids. However, the choana and nasopharynx are sometimes seen during sinus CT scans, offering insight into adenoid size.

Information about the adenoids can be gleaned from the plain sagittal scout film taken concurrently with the CT scan [4] if the CT scan does not include the nasopharynx.

Imaging studies (e.g., CT scan, MRI) are conducted to rule out a lesion other than an adenoid if the adenoids seem abnormal or if a mass is found in the nasopharynx in an older kid or an adult.

By the time someone reaches their teenage years or beyond, their adenoids have typically shrunk in size and are no longer an obstructive factor [4].

53.9 Diagnostic Procedures

Nasopharyngoscopy, either flexible or stiff.

Clinicians can examine the adenoid with a flexible or stiff nasopharyngoscopy [4].

Occasionally, a biopsy may be necessary to confirm the diagnosis of a nasopharyngeal mass in an older child or adult or in a younger kid whose nasopharyngeal tissue mass does not seem exactly like an adenoid.

A biopsy should be done in a hospital operating room if it is essential, especially in a youngster.

- Nasopharyngeal mass biopsies can be performed on adolescents and adults with proper topical anesthetic in the clinic.
- Obtain preoperative imaging with a CT scan, MRI, or magnetic resonance angiography and perform the biopsy in the operating room [4] if findings suggest the lesion may be vascular.

53.10 Treatment

53.10.1 Medical Management

53.10.1.1 Observation

Antibiotics shouldn't be given if the doctor thinks a cold or other common virus is to blame for the patient's adenoiditis. Upper respiratory virus infections that are not complex usually clear up in about 5–7 days [17].

53.10.1.2 Antibiotic Treatment

Antibiotics covering the most common pathogens are the first line of treatment if symptoms persist or the clinical presentation indicates a bacterial etiology, such as a high fever or purulent discharge from the nose or mouth. Due to its broad spectrum of activity and low incidence of adverse effects, amoxicillin is a go-to first-line antibiotic. If the patient does not react to amoxicillin, further options include cefdinir and cefuroxime. Antibiotics such as clarithromycin or azithromycin might be used if the patient has a penicillin allergy. Patients should start feeling better within 48–72 h of antibiotic treatment. Short-term treatments lead to high recurrence rates and promote antibiotic resistance development. Hence, 10 days of treatment is recommended. Amoxicillin-clavulanate should be advised to eradicate any beta-lactamase-generating organisms if the situation does not improve after a course of amoxicillin or other first-line therapies. By flushing away the irritant microorganisms and the stagnant mucous secretions that may host them, saline sprays and nasal rinses may help reduce the duration of symptoms [17].

53.10.1.3 The Allergy Treatment

Treatment with nasal steroid sprays, oral steroids, oral antihistamines, or a combination of these may be tried in patients with suspected environmental allergies causing their adenoiditis. If this helps, the patient should undergo official allergy testing and immune-modulating medication for long-term relief. It's also possible that saline sprays and nasal rinses have a role in these scenarios [3].

53.10.1.4 Reflux Treatment

Elevating the head of the bed, making dietary changes, and treating LPR/GERD with or without H2 blockers or proton-pump inhibitors may be all that's needed to alleviate the adenoiditis symptoms [15].

53.10.2 Surgical Management

53.10.2.1 Adenoidectomy

A variety of clinical manifestations can be treated by adenoidectomy in children. Regardless of the adenoid pad size, adenoidectomy may help children with recurrent or chronic otitis media. Because their adenoids may not be oversized, these youngsters may exhibit signs of nasal airway obstruction (such as nasal congestion, snoring, or sleeping with their mouths open). These kids frequently suffer from snoring or nasal congestion, though. Only somewhat older children (ages 3–4) have been included in the reliable prospective studies. Otitis media has not been studied on the efficacy of adenoidectomy in children with tiny or moderate adenoids under 3–4 years old.

Sinusitis can be chronic or recurring, and it can affect children. Some possible clinical signs are postnasal discharge, purulent anterior rhinorrhea, cough, fever, facial discomfort, and nasal congestion.

It is also possible for children to develop symptoms of a blocked nasal airway without showing evidence of acute or chronic illness. Obstruction of the nasal airways, snoring, and the need to breathe via the mouth are all signs. Chronic mouth breathing, which can develop palatal and dental abnormalities, results from an enlarged adenoid that inhibits normal airflow through the nasal cavity.

53.10.2.2 Indications

Indications for adenoidectomy [4]:

- Enlargement leading to obstructed nasal airways, which can cause obstructive breathing, obstructive sleep apnea symptoms, and chronic mouth breathing (which may cause palatal and dental abnormalities)
- Otitis media that returns or is chronic in children older than 3–4 years

- Chronic or recurrent sinusitis

As shown by Lee and Rosenfeld [9], adenoidectomy benefits children with recurrent sinusitis regardless of adenoid size. It is undeniable that adenoidectomy alleviates symptoms of chronic sinusitis in youngsters whose nasal passages were blocked by swollen adenoid pads. Some pediatric rhinologists worry that adenoidectomy alone may not help a child already in school and with a tiny adenoid pad and CT scan evidence of persistent sinusitis. However, if the adenoid was small and CT scan evidence of chronic sinusitis was present, fewer children improved, leading the authors to believe these children would benefit from initial procedures of adenoidectomy and endoscopic sinus surgery [4]. This concern was confirmed in a 1999 American Academy of Pediatrics presentation.

Two years after undergoing an adenoidectomy, children aged one to six were studied by Van den Aardweg et al. for their impact in reducing the frequency of upper respiratory infections (URIs). However, 111 youngsters from 13 hospitals were divided into two groups: those who underwent surgery and those who did not. Children who suffer from frequent respiratory infections may not benefit from adenoidectomy. However, lower rates of upper respiratory infections were seen over time in both groups, according to the study [22].

53.10.2.3 Contraindications

There are no absolute contraindications except when general anesthesia cannot be administered [4].

Limitations on complete adenoid removal

- A relative contraindication to adenoidectomy is a severe bleeding problem that cannot be managed with preoperative, intraoperative, and postoperative coagulation drugs and methods.
- A relative contraindication includes the presence of a short palate, submucous cleft palate, genuine cleft palate, muscular weakness or hypotonia due to a neurological condition, velocardiofacial syndrome, or Kabuki syndrome in the kid.
- Atlantoaxial joint laxity is found in 10% of children with Down syndrome, but can be remedied with partial adenoidectomy or prior planning for muscle speech therapy after adenoidectomy. It may be feasible to execute the operation without injuring the patient [4] if the procedure is performed while the patient is in a neutral posture or after being stabilized via neurosurgery.

References

1. Hellings P, Jorissen M, Ceuppens JL. The Waldeyer's ring. Acta Otorhinolaryngol Belg. 2000;54(3):237–41.
2. Heimroth RD, Casadei E, Salinas I. Molecular drivers of lymphocyte organization in vertebrate mucosal surfaces: revisiting the TNF superfamily hypothesis. J Immunol. 2020;204(10):2697–711.
3. Bowers I, Shermetaro C. Adenoiditis. In: StatPearls (Internet). Treasure Island (FL): StatPearls Publishing; 2023. https://www.ncbi.nlm.nih.gov/books/NBK536931/.

4. McClay JE. Adenoidectomy. In: Meyers AD, editor. . Medscape; 2019. https://emedicine.medscape.com/article/872216-overview#a7.
5. Rajeshwary A, Rai S, Somayaji G, Pai V. Bacteriology of symptomatic adenoids in children. N Am J Med Sci. 2013;5(2):113–8.
6. Pillsbury HC 3rd, Kveton JF, Sasaki CT, et al. Quantitative bacteriology in adenoid tissue. Otolaryngol Head Neck Surg. 1981;89(3 Pt 1):355–63.
7. Brodsky L, Koch RJ. Bacteriology and immunology of normal and diseased adenoids in children. Arch Otolaryngol Head Neck Surg. 1993;119(8):821–9.
8. Maw AR, Speller DC. Are the tonsils and adenoids a reservoir of infection in otitis media with effusion (glue ear)? Clin Otolaryngol Allied Sci. 1985;10(5):265–9.
9. Lee D, Rosenfeld RM. Adenoid bacteriology and sinonasal symptoms in children. Otolaryngol Head Neck Surg. 1997;116(3):301–7.
10. Brodsky L, Moore L, Stanievich JF. A comparison of tonsillar size and oropharyngeal dimensions in children with obstructive adenotonsillar hypertrophy. Int J Pediatr Otorhinolaryngol. 1987;13(2):149–56.
11. McClay JE. Resistant bacteria in the adenoids: a preliminary report. Arch Otolaryngol Head Neck Surg. 2000;126(5):625–9.
12. Shin KS, Cho SH, Kim KR, Tae K, Lee SH, Park CW, Jeong JH. The role of adenoids in pediatric rhinosinusitis. Int J Pediatr Otorhinolaryngol. 2008;72(11):1643–50.
13. Zuliani G, Carron M, Gurrola J, Coleman C, Haupert M, Berk R, Coticchia J. Identification of adenoid biofilms in chronic rhinosinusitis. Int J Pediatr Otorhinolaryngol. 2006;70(9):1613–7.
14. Cho KS, Kim SH, Hong SL, Lee J, Mun SJ, Roh YE, Kim YM, Kim HY. Local atopy in childhood adenotonsillar hypertrophy. Am J Rhinol Allergy. 2018;32(3):160–6.
15. Niu X, Wu ZH, Xiao XY, Chen X. The relationship between adenoid hypertrophy and gastroesophageal reflux disease: a meta-analysis. Medicine (Baltimore). 2018;97(41):e12540.
16. Lasisi AO, Olaniyan FA, Muibi SA, Azeez IA, Abdulwasiu KG, Lasisi TJ, Imam ZO, Yekinni TO, Olayemi O. Clinical and demographic risk factors associated with chronic suppurative otitis media. Int J Pediatr Otorhinolaryngol. 2007;71(10):1549–54.
17. American Academy of Pediatrics, Subcommittee on Management of Sinusitis and Committee on Quality Improvement. Clinical practice guideline: management of sinusitis. Pediatrics. 2001;108(3):798–808.
18. Eom TH, Jang ES, Kim YH, Chung SY, Lee IG. Articulation error of children with adenoid hypertrophy. Korean J Pediatr. 2014;57(7):323–8.
19. Koca CF, Erdem T, Bayındır T. The effect of adenoid hypertrophy on maxillofacial development: an objective photographic analysis. J Otolaryngol Head Neck Surg. 2016;45(1):48.
20. Rosenfeld RM. Clinical practice guideline on adult sinusitis. Otolaryngol Head Neck Surg. 2007;137(3):365–77.
21. Bisno AL, Gerber MA, Gwaltney JM, Kaplan EL, Schwartz RH, Infectious Diseases Society of America. Diagnosis and management of group A streptococcal pharyngitis: a practice guideline. Clin Infect Dis. 1997;25(3):574–83.
22. van den Aardweg MT, Boonacker CW, Rovers MM, Hoes AW, Schilder AG. Effectiveness of adenoidectomy in children with recurrent upper respiratory tract infections: open randomised controlled trial. BMJ. 2011;343:d5154.

Tonsillitis in Children

54

Saltuk Bugra Kilinc, Cemal Cingi, and Ljiljana Jovancevic

54.1 Introduction

Inflammation of the tonsils in the soft palate is known as tonsillitis. The tonsils, adenoids, and lingual tonsils are all commonly inflamed during a case of pharyngitis. Group A beta-hemolytic Streptococcus pyogenes (GABHS) is tonsillitis's most common bacterial cause [1].

54.2 Definitions

Inflammation of the tonsils in the soft palate is known as tonsillitis. The tonsils, adenoids, and lingual tonsils are all commonly inflamed during a case of pharyngitis. For this article, pharyngotonsillitis and adenotonsillitis are interchangeable terms. Inflammation of the lymphoid tissue at the base of the tongue is called lingual tonsillitis [2].

In the absence of an antistreptococcal immune response [2], a "carrier state" is characterized as a positive pharyngeal culture of group A beta-hemolytic Streptococcus pyogenes (GABHS).

S. B. Kilinc
Ordu State Hospital, Otorhinolaryngology Clinic, Ordu, Turkey

C. Cingi (✉)
Medical Faculty, Department of Otorhinolaryngology, Eskisehir Osmangazi University, Eskisehir, Turkey

L. Jovancevic
Department of Otorhinolaryngology, Head and Neck Surgery, University of Novi Sad, Faculty of Medicine, University Clinical Center of Vojvodina, Novi Sad, Serbia

H. Yüksel et al. (eds.), *Pediatric Airway Diseases*, Comprehensive ENT,
https://doi.org/10.1007/978-3-031-74853-0_54

54.3 Pharyngeal Anatomy

Tissue in the tonsils is lymphoid. Crypts are formed when the respiratory epithelium invaginates and covers the lymphoid contents. The palatine tonsils are meant to be the focus of attention when the term "tonsils" is used. The palatine tonsils, along with the pharyngeal tonsils (adenoids), tubal tonsils, and lingual tonsils [3], comprise Waldeyer's ring, a ring of lymphoid tissue in the throat.

Bacteria can thrive in the crypts of the tonsils. Tonsilloliths (sometimes called "tonsil stones") are solidified "plugs" that form inside the crypts. These often have an unpleasant odor and may aggravate poor breath [3].

The tonsils are graded on a scale from zero to four [3]:

Tonsils are nonexistent or have atrophy (Grade 0).

Tonsils take up less than a quarter of the oropharyngeal diameter (Grade 1+).

Tonsils comprise 25–50% of the skull (Grade 2+).

Tonsils comprise 50–75% of the head (Grade 3+).

Tonsils are between 75% and 100% complete (Grade 4).

The tonsils of a person with "kissing tonsils" occupy the whole width of the mouth (or oropharynx) and touch [3].

54.4 Etiology and Pathophysiology

Tonsillitis and related consequences are brought on by a combination of circumstances, including viral or bacterial infections and the immune system's response to them. Tonsillitis is exacerbated by living in crowded, poor environments. Viruses like the following [2] are responsible for most cases of acute pharyngitis and tonsillitis.

- Herpes simplex virus
- Epstein-Barr virus (EBV)
- Cytomegalovirus
- Other herpes viruses
- Adenovirus
- Measles virus

One research indicated that EBV was responsible for 19% of exudative tonsillitis in children [2], suggesting that EBV may induce tonsillitis even in the absence of systemic mononucleosis.

In 15–30% of patients, pharyngotonsillitis is caused by bacteria. Anaerobic bacteria primarily cause tonsillitis. Group A beta-hemolytic Streptococcus pyogenes (GABHS) is believed to be responsible for most bacterial tonsillitis cases. S pyogenes attach to the tonsillar epithelium via adhesin receptors. Bacterial tonsillitis may be triggered initially by an immune response to the pathogen's immunoglobulin coating [2].

Mycoplasma pneumoniae, Corynebacterium diphtheriae, or Chlamydia pneumoniae seldom cause acute pharyngitis. Pharyngitis can be brought on by Neisseria gonorrhea in sexually active people. Pharyngitis due to Arcanobacterium haemolyticum is common in Scandinavia and the United Kingdom but not in the United States. Haemolyticum pharyngitis is characterized by a rash that is clinically identical to scarlet fever [2].

54.4.1 Recurrent Tonsillitis

Children with recurrent GABHS tonsillitis have a distinct bacterial population than children with fewer infections, and core tonsillar cultures in cases with recurrent pharyngitis have shown a polymicrobial flora consisting of aerobic and anaerobic bacteria. The number of other microorganisms that might hinder a GABHS infection is diminished. The most frequent aerobic bacteria identified in recurrent tonsillitis are Streptococcus pneumoniae, Staphylococcus aureus, and Haemophilus influenzae; the most common anaerobic bacterium is Bacteroides fragilis [2].

Children tend to have more GABHS than adults do. In contrast, adults are more likely to have bacterial isolates, with Prevotella and Porphyromonas species and B fragilis organisms being the most commonly recovered. Beta-lactamase-producing bacteria are also more common in adulthood [2].

54.4.1.1 Chronic Tonsillitis

In most instances of chronic tonsillitis, many bacterial species are present. These include alpha- and beta-hemolytic streptococcal species, S aureus, H influenzae, and Bacteroides species. Thirty children having tonsillectomy were studied, and the results indicated that antibiotics given six months before surgery did not affect the bacteriology of the tonsils at the time of operation [4]. Chronic bacterial tonsillitis is thought to be linked to larger tonsils. Aerobic bacterial load and total B and T lymphocyte count both play a role in this correlation. Hypertrophic tonsils and adenoids are a common site for isolating the bacteria H influenzae. The microbiology of tonsils removed from patients with recurrent GABHS pharyngitis has yet to be significantly different from those of tonsils removed from patients with tonsillar hypertrophy [2] regarding penicillin resistance or beta-lactamase generation.

Chronic tonsillitis is associated with local immunologic processes. During illness, there are fewer dendritic cells on the surface epithelium and more in the crypts and extrafollicular regions, where they serve as antigen-presenting cells. Differentiating between acute and chronic tonsillitis may be possible by studying immunologic markers. One study found that these indicators made toddlers more likely to have recurrent tonsillitis. In contrast, these markers made adults who needed a tonsillectomy more likely to have chronic tonsillitis.

Chronic tonsillitis may have a connection to radiation exposure. After the Chornobyl nuclear reactor catastrophe, there was an increase in cases of persistent tonsillitis [2].

54.5 Signs and Symptoms

People with acute tonsillitis typically exhibit symptoms [2]:

- Fever
- Throat pain

Putrid odor
Trouble swallowing (dysphagia)
Painful swallowing (odynophagia)
Sore lymph nodes in the neck

Mouth breathing, snoring, sleep-disordered breathing, breathing pauses during sleep, and sleep apnea are all symptoms of airway blockage [2].

54.6 Diagnosis

A patient with symptoms of GAS pharyngitis and no signs of viral infections (such as rhinorrhea, conjunctivitis, cough, hoarseness, anterior stomatitis, discrete ulcerative lesions or blisters, and diarrhea) is supported by a positive microbiologic test (throat culture, rapid antigen detection test (RADT), or molecular point-of-care test (POC) for GAS). However, GAS pharyngitis [5] can still be diagnosed with isolated viral symptoms (such as cough or rhinorrhea).

Even though a positive test helps confirm a diagnosis of GAS, 5% and 21% of children aged 3 to 15 are pharyngeal carriers of GAS [6–8]. Patients with acute GAS pharyngitis cannot be distinguished from those with GAS carriage due to concomitant viral disease using throat culture, RADT, or a molecular point-of-care test [9]. Patients in this category may not react favorably to treatment for GAS infection [5].

54.7 Evaluation

Most patients with tonsillitis need to undergo a physical examination, score them for risk, and then undergo fast antigen testing and a throat culture. In cases with simple infections, imaging is usually unnecessary. The Centor Score can be determined after a complete history and physical examination. Fever, tonsillar enlargement and exudates, painful cervical lymphadenopathy, and the lack of a cough are the criteria used in this grading system. One point is awarded for each valid discovery. In patients scoring 0–1, no additional tests or antibiotics are required [10, 11]. This criterion was modified to incorporate an age adjustment, awarding an extra point for age groups 3–15 years and deducting an issue for patients 45 and above. Patients with a score of 2 or 3 may be candidates for quick strep testing and throat culture. Clinicians should consider testing and empiric antibiotics [1] for patients with scores of 4 or above.

Throat cultures and quick antigen tests can also be used to diagnose GABHS. As a result, clinicians should consider obtaining pharyngeal swabs in addition to rapid antigen testing for gonorrhea, chlamydia, and HIV testing in the appropriate clinical setting due to the test's low sensitivity (61–95%) but high specificity (88–100%). Rarely, tonsillitis can be caused by syphilis, and in these situations, a rapid plasma reagin (RPR) can be sent to confirm the diagnosis [13]. A mononucleosis spot test may be considered if the Ebstein-Barr virus is suspected.

Patients with unstable vital signs, a poisonous look, difficulty swallowing, an inability to accept oral intake, or trismus may need a more thorough assessment due to their infection's complexity. To rule out potentially life-threatening conditions such as abscess, Lemierre syndrome, and epiglottitis, a CT scan of the neck with intravenous contrast may be performed. Renal function should be evaluated using a basic metabolic panel and a complete blood count in the laboratory [1].

54.8 Treatment

Tonsillitis is a self-limiting condition for the vast majority of people. Supportive care, including analgesia and hydration, is the mainstay of treatment for acute tonsillitis due to the prevalence of viral etiologies; patients rarely require hospitalization [14]. Medications like NSAIDs can provide symptomatic relief [15]. Corticosteroids, typically a single dose of dexamethasone, can be considered an adjunct therapy to decrease pain scores and improve time to recovery. Holistic therapies and herbal medicines have demonstrated inconsistent and limited value, whereas studies have indicated low damage from steroids [16, 17]. Care must be used when using steroids in people with medical comorbidities such as diabetes. Treatment with zinc gluconate is not advocated [11].

Antibiotics are commonly prescribed for individuals with a high risk of bacterial pharyngitis based on Centor criteria, antigen testing, or throat culture. Most cases of bacterial tonsillitis are caused by Streptococcus pyogenes, for which penicillins are the treatment of choice if antibiotics are to be used [18]. Antibiotic therapy with azithromycin or cephalosporins is equivalent to treating penicillin in patients with penicillin allergies. However, the physician needs to assess the risks and advantages of antibiotic usage before deciding. Antibiotics may reduce suppurative complications and symptom duration, but the effect is negligible [19]. A Cochrane review found that the duration of symptoms only decreased by 16 h [15]. Antibiotics also carry risks such as increased antibacterial resistance, gastrointestinal upset, diarrhea, Clostridium difficile infection, and cost. Antibiotics are most important in patients at high risk of rheumatic heart disease, such as indigenous populations in Australia and specific lower socioeconomic status communities [20]. Rheumatic heart disease and rheumatic fever are two of the most common complications associated with rheumatic disease.

Recurrent tonsillitis is defined somewhat arbitrarily but is typically identified as five or more episodes of tonsillitis in one year [12]. Special consideration should be given to the cause; although rare, primary immunodeficiency requires care [21]. The

American Academy of Otolaryngology, Head and Neck Surgery has established guidelines for determining the need for surgical intervention. Studies show that tonsillectomy reduces school absences, painful throat days, and doctor-diagnosed illnesses, although these advantages do not last [22].

Streptococcus pyogenes (GABHS) is the most common cause of bacterial tonsillitis, and penicillins are the antibiotic of choice; these are typically a 10-day oral regimen or a single benzathine penicillin G intramuscular injection [14]. Medications like steroids and NSAIDs can provide symptomatic relief [15]. Hospital admission is rarely necessary. Azithromycin for five days is an alternative for penicillin-allergic individuals, as are cephalosporins or clindamycin for 10 days [15, 18].

54.9 Tonsillectomy

Chronic or recurrent tonsillitis associated with the streptococcal carrier state that has not responded to beta-lactamase-resistant antibiotics, or more than six episodes of streptococcal pharyngitis (confirmed by positive culture) in 1 year, five episodes in 2 consecutive years, or three or more infections in 3 years in a row, are indications for tonsillectomy. Multiple antibiotic allergies or intolerances, recurrent peritonsillar abscesses, and recurrent episodes of aphthous stomatitis, pharyngitis, and adenitis (PFAPA) indicate that a tonsillectomy should be considered for a kid.

Tonsillectomy is often recommended [2] based on the patient's age, the length of time they were sick, and other factors.

Most surgeons will remove inflamed adenoids at the time of tonsillectomy because the bacterial makeup of adenoid tissue is comparable to that of the palatine tonsils and because doing so adds minimal morbidity to the procedure. This, however, is with its detractors.

Getting tonsillitis again after having your tonsils removed is exceedingly unusual. Group A beta-hemolytic Streptococcus pyogenes (GABHS) bacterial loads are decreased after tonsillectomy, and a rise in alpha-Streptococcus, which can protect against GABHS infection, may be permitted. Excision of the tonsils is the standard treatment for chronic tonsillitis that has not responded to antibiotics [2].

Chronic tonsillitis is treated by removal of the tonsils, with or without the adenoids. Knowledge of a greater intraoperative and perioperative bleeding risk and that dissection may be more difficult due to fibrosis and scarring of the tonsillar capsule are two special technical issues for tonsillectomy patients with chronic tonsillitis. Such factors may have an impact on the choice of instruments and the timing of discharge [2].

While acute lingual tonsillitis cases seldom need surgical intervention, chronic and debilitating cases do. A tonsillectomy may be recommended if mononucleosis-related tonsillar hypertrophy causes breathing difficulties even after the infection has cleared [2].

References

1. Anderson J, Paterek E. Tonsillitis (Updated 2022 Sep 18). In: StatPearls (Internet). Treasure Island (FL): StatPearls Publishing; 2023. Available from: https://www.ncbi.nlm.nih.gov/books/NBK544342/.
2. Shah UK. Tonsillitis and peritonsillar abscess. In: Meyers AD, editor. Medscape; 2022. Updated: Feb 18, 2022. https://emedicine.medscape.com/article/871977-overview#a6 (Accessed online at June 4, 2023).
3. BuSaba N, Doron S. Tonsillectomy in adults: indications. In: Aronson MD, Deschler DG, Givens J, editors. UpToDate; 2021. last updated: Aug 24, 2021.
4. Woolford TJ, Hanif J, Washband S, Hari CK, Ganguli LA. The effect of previous antibiotic therapy on the bacteriology of the tonsils in children. Int J Clin Pract. 1999;53(2):96–8.
5. Wald ER. Group A streptococcal tonsillopharyngitis in children and adolescents: clinical features and diagnosis. In: Edwards MS, Messner AH, Blake D, editors. UpTodate; 2022. Last updated: Feb 01, 2022.
6. Shaikh N, Leonard E, Martin JM. Prevalence of streptococcal pharyngitis and streptococcal carriage in children: a meta-analysis. Pediatrics. 2010;126:e557.
7. Gunnarsson RK, Holm SE, Söderström M. The prevalence of beta-haemolytic streptococci in throat specimens from healthy children and adults. Implications for the clinical value of throat cultures. Scand J Prim Health Care. 1997;15:149.
8. Marshall HS, Richmond P, Nissen M, et al. Group A streptococcal carriage and seroepidemiology in children up to 10 years of age in Australia. Pediatr Infect Dis J. 2015;34:831.
9. Cohen JF, Pauchard JY, Hjelm N, et al. Efficacy and safety of rapid tests to guide antibiotic prescriptions for sore throat. Cochrane Database Syst Rev. 2020;6:CD012431.
10. McIsaac WJ, Kellner JD, Aufricht P, Vanjaka A, Low DE. Empirical validation of guidelines for the management of pharyngitis in children and adults. JAMA. 2004;291(13):1587–95.
11. ESCMID Sore Throat Guideline Group, Pelucchi C, Grigoryan L, Galeone C, Esposito S, Huovinen P, Little P, Verheij T. Guideline for the management of acute sore throat. Clin Microbiol Infect. 2012;18(Suppl. 1):1–28.
12. Georgalas CC, Tolley NS, Narula PA. Tonsillitis. BMJ Clin Evid. 2014;2014
13. Hamlyn E, Marriott D, Gallagher RM. Secondary syphilis presenting as tonsillitis in three patients. J Laryngol Otol. 2006;120(7):602–4.
14. Bartlett A, Bola S, Williams R. Acute tonsillitis and its complications: an overview. J R Nav Med Serv. 2015;101(1):69–73.
15. Stelter K. Tonsillitis and sore throat in children. GMS Curr Top Otorhinolaryngol Head Neck Surg. 2014;13:Doc07.
16. Wei JL, Kasperbauer JL, Weaver AL, Boggust AJ. Efficacy of single-dose dexamethasone as adjuvant therapy for acute pharyngitis. Laryngoscope. 2002;112(1):87–93.
17. Schams SC, Goldman RD. Steroids as adjuvant treatment of sore throat in acute bacterial pharyngitis. Can Fam Physician. 2012;58(1):52–4.
18. Sidell D, Shapiro NL. Acute tonsillitis. Infect Disord Drug Targets. 2012;12(4):271–6.
19. Gottlieb M, Long B, Koyfman A. Clinical mimics: an emergency medicine-focused review of streptococcal pharyngitis mimics. J Emerg Med. 2018;54(5):619–29.
20. Kocher JJ, Selby TD. Antibiotics for sore throat. Am Fam Physician. 2014;90(1):23–4.
21. Ickrath P, Morbach H, Schwaneck EC, Gehrke T, Scherzad A, Hagen R, Hackenberg S. Recurrent infections of the upper aerodigestive tract in patients with primary immunodeficiency. HNO. 2019;67(11):819–24.
22. Morad A, Sathe NA, Francis DO, McPheeters ML, Chinnadurai S. Tonsillectomy versus watchful waiting for recurrent throat infection: a systematic review. Pediatrics. 2017;139(2):e20163490.

Epiglottitis

55

Ali Budak, Cemal Cingi, and Yusuf Dundar

55.1 Introduction

Epiglottitis is characterized by the acute inflammation of the epiglottis, vallecula, arytenoids, and aryepiglottic folds, primarily affecting the supraglottic oropharynx region [1]. A historical note is that George Washington may have died from epiglottitis in 1799. In contemporary medicine, the gold standard for diagnosing suspected cases of epiglottitis is typically through nasopharyngoscopy and laryngoscopy, which enable direct visualization of the epiglottis. Radiographic assessment, which was previously used, has been largely replaced by these direct visualization techniques. It's crucial to note that the emergency airway management is imperative for critically ill patients with epiglottitis to ensure their airway is adequately maintained and to prevent life-threatening complications [2].

55.2 Etiology

Epiglottitis is typically caused by infectious agents such as bacteria, viruses, or fungi. Haemophilus influenzae type B (HIB) used to be the most common cause of epiglottitis in children, but widespread vaccination has significantly reduced this. Other bacterial culprits include Streptococcus pyogenes, Streptococcus pneumoniae, and Staphylococcus aureus [3–5]. In immunocompromised individuals,

A. Budak
Department of Otorhinolaryngology, Ankara Etlik City Hospital, Ankara, Turkey

C. Cingi (✉)
Medical Faculty, Department of Otorhinolaryngology, Eskisehir, Turkey

Y. Dundar
Department of Otolaryngology, Texas Tech University, Health Sciences Centre, Lubbock, TX, USA

H. Yüksel et al. (eds.), *Pediatric Airway Diseases*, Comprehensive ENT, https://doi.org/10.1007/978-3-031-74853-0_55

Pseudomonas aeruginosa and Candida can also lead to infections. Noninfectious causes, like injuries from heat, acid exposure, or foreign object ingestion, are another common source of illness [2]. While viruses don't directly cause epiglottitis, a preceding viral infection can create conditions conducive to bacterial superinfection. Viruses such as the Varicella-zoster virus, herpes simplex virus, and Epstein Barr virus can pave the way for secondary bacterial infections [1].

In adults, Haemophilus influenzae still accounts for some acute epiglottitis cases, along with other bacteria like H. parainfluenzae, Streptococcus pneumoniae, and group A streptococci. Other less common infectious causes include herpes simplex virus (HSV), other viruses, contagious mononucleosis, Candida (in immunocompromised patients), and Aspergillus (also in immunocompromised patients). As of 2007, methicillin-resistant Staphylococcus aureus (MRSA) had not been a common cause of epiglottitis despite its increasing importance as a pathogen in the general population [6].

Noninfectious factors can also trigger Epiglottitis, and these cases may present similarly to infectious ones. These potential causes encompass exposure to high temperatures (e.g., from smoking crack cocaine or marijuana), caustic insults (like ingesting dishwasher soap), ingestion of foreign bodies (such as accidentally swallowing and then expelling a bottle cap), and, rarely, as a side effect of chemotherapy for head and neck malignancies [7, 8].

55.2.1 Microbiology

Blood cultures can be collected in cases where the patient's overall health is compromised. In approximately 25% of adult cases of epiglottitis, blood cultures return positive results [2]. Blood culture and sensitivity testing can be precious in adults with epiglottitis because multiple infectious pathogens can lead to this condition. Specifically, 25% of individuals with acute epiglottitis have a positive blood culture for Haemophilus influenzae. In the remaining adult cases, pharyngeal cultures often identify H. parainfluenza, Streptococcus pneumoniae, and group A streptococci as causative agents [2]. If the patient's airway is clear, cultures can also be taken from the epiglottis. Some authors have reported successful aspiration of epiglottic abscesses using a spinal needle [9].

55.3 Pathophysiology

There are notable differences between the airways of children and adults. The epiglottis is higher and more forward in the neck in young children than in adults. The trachea in children also has a more horizontal orientation. The subglottis, the airway portion just below the vocal cords, is the narrowest part in infants and young children, while in adults, the narrowest part is typically at the glottis level. Moreover, the cartilage that makes up the epiglottis in newborns and young children is more flexible and malleable than in adults. This malleability is a normal part of cartilage maturation and contributes to the higher incidence of conditions like laryngomalacia in infants and toddlers. When the epiglottis is edematous (swollen), its flexibility allows it to be pulled over the laryngeal airway with each breath, which can lead to symptoms in children. The infectious process causing edema and the increased weight and mass of the epiglottis can compound these symptoms. In adults, the more rigid cartilage in the larynx and epiglottis may be better able to withstand an isolated infection in the epiglottis. However, when a disease or inflammatory process involves a more significant portion of the supraglottic tissues, causing widespread edema, it can lead to symptoms and an unstable airway in children and adults [1].

Patients of any age can develop severe edema and swelling of the epiglottis and supraglottis due to infections, often with Haemophilus influenzae (H. influenzae) or other pathogens. This can rapidly lead to airway obstruction, and although H. influenzae remains the most common pathogen, other bacteria like Streptococcus pneumoniae (S. pneumoniae), Staphylococcus aureus (S. aureus), and beta-hemolytic Streptococcus species are also frequently implicated [1]. The list of potential causative agents is more extensive in immunocompromised individuals and may include Mycobacterium tuberculosis and other pathogens.

55.4 Evaluation

Diagnosing epiglottitis is a critical and potentially life-threatening situation. Due to the risk of complications, including respiratory arrest, conducting an oropharyngeal exam, which might involve touching the throat, is typically avoided when assessing a suspected case of epiglottitis. Based on a patient's symptoms and physical examination findings, the clinical suspicion approach is the primary means of diagnosing this condition [1]. Imaging studies can help confirm the diagnosis and assess the severity. A classic finding on a lateral neck radiograph is the "thumb sign." This refers to the visible enlargement or bulging of the epiglottis, which can help the physician confirm the diagnosis. Still, it should only be attempted in cooperative, secure, and agreeable patients. Given the risk of laryngospasm, a flexible fiberoptic laryngoscopy is typically performed in a highly controlled environment, such as an operating room, and is rarely necessary. Ultrasonography has been suggested for assessing individuals with suspected epiglottitis, especially children. It can display an "alphabet P sign" in a longitudinal view, indicating epiglottal swelling. Still, it is crucial to consider the patient's clinical state and the use of ultrasonography should be guided by experienced medical professionals [1].

In cases of suspected acute epiglottitis, it's essential to promptly send the patient to the operating room for a thorough airway evaluation to determine the best course of action. Imaging techniques such as CT scans of the neck or chest X-rays are not typically part of the routine diagnostic process for epiglottitis due to the risk of worsening the patient's condition, especially if placed in a supine position [10]. In some cases, a chest X-ray might detect comorbid pneumonia, but only in patients who can be examined cautiously, as these procedures can carry risks. Ultimately, the diagnosis of epiglottitis is primarily clinical and relies on clinical suspicion, physical examination, and an understanding of the patient's symptoms and condition [11].

55.5 Prognosis

Acute adult epiglottitis can have a favorable prognosis when treated promptly and adequately. Most patients can be extubated within a few days following appropriate medical intervention. However, it's important to note that untreated epiglottitis can progress rapidly and lead to severe airway damage, respiratory failure, and death [2]. While the prognosis is generally favorable, there is still a risk of mortality in adults with acute epiglottitis, primarily due to airway complications. Patients with severe swelling of supraglottic tissues may present challenges in intubation, which can be life-threatening. In the intensive care unit (ICU), close monitoring and adequate airway protection are essential because cases of sudden cardiorespiratory arrest without a prior history of breathing obstruction have been reported. The rate of death among adults with acute epiglottitis is estimated to be around 7% [2]. Autopsies conducted on adult patients who succumbed to acute epiglottitis have revealed signs of hyperemia and edema in the epiglottis and aryepiglottic folds [12].

A retrospective study by Shapira Galitz and colleagues found that male patients, those with symptoms like dyspnea and stridor, individuals with edema in the epiglottis and aryepiglottic folds, those with elevated C-reactive protein levels, hyperglycemia, and patients with a history of recurrent episodes of epiglottitis were more likely to have a more severe or aggressive disease course [10]. This highlights the importance of prompt recognition and intervention in patients with risk factors or worsening symptoms.

55.6 Complications

The following are possible epiglottitis complications [2]:

- Meningitis.
- Epiglottic abscess.
- Cervical adenitis.
- Vocal granuloma.
- Subsequent necrotizing fasciitis of the head and neck (rare).
- Cartilaginous metaplasia of the epiglottis.
- Pneumonia.
- Pulmonary edema.
- Empyema.
- Pneumothorax.
- Pneumomediastinum (rare).

- Pericarditis.
- Septic arthritis.
- Cellulitis.
- Septic shock.
- Death (asphyxia)".

55.7 Physical Examination

The following are the possible physical manifestations of epiglottitis [13]:

- "Tripod position—Sitting up on hands, with the tongue out and the head forward
- Drooling/inability to handle secretions
- Stridor—A late finding indicating advanced airway obstruction
- Muffled voice (54%)
- Cervical adenopathy
- Fever
- Hypoxia
- Respiratory distress
- Severe pain on gentle palpation over the larynx or hyoid bone [3]
- Mild cough
- Irritability
- Tachycardia
- Toxic appearance of the patient"

55.8 Diagnosis

The introduction of the Haemophilus influenzae type b (Hib) vaccine has significantly reduced the incidence of epiglottitis. While this is a positive development in public health, it has also led to clinicians encountering this potentially life-threatening condition less frequently [14]. Consequently, there is a risk of delayed diagnosis. Given the potential causes of epiglottitis are not limited to Haemophilus influenzae, healthcare professionals need to maintain a high level of clinical suspicion and promptly recognize the condition when it does occur, particularly in adult patients. The diagnosis should rely on a combination of thorough clinical examination and any in-clinic diagnostic tools that can be employed rapidly [2].

When assessing a patient for acute epiglottitis, it's crucial to consider and rule out various conditions that may have similar presentations, such as acute angioedema, airway obstruction, bacterial laryngotracheobronchitis, caustic ingestion, thermal injuries from hot liquids or air (burns), foreign body aspiration, laryngeal diphtheria, laryngitis, laryngotracheal bronchopneumonitis, peritonsillar abscess, retropharyngeal abscess, and sepsis. A comprehensive evaluation is vital to differentiate between these conditions and accurately diagnose epiglottitis.

55.9 Differential Diagnoses

- Caustic ingestions.
- Peritonsillar abscess in emergency medicine.
- Retropharyngeal abscess must be ruled out [2].

55.10 How to Approach

Ensuring the patient's airway is of utmost importance when dealing with a suspected case of epiglottitis. Assessing the severity of the patient's distress should take precedence over further diagnostic testing. It's worth noting that adult patients often present with a lower severity level than children, but rapid deterioration can occur in any case [15]. It's crucial to involve an anesthesiologist and an ear, nose, and throat (ENT) specialist early in evaluating these patients. Having the necessary airway tools and equipment readily available is essential, including the capability to perform a cricothyrotomy if needed. Medical professionals have attempted to develop numerical scales to assess the severity of epiglottitis, which can help guide treatment [2].

The gold standard for diagnosing suspected epiglottitis in contemporary medical practice is direct visualization of the epiglottis through nasopharyngoscopy or laryngoscopy. The value of this direct visual examination, often facilitated by fiberoptic endoscopy, cannot be overstated [2]. Radiographic examination, particularly neck soft-tissue radiography, is less reliable and can miss a significant percentage of epiglottitis cases.

55.10.1 Stable Patients

A more conservative approach can be taken for patients with modest edema observed on laryngoscopy and without other critical airway signs, such as stridor, respiratory distress, or significant drooling. These patients should be closely monitored in the intensive care unit (ICU) without immediate airway intervention [2]. However, close attention to airway status is crucial due to the potential rapid progression of airway obstruction in such cases. Repeated serial examinations of airway patency should be conducted, and a low threshold for airway intervention should be maintained. Before extubating a patient, a thorough laryngoscopy examination is recommended [2]. It's crucial to have an anesthesiologist and an ear, nose, and throat (ENT) specialist readily available if rapid airway intervention is necessary during or after extubation. This careful and vigilant approach helps ensure patient safety and timely response to potential airway complications.

55.10.2 Unstable Patients

In the case of a critically ill patient with suspected epiglottitis, ensuring an open airway is paramount [2]. Several indicators signal the need for urgent intubation, including:

- Breathing problems: Patients struggling to breathe or in respiratory distress require immediate attention.
- Airway compromise on examination: When a healthcare provider observes significant obstruction or edema in the upper airway, securing the airway is crucial.
- Stridor: This high-pitched sound heard during breathing indicates a narrowed or partially blocked airway.
- Dysphagia: Difficulty swallowing, significantly if it contributes to airway compromise, warrants intervention.
- Drooling: Profuse drooling is often a sign of an inability to manage secretions and could suggest airway issues.
- Upright posture: Patients instinctively sit or stand upright to help open their airways.
- Rapid deterioration: When a patient's condition worsens significantly within 8–12 h, it strongly indicates prompt intervention.

Radiographs that reveal an enlarged epiglottis, often called the "thumb sign," can provide visual evidence of airway obstruction. If there is any uncertainty about the necessity for intervention, it's generally safer to secure the airway. In situations requiring immediate intervention, tracheostomy, cricothyrotomy, or intubation should occur in an operating room. To temporarily ventilate the patient, percutaneous transtracheal jet ventilation (PTJV) or needle-jet insufflation can be considered [16]. PTJV, in particular, may be attempted when direct laryngoscopy for tracheal intubation has already failed. PTJV can enhance the chances of success in subsequent intubation attempts by generating high intratracheal pressures, which can cause the glottis to appear lifted and opened, with the glottis' margins fluttering due to the escaping pressurized gases [2].

55.11 Treatment

Managing a patient with acute epiglottitis requires a careful and cautious approach [2]. Here are some key points to consider:

1. Comfort and Positioning: Keep the patient as comfortable as possible. Allow them to sit or position themselves in a way that feels most comfortable to them.
2. Readiness for Intubation: Be prepared for orotracheal intubation, as it might be necessary without much warning. Ensure that all intubation, cricothyroidotomy, or needle-jet ventilation equipment is readily available at the bedside.
3. Avoid Agitation: Do not agitate the patient. Avoid unnecessary procedures that could lead to agitation and respiratory distress. Sedation inhalers should be avoided.
4. Oxygen: Administer supplemental humidified oxygen if possible, but do not force the patient to use it. Forcing oxygen might agitate the patient, worsening their condition.
5. Clinical Pitfalls: Be aware of common clinical pitfalls, including underestimating the potential for sudden deterioration. Ensure adequate monitoring to detect

any changes promptly. If intubation is necessary, do not rush the procedure, and make sure there is proper support available, such as an experienced anesthesiologist for complex intubation cases.

6. Corticosteroid Therapy: Consider using dexamethasone or budesonide aerosols to treat pharyngeal edema, which can help reduce obstruction. Research suggests that corticosteroid therapy can also reduce the length of stay in the ICU and the hospital [17, 18].
7. Vaccination: Encourage vaccination, especially for children, to prevent epiglottitis. Vaccination schedules should be followed as recommended by the WHO [1]. Close contacts of patients with Haemophilus influenzae infections who are not immunized should also receive rifampin prophylaxis.

Preventative measures, including vaccination and a cautious approach to management, are critical in caring for patients with acute epiglottitis. Patients with recurrent episodes of acute epiglottitis should undergo investigation for underlying immunosuppressive conditions [1].

References

1. Guerra AM, Waseem M. Epiglottitis (Updated 2022 Oct 17). In: StatPearls. Treasure Island (FL): StatPearls Publishing; 2023. Available from: https://www.ncbi.nlm.nih.gov/books/NBK430960/.
2. Gompf SG. Epiglottitis. In: Taylor III JP, editor. Medscape; 2023. Updated: Apr 05, 2022. https://emedicine.medscape.com/article/763612-overview (Accessed online at June 4, 2023).
3. Schröder AS, Edler C, Sperhake JP. Sudden death from acute epiglottitis in a toddler. Forensic Sci Med Pathol. 2018;14(4):555–7.
4. Tsai YT, Huang EI, Chang GH, Tsai MS, Hsu CM, Yang YH, Lin MH, Liu CY, Li HY. Risk of acute epiglottitis in patients with preexisting diabetes mellitus: a population-based case-control study. PLoS One. 2018;13(6):e0199036.
5. Chen C, Natarajan M, Bianchi D, Aue G, Powers JH. Acute epiglottitis in the immunocompromised host: case report and review of the literature. Open Forum Infect Dis. 2018;5(3):ofy038.
6. Young LS, Price CS. Complicated adult epiglottitis due to methicillin-resistant Staphylococcus aureus. Am J Otolaryngol. 2007;28(6):441–3.
7. Kavanagh KR, Batti JS. Traumatic epiglottitis after foreign body ingestion. Int J Pediatr Otorhinolaryngol. 2008;72(6):901–3.
8. Wallenborn PA 3rd, Postma DS. Radiation recall supraglottitis. A hazard in head and neck chemotherapy. Arch Otolaryngol. 1984;110(9):614–7.
9. Kim SG, Lee JH, Park DJ, et al. Efficacy of spinal needle aspiration for epiglottic abscess in 90 patients with acute epiglottitis. Acta Otolaryngol. 2009;129(7):760–7.
10. Shapira Galitz Y, Shoffel-Havakuk H, Cohen O, Halperin D, Lahav Y. Adult acute supraglottitis: analysis of 358 patients for predictors of airway intervention. Laryngoscope. 2017;127(9):2106–12.
11. Solomon P, Weisbrod M, Irish JC, Gullane PJ. Adult epiglottitis: the Toronto Hospital experience. J Otolaryngol. 1998;27(6):332–6.
12. Bellis M, Herath J, Pollanen MS. Sudden death due to acute epiglottitis in adults: a retrospective review of 11 postmortem cases. Am J Forensic Med Pathol. 2016;37(4):275–8.
13. Lindquist B, Zachariah S, Kulkarni A. Adult epiglottitis: a case series. Perm J. 2017;21:16-089. https://doi.org/10.7812/TPP/16-089.

14. Mathoera RB, Wever PC, van Dorsten FR, Balter SG, de Jager CP. Epiglottitis in the adult patient. Neth J Med. 2008;66(9):373–7.
15. Ames WA, Ward VM, Tranter RM, Street M. Adult epiglottitis: an under-recognized, life-threatening condition. Br J Anaesth. 2000;85(5):795–7.
16. Chandradeva K, Palin C, Ghosh SM, Pinches SC. Percutaneous transtracheal jet ventilation as a guide to tracheal intubation in severe upper airway obstruction from supraglottic oedema. Br J Anaesth. 2005;94(5):683–6.
17. Guardiani E, Bliss M, Harley E. Supraglottitis in the era following widespread immunization against Haemophilus influenzae type B: evolving principles in diagnosis and management. Laryngoscope. 2010;120(11):2183–8.
18. Abdallah C. Acute epiglottitis: trends, diagnosis and management. Saudi J Anaesth. 2012;6(3):279–81.

Laryngitis 56

Berat Baturay Demirkiran, Nuray Bayar Muluk, and Stephan Lang

56.1 Introduction

One of the most frequent laryngeal disorders is laryngitis, a larynx inflammation. Both acute and chronic variants of this disease exist [1]. Acute laryngitis develops quickly and often resolves on its own. Chronic laryngitis is diagnosed when a patient has symptoms for more than three weeks. Acute laryngitis can be caused by abuse of the voice, exposure to toxic substances or an upper respiratory tract infection. The causative agents are usually viruses, but can also be bacteria [2]. In rare cases, inflammatory diseases such as rheumatoid arthritis, relapsing polychondritis, granulomatosis with polyangiitis, and sarcoidosis trigger laryngeal inflammation.

Acute laryngitis is not often caused by voice abuse. However, voice abuse often leads to this condition. A hoarse voice is a symptom of an underlying disease or inflammation. In most cases, the patient aggravates their dysphonia by abusing their voice in an attempt to regain their presymptomatic phonation [2].

The symptoms of chronic laryngitis last longer and the condition itself takes longer to develop. Inhaling cigarette smoke or polluted air (e.g., gaseous pollutants), irritation from asthma inhalers, voice abuse (e.g., speaking in an abnormally loud or high pitch for long periods) and gastro-oesophageal reflux are all environmental variables that can lead to chronic laryngitis. When the voice is abused, the vocal

B. B. Demirkiran
Çankiri State Hospital, ENT Clinic, Çankırı, Turkey

N. Bayar Muluk (✉)
Faculty of Medicine, Department of Otorhinolaryngology, Kırıkkale University, Kırıkkale, Turkey

S. Lang
Department of Otorhinolaryngology, Head and Neck Surgery, University Hospital Essen, Essen, Germany
e-mail: Stephan.Lang@uk-essen.de

H. Yüksel et al. (eds.), *Pediatric Airway Diseases*, Comprehensive ENT,
https://doi.org/10.1007/978-3-031-74853-0_56

folds adduct more forcefully, causing more contact and friction between them. The area of contact between the folds increases in size. Patients with persistent laryngitis due to voice abuse are the best candidates for voice therapy.

56.2 Anatomy of the Larynx

Besides its cartilaginous structure and intrinsic and extrinsic muscles, the larynx also has a mucosal coating [3].

There are three parts to the larynx: the supraglottis, the glottis, and the subglottis, respectively. The epiglottis, false vocal folds, aryepiglottic folds, and arytenoids are all components of the supraglottis, which extends above and beyond the genuine vocal folds. The glottis includes the vocal folds themselves and a 1-cm-lower region around them. The subglottis is the area below the glottis, from its inferior border to the cricoid cartilage's inferior border [4].

56.2.1 Cartilages

The larynx is held in place by soft tissue attachments to the hyoid bone and trachea in the front of the neck. The larynx is made up of a framework of nine cartilages. The thyroid, cricoid, and epiglottis cartilages are not paired, but the arytenoid, corniculate, and cuneiform cartilages are paired.

The thyroid, the largest of the laryngeal cartilages, forms a shield in front of the vocal folds. The laryngeal prominence, also known as the Adam's apple, is a midline protrusion that is more prominent in males than females and develops during puberty as a result of androgens.

Below the thyroid cartilage and above the tracheal inlet, the cricoid cartilage forms the only complete ring of the laryngeal skeleton, forming the subglottic area of the larynx. Damage to the mucosa in this area can lead to stenosis, as can occur after prolonged endotracheal intubation [4].

The arytenoids are a pair of pyramidal cartilages that lie on the posterior cricoid cartilage and are connected by a true diarthrodial articulation. The intrinsic laryngeal muscles are connected to the arytenoids, allowing complex movement and fine adjustment of the vocal folds. Vocal fold immobility and respiratory or phonatory dysfunction [4] may occur when there is interarytenoid fibrosis or fixation of the cricoarytenoid joint, as seen in rheumatoid arthritis or after trauma.

56.2.2 Vocal Folds

Muscle, fibrous ligament, Reinke's space, and mucosa form the genuine vocal folds, which run posterior from the vocal process of the arytenoid to the anterior midline of the thyroid cartilage [4].

There is a lateral depression in the laryngeal cavity, called the laryngeal ventricle, which separates the false (or "ventricular") vocal folds, which are located above, from the "true" vocal folds. The true vocal folds lack glandular components and are lubricated by mucus-producing glands in the ventricles. The false vocal folds usually adduct only during forceful glottic closure, such as during the Valsalva manoeuvre, or reflected laryngeal closure due to supraglottic irritation. Only in pathological circumstances, such as in individuals with a lack of glottic closure due to substance defects, vocal fold paralysis, neurological lesions or presbylarynx (vocal fold changes associated with ageing of the larynx), do they close together during phonation.

56.2.3 Extrinsic and Intrinsic Muscles

There are both extrinsic and intrinsic laryngeal muscles. The infrahyoid, suprahyoid, hyoglottic, and digastric muscles control laryngeal mobility. The larynx must be elevated during swallowing and fixed during the Valsalva manoeuvre. The only extrinsic laryngeal muscle is the cricothyroid muscle, which regulates the tension of the vocal folds. The intrinsic muscles are much more sensitive and regulate small changes in tension, glottal opening, and closure associated with phonation. The intrinsic muscles consist of the posterior cricoarytenoid, lateral cricoarytenoid, interarytenoid, and thyroarytenoid.

The lateral part of the vocal fold is mainly composed of the integral part of the thyroarytenoid muscle (vocal muscle). The cricoarytenoid joint enables the midline approximation (adduction) and lateral separation (abduction) of the vocal folds during phonation [4] and inspiration, respectively. The posterior cricoarytenoid muscle is only vocal fold opener.

Unlike the rest of the larynx, which is lined by respiratory epithelium (ciliated pseudostratified columnar epithelium), the mucosa of the vocal folds is composed of nonkeratinized stratified squamous epithelium, making the surface of the vocal folds more resistant to the repeated trauma of high-speed contact with the contralateral vocal fold. The subepithelial layer, called Reinke's space or superficial lamina propria, has a fluid viscosity due to mucopolysaccharides and mucoproteins. This allows the mucous membrane of the vocal folds to vibrate more quickly over the denser, fibrous tissue beneath. Damage to these layers through scarring or stiffening can lead to reduced vibration and voice quality [4].

56.2.4 Supply of Nerves

The recurrent laryngeal nerve emerges from the thoracic vagus segment and moves backwards towards the neck, winding around the aortic arch on the left and the subclavian artery on the right.

All intrinsic laryngeal muscles are innervated by the recurrent laryngeal nerve except the extrinsic cricothyroid muscle, which is innervated by the external branch of the superior laryngeal nerve. The lower pharynx and upper oesophagus also receive motor control from the vagus and recurrent laryngeal nerves via their direct pharyngeal branches. Damage to these nerves can result in paralysis of the vocal folds [4].

The internal branch of the superior laryngeal nerve provides sensory function above the vocal folds. The recurrent laryngeal nerve transmits sensory information from the area below the vocal cords. The vagus nerve also innervates the external auditory canal and hypopharynx. This can cause reflective coughing when the ear is cleaned, and irritation of the hypopharynx can cause discomfort in the ear [4].

56.3 Acute Laryngitis

Acute laryngitis typically results from inflammation in the larynx, often triggered by an upper respiratory tract infection or excessive vocal strain, and it usually resolves on its own within a three-week period. In adults with acute laryngitis, bacterial strains such as *Moraxella catarrhalis, Haemophilus influenzae*, and *Streptococcus pneumoniae* have been identified in their nasopharynx [5]. Common symptoms of an upper respiratory tract infection leading to hoarseness include a runny nose, cough, and a mild sore throat. In cases of acute vocal strain due to activities like shouting or prolonged coughing, there can also be submucosal microtrauma in the vocal folds, resulting in localized swelling and bleeding [4].

56.3.1 Etiology

Acute laryngitis can occur for a number of reasons [1].

Possible viruses of a cold include, for example, rhinovirus, parainfluenza virus, respiratory syncytial virus, different coronavirus, adenovirus, and influenza viruses. In children, the parainfluenza virus (most often parainfluenza-1) causes croup (laryngotracheobronchitis), similar to acute laryngitis in adults. A “barking” cough is a hallmark sign of this, and it can develop into inspiratory or biphasic stridor [6]. However, it can also occur as an isolated vocal symptom. Exanthematous febrile infections, including measles and chickenpox or whooping cough, can cause acute laryngitis symptoms. Therefore, it is essential to have a complete vaccination history.

If you have viral laryngitis, you might have a bacterial superinfection around a week after your symptoms first appear [1]. Streptococcus pneumoniae, Haemophilus influenzae, and Moraxella catarrhalis are the three most prevalent bacterial pathogens. Fungal infections seldom cause laryngitis in healthy people, but they frequently cause chronic laryngitis in those who are immunocompromised or who use inhaled steroid drugs [1].

Instead to infectious reasons voice abuse, overuse, allergies, laryngopharyngeal reflux, asthma, environmental toxins, smoking, inhalation trauma, and functional/conversion problems are all potential causes of acute noninfectious laryngitis [1].

Shouting and yelling for several days might cause immediate symptoms. This is a common reaction from coaches, spectators, and athletes after sporting events.. This also occurs among singers, especially those with a sudden rise in performance frequency or intensity but minimal vocal training [1].

Voice problems and laryngitis are frequently seen at patients with gastroesophageal reflux disease (GERD), especially the extraesophageal form of GERD known as laryngopharyngeal reflux (LPR). These symptoms can be severe or mild, persistent or sporadic. One third of people with gastro-oesophageal reflux experience laryngeal/voice symptoms that may not follow or accompany the usual GERD symptoms. Symptoms include a harsh or stern voice, a history of acid reflux, throat clearing or frequent coughing.

Laryngitis can be a complication of asthma because of the chemical irritation caused by inhalers, and long-term use of inhaled steroid can increase the risk of fungal laryngitis, especially if patients don't rinse their throat with water after using the inhalers. Voice changes resembling acute laryngitis can also be caused by cough-variant asthma due to repeated trauma to the vocal cords [1].

Acute laryngeal symptoms [1] can also be triggered by environmental factors such as seasonal and environmental allergies and seasonal or persistent air pollution.

Whether intentional through smoking or other drug abuse, or unintentional through exposure, the inhalation of toxic chemicals irritates the larynx, causing oedema of the vocal folds and voice problems. Patients may also be sensitive to everyday aromas such as perfumes, colognes, detergents, and more [1].

A variety of voice symptoms and physical examination findings fall under the term "functional dysphonia," which describes a group of conversion disorders. This is a diagnosis of exclusion, although it is well known that significant life stressors, such as the death of a loved one or the loss of a job, can cause symptoms [7]. It is therefore particularly important to distinguish spasmodic dysphonia of central neurological origin.

56.3.2 Pathophysiology

Acute laryngitis is diagnosed when there is inflammation of the larynx and vocal fold mucosa lasting for less than three weeks. When the vocal folds experience significant swelling, it affects the quality of their vibration, leading to potential hoarseness due to increased phonation threshold pressure. This, in turn, makes it challenging to generate sufficient phonation pressure. In cases of true aphonia, patients are unable to produce the required phonation pressure to move their vocal folds [2].

The vocal fold's membrane coating often presents with redness and swelling. This irregular thickening across the entire length of the vocal fold results in a lower pitch for individuals with laryngitis. Some authors suggest that, in certain cases, the vocal fold may become tight rather than thick. Generally, conservative treatment methods, as described below [2], can effectively resolve laryngeal inflammation, allowing the vocal folds to return to their normal vibratory function.

56.3.3 Acute Laryngitis, Symptoms, and Signs

The patient has dysphonia or a hoarse voice in addition to the typical signs of an upper respiratory tract infection (fever, cough, and rhinitis). Additionally, the following [2, 8] may occur to the person:

- Odynophonia
- Dysphagia
- Odynophagia
- Dyspnea
- Rhinorrhea
- Postnasal discharge
- Sore throat
- Nasal congestion
- Fatigue
- Malaise

56.3.4 Diagnosis

To see the larynx, direct or indirect laryngoscopy can be done. On close inspection, the inflamed vocal folds seem red with dilated capillary vessels and swollen.

Voice analysis shows vocal fold motion irregularities, including diminished mucosal waves and partial vibratory closure, asymmetry, and aperiodicity. The mucosal wave slows down as it travels [2].

56.3.5 Management of Acute Laryngitis

While waiting for laryngitis to clear up, the patient can take the following steps to make it more bearable [1, 2]:

The most important thing is to relax your voice. If you use your voice while suffering from laryngitis, your recovery will be slowed or stopped. It is recommended that you rest your voice completely. However, this isn't easy to achieve. Patients should be reminded to speak in a "confidential voice" or a normal phonatory voice at a low volume, without whispering or projecting, whenever possible.

In addition to voice preservation, voice therapy like lax vox voice therapy can support recovery.

Steam inhalation: Inhaling humidified air helps to clear secretions and exudate by increasing moisture in the upper airways. Clearing of secretions can also be supported with mucolytics such as guaifenesin [1].

It's recommended that irritants such as alcohol and tobacco are avoided. Smoking slows down the disease process and takes longer to heal.

Medication: There is no evidence to support the use of antibiotics to treat acute laryngitis in generally healthy people; however, these drugs may be prescribed for those at high risk of complications or with severe symptoms. Some authors recommend the use of broad-spectrum antibiotics without a positive gram stain and culture [1].

Oral antifungals such as fluconazole can be used to treat fungal laryngitis. A course of treatment usually lasts three weeks. However, it can be repeated if necessary. Only people with a proven fungal infection, as determined by throat examination and culture [1], should undergo this procedure.

Current data do not support antihistamine and corticosteroid usage.

Dietary and lifestyle changes, in addition to antireflux drugs, are used to treat laryngitic symptoms caused by gastroesophageal reflux. Gastroesophageal reflux disease can be effectively treated with antacid medications that inhibit acid production, such proton pump-blocking therapies [9, 10].

56.4 Chronic Laryngitis

Newly discovered etiopathogenetic variables related to the quality of environmental pollutants and hazardous products present in the workplace have rekindled interest in chronic laryngitis. Medical professionals are constantly struggling to keep up with the plethora of new hazardous and irritating products used in the industrial sector. Strategies that recognise the negative effects on the human body and provide the necessary remedial therapies are a very active area of research. Even in healthy individuals, persistent laryngitis symptoms may be present [11].

56.4.1 Pathophysiology

Chronic laryngitis is diagnosed when symptoms last over three weeks [12]. One or more long-term irritants usually cause chronic laryngitis and its accompanying inflammation. Chemical fumes and other inhaled pollutants, gastroesophageal reflux/laryngopharyngeal reflux, chronic sinusitis with postnasal drip, smoking, alcohol abuse, and prolonged use of the voice are all examples. Tobacco smoking has several adverse health effects, including an increased risk of laryngeal squamous cell carcinoma, vocal cord irritation, and benign alterations, such as hyper- and parakeratosis and polypoid chorditis [4].

The laryngeal mucosa is permanently altered by the inflammatory process that chronic laryngitis represents. The reactive and reparative processes of the larynx are the critical pathogenetic elements, and they may continue long after the triggering event has ceased. The pattern of changes is highly variable depending on the underlying factors. Levels of response to insults include inflammation, edema, hyperemia, infiltration, and mucosal proliferation [11].

Inflammation, especially in the back wall of the larynx, damages the ciliated epithelium lining the airways. As a result, the tracheobronchial tree is unable to perform its vital function of clearing mucus. When the ciliary beating of the epithelium is disrupted, mucus builds up on the back wall of the larynx and around the vocal cords, causing a reflex cough. In laryngospasm, mucus may accumulate on the vocal cords. Hyperkeratosis, dyskeratosis, parakeratosis, acanthosis, and cellular atypia [11] are all significant changes that can occur in the vocal cord epithelium.

56.4.1.1 Smoking

Cigarette smoke is linked to laryngeal inflammation via numerous proposed pathways [13]. Nicotine, carbon monoxide, formaldehyde, acetone, ammonia, and acrolein are only a few of the hundreds of chemicals included in cigarette smoke [14, 15] that cause inflammation and erythema of the laryngeal mucosa after inhalation [16, 17].

Cigarette smoke has been shown to increase the number of T lymphocytes (primarily CD8+) and macrophages within the bronchial wall [18], the number of neutrophils in bronchial secretions [19], and the number of mononuclear cells and macrophages in the periphery of the lung [20]. Furthermore, eosinophils infiltrate the submucosa at a higher rate in smokers' peripheral lung sections than in nonsmokers [20]. Despite their many roles in the immune system, eosinophils are most typically associated with asthma. Increased CD4+ T cell counts in smokers, and a correlation between higher CD4+ T cell counts and older age were found in a study of the immunologic effects of tobacco smoke on the laryngeal mucosa [21].

56.4.1.2 Laryngopharyngeal Reflux

Laryngopharyngeal reflux (LPR) is caused by the backward flow of stomach contents (acid and enzymes such pepsin) or basic duodenal bile beyond the upper esophageal sphincter, causing alterations in the larynx and pharynx's structure and function [22, 23]. Strong evidence links the development of interarytenoid mucosal hypertrophy and contact ulceration, with or without granuloma formation, to posterior laryngitis [24].

Clearing of the throat (98.3%), persistent cough (96.6%), heartburn/dyspepsia (95.7%), globus sensation (lump in the throat feeling; 94.9%), and change in voice quality (hoarseness; 94.9%) are the most prevalent symptoms associated with LPR [22]. Other symptoms include throat pain, difficulty of swallowing, and laryngospasm (the impression of choking). In most cases, signs shift and change with time. Patients who experience reflux symptoms in the laryngopharynx may not have reflux esophagitis, and tests may not show the presence of acid. Identifying LPR is addressed in greater depth elsewhere [4].

56.4.2 Chronic Laryngitis: Signs and Symptoms

Dysphonia and hoarseness of voice are common complaints. The volume and quality of one's voice may go up and down, but they only partially return [11].

Reportedly, nighttime is when chronic coughing is at its worst. Depending on how much the posterior wall of the larynx is affected, a cough caused by gastroesophageal reflux can be classified as dry or mucus-producing. Burping is possible [11].

If mucus strands pass through the vocal cords, laryngospasm might ensue, causing stridor.

Because the pharynx and the throat share innervation [11], dysphagia and otalgia can be detected when the pharynx is affected.

56.4.3 Diagnosis of Chronic Laryngitis

The following [11] are examples of laboratory experiments involving chronic laryngitis:

- If you suspect an infection, you should have a complete blood count and differential.
- Detection of bacterial, fungal, and viral pathogens using sputum culture and sensitivity.
- Laryngeal mucosa swab, bacterial, fungal, and viral culture and sensitivity.
- Autoimmune disease serological markers.
- Tests for syphilis and tuberculosis whenever such diseases are under consideration.

Imaging studies include the following [11]*:*

- Lateral plain neck radiograph
- Chest radiograph
- Computed tomography (CT) scanning and magnetic resonance imaging (MRI)
- Video fluoroscopic swallowing exam, double-contrast upper gastrointestinal (GI) series, esophageal manometry, multichannel intraluminal *impedance (MII)*-pH monitoring and pepsin and bile salt detection
- Videostrobe

If you think you have an allergy, a skin prick test can be conducted, and if you think you might have gastroesophageal reflux disease (GERD), a pH monitor can be worn for 24 h.

A bendable fiberoptic nasopharynx-laryngoscope allows for direct visualization of the larynx. For a thorough laryngeal examination, a rigid laryngoscope and direct laryngoscopy under general anesthesia may be necessary to retrieve tissue for biopsies, cultures, and smears to determine the presence of organisms. When other, less intrusive tests fail, it may be time to look closer [11].

Perform diagnostic procedures such as bronchoscopy and esophagoscopy on the aerodigestive system as needed. Mucosal stiffness due to epithelial hyperplasia, which may be produced by persistent inflammation [11], may be distinguishable by stroboscopic inspection.

56.4.4 Treatment of Persistent Laryngitis

Medication treatments primarily targeting the causal agents might be highly context-dependent. Drugs used to treat GERD fall into four categories: H2-receptor antagonists, proton pump inhibitors (PPI), alginates and prokinetics, but PPI and alginates are preferred [11].

References

1. Gupta G, Mahajan K. Acute laryngitis [Updated 2022 Sep 12]. In: StatPearls. Treasure Island (FL): StatPearls Publishing; 2023. Available from: https://www.ncbi.nlm.nih.gov/books/NBK534871/ (Accessed online at June 4, 2023).
2. Shah RK. Acute laryngitis. In: Meyers AD, editor. Medscape; 2023. Updated: Jan 05, 2023. https://emedicine.medscape.com/article/864671-overview (Accessed online at June 4, 2023).
3. Citardi MJ, Gracco CL, Sasaki CT. The anatomy of the human larynx. In: Rubin JS, Sataloff RT, Korovin GS, Gould GS, editors. Diagnosis and treatment of voice disorders. New York: Igaku-Shoin; 1995.
4. Bruch JM, Kamani DV. Hoarseness in adults. In: Deschler DG, Givens J, editors. UpToDate; 2021. Last updated: Jun 14, 2021.
5. Reveiz L, Cardona AF, Ospina EG. Antibiotics for acute laryngitis in adults. Cochrane Database Syst Rev. 2007:CD004783.
6. Mazurek H, Bręborowicz A, Doniec Z, Emeryk A, Krenke K, Kulus M, Zielnik-Jurkiewicz B. Acute subglottic laryngitis. Etiology, epidemiology, pathogenesis and clinical picture. Adv Respir Med. 2019;87(5):308–16.
7. Naunheim MR, Dai JB, Rubinstein BJ, Goldberg L, Weinberg A, Courey MS. A visual analog scale for patient-reported voice outcomes: the VAS voice. Laryngosc Investig Otolaryngol. 2020;5(1):90–5.
8. Postma GN, Koufman JA. Laryngitis. In: Bailey BJ, editor. Head and neck surgery-otolaryngology. 2nd ed. Philadelphia, PA: Lippincott-Raven; 1998. p. 731–9.
9. Modlin IM, Moss SF, Kidd M, et al. Gastroesophageal reflux disease: then and now. J Clin Gastroenterol. 2004;38(5):390–402.
10. Antunes C, Aleem A, Curtis SA. Gastroesophageal reflux disease. In: StatPearls. StatPearls Publishing; 2020.
11. Berliti S. Infectious or allergic chronic laryngitis. In: Meyers AD, editor. Medscape; 2019. Updated: Apr 17, 2019. https://emedicine.medscape.com/article/864767-overview#a5 (Accessed online at June 4, 2023).
12. Wood JM, Athanasiadis T, Allen J. Laryngitis. BMJ. 2014;349:g5827.
13. Jetté M. Toward an understanding of the pathophysiology of chronic laryngitis. Perspect ASHA Spec Interest Groups. 2016;1(3):14–25.
14. Sopori M. Effects of cigarette smoke on the immune system. Nat Rev Immunol. 2002;2:372–7.
15. Yoshida T, Tuder RM. Pathobiology of cigarette smoke-induced chronic obstructive pulmonary disease. Physiol Rev. 2007;87:1047–82.
16. Hardaker EL, Freeman MS, Dale N, Bahra P, Raza F, Banner KH, Poll C. Exposing rodents to a combination of tobacco smoke and lipopolysaccharide results in an exaggerated inflammatory response in the lung. Br J Pharmacol. 2010;160:1985–96.
17. van der Vaart H, Postma DS, Timens W, Hylkema MN, Willemse BW, Boezen HM, et al. Acute effects of cigarette smoking on inflammation in healthy intermittent smokers. Respir Res. 2005;6:22.
18. Di Stefano A, Capelli A, Lusuardi M, Caramori G, Balbo P, Ioli F, et al. Decreased T lymphocyte infiltration in bronchial biopsies of subjects with severe chronic obstructive pulmonary disease. Clin Exp Allergy. 2001;31:893–902.

19. Saetta M, Turato G. Airway pathology in asthma. Eur Respir J Suppl. 2001;34:18s–23s.
20. Lams BE, Sousa AR, Rees PJ, Lee TH. Immunopathology of the small-airway submucosa in smokers with and without chronic obstructive pulmonary disease. Am J Respir Crit Care Med. 1998;158(5 Pt 1):1518–23.
21. Rees LE, Jones PH, Ayoub O, Gunasekaran S, Rajkumar K, Stokes CR, et al. Smoking influences the immunological architecture of the human larynx. Clin Immunol. 2006;118:342–7.
22. Remacle M, Lawson G. Diagnosis and management of laryngopharyngeal reflux disease. Curr Opin Otolaryngol Head Neck Surg. 2006;14:143.
23. Koufman JA. The otolaryngologic manifestations of gastroesophageal reflux disease (GERD): a clinical investigation of 225 patients using ambulatory 24-h pH monitoring and an experimental investigation of the role of acid and pepsin in the development of laryngeal injury. Laryngoscope. 1991;101:1–78.
24. Cherry J, Margulies SI. Contact ulcer of the larynx. Laryngoscope. 1968;78:1937.

Tracheitis

57

Cem Bulut, Nuray Bayar Muluk, and Dennis Chua

57.1 Introduction

Bacterial tracheitis is a rare infectious cause of acute upper airway blockage, except in individuals with a tracheostomy or endotracheal tube. It is now more common in children who have received the Haemophilus type B immunization than acute epiglottitis. Even though patients with bacterial tracheitis may present with croup-like symptoms like barking cough, stridor, and fever, they do not respond to standard croup therapy (racemic epinephrine) and instead need antibiotic treatment and may experience acute respiratory decompensation [1–5].

57.2 Pathogenesis

Bacterial tracheitis is characterized by mucopurulent membranes that adhere or partially adhere to the tracheal mucosa and a generalized inflammatory response, including the larynx, trachea, and bronchi. Illness is most prevalent at the level of the cricoid cartilage, the narrowest section of the trachea. Subglottic edema and epithelial sloughing or mucopurulent membrane buildup within the trachea can lead to acute airway blockage. Symptoms are often milder than epiglottitis but more severe than croup [6, 7].

C. Bulut
Department of Otorhinolaryngology, Van Training and Research Hospital, Van, Turkey

N. Bayar Muluk (✉)
Department of Otorhinolaryngology, Kırıkkale University, Faculty of Medicine, Kırıkkale, Turkey

D. Chua
ENT Surgeons Medical Centre, Department of Otorhinolaryngology, Mount Elizabeth Hospital, Singapore, Singapore

H. Yüksel et al. (eds.), *Pediatric Airway Diseases*, Comprehensive ENT,
https://doi.org/10.1007/978-3-031-74853-0_57

Due to the size and structure of the subglottic airway, bacterial tracheitis may be more frequent in juvenile patients. When seen from the inside, the subglottis (the narrowest part of the pediatric airway) has funnel dimensions. Even minor edema can dramatically narrow the juvenile airway, making breathing more difficult and increasing breathing labor. Most people get well within five days [5] using breathing support and medications.

Bacterial tracheitis has an unknown cause. However, it may be related to mucosal damage or impaired local immune systems caused by a previous viral infection, tracheal injury from recent intubation, or trauma [5].

Some potentially pathogenic bacteria (such as Staphylococcus aureus, Streptococcus pneumoniae, Gram-negative enteric bacteria, and Pseudomonas aeruginosa) are found in the larynx of healthy people. Such colonization can spread into the trachea, at least temporarily [8, 9]. Babies born as early as 31 weeks gestation may already have bacteria colonizing their tracheas within the first 24 h of life [8].

Airway mucosal injury, such as that caused by a previous viral infection, is invariably present in cases of bacterial tracheitis [10, 11]. Bacterial tracheitis can also develop by aspirating bacteria-laden secretions into the trachea during an upper respiratory tract bacterial illness (such as acute bacterial sinusitis or streptococcal pharyngitis) or after a tonsillectomy [10, 12].

Since blood cultures are seldom positive [10, 13–16], tracheal infections rarely spread to the circulation.

The precise predisposing viral and bacterial etiology [17, 18] determine the pathologic findings. Edema, necrotic debris, and purulent discharges were shown to be significant contributors to the subglottic blockage that was observed in autopsies. The tracheal mucosa is swollen and red from excess blood flow. There may be necrotic or sloughed areas of mucosa. The mucosa and submucosa have cellular infiltrates of mononuclear and polymorphonuclear cells. There may be micro abscesses present [8, 19].

57.3 Microbiology

Frequently seen bacterial causes are as follows:

- S aureus: methicillin-resistant S aureus (MRSA) strains that cause tracheitis may become more common since CA-MRSA has recently emerged as a significant agent in the United States.
- The alpha-hemolytic streptococcal species, include Streptococcus pyogenes and Streptococcus pneumoniae.
- Moraxella catarrhalis has been linked to increased intubation rates and is now thought to be a primary cause of bacterial tracheitis.
- The incidence of disease caused by Haemophilus influenzae type B (Hib) has decreased with the advent of the Hib vaccination.
  - Klebsiella species.
  - Pseudomonas species.
  - Anaerobes.

- Peptostreptococcus species.
- Bacteroides species.
- Prevotella species.
- Other.
  Mycoplasma pneumoniae.
  Mycobacterium tuberculosis (endobronchial disease).
  H1N1 influenza [20].

57.3.1 Predisposing Viruses

Influenza A and B, parainfluenza, respiratory syncytial virus, rhinovirus, measles, and enterovirus have all been identified in children with bacterial tracheitis [11, 18, 21–23]. The most frequent cocirculating viruses are parainfluenza and influenza A [22, 23]. In immunocompromised people, the herpes simplex virus may predispose to and induce tracheitis [8, 24–26].

57.4 History

Bacterial tracheitis may present with symptoms that are between epiglottitis and croup. Acute or subacute manifestations have been described [5].

- Acute onset of high fever, poisonous look, stridor, tachypnea, respiratory distress, and elevated WBC counts characterize the typical presentation. Constant, nonpainful coughing fits.
- A large proportion of older children (mean age, eight y) in a study by Salamone et al. did not exhibit severe clinical symptoms [27].
- An upper respiratory infection often serves as a precursor, and then increased fever, cough, inspiratory stridor, and varied degrees of respiratory distress follow [28].
- A purulent membrane that has become loose in the airway might cause rapid decompensation, manifesting as increased respiratory discomfort in the patient.

Patients with tracheal infections caused by exotoxin-producing Staphylococcus aureus or Streptococcus pyogenes have been documented to exhibit symptoms and signs of bacterial tracheitis and multiorgan failure.

Doctors should suspect bacterial tracheitis if a kid with viral croup-like symptoms does not improve with typical croup treatment or worsens.

57.5 Clinical Characteristics

Clinical manifestations of bacterial tracheitis are mainly those of airway blockage, including stridor, cough, and respiratory distress. Controlling the airway is the first order of business in children exhibiting symptoms of severe airway blockage or impending respiratory failure (such as significant retractions, inadequate air entry, weariness, listlessness, or decreased awareness). Due to their smaller airway width, children under 2–3 years old may be at a higher risk of developing a life-threatening illness [8, 22].

57.5.1 Signs and Symptoms

Typical clinical characteristics consist of [8, 23]:

Fever (specific, though not always).
Inspiratory or biphasic stride.
Expired mucus from the respiratory tract.
Breathing problems.
Swallowing disorders, also known as odynophagia.
Drooling is unusual. However, it might be present.
Voice changes, such as hoarseness.
Increasing or sudden stridor [5].
Symptoms of respiratory distress can range in severity

- Withdrawals.
- Breathing problems.

Flaring of the nose.
To be cyanosed.
Symptoms of dysphonia.
The patient can lie in any comfortable posture, including supine [5].

Neck discomfort, orthopnea, choking, dysphagia, dysphonia, and syncope are more unusual but recorded symptoms and signs [13, 16]. Cyanosis, drowsiness, and aggressive behavior (due to hypoxemia and hypercarbia) are also possible in patients with severe blockage [29].

In most cases, a viral illness (such as parainfluenza or respiratory syncytial virus) is to blame for hoarseness and wheezing. Still, sometimes, they can be caused by a bacterial infection of the laryngeal tissues or an infection that spreads from the trachea into the bronchial tree. In addition to the above symptoms, signs of the underlying viral infection, bacterial sepsis, or toxin production may also be present, such as rhinorrhea, exanthems, pharyngitis, poor perfusion, erythroderma, lethargy, and so on [8].

S. aureus has been linked to toxic shock syndrome and scarlet fever. Germs from Staphylococcus aureus and Streptococcus group A cause bacterial tracheitis ages [30–32].

57.6 Diagnosis

Acute onset of airway obstruction with consistent clinical and radiographic characteristics in the context of a prior viral upper respiratory illness supports a presumptive diagnosis of bacterial tracheitis [22, 33–35]. Though very indicative, high fevers, a toxic look, and a poor response to therapy with nebulized epinephrine are not always present [36].

It is impossible to confirm or rule out a diagnosis using laboratory findings (such as white blood cell count or inflammatory markers) [8].

Bacterial tracheitis may only be diagnosed conclusively with a bronchoscopy involving laryngoscopy and trachea-bronchoscopy to see the airway [8] directly. Bronchoscopy is not necessary for all of the afflicted youngsters, though. The intensity of the manifestation is a significant factor in making the call [8].

Method—We use the following criteria [13, 23] to decide if a bronchoscopy is necessary.

Controlling the airway is the first order of business in children presenting with symptoms of imminent respiratory failure (such as significant airway blockage, pronounced retractions, inadequate air entry, weariness, listlessness, and a reduced state of awareness). The patient should be sent to the operating room as soon as possible so that an artificial airway may be placed. Once the youngster is stable, an operative bronchoscopy is done. The airway management is elaborated on in more depth elsewhere.

Bronchoscopy is performed in the operating room for children who do not have respiratory failure but who have a high clinical suspicion for bacterial tracheitis (for example, a child who develops sudden airway obstruction (stridor and dyspnea) after a viral upper respiratory infection, who does not respond well to inhaled epinephrine, and who has a tracheal irregularity on airway radiograph). Exudates in the trachea can be debrided using rigid bronchoscopy, which may improve the patient's condition enough to avoid intubation [13, 22].

Bedside flexible laryngoscopy is the first examination line for children presenting with less severe symptoms (such as stridor, cough, odynophagia, and fever without considerable respiratory distress). If a flexible laryngoscopy reveals purulent secretions that do not clear up with suctioning, or if the kid subsequently develops more severe airway blockage, we proceed to operational bronchoscopy.

Bronchoscopy reveals typical symptoms such as subglottic constriction (edema, erythema) and thick, purulent tracheal secretions [10, 19]. Exudate may spread into the bronchi, and pseudomembranes may be seen [15]. Endoscopy can remove purulent fluids and pseudomembranes if necessary [36]. The involvement of the neighboring laryngeal structures is uncertain. In most cases, the epiglottis looks normal. However, it occasionally becomes somewhat erythematous. Purulent exudates may also cover the rest of the larynx, which is uncommon. Mainstem bronchi involvement is common, and exudates may go lower in the bronchial tree [14, 18].

Both the quantity and nature of the identifying fluids might change. Minimal or no exudates may be seen in moderate instances. Exudates can be so thick and widespread in extreme cases that they are impossible to cough up [18]. Exudates can either remain attached to the tracheal lumen as pseudomembranes or separate from the trachea [14, 22, 37]. It has also been noted that thick, inspissated mucus casts attach to the tracheal wall [38].

The tracheal mucosa may initially seem only red and swollen. Still, if left untreated, it may eventually become coated by an exudate with a dry, glazed, gray surface, potentially reducing airflow [17]. Significant damage to the tracheal mucosa and submucosal layers is possible. There have been reports of perforation and pneumomediastinum [18].

Children suspected of having bacterial tracheitis undergo a battery of microbiological tests, which include [8]:

Patients needing ventilatory assistance should have bronchoscopy or endotracheal intubation performed to collect respiratory specimens for Gram stain and cultures (aerobic and anaerobic). Although young children typically cannot deliver an adequate expectorated sputum specimen, this does not rule out the possibility for patients who do not require these treatments.

Rapid viral antigen or polymerase chain reaction-based assays for individual agents or panels of agents should be performed on tracheal or upper respiratory specimens for viral testing. Understanding and describing the course of sickness may be aided by documenting a viral etiology.

All patients should have blood cultures taken. However, it is unusual for a kid with bacterial tracheitis to get a positive result [10, 13, 14–16].

57.6.1 Radiographic Features

Radiographic evaluation should be postponed until after airway control has been achieved [8] in patients exhibiting signs of severe airway obstruction or impending respiratory failure (such as marked retractions, poor air entry, fatigue, listlessness, or a depressed level of consciousness).

Without an artificial airway, a lateral neck or anteroposterior radiograph often reveals subglottic tracheal constriction (steeple sign). This observation, however, is not disease-specific and may be observed in healthy youngsters during inspiration. It is typical, but not universal, for the tracheal mucosa to have uneven borders below the subglottis and for there to be irregular or linear shadows (membranes) in the tracheal lumen. As the exudates or pseudomembranes move or are expectorated, a series of radiographs may show that the clouds associated with them alter or vanish [14, 37]. Foreign entities in the airway may be exudates or pseudomembranes [14, 34, 37].

Pulmonary infiltrates, atelectasis, hyperinflation, and pulmonary edema are additional signs that may be seen [12, 21, 30, 39].

57.7 Differential Diagnosis

Bacterial tracheitis can be ruled out by ruling out other causes of acute respiratory distress, such as severe obstructive dyspnea and fever [15].

Foreign body aspiration, diphtheria, and severe bacterial pneumonia (particularly with accompanying parapneumonic effusion or empyema), as well as epiglottitis, croup, peritonsillar or retropharyngeal abscess, or cellulitis, are all critical problems that are briefly covered below [8].

57.7.1 Epiglottitis

The symptoms of epiglottitis are similar to those of primary bacterial tracheitis, including a sudden onset of upper airway blockage, fever, and a poisonous look. The tripod position is preferred by children with epiglottitis, who also typically exhibit dysphagia, drooling, and discomfort. Drooling is unusual but has been reported in cases of bacterial tracheitis, which typically has a less severe appearance. Radiographic findings also vary between epiglottitis (characterized by an enlarged epiglottis, popularly known as the "thumb sign") and bacterial tracheitis. Tracheoscopy, however, may be required for diagnosis.

57.7.2 Croup

Clinical and radiological aspects of bacterial tracheitis are similar to croup (viral laryngotracheitis), especially when croup is the underlying predisposing condition. If the clinical course of croup significantly worsens (e.g., high fever, poisonous look, and increase in respiratory distress), and if the child does not respond well to nebulized epinephrine or glucocorticoids [23, 36], then bacterial tracheitis should be recognized as a consequence of croup.

57.7.3 Peritonsillar or Retropharyngeal Cellulitis/Abscess

In contrast to the absence of these symptoms in children with bacterial tracheitis, drooling, a change in voice quality, and a reluctance to move the neck are common presentations of peritonsillar or retropharyngeal cellulitis/abscess and other painful infections of the oropharynx in young children.

57.7.4 Severe Bacterial Pneumonia

Bacterial tracheitis (which may spread into the lung parenchyma) may be difficult to discern from severe bacterial pneumonia if both conditions are present. In children with pulmonary infiltrates, bacterial tracheitis should be suspected in the presence of either (1) stridor or other indications of respiratory distress disproportionate to the lung illness seen on plain radiographs or (2) irregular tracheal markings or intratracheal opacities.

57.7.5 Foreign Body Aspiration

Aspiration of a foreign body into the larynx or trachea can result in full or partial airway blockage and needs emergency care. Airway compression can be caused by a foreign body stuck in the esophagus at the cricoid cartilage or the tracheal bifurcation. Rapid onset of symptoms is expected. However, unlike bacterial tracheitis, fever is typically absent. Radiographs of the trachea may show similarities between a foreign body and tracheal exudates or pseudomembranes [34, 38]. An endoscopy may be required to tell the difference between a foreign body in the trachea and bacterial tracheitis.

57.7.6 Diphtheria

It can manifest clinically in ways that are similar to bacterial tracheitis. In most cases, symptoms develop slowly over time. Common first manifestations include fever, general malaise, and sore throat. You may see a diphtheritic membrane (it'll be gray with clear borders). Countries with high vaccination rates against diphtheria, tetanus, and pertussis have a very low incidence of diphtheria.

57.7.7 Inflammatory Bowel Disease (IBD)

Bacterial tracheitis can occasionally seem like the tracheal inflammation caused by inflammatory bowel disease (IBD). Inflammatory bowel disease often manifests in a subacute or chronic form. Bronchoscopy findings may include nodular mucosal edema, tiny erythematous lesions, and white granular lesions. Lymphocyte and plasma cell infiltrations are sometimes seen in biopsies [40–42].

57.8 Medical Care

The following [5] components make up the treatment for bacterial tracheitis:

- Airway.
  - Keeping a clear airway open is priority number one [43].
  - Do not provoke the kid. Bag-valve-mask ventilation should be beneficial if the patient's respiratory status worsens due to membrane movement.
  - When intubating a patient with subglottic inflammation, it is recommended to use an endotracheal tube that is 0.5–1 size smaller than usual. Endotracheal tube patency must be maintained with regular suctioning and high air humidity; hence, the most petite tube must be used (to avoid trauma). Between 57% and 100% of patients ultimately need intubation.
- Medication and intravenous access.
  - After breathing has been restored, an IV should be started to provide antibiotics.
  - Third-generation cephalosporins (such as cefotaxime and ceftriaxone) and penicillinase-resistant penicillins (such as oxacillin and nafcillin) have long been part of antibiotic treatment plans. For the treatment of community-acquired methicillin-resistant S. aureus (CA-MRSA), clindamycin (40 mg/

kg/d intravenously (IV), split every eighth) has recently replaced penicillinase-resistant penicillin in areas with low clindamycin resistance rates [44].

– Patients who seem toxic, those with multiorgan involvement, and those living in areas with a high prevalence of methicillin-resistant Staphylococcus aureus (MRSA) should begin treatment with vancomycin (45 mg/kg/d IV, divided every eighth).

References

1. Huang YL, Peng CC, Chiu NC, et al. Bacterial tracheitis in pediatrics: 12 year experience at a medical center in Taiwan. Pediatr Int. 2009;51(1):110–3.
2. Johnson D. Croup. Clin Evid. 2009;2009
3. Holmes A. Croup: what it is and how to treat it. US Pharm. 2013;38(7):47–50.
4. Burton LV, Lofgren DH, Silberman M. Bacterial tracheitis (Updated 2023 Jan 31). In: StatPearls. Treasure Island (FL): StatPearls Publishing; 2023. Available from: https://www.ncbi.nlm.nih.gov/books/NBK470240/ (Accessed online at June 4, 2023).
5. Rajan S. Bacterial tracheitis treatment and management. In: Steele RW, editor. Medscape; 2023. Updated: Nov 26, 2018. https://emedicine.medscape.com/article/961647-treatment (Accessed online at June 4, 2023).
6. Zoorob R, Sidani M, Murray J. Croup: an overview. Am Fam Physician. 2011;83(9):1067–73.
7. Tan AK, Manoukian JJ. Hospitalized croup (bacterial and viral): the role of rigid endoscopy. J Otolaryngol. 1992;21(1):48–53.
8. Woods CR. Bacterial tracheitis in children: Clinical features and diagnosis. In: Isaacson GC, Kaplan SL, Armsby C, editors. UpTodate; 2023. Last updated: Jan 12, 2023.
9. Hjuler IM, Hansen MB, Olsen B, Renneberg J. Bacterial colonization of the larynx and trachea in healthy children. Acta Paediatr. 1995;84:566.
10. Liston SL, Gehrz RC, Siegel LG, Tilelli J. Bacterial tracheitis. Am J Dis Child. 1983;137:764.
11. Edwards KM, Dundon MC, Altemeier WA. Bacterial tracheitis as a complication of viral croup. Pediatr Infect Dis. 1983;2:390.
12. Eid NS, Jones VF. Bacterial tracheitis as a complication of tonsillectomy and adenoidectomy. J Pediatr. 1994;125:401.
13. Gallagher PG, Myer CM 3rd. An approach to the diagnosis and treatment of membranous laryngotracheobronchitis in infants and children. Pediatr Emerg Care. 1991;7:337.
14. Henry RL, Mellis CM, Benjamin B. Pseudomembranous croup. Arch Dis Child. 1983;58:180.
15. Dudin AA, Thalji A, Rambaud-Cousson A. Bacterial tracheitis among children hospitalized for severe obstructive dyspnea. Pediatr Infect Dis J. 1990;9:293.
16. Bernstein T, Brilli R, Jacobs B. Is bacterial tracheitis changing? A 14-month experience in a pediatric intensive care unit. Clin Infect Dis. 1998;27:458.
17. Orton HB, Smith EL, Bell HO, Ford RA. Acute laryngotracheobronchitis. Arch Otolaryngol. 1941;33:926.
18. Neffson AH. Acute laryngotracheobronchitis: a 25 year review. Am J Med Sci. 1944;208:524.
19. Liston SL, Gehrz RC, Jarvis CW. Bacterial tracheitis. Arch Otolaryngol. 1981;107:561.
20. Hopkins BS, Johnson KE, Ksiazek JM, et al. H1N1 influenza A presenting as bacterial tracheitis. Otolaryngol Head Neck Surg. 2010 Apr;142(4):612–4.
21. Donnelly BW, McMillan JA, Weiner LB. Bacterial tracheitis: report of eight new cases and review. Rev Infect Dis. 1990;12:729.
22. Salamone FN, Bobbitt DB, Myer CM, et al. Bacterial tracheitis reexamined: is there a less severe manifestation? Otolaryngol Head Neck Surg. 2004;131:871.
23. Casazza G, Graham ME, Nelson D, et al. Pediatric bacterial tracheitis-a variable entity: case series with literature review. Otolaryngol Head Neck Surg. 2019;160:546.

24. Alvarez-Uria G, Surinach JM, Ventura A, et al. Herpetic tracheitis and polybacterial pneumonia in an immunocompetent young man is herpes tracheitis involved in the pathogenesis of bacterial pneumonia? J Clin Virol. 2008;41:164.
25. McCarthy DW, Qualman SJ, Rudman DT, et al. Herpetic tracheitis and brachial plexus neuropathy in a child with burns. J Burn Care Rehabil. 1999;20:377.
26. Baras L, Farber CM, Van Vooren JP, Parent D. Herpes simplex virus tracheitis in a patient with the acquired immunodeficiency syndrome. Eur Respir J. 1994;7:2091.
27. Salamone FN, Bobbitt DB, Myer CM, Rutter MJ, Greinwald JH Jr. Bacterial tracheitis reexamined: is there a less severe manifestation? Otolaryngol Head Neck Surg. 2004;131(6):871–6.
28. Casazza G, Graham ME, Nelson D, Chaulk D, Sandweiss D, Meier J. Pediatric bacterial tracheitis—a variable entity: case series with literature review. Otolaryngol Head Neck Surg. 2018:194599818808774. (QxMD MEDLINE Link)
29. Graf J, Stein F. Tracheitis in pediatric patients. Semin Pediatr Infect Dis. 2006;17:11.
30. Kasian GF, Bingham WT, Steinberg J, et al. Bacterial tracheitis in children. CMAJ. 1989;140:46.
31. Surh L, Read SE. Staphylococcal tracheitis and toxic shock syndrome in a young child. J Pediatr. 1984;105:585.
32. Naqvi SH, Dunkle LM. Bacterial tracheitis and viral croup. Pediatr Infect Dis. 1984;3:282.
33. Hopkins A, Lahiri T, Salerno R, Heath B. Changing epidemiology of life-threatening upper airway infections: the reemergence of bacterial tracheitis. Pediatrics. 2006;118:1418.
34. Friedman EM, Jorgensen K, Healy GB, McGill TJ. Bacterial tracheitis—two-year experience. Laryngoscope. 1985;95:9.
35. Walner DL, Ouanounou S, Donnelly LF, Cotton RT. Utility of radiographs in the evaluation of pediatric upper airway obstruction. Ann Otol Rhinol Laryngol. 1999;108:378.
36. Eckel HE, Widemann B, Damm M, Roth B. Airway endoscopy in the diagnosis and treatment of bacterial tracheitis in children. Int J Pediatr Otorhinolaryngol. 1993;27:147.
37. Han BK, Dunbar JS, Striker TW. Membranous laryngotracheobronchitis (membranous croup). AJR Am J Roentgenol. 1979;133:53.
38. Denneny JC 3rd, Handler SD. Membranous laryngotracheobronchitis. Pediatrics. 1982;70:705.
39. Jones R, Santos JI, Overall JC Jr. Bacterial tracheitis. JAMA. 1979;242:721.
40. Kinebuchi S, Oohashi K, Takada T, et al. Tracheo-bronchitis associated with Crohn's disease improved on inhaled corticotherapy. Intern Med. 2004;43:829.
41. Rickli H, Fretz C, Hoffman M, et al. Severe inflammatory upper airway stenosis in ulcerative colitis. Eur Respir J. 1994;7:1899.
42. Vorel ES, Mehta JJ, Russo ME, et al. A 7-year-old with persistent fever and cough. Pediatrics. 2022;150(3):e2021050751.
43. Mandal A, Kabra SK, Lodha R. Upper Airway Obstruction in Children. Indian J Pediatr. 2015;82(8):737–44.
44. Fergie J, Purcell K. The treatment of community-acquired methicillin-resistant Staphylococcus aureus infections. Pediatr Infect Dis J. 2008;27(1):67–8.

58 Peritonsillar Abscess

Berzan Haznedar, Nuray Bayar Muluk, and Suela Sallavaci

58.1 Introduction

Although peritonsillar abscess (PTA) was initially documented in the fourteenth century, the ailment was thoroughly defined in the development of antibiotics in the twentieth century. Suppurative tonsillitis can lead to a PTA, an accumulation of pus in the peritonsillar tissues. As an alternative, Weber gland abscess [1], located in the supra tonsillar fossa, is thought to cause PTA.

The center of the masform is sandwiched between the palatine tonsil capsule and the pharyngeal constrictor muscles. Boundaries of the peritonsillar space are the anterior and posterior pillars, the superior torus tubarius, and the inferior pyriform sinus. Loose connective tissue means that a severe infection here might quickly result in the development of purulent material. The base of the tongue, the lateral wall of the pharynx, and the soft palate may all become inflamed and suppurate as the infection spreads [1].

PTA is a common aftereffect of severe tonsillitis. Swallowing can be made very difficult by inflammation edema. As a result of trying to avoid the pain associated with eating and drinking, patients often end up dehydrated. Inflammation from an abscess can spread to neighboring fascial compartments in the head and neck, which can eventually block the airway [1] if the abscess grows large enough.

B. Haznedar
Gazi Yaşargil Training and Research Hospital, ENT Clinic, Diyarbakır, Turkey

N. Bayar Muluk (✉)
Faculty of Medicine, Department of Otorhinolaryngology, Kırıkkale University, Kırıkkale, Turkey

S. Sallavaci
Department of Otorhinolaryngology, University Hospital Centre "Mother Teresa", Tirana, Albania

H. Yüksel et al. (eds.), *Pediatric Airway Diseases*, Comprehensive ENT,
https://doi.org/10.1007/978-3-031-74853-0_58

58.2 Definition

Infection of the peritonsillar space is referred to by two different terminologies [2]:

Infected tissue between the palatine tonsil capsule and the pharyngeal muscles can become inflamed, resulting in peritonsillar cellulitis. An accumulation of pus does not typically accompany this condition. Cellulitis is also known as phlegmon.

Pus collects between the palatine tonsil capsule and the pharyngeal muscles, forming a peritonsillar abscess.

Needle aspiration or incision and drainage to determine the presence of pus is often necessary to ascertain the peritonsillar infection present [2].

58.3 Anatomy

Between the palatoglossal and palatopharyngeal folds of the oropharynx are a pair of lymphoid structures known as the palatine tonsils. A narrow capsule separates the tonsil from the superior and intermediate constrictor muscles [1].

The peritonsillar space is bounded on either side by the anterior and posterior pillars. This hypothetical region is connected to the superior torus tuberous and the inferior pyriform sinus. Only consisting of amorphous connective tissue, pus can quickly develop in response to a severe illness. The soft palate, the lateral wall of the pharynx, and even the base of the tongue might become inflamed and suppurative [1].

This clinical pattern of adenopathy is due to the tonsillar fossa's dense network of lymphatic arteries that drain into the parapharyngeal space and the upper cervical lymph nodes. The spread of infection to the regional lymphatics causes ipsilateral upper cervical lymphadenopathy. Particularly, in fulminant or fast-progressing instances [1], the suppurative process may become very severe that an abscess forms in the cervical region.

58.4 Pathophysiology

It has yet to be determined what causes PTA or why. The most commonly held belief is that exudative tonsillitis leads to peritonsillitis and, ultimately, an abscess. The inflammatory process can continue expanding in both treated and untreated people. It has also been shown that PTA can develop in people who have never had tonsillitis before. Epstein-Barr virus (mononucleosis) can manifest clinically as a PTA [1].

Weber glands are the supposed source of PTA, according to another idea. The tonsils are supposed to benefit from the secretions of these tiny salivary glands located in the peritonsillar area. The growth of necrotic tissue and an abscess due to an infection-caused blockage causes PTA [1].

58.5 Microbiology

In most cases, many bacteria or viruses contribute to a peritonsillar abscess. Group A streptococcus (GAS), Streptococcus anginosus, Staphylococcus aureus (including methicillin-resistant S. aureus; MRSA), and respiratory anaerobes (including Fusobacteria, Prevotella, and Veillonella species) are the most common bacterial pathogens in this area [3–7]. Rarely, you may come across a Haemophilus species. Aerobes and anaerobes are often recovered together [2] if the proper microbiologic procedures are applied.

58.6 Evaluation

Rapid assessment of the degree of upper airway obstruction is the first step in examining a patient suspected of having a deep neck space infection. Continually monitoring anxious, ill-appearing patients who are drooling and tripoding (leaning forward with the head in a sniffing position) is required in a setting where an emergency artificial airway can be introduced [2].

Clinical manifestations include severe painful throat (typically on one side), fever, and a "hot potato" or muffled voice, and these symptoms are characteristic of peritonsillar abscess (PTA). Drooling or pooling of saliva is possible. Nearly two-thirds of patients experience trismus due to irritation and reflex spasms of the internal pterygoid muscle, which helps to differentiate PTA from severe pharyngitis or tonsillitis [8, 9]. Swelling and discomfort in the neck are joint, and patients may also have pain in the ipsilateral ear [10]. Discomfort might cause fatigue, irritation, and reduced oral intake [2].

The past should inform management decisions. Frequency and severity of recurring bouts of viral pharyngitis, history of PTA, and snoring or other symptoms of obstructive sleep apnea [2] are all essential parts of the past.

58.6.1 Examination

If trismus is present, conducting a thorough physical checkup may be difficult. Drooling may indicate epiglottitis. Therefore, it's essential to check the mouth without being too rough if that's the case. Imaging or an operating room examination may be required if the diagnosis of PTA, epiglottitis, or any infection of the deep neck area is in question. Controlled insertion of an artificial airway is made possible by examination in the operating room [11].

On physical examination, extreme tonsillar swelling and fluctuation, with uvula displacement to the opposite side, are characteristics of PTA [11, 12]. Another possible symptom is a palpable, varying fullness or bulge of the posterior soft palate close to the tonsil. An erythematous pharynx and swollen tonsils with exudate are likely findings in children with peritonsillar cellulitis; uvular deviation and trismus are uncommon [9]. Children with PTA or cellulitis may also have cervical and submandibular lymphadenopathy [2].

PTAs signed by both parties are unusual. A clinical diagnosis may be more challenging if the characteristic asymmetry symptoms are lacking [13–16]. Dysphagia and trismus are two symptoms of this condition that may be present but are not diagnostic. The uvula can go forward [17]. Upper airway obstruction and snoring [13], if present, can exacerbate the symptoms of bilateral PTA.

Look at children over three who have uncomplicated streptococcal pharyngitis [2]. You'll see that their tonsils are swollen and full of exudate and that they may also have tonsillar and palatal petechiae.

Evaluation in the laboratory, although diagnostic laboratory testing is not required for PTA, may help determine the severity of the condition and guide treatment [2].

Therefore, the following [12] tests may be part of the laboratory examination of a kid with a peritonsillar infection:

The white blood cell count (WBC) is often high, with a preponderance of polymorphonuclear (PMN) leukocytes. However, this is a generic result of a complete blood count with a differential.

When oral intake is reduced, serum electrolytes become depleted.

Group A streptococcus testing (using culture or fast antigen detection) is a standard microbiologic procedure.

If an abscess drainage technique is done, the fluid should be tested using Gram stain, culture (aerobic and anaerobic), and susceptibility testing. These findings may guide antibiotic therapy in immunocompromised individuals or those with problems or infection spread, but they do not change the care of people without issues [18].

58.6.2 Imaging

Although imaging studies aren't required for a clinical diagnosis of PTA, they can assist in ruling out peritonsillar cellulitis as a possible cause of the patient's symptoms. Patients exhibiting symptoms suggestive of PTA [2] may benefit from imaging to rule out more severe disorders, such as retro- or parapharyngeal abscess or epiglottitis.

Differentiation of cellulitis from abscess is essential. To confirm the presence of an abscess before drainage [19–22], we recommend ultrasonography (US) by an expert physician for patients with a clinical diagnosis of PTA. The pooled sensitivity of the US in a metaanalysis of 17 studies (812 patients, mainly adults) for differentiating peritonsillar abscess from peritonsillar cellulitis was 86% (95% CI: 78–91%). The specificity was 76% (95% CI: 67–82%), with a positive likelihood ratio of 3.5 and a negative likelihood ratio of 0.19 [22]. Intraoral US and US conducted by a radiologist were shown to have better diagnostic features in a subgroup analysis. However, most patients got submandibular US, and operator expertise and training needed to be consistently identified among the six studies that examined point-of-care US.

The intraoral US may be less effective if the patient has trismus, discomfort, or choking. Patients who cannot tolerate an adequate oropharyngeal examination [23] might benefit significantly from submandibular or transcervical US, which circumvents these restrictions. Compared to a clinical evaluation, the US of the area appears more sensitive and specific in both cases [24, 25]. Peritonsillar abscess is a homogenous or striated region without a precise fluid collection [19, 21, 26], while peritonsillar cellulitis appears as an echo-free hollow with an uneven boundary.

58.7 Treatment

The symptoms of peritonsillar abscess (PTA) often resolve rapidly once incision and drainage (I&D) is done. Needle aspiration can be utilized for diagnosis and treatment since it pinpoints the precise location of the abscess. In rare circumstances, I&D might not be required if the aspirated fluid is cultured. Tonsillectomy may be recommended [1] if patients report persistent sore throats despite appropriate I&D.

Successful intraoral drainage is associated with few side effects. Tonsillectomy is not often recommended unless the patient has a history of recurrent tonsillitis or PTA; however, removal of the tonsils may be the sole option if the abscess is situated in an inaccessible region [1].

58.7.1 Medical Therapy

Dehydrated patients with PTAs must be given intravenous (IV) fluids until their inflammation subsides, and they may drink normally again [1].

Treating fever and pain with antipyretics and analgesics is common practice, respectively. With oral and parenteral painkillers, patients can resume eating normally. Patients can often continue oral intake with nonnarcotic analgesics after receiving I&D since the discomfort is reduced to an acceptable level [1].

After cultures are taken from the abscess, antibiotic treatment can begin. High doses of intravenous penicillin for treating PTA are still recommended. The polymicrobial character of cultured pus has also led to the recommending of medicines that target pathogens and are resistant to beta-lactamases. The most effective first-line treatment is most often cephalexin or another cephalosporin (with or without metronidazole). The following are some possible substitutes [1]:

- Cefuroxime or cefpodoxime (with or without metronidazole)
- Clindamycin
- In the absence of mononucleosis, amoxicillin-clavulanate may be prescribed

Once the patient can do so, oral antibiotics can be provided, and therapy should last 7–10 days.

58.7.1.1 Glucocorticoids

There is conflicting evidence on glucocorticoids' efficacy for treating PTA [27–29]. Patients aged 16 and up showed a significant reduction in symptoms when given glucocorticoids during needle aspiration and intravenous antibacterial treatment [28]. Another small trial found that intravenous dexamethasone reduced 24-h discomfort compared to placebo in adults receiving needle aspiration for PTA [29]. There was no evidence of benefit or harm from using glucocorticoids in 37% of 249 occurrences of PTA in children <18 years old in a retrospective case series [27]. Given the limited number of trial participants and varying findings of this research, additional data are required before routine glucocorticoid administration can be advised in managing PTA [30].

58.7.2 Surgical Therapy

Patients suspected of having PTAs should be sent to an otolaryngologist or surgeon specializing in treating PTAs. Early referral should be considered if the diagnosis is uncertain and the patient presents with airway blockage [1].

58.7.2.1 Specifics of the Process

The debate over whether or not I&D is superior to needle aspiration as a definitive treatment modality persists. If the patient is agreeable, the operation can be done while sitting in an examining chair. Both mucosalization and injection of a local anesthetic with epinephrine are used to anesthetize the supratonsillar fold and prevent further bleeding. When injecting a local drug, one must be careful not to penetrate more profoundly than the surface of the mucosa and the soft palate [1].

58.7.2.2 Needle Aspiration

Needle aspiration is safe for children as young as 7, mainly when used with conscious sedation. Because it pinpoints the exact location of the abscess cavity, needle aspiration can be utilized for diagnosis and treatment. The aspirated fluid can be submitted for culture, and I&D might not even be necessary in some instances [1].

Bleeding and the inhalation of pus and blood are among the possible complications of needle aspiration [31]. Aspiration of PTA has not been linked to carotid artery damage [30], but aspiration of a pseudoaneurysm imitating PTA or necrosis of the carotid artery can cause catastrophic bleeding [32, 33].

Needle aspiration is followed by an observation period to ensure the patient can take oral antimicrobials, painkillers, and fluids. The patient should be examined again in 24–36 h [10], even if not hospitalized.

58.7.2.3 Incision and Drainage

When doing intraoral I&D, the mucosa overlaying the abscess, typically found in the supra tonsillar fold, is incised. Following identification of the source of the abscess, loculations are broken through the use of blunt dissection. The patient is instructed to gargle with a sodium chloride solution, creating a vacuum in the abscess chamber and encouraging the collected material to drain. Immediate relief from the patient's symptoms is seen after successful aspiration or drainage [1].

Otolaryngologists are most often entrusted with incising and draining PTA [30]. Although local or procedural sedation may suffice for older kids, general anesthesia is typically necessary for younger ones [30, 34–38].

Compared to needle aspiration, incision and drainage are more painful and more likely to result in bleeding [30, 34]. A second operation may be necessary for a full recovery. Aspiration of the abscess content is a potential complication [2].

Oral antibiotic treatment, pain medicines, and drinks must be administered following the surgery, and patients must be monitored to ensure they can handle these aftercare requirements. Nonadmitted patients should be visited for follow-up in the hospital within 24–36 h [10].

58.7.2.4 Disparate Issues

The immediate removal of the tonsils as part of treatment for PTA has also been debated. Tonsillectomy for acute abscess has been demonstrated to be safe in several investigations. The excellent success rate, low recurrence rate, and minimal morbidity associated with intraoral drainage have led some to conclude that immediate or delayed tonsillectomy may not be necessary. A tonsillectomy may be required to drain an abscess if placed in an inconveniently positioned region.

No significant differences in clinical outcomes were reported between immediate and delayed tonsillectomy for PTA in a comprehensive review and metaanalysis by Tsikopoulos et al. [39].

Patients with peritonsillar abscesses are likelier to smoke, and smoking is linked to higher problems than nonsmokers [40].

References

1. Gosselin BJ. Peritonsillar abscess. In: Geibel J, editor. Medscape; 2023. Updated: Jul 25, 2022. https://emedicine.medscape.com/article/194863-overview (Accessed online at June 4, 2023).
2. Wald ER. Peritonsillar cellulitis and abscess. In: Edwards MS, Isaacson GC, Teach SJ, Calderwood SB, editors. UpToDate; 2023. Last updated: Feb 14, 2023.
3. Yellon RF, Falcone T, Roberson DW. Head and neck space infections. In: Bluestone CD, Simons JP, Healy GB, editors. Bluestone and stool's pediatric otolaryngology. 5th ed. Shelton, CT: People's Medical Publishing House; 2014. p. 1769.
4. Klug TE. Peritonsillar abscess: clinical aspects of microbiology, risk factors, and the association with parapharyngeal abscess. Dan Med J. 2017;64(3):B5333.
5. Inman JC, Rowe M, Ghostine M, Fleck T. Pediatric neck abscesses: changing organisms and empiric therapies. Laryngoscope. 2008;118:2111.
6. Ehlers Klug T, Rusan M, Fuursted K, Ovesen T. Fusobacterium necrophorum: most prevalent pathogen in peritonsillar abscess in Denmark. Clin Infect Dis. 2009;49:1467.
7. Plum AW, Mortelliti AJ, Walsh RE. Microbial flora and antibiotic resistance in peritonsillar abscesses in upstate New York. Ann Otol Rhinol Laryngol. 2015;124:875.
8. Ungkanont K, Yellon RF, Weissman JL, et al. Head and neck space infections in infants and children. Otolaryngol Head Neck Surg. 1995;112:375.

9. Szuhay G, Tewfik TL. Peritonsillar abscess or cellulitis? A clinical comparative paediatric study. J Otolaryngol. 1998;27:206.
10. Galioto NJ. Peritonsillar abscess. Am Fam Physician. 2008;77:199.
11. Goldstein NA, Hammerschlag MR. Peritonsillar, retropharyngeal, and parapharyngeal abscesses. In: Cherry JD, Demmler-Harrison GJ, Kaplan SL, Steinbach WJ, Hotez PJ, editors. Textbook of pediatric infection diseases. 8th ed. Philadelphia, PA: Elsevier; 2019. p. 119.
12. Tebruegge M, Curtis N. Infections of the upper and middle airways. In: Long SS, Prober CG, Fischer M, editors. Principles and practice of pediatric infectious diseases. 5th ed. New York, NY: Elsevier; 2018. p. 208.
13. Simons JP, Branstetter BF 4th, Mandell DL. Bilateral peritonsillar abscesses: case report and literature review. Am J Otolaryngol. 2006;27:443.
14. Safdar A, Hughes JP, Walsh RM, Walsh M. Bilateral peritonsillar abscess revisited. Ear Nose Throat J. 2005;84:791.
15. Mobley SR. Bilateral peritonsillar abscess: case report and presentation of its clinical appearance. Ear Nose Throat J. 2001;80:381.
16. Fasano CJ, Chudnofsky C, Vanderbeek P. Bilateral peritonsillar abscesses: not your usual sore throat. J Emerg Med. 2005;29:45.
17. Fiechtl JF, Stack LB. Images in clinical medicine. Bilateral peritonsillar abscesses. N Engl J Med. 2008;358:e27.
18. Herzon FS, Harris P. Mosher Award thesis. Peritonsillar abscess: incidence, current management practices, and a proposal for treatment guidelines. Laryngoscope. 1995;105:1.
19. Froehlich MH, Huang Z, Reilly BK. Utilization of ultrasound for diagnostic evaluation and management of peritonsillar abscesses. Curr Opin Otolaryngol Head Neck Surg. 2017;25:163.
20. Blaivas M, Theodoro D, Duggal S. Ultrasound-guided drainage of peritonsillar abscess by the emergency physician. Am J Emerg Med. 2003;21:155.
21. Bandarkar AN, Adeyiga AO, Fordham MT, et al. Tonsil ultrasound: technical approach and spectrum of pediatric peritonsillar infections. Pediatr Radiol. 2016;46:1059.
22. Kim DJ, Burton JE, Hammad A, et al. Test characteristics of ultrasound for the diagnosis of peritonsillar abscess: a systematic review and meta-analysis. Acad Emerg Med. 2023;30(8):859–69.
23. Zhao X, Delaney M, Breslin K, et al. Impact of transcervical ultrasound for the diagnosis of pediatric peritonsillar abscesses on emergency department performance measures. J Ultrasound Med. 2020;39:715.
24. Scott PM, Loftus WK, Kew J, et al. Diagnosis of peritonsillar infections: a prospective study of ultrasound, computerized tomography and clinical diagnosis. J Laryngol Otol. 1999;113:229.
25. Costantino TG, Satz WA, Dehnkamp W, Goett H. Randomized trial comparing intraoral ultrasound to landmark-based needle aspiration in patients with suspected peritonsillar abscess. Acad Emerg Med. 2012;19:626.
26. Lyon M, Blaivas M. Intraoral ultrasound in the diagnosis and treatment of suspected peritonsillar abscess in the emergency department. Acad Emerg Med. 2005;12:85.
27. Millar KR, Johnson DW, Drummond D, Kellner JD. Suspected peritonsillar abscess in children. Pediatr Emerg Care. 2007;23:431.
28. Ozbek C, Aygenc E, Tuna EU, et al. Use of steroids in the treatment of peritonsillar abscess. J Laryngol Otol. 2004;118:439.
29. Chau JK, Seikaly HR, Harris JR, et al. Corticosteroids in peritonsillar abscess treatment: a blinded placebo-controlled clinical trial. Laryngoscope. 2014;124:97.
30. Herzon FS, Martin AD. Medical and surgical treatment of peritonsillar, retropharyngeal, and parapharyngeal abscesses. Curr Infect Dis Rep. 2006;8:196.
31. Steyer TE. Peritonsillar abscess: diagnosis and treatment. Am Fam Physician. 2002;65:93.
32. Thomas JA, Ware TM, Counselman FL. Internal carotid artery pseudoaneurysm masquerading as a peritonsillar abscess. J Emerg Med. 2002;22:257.
33. Blum DJ, McCaffrey TV. Septic necrosis of the internal carotid artery: a complication of peritonsillar abscess. Otolaryngol Head Neck Surg. 1983;91:114.

34. Herzon FS, Nicklaus P. Pediatric peritonsillar abscess: management guidelines. Curr Probl Pediatr. 1996;26:270.
35. Apostolopoulos NJ, Nikolopoulos TP, Bairamis TN. Peritonsillar abscess in children. Is incision and drainage an effective management? Int J Pediatr Otorhinolaryngol. 1995;31:129.
36. Bauer PW, Lieu JE, Suskind DL, Lusk RP. The safety of conscious sedation in peritonsillar abscess drainage. Arch Otolaryngol Head Neck Surg. 2001;127:1477.
37. Suskind DL, Park J, Piccirillo JF, et al. Conscious sedation: a new approach for peritonsillar abscess drainage in the pediatric population. Arch Otolaryngol Head Neck Surg. 1999;125:1197.
38. Powell J, Wilson JA. An evidence-based review of peritonsillar abscess. Clin Otolaryngol. 2012;37:136.
39. Tsikopoulos A, Fountarlis A, Tsikopoulos K, Dilmperis F, Garefis K, Tsikopoulos I, et al. Immediate or interval abscess tonsillectomy? A systematic review and meta-analysis. Eur Arch Otorhinolaryngol. 2022;279(5):2245–57.
40. Marom T, Cinamon U, Itskoviz D, Roth Y. Changing trends of peritonsillar abscess. Am J Otolaryngol. 2010;31(3):162–7.

Retropharyngeal Abscess

59

Mesut Yesilova, Nuray Bayar Muluk, and Nitin R. Ankle

59.1 Introduction

A retropharyngeal abscess (RPA) is an infection in the deep neck area that can cause rapid and fatal consequences, including airway obstruction [1].

Understanding deep-space infections requires in-depth familiarity with head and neck anatomy regarding fascial planes. The cervical fascia consists of two distinct layers within the neck. Although this fascia usually adheres to neighboring tissues, genuine voids can be produced when an infection intercalates between fascial layers, leading to the fast spread of infectious inflammation and purulence between fascial planes [2].

The pharynx (nasopharynx, oropharynx, and hypopharynx), larynx, and trachea are positioned anterior to the retropharyngeal region. This area is bounded anteriorly by the visceral (buccopharyngeal) fascia, which encloses the pharynx, trachea, esophagus, and thyroid. The retropharyngeal space is bordered posteriorly by the alar fascia and on the sides by the carotid sheaths and the parapharyngeal spaces. It extends from the level of the tracheal bifurcation in the mediastinum [2] up to the skull base.

The retropharyngeal space is near two other possible spaces: the danger and prevertebral spaces. The alar fascia and the prevertebral fascia create the danger

M. Yesilova
Erdemli State Hospital, ENT Clinic, Erdemli, Mersin, Turkey

N. Bayar Muluk (✉)
Faculty of Medicine, Department of Otorhinolaryngology, Kırıkkale University, Kırıkkale, Turkey

N. R. Ankle
Department of Otorhinolaryngology, Head and Neck Surgery, KLE Academy of Higher Education and Research (KAHER), Jawaharlal Nehru Medical College, Belagavi, Karnataka, India

H. Yüksel et al. (eds.), *Pediatric Airway Diseases*, Comprehensive ENT,
https://doi.org/10.1007/978-3-031-74853-0_59

zone at the front and back of the body, respectively. The longus colli spinal muscles [2] form the posterior border of the prevertebral space, whereas the prevertebral fascia forms the anterior wall.

The prevertebral space continues to insert the psoas muscles, whereas the danger space extends along the mediastinum to the diaphragm level. Because of these anatomical connections, an infection in the retropharyngeal region can quickly move to the mediastinum, where it could cause life-threatening mediastinitis [2].

59.2 Pathophysiology

There are two potential routes of infection to the retropharyngeal area [2]:

- Contagion originating in a nearby location.
- Penetrating injuries that inflict an infection directly.

When a child develops "classic" RPA, lymph nodes in the retropharyngeal area on either side of the superior constrictor muscle have become infected due to an upper respiratory tract infection (URI). Abscesses arise [2] when these nodes degenerate or suppurate.

Henri Rouvière's nodes, a collection of lateral retropharyngeal lymph nodes near the base of the skull, are of particular significance. Despite their role as the principal lymphatic drainage of the nasopharynx, the nodes of Rouvière are usually not of considerable clinical relevance. However, in situations of nasopharyngeal cancer, they can become crucial. Because they can suppurate and cause abscesses to develop [2], they are also relevant to the issue of RPA.

Infection of the retropharyngeal lymph nodes, followed by cellulitis and abscess development, is the typical etiology of RPA in children. Around the age of four, fibrosis and atrophy begins inside these nodes, and by the age of six, the retropharyngeal nodes had typically regresses. Penetration trauma or direct transmission from a neighboring region are the most common causes of retropharyngeal space infection in older adults [2].

Mass effect, abscess rupture, and infection dissemination are the three leading causes of RPA complications. Expansion of the RPA against the pharynx or trachea, causing airway compression, is the most severe consequence. When an abscess bursts, the purulent contents might be inhaled, causing respiratory distress or even death. Adjacent tissues might become inflamed and damaged if an infection spreads [2].

Mediastinitis, purulent pericarditis and tamponade, pyopneumothorax, pleuritis, empyema, and bronchial erosion are all possible complications of infection that have spread to the mediastinum. If an infection spreads laterally, it might lodge in the carotid sheath, leading to a clot in the internal jugular vein or even a rupture of the carotid artery. Vertebral subluxation and spinal cord damage can occur if an infection spreads posteriorly and causes osteomyelitis or erosion of the spinal column. Necrotizing fasciitis, septic shock, and mortality can all result from RPA [2].

59.3 Etiology

Drainage to the retropharyngeal nodes from primary nasopharyngeal infections is the most common cause of retropharyngeal space infections. Lymphadenitis is the outcome, and it can cause cellulitis, which can swell and become an abscess. The following [2] infections are examples of those that may serve as risk factors:

- Inflammation of the pharynx.
- Tonsillitis.
- Adenoiditis.
- Otitis media.
- Acute sinusitis.
- Infections in other parts of the head and neck (such as the nose, mouth, or teeth).

Some infectious diseases of the spine, such as osteomyelitis, can spread anteriorly from the prevertebral region. Parapharyngeal, submandibular, and prevertebral gaps are adjacent anatomical locations that can transfer illness to the retropharynx [2].

Direct seeding of an infection in the retropharyngeal area from the outside can also result from penetrating trauma. Children frequently injure themselves when they put something sharp in their teeth and run around before tripping and falling on the floor. Because parents might not be aware of these risk factors, a proper diagnosis might be even more challenging. Fishbones and other foreign bodies have been linked to retropharyngeal puncture wounds.

Iatrogenic RPA occurs when the upper respiratory tract is instrumented. This area can get contaminated due to iatrogenic sources such as laryngoscopy, endotracheal intubation, surgery, endoscopy, feeding tube installation, and dental treatments.

Immune disease (HIV, diabetes, or immunosuppression) and poor dental hygiene increase the likelihood of developing RPA.

Polymicrobial infections are common, with Gram-positive and anaerobe species predominating but Gram-negative bacteria also being detected. Most bacteria come from the oropharyngeal flora, with group A beta-hemolytic streptococci being the most frequent. Also widespread is Staphylococcus aureus. Methicillin resistance is rising in Staphylococcus isolates, with 24% of all cultures and 64% of Staphylococcus-positive cultures showing resistance), as reported by Abdel-Haq et al. [3].

The genus Bacteroides is the most prevalent group of anaerobes. Haemophilus parainfluenza, Veillonella, Peptostreptococcus, Fusobacterium, and Eikenella species are some of the other organisms that might cause disease [2].

Patients who may be susceptible (immunosuppressed persons or new immigrants) should be tested for Mycobacterium tuberculosis, Bartonella henselae, and Coccidia, especially if they are not responding to standard therapy [2].

Finally, Lemierre syndrome (septic thrombophlebitis of the internal jugular vein due to RPA) should be considered while assessing these individuals. In most cases, fusobacterium necrophorum, an anaerobic Gram-negative rod [4], is the causative agent of this illness. Complicated RPA due to Lemierre syndrome may need surgical intervention, including antimicrobial treatments and anticoagulation [2].

59.4 Diagnosis and Evaluation

59.4.1 Take Care of Airway Obstruction

The first step in evaluating a kid with a possible deep neck space infection is quickly examining the degree of upper airway obstruction. Children who are anxious, ill-appearing, drooling, and posturing need continual monitoring in an environment where an emergent artificial airway may be placed [5].

Securing the airway and performing surgical drainage in the operating room are both necessary for patients with severe airway obstruction (e.g., anxiety, leaning forward with head in the "sniffing position," and marked suprasternal retractions) [5].

59.4.2 Clinical Manifestations

Retropharyngeal abscess presents differently at various stages of the disease. The symptoms and signs may be difficult to distinguish from those of uncomplicated pharyngitis. Symptoms of inflammation and blockage of the upper aerodigestive tract [5] emerge as the illness progresses.

Retropharyngeal abscess in children often manifests as a mild to moderate fever. Extra symptoms [6–9] include:

- Swallowing problems (dysphagia).
- Swallowing difficulties (odynophagia).
- Reduced saliva production and appetite.
- Stiffness in the neck, or the inability to move the neck because of discomfort (torticollis), is a common health problem.
- Sound changes (such as muffled or "hot potato" (dysphonia) quality), gurgling, or stertor.
- Stridor, tachypnea, or both; stridor often appears as the condition worsens.
- Lymphadenopathy, lump, or enlargement of the neck.
- Approximately 20% of patients have tremors.
- Mediastinal extension-associated chest discomfort.

Retropharyngeal infection symptoms often worsen more slowly than epiglottitis symptoms, although it can be difficult to tell the two apart. The youngster may have been given antibiotics for what was thought to be pharyngitis [8–10], and the symptoms may have persisted for days before the diagnosis was confirmed.

Trismus may prevent a thorough examination of the oropharynx. If epiglottitis is suspected based on drooling, careful mouth inspection must be performed without being too forceful. Imaging or inspection in the operating room may be required to confirm a diagnosis of retropharyngeal infection, epiglottitis, or other deep neck region infection. Suppose the patient is very ill or unstable. In that case, it is advised that they undergo an examination in the operating room, where an artificial airway can be placed under close medical supervision [11].

59.4.3 Radiography

Radiographs of the neck's soft tissues taken at an angle can help rule out other possible diagnoses, including RPA. The most valuable data for this investigation may be gathered while the subject inhales with the neck fully extended. Soft tissue between the radiolucent airway (pharynx and trachea) and the spine is where an RPA resides. Until shown differently [2], it is assumed that enlargement of these soft tissues is pathogenic.

Patients of any age group should have a smaller than 7 mm space between the anterior surface of the C2 vertebra and the posterior border of the airway. Young people under 15 should have a C6-T1 distance of <14 mm. The average adult has a separation of 22 mm. A less stringent (but still helpful) guideline is that the soft-tissue plane must be narrower than the corresponding vertebral body [2] in width.

Gas or a foreign body in the retropharyngeal space may also be visible on a plain film. Spinal lordosis, or natural curve, can be altered. The breadth of the soft tissue when a child's head is fully extended is no greater than the width of a child's vertebral body [2].

59.4.4 The Use of CT Scans

At the moment, CT is the gold standard for imaging pediatric RPA. A CT scan of the neck with intravenous (IV) contrast should be performed to define the lesion further and identify any potential vascular involvement. It is essential to brief the radiologist about the study's goals in advance since a routine CT scan of the neck might not utilize thin enough slices (3–5 mm) or might not scan the whole range of the retropharyngeal region (skull base to T2) [2].

Abscesses may be seen on CT, and the presence of a central lucency can assist in differentiating cellulitis from abscess. It's often a region with low attenuation and an increased ring around it. The abscess chamber may be packed with gas, and the surrounding soft tissues will be swollen and devoid of fat planes. Compression can also affect nearby structures like the airway. This analysis can also help pinpoint the abscess's precise site, measure its size, and identify any infectious issues it may be causing [2].

59.4.5 Methods Using Magnetic Resonance Imaging

However, unless there is reason to suspect that the abscess has migrated to the CNS, an MRI is often not needed and rarely used to yield pictures superior to those obtained by the other tests. In addition, the patient must spend considerable time in an unsupervised setting throughout this investigation. Finally, sedation is typically necessary for youngsters before this test, and it is risky for anybody with a compromised airway [2].

59.4.6 Ultrasonography

In cases of severe neck infections, ultrasonography (US) has been proposed as a diagnostic tool. This modality's benefits include being portable and requiring no radiation. It's also less likely to necessitate sedation, making it a better option for youngsters. Abscess development may be differentiated from cellulitis using the US, and a skilled physician can pinpoint its existence and location. However, the US can only help so much with surgical planning [2].

59.5 Treatment Strategy Factors to Consider

Patients suspected of having a retropharyngeal abscess (RPA) should have their airway assessed first. Patients who exhibit symptoms or indicators of airway compromise should have immediate access to modalities to stabilize their airway [2].

59.5.1 Surgical Versus Medical Treatment

Several research studies have focused on the debate over whether or not surgical surgery is more effective than medicinal treatment for RPA. However, 43% of patients in a nationwide series studied by Lander et al. [12] had surgical drainage. Surgical intervention and medicinal therapy resulted in the same length of hospital stay [13], according to a study by Grisaru-Soen et al. When comparing the length of hospital stays between medical and surgical treatment, Johnston et al. [14] observed that 9 of 22 patients with RPA may be released following medical therapy alone.

Since computed tomography (CT) has low specificity, researchers have been trying to define a unique set of criteria to ascertain better whether individuals need surgical drainage. The following criteria were proposed in a retrospective research that summarized the debate conducted by Page et al. [8].

- Actual abscess development, as opposed to phlegmon, was indicated by a retropharyngeal protrusion and trismus.
- Clinicians should look for alternative causes of abscess development, such as Kawasaki illness or scarlet fever if a rash is present.
- The authors discovered that cross-sectional area was the most reliable predictor of abscess formation based on radiographic criteria; however, this parameter only had a 68% likelihood of identifying purulence intraoperatively in patients with positive CT results.

- The authors noted that males are more likely to be diagnosed with RPA and that patients are typically older than five. Still, neither of these characteristics should be utilized to make a diagnosis.

59.5.2 Antimicrobial Medication

The treatment of retropharyngeal infections in children includes the use of antimicrobial medication. Children with deep neck space infections had a 7–15% death rate and as high as a 25% complication rate before the widespread use of antibiotics. Mortality and complications are now extremely rare due to the availability of antibiotic treatment.

In observational studies, antimicrobial therapy alone effectively treats suppurative retropharyngeal infection [9, 15–19]. However, 37–75% have been reported successful in retrospective series [9, 16, 18]. Ten out of eleven kids with suppurative deep neck infections larger than 1 cm^2 responded favorably to antibiotic treatment with no serious adverse effects [15].

A lengthier hospital stay, intubation or temporary tracheostomy for respiratory distress, and spontaneous rupture are all possible outcomes of nonsurgical therapy [8, 20, 21].

59.5.3 Empiric Treatment

E. coli and Streptococcus pyogenes should all be covered by empiric treatment protocols—airborne anaerobes, including Staphylococcus aureus. If drainage is conducted, culture findings and patient response to treatment might inform how the empiric treatment plan is adjusted. It is vital to remember that retropharyngeal infections are often polymicrobial when adapting treatment based on culture findings [22], as not all bacteria are routinely cultivated.

Treatments based on hunches include [5, 6]:

- Injectable ampicillin-sulbactam (50 mg/kg every 6 h) or.
- Intravenous clindamycin 15 mg/kg every 8 h (maximum single dosage 900 mg).

Methicillin-resistant S. enterocolitica is resistant to the antibiotic combination ampicillin-sulbactam. Methicillin-resistant Staphylococcus aureus (MRSA) and clindamycin may not be effective against group A Streptococcus [23], methicillin-susceptible S. aureus (S. aureus) depending on local susceptibility patterns—infections caused by S. aureus and MRSA.

To provide optimal coverage for potentially resistant Gram-positive cocci, intravenous vancomycin or linezolid should be added to empiric treatment with either ampicillin-sulbactam or clindamycin in patients who do not respond to initial therapy with the empiric regimens above or who present with moderate or severe disease.

- A maximum daily dose of 2–4 g of vancomycin (40–60 mg/kg given in three to four doses) OR.
- A maximum daily dose of 1200 mg of linezolid (for children younger than 12 years, give 30 mg/kg in three separate doses; for children older than 12 years, give 20 mg/kg in two doses).

To achieve afebrile status and clinical improvement, parenteral therapy must be continued. It's essential to finish the full 14 days of oral medication. Continuing treatment with any of the following five oral regimens is appropriate:

- Antibiotics (45 mg/kg every 12 h of amoxicillin-clavulanate), OR.
- If the patient improves while receiving parenteral clindamycin as an empiric treatment, continue with clindamycin (13 mg/kg every 8 h).
- Linezolid is an option for oral treatment when vancomycin has been added to the parenteral regimen [5]. Combined with antibiotic treatments, surgical drainage has been critical in treating retropharyngeal abscesses. Surgical drainage may be necessary for the following reasons [8, 9, 24]:

Surgical Drainage

- Compromised airway or other potentially fatal complications.
- Complete rim enhancement and scalloping on CT image and a significant hypodense region (2.5 cm^2) diagnose an advanced abscess.
- Inability to reduce fever, alleviate pain, or prevent the growth of an abscess larger than 2.5 cm^2 despite parenteral antibiotic treatment.

If surgical drainage is undertaken, obtaining specimens for aerobic and anaerobic culturing [6] is necessary.

Surgical draining is often done transorally unless the abscess is located laterally to the neck arteries or contains several deep neck space infections [6, 8, 25]. Some patients [8, 10] may need a second operation. Surgical drainage is usually safe and results in few complications.

References

1. Vieira F, Allen SM, Stocks RM, Thompson JW. Deep neck infection. Otolaryngol Clin N Am. 2008;41(3):459–83.
2. Patel VA. Pediatric retropharyngeal abscess. In: Elluru RG, editor. Medscape; 2023. Updated: Feb 14, 2023. https://emedicine.medscape.com/article/995851-overview (Accessed online at June 4, 2023).
3. Abdel-Haq N, Quezada M, Asmar BI. Retropharyngeal abscess in children: the rising incidence of methicillin-resistant Staphylococcus aureus. Pediatr Infect Dis J. 2012;31(7):696–9.
4. Chirinos JA, Garcia J, Alcaide ML, Toledo G, Baracco GJ, Lichtstein DM. Septic thrombophlebitis: diagnosis and management. Am J Cardiovasc Drugs. 2006;6(1):9–14.
5. Wald ER. Retropharyngeal infections in children. In: Edwards MS, Isaacson GC, Teach SJ, Wiley II JF, editors. UpToDate; 2023. Last updated: May 01, 2023.

6. Tebruegge M, Curtis N. Infections related to the upper and middle airways. In: Long SS, Prober CG, Fischer M, editors. Principles and practice of pediatric infectious diseases. 5th ed. New York: Elsevier Saunders; 2018. p. 208.
7. Goldstein NA, Hammerschlag MR. Peritonsillar, retropharyngeal, and parapharyngeal abscesses. In: Cherry JD, Harrison GJ, Kaplan SL, Steinbach WJ, Hotez PJ, editors. Textbook of pediatric infectious diseases. 8th ed. Philadelphia: Saunders; 2019. p. 119.
8. Page NC, Bauer EM, Lieu JE. Clinical features and treatment of retropharyngeal abscess in children. Otolaryngol Head Neck Surg. 2008;138:300.
9. Craig FW, Schunk JE. Retropharyngeal abscess in children: clinical presentation, utility of imaging, and current management. Pediatrics. 2003;111:1394.
10. Cmejrek RC, Coticchia JM, Arnold JE. Presentation, diagnosis, and management of deep-neck abscesses in infants. Arch Otolaryngol Head Neck Surg. 2002;128:1361.
11. Yellon RF, Falcone T, Roberson DW. Head and neck space infections. In: Bluestone CD, Simons JP, Healy GB, editors. Bluestone and Stool's pediatric otolaryngology. 5th ed. Shelton, CT: People's Medical Publishing House; 2014. p. 1769.
12. Lander L, Lu S, Shah RK. Pediatric retropharyngeal abscesses: a national perspective. Int J Pediatr Otorhinolaryngol. 2008;72(12):1837–43.
13. Grisaru-Soen G, Komisar O, Aizenstein O, Soudack M, Schwartz D, Paret G. Retropharyngeal and parapharyngeal abscess in children—epidemiology, clinical features and treatment. Int J Pediatr Otorhinolaryngol. 2010;74(9):1016–20.
14. Johnston D, Schmidt R, Barth P. Parapharyngeal and retropharyngeal infections in children: argument for a trial of medical therapy and intraoral drainage for medical treatment failures. Int J Pediatr Otorhinolaryngol. 2009;73(5):761–5.
15. McClay JE, Murray AD, Booth T. Intravenous antibiotic therapy for deep neck abscesses defined by computed tomography. Arch Otolaryngol Head Neck Surg. 2003;129:1207.
16. Vural C, Gungor A, Comerci S. Accuracy of computerized tomography in deep neck infections in the pediatric population. Am J Otolaryngol. 2003;24:143.
17. Shefelbine SE, Mancuso AA, Gajewski BJ, et al. Pediatric retropharyngeal lymphadenitis: differentiation from retropharyngeal abscess and treatment implications. Otolaryngol Head Neck Surg. 2007;136:182.
18. Al-Sabah B, Bin Salleen H, Hagr A, et al. Retropharyngeal abscess in children: 10-year study. J Otolaryngol. 2004;33:352.
19. Broughton RA. Nonsurgical management of deep neck infections in children. Pediatr Infect Dis J. 1992;11:14.
20. Sichel JY, Dano I, Hocwald E, et al. Nonsurgical management of parapharyngeal space infections: a prospective study. Laryngoscope. 2002;112:906.
21. Plaza Mayor G, Martínez-San Millán J, Martínez-Vidal A. Is conservative treatment of deep neck space infections appropriate? Head Neck. 2001;23:126.
22. Baum ED, Elden LM. Bacterial infections of the neck. In: Burg FD, Ingelfinger JR, Polin RA, Gershon AA, editors. Current pediatric therapy. 18th ed. Philadelphia: Saunders; 2006. p. 1117.
23. Pesola AK, Sihvonen R, Lindholm L, Pätäri-Sampo A. Clindamycin resistant emm33 Streptococcus pyogenes emerged among invasive infections in Helsinki metropolitan area, Finland, 2012–2013. Euro Surveill 2015; 20.
24. Wilkie MD, De S, Krishnan M. Defining the role of surgical drainage in paediatric deep neck space infections. Clin Otolaryngol. 2019;44:366.
25. Choi SS, Vezina LG, Grundfast KM. Relative incidence and alternative approaches for surgical drainage of different types of deep neck abscesses in children. Arch Otolaryngol Head Neck Surg. 1997;123:1271.

Submandibular Space Infections (Ludwig's Angina)

60

Taha Yasin Yildiz, Nuray Bayar Muluk, and Jeffrey C. Bedrosian

60.1 Introduction

Ludwig's angina is characterized by a "woody" or "brawny" cellulitis that spreads quickly and affects the submandibular, sublingual, and submental areas on both sides of the body. The affected tooth is usually the second or third molar in the mandible. Ludwig's angina has no lymphadenopathy or abscess development [1].

Ludwig's angina, in honor of Karl Friedrich Willhelm von Ludwig, is defined by a fast worsening of gangrenous cellulitis affecting the neck and the floor of the mouth [2]. The most dangerous consequence of Ludwig's angina is airway obstruction, caused by the gradual swelling of soft tissues and the elevation and posterior displacement of the tongue. Ludwig's angina had a mortality rate of almost 50% [3] before the discovery of antibiotics. The death rate is around 8% [2–4], thanks to advances in antimicrobial medication, imaging technologies, and surgical procedures.

Clinical diagnosis of Ludwig's angina. Most individuals also have neck edema and experience tooth pain/history of recent dental operations. Dysphonia, dysphagia, and dysarthria are among the less frequent problems. Dyspnea, tachypnea, and stridor are all signs of respiratory distress, although they only affect about a third of individuals [5]. Over 95% of people show signs of enlargement in both submandibular glands and have a tongue that is either high or protrudes on examination [3,

T. Y. Yildiz
Yozgat City Hospital, ENT Clinic, Yozgat, Turkey

N. Bayar Muluk (✉)
Faculty of Medicine, Department of Otorhinolaryngology, Kırıkkale University, Kırıkkale, Turkey

J. C. Bedrosian
Rhinology and Skull Base Surgery, Specialty Physician Associates, St. Luke's Medical Center, Bethlehem, PA, USA

H. Yüksel et al. (eds.), *Pediatric Airway Diseases*, Comprehensive ENT,
https://doi.org/10.1007/978-3-031-74853-0_60

5]. The submandibular edema is typically described as robust and stiff, with erythema overlaying it [4].

60.2 Related Anatomy

It is beyond the scope of this article to provide a full anatomic description of the main face and deep neck spaces. However, proper diagnosis and treatment of these illnesses need an in-depth understanding of this anatomy. Fascial planes separate the actual and prospective volumes of the neck, creating deep neck gaps [6, 7].

60.2.1 Facial Planes

The cervical region is divided into the superficial and deep fascia [6].

The superficial cervical fascia, located immediately under the dermis, covers and protects the face muscles. From the base of the skull (epicranium) to the shoulder blades and upper chest, this region encompasses the superficial musculoaponeurotic system (SMAS). Fat, neurovascular bundles, and lymphatics fill the area underneath this layer. It is not a system component located in the deep neck [6].

The deep cervical fascia comprises three layers—the superficial, medium, and deep layers—and surrounds the deep neck spaces [6]. The deep cervical fascia is an investing fascia that covers the neck from the surface up. It includes the submandibular and parotid glands, the masticatory muscles, and the sternocleidomastoid muscle. The nuchal ridge, the mandible, the zygomatic arch, the mastoid process, and the hyoid bone all act as upper limits. It is delimited inferiorly by the clavicles, sternum, scapula, hyoid, and acromion. It helps form the carotid sheath's lateral side and the fascia that covers the digastric muscle. As it travels from the hyoid bone to the medial table of the ramus of the mandible, it creates the floor of the submandibular cavity by enclosing the anterior belly of the digastric muscle. This fascia contributes to the later-parietal delineation of the parotid and masticator areas.

The deep cervical fascia's middle layer is split into muscular and visceral fascia. Strap muscles (sternohyoid, sternothyroid, thyrohyoid, omohyoid) and the adventitia of the significant blood arteries are encased inside the muscular division. The buccopharyngeal fascia and the anterior wall of the retropharyngeal space are structures created by the visceral division, which wraps itself around the constrictor muscles of the pharynx and esophagus. The carotid sheath is a joint effort of the muscular and visceral systems. The larynx, trachea, and thyroid gland are all encased in this intermediate layer. The carotid artery begins at the base of the skull and passes through a sheath down to the pericardium.

The prevertebral and alar layers make up the deeper layers of the deep cervical fascia. Anterior to the vertebral body and extending laterally to the transverse processes is where the prevertebral division makes its home. The posterior border of the retropharyngeal space is defined by the alar division, located between the prevertebral division and the visceral division of the middle layer.

It contributes to the carotid sheath by encasing the deep neck muscles. At the level of thoracic vertebrae 1 and 2 (T1 and T2) [6], the muscular division of the middle layer of the deep cervical fascia merges with the alar division of the deep cervical fascia.

60.2.2 The Submandibular Region

The lower border of the submandibular space is formed by the superficial layer of the deep cervical fascia that runs from the hyoid to the mandible; the body of the mandible forms the lateral border, and the mucosa of the floor of the mouth includes the superior edge.

The mylohyoid muscle separates it into two regions, the sublingual and the submaxillary spaces. The sublingual gland, hypoglossal nerve, and Wharton duct are all in the sublingual area. Pus can easily penetrate the submaxillary region through the posterior edge of the mylohyoid muscle. The anterior belly of the digastric further divides the submaxillary region into the central submental space and the lateral submaxillary space.

Dental abscesses of mandibular teeth, oral trauma, and submaxillary or sublingual sialadenitis can all lead to infection in the submandibular area.

Cellulitis and inflammation of the submandibular region, known as Ludwig angina, often extend from the submaxillary to the sublingual area by fascial planes rather than lymphatic vessels. Cellulitis or abscess can enlarge the submandibular space, leading to induration of the floor of the mouth and the subsequent forward and backward movement of the tongue, which can block the airway. There is no need for a localized abscess to diagnose Ludwig's angina. Drooling, trismus, discomfort, dysphagia, a submandibular lump, and dyspnea or airway compromise due to a displaced tongue are common symptoms, as is bilateral involvement. Tracheostomy is the only option for managing the airway in this potentially fatal illness. Ludwig's angina had a 50% fatality rate before antibiotics were discovered. The death rate is around 5% because of cutting-edge antibacterial and surgical treatments.

The parapharyngeal and retropharyngeal spaces are at risk for contamination from submandibular space infections [6].

60.3 Diffusion Mechanisms

Over two-thirds of Ludwig angina patients have an infection in one of their teeth, often the second or third mandibular molars [7, 8]. Since the roots of these teeth are situated beneath the mylohyoid muscle's attachments to the jaw, the submandibular region is initially implicated. Trauma to the mandible or floor of the mouth, sialolithiasis and infection of the submandibular or sublingual salivary glands, and contiguous spread from the peritonsillar abscess or suppurative parotitis are all potential causes of disease [7–9].

The thin lingual portions of the periodontal bone around these teeth enable the medial spread of infection. The sublingual and submental regions on both sides of the body are infected. If the illness were spreading through the lymphatic system, one side would be affected instead of both. Less frequently, an infection of the premolars and adjacent teeth or damage to the floor of the mouth [1] can cause a similar process involving the sublingual region.

Once an infection has taken hold, it changes quickly. The tongue can swell to twice or thrice its standard size, pushing back into the hypopharynx, up against the palate, and out the front of the mouth to give the patient a "double-tongue" look [10]. The epiglottis will be actively involved since it extends posteriorly immediately. The buccopharyngeal gap is a potentially life-threatening opening between the submandibular and parapharyngeal regions. The styloid process is formed when the styloglossus muscle emerges from the tongue and travels between the middle and superior constrictor muscles before attaching to the styloid. For this reason, cellulitis in the submandibular region can progress over the styloglossus muscle into the parapharyngeal area and then into the retropharyngeal space and the superior mediastinum [11].

60.4 Pathophysiology

The dental infection that causes Ludwig's angina typically begins in the subgingival pocket of the second or third mandibular molars, including partly erupted third molars [12]. The infection then travels to the floor of the mouth muscles. It has advanced to the sublingual region below the mylohyoid line. Infection of the second and third mandibular molars, which have roots below this line, can cause Ludwig's angina. The lingual aspect of the tooth socket is thinner. Therefore, the infection spreads there rather than to the buccal side of the mouth. Sublingually, it applies and then moves to the submandibular area [13].

Oral flora, including aerobes and anaerobes, are often involved in this condition. Ludwig's angina is more likely to occur in immunocompromised persons [13], and the most prevalent causative organisms are Staphylococcus, Streptococcus, Peptostreptococcus, Fusobacterium, Bacteroides, and Actinomyces.

60.5 Etiology

The submandibular space is the predominant infected area in Ludwig's angina [14, 15]. The mylohyoid muscle divides the submandibular space into the sublingual space above and the submaxillary space below. Ludwig's angina typically has an odontogenic genesis, with second and third molar infections being the most common causes. Any dental abscess or infection can easily spread to the submaxillary area because the roots of these teeth extend through the mylohyoid ridge. Once an infection has spread, it moves directly into the sublingual cavity. An infection can encircle the airway if it spreads contiguously into the pharyngomaxillary and retropharyngeal regions [4].

Over 90% of all instances [12] are due to odontogenic infections. Mandibular fracture, neck trauma, piercing of the tongue, sialadenitis, malignancy, and various parapharyngeal infections are other causes [2, 3, 15]. More than half of patients had a polymicrobial infection [15]. Staphylococcus, Streptococcus, and Bacteroides species [3] are the most frequently cultivated microorganisms. Condition from atypical organisms is dangerous for patients with immunocompromising diseases, including HIV, diabetes, transplant recipients, and alcoholics. Pseudomonas, Escherichia coli, Klebsiella, Enterococcus faecalis, Candida, and Clostridium [15] are some atypical species discovered from these individuals.

60.6 Evaluation

In terms of assessment, the airway is the most crucial factor. The patient must be intubated immediately if Ludwig's angina is suspected. As transporting a patient with an imminent airway to the CT scanner will delay treatment and may be fatal, imaging plays no role in the patient's initial evaluation [13].

Although an emergent awake tracheostomy should be prepared before any airway intervention [13], awake fiberoptic intubation is the safest technique to secure the airway.

Once the airway has been secured, a computed tomography (CT) scan of the neck with intravenous (IV) contrast can be utilized to determine the severity of the infection and assess for any abscess [16]. CT scans and MRIs can also identify mediastinal fluid cumulus and confirm airway edema. In cases of infections caused by anaerobic bacteria, X-rays of the neck and chest may reveal gas in the tissues. Finally, ultrasonography can detect metastatic abscesses and pus [17].

Since this is a clinical diagnosis, laboratory testing is usually irrelevant at the outset. Hematogenous spread of the virus can be detected by taking blood cultures [13].

60.7 Treatment

60.7.1 Controlling the Airway

Patients with Ludwig's angina should begin therapy with airway control. The choice to perform airway-securing procedures still relies on the clinician's discretion and experience. There are currently no accepted airway management standards for individuals with Ludwig's angina. Now, advice is mainly gleaned from an individual's or group's experience and the resources available inside a given organization [18]. Any patient who presents with respiratory distress or who is at risk for airway blockage needs to be intubated right away. Intubation using either the oral route (orotracheal intubation) or the nasal route (fiber-optic nasotracheal intubation) is advised. Patients with Ludwig's angina should not undergo blind nasotracheal intubation due to the risk of hemorrhage and abscess rupture [15, 18, 19]. Ludwig's angina patients who are not intubated require airway devices such as tracheostomy and cricothyroidotomy tools [4].

Most cases may be handled initially with close monitoring and intravenous antibiotics, even if the critical issue is maintaining a sufficient airway, which may need immediate tracheostomy [20, 21]. Before stridor, cyanosis, and asphyxia set in, mechanical airway control must be obtained if cellulitis and edema continue progressing or if dyspnea begins. These patients can rapidly worsen and are best addressed in the operating room. Therefore, consulting with otolaryngology and anesthesia is preferable as soon as possible. In extreme instances, an emergency tracheostomy may be necessary [1].

Fiberoptic intubation through the nasal route is advised if airway compromise is suspected. To evaluate the airway and facilitate the nasal intubation of an endotracheal tube under direct observation [22], fiberoptic laryngoscopy is performed. To avoid this problem, a nasopharyngeal airway may be used. In advanced Ludwig angina, blind oral or nasotracheal intubation is painful and hazardous due to the risk of generating severe laryngospasm. If intubation is unsuccessful, tracheostomy is the most common alternative [1].

60.7.2 Antibiotics

As soon as feasible, antibiotic treatment should begin. Initially, it is best to use antibiotics that are effective against aerobic and anaerobic bacteria. Antibiotics are frequently prescribed in combinations, such as penicillin, clindamycin, and metronidazole [3]. Intravenous steroids have been recommended in recent case studies [2, 15, 23]. According to these accounts, the requirement for airway management may have been averted if corticosteroids had been administered instead. In randomized controlled studies, corticosteroids are ineffective in individuals with Ludwig's angina [4].

Because airway obstruction is the leading cause of mortality in patients with Ludwig's angina, antibiotic treatment and, in severe instances, surgical drainage of the infection are primary therapeutic goals [13].

Although flexible fiberoptic nasal intubation is the preferred form of intubation, preparations for emergency awake tracheostomy must be made before any airway intervention is attempted [24]. Because of the late nature of stridor and cyanosis, it is crucial to address the airway first. The following procedure would be an emergency tracheotomy if the patient could not be intubated [19].

Once an airway has been established and cultures obtained, broad-spectrum intravenous antibiotics are the first line of treatment [3]. Antibiotics should cover Gram-positive bacteria, Gram-negative bacteria, and anaerobes [12]. The most commonly prescribed antibiotics are ampicillin-sulbactam or clindamycin. Pseudomonads should be included in the expanded coverage for immunocompromised individuals. Cefepime, meropenem, and piperacillin-tazobactam are the only antibiotics available. Doctors should consider methicillin-resistant Staphylococcus aureus (MRSA) coverage for immunocompromised patients, high-risk patients, and those with a history of MRSA infection [13].

It's debatable whether or not to give patients intravenous steroids. Steroids have been proven in a few case reports [25] to reduce the need for airway control. Still, more research is needed before it becomes a standard of therapy, and the decision is left to the treating physician's discretion. Antibiotic treatment typically lasts for 2 weeks. Close attention must be paid to the number of white blood cells and the temperature [13].

If the infection is odontogenic, a tooth should be removed to eliminate the cause of the problem. Patients who do not improve after antibiotic treatment or show signs of a fluid accumulation on imaging may have needle aspiration or surgical incision and drainage [13].

60.7.3 Surgery

Early surgical decompression has not been found to enhance results. Therefore, it is often reserved for patients who have failed medicinal therapy [3]; however, early tooth extraction and cultures are indicated in patients requiring intubation due to odontogenic infections.

When a suppurative infection is present, such as with a purulent needle aspirate, crepitus, fluctuance, or soft tissue air, surgical drainage may be necessary to relieve pressure on the neck's fascial compartments and drain the pus. The incision is typically made perpendicular to the skin and two fingerbreadths inferior to the mandibu lar angle. The surgeon will displace the submandibular gland and divide the mylohyoid muscles to decompress the afflicted fascial compartments [17].

Surgical decompression performed early on is not likely to reveal the presence of pus and may only mildly enhance airflow. Abscesses typically don't appear until after the first 24–36 h [1] and can be hard to spot in the clinic.

After this first period, we repeat computed tomography imaging to search for an abscess if the patient is not responding well to antibiotics alone or if visible fluctuation is present. If an accumulation is seen on imaging, the patient should undergo needle aspiration or an incision and drainage treatment while under general anesthetic [26]. A tracheostomy or endotracheal tube with a cuff should be used for this procedure. In addition, if a tooth is suspected of being the infection's origin, it must be removed [1].

Samples should be taken for Gram stain and culture for aerobic and anaerobic bacteria [1] when needle aspiration, incision, and drainage are necessary.

References

1. Chow AW. Ludwig angina. In: Durand ML, Bogorodskaya M, editors. UpToDate; 2022. Last updated: Oct 04, 2022.
2. Saifeldeen K, Evans R. Ludwig's angina. Emerg Med J. 2004;21:242–3.
3. Bansal A, Miskoff J, Lis RJ. Otolaryngologic critical care. Crit Care Clin. 2003;19:55–72.
4. Winters M. Evidence-based diagnosis and management of ENT emergencies. American Academy of Emergency Medicine. Medscape Emerg Med. 2007; https://www.medscape.com/viewarticle/551650_4 (Accessed online at June 4, 2023)

5. Moreland LW, Corey J, McKenzie R. Ludwig's angina. Report of a case and review of the literature. Arch Intern Med. 1988;148:461–6.
6. Murray AD. Deep neck infections. In: Meyers AD, editor. Medscape; 2023. Updated: April 07, 2022. https://emedicine.medscape.com/article/837048-overview (Accessed online at June 4, 2023).
7. Boscolo-Rizzo P, Da Mosto MC. Submandibular space infection: a potentially lethal infection. Int J Infect Dis. 2009;13:327.
8. Bridwell R, Gottlieb M, Koyfman A, Long B. Diagnosis and management of Ludwig's angina: an evidence-based review. Am J Emerg Med. 2021;41:1.
9. Kovalev V. A severe case of Ludwig's angina with a complicated clinical course. Cureus. 2020;12:e7695.
10. Mohamad I, Narayanan MS. "Double Tongue" appearance in Ludwig's angina. N Engl J Med. 2019;381:163.
11. Furst IM, Ersil P, Caminiti M. A rare complication of tooth abscess—Ludwig's angina and mediastinitis. J Can Dent Assoc. 2001;67:324.
12. Quinn FB. Ludwig angina. Arch Otolaryngol Head Neck Surg. 1999;125(5):599.
13. An J, Madeo J, Singhal M. Ludwig angina (Updated 2022 Oct 10). In: StatPearls. Treasure Island (FL): StatPearls Publishing; 2023. Available from: https://www.ncbi.nlm.nih.gov/books/NBK482354/ (Accessed online at June 4, 2023).
14. Brook I. Microbiology and principles of antimicrobial therapy for head and neck infections. Infect Dis Clin N Am. 2007;21(2):355–91.
15. Spitalnic SJ, Sucov A. Ludwig's angina: case report and review. J Emerg Med. 1995;13:499–503.
16. Saifeldeen K, Evans R. Ludwig's angina. Emerg Med J. 2004;21(2):242–3.
17. Barakate MS, Jensen MJ, Hemli JM, Graham AR. Ludwig's angina: report of a case and review of management issues. Ann Otol Rhinol Laryngol. 2001;110(5 Pt 1):453–6.
18. Marple BF. Ludwig angina: a review of current airway management. Arch Otolaryngol Head Neck Surg. 1999;125:596–9.
19. Shockley WW. Ludwig angina: a review of current airway management. Arch Otolaryngol Head Neck Surg. 1999;125:600.
20. Vieira F, Allen SM, Stocks RM, Thompson JW. Deep neck infection. Otolaryngol Clin N Am. 2008;41:459.
21. Ovassapian A, Tuncbilek M, Weitzel EK, Joshi CW. Airway management in adult patients with deep neck infections: a case series and review of the literature. Anesth Analg. 2005;100:585.
22. Barton ED, Bair AE. Ludwig's angina. J Emerg Med. 2008;34:163.
23. Freund B, Timon C. Ludwig's angina: a place for steroid therapy in its management? Oral Health. 1992;82:23–5.
24. Crespo AN, Chone CT, Fonseca AS, Montenegro MC, Pereira R, Milani JA. Clinical versus computed tomography evaluation in the diagnosis and management of deep neck infection. Sao Paulo Med J. 2004;122(6):259–63.
25. Wolfe MM, Davis JW, Parks SN. Is surgical airway necessary for airway management in deep neck infections and Ludwig angina? J Crit Care. 2011;26(1):11–4.
26. Shi H, Yang Z, Li H, et al. Efficacy of needle aspiration in patients with oral-maxillofacial abscesses: a retrospective study of 15 consecutive patients. Am J Otolaryngol. 2022;43:103216.

Part VI

Surgical Interventions for Upper Airway Management

Choanal Atresia Management

61

Rezzan Budak, Cemal Cingi, and Mario Milkov

61.1 Introduction

Choanal atresia is the congenital closure of the posterior nasal aperture. It is seen approximately once in 5000/8000 births [1]. It may be unilateral or bilateral. Unilateral atresia is twice as common as bilateral atresia [1]. Choanal atresia is twice as common in women than in men. Its etiology needs to be clarified, and there are various theories. Persistent bucconasal membrane, persistent buccopharyngeal membrane, congenital adhesions in mucous membranes, and anomalies in the migration of the cephalic neural crest may be the cause of choanal atresia. Computed tomography and histopathological examinations of choanal atresia cases showed that the atresia was 10% bone and 90% bone and membranous type. Familial predisposition is 20% [2, 3]. The boundaries of choanal atresia are the sphenoid bone superiorly, the vomer medially, the medial pterygoid lamina laterally, and the horizontal part of the maxilla palatum inferiorly. The pterygoid lamina may be medialized in bilateral choanal atresia, and the vomer may be thickened.

Choanal atresia can be seen with many craniofacial anomalies and systemic malformations, including skull base defects. The frequency of cooccurrence of another anomaly with choanal atresia is 73.6%. Congenital anomalies in which choanal atresia can occur together are CHARGE 25.6% (C: coloboma, H: heart defect, A: atresia choanae,

R. Budak
Department of Otorhinolaryngology, Etimesgut Şehit Sait Ertürk State Hospital, Ankara, Turkey

C. Cingi (✉)
Medical Faculty, Department of Otorhinolaryngology, Eskisehir Osmangazi University, Eskisehir, Turkey

M. Milkov
Faculty of Dental Medicine, Department of Dental Materials Science and Biomaterials, Prof. Paraskev Stoyanov Medical University, Varna, Bulgaria

H. Yüksel et al. (eds.), *Pediatric Airway Diseases*, Comprehensive ENT, https://doi.org/10.1007/978-3-031-74853-0_61

R: retarded growth and development, G: genital hypoplasia, E: ear anomalies, deafness, extremity abnormalities), branchial anomalies, Treacher-Collins syndrome, Down syndrome, Apert syndrome, Crouzon syndrome, craniosynostosis, meningocele, humeroradial synostosis, mandibular facial synostosis, microcephaly, micrognathia, nasopharyngeal anomalies, and palatal defects can be given as examples [2–4].

61.2 Embryology

There are various theories about the biology of choanal atresia. It is thought to most commonly develop due to the rupture of the nasobuccal membrane. Between the third and fourth weeks of pregnancy, the lateral nasal ectodermal plates fold inward to form the nasal sulci. The thin bucconasal membrane that forms the base of these sacs separates the nasal cavity from the oral cavity. Choana occurs due to the rupture of the bucconasal membrane between the fifth and sixth weeks of pregnancy. Another hypothesis for the formation of choanal atresia is the different migration of neural crest cells [5–7].

61.3 Symptoms

Choanal atresia can be bilateral or unilateral. While bilateral choanal atresia is diagnosed in the neonatal period, unilateral choanal atresia is diagnosed at later ages. It should not be forgotten that bilateral choanal atresia is the most common cause of respiratory distress in newborns [8]. Bilateral atresia should be considered a newborn emergency. Oral breathing in the neonatal period begins in the second–fourth period. In bilateral choanal atresia, cyclic cyanosis improves with crying and increases while sucking and when the mouth is closed. In unilateral cases, patients present with nasal discharge and nasal congestion on the side where the choanae is blocked later in life.

61.4 Diagnosis

Failure to advance the 6 F aspiration catheter from the nasal passage to the oropharynx during the first examination should suggest choanal atresia. Nasal passage length is approximately 3 cm in the newborn period. Inability to advance the catheter more than 3 cm or if the cotton placed in front of the nose does not move with respiration requires endoscopic examination for differential diagnosis. A closed choana opening during nasal endoscopic examination is diagnostic. Computed tomography: It is used to support the diagnosis, see the presence of additional pathology, and determine the type of atresia. In CT images taken in the axial and coronal planes, it is determined that the air passage does not continue at the mouth of the choana and that the posterior part of the nasal passage is blocked by bone or mucous membrane. Vomer thickness increases in osseous choanal atresia [8]. CT has an essential place in the planning of surgical intervention. Accurate analysis of the relationship of atresia with the turbinates, lateral nasal wall, and vomer will be guiding during the surgery (Figs. 61.1, 61.2, 61.3, 61.4, and 61.5).

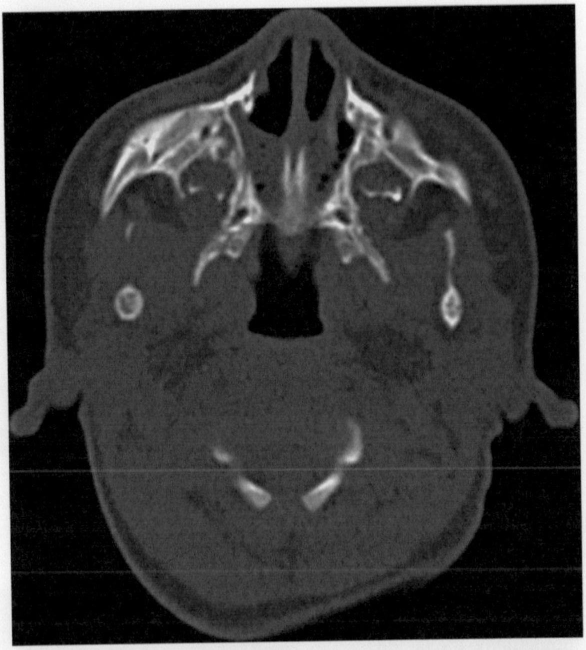

Fig. 61.1 In axial sectioned computed tomography, the lateral nasal wall is bent inward, the vomer is thickened, and mucosal thickening is seen just in front of the choanal level, where the bone structure continues

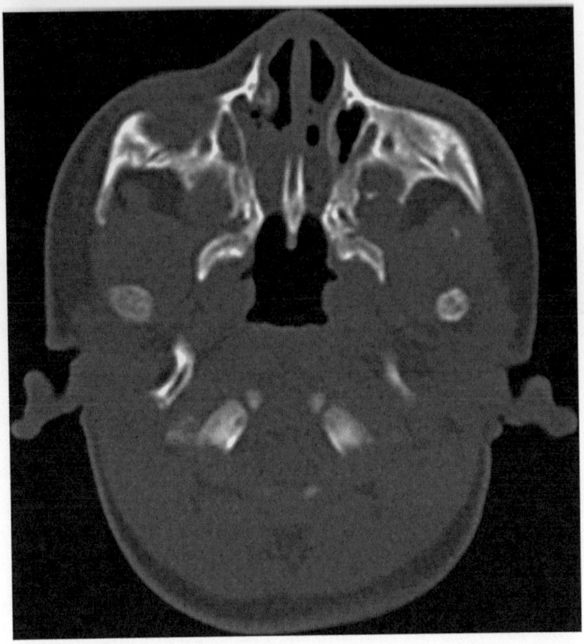

Fig. 61.2 Axial cross-sectional computed tomography shows that the lateral nasal wall is slightly bent inwards, there is no thickening in the vomer, and the bone structure at the choanal level continues in thin lamellar form

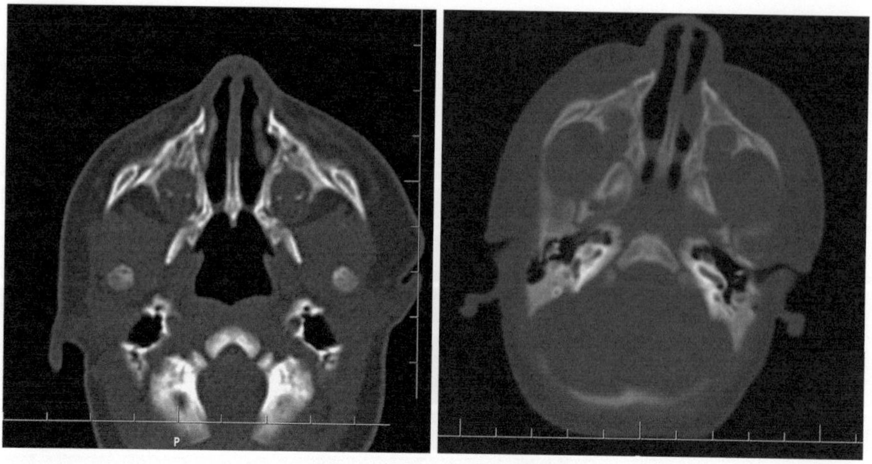

Figs. 61.3 and 61.4 Only membranous atresia is seen at the choanal level in axial sectioned computed tomographies

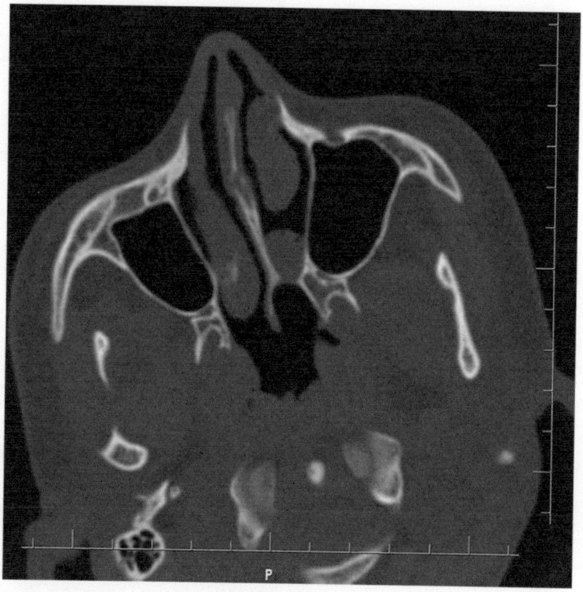

Fig. 61.5 In axial sectioned computed tomography, the lateral nasal wall is bent inward, the vomer is thickened, and bony and membranous stenosis are seen together at the choanal level

61.5 Treatment

Choanal atresia patients are cases that require multidisciplinary follow-up due to both low birth weight and the presence of congenital anomalies. With the joint work of neonatal, anesthesia, and ENT clinics, positive results can be achieved during surgical intervention and postoperative follow-up. The patient is monitored in the neonatal unit with oral airway, McGovern pacifier (Fig. 61.6), or endotracheal intubation. McGovern pacifier is the first preferred method for ease of use. If the patient

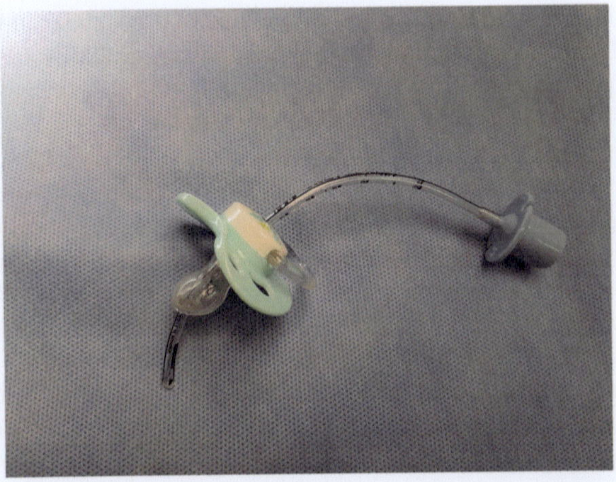

Fig. 61.6 McGovern pacifier; It can be easily prepared by puncturing both ends of a regular pacifier and passing a size 2.5 intubation tube through it

cannot breathe adequately with the McGovern pacifier, then the oral airway is followed by endotracheal intubation if ventilation is still inadequate. During the patient's preoperative evaluation, vital organ failures must be considered, and the operation must be planned by paying attention to the priority order.

For example, choanal atresia surgery may be required for newborns with common neurological, gastrointestinal, or cardiac defects.

Choanal atresia surgery can be examined under endonasal and transpalatal approaches. In determining the surgical method in congenital choanal atresia, factors such as the patient's nasopharynx width, the thickness of the atresia, the vomer thickness, whether it is unilateral or bilateral, the need for postoperative stents, the presence of additional anomalies, and the surgeon's experience should be taken into consideration. Until recently, transpalatal approaches were preferred in the treatment of congenital choanal atresia, but in recent years, endoscopic transnasal procedures have gained more importance in the treatment of choanal atresia, especially with the introduction of rigid endoscopes and advanced endoscopic instruments such as drills, lasers, and microdebriders [9, 10] (transnasal surgery, transpalatal surgery). It is less invasive, but restenosis is a common complication after this surgery [11]. Although placing a stent in the choana after transnasal surgery is still a commonly used method to prevent restenosis, it is now more preferred to complete the surgery without placing a stent using different surgical techniques due to the risk of the stent becoming a focus of infection and the risk of necrosis in the turbinate and septa due to pressure [12–17].

61.5.1 Surgery

In transpalatal surgery, as in cleft palate operations, the choanal region is reached through an incision made at the level of the alveolar arch, and the process is based on the principle of removing the obliterated part of the choanal mouth from the posterior, remaining in the inferior and medial lines. Although it can be preferred in terms of not damaging the nasal mucosa and making manipulation easier, especially in bone-type choanal atresia, publications report that 52% of the patients operated on with this method developed a growth problem in the palate [18, 19]. The transpalatal method is used in patients who have completed their facial development or in patients with resistant restenosis. It may be preferred in such cases.

Having a good view in transnasal endoscopic surgery is the most important factor that protects the patient from surgical complications. The 0-degree, 2.7-mm diameter, 90-mm long nasal endoscope is frequently preferred in choanal atresia surgery due to its ease of use and manipulation in narrow areas (Fig. 61.7). The instruments used mostly for tympanomastoidectomy surgery in ENT clinics can be easily used in choanal atresia repair. Successful decongestion before transnasal endoscopic surgery is essential for both field of view and bleeding control. Placing pads impregnated with 1/10,000 adrenaline solution into the nasal passage and waiting for 7–10 minutes provides decongestion and expands the field of view. Local anesthetic containing epinephrine and lidocaine (2%) used in regional anesthesia is applied to the tail part of the inferior turbinate, choana mucosa, septum posterior, sphenopalatine region, and middle turbinate posterior adhesion site. The total dose should be at most 7 mg/kg. It should be remembered that the patient will be affected cardiologically by applying epinephrine to the nasal passage, and the anesthesia team should be informed about the procedure performed.

In some cases, in endoscopic examination, the choana opening, which should typically be present in the area indicated by the tail of the inferior turbinate, can be seen as a slight niche (Fig. 61.8). This niche suggests the starting point of the operation. Staying below the lower line of the middle turbinate during surgery significantly reduces the complication rate. Most of the choanal arteries have a membranous and bony membranous structure, and the remaining part has a pure skeletal system, so that the visible niche can be easily perforated with the help of an aspirator. The

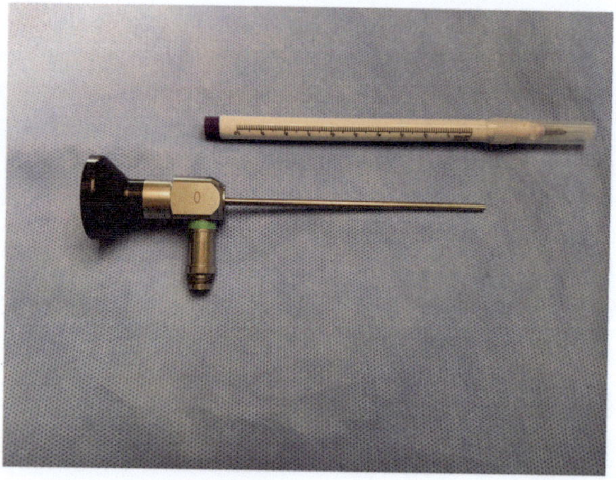

Fig. 61.7 Nasal endoscope used in surgery

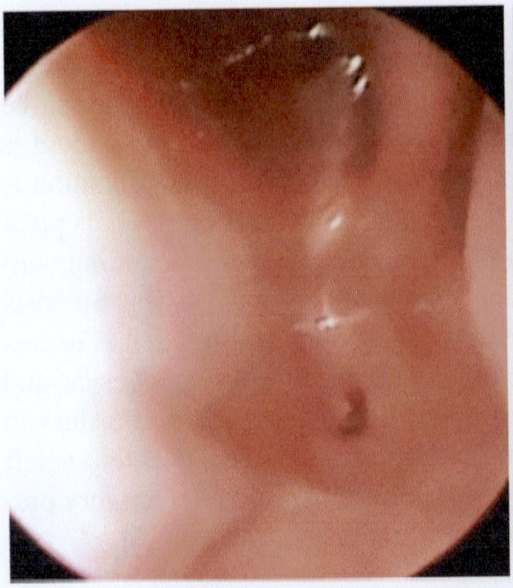

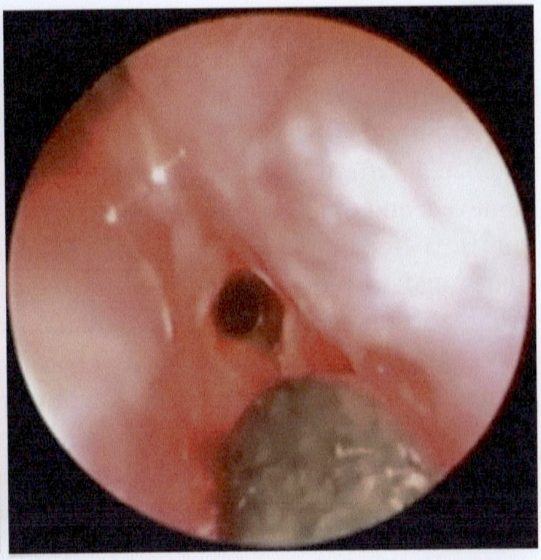

Figs. 61.8 and 61.9 The area where the niche is usually located and its opening with the help of an aspirator can be seen

intervention should be done very gently. The immediate neighborhood of the area that fits the choanae is vital, so one should move as close to the septum and the bottom of the nasal passage as possible. In osseous-type choanal atresia, if the niche cannot be seen, an ostium of approximately 2–3 mm is opened from the tail part of the inferior turbinate to the choanal region with the help of a tourniquet (Fig. 61.9). After the nasopharynx wall is seen in the posterior, the ostium found is accepted as the starting point, starting from the posterosuperior position on the septum in both nasal passages.

A 5-mm transverse incision is made, and the incision is extended anteriorly to the base. After the mucosal flap is created, the area around the ostium is expanded by checking it regularly with the help of a stylet. It should be kept mainly in the medial and inferior regions. Approximately 1 mm of mucosal flap is left in front of the torus tubarius on the superiolateral side. An incision made on the posterior septum releases about 0.5 cm of the vomer with the help of an elevator and removes it to be combined with the newly created ostia. During excision, the patient should remain inferior to the middle turbinate. Then, the posterior 0.5-cm horizontal part of the hard palate is removed with the help of a tourniquet or bone curette. After the bone parts are removed, the mucosal flap of the posterior aspect of the resulting closed choana is excised. Septal flaps are laid inferomedially to prevent bone structures from being exposed. The fact that mucosal flaps cover the bone structures, in other words, not leaving an exposed bone or cartilage surface, reduces the risk of infection and necrosis. Injury to opposing surfaces during surgery increases the possibility of synechiae; it is essential to exercise utmost care. When posterior septal excision is performed in the transnasal endoscopic method, nasal stent placement is generally unnecessary. Therefore, there is no risk of stent-related complications. In postoperative care, the patient is recommended nasal irrigation and nasal moisturizing drops to keep the nasal mucosa moist for 1 week.

Bilateral choanal atresias are generally operated on in the first few days of life, so patients are followed in neonatal intensive care conditions. If there is postoperative bleeding, nasal tampons impregnated with antibiotics + decongestant can be placed in both nasal passages, and the tampons are removed before the patient is extubated. After the patient's nasal breathing begins, postoperative stabilization is achieved, and oral feeding is recommended, especially if the sucking reflex is present. Breastfeeding is recommended. The aim is to ensure that nasal breathing continues and to prevent synechiae by reducing edema in mutual tissues. Stenosis usually occurs within the first month, so weekly endoscopic examination is necessary in the first month. Postoperatively, it is followed by antibiotics, analgesics, and antiinflammatory drugs for 1 week. Postoperative follow-up is more effortless in patients without a stent. In cases where stent placement is required, the stent is left in place for 8–12 weeks. Studies show that applying mitomycin-c after surgery prevents the development of stenosis in cases where a stent is not placed [20].

61.6 Complications

Choanal atresia is the most common cause of respiratory failure in newborns. It is a disease that can develop complications from diagnosis to the postoperative period and requires a multidisciplinary approach. The patient may be arrested due to respiratory distress at the time of diagnosis, so the baby with choanal atresia should be immediately fitted with a McGovern pacifier at the time of diagnosis. If the baby cannot breathe with a pacifier, oral airway should be tried; if he still cannot breathe, he should be intubated. Feeding should be done with the help of an orogastric tube. Food aspiration may occur when oral feeding is attempted because the patient cannot breathe nasally. Cardiac complications such as tachycardia and hypertension may develop due to the topical decongestants used during the examination. Therefore, it is recommended that the test be performed under the monitoring and supervision of a neonatal physician, considering the possibility of emergency intervention. Bleeding, skull base penetration, circulation and rhythm disturbances, and hypothermia may occur during surgery. Therefore, the operating room temperature should be between 21 and 24 degrees, and the patient should be covered to keep warm. Bleeding may occur due to not waiting enough time after local anesthesia at the beginning of the operation or due to significant vessel injury due to variations. The possibility of bleeding due to vascular damage can be reduced by staying below the lower edge of the middle turbinate, checking the presence of space that can be expanded at the mouth of the choana with the help of a continuous stylet, and working anteromedially. Skull base penetration is a complication whose risk can be reduced by staying below the lower edge of the middle turbinate. Possible difficulties in the postoperative period are bleeding, cardiac complications due to topical decongestion, anesthesia complications (hypotonia, hyponatremia, failure to wake up, etc.), synechiae, nasal mucosa necrosis in patients with nasal stents, and stent-related infection. Synechiae is a condition that needs to be treated when noticed. It is a less common complication when atraumatic surgery is performed. Choana stenosis is another common postoperative complication. Stenosis manifests as the baby's oral intake decreases and its duration increases during follow-ups. When stenosis is observed, repair is planned without delay. The most common cause of choanal stenosis is inadequate bone and mucosa excisions.

Experience and suitability of surgical instruments are the most critical factors in repairing and following choanal atresia. It is possible to prevent complications with appropriate surgical equipment and experience. Bilateral choanal atresia is a neonatal emergency, and satisfactory results can be obtained in treatment with a multisplinter approach.

References

1. Leclerc JE, Fearon B. Choanal atresia and associated anomalies. Int J Pediatr Otorhinolaryngol. 1987;13:265–72. https://doi.org/10.1016/0165-5876(87)90107-8.
2. Hengerer AS, Brickman TM, Jeyakumar A. Choanal atresia: embryologic analysis and evolution of treatment, a 30-year experience. Laryngoscope. 2008;118:862–6.
3. Brown OE, Pownell P, Manning SC. Choanal atresia: a new anatomic classification and clinical management applications. Laryngoscope. 1996;106:97–101. https://doi.org/10.1097/00005537-199601000-00019.
4. Burrow TA, Saal HM, de Alarcon A, Martin LJ, Cotton RT, Hopkin RJ. Characterization of congenital anomalies in individuals with choanal atresia. Arch Otolaryngol Head Neck Surg. 2009;135:543–7.
5. Dunham ME. Miller RP: Bilateral canal atresia and associated with malformation of the anterior skull base, embryogenesis and clinical complications. Ann Otol Rhinol Laringol. 1992;101:916.
6. Hengerer AS, Strome M. Chonal atresia: a new embriyologic theory and ıts influence surgical manegment. Laryngscope. 1982;92:913.
7. Gujrathi CS, Daniel SJ, James AL, Forte V. Management of bilateral choanal atresia in the neonate: an institutional review. Int J Pediatr Otorhinolaryngol. 2004;68(4):399–407.
8. Slovis TL, Egli DF. Congenital anomalies and acquired lesions. In: Kuhn JP, Slovis TL, Haller JO, editors. Caffey's pediatric diagnostic imaging, vol. 1. 10th ed. USA: Elsevier; 2004. p. 22–8.
9. Teissier N, Kaguelidou F, Couloigner V, François M, Van Den Abbeele T. Predictive factors for success after transnasal endoscopic treatment of choanal atresia. Arch Otolaryngol Head Neck Surg. 2008;134(1):57–61.
10. Van Den Abbeele T, François M, Narcy P. Transnasal endoscopic treatment of choanal atresia without prolonged stenting. Arch Otolaryngol Head Neck Surg. 2002;128(8):936–40.
11. Sharma RK, Lee CA, Gunasekaran S, Knight LC, Bielby M. Stenting for bilateral congenital choanal atresia—a new technique. Int J Pediatr Otorhinolaryngol. 2006;70(5):869–74.
12. Ibrahim AA, Magdy EA, Hassab MH. Endoscopic choanoplasty without stenting for congenital choanal atresia repair. Int J Pediatr Otorhinolaryngol. 2010;74(2):144–50.
13. Karaagac AT, Yıldırım A, Oner CN. A 2-month-old baby with CHARGE syndrome. Marmara Med J. 2013;26(1):39–42.
14. Schoem SR. Transnasal endoscopic repair of choanal atresia: why stent? Otolaryngol Head Neck Surg. 2004;131(4):362–6.
15. Durmaz A, Tosun F, Yldrm N, Sahan M, Kvrakdal C, Gerek MJ. Transnasal endoscopic repair of choanal atresia: results of 13 cases and meta-analysis. Craniofac Surg. 2008;19(5):1270–4.
16. Yaniv E, Hadar T, Shvero J, Stern Y, Raveh E. Endoscopic transnasal repair of choanal atresia. Int J Pediatr Otorhinolaryngol. 2007;71(3):457–62.

17. Stankiewicz JA. The endoscopic repair of choanal atresia. Otolaryngol Head Neck Surg. 1990;103(6):931–7.
18. Gök Ü, Kaygusuz İ, Özer N, Keleş E. Erişkinlerde unilateral koanal atrezi. KBB ve Baş Boyun Cerrahisi Dergisi. 1999;7:209–12.
19. Freng A. Surgical treatment of congenital cohanal atresia. Ann Otol Rhinol Laryngol. 1978;87:346–50.
20. Aksoy F, Demirhan H, Yildirim YS, Ozturan O. Bilateral choanal atresia in an adult - management with mitomycin C and without stents: a case report. Cases J. 2009;2:9307.

62 Pediatric Functional Endoscopic Sinus Surgery

Ali Budak, Cemal Cingi, and Hesham Negm

62.1 Introduction

Nowadays, endoscopic methods are frequently preferred in diagnosing and treating nasal pathologies. External open surgical approaches are more invasive than functional endoscopic sinus surgery, and available surgical interventions have high mortality and morbidity. Endoscopic methods are mainly used to diagnose and treat nasal pathologies seen in the pediatric period [1]. Endoscopic procedures are successfully used in the treatment of many pathologies such as acute sinusitis, chronic sinusitis, nasal polyps, sinus benign tumors, skull base tumors, congenital or traumatic encephaloceles or CSF fistulas and lacrimal duct obstructions, orbital decompression, choanal atresia, subperiosteal abscesses, and so on.

In the diagnosis of nasal pathologies, anamnesis, detailed ENT examination are used. Endoscopic examination, computed tomography, and laboratory tests may be needed in some cases. It is difficult to perform an endoscopic analysis in children, so topical anesthesia, nasal decongestion, sedation, and even general anesthesia may sometimes be required.

A. Budak
Department of Otorhinolaryngology, Ankara Etlik City Hospital, Ankara, Turkey

C. Cingi (✉)
Medical Faculty, Department of Otorhinolaryngology, Eskisehir Osmangazi University, Eskisehir, Turkey

H. Negm
Faculty of Medicine, Department of Otorhinolaryngology, Cairo University, Cairo, Egypt

H. Yüksel et al. (eds.), *Pediatric Airway Diseases*, Comprehensive ENT, https://doi.org/10.1007/978-3-031-74853-0_62

62.2 Anatomy

Understanding the nasal cavity and the development of the paranasal sinuses is crucial for effective endoscopic sinus surgery (ESS) in children. The uncinate process, ethmoid infundibulum, hiatus semilunaris, bulla ethmoidalis, and their primary connections are present at birth in humans. These are a few of the few constants in life. These sinuses and the lateral nasal wall are expanding and becoming pneumatized for the most part. The sphenoid and frontal sinuses do most of their development between the ages of 4 and 14 [2].

All newborns have sinuses in their maxillae and ethmoids. The average youngster has 3–15 ethmoid air cells on each side. However, throughout the first 3–4 years of life, the cells expand and pneumatize at a high rate. As a shallow sac in the lateral nasal wall, the maxillary sinus undergoes fast growth in the first 4 years of life. The maxillary sinus develops at around 4 years of age, reaching laterally to the infraorbital canal and inferiorly to the attachment of the inferior turbinate [2].

Neither the frontal nor the sphenoid sinus is present at birth; the sphenoid sinus is a blind mucosal sac that does not extend to the sphenoid bone or cartilage. By the time a child is 4 years old, the sphenoid sinus is the size of a pea and can be identified, and the frontal sinus has begun to extend from the frontal recess. The ethmoid stops developing between the ages of 4 and 8. The maxillary sinus floor has reached the middle of the inferior meatus by the time a child is 7 years old. The permanent teeth have not yet entirely erupted, and the nose floor is still lower than the maxillary sinus floor. Permanent tooth buds might be harmed if a Caldwell Luc operation or inferior meatal window was done on a preschooler. During this stage of development, the sphenoid and frontal sinuses enlarge [2].

The paranasal sinuses reach their full adult size and complete pneumatization between the ages of 8 and 14. The maxillary sinus has grown and spread to the nasal floor. Minor changes in pneumatization and sphenoid sinus configuration [2] are possible during the next decade.

Surgical procedures for sinus surgery, particularly for the anterior ethmoid and maxillary sinuses, remain primarily stable throughout a child's development due to the stability of the linkages between the paranasal sinuses. The procedure is technically safe for use on youngsters. The author performed endoscopic drainage of a subperiosteal abscess on a 7-week-old newborn by opening the lamina papyracea to a considerable degree. The lamina papyracea and ethmoid bulla seemed higher regarding the middle turbinate [2] despite the lateral nasal wall markers being in the same locations as in older children.

To perform effective surgery and avoid difficulties, it is crucial to have a thorough understanding of the endoscopic anatomic linkages between the nasal cavity, the lateral nasal wall, and the paranasal sinuses. Anatomical features of the lateral nasal wall were given new names during the evolution of endoscopic sinus surgery. A worldwide conference on the terminology, staging, and treatment of sinus illness was conducted to standardize the language used to describe the paranasal sinuses. Experts in endoscopic sinus surgery practically dominated the room. This architecture is essential for the endoscopic sinus surgeon to understand in patients of all ages [2].

62.3 Indications

Rhinosinusitis is a common disease in childhood [3, 4]. In treatment, medical treatments are preferred before endoscopic surgery. In cases where there is no response to medical therapy, conventional surgical interventions are tried. Thanks to the development of nasal endoscopic instruments in recent years, these diseases can be treated more effectively and efficiently in the pediatric age group [1]. Endoscopic surgery has many possible complications. Publications report that endoscopic sinus surgery affects facial development, especially in young children [5, 6].

In children with chronic or frequently recurring sinusitis, a complete systemic examination should be performed, and the decision for surgery should be made. It was found that 64% of children with chronic sinusitis had hypersensitivity to allergens in allergy tests [7]. In pediatric patients with chronic or recurrent sinusitis, allergic rhinitis, adenoid vegetation, tonsillar hypertrophy, cystic fibrosis, immune system disorders, immotile cilia syndrome, and cyanotic heart diseases should be excluded.

Endoscopic sinus surgery (ESS) in youngsters requires an in-depth familiarity with the nasal cavity and the maturation of the paranasal sinuses. Humans are born with an uncinate process, an ethmoid infundibulum, a hiatus semilunaris, and a bulla ethmoidalis, all of which have their essential connections in place. You can count on these few things in life. Pneumatization and enlargement of these sinuses and the lateral nasal wall are occurring. Between the ages of 4 and 14, most growth occurs in the sphenoid and frontal sinuses [2].

Sinuses in the maxillae and ethmoids are present in every birth. Children typically have between 3 and 15 ethmoid air cells on each side. Cells grow and pneumatize rapidly throughout the first 3–4 years of life. The maxillary sinus, a small sac on the side of the nose, develops quickly in the first 4 years of life. During its formative years (ages 4–8), the maxillary sinus expands laterally to the infraorbital canal and inferiorly to the attachment of the inferior turbinate [2].

The sphenoid sinus is a blind mucosal sac that does not extend to the sphenoid bone or cartilage, and the frontal sinus does not exist in newborns. The frontal sinus will have begun to expand from the frontal recess, and the sphenoid sinus will be the size of a pea and easily identifiable when a kid is 4 years old. From the ages of 4–8, the ethmoid ceases to grow. When a child is seven, the maxillary sinus floor has developed to the middle of the inferior meatus. Due to incomplete permanent tooth eruption, the nasal base is still lower than the maxillary sinus. A Caldwell Luc procedure or an inadequate meatal window could affect a preschooler's developing permanent teeth. The sphenoid and frontal sinuses get more prominent [2] as a child matures.

Between ages 8 and 14, the paranasal sinuses develop to their full adult size and are fully pneumatic. The maxillary sinus has expanded into the nasal cavity and reached the floor. Over the next decade, the pneumatization and sphenoid sinus configuration [2] will shift slightly.

The paranasal sinuses' solid connections make it possible to perform sinus surgery on children at any point in their development, with the anterior ethmoid and maxillary sinuses being the most commonly operated on. The technique poses no known risks for children. The author accomplished endoscopic drainage of a subperiosteal abscess in a 7-week-old baby by extensively opening the lamina papyracea. Although the lateral nasal wall markers were in the same places as in older children, the lamina papyracea and ethmoid bulla seemed higher about the middle turbinate [2].

Understanding the endoscopic anatomic connections between the nasal cavity, the lateral nasal wall, and the paranasal sinuses is vital for efficient surgery and avoiding complications. During the development of endoscopic sinus surgery, formerly unnamed structures of the lateral nasal wall were given new identities. A worldwide conference on sinus sickness terminology, staging, and management was held to standardize the vocabulary used to define the paranasal sinuses. Sinus specialists who do endoscopic procedures nearly took over the discussion. The endoscopic sinus surgeon should be familiar with this structure in patients of all ages [2].

Pediatric sinusitis diagnosis: It should be determined based on a good anamnesis, anterior rhinoscopic examination, nasal endoscopic examination, laboratory, and radiological imaging. The most common examination findings are runny nose and postnasal drip. Discharge is present in 77% of patients. In total, 61% of sinusitis patients have otitis media, and 48% have cough [7]. In the differential diagnosis, paranasal tomography taken in axial and coronal planes shows inflammatory soft tissue densities in the paranasal sinuses, mucosal thickening, and obstruction in the osteomeatal complex (Figs. 62.1, 62.2, 62.3, 62.4, 62.5, 62.6 and 62.7).

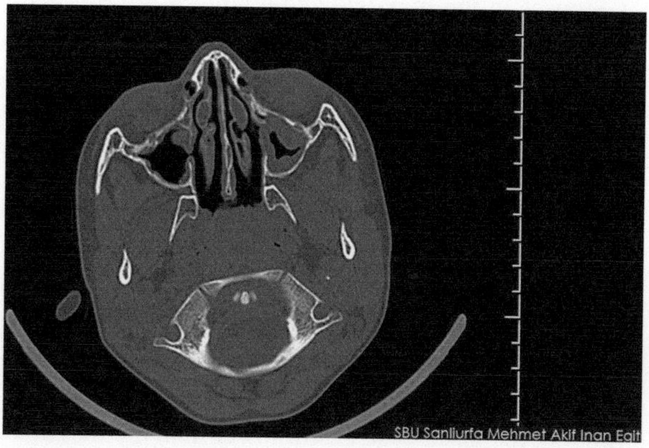

Fig. 62.1 Paranasal CT taken in axial plane shows that the bilateral maxillary sinus ostium is obliterated. Chronic sinusitis case

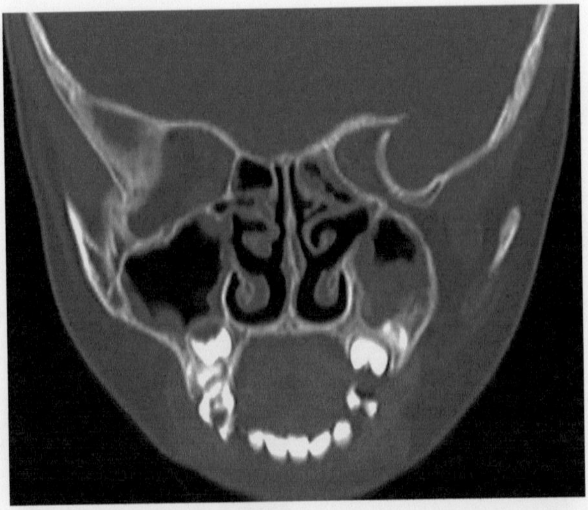

Fig. 62.2 Coronal Paranasal CT showing sinusitis

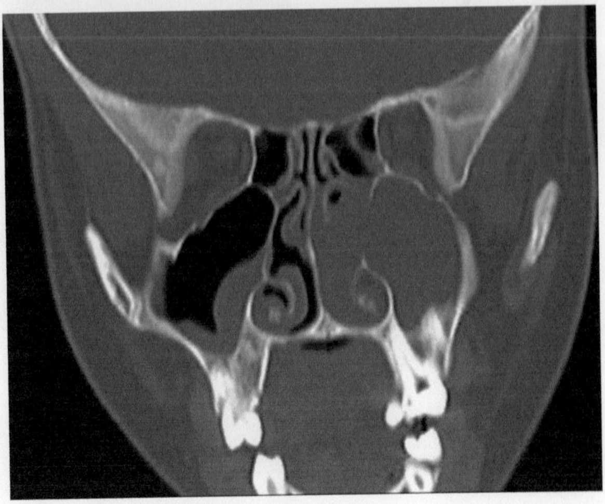

Fig. 62.3 Coronal Paranasal CT showing sinusitis

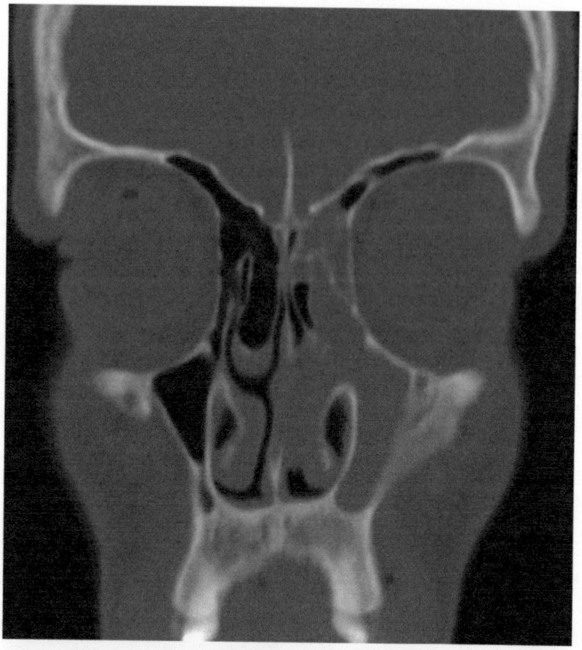

Fig. 62.4 Coronal Paranasal CT showing sinusitis

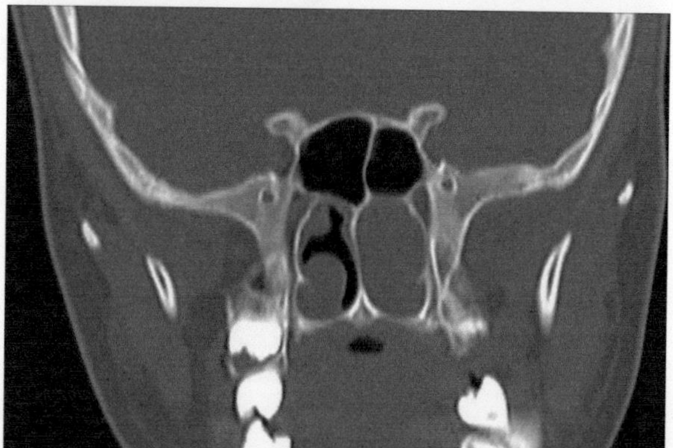

Fig. 62.5 Coronal Paranasal CT showing sinusitis

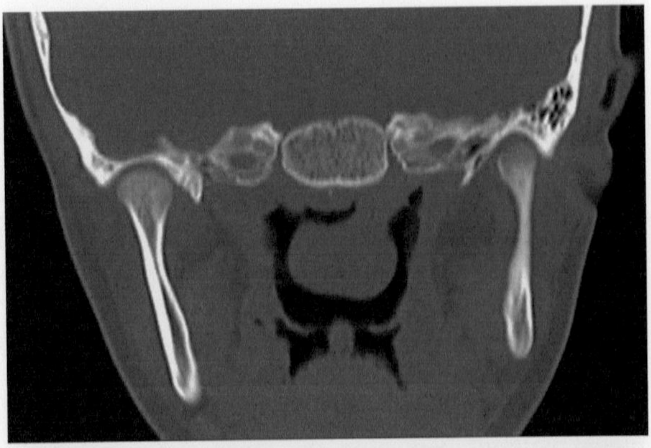

Fig. 62.6 Coronal Paranasal CT showing sinusitis

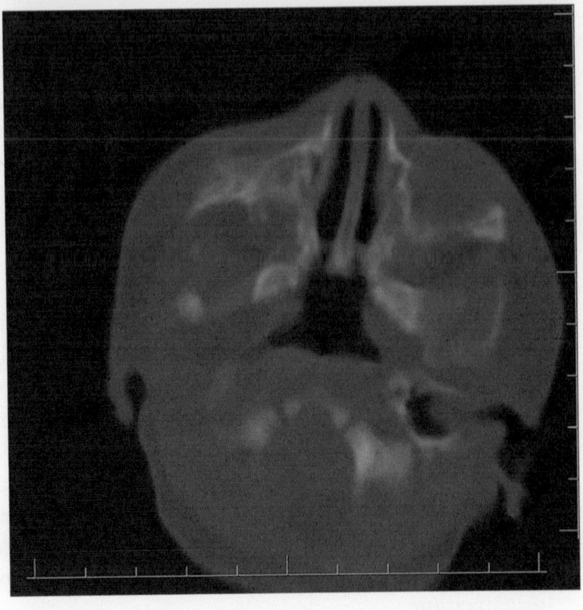

Fig. 62.7 Axial Paranasal CT showing sinusitis

62.4 Treatment

Most cases of pediatric sinusitis benefit from medical treatment. Surgical treatment is recommended to prevent complications and control symptoms in patients who do not respond to medical treatment. The most frequently applied surgical procedures in children are sinus lavage, adenoidectomy, and functional endoscopic sinus surgery. Caldwell-Luc and open surgical methods are rarely used in the pediatric period because they affect facial development. Publications report that adenoidectomy is the first surgical method to treat chronic sinus infections in children due to its low morbidity, affordability, no need for exceptional surgical experience, and effectiveness [8–11].

Functional endoscopic sinus surgery (FESC) is rarely preferred in treating sinusitis, especially in young children. Adenoidectomy and inferior meatus antrostomy are the first preferred surgical approaches in pediatric cases.

In pediatric sinusitis, obstruction of the osteomeatal complex is blamed as the primary source of sinusitis due to anatomical variations and congenital problems. Treating the osteomeatal complex provides satisfactory results in the treatment of sinusitis. The purpose of opening the osteometal complex is to correct the pathologies that prevent the mucociliary activity of the sinus [12–15]. Messerklinger's limited functional approach should be preferred instead of Vigand's posterior approach [15] in children [13]. The limited functional approach aims to correct only the pathologies that are thought to cause the disease after an accurate diagnosis. The natural anatomical structure should be preserved, and the surgery should be completed without damaging the sinus and nasal mucosa's drainage and ventilation areas.

All patients should have a computed tomography (CT) in preoperative evaluation. Since pediatric patients' compliance with the operation will be low, the process should be performed under general anesthesia, not locally. Preoperative decongestion is vital for both bleeding control and the visual field. Before applying local anesthesia, the nasal mucosa is decongested with oxymetazoline spray (0.05%).

62.4.1 Surgical Therapy

The following recommendations for endoscopic sinus surgery [16] were included in the clinical consensus statement on juvenile chronic rhinosinusitis.

- After medical therapy and adenoidectomy have failed, endoscopic sinus surgery effectively treats pediatric chronic rhinosinusitis.
- Before endoscopic sinus surgery, a CT scan of the paranasal sinuses is indicated to assess the disease's structure, development, and extent.
- Image-guided endoscopic sinus surgery is helpful for revision endoscopic sinus surgery cases and patients with extensive nasal polyposis that can obstruct visualization.
- There are insufficient data to suggest that endoscopic sinus surgery for chronic rhinosinusitis in children significantly stunts their face development.
- Postoperative debridement is not required to manage this condition effectively in chronic rhinosinusitis cases in children.

62.4.1.1 Minimally Invasive Technique

There is little doubt that the criteria for surgery and the quantity of surgery performed for juvenile sinus illness have gotten more conservative over time. Surgical draining of the sinuses should be considered only when CT scans reveal the presence of disease. Many pediatric sinus surgeons have recommended merely doing a mini-FESS because the OMC is the bottleneck for outflow of the anterior sinuses (the OMC consists of the uncinate process and the infundibular region around the ethmoid complex). The uncinate process is excised, the maxillary ostia is located and opened, and an ethmoid bullectomy or anterior ethmoidalectomy is performed. Success rates are comparable or even more significant, with fewer problems reported. While Talbot recommended simply removing OMC illness to free the frontal sinus and frontal recess, Smith found that opening the ethmoids cleared the sphenoid [17].

Setliff recommended a small-hole or minimally invasive approach [18, 19]. The uncinate process's mucosa and bone are removed during this procedure for maxillary sinus disease, but the ostia are left alone. He does not drill a big hole in the skull to clear up the maxillary sinus. Since the maxillary, ethmoid bulla and frontal sinus ostia are pretty large, the assumption behind minimally invasive surgery is that narrow mucous membrane-lined clefts are the predisposing factor to clinical illness. A significant drain isn't necessary for the sinuses. The extent of the convoluted and limited draining channel for the anterior sinuses is unexpected when seen on a routine CT scan [2]. This minimally invasive procedure has been successfully used on adult and pediatric patients. The infundibulum, the sinuses' natural drainage system, was widened with an uncinectomy using a pediatric backbiter and surgical microdebrider. The maxillary ostia's appearance (normal, polypoid, or edematous) did not influence the decision not to do an antrostomy [2].

Most patients had maxillary sinus ostium edema or obscuration, with or without polyps, pus, or cysts, as reported by Setliff in 1996. He did not elaborate on his ethmoid, sphenoid, or frontal sinus surgical approach. In 300 patients, he operated on just one needed further surgery to open their maxillary sinus after his initial operation. Since he started using the MIS method, his overall rate of surgical redos has decreased from 15% to 7%. For the maxillary ostia to drain, the whole uncinate must be removed. On the other hand, Mendelsohn and Gross [20] argued for enlarging the Ostia to three to five times its usual size and even making a mega-ostia for individuals with ciliary abnormalities.

62.4.1.2 Technique for Nasal Polyps in Children

Changing typical landmarks, the propensity for copious bleeding, and the potential for recurrence make nasal polyposis a challenging illness to treat in both adults and children. Cystic fibrosis (CF) is a disease that has to be checked out in youngsters. Nasal polyps in kids can also be caused by other conditions, such as allergic polyposis or fungal sinusitis (AFS). Endoscopic sinus surgery (ESS) principles must be used to remove polypoid illness. The Messerklinger procedure is recommended for the removal of polyps and the opening of the sinuses. Steroids, both preoperatively and postoperatively, can reduce the fibrovascular character of the polyps, leading to less bleeding during surgery and better recurrence prevention [2].

However, the surgical microdebrider has been the most significant development in endoscopic sinus surgery (ESS) for children with nasal polyposis. While the polyps are being resected and eliminated effectively, any bleeding is suctioned away. Several writers highlight the improved patient safety afforded by the surgical microdebrider. Nevertheless, a thorough understanding of the typical architecture and anatomic variations of the nasal cavity, lateral nasal wall, and paranasal sinus in children of varying ages is essential. Preoperative CT scanning is highly recommended to assess the severity of the illness and the modifications the polyps have made to the nasal cavity and the paranasal sinuses [21].

Nasal and sinus infections are common in children with CF. Symptoms include a buildup of thick, inspissated mucus from the exocrine glands. Sinus drainage is obstructed due to the vast, sticky mucus produced by people with cystic fibrosis. As a result, the surgical approach taken with patients who suffer from CF and chronic sinusitis is the same as that taken with individuals who suffer from chronic sinusitis alone. However, because part of the viscous mucus must be manually drained regularly to help clean the sinuses [2], a minimally invasive or small-hole approach may give inadequate access to the sinuses.

62.4.1.3 Lasers

Endoscopic sinus surgery (ESS) using lasers has been documented in adults, not children. Carbon dioxide (CO2), argon, potassium titanyl phosphate (KTP), erbium yttrium aluminum garnet (YAG), and holmium yttrium aluminum garnet (YAG) are only some of the lasers that fall into this category. The holmium yttrium aluminum garnet laser has the most significant practical uses. It works well for removing bone or shaping existing bone. It stops bleeding adequately, however, only at the capillary level. Improved hemostasis and more accurate bone shaping are two benefits of laser surgery [2].

Increased collateral thermal deposition leading to increased synechia and scarring; decreased visualization through the endoscope due to the splatter effect of the tissue upon contact with the laser pulse; increased length of surgery. More elaborate surgical setup, increased cost, increased collateral thermal deposition. The KTP/532 laser has shown promising results in treating vascular conditions such as inherited hemorrhagic telangiectasia and turbinate reduction. When treating chronic sinusitis in children, endoscopic sinus surgery (ESS) typically does not need lasers [2].

62.5 Computer-Assisted Sinus Surgery

Sinus surgery using a computer has increased in popularity over the past several years. Sinus surgeons often only perform this procedure on patients undergoing a second surgery or those whose anatomy has been severely altered [2].

Data from a mechanical sensor wand is integrated by stereotactic software on the computer. The patient's face and forehead will have several sensors attached to it. CT scans are taken from the top of the head down to the upper incisors using a 3-mm slice thickness and 3-mm increments. Information from a CT scan is sent to the computer and sensing device. After that, you touch a sensor to designate the CT scan pictures you uploaded into the computer [2], and registration may commence.

Another option for matching patients to their digital photographs is to use landmarks on their faces, such as the lateral canthus. Once registration is done, a 3D reconstruction of sagittal, coronal, and axial pictures may be viewed on a screen. The probe tip has a range of 0–3.7 mm and an accuracy of about 2 mm. A 3D representation of the wand's position is displayed on the screen when it is put intranasally during surgery. This method has been helpful in adult revision and extensive sinonasal lesions, where normal anatomy is covered or changed. It has been proven beneficial in the pediatric population in recent studies. As technology has advanced, different systems have become accessible, simplifying the process further [2].

References

1. Eviatar E, Pitaro K, Gavriel H, Krakovsky D. Complications following powered endoscopic sinus surgery: an 11-year study on 1190 patients in a single institute in Israel. Isr Med Assoc J. 2014;16:338–40.
2. McClay JE. Pediatric sinusitis surgery treatment & management. In: Meyers AD, editor. Medscape; 2023. Updated: Apr 04, 2023. https://emedicine.medscape.com/article/873298-treatment#d12 (Accessed online at October 26, 2023).
3. Siedek V, Stelter K, Betz CS, Berghaus A, Leunig A. Functional endoscopic sinus surgery—a retrospective analysis of 115 children and adolescents with chronic rhinosinusitis. Int J Pediatr Otorhinolaryngol. 2009;73:741–5.
4. Rastatter JC, Snyderman CH, Gardner PA, Alden TD, TylerKabara E. Endoscopic endonasal surgery for sinonasal and skull base lesions in the pediatric population. Otolaryngol Clin N Am. 2015;48:79–99.
5. Makary CA, Ramadan HH. The role of sinus surgery in children. Laryngoscope. 2013;123:1348–52.
6. Min HJ, Chung HJ, Seong SY, Sim NS, Yoon JH, Lee JG, Kim CH, Cho HJ. Differential characteristics of pediatric sinusitis who underwent endoscopic sinus surgery: children vs. adolescents. Clin Otolaryngol. 2016;41:579–84.
7. Gross CW, Winther B. Functional endonasal sinus surgery in children: practical considerations and technical aspects. Pediatr Funct Surg. 1990:109–12.
8. Manning SC. Pediatric sinusitis. Otoloryngol Clin North Anı. 1993;26(4):623–38.
9. Vandenberg SJ, Heatley DG. Efficacy of adenoidectomy in relieving symptoms of chronic sinusitis in children. Arch Otolaryngol Head Neck Surg. 1997;135:675–8.
10. Paul D. Sinus infection and adenotonsillitis in pediatric patients. Laryngoscope. 1981;91:997–1000.
11. Takahashi H, Fujita A. Honjol: effect of adenoidectomy on otitis media with effusion, tuba! function and sinusitis. Am J Otolaryngol. 1989;10:208–13.
12. Kennedy DW, Zinreich SJ, Rosenbaum AE, et al. Functional endoscopic sinus surgery: theory and diagnostic evaluation. Arch Otolaryngol. 1985;111:576.
13. Önerci M, Bayar N. Functional endoskopik sinus surgery in children. KBB ve Baş Boyun Cerrahisi Dergisi. 1993;1:149–51.
14. Stammberger H. Endoscopic endonasal surgery. Concepts in treatment of recurring rhinosinusitis. Part I. Anatomic and pathophysiologic considerations. Otolaryngol Head Neck Surg. 1986;94:143–6.
15. Wigand ME, Steiner W, Jauman MP. Endonasal sinus surgery with endoscopic control: From radical operation to rehabilitation of the sinüs mucosa. Endoscopy. 1978;10:255–60.
16. Brietzke SE, Shin JJ, Choi S, et al. Clinical consensus statement: pediatric chronic rhinosinusitis. Otolaryngol Head Neck Surg. 2014;151(4):542–53.
17. Talbot AR. Frontal sinus surgery in children. Otolaryngol Clin N Am. 1996;29(1):143–58.
18. Setliff RC. The hummer: a remedy for apprehension in functional endoscopic sinus surgery. Otolaryngol Clin N Am. 1996;29:93.
19. Setliff RC 3rd. Minimally invasive sinus surgery: the rationale and technique. Otolaryngol Clin N Am. 1996;29:115–29.

20. Mendelsohn MG, Gross CW. Soft-tissue shavers in pediatric sinus surgery. Otolaryngol Clin N Am. 1997;30(3):443–9.
21. Tsukidate T, Haruna S, Fukami S, Nakajima I, Konno W, Moriyama H. Long-term evaluation after endoscopic sinus surgery for chronic pediatric sinusitis with polyps. Auris Nasus Larynx. 2012;39(6):583–7.

Septoplasty to Provide Nasal Breathing in Children

63

Soner Taşar, Cemal Cingi, and Jeffrey C. Bedrosian

63.1 Introduction

Since the 1950s, pediatric septoplasty has been controversial because of fears that the treatment may stunt the development of the nose and face. However, newer research shows that septoplasty may be performed safely in the right pediatric patient [1] without compromising nasal and facial growth.

We found three studies with long-term follow-up utilizing anthropometric measurements that all concluded that septoplasty in children had no adverse effects on nasal or face development. Another comparable study found that external septoplasty does not affect overall face or nasal growth but may hinder dorsal strut development. One research showed that the incidence of facial and dental malformations was significantly higher in children with symptomatic uncorrected deviated nasal septum compared with age- and sex-matched controls, lending credence to the use of septoplasty in these cases [1].

S. Taşar
Department of Otorhinolaryngology, Afyon State Hospital, Afyon, Türkiye

C. Cingi (✉)
Faculty of Medicine, Department of Otorhinolaryngology, Eskişehir Osmangazi University, Eskisehir, Türkiye

J. C. Bedrosian
Rhinology and Skull Base Surgery, Specialty Physician Associates, St. Luke's Medical Center, Bethlehem, PA, USA

H. Yüksel et al. (eds.), *Pediatric Airway Diseases*, Comprehensive ENT,
https://doi.org/10.1007/978-3-031-74853-0_63

63.2 Children's Nasal Development

Adolescent nasal development may be seen in white females between the ages of 8 and 12. In boys, peak height was reached around age 13. The development velocity curve displayed its most significant decreasing slope at 13.4 for teenage girls and 14.7 for adolescent boys (ages 2–5). Sixteen-year-old girls and 17-year-old boys are said to be the youngest patients for rhinoplasty. Nose development is finished around age 16 in girls and 18 in boys [2] in height, depth, and inclination. It has been stated that the nasal size and nasal bridge mature at 12 in girls and 15 in boys [3]. In Switzerland, both sexes had continued nose development and lengthening until age 20 [4, 5].

63.2.1 Nasal Skeleton Growth in Children

As kids become older, their noses get bigger. The nasal bones and cartilage will develop as follows [4, 6]:

- Backwards developments. The dorsolateral cartilages may be expressed within the skull, with the skeletal cribriform plate taking its place at the skull's anterior base. Even in 4-year-old children, it is possible to find dorsolateral cartilages that reach the nasofrontal suture while investigating nasal dorsum fistulas.
- Ossification over time. The cartilaginous septum ossifies progressively, and the perpendicular plate grows caudoventrally from a region near the anterior cranial base [7, 8].

63.2.2 Progressive Ossification

After the age of 10 years [9], the vomeral alae on both sides of the septal cartilage have undergone ossification. Adolescents have an overlap of the vomeral wings and perpendicular plate [10].

63.2.3 Nasal Dorsum

The nasal dorsum relies heavily on the septodorsal cartilage, which is rooted in the sphenoid in early children. Following the growth of the perpendicular plate [9], the septal cartilage detaches from the sphenoid. The spinoseptal ligament [10] links the septum in children and adults to the premaxilla.

63.2.3.1 Choanae and Nasal Septum

The vomer's inferior (medial) portion forms the nasopharyngeal border of the nasal septum. The choanal rim of the septum does not reflect the cartilaginous nasal septum or the perpendicular plate derived from the sphenoid [10].

63.2.3.2 Septovomeral Junction

The septal cartilage still resides in the encircling bone. The vomeral wings and the perpendicular plate combine to produce the vomeral tunnel, which can extend to the sphenoid [7]. Eventually, this "sphenoid tail" will ossify [11, 12] in most people. If the vomer ala is only present on one side, then the incomplete vomer bone will be accompanied by a sphenoid tail made of cartilage [10]. Deformity of the posterior septum occurs in around 25% of human embryos. At birth, there is a rise to 37% [13] at the cartilaginous septum's intersection with the vomer and perpendicular plate. The mismatch between "the overdeveloping septum and the pressure of the surrounding structures," i.e., the bony face skeleton, has been cited as the cause. In a different research, the percentage of those with anterior and posterior septal deformities was 57% [14].

63.3 Postnatal Growth of the Human Nasal Septum

Nasal septum development, excluding the vomer, is fastest in newborns and eventually slows to a plateau at 20. The size of the cartilaginous component shows a sharp growth that peaks around the age of two. The ossification of septal cartilage at the septoethmoidal junction causes the perpendicular plate to form, allowing the entire septum to expand later. The production of new cartilage counteracts the ossification. To make up for the cartilage that is lost due to ossification, mitotic activity, and intercellular matrix expansion are involved [15].

63.4 Nasal Skeleton Growing after Nasal Fractures

Septum fractures, sometimes accompanied by breaks in the bony nasal pyramid, are surprisingly common in youngsters. The long-term consequences of these breaks on the face are rarely discussed. A closed reduction of the displaced bony pyramid and fragmented sections of the septum [10] was part of the therapy for nasal injuries in a 4-year-old child. A year later, the dorsum of the nose seemed normal, but further development caused a gradual deviation of the septum and dorsum by age 8 [4, 10], and the deformity worsened over the teen years.

63.5 Pathophysiology

Septal cartilage is very elastic despite its role as a structural support for the nasal dorsum. It can take on a lot of pressure without being permanently distorted. Cartilage fractures when an external force surpasses the biomechanical stress point [16].

Septal cartilage, barring injury, is typically aligned. The intrinsic tension of the cartilage is balanced on both sides. Due to the asymmetric nature of cartilage destruction following trauma, one side of the joint is typically more affected than the other. Septal cartilage shows considerable proliferation on the dominant side during time, compared to the contralateral side. There is a shift, with the convex side showing more rapid expansion. This is often the uninjured side of the body [16].

Minor nose injuries, especially during puberty, can result in unilateral microfractures that significantly alter the patient's septal cartilage growth pattern in the midface [16].

63.6 Indications for Pediatric Septoplasty

Septal abscess, septal hematoma, severe deformity following acute nasal fracture, cleft lip and nose, and severe obstructive sleep apnea with complete occlusion of the nasal route are all indications of pediatric septoplasty.

Nasal blockage due to a significantly deviated septum (where feasible, rhinomanometry should be used to determine the severity of the obstruction) [4, 17].

63.7 Pediatric Nasal Septal Deformities: Diagnosis and Treatment

Congenital disabilities of the nasal septum are possible. These can occur alone or with other congenital midface defects such as cleft lip and palate [18, 19]. Normal vaginal births are more likely to result in intrapartum trauma than cesarean sections, hypothesized to cause anterior deviations in an otherwise well-formed nasal septum [20].

The decision to operate on a child born with a nasal septal deformity is fraught with debate [21]. When developing, the midface relies heavily on the nasal septum [22]. Maxillary hypoplasia has been linked to the disruption of this growth center, as suggested by both animal studies [23] and longitudinal clinical observations. Given this knowledge, remedial surgery must minimize interference with the patient's natural growth patterns.

Nasal tip deviations caused by intrapartum pressure effects may correct themselves after delivery. Infants are obligatory nasal breathers. Therefore, severe nasal septal abnormalities might block their airways. In such cases, surgical repair in the newborn period may be required. The nasal septum may be repositioned on the maxillary crest by intranasal stenting or surgical manipulation of the cartilage lining the nasal passages. Some writers, however, have suggested a more cautious approach, such as septoplasty with the removal of cracked or malformed cartilage, for more severe instances [24].

The cartilaginous anterior nasal septum or the bone posterior vomer may be seldom missing from birth [18, 25, 26].

Unilateral or bilateral mucoperichondrial elevation during septoplasty does not stunt facial development. Unilateral mucosal elevation may facilitate septal stabilization. The nasal floor mucosa should not be raised to protect the incisive nerves. The cartilaginous septum can be reshaped and have small portions removed if necessary. Since the length and height of the nasal septum and nasal dorsum depend on this area, separating the septal cartilage from the perpendicular plate should be avoided, especially at the dorsal portion. Making incisions or removing tissue from the sphenoethmoid dorsal zone [4] is not recommended, which is a growing and supporting area.

Septoplasty is recommended if the breathing difficulties caused by the septal deviation are severe. Children as young as six can often undergo septal surgery. However, septal surgery is an option even for newborns and younger children [4].

Unilateral or bilateral elevation of the mucoperichondrium may not hurt facial development, according to research by Verwoerd and Verwoerd-Verhoef [10]. In youngsters, a secondary deformity is more likely to occur when a unilateral mucosal elevation is performed for septal stability. The nasal floor mucosa should not be lifted to protect the incisive nerves. The septum can be moved once the overlapping or crooked pieces of cartilage have been disentangled from the adhering fibrous tissue. Then, the midline will be used to repair the septum. In this context, alterations and small-scale removals may be made. No surgeries, including incisions and excisions, should be performed in the sphenoethmoid dorsal zone, a critical growth and support area.

Since the length and height of the nasal septum and nasal dorsum depend on this area, separating the septal cartilage from the perpendicular plate should be avoided, especially at the dorsal portion. Nasal dorsum outgrowth is not seen when an excision is conducted at the cartilaginous septum's base. However, the septospinal ligament should be unbroken, and anterior septal excision should be avoided. Nasal growth may be impacted by resections of the crista septi or spina vomeri [10].

References

1. Lawrence R. Pediatric septoplasy: a review of the literature. Int J Pediatr Otorhinolaryngol. 2012;76(8):1078–81.
2. Meng HP, Goorhuis J, Kapila S, Nanda RS. Growth changes in the nasal profile from 7 to 18 years of age. Am J Orthod Dentofacial Orthop. 1988;94:317–26.
3. Akgüner M, Barutçu A, Karaca C. Adolescent growth patterns of the bony and cartilaginous framework of the nose: a cephalometric study. Ann Plast Surg. 1998;41:66–9.
4. Cingi C, Muluk NB, Ulusoy S, Lopatin A, Şahin E, Passali D, Bellussi L, Atilla H, Hanci D, Altıntoprak N, Rusetski Y, Sarafoleanu C, Mladina R, Kalogjera L, Manea C. Septoplasty in children. Am J Rhinol Allergy. 2016;30(2):e42–7.
5. Zankl A, Eberle L, Molinari L, Schinzel A. Growth charts for nose length, nasal protrusion, and philtrum length from birth to 97 years. Am J Med Genet. 2002;111:388–91.
6. Bosma JF. Anatomy of the infant head. Baltimore: Johns Hopkins University Press; 1985.
7. Peter K. Die Nase des Kindes. In: Handbuch der Anatomie des Kindes, Bd 2. München: Bergmann Verlag; 1938.
8. Entwicklung HK. Bau und Form Veränderungen der menschlichen Nasenscheidewand in fetalen Leben. Arch Ohr-Nasen-Kehl Heilk. 1933:1–24.
9. Verwoerd CD, van Loosen J, Schütte HE, Verwoerd-Verhoef HL, van Velzen D. Surgical aspects of the anatomy of the vomer in children and adults. Rhinol Suppl. 1989;9:87–96.
10. Verwoerd CD, Verwoerd-Verhoef HL. Rhinosurgery in children: developmental and surgical aspects of the growing nose [in German with English abstract]. Laryngorhinootologie. 2010;89(Suppl. 1):S46–71.

11. Scott JH. The cartilage of the nasal septum. Br Dent J. 1953;95:37–43.
12. Melsen B. Histological analysis of the postnatal development of the nasal septum. Angle Orthod. 1977;47:83–96.
13. Takahashi R. The formation of the nasal septum and the etiology of septal deformity. The concept of evolutionary paradox. Acta Otolaryngol Suppl. 1987;443:1–160.
14. Gray LP. Deviated nasal septum. Incidence and etiology. Ann Otol Rhinol Laryngol Suppl. 1978;87(Pt. 3., Suppl. 50):3–20.
15. Vetter U, Pirsig W, Helbing G, et al. Patterns of growth in human septal cartilage: a review of new approaches. Int J Pediatr Otorhinolaryngol. 1984;7:63–74.
16. Watson D. Septoplasty. In: Meyers AD, editor. Medscape; 2023. Updated: Jan 21, 2021. https://emedicine.medscape.com/article/877677-overview#a9 (Accessed online at June 4, 2023).
17. Christophel JJ, Gross CW. Pediatric septoplasty. Otolaryngol Clin N Am. 2009;42:287–94.
18. Isaacson GC. Congenital anomalies of the nose. In: Messner AH, Armsby C, editors. UpToDate; 2022. Last updated: Jan 10, 2022.
19. Yoon YJ, Perkiomaki MR, Tallents RH, et al. Association of nasomaxillary asymmetry in children with unilateral cleft lip and palate and their parents. Cleft Palate Craniofac J. 2003;40:493.
20. Alpini D, Corti A, Brusa E, Bini A. Septal deviation in newborn infants. Int J Pediatr Otorhinolaryngol. 1986;11:103.
21. Béjar I, Farkas LG, Messner AH, Crysdale WS. Nasal growth after external septoplasty in children. Arch Otolaryngol Head Neck Surg. 1996;122:816.
22. Grymer LF, Bosch C. The nasal septum and the development of the midface. A longitudinal study of a pair of monozygotic twins. Rhinology. 1997;35:6.
23. Meeuwis J, Verwoerd-Verhoef HL, Verwoerd CD. Normal and abnormal nasal growth after partial submucous resection of the cartilaginous septum. Acta Otolaryngol. 1993;113:379.
24. Emami AJ, Brodsky L, Pizzuto M. Neonatal septoplasty: case report and review of the literature. Int J Pediatr Otorhinolaryngol. 1996;35:271.
25. Robinson B, Hilger P. Hereditary agenesis of nasal cartilage. Surgical implications. Arch Otolaryngol Head Neck Surg. 1989;115:985.
26. Yan DJ, Lenoir V, Chatelain S, et al. Congenital vomer agenesis: a rare and poorly understood condition revealed by cone beam CT. Diagnostics (Basel). 2018;8(1):15.

64 Tracheostomy to Eliminate Upper Airway Obstruction in Children

Murat Gumussoy and İbrahim Çukurova

64.1 Introduction

Respiratory distress and stridor due to upper respiratory tract infections are among the top reasons pediatric patients visit the emergency department. The clinical course and severity of symptoms related to respiratory tract infections can vary significantly in patients presenting to the emergency department. It ranges from mild, self-limited to life-threatening airway obstruction. For this reason, emergency physicians need to evaluate children with respiratory distress originating from the upper respiratory tract with a multidisciplinary approach to maintain the patency and continuity of the airway [1–3].

In the pediatric emergency department, retropharyngeal abscess, characterized by retropharyngeal space infection with rapidly worsening clinical findings and aggravation by respiratory distress, is a true airway emergency. The basic approach in these patients is to plan surgical drainage without delay and ensure airway patency. Tracheotomy should primarily be considered among the options [4, 5]. Epiglottitis is an acute bacterial infection of the supraglottic region and is another airway emergency. The most common cause of airway obstruction of viral origin in the glottic and subglottic regions is viral croup or laryngotracheobronchitis. Viral croup is also the most common cause of infectious airway obstruction in children. Bacterial tracheitis, also known as bacterial croup, is a potentially life-threatening, fatal infection of the subglottic trachea. It is a bacterial infection secondary to a viral infection (croup) that seriously affects breathing in children and is a clinical condition that produces mucopurulent exudates that can acutely obstruct the upper airway [6–8].

M. Gumussoy · İ. Çukurova (✉)
Department of Otolaryngology-Head and Neck Surgery, University of Health Sciences, Izmir Tepecik Training and Research Hospital, Izmir, Turkey

H. Yüksel et al. (eds.), *Pediatric Airway Diseases*, Comprehensive ENT,
https://doi.org/10.1007/978-3-031-74853-0_64

The main goal in the treatment of diseases that cause upper airway obstruction caused by infection is to ensure the continuity of the airway. Airway obstruction is life-threatening and requires urgent intervention. It is vital that a team consisting of an emergency room doctor, a pediatrician, an ear, nose, and throat specialist, and a pediatric pulmonologist evaluate the child with airway obstruction and plan his or her treatment with a multidisciplinary approach [9, 10].

As Ear, Nose, and Throat Physicians, we provide advantages with endoscopic imaging (flexible and rigid endoscopy) methods that provide practical and rapid vision in diagnosing upper airway obstruction and direct vision in the differential diagnosis of upper airway obstruction [11]. We also perform emergency tracheotomy in children to maintain patency of the acute airway and elective tracheotomy in cases of prolonged intubation despite appropriate medical treatment. With this airway surgery, we both ensure the patency of the airway and reduce the dead space in the airway, allowing tracheal secretions to be removed easily. Pediatric tracheotomy also contributes positively to reducing effortful breathing in pediatric patients, protecting them from the side effects of prolonged intubation, facilitating intensive care services, and reducing bed occupation times [12].

This section lists infections causing acute upper respiratory tract obstruction according to their anatomical location. Diagnosis and treatment approaches such as retropharyngeal abscess, epiglottitis, viral croup, and bacterial tracheitis are mentioned, as well as indications, techniques, and complications of pediatric tracheotomy applied in surgical treatment.

64.2 Airway Differences in Children

The airway in children differs anatomically, physiologically, and histologically compared to adults. These developmental disadvantages make children more prone to airway obstruction during infection [1–3]. So much so that, due to the differences in airway pathophysiology mentioned below, the spread of infection and edema formation in the respiratory mucosa during acute airway infections in children are more exaggerated and severe compared to adults.

[4–7].

Anatomical, physiological, and histological differences of the airway in children [8–10, 13–15]:

1. Nasal breathing is more dominant in children during the neonatal period.
2. They may have breathing problems in the first 2 years of their lives because they cannot achieve oral/nasal breathing coordination.
3. The epiglottis is U-shaped and at the hard and soft palate level.
4. The larynx is located upwards and anteriorly.
5. Vocal cords are located anteriorly.
6. These differences in the epiglottis and laryngeal region separate the air and digestive tract from each other. However, allowing the child to feed and breathe

simultaneously by separating. It also increases the possibility of transmission of oral cavity infections.
7. The airway diameter is narrow in the neonatal period.
8. The diameter is approximately 4 mm in children and 20 mm in adults.
9. In the first 5 years after birth, the upper respiratory tract lumen diameter changes longitudinally rather than transversely.
10. The trachea is shorter and narrower in children than in adults.
11. The subglottic region in children is the narrowest part of the upper respiratory tract (cricoid cartilage), and in adults, it is the glottic region.
12. Histologically, children's upper respiratory tract mucous membranes are cartilaginous. It is loosely attached to the rings and is rich in soft tissue.
13. The subglottic region is surrounded by hard cricoid cartilage, and its mucosa allows the formation of submucosal edema with its loose structure.
14. Any infection at the subglottic level increases the risk of airway edema, narrowing of the airway diameter, and thus obstruction.
15. A 1 mm edema in the respiratory mucosa in a newborn can cause emergency airway problems by obstructing 60% of the airway, especially at the cricoid level.
16. Since the essential criteria determining airway resistance depend on the airway length, diameter, and viscosity of the gas, an increase in airway resistance due to inflammation, secretion, and edema also causes increased respiratory load.

It should not be forgotten that upper respiratory tract diseases are more common in school-aged children due to the above-mentioned differences and that acute exacerbations and sudden respiratory distress may result in intubation and tracheotomy, especially in children under the age of 6 [16–18].

64.3 Stridor

It is a high-frequency sound due to the swirling of respiratory air while passing through a narrow area. The characteristic and most crucial auscultation finding of upper airway obstruction is stridor. Although it is clinically significant in diagnosis, it is a symptom, not a diagnosis. Infectious causes come to the fore in the acute occurrence of stridor. Physiologically, when an obstruction occurs in the airway, the stridor appears as high-frequency noisy breathing, especially in the inspiration phase of the respiratory period, due to the airflow, which normally progresses laminarly, experiencing turbulence in the area where the obstruction occurs, according to Bernoulli's principle. In a child with stridor, the primary pathology is at the level of the larynx or trachea. In the laryngeal region, supraglottic and glottic obstructions, it is inspiratory, in the trachea or main bronchi, it is expiratory, and in case of obstruction in both the glottic and subglottic areas, it is biphasic (inspiratory and expiratory). It can often be accompanied by restlessness, drowsiness, hoarse voice, and withdrawal symptoms. In the early stage of the disease, the inspiratory character of stridor due to infection in the glottic area appears in a biphasic character as the infection exceeds the cricoid level and progresses to the subglottic area. This picture is important in understanding the disease's level and localization [14, 19–21].

64.4 Infections That Cause Upper Respiratory Obstruction

Clinical symptoms of infections causing upper respiratory tract obstruction are related to the anatomical location and degree of obstruction [14, 15, 18–23]. Infections are listed according to their anatomical location:

4.1 Retropharyngeal abscess (pharynx)
4.2 Epiglottitis (larynx-supraglottic region)
4.3 Viral croup (larynx-glottic-subglottic region)
4.4 Bacterial tracheitis (trachea-subglottic region)

64.4.1 Retropharyngeal Abscess

Retropharyngeal abscess is an uncommon but important cause of airway obstruction in childhood. The retropharyngeal area is located between the middle and deep layers of the deep cervical fascia and extends towards the posterior of the larynx. This area is divided into right and left, where the superior constrictor pharyngeus muscle attaches to the prevertebral fascia. In children younger than 1 year, the lymphoid tissue is abundant in the retropharyngeal region. Retropharyngeal abscesses are the result of suppurative adenoids, which often occur in early childhood in the nasopharynx, oropharynx, nose, paranasal sinuses, adenoids, tonsils, and retropharyngeal lymph nodes that drain from the middle ear. The most common cause of retropharyngeal area infections is the infection of the lymph nodes in this area, secondary to upper respiratory tract infections and usually following bacterial pharyngitis and then abscessing with suppuration. This potential space, which starts from the skull base, extends down to the mediastinum, and infections can spread primarily to the chest and mediastinum in this way [24–26].

More than 95% of retropharyngeal abscesses are seen in children younger than 6 years, most commonly between 3 months and 3 years of age. It develops less frequently in older children, where the lymphoid tissue gradually atrophies. The most common causative agents are *Staphylococcus aureus*, group A streptococci, and oral anaerobic microorganisms. *Hemophilus influenzae*, Klebsiella, and *Mycobacterium avium* intracellulare may also be causative agents [25–27].

Clinically, the disease may present with symptoms and findings such as fever, dyspnea, sore throat, dysphagia, odynophagia, trismus, neck pain, and limitation of neck movements, or it may have no specific findings. Classic symptoms are dysphagia, dyspnea and neck stiffness. Craig and Schunk [28] reported that the patient's inability to hyperextend his head, called the "Bolte sign" in patients with retropharyngeal abscess, is particularly important in diagnosis. Unfortunately, young children cannot fully express their complaints without being restless or fully cooperating during a physical examination. This makes diagnosis difficult.

Lateral neck radiography (LBG), computed tomography (CT), and magnetic resonance imaging (MRI) can be performed as imaging methods. Chest radiographs should also be included when mediastinitis is considered. LBG is very useful in diagnosis [28, 29] (Fig. 64.1).

However, LBG must be taken in a sitting position, with the neck hyperextended and inspired. Retropharyngeal wall thickness at the level of the cervical second vertebra being more than 7 mm (normally 3.5 mm) or soft tissue thickness at the level of the sixth cervical vertebra being more than 14 mm in children is pathological, and a space-occupying lesion in the retropharyngeal area should be considered. However, it should be remembered that there may be errors in LBG due to crying, swallowing, breathing, and position. CT is the gold standard imaging technique for identifying abscesses, evaluating potential complications, and planning surgical intervention [28–31] (Fig. 64.2).

Diagnosis in ear, nose, and throat (ENT) is the presence of a fluctuating and palpable mass on the posterior wall of the pharynx. An important finding is an observation of an abscess collection on the posterior wall of the pharynx during endoscopic examination. By evaluating the location, size, and patency of the airway of the abscess in patients, the diagnosis can be easily made using endoscopy and clinical findings. Emergency and surgical interventions are valuable in direct proportion to the size of the airway obstruction and abscess [29–31] (Fig. 64.3).

Delay in diagnosis and treatment is a condition that can lead to potentially lethal complications involving the respiratory tract. The potential danger is that the infection passes from the alar fascia to the dangerous area, causing potentially lethal, life-threatening mediastinitis and related complications involving vital structures. In addition, they can cause thrombosis of the adjacent structures, the jugular veins, and erosion of the internal carotid artery, and mortality rates can reach up to 80%. Be sure to consider epiglottitis in the differential diagnosis should be taken [27, 29, 31].

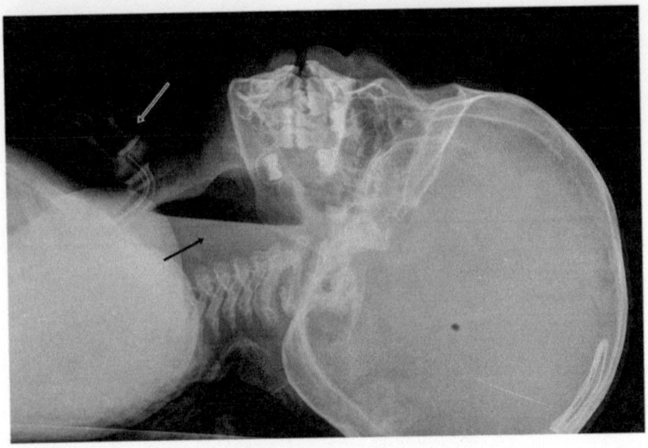

Fig. 64.1 Preoperative lateral neck radiography (black arrow retropharyngeal abscess) and a tracheotomy were performed on the patient, and the cannula can be seen in the picture (white arrow)

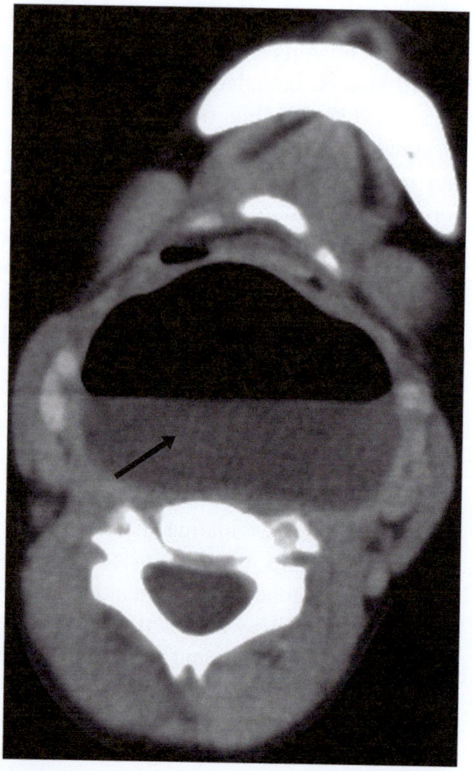

Fig. 64.2 Preoperative neck axial CT (black arrow retropharyngeal abscess)

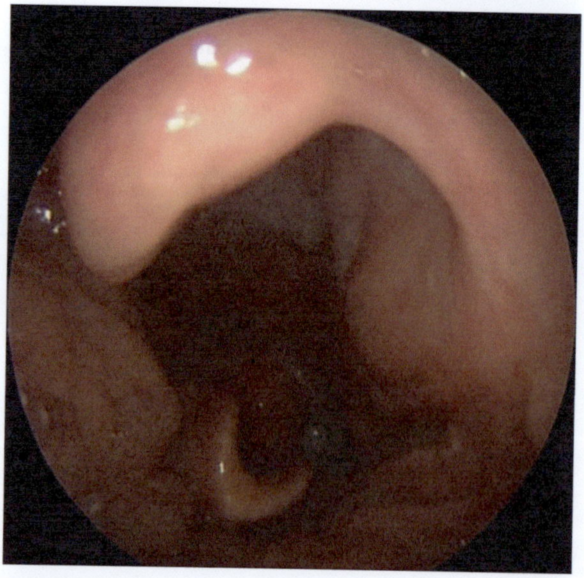

Fig. 64.3 Six-year-old boy, endoscopic examination showing retropharyngeal abscess formation on the left

Ensuring airway safety, antibiotic treatment, and surgical drainage are the three most important steps in treating patients with retropharyngeal abscesses. The diagnosed child should be hospitalized and kept under surveillance, and especially respiratory distress should be closely monitored. Intravenous antibiotic therapy should be added [32–34].

To decide on surgical drainage of the abscess and tracheotomy, the following points are to be followed:

1. Routine ENT examination and endoscopic imaging of the oropharynx, nasopharynx, and larynx,
2. Evaluation of airway patency for the need for tracheotomy,
3. Visualizing the size of the abscess in the retropharyngeal area,
4. Retropharyngeal wall thickness at the level of the second cervical vertebra in the lateral neck radiograph is more than 7 mm,
5. Soft tissue thickness at the level of the sixth cervical vertebra is more than 14 mm,
6. The presence of an abscess larger than 2 cm on computed tomography.

Surgical drainage provides a high recovery rate if applied within the above criteria. A study observed that the cure rate was 12% with antibiotic treatment alone and 88% with surgical treatment [35]. Figure 64.4 shows the flexible endoscopic view after drainage.

Surgical drainage must be performed under operating room conditions. During intubation, care should be taken not to rupture the abscess, and the patient should be

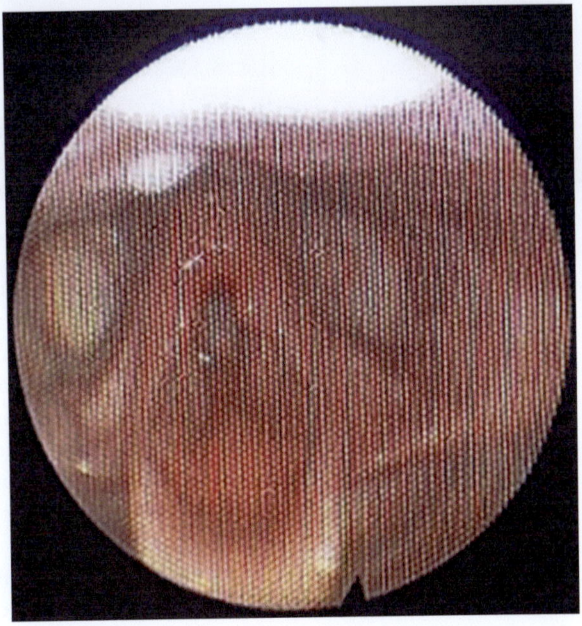

Fig. 64.4 Flexible endoscopic larynx examination after retropharyngeal abscess drainage

placed in the Trendelenburg position. If intubation is risky, tracheotomy should be prepared. Culture should be taken.

64.4.2 Epiglottitis (Supraglottitis)

It is the most severe form of acute upper respiratory tract obstruction caused by infectious causes. *Hemophilus influenzae* type b (Hib) is the most common cause of acute epiglottitis in children and adults. It is a life-threatening infection of the supraglottic larynx that usually occurs in children under 6 years of age [36]. Michel first described it in 1878 as angina epiglottitis anterior and represented a true airway emergency. The infection is bacterial cellulitis that affects the lingual surface of the epiglottis and aryepiglottic folds, which are supraglottic structures. As supraglottic edema increases, the epiglottis expands anteriorly and posteriorly, causing progressive airway obstruction. While Hib was the most common causative agent before widespread vaccination, the incidence of epiglottitis decreased after vaccination [37, 38].

Clinically, it is characterized by high fever, irritability, sore throat, difficulty in swallowing, and rapidly progressive (within hours) respiratory difficulties in children. Inspiratory stridor is observed due to epiglottis edema and airway obstruction. Its course is very rapid, with no complaints, and the condition settles in 3–8 h. The child prefers the tripod position (sitting leaning forward, supporting with hands, chin up, and mouth open) to keep the airway open. The child does not want to talk due to pain. There is salivation from the mouth. Fever is over 40 °C [36, 38].

Blackstock et al. [39] defined the 4D findings for the diagnosis of epiglottitis as

1. Drooling
2. Dysphonia
3. Dysphagia

Cervical tenderness and lymphadenopathy can be found at any age. Compared to croup, stridor and hoarseness are less common. Stridor is a late finding and should suggest that airway obstruction is progressing. In 50% of cases, other infections such as otitis, cellulitis, pneumonia, and meningitis may accompany the disease.

Regarding ENT, the diagnosis is made by directly visualizing the supraglottic region and epiglottis. Manipulations to the upper respiratory tract, pharynx examination with a tongue depressor, painful procedures such as bloodletting, flexible endoscopic examination, and even small changes in body position may aggravate respiratory distress as they may cause complete obstruction. For this reason, the patient should be evaluated with direct laryngoscopy under operating room conditions. Operating room conditions provide us with imaging opportunities for diagnosis and evaluation and application opportunities for emergency tracheotomy. Observation of the swollen cherry red epiglottis during direct laryngoscopy is sufficient for diagnosis [40–42] (Fig. 64.5).

A radiological examination is performed to support the diagnosis and to exclude diagnoses such as croup and retropharyngeal abscess. A thick and rounded

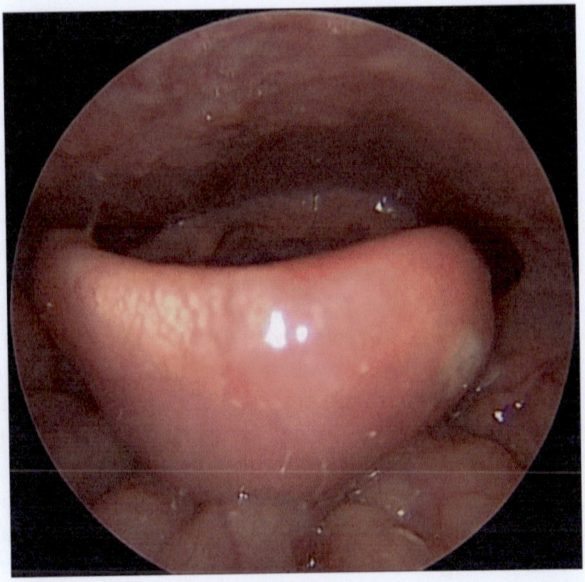

Fig. 64.5 In the endoscopic image of the patient with suspected acute epiglottitis, the epiglottis is seen as swollen and edematous

epiglottis (thumb sign), loss of air space, and thickening of the aryepiglottic folds may be seen on the lateral neck radiograph.

The most important step in treatment is to ensure adequate airway and maintain patency. When epiglottitis is considered, the patient should be monitored by a team experienced in approaching the difficult airway. Historically, patients underwent tracheotomy when diagnosed with supraglottitis. Today, tracheotomy is still valid. Emergency airway surgery is required if the infection does not subside within 48–72 h with tracheotomy antibiotic treatment.

It is indicated when there is tract obstruction and intubation is impossible. Although modern techniques are used for intubation (video laryngoscopy), failure during intubation will require an emergency tracheotomy, so the ENT team must be ready at the patient's bedside in all cases. Antibiotic treatment starts once the airway is guaranteed and the patient is transferred to the intensive care unit. Traditionally, chloramphenicol and ampicillin have been the antibiotics of choice. Antibiotic sensitivity is determined based on culture and sensitivity results. The patient can be extubated when there is air leakage with positive pressure or when a repeat endoscopic examination shows resolution of the supraglottic swelling. Flexible laryngoscopy in the intensive care unit is usually sufficient to evaluate recovery and follow-up. Extubation can usually be done within 48 h since the response to antibiotics is rapid [37, 39–42].

64.4.3 Viral Croup (Laryngotracheobronchitis)

Viral croup is the most common cause of infective upper respiratory tract obstruction in the pediatric age group. It is 15 times more common than acute epiglottitis. Many parents have encountered croup in their children and have spent an anxious night due to the acute clinical picture. The most common etiological agents are parainfluenza type 1, influenza, and respiratory syncytial virus. Affected children are usually at preschool age, with a male predominance between 18 and 24 months, with a prevalence under 3 years of age. Croup is more common in autumn and winter. Reported incidence rates vary between 1.5 and 6%, with less than 5% of children requiring hospital monitoring and only 1–2% of those monitored in hospitals requiring endotracheal intubation and fewer requiring tracheotomy and intensive care [43–45].

The subglottic larynx epithelium has abundant mucous glands containing secretions that can further narrow the airway lumen in response to infection. The primary pathology is airway obstruction due to subglottic edema and secretions [43, 45].

Clinical Findings: Initially, patients have a prodromal period of upper respiratory tract infection-like symptoms such as nasal congestion, runny nose, and cough, lasting 1–2 days. A barking cough and inspiratory stridor follow this. Croup is a clinical diagnosis. Laboratory findings are primarily average in patients. Radiological imaging is mainly used to make the differential diagnosis of diseases such as epiglottitis and retropharyngeal abscess. The classic radiological finding of Viral Croup is the pencil-point appearance of hypopharyngeal widening and typical narrowing in the subglottic area on the lateral neck radiograph. However, the absence of these findings does not rule out the diagnosis of croup. Radiography may be normal in approximately half of the patients [44–47].

In treatment, the main goal is primarily to ensure airway patency. Traditionally, cold steam therapy reduces cough due to mucosal irritation. However, studies have shown that cold steam therapy does not affect improving clinical symptoms in moderate croup. However, the use of glucocorticoids has been shown to improve symptoms. Since corticosteroid use became routine, intubation and tracheotomy rates have dropped significantly. If airway obstruction symptoms are severe despite all these treatments (in 1% of cases), endotracheal intubation and rarely tracheotomy can be performed [43, 46, 48, 49].

64.4.4 Bacterial Tracheitis

Bacterial tracheitis was first described as acute laryngotracheobronchitis in the medical literature in the late 1920s [50]. It is a bacterial infection of the trachea that occurs after a viral infection. Clinically, it resembles a severe viral croup. However, the fever is higher, and there is a toxic appearance. There are dark and sticky secretions in the trachea. Its physiopathology is characterized by the formation of mucopurulent exudates that can acutely obstruct the upper airway [49–51].

Bacterial tracheitis without tracheotomy is also known as membranous laryngotracheobronchitis, bacterial laryngotracheobronchitis, and pseudomembranous croup. As these alternative names suggest, bacterial tracheitis is the ulceration and pseudomembrane formation of the trachea, mucopurulent exudate, and sloughing of the mucosa that obstructs the tracheal lumen and can lead to significant airway obstruction. It should be considered in the differential diagnosis of every child with viral croup that does not respond to conventional treatment [51, 52].

Bacterial tracheitis most commonly affects preschool and early school-age children. The average age at diagnosis is 5 years. Its incidence is 4–8 per 1,000,000 children and peaks mostly in autumn and winter. It is more common in children with tracheostomy or endotracheal tubes than in other children [50–52].

The clinical features of bacterial tracheitis are similar to the clinical features of both common viral croup and epiglottitis. The most common etiology is *Staphylococcus aureus*, *Hemophilus influenzae*, v. e anaerobic organisms are held responsible. Additionally, *Moraxella catarrhalis* has recently been playing a role with increasing frequency and is associated with a more severe course [53].

Clinical findings: Initially, children typically have upper respiratory tract symptoms such as croup-like barking cough, stridor, and low-grade fever. Clinical signs are not as rapid as supraglottitis. After a few days, respiratory distress and clinical deterioration develop, along with high fever and toxicity. Children with bacterial tracheitis can lie flat and swallow their saliva, and the dysphagia seen in epiglottitis is not observed in children. Some children may have concurrent pneumonia, sinusitis, otitis media, or pharyngitis. Differential diagnoses include croup, viral laryngotracheobronchitis, epiglottitis, bronchiolitis, angioedema, and diphtheria in unvaccinated patients. However, suspicion of bacterial tracheitis should be investigated when a patient with respiratory distress does not respond to racemic epinephrine and/or systemic corticosteroids, which typically improve croup and viral laryngotracheobronchitis [53, 54].

Bacterial tracheitis mainly affects pediatric patients: Those with a natural, intact airway and those with an artificial airway with an endotracheal tube or tracheotomy tube. Patients with stable airways should be examined with flexible laryngoscopy. In this way, mucopurulent secretions in the glottic or subglottic regions can be easily seen. If symptoms worsen, the patient should be evaluated with direct laryngoscopy and rigid bronchoscopy under general anesthesia. Direct laryngoscopy reveals edematous structures, erythema of the subglottis, mucopurulent tracheal secretions, and thick pseudomembranes along the trachea [50, 53].

Radical treatment intervention requires aggressive debridement. Debridement is performed with aspiration and forceps. Appropriate material taken from debris and tracheal secretions is used for culture. The risk of tracheitis is increased for children with previous intubation or tracheotomy. The reason is that the intubation tube or tracheotomy cannula provides an easy entry route for bacteria. In addition, the risk of infection increases due to the ulceration caused by the tube to the trachea. Additionally, it has been shown that bacterial biofilms colonized by bacteria colonize the inner surface of tracheotomy tubes [52–55].

Approximately 80% of patients with bacterial tracheitis require intubation or tracheotomy, and 94% are followed in the intensive care unit. Intubation is usually required between 3 and 7 days. Broad-spectrum antibiotic treatment should be started immediately. Cefuroxime and Ampicillin/Sulbactam can be used for initial treatment. For coverage of Gram-negative organisms, a third-generation Cephalosporin (Ceftriaxone, Cefotaxime) and a semisynthetic penicillin such as Nafcillin should be preferred. Ultimately, antibiotic coverage should be determined by Gram stain, culture, and sensitivity results. The treatment duration is 10–14 days [53–56].

64.5 Pediatric Tracheotomy Management in Upper Airway Infections

Tracheotomy is defined as creating a surgical opening in the anterior wall of the trachea to ensure airway patency. Evidence shows that tracheotomy, thought to date back to before Christ, was first applied in the Ancient Egyptian and Ancient Greek civilizations. The first elective tracheotomy in history was performed by the Greek physician Asclepiades in the 100s BC, and emergency tracheotomy gained a different meaning when Trousseau, a French physician, reported that he performed a tracheotomy and treated 47 of 215 children during the diphtheria epidemic in 1833 [57, 58].

Tracheotomy has historically been a life-saving surgical procedure, almost always with the indication of acute airway obstruction (trauma, infections, and foreign body aspiration). In the 1950s, the indication and need for pediatric tracheotomy due to airway obstruction caused by upper respiratory tract infections such as Polio, Ludwing angina, diphtheria, tetanus, and laryngotracheobronchitis have changed over time. The main contribution to this change has been the control of infections following the application and widespread use of modern treatment methods, especially antibiotics. A relative decrease in pediatric tracheotomies in infectious diseases is noteworthy, with the application of intubation techniques and the development of intensive care conditions in patients with airway obstruction and respiratory distress despite medical treatment [57–59].

As upper respiratory tract diseases of infectious origin, epiglottitis and retropharyngeal abscess are real airway emergencies. In a pediatric patient evaluated in the emergency department with suspicion of retropharyngeal abscess, the ENT team can evaluate airway patency and abscess formation in a short time with flexible endoscopic imaging. The pharynx, larynx, and vocal cords are evaluated with endoscopic examination. The aim is to see the infection's focus and clarify the airway. If the patient is evaluated multidisciplinary and decides to drain the abscess, the procedure should be performed under operating room conditions. Intubation may damage the wall of the abscess and cause drainage. The patient should be placed in the Trendelenburg position at this stage if purulent abscess material is aspirated. Tracheotomy should be performed to guarantee the airway [23, 25–27, 29–31, 34, 35].

Similarly, endoscopic evaluation is the gold standard for the diagnosis of epiglottitis. When the child is in a life-threatening situation with an infected and swollen epiglottis blocking the airway, it is precious to evaluate the airway and make diagnostic observations. Intubation is risky in a child with respiratory distress if the epiglottis is infected and obstructs the supraglottic area or prevents visibility of the vocal cords. If the child cannot be intubated, the critical process begins, and a vital struggle begins for the ENT team, who are waiting for an emergency tracheotomy. The airway is opened, and the tracheotomy cannula is placed in the trachea to ensure airway continuity [38, 40–42]. In cases of viral croup, only 1% of children are intubated and followed in intensive care, thanks to clinical findings, radiological evaluation, and endoscopic examination.

For this reason, pediatric tracheotomy is performed for very few patients. The main problem is whether to intubate the children safely under close monitoring or perform a tracheotomy [43–45]. Despite all these positive developments, it should not be forgotten that the incidence of tracheotomy is higher in pediatric patients than in adults in respiratory tract infections. This situation is probably related to a higher frequency of infection and the vulnerability of the child's trachea to edema and inflammation. Today, tracheotomy continues to be an effective intervention with its life-saving role in ensuring airway control in respiratory tract infections, eliminating emergency airway problems, or after prolonged intubation [46–48]. Bacterial tracheitis is different from the diseases mentioned above. Bacterial tracheitis is more common in intubated children or those with a tracheotomy. It is an example of a secondary infection in children with artificial airways. It is the severe form of the viral croup-like condition and has a better prognosis in children without a history of intubation or tracheotomy. However, tracheotomy is performed during the disease due to the dark, sticky mucopurulent exudate. This situation is ironic [49–56].

64.6 Pediatric Tracheotomy

The most critical factor determining the prognosis of children who undergo tracheotomy is the indication that causes the need for airway surgery. It has become an increasingly important option with its life-saving advantages and shortening the duration of pediatric intensive care unit treatment after sudden and fatal airway obstruction in children due to oral cavity, nasal passage, and upper airway infections. This allows children to receive adequate treatment, be discharged with a short hospital stay, and return home healthy [59, 60]. Tracheotomy has many reported advantages: patient comfort, less need for sedation, less respiratory effort, better long-term laryngeal function, faster weaning from mechanical ventilation, lower risk of ventilator-associated pneumonia, shorter intensive care stay, and shorter This can be considered as ensuring good oral hygiene. It is a known fact that tracheotomy performed in children due to upper airway obstruction due to upper respiratory tract infections always has better clinical results than prolonged ventilation. Namely, if children are older than 1 year, do not have a chronic disease, or have undergone a tracheostomy due to an upper airway obstruction, their survival rates and chances of leaving the ventilator are higher. This way, pediatric intensive care units achieve a higher bed turnover rate after tracheotomy [61, 62].

64.6.1 Indications

Tracheotomy indications can be examined in six main groups [61–63]:

1. Obstruction of the upper respiratory tract
   (a) Syndromes with airway anomalies
   (b) Bilateral vocal cord paralysis, laryngomalacia, and subglottic web

(c) Infections that cause upper respiratory obstruction
(d) Tumors

2. To provide access to ventilation in cases with difficult intubation, such as retropharyngeal abscess, bleeding after tonsillectomy, obstructive sleep apnea, foreign body in the trachea, and facial burn.
3. Clearing lung secretions and preventing aspiration.
4. To assist weaning from the ventilator.
5. Preventing laryngotracheal stenosis in long-term intubation for.
6. In respiratory failure due to central or neuromuscular reasons.

64.6.2 Contraindications

Because of the continuity of the emergency airway, there is no absolute contraindication to tracheostomy. Some relative contraindications are as follows [64, 65]:

1. Coagulopathy
2. Local infection
3. Anatomical problems
4. Surgical approach difficulties

64.7 Pediatric Tracheotomy Surgical Technique

Pediatric tracheotomy has challenges specific to pediatric patients. These are technically a more complicated and risky procedure than adult tracheotomy due to combined anomalies, short fatty neck, small anatomical dimensions, and proximity to important vital organs. Therefore, the aim of pediatric tracheotomy surgery should be to create a safe airway with minimal morbidity and mortality [66].

Pediatric tracheostomy presents the surgeon with a complex problem not only because of the relative difference in size but also because of the variation in the anatomy. The hyoid bone, thyroid cartilage, and cricoid cartilage are higher in the neck in pediatric patients. Additionally, these structures in the neck, especially the cricoid cartilage, may be difficult to separate or palpate from the first tracheal ring or thyroid cartilage.

A layer of pretracheal fat makes it difficult for the surgeon to palpate typical structures. Other structures lower in the neck or in the superior mediastinum that are not frequently seen in the adult tracheostomy procedure may be more easily encountered in children, such as the innominate artery, left brachiocephalic vein, and the

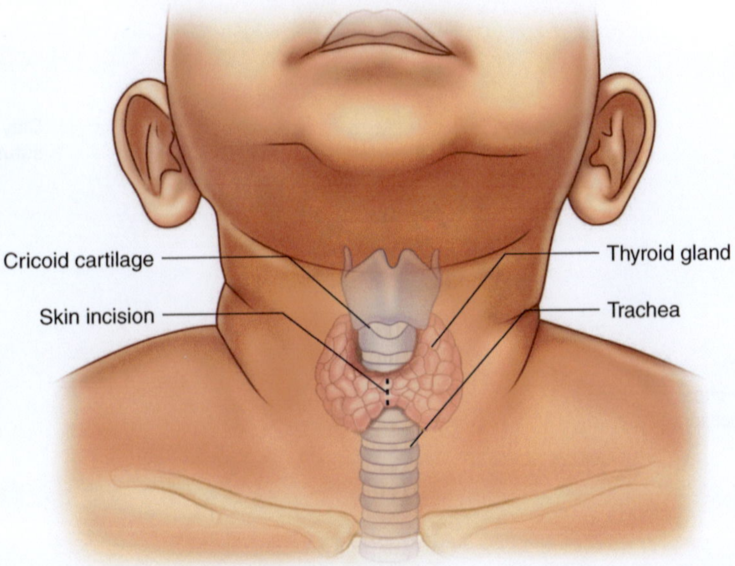

Fig. 64.6 Skin incision. (1) Skin incision illustration: A vertical incision is made in the midline between the cricoid cartilage and the suprasternal notch through the trachea. (2) Removal of subcutaneous fat tissue. (3) Removing the thyroid from the field of view. (4) Tracheal incision

apices of the lungs. The presence of such structures in the neck can be accentuated by hyperextension of the neck, and as a result, low tracheostomy in a child rarely occurs. Interestingly, recurrent laryngeal nerves are located right next to the trachea in the child and are more easily encountered during the procedure, especially if the dissection accidentally moves laterally from the midline [62–66].

Surgical Technique:

The aim is to ensure respiratory safety.

The patient is placed on the operating table, and a pillow-like elevation is placed under the back to hyperextend the neck. Sterile conditions are created for surgery. The anterior neck from the mandible to the breasts is stained with betadine. Appropriate tracheostomy tubes are prepared along with surgical sets, and their balloons are checked [66–69].

If the surgery is elective, the patient is intubated; if it is urgent, a local tracheotomy is performed.

Stages in the application of the surgical technique is shown in Figs. 64.6, 64.7 and 64.8.

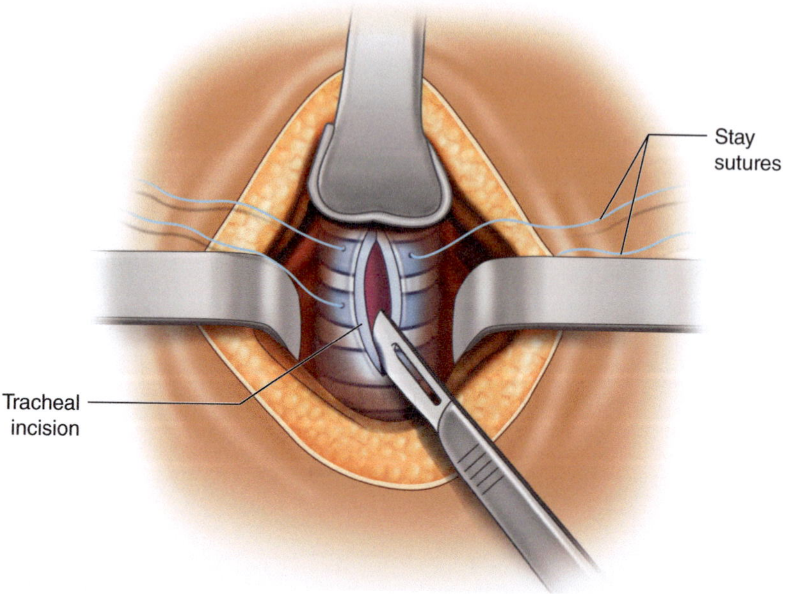

Fig. 64.7 Tracheal incision illustration: vertical incision and stay sutures between trachea 2–3 rings (to ensure patency of the trachea in case of unwanted decannulation). Stay Sutures. Inserting the cannula into the trachea. Fixing the cannula and staying sutures to the neck

Fig. 64.8 Illustration of longitudinal fixation of the cannula and stay sutures: The cannula is fixed to the neck with a necktie. Stay sutures are fixed to the right and left longitudinally with tape

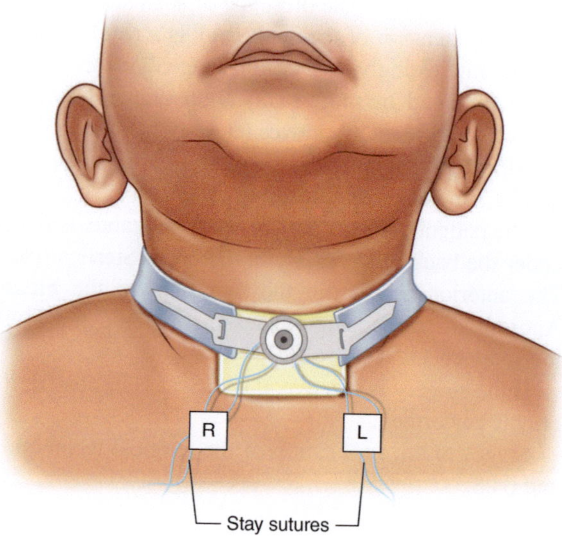

64.8 Pediatric Tracheotomy Complications

Complications in tracheotomy are multifactorial. The child's age, indication and intubation duration, surgeon's tracheotomy experience, and surgical technique selection and management can be listed. In publications, mortality rates related to tracheotomy vary between 0.5 and 3.6%. In our survey study regarding the pediatric tracheotomy technique for ENT physicians in our country in 2019, 3.9% of the participants stated that they encountered death while performing tracheotomy [69]. Pediatric tracheotomy complication rates vary widely in the literature, from 10 to 51% [66–69].

8.1 Early complications: tube obstruction, unintended decannulation, bleeding, pneumonia, pneumothorax, subcutaneous emphysema.

8.2 Late complications include stomal granulation, tracheomalacia, tracheal stenosis, tracheal-cutaneous fistula, tracheoesophageal fistula, and innominate artery bleeding.

The most common potential early complications of pediatric tracheotomy are undesirable decannulation and tracheostomy tube obstruction. Late complications: Stomal granulation, Subglottic stenosis, and Tracheomalacia [69, 70].

Again, in our national survey study, the early complication rate of ENT physicians is 32.7% and the late complication rate is 21.2%. The most common complication in the early period is the Cannula problem at 42.5%, then undesirable decannulation at 27.9%, in the late period, Stomal granulation at 15.6%, and Tracheomalacia at 19.2% [69].

In our experience, some families needed more time to feel comfortable signing the consent form. These families have to pay a large amount of money for their tracheostomy-dependent children due to the difficulties of home care, high costs, and lack of suitable space for equipment.

They experience stress. We believe that for the success of airway control and appropriate treatment in children, it is necessary, from a legal and medical perspective, to resolve the concerns of parents quickly, encourage them to consider the decision of tracheotomy as soon as possible, and then stabilize the clinical condition and provide them with the necessary information and training on how to take good care of their children at home [5, 8, 71].

References

1. Richards AM. Pediatric respiratory emergencies. Emerg Med Clin N Am. 2016;34:77–96.
2. Choi J, Lee GL. Common pediatric respiratory emergencies. Emerg Med Clin N Am. 2012;30(2):529–63.
3. Black AE, Flynn P, Smith HL, Thomas ML, Wilkinson KA, Wilkinson T. Development of a guideline for the management of the unanticipated difficult airway in pediatric practice. Pediatr Anesth. 2015;25:346–62.
4. Sunder RA, Haile DT, Farrell PT, Sharma A. Pediatric airway management: current practices and future directions. Paediatr Anaesth. 2012;22:1008–15.
5. Can FK, Anıl AB, Anıl M, Gumussoy M, Çitlenbik H, Kandoğan T, Zengin N. The outcomes of children with tracheostomy in a tertiary care pediatric intensive care unit in Turkey. Turk Pediatri Ars. 2018;53(3):177–84. https://doi.org/10.5152/TurkPediatriArs.2018.6586.

6. Barch B, Rastatter J, Jagannathan N. Difficult pediatric airway management using the intubating laryngeal airway. Int J Pediatr Otorhinolaryngol. 2012;76:1579–82.
7. Long S. Respiratory tract symptom complexes. In: Long S, Pickering LK, Prober CG, editors. Principles and practice of pediatric infectious diseases. 4th ed. Elsevier; 2012. p. 162–71.
8. Cherry JD. Croup (laryngitis, laryngotracheitis, spasmodic croup, laryngotracheo-bronchitis, bacterial tracheitis, and laryngotracheobronchopneumonitis) and epiglottitis (supraglottitis). In: Chery JD, Harrison GJ, Kaplan SL, et al., editors. Feigin and Cherry's textbook of paediatric infectious diseases. 7th ed. Philadelphia: Elsevier Saunders; 2014. p. 241–60.
9. Pfleger A, Eber E. Management of acute severe upper airway obstruction in children. Paediatr Respir Rev. 2013;14(2):70–7.
10. Adewale L. Anatomy and assessment of the pediatric airway. Paediatr Anaesth. 2009;19:1–8.
11. Wellenstein DJ, de Witt JK, Schutte HW, Honings J, van den Hoogen FJA, Marres HAM, Takes RP, van den Broek GB. Safety of flexible endoscopic biopsy of the pharynx and larynx under topical anesthesia. Eur Arch Otorrinolaringol. 2017;274(9):3471–6.
12. Campisi P, Forte V. Pediatric tracheostomy. Semin Pediatr Surg. 2016;25(3):191–5.
13. Dalal PG, Murray D, Messner AH, et al. Pediatric laryngeal dimensions: an age based analysis. Anesth Analg. 2009;108(5):1475–9.
14. Stroud RH, Friedman NR. An update on inflammatory disorders of the pediatric airway: epiglottitis, croup, and tracheitis. Am J Otolaryngol. 2001;22(4):268–75.
15. Lerner EB, Dayan PS, Brown K, et al. Characteristics of the pediatric patients treated by the pediatric emergency care applied research network's affiliated EMS agencies. Prehosp Emerg Care. 2014;18(1):52–9.
16. Fiadjoe JE, Nishisaki A, Jagannathan N, et al. Airway management complications in children with difficult tracheal intubation from the pediatric difficult intubation (PeDI) registry: a prospective cohort analysis. Lancet Respir Med. 2016;4(1):37–48.
17. Jeff H, Ramesh R, Bhananker SM. Pediatric airway management. Int J Crit Illn Inj Sci. 2014;4(1):65–70.
18. Wani TM, Bissonnette B, Rafiq Malik M, et al. Age-based analysis of pediatric upper airway dimensions using computed tomography imaging. Pediatr Pulmonol. 2016;51(3):267–71.
19. Pfleger A, Eber E. Assessment and causes of stridor. Paediatr Respir Rev. 2016;18:64–72.
20. Ida JB, Thompson DM. Pediatric stridor. Otolaryngol Clin N Am. 2014;47(5):795–819.
21. Mandal A, Kabra SK, Lodha R. Upper airway obstruction in children. Indian J Pediatr. 2015;82(8):737–44.
22. Petrocheilou A, Tanou K, Kalampouka E, et al. Viral croup: diagnosis and a treatment algorithm. Pediatr Pulmonol. 2014;49(5):421–9.
23. Leboulanger N, Garabedian EN. Airway management in pediatric head and neck infections. Infect Disord Drug Targets. 2012;12(4):256–60.
24. LeRiger MM, Miler V, Tobias JD, Raman VT, Elmaraghy CA, Jatana KR. Potential for severe airway obstruction from pediatric retropharyngeal abscess. Int Med Case Rep J. 2017;10:381–4.
25. Jain A, Singh I, Meher R, Raj A, Rajpurohit P, Prasad P. Deep neck space abscesses in children below 5 years of age and their complications. Int J Pediatr Otorhinolaryngol. 2018;109:40–3.
26. Gumussoy ÇI. Retropharyngeal abscess as a potentially mortal complication of tonsillitis: case report. Turkiye Klinikleri J Case Rep. 2013;21(4):204–7.
27. Elsherif AM, Park AH, Alder SC. Indicators of a more complicated clinical course for pediatric patients with retropharyngeal abscess. Int J Pediatr Otorhinolaryngol. 2010;74:198–201.
28. Craig FW, Schunk JE. Retropharyngeal abscess in children: clinical presentation, utility of imaging, and current management. Pediatrics. 2003;111:1394–8.
29. Chuler PJ, Cohnen M, Greve J, et al. Surgical management of retropharyngeal abscesses. Acta Otolaryngol. 2009;129:1274–9.
30. Martin CA, Gabrillargues J, Louvrier C, Saroul N, Mom T, Gilain L. Contribution of CT scan and CT-guided aspiration in the management of retropharyngeal abscess in children based on a series of 18 cases. Eur Ann Otorhinolaryngol Head Neck Dis. 2014;131(5):277–82.
31. Gottlieb M, Long B, Koyfman A. Clinical mimics: an emergency medicine-focused review of streptococcal pharyngitis mimics. J Emerg Med. 2018;54(5):619–29.

32. Argintaru N, Carr D. Retropharyngeal abscess: a subtle presentation of a deep space neck infection. J Emerg Med. 2017;53(4):568–9.
33. Bochner RE, Gangar M, Belamarich PF. A clinical approach to tonsillitis, tonsillar hypertrophy, and peritonsillar and retropharyngeal abscesses. Pediatr Rev. 2017;38(2):81–92.
34. Lorrot M, Haas H, Hentgen V, Van Den Abbeele T, Bonacorsi S, Doit C, Cohen R, Grimprel E. Antibiotherapy of severe ENT infections in children: peripharyngeal abscesses. Arch Pediatr. 2013;20(Suppl 3):e1–4.
35. Levitt GW. Cervical fascia and deep neck infections. Otolaryngol Clin N Am. 1976;93:703–16.
36. Isaacson G, Isaacson DM. Pediatric epiglottitis caused by group G beta-hemolytic streptococcus. Pediatr Infect Dis J. 2003;22:846–7.
37. Baird SM, Marsh PA, Padiglione A, Trubiano J, Lyons B, Hays A, Campbell MC, Phillips D. Review of epiglottitis in the post *Haemophilus influenzae* type-b vaccine era. ANZ J Surg. 2018;88(11):1135–40.
38. McEwan J, Giridharan W, Clarke RW, et al. Paediatric acute epiglottitis: not a disappearing entity. Int J Pediatr Otorhinolaryngol. 2003;67:317–21.
39. Blackstock P, Adderhey RJ, Steward DJ. Epiglottitis in young infants. Anesthesiology. 1987;67(1):97–100.
40. Shah RK, Stocks C. Epiglottitis in the United States: national trends, variances, prognosis, and management. Laryngoscope. 2010;120:1256–62.
41. Slijepcevic A, Strigenz D, Wiet G, et al. EBV epiglottitis: primary supraglottic viral infection in a pediatric immunocompetent host. Int J Pediatr Otorhinolaryngol. 2015;79:1782–4.
42. Acevedo JL, Lander L, Choi S, et al. Airway management in pediatric epiglottitis: a national perspective. Otolaryngol Head Neck Surg. 2009;140:548–51.
43. Bjornson CL, Johnson DW. Croup in children. CMAJ. 2013;185(15):1317–23.
44. Smith DK, McDermott AJ, Sullivan JF. Croup: diagnosis and management. Am Fam Physician. 2018;97(9):575–80.
45. Loftis L. Acute infectious upper airway obstructions in children. Semin Pediatr Infect Dis. 2006;17:5–10.
46. Bagwell T, Hollingsworth A, Thompson T, Abramo T, Huckabee M, Chang D, Crawley L, Robbins JM. Management of Croup in the emergency department: the role of multidose nebulized epinephrine. Pediatr Emerg Care. 2020;36(7):e387–92.
47. Hester G, Barnes T, O'Neill J, Swanson G, McGuinn T, Nickel A. Rate of airway intervention for croup at a tertiary children's hospital 2015–2016. J Emerg Med. 2019;57(3):314–21.
48. Hodnett BL, Simons JP, Riera KM, et al. Objective endoscopic findings in patients with recurrent croup: 10-year retrospective analysis. Int J Pediatr Otorhinolaryngol. 2015;79:2343–7.
49. Milla CE, Zirbes J. Pulmonary complications of endocrine and metabolic disorders. Paediatr Respir Rev. 2012;13:23–8.
50. Casazza G, Graham ME, Nelson D, Chaulk D, Sandweiss D, Meier J. Pediatric bacterial tracheitis—a variable entity: case series with literature review. Otolaryngol Head Neck Surg. 2019;160(3):546–9.
51. Martin-Loeches I, Povoa P, Rodríguez A, Curcio D, Suarez D, Mira JP, Cordero ML, Lepecq R, Girault C, Candeias C, Seguin P, Paulino C, Messika J, Castro AG, Valles J, Coelho L, Rabello L, Lisboa T, Collins D, Torres A, Salluh J, Nseir S. TAVeM study. Incidence and prognosis of ventilator-associated tracheobronchitis (TAVeM): a multicentre, prospective, observational study. Lancet Respir Med. 2015;3(11):859–68.
52. Alves AE, Pereira JM. Antibiotic therapy in ventilator-associated tracheobronchitis: a literature review. Rev Bras Ter Intensiva. 2018;30(1):80–5.
53. Russell CJ, Mack WJ, Schrager SM, Wu S. Care variations and outcomes for children hospitalized with bacterial tracheostomy-associated respiratory infections. Hosp Pediatr. 2017;7(1):16–23.
54. Yamamoto K, Ohmagari N. Bacterial tracheitis caused by *Haemophilus influenzae* after influenza. Intern Med. 2016;55(8):1031.
55. Tebruegge M, Pantazidou A, Thorburn K, et al. Bacterial tracheitis: a multi-centre perspective. Scand J Infect Dis. 2009;41:548–57.

56. Hopkins A, Lahiri T, Salerno R, et al. Changing epidemiology of life-threatening upper airway infections: the reemergence of bacterial tracheitis. Pediatrics. 2006;118:1418–21.
57. Pratt LW, Ferlito A, Rinaldo A. Tracheotomy: historical review. Laryngoscope. 2008;118:1597–606.
58. Pierson DJ. Tracheostomy from A to Z: historical context and current challenges. Respir Care. 2005;50(4):473–5.
59. Cochrane LA, Bailey CM. Surgical aspects of tracheostomy in children. Paediatr Respir Rev. 2006;7(3):169–74.
60. Dal'Astra AP, Quirino AV, Caixeta JA, Avelino MA. Tracheostomy in childhood: review of the literature on complications and mortality over the last three decades. Braz J Otorhinolaryngol. 2017;83(2):207–14.
61. Mahadevan M, Barber C, Salkeld L, Douglas G, Mills N. Pediatric tracheotomy: 17 year review. Int J Pediatr Otorhinolaryngol. 2007;71:1829–35.
62. Scurry WC, McGinn JD. Operative tracheotomy. Oper Tech Otolaryngol Head Neck Surg. 2007;18:85–9.
63. Yoon PJ. The infant tracheostomy. Oper Tech Otolaryngol Head Neck Surg. 2005;16:183–6.
64. Gallagher TQ, Hartnick CJ. Pediatric tracheotomy. Adv Otorhinolaryngol. 2012;73:26–30.
65. Cheung NH, Napolitano LM. Tracheostomy: epidemiology, indications, timing, technique, and outcomes. Respir Care. 2014;59(6):895–915. discussion 916–9.
66. Zhu H, Das P, Brereton J, Roberson D, Shah RK. Surveillance and management practices in tracheotomy patients. Laryngoscope. 2012;122(1):46–50.
67. Atmaca S, Bayraktar C, Aşilioğlu N, Kalkan G, Ozsoy Z. Pediatric tracheotomy: 3-year experience at a tertiary care center with 54 children. Turk J Pediatr. 2011;53(5):537–40.
68. Gumussoy M. Pediatric tracheotomy: comparison of surgical technique with early and late complications in 273 cases. Pak J Med Sci. 2019;35(1):247–51.
69. Gumussoy M, Cukurova I, Atmaca S. National questionnaire on skills and techniques in pediatric tracheotomy surgery in Turkey. Int J Pediatr Otorhinolaryngol. 2020;130:109791.
70. Kremer B, Botos-Kremer AI, Eckel HE, Schlöndorff G. Indications, complications, and surgical techniques for pediatric tracheostomies—un update. J Pediatr Surg. 2002;37(11):1556–62.
71. Rai SK, Holler T, Propst E, Wolter NE, Amin R. Tracheostomy care: clinical practice patterns of pediatric otolaryngologistshead and neck surgeons in a publicly funded (Canadian) health care system. Int J Pediatr Otorhinolaryngol. 2018;115:177–80.

65 Adenoidectomy and Tonsillectomy to Eliminate Airway Obstruction

Omer Çağatay Ertugay and Sema Zer Toros

65.1 Introduction

Airway obstruction is a multifaceted clinical entity with numerous underlying etiologies, capable of compromising one's quality of life and posing potential life-threatening situations. In otolaryngological diseases, especially in the pediatric cohort, hypertrophy of the adenoid and tonsillar tissues is a predominant factor responsible for airway obstruction. Such hypertrophy can impede airflow, interfere with normal speech and swallowing, and disrupt sleep architecture, leading to secondary complications ranging from poor academic performance in children to cardiovascular anomalies.

Nasal breathing is of vital importance in children when compared with adults. Elevated larynx position is the main factor that makes mouth breathing difficult. Nasal congestion and obstruction strongly trigger respiratory distress in pediatric cases. For example, severe systemic hypoxic effects may be seen in cases of choanal atresia in neonates, especially when it is bilateral. Therefore, the blockage of the nasal airway by adenoid hypertrophy can lead to various complications which may adversely affect the growth process.

Adenotonsillectomy—the surgical removal of both adenoids and tonsils—is a procedure steeped in historical significance and has undergone myriad evolutions over the past century. From primarily a procedure to combat recurrent infections, its indication has significantly broadened to address airway obstruction. Today, it remains one of the most commonly performed surgeries worldwide.

In this chapter, we shall delve into the nuances of adenotonsillectomy concerning airway obstruction. Through a comprehensive overview, we will explore its indications, technical aspects, and post-operative care and evaluate its therapeutic

O. Ç. Ertugay · S. Z. Toros (✉)
Haydarpaşa Numune Training and Research Hospital, Department of Otorhinolaryngology, Istanbul, Türkiye

H. Yüksel et al. (eds.), *Pediatric Airway Diseases*, Comprehensive ENT,
https://doi.org/10.1007/978-3-031-74853-0_65

outcomes. Our focus remains on providing an analytical perspective, leveraging existing evidence and experience, to illuminate the pivotal role of adenotonsillectomy in managing airway obstructions resulting from adenotonsillar hypertrophy.

65.2 Anatomy and Pathophysiology Review

Adenoids (Pharyngeal Tonsils): Positioned posterior to the nasal cavity, adenoids can obstruct the nasopharynx when hypertrophic, impeding normal nasal breathing and predisposing to otitis media due to Eustachian tube dysfunction [1]. The vertical position of adenoid hypertrophy varies when it is visualized by an endoscopic approach, ranging from a partial blockage over the openings of the Eustachian tubes to a complete blockage of the nasopharyngeal airway. Recurrent upper respiratory tract infections mainly cause hypertrophy. Children of school and preschool age are exposed to many microorganisms in the crowd, which leads to a hyperreaction of Waldeyer Ring, resulting in airway obstruction. The contribution of allergy remains a controversial issue. It is mainly related to concha hypertrophy and swelling of the nasal mucosa with or without polyps.

Palatine Tonsils: Situated between the palatoglossal and palatopharyngeal arches, enlarged palatine tonsils can obstruct the oropharynx, causing sleep disturbances and swallowing difficulties [2]. As mentioned above, recurrent infections compromise the leading cause. Malignancies of the lymphoid tissue should also be considered. Tonsillar hypertrophy is graded according to its occupation size in the oropharynx, ranging from a partial to a complete blockage. The obstruction should be evaluated with the position of the soft palate, posterior pharyngeal wall, and tongue base. However, it is rare in children. Some patients may demonstrate a circular collapse; therefore, tonsillectomy alone may not be a sufficient treatment.

Pharyngeal and palatine tonsils are the components of the Waldeyer ring. There are also tubal and lingual tonsils, which may also be hypertrophied, thereby participating in the obstruction. The lingual tonsil is located in the base of the tongue, having a network with other cervical lymphatic drainage.

65.3 Indications for Adenotonsillectomy

Obstructive Sleep Apnea (OSA): Enlarged tonsils and adenoids can lead to partial or complete pharyngeal obstruction during sleep, resulting in OSA [3]. Hypoxia during sleep can interfere with hormonal disturbances such as inappropriate growth factor secretion, psychosocial status, and cognitive improvement. The main indications are recurrent tonsil infections, as well as airway obstruction, febrile convulsions, peritonsillar abscess, PFAPA syndrome (Periodic fever, Aphthous stomatitis, Pharyngitis, and Adenitis), speech abnormalities, acute rheumatic fever, and post-streptococcal glomerulonephritis.

Recurrent or Persistent Infection: Chronic or recurrent episodes of tonsillitis or adenoiditis, not amenable to medical therapy, may necessitate surgical intervention

[4]. Besides the complications of infections, frequent use of antibiotics can also be prevented.

Dysphagia and Feeding Difficulties: Especially prevalent in children, where hypertrophied tissues can cause mechanical obstruction during swallowing [4]. The oral and pharyngeal phases of swallowing are affected by excessive tissue, and the remnants of food can deteriorate oral hygiene.

Speech Abnormalities and Dental Malocclusions: Due to chronic mouth breathing, secondary to adenoidal hypertrophy [5]. Dryness of the oral mucosa is a typical result of mouth breathing and dental and maxillomandibular abnormalities due to lack of tactile stimulus of the tongue.

Peritonsillar Abscess: Involvement of the peritonsillar space in children is presented with fever, pain, and difficulty swallowing. Mastication can also be impaired. Two or more episodes of abscess is favored to undergo surgery.

PFAPA syndrome (Periodic fever, Aphthous stomatitis, Pharyngitis, and Adenitis): An autoimmune disorder of the lymphoid tissue presented with periodic episodes and mainly accompanied by tonsillar hypertrophy. Fever is mainly managed by steroid use.

65.4 Contraindications

Age: Although not an absolute contraindication, children under 3 years of age pose an increased risk due to anesthesia sensitivity and postoperative respiratory concerns [6]. Any signs of severe obstruction should address surgical intervention regardless of the age.

Bleeding Disorders: Patients with coagulopathies or those on anticoagulants have a heightened risk of post-operative bleeding [7]. Appropriate replacement before surgery is mandatory.

Cervical Spine Abnormalities: Conditions such as atlantoaxial instability in Down syndrome patients may complicate intubation [8].

65.5 Surgical Techniques

Two primary methods dominate the landscape:

Cold Dissection: Uses scalpel, scissors, or curette. The tonsil is dissected from the tonsillar bed, preserving the muscle layer underneath [9]. The advantages and disadvantages of all techniques still remain controversial.

Electrocautery or Diathermy: This technique simultaneously deploys an electrical current to cut and coagulate tissues [9]. Electrocautery provides surgery with diminished hemorrhage but emits a high level of heat compared to diathermy. Postoperative pain is the main disadvantage.

Regardless of the method chosen, the primary goal remains the same: Complete removal of adenoid and tonsillar tissues with minimal damage to surrounding structures. Lately, tonsillar reduction rather than complete removal has been postulated in the literature. Patients with obstructive complaints, without any history of recurrent tonsillar infections, could be candidates for this kind of surgery. On the other hand, the possibility of refractory hypertrophy and reobstruction should be kept in mind. Further long-term studies will clarify the contradiction.

65.6 Postoperative Care and Complications

Pain Management: Opioids, NSAIDs, and paracetamol constitute the analgesic arsenal. However, concerns about opioid-induced respiratory depression, especially in children with residual obstructive symptoms, necessitate judicious use [10]. Paracetamol is the first level of choice.

Bleeding: The most dreaded complication, posttonsillectomy hemorrhage, mandates immediate medical or surgical intervention [11]. The most common etiology is trauma during oral intake. Diet adherence is significant in preventing traumatic hemorrhage.

Dehydration: Secondary to dysphagia. Encourage oral intake, and in severe cases, intravenous fluids might be required [12].

Infection: Though uncommon, peritonsillar abscesses can develop postoperatively as a complication. Postoperative antibiotic use is still not recommended unless a complication occurs.

65.7 Outcomes and Efficacy

Adenotonsillectomy's efficacy in addressing airway obstruction stemming from adenotonsillar hypertrophy has been a focal point of numerous clinical studies over the past decades. A robust body of evidence, both quantitative and qualitative, supports its therapeutic advantages, especially in pediatric patients. Elimination of the obstruction recovers the hypoxic process, therefore reducing the effects of respiratory distress.

Resolution of Obstructive Sleep Apnea (OSA) Studies have consistently demonstrated a marked reduction in the Apnea-Hypopnea Index (AHI) postoperatively. A significant proportion of patients, particularly children, who undergo adenotonsillectomy for OSA experience complete resolution or a drastic reduction in their symptoms. This enhances sleep quality and augments daytime functioning, concentration, and overall cognitive performance [13–15]. Concerning the long-term effects of OSA, the life-long benefits of the surgery is predictable.

Cardiovascular Benefits Chronic airway obstruction, especially OSA, can place undue stress on the cardiovascular system. Adenotonsillectomy can decrease the risk of pulmonary hypertension, right-sided heart failure, and other cardiovascular complications associated with chronic upper airway obstruction by rectifying this obstruction [16]. Elevated intrathoracic pressure impairs venous blood return from the head, resulting in congestion of the upper airway mucosa.

Neurocognitive and Behavioral Outcomes In pediatric populations, untreated airway obstruction has been linked with neurocognitive deficits, learning difficulties, and behavioral issues. During the post-adenotonsillectomy period, many children demonstrate notable improvements in attention span, academic performance, and a reduction in behavioral problems, offering them a renewed chance for optimal developmental progress [17].

Improved Quality of Life Beyond the tangible physiological benefits, adenotonsillectomy contributes to a qualitative elevation in the affected individuals' lives. This includes improved self-esteem, reduced anxiety from breathing difficulties, and better social interactions, especially pertinent for adolescents [18]. Shortness of breath during daytime exercises and mouth-breathing decrease the quality of life, both of which are eliminated by the surgery.

Reduction in Recurrent Infections Although our primary focus is airway obstruction, it's worth noting that adenotonsillectomy also curtails the frequency of recurrent throat infections in those predisposed, further diminishing the morbidity and healthcare costs associated with recurrent episodes of illness [19]. Any possibility of increased rate of lower respiratory tract infections postoperatively is highly discussed in the literature, and no significant result has been reported.

Long-Term Efficacy While immediate postoperative benefits are undeniable, long-term follow-ups have cemented adenotonsillectomy's standing as a durable solution for adenotonsillar-induced airway obstruction. The majority of patients maintain the initial benefits of surgery years after the procedure, underscoring its lasting impact [20].

However, like any medical intervention, the outcomes vary based on individual patient factors, including age, comorbidities, severity of the initial obstruction, and the surgical technique employed. It remains crucial for clinicians to engage in a holistic preoperative evaluation and set realistic post-operative expectations.

65.8 Conclusion

Adenotonsillectomy is a cornerstone in the surgical management of airway obstruction due to adenotonsillar hypertrophy. While the procedure has its associated risks, in the hands of a skilled otolaryngologist and with judicious patient selection, the outcomes can be transformative, substantively elevating the quality of life of the affected individual.

References

1. Rout MR, Mohanty D, Vijaylaxmi Y, Bobba K, Metta C. Adenoid hypertrophy in adults: a case series. Indian J Otolaryngol Head Neck Surg. 2013;65(3):269–74. https://doi.org/10.1007/s12070-012-0549-y.

2. Sağıroğlu A, Acer N, Okuducu H, et al. Palatine tonsil volume estimation using different methods after tonsillectomy. Anat Sci Int. 2017;92(4):500–8. https://doi.org/10.1007/s12565-016-0350-1.
3. Mitchell RB. Adenotonsillectomy for obstructive sleep apnea in children: outcome evaluated by pre- and postoperative polysomnography. Laryngoscope. 2007;117(10):1844–54. https://doi.org/10.1097/MLG.0b013e318123ee56.
4. Burton MJ, Glasziou PP. Tonsillectomy or adeno-tonsillectomy versus non-surgical treatment for chronic/recurrent acute tonsillitis. Cochrane Database Syst Rev. 2009;(1):CD001802. https://doi.org/10.1002/14651858.CD001802.pub2.
5. Alzahrani HA, Alkhaldi RO, Alsufyani DH, Alghamdi SA, Althobity TA, Fageeh YA. Adenoid hypertrophy and orthodontic complications: an assessment of parental knowledge in Saudi Arabia. Cureus. 2023;15(7):e41692. https://doi.org/10.7759/cureus.41692.
6. Ing C, Sun M, Olfson M, et al. Age at exposure to surgery and anesthesia in children and association with mental disorder diagnosis. Anesth Analg. 2017;125(6):1988–98. https://doi.org/10.1213/ANE.0000000000002423.
7. Liu JH, Anderson KE, Willging JP, et al. Posttonsillectomy hemorrhage: what is it and what should be recorded? Arch Otolaryngol Head Neck Surg. 2001;127(10):1271–5. https://doi.org/10.1001/archotol.127.10.1271.
8. Crosby ET, Lui A. The adult cervical spine: implications for airway management. Can J Anaesth/Journal canadien d'anesthésie. 1990;37:77–93.
9. Verma R, Verma RR, Verma RR. Tonsillectomy-comparative study of various techniques and changing trend. Indian J Otolaryngol Head Neck Surg. 2017;69(4):549–58. https://doi.org/10.1007/s12070-017-1190-6.
10. Jensena DR. Pharmacologic management of post-tonsillectomy pain in children. World J Otorhinolaryngol Head Neck Surg. 2021;7(3):186–93. https://doi.org/10.1016/j.wjorl.2021.03.004.
11. Allareddy V, Martinez-Schlurmann N, Rampa S, et al. Predictors of complications of tonsillectomy with or without adenoidectomy in hospitalized children and adolescents in the United States, 2001-2010: a population-based study. Clin Pediatr (Phila). 2016;55(7):593–602. https://doi.org/10.1177/0009922815616885.
12. Khasawneh L, Al-Mashakbeh Y, Al Katatbeh M. Predictors of dehydration following adenotonsillectomy in Jordanian pediatric cases. Med J Islam Repub Iran. 2022;36:114.
13. Gorman D, Ogston S, Hussain SSM. Improvement in symptoms of obstructive sleep apnoea in children following tonsillectomy versus tonsillotomy: a systematic review and meta-analysis. Clin Otolaryngol. 2017;42:275–82.
14. Camacho M, Dongcai L, Kawai M, et al. Tonsillectomy for adult obstructive sleep apnea: a systematic review and meta-analysis. Laryngoscope. 2016;126:2176–86.
15. Reckley LK, Song SA, Chang ET, Cable BB, Certal V, Camacho M. Adenoidectomy can improve obstructive sleep apnoea in young children: systematic review and meta-analysis. J Laryngol Otol. 2016;130:990–4.
16. Cincin A, Sakalli E, Bakirci EM, Dizman R. Relationship between obstructive sleep apnea-specific symptoms and cardiac function before and after adenotonsillectomy in children with adenotonsillar hypertrophy. Int J Pediatr Otorhinolaryngol. 2014;78(8):1281–7. https://doi.org/10.1016/j.ijporl.2014.05.011.
17. Goldstein NA, Post C, Rosenfeld R. Impact of tonsillectomy and adenoidectomy on child behavior. Arch Otolaryngol Head Neck Surg. 2000;126:494–8.
18. Argiris K. Improvement in quality of life by adenotonsillectomy in children with adenotonsillar disease. Clin Otolaryngol. 2011;36(3):280; author reply 281. https://doi.org/10.1111/j.1749-4486.2011.02263.x.
19. Burton MJ, Glasziou PP, Chong LY, Venekamp RP. Tonsillectomy or adenotonsillectomy versus non-surgical treatment for chronic/recurrent acute tonsillitis. Cochrane Database Syst Rev. 2014;2014(11):CD001802. https://doi.org/10.1002/14651858.CD001802.pub3.
20. Lim J, McKean MC. Adenotonsillectomy for obstructive sleep apnoea in children. Cochrane Database Syst Rev. 2009;(2):CD003136. https://doi.org/10.1002/14651858.CD003136.pub2.

Management of Laryngeal Webs in Children

66

Perçin Serhat Yergin and Sema Zer Toros

66.1 Introduction

Laryngeal webs, anatomically situated at the level of the glottis or subglottis, are a consequential etiological constituent of laryngeal anomalies in the pediatric population. Laryngeal webs are either congenital or acquired. They are complex malformations that engender a spectrum of respiratory and phonatory difficulties, with immediate and long-term repercussions. These webs are generally constituted of membranous tissue and can be differentiated based on location, thickness, and extent of the glottic aperture they cover. Webs may range from thin and limited, hardly influencing the airway patency, to thick and extensive, potentially leading to significant airway obstruction.

The rarity and heterogeneity of these webs, coupled with their potential to compromise the pediatric airway and voice, necessitate detailed understanding and prudent clinical management. Although advances in diagnostic imaging and surgical intervention techniques have significantly enhanced the management of laryngeal webs, they pose considerable clinical challenges. This chapter provides a comprehensive overview of laryngeal webs, exploring their etiology, epidemiology, clinical presentation, diagnostic methodologies, management strategies, and long-term prognosis. The goal is to arm practitioners with a robust, up-to-date knowledge base, enabling them to optimally manage this complex congenital condition and provide the best care to the affected pediatric population.

P. S. Yergin
Uskudar Aktif International Hospital, Istanbul, Türkiye

S. Z. Toros (✉)
Department of Otorhinolaryngology, Haydarpaşa Numune Training and Research Hospital, Istanbul, Türkiye

H. Yüksel et al. (eds.), *Pediatric Airway Diseases*, Comprehensive ENT,
https://doi.org/10.1007/978-3-031-74853-0_66

66.2 Etiology and Epidemiology

Laryngeal webs constitute approximately 5% of all congenital laryngeal anomalies, placing them among the rarer monsters encountered in pediatric otolaryngology [1]. The formation of these webs is speculated to be multifactorial, with various etiological theories being proposed. It is generally agreed that they arise during embryogenesis due to an interruption of the normal development process of the laryngotracheal tube.

Congenital laryngeal webs arise from perturbations in the embryological development of specific laryngeal structures, specifically the epithelial lamina, laryngeal cecum, or the vestibulotracheal duct [2]. Several hypotheses propose mechanisms to elucidate the aberrant laryngeal anatomy observed in patients. One postulation posits an atypical inferior elongation of the epithelial lamina during embryonic development, which extends into the primitive subglottis and retains its structural integrity postembryogenesis [3]. Alternatively, Sanudo's description offers another perspective, pointing toward a ventral extension of the infraglottis termed the vestibulotracheal duct. If, for any reason, the vestibulotracheal duct [2] fails to manifest that the resulting ventral and caudal displacement of the epithelial lamina might encourage the induction or migratory patterns of cartilaginous cells, predisposing them to populate the region slated to mature into the anterior subglottis [3].

On the genetic front, evidence suggests that certain forms of laryngeal webs may be associated with specific genetic disorders. One such disorder is 22q11.2 deletion syndrome, also known as DiGeorge Syndrome, characterized by various congenital malformations, including laryngeal webs. Digeorge's syndrome can be seen in up to 65% of anterior glottic webs, necessitating genetic evaluation [4]. However, it is essential to note that the definitive pathogenetic mechanisms responsible for laryngeal web formation remain elusive.

Acquired laryngeal webs are less standard than congenital ones. Neck traumas and iatrogenic causes constitute two leading causes. Although it is usually associated with anterior laryngeal papillomatosis surgery as iatrogenic causes, it can rarely be induced by prolonged intubation [5].

66.3 Clinical Presentation and Diagnosis

The clinical presentation is heterogeneous, primarily contingent on the web's size, thickness, and position within the larynx. Infants with thin, anteriorly positioned webs may be asymptomatic or present with mild stridor. In contrast, those with thicker, more posteriorly situated webs can present with severe respiratory distress shortly after birth.

Severe cases require urgent airway intervention in infants, but subtle airway symptoms are usually present. In infants, biphasic stridor and chest wall retraction are observed, which are more prominent in situations requiring effort, such as feeding and crying.

Diagnosis is often made via transnasal flexible laryngoscopy or direct laryngoscopy. However, advances in imaging techniques like high-resolution computed tomography (HRCT) and magnetic resonance imaging (MRI) are increasingly being employed. Endoscopic examination provides a more precise assessment of both arytenoid mobility and subglottic extension of the web. Differential diagnosis should consider other causes of upper airway obstruction, like laryngeal atresia, laryngomalacia, and subglottic stenosis.

In Cohen's [6] sophisticated classification of glottic webs, there exists a precise categorization delineating the extent of glottic involvement and its subsequent clinical manifestations. (Fig. 66.1) This taxonomy comprises four distinct categories, each reflecting the depth and progression of the web, as well as its associated clinical sequelae:

1. Type I
   - Morphology: A slender anterior web with <35% glottic involvement.
   - Clinical Manifestations: Patients present with subtle hoarseness while largely devoid of respiratory distress or airway obstruction.
2. Type II
   - Morphology: This continuum encompasses thin to moderately thick web formations involving 35–50% of the glottic space.
   - Clinical Manifestations: Clinically, these patients may exhibit a faint and husky vocal quality. Concurrently, they might experience a mild compromise in their airway, though not critically threatening.
3. Type III
   - Morphology: A robust web that is thickened and possesses anterior extensions. In certain circumstances, these extensions might be of cartilaginous subglottic nature, spanning 50–75% of the total glottic length.
   - Clinical Manifestations: The repercussions of such an extensive web are notable, manifesting as a highly feeble voice and intermediate-grade airway symptoms. These symptoms, while significant, typically fall short of necessitating immediate surgical interventions.
4. Type IV
   - Morphology: A pervasive, uniformly thick web occupying 75–90% of the glottic expanse. This category is also distinctively marked by a cartilaginous subglottic extension.

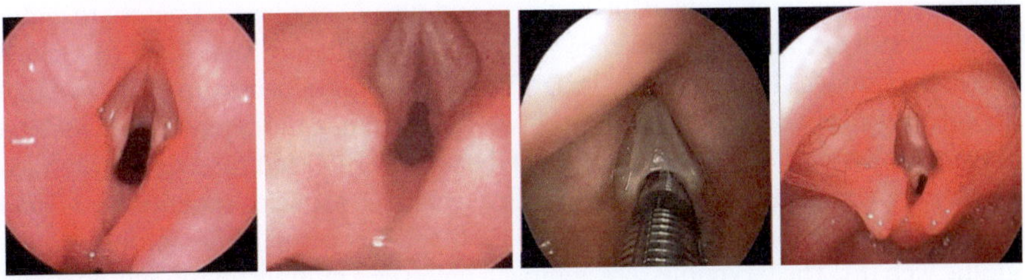

Fig. 66.1 Types 1, 2, 3, and 4 laryngeal webs by Cohen classification, respectively

- Clinical Manifestations: The clinical scenario with this category is rather dire. Patients not only present with aphonia but also experience acute respiratory distress, often necessitating surgical intervention, most commonly in a tracheotomy.

This nuanced classification is instrumental in guiding clinicians toward a more informed diagnostic and therapeutic approach, contingent upon the distinct morphological and clinical characteristics intrinsic to each category.

66.4 Management and Treatment

The management of laryngeal webs is primarily tailored according to the severity of symptoms, the web's anatomical characteristics, and the patient's overall health status. For asymptomatic or minimally symptomatic patients with small, thin webs, conservative management is often sufficient, comprising careful observation and voice therapy.

However, surgical intervention becomes the cornerstone for managing symptomatic laryngeal webs, with the approach heavily relying on the web's thickness, subglottic extension, and associated laryngeal anomalies. The principal surgical modalities can be broadly classified into endoscopic and open procedures.

Endoscopic approaches are generally preferred for thinner, anteriorly located webs due to their lesser invasiveness and fewer complications (Cohen type 1 and type 2). These techniques include laser excision, microlaryngeal surgery, and dilation with or without placement of a laryngeal keel.

Laser excision, primarily utilizing CO2 lasers, is often preferred due to its precision and excellent hemostatic properties. The laser vaporizes the web tissue layer by layer, ensuring minimal collateral damage to the surrounding structures. In the case of microlaryngeal surgery, cold steel instruments are used to cut and remove the web, with concurrent or subsequent balloon dilation often employed to restore the glottic aperture.

Laryngeal keels, made of silicone or metal, can be placed postoperatively, straddling the anterior commissure to prevent restenosis, particularly in more extensive webs. They are usually put through a small anterior subglottic incision and secured with sutures, with removal scheduled after a few weeks once sufficient healing has occurred [7].

For extensive, thick webs (Cohen type 3 and type 4) or those refractory to endoscopic treatment, open approaches such as laryngofissure and laryngotracheal reconstruction (LTR) are employed. These techniques necessitate an external approach via a neck incision. In the mid-twentieth century, the external open method via laryngofissure was detailed, first by McNaught in 1950 and subsequently refined by Montgomery and Gamble. This operative technique provides superior access and facilitates the meticulous excision of the cartilaginous components intrinsic to the glottic web [8]. The laryngofissure approach involves a midline thyrotomy, allowing direct access to the laryngeal lumen to excision the web and subsequent suture closure. LTR is often reserved for severe cases involving subglottic extension, requiring cartilage grafting to augment the subglottic lumen [9].

These open surgical techniques are more invasive and carry inherent risks such as potential voice changes, wound complications, and subglottic stenosis. However, they are indispensable in managing severe or recalcitrant laryngeal webs.

Postoperative management is equally crucial in all surgical interventions, characterized by close monitoring for recurrence, the potential need for repeat interventions, and the provision of voice therapy for optimal phonatory outcomes. Recurrence of the web could be seen in almost half of the patients who underwent procedures, and the recurrence rate is similar between Cohen type 1/2 cases and Cohen type 3/4 cases [10]. Hence, managing laryngeal webs represents a continuum of care, where surgical intervention is just one part of a comprehensive treatment strategy.

Evaluating voice quality in the pediatric demographic presents significant complexities. Clary et al. reported that children's voices improved after surgery, and their voice results were satisfactory [11]. De Trey et al. advocate for the subsequent meticulous procedures to enhance vocal outcomes in Cohen type 3/4 cases: (1) In the process of comprehensive laryngofissure and web segmentation, engage in a rigorous division of the web, either utilizing endoscopic methods or by leveraging intraoperative flexible endoscopy, avoid inflicting damage upon the vocal ligaments and prioritize the retention of the integral glottic mucosa. (2) Throughout the phase of airway expansion and laryngofissure sealing, uphold a pronounced angle at the anterior commissure and strive for the most optimal mucosal juxtaposition of the vocal ligaments, thus deterring scar-induced misshaping of the emergent anterior commissure and refrain from excessive dilation of the posterior commissure [12].

66.5 Prognosis and Long-Term Outcomes

The prognosis of pediatric laryngeal webs is primarily influenced by the initial severity of the web, associated anomalies, and the need for multiple surgical interventions. While the immediate postoperative period may witness a resolution of airway symptoms, long-term voice outcomes can be variable. Phonatory difficulties, including dysphonia and hoarseness, may persist or develop later in life, requiring ongoing voice therapy.

66.6 Conclusion

In conclusion, laryngeal webs in the pediatric population present unique diagnostic and therapeutic challenges. While surgical intervention can effectively alleviate airway symptoms, managing laryngeal webs is complex, often requiring multiple interventions, comprehensive postoperative follow-up, and voice therapy to optimize long-term outcomes.

References

1. Avelino MAG, Pazinatto DB, Rodrigues SO, Maunsell R. Congenital laryngeal webs: from diagnosis to surgical outcomes. Braz J Otorhinolaryngol. 2022;88:497–504. https://doi.org/10.1016/j.bjorl.2020.06.018.
2. Sanudo JR, Domenech-Mateu JM. The laryngeal primordium and epithelial lamina. A new interpretation. J Anat. 1990;171:207–22.
3. Milczuk HA, Smith JD, Everts EC. Congenital laryngeal webs: surgical management and clinical embryology. Int J Pediatr Otorhinolaryngol. 2000;52:1–9. https://doi.org/10.1016/S0165-5876(99)00284-0.
4. Miyamoto RC, Cotton RT, Rope AF, et al. Association of anterior glottic webs with velocardiofacial syndrome (chromosome 22q11.2 deletion). Otolaryngol Head Neck Surg. 2004;130:415–7. https://doi.org/10.1016/j.otohns.2003.12.014.
5. Scadding GK, Bull PD, Graham JM. Laryngeal webs and subglottic hemangiomas. In: Pediatric ENT. Berlin, Heidelberg: Springer; 2007. p. 211–22.
6. Cohen SR. Congenital glottic webs in children. A retrospective review of 51 patients. Ann Otol Rhinol Laryngol Suppl. 1985;121:2–16.
7. Paniello RC, Desai SC, Allen CT, Khosla SM. Endoscopic keel placement to treat and prevent anterior glottic webs. Ann Otol Rhinol Laryngol. 2013;122:672–8. https://doi.org/10.1177/000348941312201102.
8. Alkan U, Nachalon Y, Vaisbuch Y, Katz O, Hamzany Y, Stern Y. Treating paediatric anterior glottic web: single-Centre experience of 20 patients with comparison among techniques. Clin Otolaryngol. 2017;42:893–7. https://doi.org/10.1111/coa.12749.
9. Cotton RT, Myer CM, O'Connor DM, Smith ME. Pediatric laryngotracheal reconstruction with cartilage grafts and endotracheal tube stenting: the single-stage approach. Laryngoscope. 1995;105:818–21. https://doi.org/10.1288/00005537-199508000-00009.
10. Lawlor CM, Dombrowski ND, Nuss RC, Rahbar R, Choi SS. Laryngeal web in the pediatric population: evaluation and management. Otolaryngol Head Neck Surg. 2020;162:234–40. https://doi.org/10.1177/0194599819893985.
11. Clary RA, Pengilly A, Bailey M, et al. Analysis of voice outcomes in pediatric patients following surgical procedures for laryngotracheal stenosis. Arch Otolaryngol Head Neck Surg. 1996;122:1189–94. https://doi.org/10.1001/archotol.1996.01890230035008.
12. De Trey LA, Lambercy K, Monnier P, Sandu K. Management of severe congenital laryngeal webs—a 12 year review. Int J Pediatr Otorhinolaryngol. 2016;86:82–6. https://doi.org/10.1016/j.ijporl.2016.04.006.

Management of Laryngeal Papillomatosis in Children

67

Mustafa Nuhut and Sema Zer Toros

67.1 Introduction

Rarely, any part of the airway, from the nasal vestibule to the terminal bronchi, can become infected with low-risk human papillomavirus (HPV) types 6 and 11. The tonsillar pillars, uvula, and laryngeal commissure epithelium are commonly affected by exophytic papillomas. Laryngeal papillomatosis affects an estimated 4.3 out of every 100,000 children and 1.8 out of every 100,000 adults [1, 2]. When diagnosed before 12, JoRRPs are said to be juvenile-onset. Approximately equal numbers of males and females are present between the ages of 2 and 6 [3]. In contrast to Europe and South America, where RRP is more common in adults, it is more common in children and adolescents in sub-Saharan Africa [4, 5]. JoRRP is transmitted from mother to child during pregnancy or acquired from an HPV-positive mother at birth. Unlike in adults, the disease typically progresses more rapidly in children [6].

67.2 Etiology

Human papillomavirus is a member of the papovavirus family; it is an icosahedral-shaped, naked virus with a circular, supercoiled double-stranded DNA genome. Southern blot hybridization confirmed the presence of HPV DNA in laryngeal

M. Nuhut
Medient Ear Nose Throat Medical Center, Istanbul, Türkiye

S. Z. Toros (✉)
Department of Otorhinolaryngology, Haydarpasa Numune Training and Research Hospital, Istanbul, Türkiye

H. Yüksel et al. (eds.), *Pediatric Airway Diseases*, Comprehensive ENT,
https://doi.org/10.1007/978-3-031-74853-0_67

papillomas. It allowed for identifying HPV types 6 and 11 in the papillomas, proving the link between HPV and papillomas [7].

Although HPV types 6 and 11 account for the vast majority of JoRRP cases, other HPV types, including high-risk kinds, have been discovered [8–10]. HPV strains 6 and 11 relate to condyloma acuminata (genital warts). Particularly in squamous cell carcinoma of the head and neck and the cervix of the uterus, types 16 and 18 have been linked to carcinogenesis. Juvenile-onset papillomatosis is often passed from mother to child through the placenta. First-born children, mothers who have given birth before, and those who have genital warts all increase their chances [11–13]. Despite claims that the HPV 11 subtype is linked to more severe disease than HPV 6, research reveals that the age at the disease beginning is more closely connected to the clinical course than the HPV subtype [8, 14]. In addition, research suggests that 2% of RLP patients may develop malignant degeneration. The majority of documented cases of malignant transformation have involved adults, and additional risk factors, including smoking and prolonged illness, have been linked to these cases [15].

67.3 Clinical Presentation

The larynx is the most common site of initial presentation for respiratory papillomas. However, they can develop anywhere on the respiratory mucosa. As the second most common benign tumor of the larynx in children, laryngeal papilloma is also a prevalent cause of hoarseness in young people [3, 16]. The loud cords represent the pseudostratified and stratified epithelium boundary. As a result, papillomas populate the voice chords often. Dysphonia is the most prevalent presenting issue in children diagnosed with RRP, which often occurs between the ages of 2 and 4. Seventy-five percent of people with JoRRP have a diagnosis before they turn 5 [8, 17].

Progressive dysphonia, stridor, and respiratory distress are the presenting signs. Symptoms may include dysphonia, stridor, a persistent cough, choking fits, frequent respiratory infections, and even hemoptysis [18]. Asthma, laryngotracheobronchitis, foreign body aspiration, and laryngomalacia are common incorrect diagnoses [19].

The clinical course of laryngeal papillomatosis cannot be predicted with any degree of accuracy. This condition is notoriously difficult to cure because it frequently returns and spreads throughout the aerodigestive tract. Although the larynx is the most common site of involvement, the entire aerodigestive tract is at risk when RRP is present. The rate of yearly and lifetime procedures and distal dissemination are indicators of the disease's virulence. HPV 11 subtypes, involvement of different levels of the larynx, younger age, and maternal genital warts have been related to more severe illness [8, 12, 20]. In children with JoRRP, distal spread occurs between 5 and 48% of cases [21, 22]. Subglottic involvement, tracheostomy status, and prolonged illness duration are risk factors for tracheobronchial disease. Pneumonia, atelectasis, fever, and septic shock can all result from lung involvement [23, 24].

Derkay suggested an RRP staging system that considers lesions' anatomical location and severity. The most widely used method for illness staging is Derkay's. Using this method, you may assess the anatomical distribution of illness and the functional evaluation of clinical aspects [25]. This staging system's weakness is that it cannot differentiate between varying degrees of severity within a given location despite being competent for defining the presence of illness, the number of sites implicated, and the bulkiness of each lesion [26]. The time between surgeries tends to decrease in tandem with the patient's anatomical score [27].

Laryngeal papillomatosis exhibits erratic activity in the clinic. Surgery is performed less often over time for most patients, but for about a third of those people, it either stays the same or gets more frequent [27–29].

Papilloma malignant degeneration occurs seldom and has a dismal prognosis when it does. It often manifests earlier and causes tracheal involvement in youngsters [30]. Oncoproteins E6 and E7 are essential to the process by which normal cells become cancerous. Through direct interactions with cell cycle regulatory proteins, E6 and E7 proteins induce cancer [31].

67.4 Diagnosis

A flexible fiberoptic laryngoscope examination is recommended for all individuals suspected of having laryngeal papillomatosis. In severe cases, a biopsy taken by direct laryngoscopy may be required. Papillomas can be either pedunculated or sessile exophytic aggregates at the macroscopic level. On microscopic examination, papillomas are shown to be exophytic projections of stratified squamous epithelium, with aberrant keratinization and basal cell hyperplasia within the connective tissue stroma that supports them. You may have dyskeratosis, parakeratosis, or dysplasia.

Patients with a clinical presentation suggestive of pulmonary involvement warrant chest imaging [32].

67.5 Treatment

Until the condition is in remission, surgical removal of laryngeal papillomas remains the gold standard therapy. During surgery, your surgeon will work to remove any formed papillomas and restore a clear airway while protecting your vocal cords and other mucosal tissue as much as possible. This is why cold instruments, laser (CO_2, KTP, or flash dye), microdebrider, or coblation are favored in the surgical treatment of papillomas [15, 33, 34]. Latent virus can persist in surrounding tissue even after removing all clinically apparent papillomas.

Vocal cord trauma is reduced to a minimum, and heat damage to neighboring tissues is avoided with the microflap approach for surgical treatment of the condition employing microlaryngeal devices. When dealing with a highly vascular lesion, cold steel surgery has the obvious drawback of being unable to perform direct hemostasis. Using a powered microdebrider in the surgical excision of laryngeal papillomas is a recent but rapidly growing trend. The laryngeal debridement blade facilitates thorough and accurate papilloma removal. There is little danger of heat injury from contamination of the lower respiratory system.

For a long time, surgeons have been using a carbon dioxide (CO_2) laser to treat JORRP. Many surgeons use this method because it effectively removes papillomas while causing minimum bleeding. Papillomas of the trachea and bronchi are often treated with fiber-delivered laser systems. Regarding papilloma ablation and hemostasis, KTP and Nd:YAG lasers are on par with CO_2 lasers. Using a laser or microdebrider does not correlate with longer times between procedures [27]. Publications claim that laser surgery is more effective than cold tools, and microdebrider surgery is more effective than CO_2 laser. However, the actual results may vary from surgeon to surgeon [35, 36]. When compared to lasers and cold instruments, microdebriders provide several benefits, including decreased operation time and the absence of thermal harm [36]. Coblation® is a low-heat method that uses a plasma layer to disintegrate tissue with minor tissue damage. Coblation® for JORRP has seen relatively little research because of the lack of available data [37]. Many potential problems have been associated with laryngeal airway operations. Iatrogenic squamous metaplasia, the most frequent and initial consequence, occurs when the lesion returns or the illness spreads to other tissues. It is possible to develop glottic stenoses, granulomas, and synechia after undergoing repeated surgical removal of papillomas. Long-term exposure to these factors leads to diminished vocal quality [38–40].

Lesions that produce significant blockage of the respiratory system and are linked with aggressive illness may necessitate tracheotomy. In this case, decannulation should be considered as soon as feasible after verifying airway safety [41]. It is debatable whether or not the lesion will extend to the lower airways after tracheostomy. However, a tracheotomy is to be avoided if at all feasible [42].

RRPs are often treated by surgical excision. Patients who require more than three to four operations each year are often candidates for adjuvant treatment, while the precise circumstances under which this is warranted remain unclear to physicians. JORRP generally needs more than four procedures each year; consequently, children are more likely to need adjuvant therapy [20]. Adjuvant therapy has made use of antiviral, antiproliferative, and immunomodulatory drugs. Several of these medicines' efficacy in RRP must be examined in rigorous, randomized, controlled research.

One of the earliest systemic medications used as adjuvant therapy for RRPs is interferon therapy. Natural alpha interferons are polypeptides with antiviral and antiproliferative properties due to their influence on the immune system. Interferon treatment, however, is not typically chosen because of its debatable efficiency and severe side-effect profile, which includes pancytopenia, hepatorenal failure, and cardiac dysfunction [43, 44].

Cidofovir and bevacizumab are two intralesional treatments. Bevacizumab is a recombinant humanized monoclonal antibody that prevents angiogenesis by inhibiting human vascular endothelial growth factor A. This antibody treats malignancies that have spread to other parts of the body. Using Bevacizumab systemically or intralesionally successfully manages aggressive papillomatosis, allowing patients to go longer between surgical procedures [24, 45]. Cidofovir or the KTP laser's adjuvant status makes them both viable options for achieving this goal [46].

Cidofovir is a cytosine nucleotide analog that inhibits viral DNA polymerase, preventing the replication of DNA viruses. Intralesional administration of cidofovir resulted in regression of lesions, reduction in recurrence rates, and complete remission [47, 48]. The maximum safe dose of cidofovir is 3 mg/kg, although there is still no agreement on the best delivery schedule for this drug [32, 47–49].

In addition, no randomized controlled studies on the effectiveness of medicines such as ribavirin, acyclovir, cimetidine, and indole-3-carbinol have been used in adjuvant therapy [50–53]. There is a wide variety of reactions to treatment with many of these adjuvant medicines, and their usage is often off-label.

In 2004, Cervarix (manufactured by GlaxoSmithKline Biological) became the first human papillomavirus (HPV) vaccination available, and its primary purpose was to protect against cervical cancer caused by oncogenic HPV strains 16 and 18 [54]. In 2006, Merck Sharp & Dohme introduced Gardasil. This vaccination protects against not just cervical cancer but also less severe conditions such as genital warts of the cervix, vulva, vagina, and anus, as well as recurrent respiratory papillomatosis (RRP) [55, 56]. The 9-valent HPV vaccination (Gardasil9; Merck Sharp & Dohme) was developed as a follow-up to the earlier vaccines, and it protects against 31 additional carcinogenic subtypes (types 31, 33, 45, 52, and 58). It is possible that the prevalence of HPV-related illnesses, including cervical cancer, oropharyngeal cancer, genital warts, and RRP, will decrease now that preventive HPV vaccination has been implemented in several countries [56, 57].

A favorable benefit in individuals with diverse clinical symptoms of HPV has been indicated. However, the therapeutic use of the HPV vaccination is contentious [57]. Several case studies describing using 9-valent Gardasil in conjunction with primary surgical debridement have been reported in several years, and the outcomes have been encouraging. It was hypothesized in early cases that lengthening the time between JoRRP surgeries might be beneficial, especially for patients with chronic illness [58, 59]. Rosenberg and coworkers conducted a meta-analysis of 11 studies that included 63 RRP individuals treated with Gardasil-9. The number of monthly operations dropped by a statistically significant amount following HPV vaccination, according to a meta-analysis of the available data [59]. The HPV-9 vaccination is effective. However, it needs to be clarified how. However, it is thought that this is because of the vaccine-mediated humoral response that blocks latent HPV infection in the area around the incision, hence decreasing the likelihood of a recurrence [60, 61].

67.6 Conclusions

Although RRP only affects a small percentage of the population, it requires many surgeries. Hoarseness is the first symptom of JoRRP, but the disorder can progress to dangerous upper airway blockage and even death. Laryngeal papillomatosis is incurable. Surgery to remove the papillomas while leaving the normal mucosa intact is considered the gold standard of therapy. About 20% of individuals with RRP need adjuvant treatment since the illness cannot be controlled with surgery alone. Despite their widespread usage, the evidence base for adjuvant therapy is weak. These treatments often involve immunological modulation, HPV replication disruption, inflammatory management, and angiogenesis suppression. The current results imply that RRP can be prevented with HPV vaccinations. More research on the HPV vaccine's therapeutic potential is required, particularly for JoRRP.

References

1. Derkay CS, Wiatrak B. Recurrent respiratory papillomatosis: a review. Laryngoscope. 2008;118:1236–47. https://doi.org/10.1097/MLG.0b013e31816a7135.
2. Derkay CS. Recurrent respiratory papillomatosis. Laryngoscope. 2001;111:57–69. https://doi.org/10.1097/00005537-200101000-00011.
3. Larson DA, Derkay CS. Epidemiology of recurrent respiratory papillomatosis. APMIS. 2010;118:450–4. https://doi.org/10.1111/j.1600-0463.2010.02619.x.
4. Seedat RY, Schall R. Age of diagnosis, incidence and prevalence of recurrent respiratory papillomatosis—a South African perspective. Clin Otolaryngol. 2018;43:533–7. https://doi.org/10.1111/coa.13016.
5. San Giorgi MRM, Van Den Heuvel ER, Tjon Pian Gi REA, et al. Age of onset of recurrent respiratory papillomatosis: a distribution analysis. Clin Otolaryngol. 2016;41:448–53. https://doi.org/10.1111/coa.12565.
6. Rodier C, Lapointe A, Coutlée F, et al. Juvenile respiratory papillomatosis: risk factors for severity: risk factors for severe juvenile respiratory papillomatosis. J Med Virol. 2013;85:1447–58. https://doi.org/10.1002/jmv.23615.
7. Mounts P, Shah KV, Kashima H. Viral etiology of juvenile- and adult-onset squamous papilloma of the larynx. Proc Natl Acad Sci USA. 1982;79:5425–9. https://doi.org/10.1073/pnas.79.17.5425.
8. Buchinsky FJ, Donfack J, Derkay CS, et al. Age of child, more than HPV type, is associated with clinical course in recurrent respiratory papillomatosis. PLoS One. 2008;3:e2263. https://doi.org/10.1371/journal.pone.0002263.
9. Ushikai M, Fujiyoshi T, Kono M, et al. Detection and cloning of human papillomavirus DNA associated with recurrent respiratory papillomatosis in Thailand. Jpn J Cancer Res. 1994;85:699–703. https://doi.org/10.1111/j.1349-7006.1994.tb02417.x.
10. Sanchez GI, Jaramillo R, Cuello G, et al. Human papillomavirus genotype detection in recurrent respiratory papillomatosis (RRP) in Colombia. Head Neck. 2013;35:229–34. https://doi.org/10.1002/hed.22953.
11. Abramson AL, Steinberg BM, Winkler B. Laryngeal papillomatosis: clinical, histopathologic and molecular studies. Laryngoscope. 1987;97:678–85. https://doi.org/10.1288/00005537-198706000-00005.
12. Silverberg M. Condyloma in pregnancy is strongly predictive of juvenile-onset recurrent respiratory papillomatosis. Obstet Gynecol. 2003;101:645–52. https://doi.org/10.1016/S0029-7844(02)03081-8.
13. Gerein V, Schmandt S, Babkina N, et al. Human papilloma virus (HPV)-associated gynecological alteration in mothers of children with recurrent respiratory papillomatosis during long-term observation. Cancer Detect Prev. 2007;31:276–81. https://doi.org/10.1016/j.cdp.2007.07.004.
14. Buchinsky FJ, Valentino WL, Ruszkay N, et al. Age at diagnosis, but not HPV type, is strongly associated with clinical course in recurrent respiratory papillomatosis. PLoS One. 2019;14:e0216697. https://doi.org/10.1371/journal.pone.0216697.

15. Ivancic R, Iqbal H, deSilva B, et al. Current and future management of recurrent respiratory papillomatosis. Laryngosc Investig Otolaryngol. 2018;3:22–34. https://doi.org/10.1002/lio2.132.
16. Wiatrak BJ, Wiatrak DW, Broker TR, Lewis L. Recurrent respiratory papillomatosis: a longitudinal study comparing severity associated with human papilloma viral types 6 and 11 and other risk factors in a large pediatric population. Laryngoscope. 2004;114:1–23. https://doi.org/10.1097/01.mlg.000148224.83491.0f.
17. Cohn AM, Kos JT, Taber LH, Adam E. Recurring laryngeal papillopa. Am J Otolaryngol. 1981;2:129–32. https://doi.org/10.1016/s0196-0709(81)80030-0.
18. Hawkes M, Campisi P, Zafar R, et al. Time course of juvenile onset recurrent respiratory papillomatosis caused by human papillomavirus. Pediatr Infect Dis J. 2008;27:149–54. https://doi.org/10.1097/INF.0b013e318159833e.
19. Ilboudo M, Zohoncon TM, Traore IMA, et al. Implication of low risk human papillomaviruses, HPV6 and HPV11 in laryngeal papillomatosis in Burkina Faso. Am J Otolaryngol. 2019;40:368–71. https://doi.org/10.1016/j.amjoto.2019.02.003.
20. Schraff S, Derkay CS, Burke B, Lawson L. American Society of Pediatric Otolaryngology Members' experience with recurrent respiratory papillomatosis and the use of adjuvant therapy. Arch Otolaryngol Head Neck Surg. 2004;130:1039. https://doi.org/10.1001/archotol.130.9.1039.
21. Armstrong LR, Derkay CS, Reeves WC. Initial results from the National Registry for juvenile-onset recurrent respiratory papillomatosis. Arch Otolaryngol Head Neck Surg. 1999;125:743. https://doi.org/10.1001/archotol.125.7.743.
22. Lindeberg H, Elbrçnd O. Laryngeal papillomas: clinical aspects in a series of 231 patients. Clin Otolaryngol. 1989;14:333–42. https://doi.org/10.1111/j.1365-2273.1989.tb00381.x.
23. Blackledge FA, Anand VK. Tracheobronchial extension of recurrent respiratory papillomatosis. Ann Otol Rhinol Laryngol. 2000;109:812–8. https://doi.org/10.1177/000348940010900905.
24. Fortes HR, von Ranke FM, Escuissato DL, et al. Recurrent respiratory papillomatosis: a state-of-the-art review. Respir Med. 2017;126:116–21. https://doi.org/10.1016/j.rmed.2017.03.030.
25. Derkay CS, Malis DJ, Zalzal G, et al. A staging system for assessing severity of disease and response to therapy in recurrent respiratory papillomatosis. Laryngoscope. 1998;108:935–7. https://doi.org/10.1097/00005537-199806000-00026.
26. Lee AS, Rosen CA. Efficacy of cidofovir injection for the treatment of recurrent respiratory papillomatosis. J Voice. 2004;18:551–6. https://doi.org/10.1016/j.jvoice.2003.07.007.
27. Campisi P, Hawkes M, Kim Simpson RN, Canadian Juvenile Onset Recurrent Respiratory Papillomatosis Working Group. The epidemiology of juvenile onset recurrent respiratory papillomatosis derived from a population level national database. Laryngoscope. 2010;120:1233–45. https://doi.org/10.1002/lary.20901.
28. Silverberg MJ, Thorsen P, Lindeberg H, et al. Clinical course of recurrent respiratory papillomatosis in Danish children. Arch Otolaryngol Head Neck Surg. 2004;130:711. https://doi.org/10.1001/archotol.130.6.711.
29. Ongkasuwan J, Friedman EM. Juvenile recurrent respiratory papilloma: variable intersurgical intervals. Laryngoscope. 2012;122:2844–9. https://doi.org/10.1002/lary.23534.
30. Karatayli-Ozgursoy S, Bishop JA, Hillel A, et al. Risk factors for dysplasia in recurrent respiratory papillomatosis in an adult and pediatric population. Ann Otol Rhinol Laryngol. 2016;125:235–41. https://doi.org/10.1177/0003489415608196.
31. Go C, Schwartz MR, Donovan DT. Molecular transformation of recurrent respiratory papillomatosis: viral typing and P53 overexpression. Ann Otol Rhinol Laryngol. 2003;112:298–302. https://doi.org/10.1177/000348940311200402.
32. Lawlor C, Balakrishnan K, Bottero S, et al. International Pediatric Otolaryngology Group (IPOG): juvenile-onset recurrent respiratory papillomatosis consensus recommendations. Int J Pediatr Otorhinolaryngol. 2020;128:109697. https://doi.org/10.1016/j.ijporl.2019.109697.
33. Goon P, Sonnex C, Jani P, et al. Recurrent respiratory papillomatosis: an overview of current thinking and treatment. Eur Arch Otorrinolaringol. 2008;265:147–51. https://doi.org/10.1007/s00405-007-0546-z.

34. Wilcox LJ, Hull BP, Baldassari CM, Derkay CS. Diagnosis and management of recurrent respiratory papillomatosis. Pediatr Infect Dis J. 2014;33:1283–4. https://doi.org/10.1097/INF.0000000000000551.
35. Ilmarinen T, Nissilä H, Rihkanen H, et al. Clinical features, health-related quality of life, and adult voice in juvenile-onset recurrent respiratory papillomatosis. Laryngoscope. 2011;121:846–51. https://doi.org/10.1002/lary.21332.
36. Holler T, Allegro J, Chadha NK, et al. Voice outcomes following repeated surgical resection of laryngeal papillomata in children. Otolaryngol Head Neck Surg. 2009;141:522–6. https://doi.org/10.1016/j.otohns.2009.06.080.
37. Rachmanidou A, Modayil PC. Coblation resection of paediatric laryngeal papilloma. J Laryngol Otol. 2011;125:873–6. https://doi.org/10.1017/S0022215111001253.
38. Hermann JS, Pontes P, Maurice Weckx LL, et al. Laryngeal sequelae of recurrent respiratory papillomatosis surgery in children. Rev Assoc Med Bras. 2012;58:204–8. https://doi.org/10.1016/S0104-4230(12)70181-1.
39. Soldatski IL, Onufrieva EK, Steklov AM, Schepin NV. Tracheal, bronchial, and pulmonary papillomatosis in children. Laryngoscope. 2005;115:1848–54. https://doi.org/10.1097/01.mlg.0000173155.57491.2a.
40. Crockett DM, McCabe BF, Shive CJ. Complications of laser surgery for recurrent respiratory papillomatosis. Ann Otol Rhinol Laryngol. 1987;96:639–44. https://doi.org/10.1177/000348948709600604.
41. Venkatesan NN, Pine HS, Underbrink MP. Recurrent respiratory papillomatosis. Otolaryngol Clin N Am. 2012;45:671–94. https://doi.org/10.1016/j.otc.2012.03.006.
42. Shapiro AM, Rimell FL, Shoemaker D, et al. Tracheotomy in children with juvenile-onset recurrent respiratory papillomatosis: the Children's Hospital of Pittsburgh experience. Ann Otol Rhinol Laryngol. 1996;105:1–5. https://doi.org/10.1177/000348949610500101.
43. Leventhal BG, Kashima H, Levine AS, Levy HB. Treatment of recurrent laryngeal papillomatosis with an artificial interferon inducer (poly ICLC). J Pediatr. 1981;99:614–6. https://doi.org/10.1016/S0022-3476(81)80274-0.
44. Healy GB, Gelber RD, Trowbridge AL, et al. Treatment of recurrent respiratory papillomatosis with human leukocyte interferon. N Engl J Med. 1988;319:401–7. https://doi.org/10.1056/NEJM198808183190704.
45. Rogers DJ, Ojha S, Maurer R, Hartnick CJ. Use of adjuvant intralesional bevacizumab for aggressive respiratory papillomatosis in children. JAMA Otolaryngol Head Neck Surg. 2013;139:496–501. https://doi.org/10.1001/jamaoto.2013.1810.
46. Maturo S, Hartnick CJ. Use of 532-nm pulsed potassium titanyl phosphate laser and adjuvant intralesional bevacizumab for aggressive respiratory papillomatosis in children: initial experience. Arch Otolaryngol Head Neck Surg. 2010;136:561–5. https://doi.org/10.1001/archoto.2010.81.
47. Graupp M, Gugatschka M, Kiesler K, et al. Experience of 11 years use of cidofovir in recurrent respiratory papillomatosis. Eur Arch Otorrinolaringol. 2013;270:641–6. https://doi.org/10.1007/s00405-012-2221-2.
48. Chadha NK, James A. Adjuvant antiviral therapy for recurrent respiratory papillomatosis. Cochrane Database Syst Rev. 2012;12:CD005053. https://doi.org/10.1002/14651858.CD005053.pub4.
49. McMurray JS, Connor N, Ford CN. Cidofovir efficacy in recurrent respiratory papillomatosis: a randomized, double-blind, placebo-controlled study. Ann Otol Rhinol Laryngol. 2008;117:477–83. https://doi.org/10.1177/000348940811700702.
50. Kimberlin DW. Current status of antiviral therapy for juvenile-onset recurrent respiratory papillomatosis. Antivir Res. 2004;63:141–51. https://doi.org/10.1016/j.antiviral.2004.06.013.
51. Morrison GA, Kotecha B, Evans JN. Ribavirin treatment for juvenile respiratory papillomatosis. J Laryngol Otol. 1993;107:423–6. https://doi.org/10.1017/s0022215100123321.
52. Rosen CA, Bryson PC. Indole-3-carbinol for recurrent respiratory papillomatosis: long-term results. J Voice. 2004;18:248–53. https://doi.org/10.1016/j.jvoice.2003.05.005.

53. Harcourt JP, Worley G, Leighton SE. Cimetidine treatment for recurrent respiratory papillomatosis. Int J Pediatr Otorhinolaryngol. 1999;51:109–13. https://doi.org/10.1016/s0165-5876(99)00279-7.
54. Harper DM, Franco EL, Wheeler C, et al. Efficacy of a bivalent L1 virus-like particle vaccine in prevention of infection with human papillomavirus types 16 and 18 in young women: a randomised controlled trial. Lancet. 2004;364:1757–65. https://doi.org/10.1016/S0140-6736(04)17398-4.
55. Garland SM, Kjaer SK, Muñoz N, et al. Impact and effectiveness of the quadrivalent human papillomavirus vaccine: a systematic review of 10 years of real-world experience. Clin Infect Dis. 2016;63:519–27. https://doi.org/10.1093/cid/ciw354.
56. Freed GL, Derkay CS. Prevention of recurrent respiratory papillomatosis: role of HPV vaccination. Int J Pediatr Otorhinolaryngol. 2006;70:1799–803. https://doi.org/10.1016/j.ijporl.2006.06.006.
57. Dion GR, Teng S, Boyd LR, et al. Adjuvant human papillomavirus vaccination for secondary prevention: a systematic review. JAMA Otolaryngol Head Neck Surg. 2017;143:614–22. https://doi.org/10.1001/jamaoto.2016.4736.
58. Young DL, Moore MM, Halstead LA. The use of the quadrivalent human papillomavirus vaccine (gardasil) as adjuvant therapy in the treatment of recurrent respiratory papilloma. J Voice. 2015;29:223–9. https://doi.org/10.1016/j.jvoice.2014.08.003.
59. Rosenberg T, Philipsen BB, Mehlum CS, et al. Therapeutic use of the human papillomavirus vaccine on recurrent respiratory papillomatosis: a systematic review and meta-analysis. J Infect Dis. 2019;219:1016–25. https://doi.org/10.1093/infdis/jiy616.
60. Makiyama K, Hirai R, Matsuzaki H. Gardasil vaccination for recurrent laryngeal papillomatosis in adult men: first report: changes in HPV antibody titer. J Voice. 2017;31:104–6. https://doi.org/10.1016/j.jvoice.2016.01.008.
61. Buchinsky FJ, Ruszkay N, Valentino W, et al. In RRP, serologic response to HPV is frequently absent and slow to develop. PLoS One. 2020;15:e0230106. https://doi.org/10.1371/journal.pone.0230106.

Part VII

Miscellaneous

The Role of the Critical Airway Team 68

Zeynel Öztürk, Nuray Bayar Muluk, and Felicia Manole

68.1 Introduction

A critical airway is a life-threatening scenario of hypoxemia about to become hypoxia following failed or inadequate ventilation. In such systems, esophageal intubation compounds the criticality of the situation as, besides the loss of oxygenation, the risk of stomach contents being aspirated into the airways is enhanced by ventilating into the stomach [1, 2]. Cervical spine injury or non-exclusion is not an issue, as almost always endotracheal intubation (ETI) can be done with little head manipulation and without neck manipulation; the problem would lie, in the end, on whether the patient can be ventilated or not [3–7].

Indications for surgical airway in elective scenarios, specifically for tracheostomy, are well established in the intensive care unit (ICU). It is required for medium-to-long-term ventilation and advised as an early procedure in head injury with coma expected not to recover in the short term; in patients with any cancer in the neck compressing the trachea, and it is often the only practicable procedure for inoperable cancer or as an airway control procedure before or during surgery; after thyroid surgery in patients with longstanding goiter and tracheomalacia, as a tracheostomy prevents postoperative airway obstruction; before surgery in some neck abscesses, as it protects the lower airways from accidental or spontaneous pus release into the lungs during the procedure [8].

Z. Öztürk
Department of Otorhinolaryngology, Private Florya Hospital, Istanbul, Turkey

N. Bayar Muluk (✉)
Department of Otorhinolaryngology, Kırıkkale University, Faculty of Medicine, Kırıkkale, Turkey

F. Manole
Department of ENT, University of Oradea, Faculty of Medicine, Oradea, Romania

H. Yüksel et al. (eds.), *Pediatric Airway Diseases*, Comprehensive ENT,
https://doi.org/10.1007/978-3-031-74853-0_68

68.2 Causes of the Difficult Pediatric Airway

68.2.1 Normal Pediatric Airway

Predictable differences in the pediatric airway (compared to adult airway anatomy) may make management difficult. These differences, most evident in children less than 2–3 years of age, include the following [9]:

- A prominent occiput affects positioning
- A large tongue and small mouth may make laryngoscopy difficult
- The larynx may be harder to locate with the laryngoscope because it is higher and more anterior than in an adult
- The epiglottis is large and floppy and may be difficult to control

Anatomic features of the standard pediatric airway are reviewed separately [9].

68.2.1.1 Normal Pediatric Physiology

Young children are prone to desaturation, even when optimally oxygenated, due to their high native metabolic rate and small pulmonary functional reserve capacity. Thus, airway management in children with compromised pulmonary function, as is seen with obstructive lung disease, pneumonia, sepsis, and acute respiratory distress syndrome (ARDS), can be accompanied by rapid desaturation during intubation attempts even with meticulous attention to pre-procedure oxygenation [9].

68.2.2 Congenital Abnormalities

Numerous congenital conditions have features that may make airway management difficult. In addition, children with underlying airway abnormalities who acquire an acute illness (such as croup or an upper respiratory tract infection) may quickly develop respiratory compromise. Congenital features that may interfere with airway management include the following [9]:

- **Misshapen head**—Positioning of the head to optimally align the pharyngeal and tracheal axes may be difficult if the head is misshapen, as can occur with craniosynostosis (such as Apert or Crouzon syndrome) or macrocephaly.
- **Facial abnormalities**—Facial asymmetry or underdevelopment may make it difficult to achieve a good seal between the face and a mask, creating difficulties with bag-mask ventilation. For example, maxillary hypoplasia is a feature of Apert syndrome, while Goldenhar syndrome includes unilateral hypoplasia of the mandible.
- **Abnormal neck mobility**—Limited neck mobility (as occurs with Klippel-Feil syndrome) or cervical spine instability (which can occur with Down syndrome and the mucopolysaccharidoses) may interfere with the positioning of the head.

- **Small oral aperture**—Opening the mouth for laryngoscopy may be difficult in children with microstomia, a feature of Freeman-Sheldon and Hallermann-Streiff syndromes.
- **Small oral cavity**—Children with small mandibles or palatal abnormalities (such as high arched or cleft palates) have a smaller oral cavity. This may make laryngoscopy and control of oral structures difficult. For instance, mandibular hypoplasia is a feature of the Robin sequence and Treacher-Collins syndrome.
- **Large tongue**—A large tongue may obstruct the airway during bag-mask ventilation or be challenging to control during laryngoscopy. Macroglossia occurs in several conditions (such as hypothyroidism, Beckwith–Wiedeman syndrome, and Down syndrome). It is also a feature of infiltrative diseases such as mucopolysaccharidoses.
- **Masses**—Masses in the neck (such as cystic hygromas) may interfere with positioning. Masses within the airway (such as teratomas or hemangiomas) may obstruct the airway and interfere with the visualization of the larynx. Mediastinal masses may make tube placement difficult and interfere with ventilation after successful intubation [10].
  - **Laryngeal and subglottic abnormalities**—Abnormalities of the larynx or subglottic trachea may interfere with bag-mask ventilation, supraglottic airway placement and ventilation, and endotracheal intubation.

68.2.3 Acquired Conditions

Acquired conditions that can cause difficulties with airway management may develop due to infection, allergic reactions, trauma, or aspiration of a foreign body [9].

Infection—The specific difficulties in airway management arising from illness depend upon where the disease is located within the airway [9].

Anaphylaxis—Edema involving the tongue, oropharynx, and larynx that can interfere with laryngoscopy and visualization of the larynx may develop due to anaphylaxis. Symptoms typically respond to aggressive medical management [9].

Trauma—Injury to the face or airway (as the result of blunt or penetrating trauma, thermal burns, or caustic ingestions) may complicate airway management [9]:

- Facial burns may make it challenging to deliver bag-mask ventilation because an adequate seal between the mask and face cannot be achieved.
- An expanding hematoma in the pharynx can interfere with laryngoscopy.
- Injury to the midface (e.g., LeFort fracture), larynx, or subglottic trachea may be exacerbated by intubation, making securing the airway difficult.
- Spinal immobilization with a rigid cervical collar, regardless of the injury, can make direct laryngoscopy difficult because the clinician cannot optimally position the patient in the sniffing position and adequately align the visual axis [9].

Foreign body—A foreign body in the airway may cause significant obstruction and require immediate treatment. Identification and removal of the foreign body during laryngoscopy can be challenging. In addition, typical anatomic landmarks may be distorted by the foreign body.

Piercings around the mouth and tongue may interfere with or become dislodged during laryngoscopy [11]. The average shedding of primary teeth creates a potential airway foreign body in children ≥6 years old.

Other causes—Other acquired conditions in children that may make airway management difficult include tumors, previous surgery, radiation treatment, or obesity [12].

68.3 Airway Assessment in Children

In children and adults undergoing anesthesia or sedation, the airway evaluation remains integral to the preoperative assessment [13, 14]. The airway-focused history may help identify issues encountered in previous perioperative or intensive care unit (ICU) admissions. Medical records of earlier encounters should be reviewed to determine the ease of mask ventilation, the need for airway adjuncts, the type of laryngoscope used, the number of attempts at direct laryngoscopy, and the plain laryngoscopic view achieved. The latter is generally classified using the Cormack and Lehane scale. This should be followed by an assessment of the airway, including an evaluation of the symmetry of the head, face, and neck, degree of mouth opening, presence or absence of oral pathology, oral hygiene, measurement of mentohyoid and thyromental distance, adequacy of neck flexion/extension, and neck circumference [15, 16]. Concerns in one or more of these parameters may indicate the potential for difficulties with airway management. The Mallampati score is commonly used in adults to predict endotracheal intubation problems and may also apply to cooperative children [17]. Unlike adult patients, neck circumference and body mass index are not independent predictive factors in children [16, 18].

In general, patients with a higher ASA physical status (III and IV), Mallampati airway score of III or IV, infants, and those undergoing oromaxillofacial, otolaryngologic, and cardiac surgery are more likely to have airway management issues [19–21]. Additionally, there is a higher incidence of airway difficulties in patients with external ear anomalies (microtia), micrognathia, and certain congenital anomalies and syndromes, including Pierre Robin sequence, Treacher Collins syndrome, and Goldenhar syndrome [22–24]. Another unique and increasingly common comorbid condition, obstructive sleep apnea (OSA), may be associated with airway management issues [13, 24].

68.3.1 Complex Airway Assessment (LEMON)

The mnemonic LEMON has been developed by researchers in emergency airway management to rapidly identify adult patients in whom direct laryngoscopy may be difficult. Although widely used in adults with good predictive value, evidence in children is lacking [9].

Components of the mnemonic include the following [9]:

- **L**: Look externally for indicators of a difficult airway (such as a misshapen head, facial abnormalities, or neck masses).
- **E**: Evaluate mouth opening, thyromental distance, and the distance between the mandible and the thyroid cartilage (this correlates with the distance between the base of the tongue and the larynx). Adequate mouth opening and thyromental distance should be the width of three of the patient's fingers. The distance between the mandible and thyroid cartilage should be the width of two fingers.
- **M**: Mallampati score: Assigning a Mallampati score may be difficult in young children. For the obtunded, supine patient, a crude assessment can be made using a tongue blade [25].
- **O**: Obstruction: Signs of airway obstruction (such as stridor, a muffled voice, or difficulty handling secretions) always indicate that airway management may be complex. Upper airway obstruction can interfere with bag-mask ventilation, as well as with laryngoscopy and intubation.
- **N**: Neck mobility: Conditions that limit neck mobility (such as congenital anomalies or cervical spine immobilization) can usually be identified by observation.

68.4 Timing

In a life-threatening situation such as a critical airway, the time window for sound decision-making is often very narrow, and any delay in recognizing the need for the most demanding of emergency surgical airways (ESAs), i.e., a tracheostomy, affects patients' outcome in terms of exits and severe neurological or cardiac damage. While definitions of emergency and urgent are evident in case of bleeding or hemorrhagic shock, in airway compromise, such reports cannot be used due to the impossibility of predicting how many minutes to hours of fatigue endurance a patient can tolerate in hypoxemia from incomplete airway obstruction. Actual (complete) airway obstruction causes cardiac arrest by acute severe vagal reflex or respiratory arrest, soon followed by cardiac arrest (respiratory-cardiac arrest), depending on functional residual capacity (FRC) and cardiac physiological reserve. Impending (incomplete or partial) airway obstruction is killed by exhaustion from hypoxemia or damage from relative hypoxia to organs like the heart and brain. Signs suggesting an impending airway obstruction warranting ESA must, therefore, be recognized clearly and unmistakably [7].

68.5 Management of Difficult Pediatric Airway

General emergency medicine specialists and anesthesiologists have used bedside evaluation tools to identify patients for whom airway management may be complex. However, the applicability of these indicators for children needs to be clarified.

Nevertheless, a reasonable approach can be developed using evidence from the operating room and clinical experience in the emergency department to identify children with difficult airways [9].

Bag-mask ventilation—Bag-mask ventilation may be difficult in children with the following features [9]:

- A misshapen head (due to trauma or a congenital anomaly) or limited neck mobility (such as a patient whose cervical spine is immobilized) can interfere with proper positioning.
- Facial burns or any disruption of lower facial continuity (as can occur with facial trauma or a congenital anomaly with facial asymmetry) can make achieving an adequate seal between the face and the mask challenging.
- Patients who are obese, have significant lung disease (such as severe asthma), upper airway swelling, or tracheal narrowing may be difficult to ventilate with a bag and mask [26].

Laryngoscopy and intubation—Several clinical features appear to be sensitive predictors of difficult laryngoscopy and intubation for adults, as described separately [9].

Features potentially useful in children include [9]:

- Smallmouth opening (<3 patient fingers)
- Mallampati score
- Thyromental distance (3 patient finger-widths); difficulty visualizing the larynx may occur when the distance is longer or shorter
- Difficult bag-mask ventilation [27]

Cricothyroidotomy—Needle cricothyroidotomy, which permits percutaneous transtracheal oxygenation, should always be considered a problematic technique in children because typical landmarks are difficult to identify, and the caliber of the airway is small. In addition, few practitioners can gain proficiency with this technique because children rarely require it [9].

68.6 Alternative Techniques

Alternative techniques for providing oxygenation and ventilation must be considered for the child who may be difficult to intubate. These techniques may be temporizing, such as a supraglottic airway (e.g., laryngeal mask airway, i-gel) or a percutaneous needle cricothyrotomy or provide alternative procedural approaches to endotracheal intubation (e.g., intubating introducers or fiberoptic intubation). Several factors impact the choice of device, including the clinical situation, type of airway difficulty, and operator experience [9].

Video laryngoscopy—Video laryngoscopes (VLs) display the glottic view on a video monitor during endotracheal intubation and allow indirect or, when fitted with standard geometry blades, either indirect or direct laryngoscopy. Video laryngoscopy is becoming widely used by emergency medicine providers for pediatric endotracheal intubation. For children with difficult airways undergoing endotracheal intubation in the operating room, video laryngoscope has a higher first-pass success rate than direct laryngoscopy. Practitioners with airway training and experience, including those early in their careers, can use these advanced laryngoscopes effectively with little additional training and orientation. Acute angle scopes may be challenging to use in young infants because of the size of the blade. A common problem is the inability to pass the endotracheal tube (ETT) through the vocal cords despite having an adequate view of the glottic opening. This is a more common problem in infants, in whom the bulky VL blade may make maneuvering the ETT into the pharynx more complex, leading to lower rates of successful intubation with VL than in older children. Several devices are available in sizes appropriate for infants and children. The technique of video laryngoscopy for standard and acute angle blades is described separately [9].

Intubating introducers (gum elastic bougie) are helpful when visualizing the epiglottis, but the vocal cords cannot be seen. They are contraindicated in patients with laryngeal or tracheal injury. These devices are semi-rigid solid or hollow rods with the distal tip bent at a 30° angle. Pediatric-sized introducers permit the placement of endotracheal tubes as small as 4.0 mm (internal diameter) [9].

Supraglottic airway—A supraglottic device [e.g., laryngeal mask airway (LMA), i-gel, or AirQ] should be used as the initial rescue device for a child with a failed intubation unless they have upper airway obstruction or an airway condition that would impede successful placement or could be worsened by injury [9].

The LMA should be avoided in patients with airway obstruction (e.g., croup, asthma) or distorted airway anatomy (e.g., laryngeal trauma, congenital anomalies of the larynx, or epiglottitis) [9].

Supraglottic airways [e.g., Laryngeal Mask Airway (LMA), i-gel, and others] are available in multiple sizes suitable for infants, children, and adults. The appropriate size is based on the patient's weight. The Classic LMA is a scaled-down version of the adult LMA. At the same time, the pediatric ProSeal LMA has specific design features that may permit a better seal and more excellent protection against aspiration, especially in infants and young children, including a gastric channel that allows passage of a nasogastric tube and gastric decompression, while the LMA is in place [9].

In anesthesia studies in children, LMAs can be successfully inserted on the first attempt 80–100% of the time, depending upon the technique (rotational, lateral, or standard placement) and specific device (Classic LMA or ProSeal LMA) used. Although experience with the device as a rescue airway in children is limited [28], case series and reports suggest that an adequate airway can be achieved with an LMA in neonates when bag-mask ventilation and tracheal intubation have failed [29].

Flexible intubating scope—In the hands of a clinician with extensive training and experience with the device, using a flexible intubating content is an excellent method for endotracheal intubation for a patient with a problematic airway who is breathing spontaneously. Flexible intubation should be considered in cases where the pre-intubation assessment suggests that orotracheal intubation via rapid sequence intubation (preferred in most emergency department intubation scenarios) is unlikely to be successful and the patient can tolerate a longer intubation attempt. Examples include congenital airway anomalies such as micrognathia or conditions where difficulty aligning the oral, pharyngeal, and laryngeal axes is predicted (such as when neck mobility is limited). The small size of the nasal passages in very young children often precludes the nasal route for intubation; patient cooperation and compliance may limit its utility for awake intubation [9].

68.7 Surgical Airway

Rarely do the techniques and devices discussed above need to provide an airway. As a result, emergency healthcare providers should be familiar with surgical airway techniques, such as a needle or surgical cricothyroidotomy; in reality, few practitioners have enough opportunities with these approaches to gain proficiency [30]. Surgical cricothyroidotomy should be avoided in children <10 years old [9].

Equipment required for needle and surgical cricothyroidotomy should be organized in advance and readily available in locations where emergency airway procedures are performed [9].

The time available and the ease of surgical airway intervention decrease as the child ages. Four independent risk factors were found to be associated with an increased risk of serious complications [13]: (1) more than two endotracheal intubation attempts; (2) weight less than 10 kg; (3) short thyromental distance (micrognathia); and (4) three direct laryngoscopy attempts before an indirect technique [24]. After the exclusion of upper airway obstruction, there may be a role for using neuromuscular blockade to relieve undiagnosed laryngospasm (see above). This can be combined with epinephrine to relieve an undiagnosed or coexistent bronchospasm. Invasive airway access is the next option when these rescue attempts and alternative airway devices fail. As open surgical access is beyond the realm of most pediatric anesthesiologists, a surgeon is the preferred candidate to perform an open surgical airway, and surgical help should be immediately requested for invasive airway access. Severe complications may result from improperly performed emergent surgical airway access or high-pressure rescue jet ventilation through a wrongly positioned tracheostomy tube [31–33].

References

1. Ghafour AU, Martin TW. "RSI"—is it rapid sequence induction or rapid sequence intubation? Pediatr Emerg Care. 2004;20:803.
2. Nolan J. Strategies to prevent unrecognized oesophageal intubation during out-of hospital cardiac arrest. Resuscitation. 2008;76:11–23.
3. Wahlen BM, Gercek E. Three-dimensional cervical spine movement during intubation using Macintosh and Bullard laryngoscopes, the Bonfils fibrescope, and the intubating laryngeal mask airway. Eur J Anaesthesiol. 2004;21:907–13.

4. Manoach S, Paladino L. Manual-in-line stabilization for acute airway management of suspected cervical spine injury: review and current questions. Ann Emerg Med. 2007;50:236–45.
5. Ford P, Nolan J. Cervical spine injury and airway management. Curr Opin Anaesthesiol. 2002;15:193–201.
6. Ghafour AU, Martin TW, Gopalakrishnan S, Visvanitra S. Caring for the patients with cervical spine injuries: what have we learned? J Clin Anaesth. 2005;17:640–9.
7. Bonanno FG. The critical airway in adults: the facts. J Emerg Trauma Shock. 2012;5(2):153–9. https://doi.org/10.4103/0974-2700.96485. PMID: 22787346; PMCID: PMC3391840.
8. Altman KW, Waltonen JD, Kern RC. Urgent surgical airway intervention: a 3 year county hospital experience. Laryngoscope. 2005;115:2101–4.
9. Mick NW. The difficult pediatric airway for emergency medicine. In: Nagler J, Wiley II JF, editors. . UpToDate; 2023.
10. Blank RS, de Souza DG. Anesthetic management of patients with an anterior mediastinal mass: continuing professional development. Can J Anaesth. 2011;58:853.
11. DeBoer S, McNeil M, Amundson T. Tongues, tubes, and teens: body piercing and airway management. Pediatr Emerg Care. 2006;22:755.
12. Nafiu OO, Burke CC, Gupta R, et al. Association of neck circumference with perioperative adverse respiratory events in children. Pediatrics. 2011;127:e1198.
13. Krishna SG, Bryant JF, Tobias JD. Management of the difficult airway in the pediatric patient. J Pediatr Intensive Care. 2018;7(3):115–25.
14. Sunder RA, Haile DT, Farrell PT, Sharma A. Pediatric airway management: current practices and future directions. Paediatr Anaesth. 2012;22(10):1008–15.
15. Apfelbaum JL, Hagberg CA, Caplan RA, et al. Practice guidelines for management of the difficult airway: an updated report by the American Society of Anesthesiologists Task Force on Management of the Difficult Airway. Anesthesiology. 2013;118(02):251–70.
16. Gonzalez H, Minville V, Delanoue K, Mazerolles M, Concina D, Fourcade O. The importance of increased neck circumference to intubation difficulties in obese patients. Anesth Analg. 2008;106(04):1132–6.
17. Santos AP, Mathias LA, Gozzani JL, Watanabe M. Difficult intubation in children: applicability of the Mallampati index. Rev Bras Anestesiol. 2011;61(02):156–8.
18. Sheff SR, May MC, Carlisle SE, Kallies KJ, Mathiason MA, Kothari SN. Predictors of a difficult intubation in the bariatric patient: does preoperative body mass index matter? Surg Obes Relat Dis. 2013;9(03):344–9.
19. Heinrich S, Birkholz T, Ihmsen H, Irouschek A, Ackermann A, Schmidt J. Incidence and predictors of difficult laryngoscopy in 11,219 pediatric anesthesia procedures. Paediatr Anaesth. 2012;22(08):729–36.
20. Heinrich S, Birkholz T, Irouschek A, Ackermann A, Schmidt J. Incidences and predictors of difficult laryngoscopy in adult patients undergoing general anesthesia: a single-center analysis of 102,305 cases. J Anesth. 2013;27(06):815–21.
21. Heinrich S, Ackermann A, Prottengeier J, Castellanos I, Schmidt J, Schüttler J. Increased rate of poor laryngoscopic views in patients scheduled for cardiac surgery versus patients scheduled for general surgery: a propensity score-based analysis of 21,561 cases. J Cardiothorac Vasc Anesth. 2015;29(06):1537–43.
22. Butler MG, Hayes BG, Hathaway MM, Begleiter ML. Specific genetic diseases at risk for sedation/anesthesia complications. Anesth Analg. 2000;91(04):837–55.
23. Uezono S, Holzman RS, Goto T, Nakata Y, Nagata S, Morita S. Prediction of difficult airway in school-aged patients with microtia. Paediatr Anaesth. 2001;11(04):409–13.
24. Fiadjoe JE, Nishisaki A, Jagannathan N, et al. Airway management complications in children with difficult tracheal intubation from the pediatric difficult intubation (PeDI) registry: a prospective cohort analysis. Lancet Respir Med. 2016;4(01):37–48.
25. Brown CA. Identification of the anatomically difficult airway. In: Brown CA, Sakles JC, Mick NW, Mosier JM, Braude DA, editors. Walls manual of emergency airway management. 6th ed. Philadelphia: Wolters Kluwer; 2023.
26. Kheterpal S, Han R, Tremper KK, et al. Incidence and predictors of difficult and impossible mask ventilation. Anesthesiology. 2006;105:885.

27. Daigle CH, Fiadjoe JE, Laverriere EK, et al. Difficult bag-mask ventilation in critically ill children is independently associated with adverse events. Crit Care Med. 2020;48:e744.
28. Dingeman RS, Goumnerova LC, Goobie SM. The use of a laryngeal mask airway for emergent airway management in a prone child. Anesth Analg. 2005;100:670.
29. Qureshi MJ, Kumar M. Laryngeal mask airway versus bag-mask ventilation or endotracheal intubation for neonatal resuscitation. Cochrane Database Syst Rev. 2018;3:CD003314.
30. Nagler J, Auerbach M, Monuteaux MC, et al. Exposure and confidence across critical airway procedures in pediatric emergency medicine: an international survey study. Am J Emerg Med. 2021;42:70.
31. Stacey J, Heard AM, Chapman G, et al. The 'Can't intubate Can't Oxygenate' scenario in pediatric anesthesia: a comparison of different devices for needle cricothyroidotomy. Paediatr Anaesth. 2012;22(12):1155–8.
32. Coté CJ, Hartnick CJ. Pediatric transtracheal and cricothyrotomy airway devices for emergency use: which are appropriate for infants and children? Paediatr Anaesth. 2009;19(01):66–76.
33. Johansen K, Holm-Knudsen RJ, Charabi B, Kristensen MS, Rasmussen LS. Cannot ventilate-cannot intubate an infant: surgical tracheotomy or transtracheal cannula? Paediatr Anaesth. 2010;20(11):987–93.

Epidermolysis Bullosa: ENT Involvement 69

Oğuzhan Oğuz, Nuray Bayar Muluk, and Gabriela Kopacheva-Barsova

69.1 Definition

Increased cutaneous vulnerability to mechanical stress is the hallmark of epidermolysis bullosa (EB), a clinically and genetically heterogeneous inherited skin fragility disorder characterized by structural anomalies that disrupt the dermo-epidermal junction or the basal layer of the epidermis [1]. Clinical hallmarks include blisters, erosions, nonhealing ulceration, and scars after modest trauma [2], but these vary depending on the precise genetic abnormality and its molecular sequelae.

Blistering in reaction to mechanical trauma characterizes the epidermolysis bullosa (EB) syndrome of inherited bullous illnesses. Epidermolysis bullosa subtypes have traditionally been categorized based on skin appearance [3, 4].

Diagnostic methods, including prenatal and preimplantation screening, have been developed thanks to research into the molecular basis of epidermolysis bullosa. Newer treatments (e.g., gene or protein therapy) may alleviate the skin fragility experienced by individuals with epidermolysis bullosa [3] based on a greater understanding of the basement membrane zone (BMZ) and the genes responsible for its components.

O. Oğuz
Department of Audiology, Istanbul Nişantaşı University, Health Services Vocational School, Istanbul, Turkey

Dr. Oğuzhan Oğuz Wellnose Clinic, Istanbul, Turkey

N. Bayar Muluk (✉)
Department of Otorhinolaryngology, Kırıkkale University, Faculty of Medicine, Kırıkkale, Turkey

G. Kopacheva-Barsova
Department of Otorhinolaryngology, Cyril and Methodius University of Skopje, Faculty of Medicine, Skopje, Republic of North Macedonia

H. Yüksel et al. (eds.), *Pediatric Airway Diseases*, Comprehensive ENT,
https://doi.org/10.1007/978-3-031-74853-0_69

69.2 Symptoms and Signs

The severity of pain or pruritus, the age at which symptoms first appeared, the number of blisters, where they occurred, and what might have caused them are all important broad considerations [3].

Evidence of mucosal involvement, such as oral, nasopharyngeal, ophthalmic, genitourinary, gastrointestinal, or respiratory problems, and alterations in growth or development are two examples of the types of systemic information that may be related to epidermolysis bullosa (EB). Identifying a history of blistering disease in a family is crucial [3].

Examine all visible areas of skin and mucosal surfaces, including the eyes, mouth, and genitalia. Examine blisters for size, location, and type. Determine to what extent you can generalize lesions' propensity to divide. Blisters can be classified as either superficial (presenting as crusted erosions), intraepidermal (flabby and perhaps expanding with pressure), or intralamina lucida (tight, healing with atrophy but no scarring). Milia and scar tissue occur as blisters heal in the sublamina densa. Check for nail, hair, and tooth involvement [3].

69.3 Pathophysiology

Genetic defects in the basement membrane generate the bullous disorder known as epidermolysis bullosa. There are four main types of epidermolysis bullosa, including type 1 (intraepidermal skin separation), type 2 (skin separation in lamina lucida or central BMZ), type 3 (sublamina densa BMZ separation, as seen in the images below), and type 4 (sporadic, blistering at any level) Kindler syndrome [5, 6].

69.4 Etiology

The basement membrane zone (BMZ) is a complex structure in many stratified squamous epithelial tissues like skin and oral mucosa. Various specialized parts come together to build anchoring complexes in the BMZ. Basal cell cytoskeleton intermediate filaments containing keratin insert on hemidesmosomes, condensations of the basal cell plasma membrane, at the top of the BMZ. Anchoring filaments cross the lamina lucida from the plasma membrane of the basal cell out into the extracellular environment, tying together the lamina densa and the hemidesmosomes. Anchoring fibrils rich in type VII collagen stretch from the lamina densa into the papillary dermis at the most inferior part of the BMZ, linking the lamina densa to anchoring plaques and entrapping interstitial collagen fibrils. Therefore, the cutaneous BMZ connects the dense network of interstitial collagen fibrils in the dermis to the vast cytoskeletal network of basal cells [3].

69.4.1 Keratin Filaments

Basal keratinocytes use a combination of keratins 5 and 14 to construct intermediate filaments. Keratins have a nonhelical carboxyterminal and aminoterminal area and a nonhelical core alpha-helical rod with multiple nonhelical discontinuities. The helix boundary motifs at the ends of the keratin rod contain the regions of maximum conservation between the keratins. Electron-dense structures, known as hemidesmosomes [3], are anchor points for inserting keratin intermediate filaments.

69.4.2 Hemidesmosomes

Peptin and BP230 are two examples of intracellular proteins found in these structures. Intermediate filaments are bound by the 500-kilodalton protein lectin (HD1). Its alternative name, BPAG1, also knows a 230-kD protein similar to desmoplakin and plectin, BP230. In the same way that plectin does, BP230 helps to link hemidesmosomes to intermediate filaments. Collagen XVII (BP180) and alpha-6-beta-4 integrin, both found in the plasma membrane, also have their intracellular domains in hemidesmosomes. The beta-4 integrin subunit has a wide cytoplasmic domain that interacts with other proteins in the hemidesmosomal plaque and plays a crucial role in hemidesmosome formation. Collagen XVII is a transmembrane collagenous protein that binds laminin-332 extracellularly and interacts with alpha 4 integrin and BP230 within cells [3].

69.4.3 Anchoring Filaments

Collagen XVII (BP180) and alpha-6-beta-4 integrin are found in their extracellular domains in these structures. Laminin-332 and laminin-6 are also found in anchoring filaments. Laminin-332 is a big heterotrimeric molecule consisting of alpha-3, beta-3, and gamma-2 chains, just like the other laminin proteins. The alpha-3, beta-1, and gamma-1 chains of laminin-332 disulfide-bond to those of laminin-311, the other known anchoring filament laminin. To link anchoring filaments to anchoring fibrils, laminin-332 develops a strong connection with type VII collagen [3].

69.4.3.1 Anchoring Fibrils

Fibrous anchors are mostly made up of collagen type VII. During the process of forming anchoring fibrils, type VII collagen undergoes proteolytic cleavage at its C-terminal globular domain (NC-2), leaving behind its massive N-terminal globular domain (NC-1), which interacts with laminin-332 in the lamina densa. Triple-helical chains of type VII collagen are joined by antiparallel joining of two molecules. After that, antiparallel dimer lateral interactions produce anchoring fibrils. The BMZ is attached to the dermis below it by anchoring fibrils that wrap around the collagen fibers in the dermal interstitium and insert back into the lamina densa [3].

69.4.3.2 The Molecular Basis of Simplex Epidermolysis Bullosa

Mutations in the keratin five and keratin 14 genes account for most instances of epidermolysis bullosa simplex [7]. Mid-basal cell separation is linked to intermediate filament clumping variability [3] in the skin.

Most keratin gene mutations that cause epidermolysis bullosa simplex are dominantly inherited and disrupt the formation of keratin filaments. Recessively inherited diseases can range in severity and affect a smaller subset of patients [3].

Epidermolysis bullosa simplex is most severe when mutations occur in the areas of keratins 5 and 14 that are the most conserved (helix boundary domains). The Dowling-Meara subtype shows intermediate filament clumping and is one of the severe variants. The Weber-Cockayne subtype, on the other hand, is linked to mutations in the less conserved areas of keratin five and keratin 14 genes [8].

69.5 Oral Manifestations of Epidermolysis Bullosa

Soft tissue and dental abnormalities are among the oral symptoms of EB [9]. Patients with epidermolysis bullosa simplex (EBS) typically only experience mild intraoral blistering and superficial erosions. Most people with JEB or DEB will develop scarring and lose the typical architecture of their intraoral soft tissues. Dental cavities and eventual tooth loss are expected outcomes of JEB, and enamel hypoplasia with pitting and furrowing is a hallmark of this disease. Dental cavities and early tooth loss are also influenced by [2].

Constraints (microstomia, ankyloglossia), aberrant mobility of the tongue, and the obliteration of the oral vestibules contribute to reduced food clearance, leading to poor oral hygiene and pain.

Constant consumption of high-calorie and cariogenic soft diets were recommended.

69.5.1 Intraepidermal Epidermolysis Bullosa

The EB Simplex subtypes are caused by mutations in the "PKP1, DSP, KRT5, KRT14, PLEC1, ITGA6, and genes" [5, 10]. The oral mucosa, composed of a stratified epithelium like the skin [11–13], expresses all of the genes responsible for intra-epidermal cleavage in the skin. As could be expected, those with EB Simplex also have an abnormally delicate oral mucosa, with a high prevalence of oral mucosal blistering and ulceration [14]. However, some people can have serious oral blisters and extensive mucosal involvement, which is uncommon but can occur due to trauma or tissue manipulation. Usually, oral soft tissue lesions heal without scarring. However, some severely affected forms of EB Simplex (e.g., Dowling Meara) [10] might show oral scarring.

69.5.2 Junctional Epidermolysis Bullosa

Mutations in genes involved in basement membrane-mediated cell adhesion, including LAMA3, LAMB3, LAMC3, COL17A1, ITG6A, and ITGB4, induce Junctional types of EB [5, 10, 15, 16]. Epithelial cell adhesion is critical in both the oral mucosa and the developing tooth bud, and the proteins produced from these genes play a vital role in this process [17, 18]. Although the degree of tissue fragility caused by these mutations varies from person to person, nearly everyone affected by Junctional EB experiences increased fragility of the oral mucosa, marked by blister formation and ulceration [14, 19]. This can be pretty serious for some people. Oral soft tissue lesions are common among Junctional EB subtypes. However, most people who have them do not develop noticeable scarring. The flexibility and structure of the soft tissues are unaltered. Herlitz EB stands out because it often has excessive granulation tissue around the mouth. Reduced mouth opening (microstomia) and decreased lip and perioral tissue mobility are expected outcomes [10, 14].

The genes responsible for the Junctional EB subtypes are essential for proper tooth development [17, 18]. In particular, the odontogenic epithelium, the precursor of the cells that create tooth enamel, the ameloblasts, uses the proteins produced by these genes to adhere to one another. Ameloblasts secrete an extracellular matrix to ensure proper enamel mineralization, stay in close contact with and adhere to neighboring ameloblasts, and regulate the local environment. Enamel abnormalities develop when ameloblasts lose their ability to stick to one another. Leakage of blood fluids into the growing enamel due to dysfunctional ameloblast adhesion might lead to albumin retention and impaired mineralization [20]. Lesions to the enamel in Junctional EB patients can range from widespread pitting to complete enamel loss, exposing the dentin beneath. Abnormal tooth eruption has been documented in certain patients with the Herlitz EB subtype [10, 21].

69.5.3 Dermolytic Epidermolysis Bullosa

Mutations in the COL7A1 gene, which codes for anchoring fibril protein in the dermal–epidermal basement membrane zone [10, 22], induce dystrophic EB. The severity of the dominant subtype is inversely proportional to the amount and functionality of the anchoring fibril protein present, making it less severe than the generalized recessive subtype. In the earliest phases of tooth development, type VII collagen can be seen in the basement membrane zone of the oral mucosa [23]. Expression of the COL7A1 gene is absent in ameloblasts [10].

Dystrophic EB can cause mild to severe soft tissue symptoms [14, 24–27]. Blistering is a rare symptom of Dominant Dystrophic EB, which can cause greater tissue fragility in the mouth. It is not hard to get a patient to start blistering, and those with even modest anxiety about dental procedures may avoid them. Soft tissue damage should be minimal while dealing with dominant dystonic EB. The oral and perioral mucosa of people with severe generalized recessive dystrophic EB tend to be highly fragile. This is usually seen right after birth and can hinder the newborn's breastfeeding ability. The tongue is not immune to oral ulcerations that can damage the entire oral mucosa. Scarring forms as the lesions heal. Repeated blistering and subsequent scarring significantly alter the appearance of the mouth. Ankyloglossia occurs when the tongue loses its lingual papillae and becomes stuck flat on the bottom of the mouth. The palatal rugae are one of the anatomical features that are removed. The soft tissue connection moves up until it is just below the crowns of the teeth, eliminating the oral vestibules that ordinarily provide corridors for food clearing between the teeth and the lips and cheeks. Scarring prevents the soft tissues that define the mouth opening from developing correctly, resulting in a significantly narrowed oral aperture. Individuals with severe microstomia may be unable to open their mouths fully, and even when they can, the space between their teeth may be minimal [10].

Milia are commonly seen on the skin of people with EB and can also appear in the mouth. Milia, or intra-oral keratocysts, are more prevalent in the dermolytic variants of EB than in EB Simplex [10, 14]. About half of people with the dominant and recessive types of EB have milia.

References

1. Has C, Bauer JW, Bodemer C, et al. Consensus reclassification of inherited epidermolysis bullosa and other disorders with skin fragility. Br J Dermatol. 2020;183:614.
2. Laimer M, Bauer J, Murrell DF. Epidermolysis bullosa: epidemiology, pathogenesis, classification, and clinical features. In: Hand JL, Corona R, editors. . UpToDate; 2022.
3. Marinkovich MP. Epidermolysis bullosa. In: James WD, editor. . Medscape; 2023. https://emedicine.medscape.com/article/1062939-overview.
4. Sawamura D, Nakano H, Matsuzaki Y. Overview of epidermolysis bullosa. J Dermatol. 2010;37(3):214–9.
5. Fine JD, Eady RA, Bauer EA, et al. The classification of inherited epidermolysis bullosa (EB): report of the third international consensus meeting on diagnosis and classification of EB. J Am Acad Dermatol. 2008;58(6):931–50.
6. McGrath JA, Mellerio JE. Epidermolysis bullosa. Br J Hosp Med (Lond). 2006;67(4):188–91.
7. Gong Z, Zou X, Xue R, et al. Large intragenic deletion of KRT14 causes autosomal-dominant epidermolysis bullosa simplex with generalized hyperpigmentation. J Dermatol Sci. 2023;13:27.
8. Kotalevskaya YY, Stepanov VA. Molecular genetic basis of epidermolysis bullosa. Vavilovskii Zhurnal Genet Selektsii. 2023;1:18–27.
9. Fine JD, Mellerio JE. Extracutaneous manifestations and complications of inherited epidermolysis bullosa: part II. Other organs. J Am Acad Dermatol. 2009;61:387.
10. Wright JT. Oral manifestations in the epidermolysis bullosa spectrum. Dermatol Clin. 2010;28(1):159–64.
11. Pelissier A, Ouhayoun JP, Sawaf MH, Forest N. Evolution of cytokeratin expression in developing human tooth germ. J Biol Buccale. 1990;18:99–108.
12. Modolo F, Martins MT, Loducca SV, de Araujo VC. Expression of integrin subunits alpha2, alpha3, alpha5, alphav, beta1, beta3 and beta4 in different histological types of ameloblastoma compared with dental germ, dental lamina and adult lining epithelium. Oral Dis. 2004;10(5):277–82.

13. Kieffer-Combeau S, Meyer JM, Lesot H. Cell–matrix interactions and cell–cell junctions during epithelial histo-morphogenesis in the developing mouse incisor. Int J Dev Biol. 2001;45(56):733–42.
14. Wright JT, Fine JD, Johnson LB. Oral soft tissues in hereditary epidermolysis bullosa. Oral Surg Oral Med Oral Pathol. 1991;71:440–6.
15. Uitto J, Pulkkinen L, Christiano AM. Molecular basis of the dystrophic and junctional forms of epidermolysis bullosa: mutations in the type VII collagen and kalinin (laminin 5) genes. J Invest Dermatol. 1994;103:39S–46S.
16. McGrath JA, Gatalica B, Christiano AM, et al. Mutations in the 180-kD bullous pemphigoid antigen (BPAG2), a hemidesmosomal transmembrane collagen (COL17A1), in generalized atrophic benign epidermolysis bullosa. Nat Genet. 1995;11(1):83–6.
17. Aberdam D, Aguzzi A, Baudoin C, Galliano MF, Ortonne JP, Meneguzzi G. Developmental expression of nicein adhesion protein (laminin-5) subunits suggests multiple morphogenic roles. Cell Adhes Commun. 1994;2:115–29.
18. Asaka T, Akiyama M, Domon T, et al. Type XVII collagen is a key player in tooth enamel formation. Am J Pathol. 2009;174(1):91–100.
19. Sedano HO, Gorlin RJ. Epidermolysis bullosa. Oral Surg Oral Med Oral Pathol. 1989;67:555–63.
20. Kirkham J, Robinson C, Strafford SM, et al. The chemical composition of tooth enamel in junctional epidermolysis bullosa. Arch Oral Biol. 2000;45(5):377–86.
21. Brooks JK, Bare LC, Davidson J, Taylor LS, Wright JT. Junctional epidermolysis bullosa associated with hypoplastic enamel and pervasive failure of tooth eruption: oral rehabilitation with use of an overdenture. Oral Surg Oral Med Oral Pathol Oral Radiol Endod. 2008;105(4):e24–8.
22. Christiano AM, Greenspan DS, Hoffman GG, et al. A missense mutation in type VII collagen in two affected siblings with recessive dystrophic epidermolysis bullosa. Nat Genet. 1993;4(1):62–6.
23. Heikinheimo K, Morgan PR, Happonen RP, Stenman G, Virtanen I. Distribution of extracellular matrix proteins in odontogenic tumors and developing teeth. Virchows Arch B Cell Pathol. 1991;61:101–9.
24. Album MM, Gaisin A, Lee KWT, Buck BE, Sharrar WG, Gill FM. Epidermolysis bullosa dystrophica polydysplastica. Oral Surg Oral Med Oral Pathol. 1977;43:859–72.
25. Crawford E, Burkes EJ, Briggaman R. Hereditary epidermolysis bullosa: oral manifestations and dental therapy. Oral Surg. 1976;42:490–500.
26. Winter G. Dental problems in epidermolysis bullosa. In: Priestley GC, Tidman MJ, Weiss JB, Eady RAJ, editors. Epidermolysis bullosa: a comprehensive review of classification, management and laboratory studies. Berkshire: D.E.B.R.A; 1990. p. 21–7.
27. Wright JT, Fine JD, Johnson LB, Steinmetz TT. Oral involvement of recessive dystrophic epidermolysis bullosa inversa. Am J Med Genet. 1993;47:1184–8.

Pierre Robin Sequence: Controversies in Management

70

Zeynel Öztürk, Nuray Bayar Muluk, and Felicia Manole

70.1 Definition

Multiple factors [1–3] contribute to the Pierre Robin sequence (PRS), also called Pierre Robin syndrome. Hypoplasia of the mandible before the ninth week of development is assumed to be the underlying cause in most cases. The tongue blocks the space between the palatal shelves when they develop until about week 8. The palatal shelves fuse once the tongue is retracted between the tenth and eleventh weeks of development. Hypoplasia of the mandible in the Pierre Robin sequence causes the tongue to shift backward, preventing the palate from closing. The Pierre Robin sequence has a mysterious origin. Chin growth restriction during pregnancy due to oligohydramnios, myotonia, or connective tissue disease [1] are all possible causes.

In most cases, the Pierre Robin sequence occurs in isolation. However, in rare instances (37% in one cohort of 74 individuals), numerous abnormalities develop as part of a syndrome. About a third of those with congenital anomalies also suffered from Stickler or velocardiofacial syndrome (VCFS). Therefore, developmental misexpression of SOX9 (sex-reversed Y chromosome [SRY]-box 9), a transcription factor crucial for sex and skeletal development, might account for some occurrences of Pierre Robin sequencing [4]. Because of the correlation between Stickler syndrome and VCFS [1], patients with the Pierre Robin sequence should undergo ophthalmologic testing and a fluorescence in situ hybridization (FISH) study to look for chromosome 22 deletion.

Z. Öztürk
Department of Otorhinolaryngology, Private Florya Hospital, Istanbul, Turkey

N. Bayar Muluk (✉)
Department of Otorhinolaryngology, Kırıkkale University, Faculty of Medicine, Kırıkkale, Turkey

F. Manole
Department of ENT, University of Oradea, Faculty of Medicine, Oradea, Romania

H. Yüksel et al. (eds.), *Pediatric Airway Diseases*, Comprehensive ENT,
https://doi.org/10.1007/978-3-031-74853-0_70

70.2 Pathophysiology

There is no single cause for PRS. These varying causes of malformations and deformities and connective tissue dysplasia point to a wide range of pathogenetic heterogeneity and phenotypic variability. Patients with PRS should be classified into one of three groups: those with isolated PRS, those with PRS as part of a recognized syndrome, and those with isolated PRS as part of a complex of numerous defects.

Intrauterine pressures that act on the mandible to restrict its growth and impact the tongue between the palatal shelves are typically to blame for isolated PRS. Oligohydramnios has been linked to deformed PRS in some cases. Since intrauterine molding causes micrognathia, mandibular catchup growth after delivery is to be anticipated after intrauterine pressures are no longer present. Isolated deformational PRS is not likely to be the only cause of the most severe cases of micrognathia. There is little chance of a growth acceleration [5].

Patients with PRS have a family history of cleft lip and/or cleft palate in the range of 13–27.7% [6, 7]. By comparing data from several sources, Jakobsen et al. [8] suggested that GAD67 on 2q31, PVRL1 on 11q23–q24, and SOX9 on 17q24.3–q25.1 might all play a role in the etiology of PRS. Some patients with nonsyndromic PRS were found to have disease-causing mutations in the COL11A1 and COL11A2 genes [9], discovered by Melkoniemi et al. [9].

Nonsyndromic PRS may be caused by SOX9 and KCNJ2 dysregulation, as suggested by the screening of 10 unrelated patients for these mutations by Jakobsen et al. [10]. Linkage analysis results, a clustering of translocation breakpoints 1.06–1.23 Mb upstream of SOX9, and microdeletions both approximately 1.5 Mb centromeric and approximately 1.5 Mb telomeric of SOX9 were reported by Benko et al. [11] as supporting the existence of a 17q24 locus underlying PRS.

Studies differ on what percentage of patients have isolated PRS. Only 25% of PRS cases were determined to have identifiable syndromes; 35% had numerous abnormalities without a known cause, and 40% were considered to be sporadic. Similarly, a study indicated that 74% of PRS cases were solitary.

Stickler syndrome is the most frequent syndromic form of PRS, accounting for 20–25% of all cases. Velocardiofacial syndrome is the second most frequent PRS syndrome, occurring in around 15% of all PRS patients. The remaining six cases of syndromic PRS are attributable to a variety of different syndromes, including Treacher Collins syndrome (mandibulofacial dysostosis), Nager syndrome, spondylo-epiphyseal dysplasia congenita (SEC), and others.

Cohen correlated PRS with 46 diseases. This list is not exhaustive, but it does cover the basics. A variety of abnormalities, including those of the eye, ear, heart, and limb, have been linked to PRS [12].

For this reason, the Pierre Robin sequence (formerly known as Pierre Robin syndrome) is now properly referred to as a sequence rather than a syndrome. In contrast, a syndrome is a collection of abnormalities that share a common pathophysiology but manifest in distinct ways. The progression from micrognathia to glossoptosis and, perhaps, airway obstruction and/or a cleft palate is a hallmark of PRS. Common explanations for hypoplastic mandibular development are as follows [13].

70.2.1 Mechanical Theory

Around the seventh week of pregnancy, the mandible begins to develop dorsally and inferiorly. As early as the 11th week of gestation, the palatal gap cannot close normally if the mandible does not develop normally. Upper airway blockage [14] is the end result of glossoptosis, which is caused by aberrant mandibular development.

70.2.2 Neurological Maturation Theory

This theory claims that the mandible and palatal shelves fail to fuse and expand at the proper rates because the neuromuscular development of the tongue is delayed [14].

70.2.3 The Theory of Mandibular Compression

According to this view, the fetal head becomes flexed due to external factors, which then presses the mandible against the chest and prevents it from developing typically. Possible causes include oligohydramnios, uterine abnormalities, and pregnancies with multiple babies. If the tongue develops typically, it will eventually shift backward, blocking the patient's upper airway. A cleft palate can be caused by the tongue's tip blocking blood flow to the palatal shelves during development [13, 14].

70.3 Pierre-Robin-Sequence Clinical Characteristics

Micrognathia, glossoptosis, and cleft palate are the clinical hallmarks of the Pierre Robin syndrome. When the tongue prolapses backward, it blocks the airway and can be fatal. Failure to thrive, coma, and pulmonary hypertension can all result from respiratory impairment. Eating concerns are prevalent [15].

In most situations, airway issues disappear around the third to the twelfth month of life, thanks to the rapid face growth. Prematurity and airway impairment significantly contribute to the high mortality rate in patients with the Pierre Robin sequence. Premature newborns with Pierre Robin sequences had a mortality rate between 1.7 and 11.3% [3, 16]. However, when additional abnormalities are present, the observed mortality rate rises to 26% [1, 3].

70.4 Differential Diagnoses

The most common diseases that need to be ruled out are listed below [5]:

Beckwith–Wiedemann Syndrome
CHARGE Syndrome
Childhood Sleep Apnea

DiGeorge Syndrome
Fetal Alcohol Syndrome
Mandibulofacial Dysostosis (Treacher Collins Syndrome)
Multiple Births
Pectus Excavatum
Pediatric Cleft Lip and Palate
Stridor
Velocardiofacial Syndrome [5]

70.5 Physical Examination

The three main parts [5] of the Pierre Robin sequence are as follows:

- Retrognathia and micrognathia
- Cleft palate, which can be either U- or V-shaped.
- Glossoptosis frequently occurs alongside airway obstruction; the tongue is not truly larger than expected, but due to the short mandible, the tongue is huge for the airway and hence causes obstruction; infrequently, the tongue is smaller than usual.

PRS is a cluster of abnormalities that begins with a single developmental glitch. Some have proposed alternative classifications that consider the occurrence of a cleft palate in either the U or V shape and the airway obstruction [5].

Hypoxia, cor pulmonale, failure to thrive, and brain damage can result from airway blockage due to PRS if it is severe or not appropriately handled. There is a correlation between a syndromic pattern and a worse prognosis in patients with PRS. There may be a 30% mortality rate [17]. Newborns with PRS need close observation because of the risk of severe airway blockage during the first 4–8 weeks of life [5].

PRS might result from a single chromosome abnormality, a known disease, or a cluster of other birth defects. Correct management of an infant affected by PRS generally hinges on correctly diagnosing a suspected condition [2, 18]. Stickler syndrome accounts for 20–25% of all occurrences of PRS [5] and is the most common syndromic disorder.

70.5.1 Micrognathia

Clinical evidence of a malformed mandible. As a rule, this entails an increased mandibular angle and a shorter mandibular body length. Micrognathia has been diagnosed in the past using defined indicators. However, none has proven beneficial in identifying patients with breathing difficulties [13].

70.5.2 Glossoptosis

The hallmark of this condition is the forward movement of the tongue's base toward the throat. Respiratory discomfort can range in intensity from mild to severe. Endoscopy and computed tomography (CT) imaging may be helpful in assessing the level of obstruction present in glossoptosis, but there is no gold standard for diagnosis of this condition [13].

70.5.3 Congestion of the Airway

Airway blockage can range in clinical severity from mild malfunction not requiring intervention to severe ventilatory impairment necessitating intubation soon after birth. Abnormal breathing sounds, increased use of respiratory accessory muscles, desaturations, trouble feeding/swallowing, reflux, and aspiration are all possible clinical indicators of airway obstruction. Chronic symptoms of airway obstruction include inability to gain weight, difficulties communicating, cognitive impairments, and, in the end, pulmonary hypertension and cor pulmonale [13].

70.5.4 *Cleft* Palate

Cleft palate is common but is not a necessary part of the PRS triad. While U-shaped cleft palates are the norm, V-shaped ones have also been documented [14].

70.6 Diagnosis

70.6.1 Studies in Radiology

Diagnostic studies, such as bone radiography, are appropriate when Pierre Robin sequence (PRS) is diagnosed to evaluate for other possible disorders.

Mandibular osteotomies can be more precisely planned with the help of preoperative computed tomography (CT) [5, 19].

70.6.2 Variants Tests

Complete genetic testing (fluorescence in situ hybridization [FISH] for 22q deletion, test for mutation in Treacle [TCOF1] gene) should be performed when PRS is suspected or diagnosed. If you suspect a syndrome, you should get an ophthalmologic evaluation as well [5].

Polysomnography and an airway examination with bedside nasopharyngoscopy [5] are recommended for children with suspected PRS because of the tiny jaw and the increased risk of upper-airway obstruction.

Finally, a feeding specialist (a speech pathologist) should assess children with PRS who are having trouble eating [5].

70.7 Management of Pierre Robin Sequence

Upper airway obstruction and eating difficulties are the two most common complications in patients with the Pierre Robin sequence [3, 20]. Patients with this condition need to be monitored for signs of apnea and airway blockage. If you want to keep your airway clear while still eating, you should lay prone. While waiting for compensatory growth, the airway may be protected with a rubber tube inserted through the nose (nasopharyngeal trumpet). If conservative treatments for respiratory blockage fail [1], more intrusive temporizing techniques will be required.

Upper airway blockage can be treated non-surgically with noninvasive respiratory support (NRS) or a nasopharyngeal airway (NPA). Both mandibular distraction osteogenesis and glossopexy can be performed surgically. If these methods fail to relieve airway obstruction, a tracheostomy may be necessary [15].

Noninvasive positive pressure ventilation or continuous positive airway pressure are used in

- NRS to treat airway blockage. Over the course of a decade, 81 patients were treated with either NRS (9 patients) or positioning and medical care (63%), temporary intubation and positioning (12 patients), tracheotomy (16 patients), or both (12 patients) [21]. In newborns with severe upper airway blockage due to Pierre Robin sequence, NRS was demonstrated to improve breathing patterns, respiratory attempts, and transcutaneous carbon dioxide pressures. There was no need for tracheostomy in any of the seven infants who were given NRS, and six of them were able to wean themselves off of nutritional support.
- NPA implantation is a further nonsurgical choice for airway blockage relief [22–24]. There is evidence that this technique can increase oxygen saturation and lead to weight gain [1].

An external fixator is typically utilized to open the mouth cavity after an osteotomy or fracture of the mandible has been performed [25–27]. The mandibular size can be permanently altered via distraction, allowing for more room for the tongue. Many patients have been spared the trauma of a tracheostomy as a result [1].

Glossopexy, also known as tongue-lip adhesion, is a surgical procedure in which the tongue is sutured to the lip in order to prevent retrusion. Although glossopexy has fallen out of favor, it is still viable due to its positive effects on morbidity and weight gain normalization [1, 28, 29].

70.7.1 Approach Considerations

Medical professionals have cause for grave anxiety while caring for a newborn with Pierre Robin sequence (PRS).

There are three main parts [5] to PRS:

- **Micrognathia/retrognathia**
- **Palate split**
- **Glossoptosis in comparison**

Many newborns experience airway discomfort due to micrognathia and relative glossoptosis [30]. Possible need for immediate medical attention. Infants have a hard time getting enough calories since their bodies will always put breathing first. Problems with eating are compounded by a cleft palate [5].

70.7.1.1 Care for Newborns

The potential for death is the most significant cause for alarm in cases of airway impairment [30]. The breathing and feeding issues for neonates with PRS are typically more severe because most infants have an isolated impairment rather than a syndrome. Most newborns can be cared for while lying flat on their backs. Mechanical ventilation, tracheostomy, and invasive devices such as oral airways and palatal prostheses may be prevented [5].

These newborns likewise require a prone feeding posture but can get oral nutrition. Again, relatively few newborns will require gavage feeding tubes or other devices for an extended period. The optimum method in the complicated care of infants affected by PRS and Robin complexes [5] is multidisciplinary care that includes a neonatologist, a neonatal nurse specialist, members of the craniofacial team, and the parents.

Babies with nonsyndromic PRS who feed orally while prone and breathe independently typically go home within a few days. The significant airway blockage and feeding problems are predicted to lessen as the mandible grows. Continued examinations of feeding and speaking are required, as are checks of respiratory capacity. Some newborns have much more severe immediate or long-term medical difficulties [5], but the cleft palate must be closed eventually and long-term orthodontic care is required.

70.7.1.2 Postneonatal Care

Airway

Airway obstruction due to micrognathia/retrognathia can range from minor to severe [30]. In cases of severe obstruction, prompt treatment may be necessary, including a highly challenging intubation. Many newborns with airway issues have only moderate symptoms at birth but often worsen in the first 4–8 weeks of life. This could be because a newborn has minimal breathing requirements. The barrier becomes more formidable as the infant's needs increase.

It is usually best to take things slowly and try several positions when dealing with a mild obstruction. Breathing difficulties might occur when the mandible is too tiny concerning the tongue. When a newborn is placed in the prone position, gravity pulls the tongue forward, opening the airway. Babies whose blockage has a nonsyndromic cause usually grow out of it by the time they are one.

Many medical professionals recommend using a nasopharyngeal airway if other measures, such as changing the patient's position, have failed to alleviate the obstruction. Airway obstruction caused by relative glossoptosis can be avoided using a nasopharyngeal airway. Effective short-term management of airway blockage can be achieved with this method in the neonatal intensive care unit (ICU). Dislodgement of a nasopharyngeal airway can induce an acute airway obstruction, so most hospitals are reluctant to let patients go home with one.

Patients who can sustain a CO_2 level of 50 or above should consider surgery. PRS [31] can be treated with one of three different types of surgical procedures:

Adhesion/Glossopexy of the Tongue to the Lip

- ***Tracheostomy**
- **Mandibular distraction osteogenesis**

In newborns with PRS and upper-airway obstruction, the Tübingen palatal plate (TPP) has been argued as a less invasive alternative [32].

Glossopexy (Adhesion of the Tongue to the Lips)

When the lower lip and the tongue are sutured together, the tongue is pulled forward, and the airway is widened. This attachment between the tongue and lip is broken later, probably once the youngster has shown signs of catchup growth. The consequence is a minor aesthetic change to the lip and tongue [5].

In a glossopexy, the base of the tongue is surgically attached to the jaw to move it forward. The tongue-lip adhesion/glossopexy has been debated because it is difficult to place a suture that permanently binds the base of the tongue ahead on the jaw, which is somewhat soft. However, some maxillofacial surgeons support it [5].

Tracheostomy

With a tracheostomy tube in place, airflow can avoid the blocked oropharynx and hypopharynx. The tracheostomy tube can be removed [5] if the infant's airway blockage resolves.

Tracheostomy tubes, sadly, call for constant surveillance. Acute respiratory arrest can occur if the tracheostomy tube becomes obstructed or dislodged. However, a tracheostomy tube inserted in a baby is unlikely to be in situ for less than a year. Care for a tracheostomy tube might be complex for the family, but there are established ways to teach them what they need to know. Even now, the gold standard for treating children with life-threatening airway obstruction is a tracheostomy [5].

Distraction-Induced Bone Growth

Sidman popularized distraction osteogenesis, a more modern treatment designed to treat airway obstruction in PRS [33], as he had the most experience treating patients with PRS anywhere in the world with this method [34].

Many institutions have developed specialized knowledge in this field. This method divides the mandible on both sides, close to the angle. The two halves of the mandible are separated by about 1.5–2 mm per day using a mechanical device. The mandible lengthens over 2–3 weeks as new bone is created at the fracture sites. Newborns can undergo distraction to avoid having a tracheostomy, and adults can have a distraction to have a tracheostomy tube removed [5].

70.7.1.3 Feeding

Many kids with PRS struggle to eat properly. A patient with airway issues will likely experience feeding difficulties [5] because of the body's natural tendency to prioritize breathing over eating.

Feeding may be managed using particular measures, such as raising the child's head and using special cleft nursing bottles if the kid displays catchup growth. Gavage or feeding tubes can offer enough nutrients for the time being if this is not enough. Many newborns need gastrostomy tubes if they have trouble feeding even after several months. These tubes can be removed after the youngster eats normally [5].

70.7.1.4 Palate Split

Infants in the United States usually have their cleft palates corrected between the ages of 10 and 18 months, though this age range can be pushed back if there are airway problems. Current medical consensus holds that earlier intervention increases a child's chances of a successful surgical outcome and, by extension, of normal palate function and everyday speech. Palate repair can be done anytime [5] if the child already has a tracheostomy tube.

70.7.1.5 Micrognathia/Retrognathia

If there is considerable airway obstruction and the family chooses distraction osteogenesis of the jaw, micrognathia can be treated in the perinatal period. In most cases, micrognathia's functional and aesthetic defects are not addressed until the newborn has reached complete growth of the facial bones. Surgery to correct a tooth occlusion problem is rarely necessary in infants born with retrognathia. However, newborns with micrognathia or retrognathia may benefit from a chin augmentation treatment for cosmetic reasons.

70.7.1.6 40-Year-Olds Hilaire and Buchbinder

Patients with syndromic PRS and Robin complexes may not benefit from the use of various obstruction, placement, and traction devices. Patients with PRS who have the syndromic form are more likely to require tracheostomy, tongue-lip adhesion, other glossopexy procedures, and a nasopharyngeal airway [5].

When deciding on a course of treatment for a patient, it is usually beneficial to consult with experts from multiple fields. Postponing palatal closure may improve treatment outcomes in patients with both syndromic and nonsyndromic PRS. Given the enormous heterogeneity between syndromes and within each clinical state, the timing and choice of procedures must be carefully considered based on an accurate diagnosis and the particulars of the specific case [5].

Airway blockage or narrowing is the primary issue [35, 36]. Different factors contributing to airway obstruction are associated with PRS and Robin complexes, as was described earlier. Therefore, to effectively manage PRS in an infant, a precise diagnosis must be made as soon as feasible [5].

Most infants with nonsyndromic PRS and a typically sized tongue have some degree of micrognathia, which can cause airway obstruction. Gravity forces the tongue forward and keeps the airway open if the newborn is prone (face down). This may not be enough for more severe situations, in which case tongue-lip adhesion or glossopexy may be required [5].

References

1. Buchanan EP. Syndromes with craniofacial abnormalities. In: Firth HV, TePas E, editors. . UpToDate; 2022.
2. Shprintzen RJ. The implications of the diagnosis of Robin sequence. Cleft Palate Craniofac J. 1992;29:205.
3. Evans KN, Sie KC, Hopper RA, et al. Robin sequence: from diagnosis to development of an effective management plan. Pediatrics. 2011;127:936.
4. Benko S, Fantes JA, Amiel J, et al. Highly conserved non-coding elements on either side of SOX9 associated with Pierre Robin sequence. Nat Genet. 2009;41:359.
5. Tolarova MM. Pierre Robin sequence treatment and management. In: Elluru RG, editor. . Medscape; 2022. https://emedicine.medscape.com/article/995706-treatment#d10.
6. Marques IL, Barbieri MA, Bettiol H. Etiopathogenesis of isolated Robin sequence. Cleft Palate Craniofac J. 1998;35(6):517–25.
7. Holder-Espinasse M, Abadie V, Cormier-Daire V, Beyler C, Manach Y, Munnich A, et al. Pierre Robin sequence: a series of 117 consecutive cases. J Pediatr. 2001;139(4):588–90.
8. Jakobsen LP, Knudsen MA, Lespinasse J, García Ayuso C, Ramos C, Fryns JP, et al. The genetic basis of the Pierre Robin sequence. Cleft Palate Craniofac J. 2006;43(2):155–9.
9. Melkoniemi M, Koillinen H, Männikkö M, Warman ML, Pihlajamaa T, Kääriäinen H, et al. Collagen XI sequence variations in nonsyndromic cleft palate, Robin sequence and micrognathia. Eur J Hum Genet. 2003;11(3):265–70.
10. Jakobsen LP, Ullmann R, Christensen SB, Jensen KE, Mølsted K, Henriksen KF, et al. Pierre Robin sequence may be caused by dysregulation of SOX9 and KCNJ2. J Med Genet. 2007;44(6):381–6.
11. Benko S, Fantes JA, Amiel J, Kleinjan DJ, Thomas S, Ramsay J, et al. Highly conserved non-coding elements on either side of SOX9 associated with Pierre Robin sequence. Nat Genet. 2009;41(3):359–64.
12. Hennekam RCM, Krantz ID, Allanson JE, editors. Gorlin's syndromes of the head and neck. 5th ed. New York: Oxford University Press; 2010. p. 955–61.
13. Baxter D, Shanks AL. Pierre Robin syndrome. In: StatPearls [Internet]. Treasure Island (FL): StatPearls Publishing; 2023. https://www.ncbi.nlm.nih.gov/books/NBK562213/.
14. Giudice A, Barone S, Belhous K, Morice A, Soupre V, Bennardo F, Boddaert N, Vazquez MP, Abadie V, Picard A. Pierre Robin sequence: a comprehensive narrative review of the literature over time. J Stomatol Oral Maxillofac Surg. 2018;119(5):419–28.
15. van den Elzen AP, Semmekrot BA, Bongers EM, et al. Diagnosis and treatment of the Pierre Robin sequence: results of a retrospective clinical study and review of the literature. Eur J Pediatr. 2001;160:47.
16. Bütow KW, Hoogendijk CF, Zwahlen RA. Pierre Robin sequence: appearances and 25 years of experience with an innovative treatment protocol. J Pediatr Surg. 2009;44:2112.
17. Jones KL, Jones MC, del Campo M, Robin sequence. Smith's recognizable patterns of human malformation. 8th ed. Philadelphia: Elsevier; 2022. p. 334–6.
18. Olasoji HO, Ambe PJ, Adesina OA. Pierre Robin syndrome: an update. Niger Postgrad Med J. 2007;14(2):140–5.

19. Siska RC, Prabhu SS, Lor LS, Emmerich V, Massary D, Pan BS, et al. Safety of mandibular osteotomies in infants with Pierre Robin sequence: computer-aided modeling to characterize the risks of various techniques. Plast Reconstr Surg. 2022;149(5):1169–77.
20. Poets CF, Bacher M. Treatment of upper airway obstruction and feeding problems in Robin-like phenotype. J Pediatr. 2011;159:887.
21. Leboulanger N, Picard A, Soupre V, et al. Physiologic and clinical benefits of noninvasive ventilation in infants with Pierre Robin sequence. Pediatrics. 2010;126:e1056.
22. Wagener S, Rayatt SS, Tatman AJ, et al. Management of infants with Pierre Robin sequence. Cleft Palate Craniofac J. 2003;40:180.
23. Parhizkar N, Saltzman B, Grote K, et al. Nasopharyngeal airway for management of airway obstruction in infants with micrognathia. Cleft Palate Craniofac J. 2011;48:478.
24. Abel F, Bajaj Y, Wyatt M, Wallis C. The successful use of the nasopharyngeal airway in Pierre Robin sequence: an 11-year experience. Arch Dis Child. 2012;97:331.
25. Denny AD, Talisman R, Hanson PR, Recinos RF. Mandibular distraction osteogenesis in very young patients to correct airway obstruction. Plast Reconstr Surg. 2001;108:302.
26. Denny A, Kalantarian B. Mandibular distraction in neonates: a strategy to avoid tracheostomy. Plast Reconstr Surg. 2002;109:896.
27. Denny AD. Distraction osteogenesis in Pierre Robin neonates with airway obstruction. Clin Plast Surg. 2004;31:221.
28. Denny AD, Amm CA, Schaefer RB. Outcomes of tongue-lip adhesion for neonatal respiratory distress caused by Pierre Robin sequence. J Craniofac Surg. 2004;15:819.
29. Cozzi F, Totonelli G, Frediani S, et al. The effect of glossopexy on weight velocity in infants with Pierre Robin syndrome. J Pediatr Surg. 2008;43:296.
30. Zaballa K, Singh J, Waters K. The management of upper airway obstruction in Pierre Robin sequence. Paediatr Respir Rev. 2022;45:11–5.
31. Lee JH, Kim YH. Temporary tongue-lip traction during the initial period of mandibular distraction in Pierre Robin sequence. Cleft Palate Craniofac J. 2009;46(1):19–23.
32. Poets CF, Koos B, Reinert S, Wiechers C. The Tübingen palatal plate approach to Robin sequence: summary of current evidence. J Craniomaxillofac Surg. 2019;47(11):1699–705.
33. Hong P. A clinical narrative review of mandibular distraction osteogenesis in neonates with Pierre Robin sequence. Int J Pediatr Otorhinolaryngol. 2011;75(8):985–91.
34. Sidman JD, Sampson D, Templeton B. Distraction osteogenesis of the mandible for airway obstruction in children. Laryngoscope. 2001;111(7):1137–46.
35. Han KD, Seruya M, Oh AK, Zalzal GH, Preciado DA. "Natural" decannulation in patients with Robin sequence and severe airway obstruction. Ann Otol Rhinol Laryngol. 2012;121(1):44–50.
36. Glynn F, Fitzgerald D, Earley MJ, Rowley H. Pierre Robin sequence: an institutional experience in the multidisciplinary management of airway, feeding and serous otitis media challenges. Int J Pediatr Otorhinolaryngol. 2011;75(9):1152–5.

Herpes Simplex Viruses in Children

71

Rahime Koca and Erdem Atalay Çetinkaya

71.1 General Characteristics and Classification

According to the latest update by the International Committee on Taxonomy of Viruses, eight types of herpesviruses infecting humans are defined as Human Herpesviruses (HHV) which are divided into three subgroups [1]. Herpes simplex virus types 1 and 2 (HSV-1 and HSV-2) are included in the alphaherpesvirinae subfamily. Varicella zoster virus (Human Herpesvirus Type 3) is also in this subfamily. Cytomegalovirus (CMV—Human Herpesvirus Type 5), HHV 6 variant A and variant B, and HHV-7 make up the betaherpesvirinae subfamily. The third subfamily, namely, the gammaherpesvirinae, comprises Epstein–Barr virus (EBV-Human herpes virus type 4) and Kaposi's Sarcoma-associated herpes virus (Human herpes virus type 8) [2–4].

Herpes viruses are typically spherical, enveloped DNA viruses 150–300 nm in diameter. Their double-stranded DNA which is approximately 120–230 kb in size is linear in the virion and circular in the host cell during latent infection. Although the genome organization of human herpes viruses is quite similar, their genome lengths and sequences are different. Structural proteins such as envelope, tegument, and capsid proteins and non-structural proteins such as thymidine kinase, thymidylate synthetase, helicase, primase, and DNA polymerase are encoded; the number of encoded proteins (ranging from 70 to 200) vary depending on the type of virus [1, 5]. Herpes viruses have icosahedral nucleocapsids consisting of 162 hexagonal capsomers. Outside this capsid which is 95–110 nm in size lies the tegument layer consisting of amorphous proteins. The tegument layer is surrounded by a lipid envelope that originates from the outermost host cell membrane and contains various viral glycoproteins. While some of the tegument proteins are responsible for the

R. Koca · E. A. Çetinkaya (✉)
Department of Otorhinolaryngology, University of Health Sciences, Antalya Training and Research Hospital, Antalya, Turkey

H. Yüksel et al. (eds.), *Pediatric Airway Diseases*, Comprehensive ENT, https://doi.org/10.1007/978-3-031-74853-0_71

connection between the envelope and the capsid, others are in charge of initiating the replication in the infected cell. Envelope glycoproteins form protrusions on the virus surface and play a role in the attachment of the virus to the host cell, the formation of neutralizing antibodies, and the escape of the virus from the immune response [5, 6].

Before binding strongly between envelope glycoproteins and cellular receptors, the virus attaches to glycosaminoglycans on the cell surface with a low affinity [5]. These specific interactions determine the cell's susceptibility to infection, i.e., viral tropism and host diversity, to a great extent. The envelopes of herpes viruses fuse with the cell membrane which is followed by the release of tegument and nucleocapsid proteins into the cell cytoplasm. The virus may also enter the cell by endocytosis after which the virus envelope fuses with the endosomal membrane [7, 8]. Released into the cytoplasm, the nucleocapsid is carried by dynein transport proteins to the host cell nucleus via the tubulin microtubule network. Upon reaching the host cell nucleus, the viral nucleocapsid along with viral nucleic acid is discharged into the nuclear pore. The viral genome is linear outside the nucleus but takes a circular form once inside the nucleus. Transcription of the herpes virus genome begins. Capsid proteins are synthesized in the cytoplasm and transported to the nucleus. In the nucleus, the capsid is assembled together with the viral genome. Viral genome transcription occurs in three main phases. Initially, "immediate early" or alpha genes are transcribed, followed by the transcription of "early" or beta genes and "late" or gamma genes. Varying theories suggest that nucleocapsids are enveloped from either the inner nuclear membrane or the Golgi apparatus and mature virions are released from the cell surface by exocytosis [5, 7].

Primary infections often exhibit more severe symptoms than reactivated latent infections because no immunity has been developed previously. Still, a mild or asymptomatic primary infection may also continue with recurrent infections with more severe symptoms. Despite the possibility of viral replication and transmission, herpes infections reactivated from the latent phase may remain asymptomatic [9]. Although the cell latently infected with herpes viruses does not exhibit any infectious virus, the latent genome is transcriptionally active and there is protein expression, albeit limited, in some herpes viruses [10]. In some infected cells, viral reactivation is induced by radiation, fever, UV, nerve trauma, stress, or hypoxia. The development and reactivation of life-threatening herpes virus infections are observed more frequently in immunosuppressed and immunodeficient hosts with suppressed T-cell immunity. Thus, cellular immunity is thought to be critical in controlling severe herpes virus infections [5, 11]. Humoral immunity is crucial against primary infections of herpes viruses. Transplacental transfer of antibodies protects the neonate against Herpes simplex virus (HSV), Varicella zoster virus (VZV), and CMV infections. Exposure of the fetus to VZV or CMV during development causes congenital sequelae and inhibits fetal development. If the mother suffers from primary infection, especially in the last trimester, very serious neonatal herpes virus infections may develop because the mother cannot develop immunity and pass it to the newborn and the existing viral load is high [5]. In immunocompromised individuals, VZV immunoglobulin and CMV hyperimmunoglobulin reduce the severity of primary herpes infections. However, as most herpes viruses in the body spread through cell-to-cell transmission, once the infection has occurred, the role of antibodies in protection is limited, and cellular immunity becomes dominant thereafter. This is why patients with hypogammaglobulinemia do not develop severe herpes virus infections [5]. Most herpes viruses encode many anti-apoptotic proteins as well as a variety of proteins preventing the recognition of infected cells by CD4+, CD8+, and NK cells and the formation of interferon response [11]. Moreover, CMV, HHV-6, and HHV-7 can encode host chemokines and chemokine receptors and the spread of infected cells is managed through chemokine receptors expressed as such [10]. For HSVs, which establish latency in the dorsal root ganglia, neurons are significant for escape from the immune response. Furthermore, binding of HSV envelope glycoproteins to the Fc portions of immunoglobulins and complement (C3b) receptors is one of the viral strategies hindering effective host response to infection. CMV inhibits the production of MHC class I and II molecules in the host cell. EBNA-1 (Epstein-Barr virus nuclear antigen-1), which is synthesized only in latently EBV-infected cells, plays an active role in the escape of the virus from the immune response by inhibiting viral peptide presentation of the infected cell through MHC class I molecules [5, 10]. Thanks to all these mechanisms, herpes viruses successfully protect themselves by escaping from the influence of the host immune system.

All oral and intravenous drugs approved by the US Food and Drug Administration (FDA) for herpes virus infections exert their anti-viral effects by inhibiting DNA polymerase. Antiviral therapy targets DNA polymerase, thymidine kinase, and ribonucleotide reductase. As such, these drugs are only effective against lytic replication and not in the latent phase. Varicella zoster vaccines developed against VZV to prevent herpes virus infections have been licensed. Being live attenuated vaccines, both of these induce humoral and cellular immune responses. They differ by the amount of virus they contain. Varicella immunoglobulin can be employed to reduce the severity of the disease in immunocompromised patients while CMV immunoglobulin can be used in high-risk organ transplant patients. Additionally, ganciclovir and foscarnet are used in organ transplant patients and drug-resistant patients with HSV, VZV, and CMV [5].

In conclusion, human herpes viruses whose natural hosts are humans are found all over the world. Geographical location, socioeconomic level, and age are the main factors influencing the transmission of herpes virus infection [5, 10].

71.2 Herpes Simplex 1 and 2

HSV-1 is the prototype of the alphaherpesvirinae subfamily and is common across the world together with HSV-2, another member of the same subfamily [6]. They cause infections in mucocutaneous surfaces, central nervous system, and visceral organs. The most important characteristics of HSVs are that they are neurotropic and that they establish latency in sensory ganglia. They, therefore, cause recurrence and persistent infections with periodic reactivations. People infected with HSV-1 and HSV-2 may not show clinical symptoms during initial transmission or reactivation episodes. Once herpes simplex viruses lead to clinical symptoms, a wide spectrum of diseases can be observed, ranging from minor diseases such as herpes labialis (cold sores) to life-threatening conditions such as herpes simplex encephalitis or neonatal herpes simplex infection. Accordingly, the proper management of HSV-1 and HSV-2 infections depends on the clinical recognition of common and at times atypical syndromes caused by these viruses, the accurate application of the laboratory tests required to establish the diagnosis, and the early initiation of appropriate antiviral treatment [12, 13].

71.2.1 Etiology

HSVs are enveloped, double-stranded, linear DNA viruses approximately 160 nm in diameter (between 120–200 nm) [14, 15]. Complete DNA sequencing has revealed over 90% homology between HSV-1 and HSV-2. It has an icosahedral capsid consisting of 162 capsomeres, a tegument layer, and an envelope containing phospholipid-rich glycoproteins. These glycoproteins play an important role in the virulence of the virus. They are involved in the adhesion of the virus to the cell, its entry into the cell, and the expression of late genes. The binding of HSV to cell surface receptors starts the infection; subsequently, the HSV envelope fuses with the host cell plasma membrane. Thereafter, the viral capsid is carried to the nucleus where viral DNA is released [15]. Immediate early proteins consisting of six proteins regulate the replication cycle of the virus while also blocking the presentation of antigenic peptides on the cell surface. Early proteins contain enzymes primarily responsible for the synthesis of viral nucleic acids, such as thymidine kinase and DNA polymerase, which are also the main targets of antiviral therapy. Late proteins are those involved in the formation of capsid, tegument, and envelope [16].

In some neurons, HSV infection does not cause cell death and the cell continues to function normally. The viral genomes remain in the cell. This is called latent infection. In latency, RNAs encoded by a limited number of viruses are replicated. Over time, the viral genome can be reactivated which will lead to the release of the virus from infected neurons without causing significant damage. Viral replication starts when HSV exits neurons and re-enters capital cells. This is called reactivation. Enzymes called latency-associated transcript RNAs prevent reactivation [17, 18]. HSV maintains its viability for at least 48 h at 4 °C in liquids. It is not resistant to dry environments and is rapidly destroyed. It can survive for months at −70 °C and is inactivated by moist heat at 52 °C in 30 min and by dry heat at 90 °C in 30 min. Optimum pH values are between 5.5 and 9.5 [19].

71.2.2 Epidemiology

The only natural host for HSV is humans, and it is common worldwide. HSV infections are mostly asymptomatic or non-specific. Typically, the transmission of HSV-1 occurs orally while HSV-2 is transmitted through sexual contact. Routes of transmission are intimate and direct contact with infected secretions and sexual contact as well as perinatal transmission. Infection begins when the virus contacts the mucosal surfaces of the susceptible host such as the oropharynx, cervix, and conjunctiva or skin with compromised integrity. Because HSV becomes quickly inactivated at room temperature and in dry environments, airborne transmission is not possible [16, 17]. Primary infections start in the first years of life (between 6 months and 2 years of age) following the waning of maternal antibodies. Despite the formation of antibodies after recovery, the virus does not leave the organism. As a result, the host becomes a lifelong carrier [14]. Among healthy individuals, children from 6 months to 3 years of age are frequently observed to carry HSV-1 in the oral cavity [19]. HSV-1 antibody positivity is in direct proportion to age. More than 90% of adults up to 50 years of age are seropositive. On the other hand, HSV-1 antibody positivity is inversely proportional to socioeconomic status [17, 20]. Furthermore, HSV-2 antibody positivity starts emerging in puberty and increases with the onset of sexual activity. HSV-2 is twice as common in women as in men and is common among individuals with HIV and homosexual men. Co-infections of HSV-1 and HSV-2 are possible, although rare. Antibodies developed as a result of previous HSV-1 infection may provide protection against HSV-2, albeit to a lesser degree. Therefore, HSV-2 infection in the presence of HSV-1 infection is subclinical. However, whether or not HSV-2 antibodies protect HSV-1 is not yet known [17, 21].

HSV is a cause of high morbidity and mortality especially for neonates. If primary infection occurs before the 20th week of pregnancy, spontaneous abortion may occur. The most common route of transmission in neonates is the birth canal. On the other hand, transplacental or postnatal transmission is less common. Despite the very low incidence of neonatal infections, the issue is important because the mortality risk is higher than 50% and among surviving infants, 50% may develop severe sequelae. The mothers of 60% of infants with HSV infection do not demonstrate any HSV symptoms [17, 19, 21].

71.2.3 Pathogenesis and Pathology

Primary HSV infections are first-episode infections in susceptible individuals who have never been infected with HSV-1 or HSV-2. Primary HSV infections can be severe because patients are seronegative and have not previously developed immunity. In contrast, non-primary first-episode infection is when a person previously infected with one type of HSV becomes infected with the other type for the first time. Non-primary first infections may be milder as there may be even a low level of cross-immunity. Recurrent infections develop due to latent infection in the sensory ganglia and periodic reactivation of the latent infection. Recurrent infections may often be asymptomatic and nonetheless highly infectious [22]. The virus enters the body through epidermis and dermis cells on mucosal surfaces or skin with compromised integrity. The virus is attached to specific receptors on the cell membrane of the epidermis and dermis through the glycoproteins in its envelope, thereby entering the cell [16, 17]. HSV-1 and HSV-2 display marked tropism for cells of ectodermal origin such as skin and neural cells. The first viral replication happens here. In symptomatic primary infection cases, the incubation period can last between 2 and 20 days [23, 24]. After growth in the epidermis and dermis cells in the inoculation area, infection occurs in cutaneous sensory nerve endings. The viral nucleocapsid that reaches the nerve cell travels along the axon and reaches the cranial nerve and dorsal root ganglia. While HSV-1 most commonly involves the trigeminal nerve and cranial nerve ganglia, lumbosacral ganglia are involved in genital herpes infections. In cases of cranial nerve ganglia involvement, infection may also spread to the superior and inferior cervical ganglia. A second replication and latent infection occurs in the dorsal root ganglia [16, 17, 21]. The latency of HSV-1 and HSV-2 in neural cells can be revealed by the identification of latency-associated transcripts (LAT). LAT is the only highly expressed viral gene product during latent infection. It is a non-protein coding RNA that strongly regulates HSV-1 gene expression [25]. Some animal models have shown that LAT is needed for the establishment of latent infection and the actualization of efficient viral reactivation [26].

Latent infection persists for life and in some circumstances may turn into cytolytic infection. They cannot be eradicated by currently available antiviral medications or by the host's immune response. Since latency means no virus replication, DNA synthesis, which is the main target of antiviral therapy, does not occur, hence the inefficiency of drugs. In latent infection, the HSV genomes are kept latent in the cell nucleus in episomal or extrachromosomal form, and this is how the host cell survives [16, 19, 27].

Like the mechanism of latency, the mechanism of reactivation of primary HSV infection has not been fully revealed. When reactivation is triggered, HSV-1 and HSV-2 travel along the axons to the periphery and reach the mucocutaneous areas. The latent virus goes into the reactivation phase when nerve cells are stimulated by internal and external influences such as infection, hormones, and nutrition; mechanical factors such as trauma, UV radiation, and sunlight; hormonal factors such as menstruation and emotional stress, and stimuli such as epinephrine and corticosteroids that are dependent on or independent from hormonal factors; altered immune response; and decreased nerve growth factor. Whether or not the clinical disease will occur in recurrent infections after the reactivation depends on the immunity of the host. Recurrent infection may lead to the formation of vesicles on a wider area compared to the primary infection. It is found that recurrent HSV infection is localized to the original site, not to the original skin [16, 17]. When the virus starts replicating in the epithelial cells at the site of re-inoculation in case of recurrence, it causes pathological changes in these cells and leads to destruction. Infected cells are characterized by cytoplasmic enlargement, ballooning degeneration, nuclear chromatin condensation, and eosinophilic intranuclear inclusions. Plasma membrane degeneration in infected cells leads to cell fusion and multinucleated giant cell formation. Because of the local inflammatory response, intracellular edema develops, and vesicles form between the epidermis and dermis. These vesicles contain large amounts of virus, cell debris, and inflammatory cells. As the vesicles enlarge, they become visible and are surrounded by an erythematous border. Lesions of mucosal membranes are more ulcerative than skin lesions. This is because the epithelium on mucosal surfaces is thinner and therefore ruptures more easily. In the later stages of the disease, vesicles turn into pustules, and thereafter they dry and scab over. HSV lesions are typically superficial and do not leave scarring [9, 13].

In cases of primary HSV infection, a cellular and humoral immune response develops in symptomatic patients shortly after the outbreak of lesions. Some human and animal studies have revealed that a normal host attempts to limit the infection by use of non-specific immune mechanisms. Virus-specific adaptive immunity then follows [28]. Non-specific immune response consists of the mobilization of polymorphonuclear leukocytes and monocytes to the site of infection, the release of interferon-gamma and other cytokines, and the activation of macrophages and NK cells. Among the cytokines, IL-2 in particular plays a role in early defense. Antibodies that have been produced following the initial immune response can still be detected 2–12 weeks after the development of infection [29]. Viruses residing in the ganglia of the sensory nerves are prevented from reaching the central nervous system, again thanks to the immune response. B lymphocytes and helper and cytotoxic T cells limit the growth of the virus in the central nervous system. $CD8^+$ T lymphocytes exert their effects by releasing interferon-gamma and granzyme B from the ganglia, which is crucial since the cellular immune response is more important in HSV infections. HSV-2 reactivation occurs frequently in cases where $CD8^+$ T lymphocyte response is absent or lower than $CD4^+$ T lymphocyte response. Additionally, the course of the disease is more severe [30, 31]. Cell-mediated virus-specific immunodeficiency may lead to life-threatening disseminated HSV-1 and HSV-2 infections in neonates, children with genetic immunodeficiencies, immunocompromised children, organ transplant recipients, or high-risk populations such as people with HIV. Disseminated HSV infection spreads to multiple organs such as the lung, liver, and brain, leading to cell destruction and progressing with multiple organ hyperinflammation causing massive apoptosis. It results in Systemic inflammatory response syndrome (SIRS) with lethal consequences [29].

The most serious HSV infection is viral encephalitis for which HSV-1 is the most common etiology. Here the pathological mechanism is the ascending spread of infection from the cranial nerves to the brain via neural pathways. Encephalitis may occur together with primary infection as well as developing after primary infection or with reactivation of latent virus. Hematogenous transmission of the virus to the central nervous system is observed only in neonates. Upon reaching brain parenchyma cells, the virus triggers widespread hemorrhagic necrosis and vascular compromise. Activated glial cells such as astrocytes and microglia enable the production of cytokines and chemokines in response to HSV infection. Neuroimmune response to infection contributes to the development of inflammation and sequelae in the brain [32]. Acute phase reactants including beta-2 microglobulin, neopterin, IL-6, and interferon-gamma are observed to increase in the cerebrospinal fluid [33, 34]. On the other hand, elevated levels of soluble CD8, beta microglobulin, neopterin, and specific anti-HSV IgG have been detected in the convalescent period. Studies with a small number of pediatric patients with herpes encephalitis showed that they lacked signal transducer and activator of transcription-1 (STAT-1), UNC93B, Toll-like receptor-3 (TLR3), TNF receptor-associated factor-3 (TRAF3) and experienced nuclear factor-κβ (NF-κβ) mutations [35–37]. Furthermore, a number of genetic studies reported that in some pediatric patients with childhood HSV encephalitis, although sporadic, Mendelian—especially autosomal recessive—transmission was suspected [38]. HSV infection spreads from cell to cell in the presence of antibodies against virus tegument, capsid, and surface glycoproteins. Antibody-dependent cell-mediated cytotoxicity is a vital mechanism of destruction of HSV-infected cells; however, HSV infections are severe in neonates because the mechanism has not fully developed in individuals in this age group [17, 19].

HSV infections are also associated with the development of malignancy. HSV-2 is associated with cervical cancer and seroepidemiological studies have found high antibody titers against HSV-2 in women with cervical dysplasia and carcinoma in situ [19].

71.2.4 Herpes Simplex Virus Infections

71.2.4.1 Herpetic Gingivostomatitis

Gingivostomatitis is the most common HSV-related primary infection in children. While both HSV-1 and HSV-2 may be the etiologic agents, it is most frequently caused by HSV-1. It is typically observed in children between 6 months and 5 years of age. However, it can also be seen in adults. The disease is symptomatic in 10–30% of cases. In symptomatic cases, the disease continues for 5–12 days after an incubation period of 3–5 days on average. Symptoms include tenderness, burning, and pain in the lesion area; difficulty in eating; malaise; fever up to 40 °C; vesicles on the gingiva, hard and soft palate, oral mucosa, and tongue. Painful cervical lymphadenopathies may also be observed [9, 39, 40] (Fig. 71.1). The analysis of HSV DNA in whole blood or plasma by PCR in children with HSV-1 gingivostomatitis

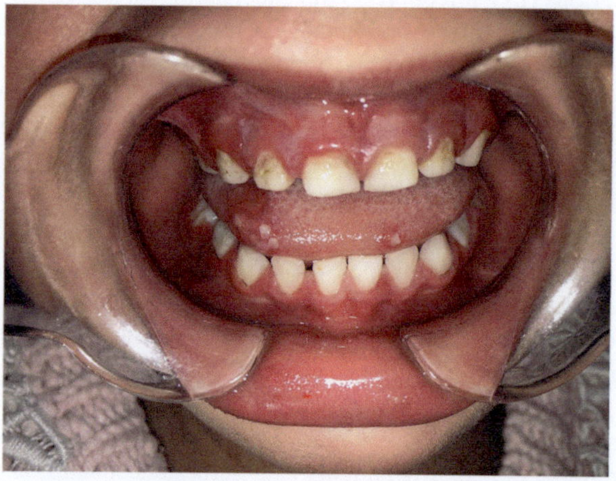

Fig. 71.1 Herpetic gingivostomatitis with vesicles on tongue due to herpes simplex virus type 1. (Picture taken from the archive of Rahime Koca, MD)

showed positivity in one-third of the patients [41]. Vesicles rupture in a short time and painful superficial ulcers develop on the oral mucosa and gingiva. The most typical manifestation is acute gingivitis characterized by erythema and edema. In healthy individuals, fever resolves in 2–7 days on average, but it may take up to 14 days for complete resolution of all symptoms [20] (Fig. 71.2).

Herpetic epiglottitis, acute otitis media, and hepatitis are not very common complications. On the other hand, transverse myelitis and acute disseminated encephalomyelitis are complications that may follow herpetic gingivostomatitis [13, 42].

A differential diagnosis should be made by considering herpangina and hand, foot, and mouth disease caused by enteroviruses, impetigo caused by *Staphylococcus aureus* and beta-hemolytic streptococci, and Steven-Johnson Syndrome (erythema multiforme) [13, 43].

71.2.4.2 Herpes Labialis

Herpes simplex labialis (cold sores) is the most common recurrent HSV-1 infection. Recurrent HSV-1 infections have a shorter and milder course compared to primary infections. Lesions are typically unilateral as reactivation usually develops from a single latent source. While they most commonly occur on the vermillion border of

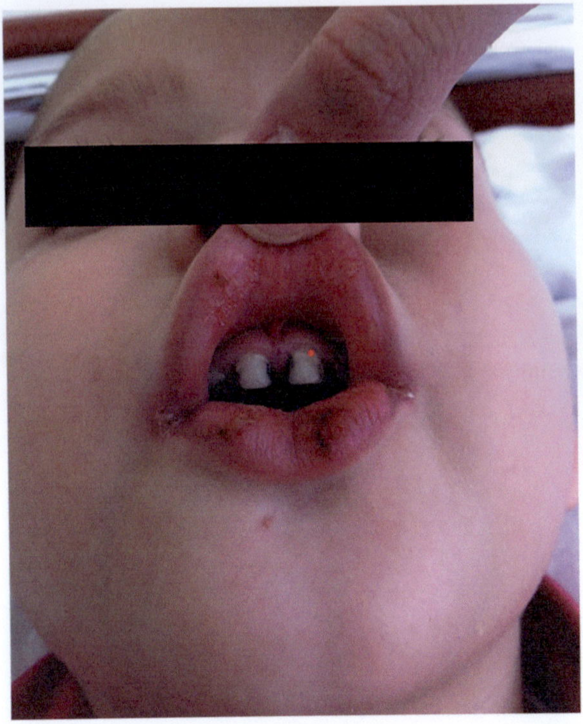

Fig. 71.2 Toddler with orolabial lesions of herpetic gingivostomatitis and herpes labialis. (Picture taken from the archive of Bilge Aldemir Kocabaş, MD)

the lip, lesions may also be observed on the nose, nasal septum, chin, and cheek [14, 22]. Infection frequently develops after exposure to stimuli such as fever, menstruation, dental procedures affecting the trigeminal nerve, sunlight, and UV rays. Vesicular lesions appear after the burning, pain, and itching on the lips that occur in the first 3–6 h. Vesicles turn first into pustules, then ulcerated lesions, and eventually, in 72–96 h, scabs (Fig. 71.3). The virus remains contagious until the lesions heal. Healing occurs in 8–10 days on average without scarring [9, 14, 16, 17, 39, 40].

71.2.4.3 Tonsillopharyngitis, Epiglottitis, Supraglottitis, Laryngotracheitis

In older children and adolescents, primary HSV-1 infection usually presents as ulcerative, exudative tonsillopharyngitis. It may involve dysphagia, sore throat, and high fever. Typically, vesicles on the posterior pharyngeal wall and tonsils rupture and cause the formation of ulcers and gray exudates. In healthy individuals, fever resolves in 2–7 days and patients recover completely in 14 days. Under normal conditions, there is no sequelae after the infection [20, 44]. In studies conducted on college students from high socioeconomic status backgrounds, HSV has been shown to be the most common cause of acute pharyngitis with an

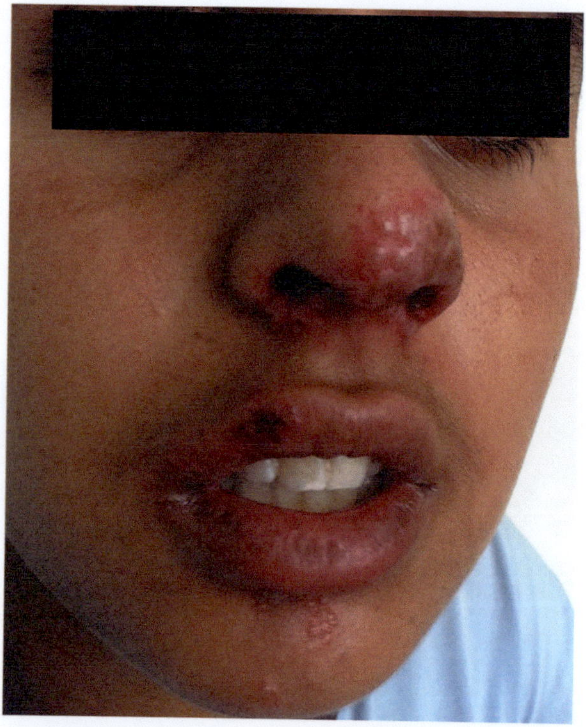

Fig. 71.3 Herpes labialis with ulcerated and pustular lesions on orolabial region and nose. (Picture taken from the archive of Bilge Aldemir Kocabaş, MD)

incidence ranging from 5 to 24% [44, 45]. In some cases, the etiologic agent of acute pharyngitis is HSV-2 while symptoms and clinical course are similar to those of HSV-1. Virus isolation and culture or PCR tests are required to differentiate the virus type [46]. Differential diagnosis includes streptococcal and EBV infections, diphtheria, HIV, and pharyngitis due to tularemia, although the last three are rare [45].

Acute, prolonged, atypical laryngotracheitis or herpetic croup can develop due to HSV-1 and HSV-2 at all ages in healthy or immunocompromised patients. In such cases, symptoms usually do not respond to steroid treatment. Diagnosis then is made by using appropriate viral HSV culture and PCR or tissue immunohistochemistry for HSV antigens obtained with laryngoscopy. Herpetic epiglottitis is also a rare clinical manifestation in neonates and older children [47].

In immunocompromised patients, the infection may spread under the mucosa and into deeper tissues. In such cases, HSV and candida infection often coexist. The use of systemic acyclovir accelerates recovery. Moreover, HSV-1 and varicella zoster virus infections have been implicated as common causes of Bell's palsy. Antiviral treatment is also recommended in such cases [48].

71.2.4.4 Other Cutaneous Infections

Other cutaneous infections include herpes infections in healthy children and adolescents which are usually caused by inoculation of infected secretions into sites of skin trauma such as a small cut or abrasion (Fig. 71.4).

In herpetic whitlow, lesions are generally found on the terminal phalanx including the nailbed, and the affected finger is characterized by edema, erythema, and localized tenderness. Vesicular and pustular lesions develop [17, 19]. In neonates and infants with symptomatic or subclinical oral HSV-1 infection, autoinoculation is observed especially due to finger sucking and nail biting [22, 49]. In adolescents and older children, however, autoinoculation develops due to genital secretions during the first episode of HSV-2 infection [50]. Lymphadenitis and axillary lymphadenopathy are common, and surgical intervention is contraindicated [9]. Contrary to other recurrent herpes infections, recurrent herpetic whitlow has a course as painful as primary infection. In primary infection, complete recovery takes 18–20 days. The course of the disease is shorter in recurrent infections [22].

Herpes gladiatorum, which is more common in adolescent and high school athletes and wrestlers, is a form of HSV-1 infection characterized by vesicular lesions on hands, shoulders, face, and trunk. Healing occurs within 6–10 days without scarring [19, 22, 51].

Eczema herpeticum, which develops in case of thermal or chemical burns, diaper dermatitis, and skin damage caused by atopic dermatitis, is a form of herpes with a potential for a serious course due to rapidly spreading vesicles and the risk of visceral disseminated infection [9].

In studies with patients having recurrent erythema multiforme, also a skin disease, skin biopsies demonstrated HSV antigen (HSV type-common glycoprotein antigen) in approximately 75% of cases [48, 52].

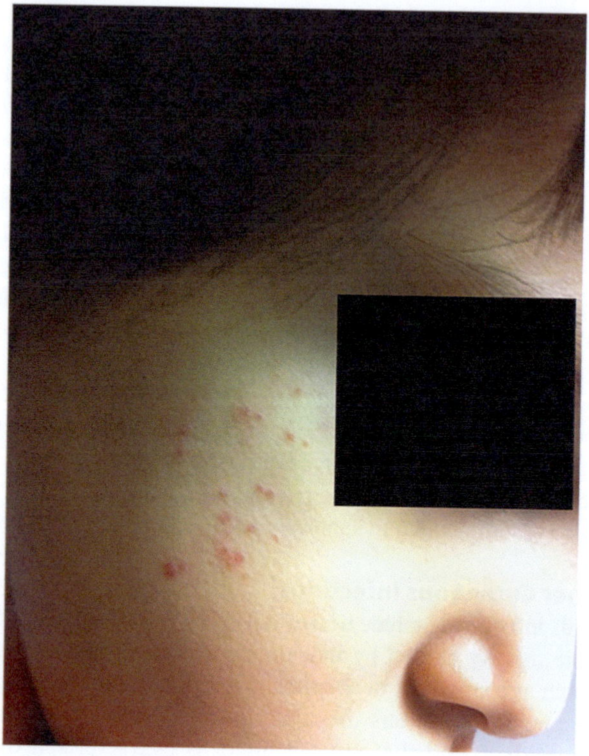

Fig. 71.4 Herpetic lesions on cheek after a skin trauma. (Picture taken from the archive of Bilge Aldemir Kocabaş, MD)

71.2.4.5 Eye Infections

The most significant cause of corneal blindness is HSV infection in the eye [17]. HSV-1 is the etiologic agent in most cases with the exception of neonates. Eye infections caused by HSV-2 tend to have a more severe course [14]. Conjunctivitis or keratoconjunctivitis is often unilateral and is accompanied by blepharitis and unilateral preauricular lymphadenopathy [22]. Infections may be primary or occur as a result of reactivation from the trigeminal ganglion. Acute pain in the eye, blurred vision, and dendritic lesions in the cornea are observed. While it first presents as diffuse punctate keratitis, later a diffuse scattered microdendritic appearance develops. In primary ocular herpes infection, if there are no herpetic vesicles on the skin, the presence of herpetic vesicles on the eyelid provides differentiation from other viral keratoconjunctivitis. Spontaneous recovery without any corneal sequelae typically occurs within 14–21 days. Topical antiviral use combined with interferon therapy or debridement accelerates healing. Recurrence is common, and attacks may present with pain, chemosis, excessive tearing, loss of vision, and photophobia [17, 19]. Identified in neonates or immunocompromised patients, chorioretinitis is usually observed in individuals with disseminated HSV infections [14].

71.2.4.6 Genital Herpes Infections

Genital HSV infections are seen in adolescents and young adults but are rare in infants and children. Almost 90% of infections go undetected. As viral shedding continues in symptomatic and asymptomatic individuals, pregnant women can transmit the virus to their newborns or sexual partners to each other. In primary genital herpes infections, a brief prodromal period of local burning and pain may precede the development of vesicular lesions on the genital mucosal surfaces, keratinized skin, or anus. Vesicles on mucosal surfaces rupture to form painful ulcers. Yellow-grayish exudates are visible on the surface of the ulcers and they spread on an erythematous surface. In a few days, vesicles turn into pustules, and then crusts develop on them. Patients may present with urethritis, dysuria, urinary retention, and inguinal and pelvic lymphadenopathy [16, 17, 22]. 15% of patients may develop aseptic meningitis with systemic symptoms including fever, headache, and myalgia accompanying local symptoms [22]. Primary genital herpes resolves in 14–21 days. Genital HSV infections increase the risk of being infected with HIV. Despite being rare, pediatric genital HSV infections may develop due to autoinoculation or sexual abuse. Transverse myelitis, disseminated infection, extragenital lesions, and superinfections are other complications resulting from genital herpes infections [17, 21].

71.2.4.7 Central Nervous System Infections

HSV is the most common cause of sporadic, non-epidemic, fatal encephalitis in children and adults in developed countries. It accounts for approximately 10–20% of viral encephalitis. HSV-1 is the causative agent in more than 95% of cases. Self-limited aseptic meningitis can also follow primary infections of genital HSV infections. Clinical symptoms of encephalitis are severe with a mortality rate of 75% [22, 53, 54]. It is an acute necrotizing infection involving mostly the temporal lobe but also the limbic system and the orbital region of the frontal lobe [22]. Hemorrhagic encephalitis is suggestive to HSV encephalitis since it leads to tissue damage in a manner that also affects the vascular walls. Typically, the virus reaches the CNS by neurotropic spread from the periphery via the olfactory bulb. It can either spread from the infected nasopharyngeal mucosa through the cribriform plate or reach the central nervous system during latent HSV reactivation in the trigeminal or autonomic nerve roots. Hematogenous spread may also be seen in disseminated infections [13, 48, 55]. Infection may begin with non-specific symptoms such as fever, nausea, vomiting, generalized seizures, confusion, and neck stiffness. More specific symptoms indicating temporal and frontal lobe involvement such as speech impairment and aphasia, hallucinations, focal seizures, behavioral changes, and anosmia may also be observed [22]. When it comes to diagnosis, MR (magnetic resonance) is a more sensitive imaging technique and provides findings in the earlier period. Paroxysmal lateralized epileptiform discharges (PLEDs) are a finding characteristic of HSV encephalitis seen in EEG (electroencephalogram) [56]. In the cerebrospinal fluid, there may be a mild increase in protein levels in the first week followed by more serious elevation, mild increases in polymorphonuclear leukocytes and mononuclear cells, and a mild decrease in glucose. Erythrocyte levels in CSF may also be elevated [22]. HSV-specific antibody production starts in CSF from the second week of the disease. Detection of HSV DNA in CSF by PCR is the most sensitive method for the diagnosis [55]. HSV is also the most common cause of recurrent aseptic meningitis (Mollaret's meningitis). It may also be identified as the causative agent of many other neurological syndromes including atypical pain syndromes, trigeminal neuralgia, vestibular neuritis, temporal lobe epilepsy, and acute disseminated encephalomyelitis [57].

71.2.4.8 Perinatal Herpes Infections

In the neonatal period, HSV infections can be transmitted in the birth canal during labor or in utero. Congenital herpes infection due to intrauterine transmission is rare. Congenital infection cases present symptoms resulting from cutaneous, ocular, and central nervous system involvement. Skin manifestations include scarring and active vesicles; ocular findings include chorioretinitis, keratoconjunctivitis, and microphthalmia while central nervous system findings include microcephaly and hydrocephalus [22, 58]. In the postpartum period, infection can be transmitted from the mother or another adult via non-genital contact as in the case of herpes labialis, and the causative agent is often HSV-1.

Neonatal herpes develops largely as a result of contact of the child with infected secretions from the mother with asymptomatic genital herpes infection in the birth canal. The risk of neonatal infection is associated with the mother's HSV antibody rate at the time of delivery [17, 59]. The risk of transmission of infection to the neonate varies between 30 and 50% in women who had the primary infection within 6 weeks before delivery while the rate of transmission is 1% in women who had the first episode of infection in the first half of pregnancy. The risk of infection has been reported as lower than 2% in recurrent HSV infections. The risk of infection drops significantly in cesarean section without rupture of the membrane [17, 19, 22].

The causative agent in neonatal herpes infections is HSV-2 with a 70% rate. Neonatal herpes mainly presents with three types of infection [17].

1. Skin, Eyes, and Mouth Disease (SEM): This type accounts for 45% of all cases. It is characterized by vesicles on the erythematous base and conjunctivitis. It is seen in the first 5–11 days. Vesicles mostly develop in trauma sites such as the scalp or inside the mouth in neonates. If left untreated, encephalitis or disseminated infection develops in 80% of cases. Treatment prevents mortality [22, 60, 61].
2. Encephalitis: It accounts for 30% of all neonatal herpes cases [60]. It is seen in the first 14–21 days and presents with lethargy, irritability, fever, loss of tonus, and seizures. Mortality rate is 5% and 50% with treatment and without treatment, respectively [62].
3. Disseminated Infection: It constitutes 25% of cases [60]. It is seen in the first 5–11 days and may be mistaken for bacterial sepsis. Symptoms include hyperthermia, hypothermia, irritability, cyanosis, apnea, respiratory failure, bleeding, hepatomegaly, cardiovascular failure, and seizures. The disease progresses rapidly. If treatment is not administered, disseminated intravascular coagulopathy (DIC) develops. Patients die due to shock, DIC, and viral pneumonia.

Mortality rate is 30% and about 90% with treatment and without treatment, respectively. Severe neurological sequelae may develop in surviving infants [17, 22, 48, 61].

71.2.4.9 Herpes Infections in Immunodeficient Patients

HSV infection is common in patients infected with HIV. It is particularly associated with HSV-2. HSV-2 infection may increase mother-to-child transmission of HIV [17]. The rate of development of disseminated HSV infection in children who underwent organ transplantation, renal in particular, was found to be 25%. Moreover, the rate of development of disseminated HSV in children who received bone marrow is 10% [13, 63, 64]. HSV infections are also common in individuals with burns and in children receiving cancer treatment. Infections in the liver, kidney, lung, bone marrow, and gastrointestinal system may develop along with disseminated mucocutaneous infections [17]. Esophageal, tracheal, and pulmonary involvement is seen as a result of severe diffuse ulcerations caused by HSV on keratinized and non-keratinized mucosal surfaces [65]. HSV pneumonia may occur following dissemination or aspiration of tracheobronchial or esophageal infection. This type of pneumonia may be focal or multifocal. Interstitial infiltrations result from hematogenous spread of HSV infection in other areas.

In immunosuppressed individuals, necrotizing hepatitis with high mortality can be observed [19, 48].

71.2.5 Laboratory Findings and Diagnosis

Detection of HSV infections in neonatal and pediatric populations through the use of diagnostic techniques is especially important to prevent mortality and morbidity. Virus isolation and detection of viral DNA by PCR are the most sensitive methods. Histological findings and imaging methods support the diagnosis but are not diagnostic.

Cytological examinations can show giant cells and intranuclear inclusions in samples obtained from the lesion site through Wright's, Giemsa, or Papanicolaou's staining methods or the Tzanck test, albeit non-specific [19, 22].

Virus isolation and subsequent cell culture is the most specific method in the diagnosis of active HSV infection [9, 66]. Various factors influence the success of virus isolation. Isolation from vesicular lesions proves more successful than isolation from lesions in the ulcerative phase. A swab sample should be collected from the base of the skin lesion or the contents of an intact vesicle should be aspirated. Chances of isolation are better in primary infections compared to recurrent infections. There is a higher chance of isolation in immunocompromised patients as virus antigen release is greater. HSV grows by cytopathic effect in 18–72 h in cell culture prepared with the eligible sample. The agent grown is identified by a neutralization test using specific antiserum or immunohistochemical staining which is the most common method [19, 67, 68].

With regards to central nervous system involvement in HSV, especially in HSV encephalitis, the gold standard diagnostic method is the detection of HSV DNA in CSF by PCR. PCR method is also used in blood and swab samples [19, 21, 55, 69].

For the diagnosis of HSV infection, antibodies formed during infection can also be detected by various methods such as neutralization, passive hemagglutination, Radioimmunoassay (RIA), ELISA, and antibody-dependent cellular cytolysis. IgM and IgG antibodies begin to form on days 4–7 of primary infection and reach the highest level in weeks 2–4. Then, their titers start decreasing. Generally, IgM antibodies disappear within 4–6 months. IgG antibodies, on the other hand, remain positive throughout the host's lifetime, despite their low titers. Determination of the type of HSV is needed for clinical and epidemiologic differentiation. Serological methods cannot be used for type differentiation. Western blot method has over 98% sensitivity and specificity in differentiating anti-HSV-1 and anti-HSV-2 antibodies. In primary infection, a four-fold titer increase in IgM antibodies in acute and convalescent period sera enables the diagnosis of HSV even though type differentiation cannot be made [17, 19, 21].

71.2.6 Treatment

Currently, none of the drugs used for HSV infection can eradicate the infection. The antivirals used for treatment are mainly acyclovir, famciclovir, and valacyclovir. Valacyclovir is the prodrug of acyclovir while famciclovir is the prodrug of penciclovir. Acyclovir has low oral bioavailability and is administered in frequent doses. On the other hand, valacyclovir and famciclovir have high oral bioavailability and can be given once daily or twice daily during treatment. Only acyclovir is available as a suspension and an intravenous drug. Penciclovir and acyclovir are available in topical forms. Drug resistance to acyclovir and penciclovir is observed in immunosuppressed patients; foscarnet or cidofovir is employed in treatment in such cases [22, 48].

Acyclovir is first converted into acyclovir monophosphate by viral thymidine kinase in the infected cell and then further converted into acyclovir triphosphate by secondary and tertiary phosphorylation by host cell enzymes. Acyclovir triphosphate works by suppressing DNA polymerase. It binds to the replicating DNA strand, thereby preventing the completion of the strand. It is therefore only effective in active infections and does not work in case of latent infection. Ganciclovir is also one of the antivirals effective against HSV-1 and HSV-2 and is used topically in herpes keratitis because of its high toxicity compared to others [48].

In gingivostomatitis, treatment initiated within the first 72 h of the disease with a regimen of oral acyclovir 15 mg/kg/dose 5 times/day for 7 days reduces the duration and severity of the disease. In the treatment of recurrent herpes labialis in adolescents, the following regimens may be applied: oral valacyclovir 2000 mg 1 day peroral; acyclovir 200–400 mg 5 times/day peroral for 5 days; famciclovir 1500 mg one dose 1 day. Treatment reduces the duration of recurrent infection. Long-term prophylactic oral acyclovir or valacyclovir treatment can be administered in patients with severe and frequent recurrent episodes.

Oral acyclovir and valacyclovir are given perorally also in other cutaneous infections to reduce the recurrence and severity of the disease. High-dose acyclovir (1600–2000 mg/day peroral divided into 2–3 doses for 10 days) is administered to treat herpetic whitlow.

HSV infections can be severe in patients with burns for whom intravenous acyclovir (10–20 mg/kg/day divided into doses over 8 h) is used in therapy.

Despite the fact that antiviral drugs are not effective in the treatment of HSV-associated erythema multiforme, daily use of these for herpes labialis prophylaxis prevents erythema multiforme attacks.

Primary genital herpes in pediatric patients is treated with antiviral agents (acyclovir, valacyclovir, famciclovir) [22].

In ocular infections, topical trifluridine is used together with topical ganciclovir. In neonates, parenteral treatment is combined with topical treatment. Oral acyclovir prophylaxis has been observed to decrease scarring in the long term in recurrent keratitis [70].

In HSV encephalitis, a dose of 10–15 mg/kg of intravenous acyclovir is given as a 1-h infusion every 8 h for 14–21 days in children aged 3 months to 12 years. On the other hand, in children over 12 years of age, a dose of 10 mg/kg every 8 h is recommended [71].

Severe disseminated and mucocutaneous infections in immunodeficient patients are treated with intravenous acyclovir. 30 mg/kg is administered in three divided doses for 7–14 days.

In perinatal infections, however, all infants with suspected neonatal HSV infection should be treated with high-dose intravenous acyclovir. Treatment is planned to include 60 mg/kg/day every 8 h. Neutrophil levels and renal function should be followed and monitored. Treatment lasts 14 days in skin, eyes, and mouth disease and 21 days in disseminated and central nervous system infections. Suppressive oral acyclovir treatment for 6 months after the completion of intravenous treatment prevents recurrence and improves neural development [22].

71.2.7 Prevention

Avoiding contact with people with HSV-associated lesions reduces the risk of transmission; however, the virus can still spread through saliva and urethral and cervical secretions from some asymptomatic individuals. Partners with active genital lesions or a history of HSV infection should use condoms during sexual intercourse. Considering the high mortality and morbidity of neonatal infection, measures should be adopted to prevent transmission, especially during delivery [14, 17, 19]. Recombinant virus glycoproteins, DNA-based vaccines, and infected cell extracts have been studied in many HSV vaccine trials. However, there is still no vaccine with proven efficacy to protect oneself against HSV infections and to prevent transmission, reactivation, and latency [72, 73].

References

1. Szpara ML, Gatherer D, Ochoa A, Greenbaum B, et al. Evolution and diversity in human herpes simplex virus genomes. J Virol. 2014;88:1209–27.
2. Pellet PE, Roizman B. The family Herpesviridae: a brief introduction. In: Knipe DM, Howley PM, editors. Fields virology. 5th ed. Philadelphia: Lippincott Williams and Wilkins; 2005. p. 2479.
3. Davison AJ. Herpesvirüs systematics. Vet Microbiol. 2010;143:52–69.
4. Pellett PE, Roizman B, et al. Herpesviridae. In: Knipe DM, Howley PM, Cohen JI, editors. Fields virology, vol. 2. 6th ed. Philadelphia: Lippincott Williams and Wilkins; 2013. p. 1802–22.
5. Cohen JI. Introduction to Herpesviridae. In: Bennett JE, Dolin R, Blaser MJ, editors. Mandell, Douglas, and Bennett's principle and practice of infectious diseases. 8th ed. Philadelphia: Elsevier Saunders; 2015. p. 1707.
6. Shukla D, Spear PG. Herpesviruses and heparan sulfate: an intimate relationship in aid of viral entry. J Clin Invest. 2001;108:503–10.
7. http://orbi.ulg.ac.be/bitstream/2268/135768/1/INTRO_S.FRANCOIS.pdf.
8. Eisenberg RJ, Atanasiu D, Cairns TM, Gallagher JR, et al. Herpes virus fusion and entry: a story with many characters. Viruses. 2012;4:800–32.
9. Prober CG, Kimberlin DW. Herpes simplex virus. In: Long SS, Prober CG, Fischer M, editors. Principle and a practice of pediatric infectious diseases. 5th ed. Elsevier; 2018. p. 5481–525.
10. Hengel H. Common characteristics and distinct features of human pathogenic Herpesviruses. In: Sundmacher R, editor. Color atlas of herpetic eye disease: a practical guide to clinical management. Berlin: Springer Science & Business Media; 2009. https://doi.org/10.1007/978-3-540-694463-2_1.
11. Hasdemir MU. Herpes Virüslerin Genel Özellikleri. In: Topçu AW, Söyletir G, Doğanay M, editors. Enfeksiyon Hastalıkları ve Mikrobiyolojisi. 3rd ed. Nobel Tıp Kitapevleri: İstanbul; 2008. p. 1174.
12. Roizman B, Knipe DM, Whitley RJ. Herpes simplex viruses. In: Knipe DM, Howley PM, editors. Fields' virology. 5th ed. Lippincott Williams and Wilkins: Philadelphia; 2007. p. 2502.
13. Harrison GJ, Pinsky AB, Arvin AM. Herpes simplex viruses 1 and 2. In: Cherry JD, Harrison GJ, Kaplan SL, Steinbach WJ, Hotez PJ, editors. Feigin and Cherry's textbook of pediatric infectious diseases, vol. 1. 8th ed. Elsevier; 2019. p. 1403–29.
14. Demirdağ K, Denk A. Herpes Simpleks Virüs Enfeksiyonları. In: Kurt H, Gündeş S, Geyik MF, editors. Enfeksiyon Hastalıkları. İstanbul: Nobel Tıp Kitabevleri; 2016. p. 154–7.
15. Roizman B, Knipe DM, Whitley RJ. Herpes simplex viruses. In: Knipe D, Howley P, Cohen JI, editors. Fields virology, vol. 2. 6th ed. Philadelphia: Lippincott Williams and Wilkins; 2013. p. 1823–97.
16. Whitley RJ, Roizman B. Herpes simplex virüs infections. Lancet. 2001;357:1513–8.
17. Schiffer JT, Corey L. Herpes simplex virus. In: Mandell GL, Bennet JE, Dolin R, editors. Principles and practice of infectious diseases. 7th ed. Philadelphia: Churchill Livingstone; 2010. p. 1943.
18. Yoshikawa T, Hill JM, Stanberry LR, et al. The characteristic site-specific reactivation phenotypes of HSV-1 and HSV-2 depend upon latency-associated transcript region. J Exp Med. 1996;184:659.
19. Serter D. Herpes Simpleks Virüsleri (HSV-1 ve HSV-2). In: Topçu AW, Söyletir G, Doğanay M, editors. Enfeksiyon Hastalıkları ve Mikrobiyolojisi. 3rd ed. Nobel Tıp Kitapevleri: İstanbul; 2008. p. 1655–66.
20. Simmons A. Clinical manifestations and treatment considerations of herpes simplex virus infection. J Infect Dis. 2002;186(Suppl 1):71–7.
21. Jawetz M. Adelberg's medical microbiology. In: Brooks GF, Butel JS, Morse SA, editors. Herpes simplex viruses. 23rd ed. McGraw Hill Comp. Inc. Lange; 2004. p. 429.

22. Stanberry LR. Herpes simplex virus. In: Kliegman RM, St Geme III JW, Blum NJ, Shah SS, Tasker RC, Wilson KM, Behrman RE, editors. Nelson textbook of pediatrics. 21st ed. Elsevier; 2020. p. 1701–8.
23. Halperin SA, Shehab Z, Thacker D, et al. Absence of viremia in primary herpetic gingivostomatitis. Pediatr Infect Dis. 1983;2:452–3.
24. Stanberry LR, Floyd-Reising SA, Connelly BL, et al. Herpes simplex viremia: report of eight pediatric cases and review of the literature. Clin Infect Dis. 1994;18:401–40.
25. Nicoll MP, Hann W, Shivkumar M, Harman LE, Connor V, Coleman HM, Proença JT, Efstathiou S. The HSV-1 latency associated transcript functions to repress latent phase lytic gene expression and suppress virus reactivation from latently infected neurons. PLoS Pathog. 2016;12(4):e1005539. https://doi.org/10.1371/journal.ppat.1005539.
26. Perng GC, Dunkel EC, Geary PA, et al. The latency-associated gene of herpes simplex virus type 1 (HSV-1) is required for efficient in vivo spontaneous reactivation of HSV-1 from latency. J Virol. 1994;68:8045–55.
27. Lycke E. The pathogenesis of genital herpes simplex virus infection. Scand J Infect Dis. 1991;78(suppl):7.
28. Koelle DM, Corey L. Recent progress in herpes simplex virus immunobiology and vaccine research. Clin Microbiol Rev. 2003;16:96–113.
29. Nagamori T, Koyano S, Asai Y, et al. Sequential changes in pathophysiology of systemic inflammatory response in a disseminated neonatal herpes simplex virus (HSV) infection. J Clin Virol. 2012;53(3):265–7.
30. Manickan E, Rouse BT. Roles of different T-cell subsets in control of herpes simplex virus infection determined by using T-cell-deficient mouse models. J Virol. 1995;69:8178–9.
31. Hoshino Y, Pesnicak L, Cohen JI, et al. Rates of reactivation of latent herpes simplex virus from mouse trigeminal ganglia ex vivo correlate directly with viral load and inversely with number of infiltrating CD8+ T cells. J Virol. 2007;81:8157–64.
32. Lokensgard JR, Cheeran MC, Hu S, et al. Glial cell responses to herpesvirus infections: role in defense and immunopathogenesis. J Infect Dis. 2002;186(suppl 2):171–S179.
33. Aurelius E, Andersson B, Forsgren M, et al. Cytokines and other markers of intrathecal immune response in patients with herpes simplex encephalitis. J Infect Dis. 1994;170:678–80.
34. Aurelius E, Forsgren M, Skoldenberg B, et al. Persistent intrathecal immune activation in patients with herpes simplex encephalitis. J Infect Dis. 1993;168:1248–52.
35. Audry M, Ciancanelli M, Yang K, et al. NEMO is a key component of NF-κβ- and IRF-3-dependent TLR3-mediated immunity to herpes simplex virus. J Allergy Clin Immunol. 2011;128:610–7.
36. Casrouge A, Zhang SY, Eidenschenk C, et al. Herpes simplex virus encephalitis in human UNC-93B deficiency. Science. 2006;314:308–12.
37. Zhang SY, Jouanguy E, Ugolini S, et al. TLR3 deficiency in patients with herpes simplex encephalitis. Science. 2007;317:1522–7.
38. Abel L, Plancoulaine S, Jouanguy E, et al. Age-dependent Mendelian predisposition to herpes simplex virus type 1 encephalitis in childhood. J Pediatr. 2010;157:623–9.
39. Nadelman CM, Newcomer VD. Herpes simplex virus infections. Postgrad Med. 2000;107:189–200.
40. Fatahzadeh M, Schwartz RA. Human herpes simplex virus infections: epidemiology, pathogenesis, symptomatology, diagnosis and management. J Am Acad Dermatol. 2007;57:737–63.
41. Harel L, Smetana Z, Prais D, et al. Presence of viremia in patients with primary herpetic gingivostomatitis. Clin Infect Dis. 2004;39:636–40.
42. Sarioglu B, Kose S, Saritas S, et al. Severe acute disseminated encephalomyelitis with clinical findings of transverse myelitis after herpes simplex virus infection. J Child Neurol. 2014;29(11):1519–23.
43. Parrott RH, Wolf SI, Nudelman J, et al. Clinical and laboratory differentiation between herpangina and infectious (herpetic) gingivostomatitis. Pediatrics. 1954;14:122–9.
44. McMillan JA, Weiner LB, Higgins AM, et al. Pharyngitis associated with herpes simplex virus in college students. Pediatr Infect Dis J. 1993;12:280–4.

45. Glezen WP, Fernald GW, Lohr JA. Acute respiratory disease of university students with special reference to the etiologic role of herpesvirus hominis. Am J Epidemiol. 1975;101:111–21.
46. Rosain J, Froissart A, Estrangin E, et al. Severe acute pharyngotonsillitis due to herpes simplex virus type 2 in a young woman. J Clin Virol. 2015;63:63–5.
47. Machin N, Morgan D, Turner A, et al. Neonatal herpes simplex 2 infection presenting with supraglottitis. Arch Dis Child. 2013;98(8):611–2.
48. Büke Ç. Herpes Simplex Virüsleri (HSV-1 ve HSV-2). In: Topçu AW, Söyletir G, Doğanay M, editors. Enfeksiyon Hastalıkları ve Mikrobiyolojisi. 4th ed. Nobel Tıp Kitapevleri: İstanbul; 2017. p. 1466–74.
49. Feder HM Jr, Long SS. Herpetic whitlow: epidemiology, clinical characteristics, diagnosis, and treatment. Am J Dis Child. 1983;137:861–3.
50. Wu IB, Schwartz RA. Herpetic whitlow. Cutis. 2007;79:193–6.
51. Becker TM, Kodsi R, Bailey P, et al. Grappling with herpes: herpes gladiatorum. Am J Sports Med. 1988;16:665–9.
52. Orton PW, Huff JC, Tonnesen MG, et al. Detection of a herpes simplex viral antigen in skin lesions of erythema multiforme. Ann Intern Med. 1984;101:48–50.
53. Schmutzhard E. Viral infections of the CNS with special emphasis on herpes simplex infections. J Neurol. 2001;248:469–77.
54. Huppatz C, Durrheim DN, Levi C, et al. Etiology of encephalitis in Australia, 1990–2007. Emerg Infect Dis. 2009;15:1359–65.
55. Lakeman FD, Whitley RJ, National Institute of Allergy and Infectious Diseases Collaborative Antiviral Study Group. Diagnosis of herpes simplex encephalitis: application of polymerase chain reaction to cerebrospinal fluid from brain-biopsied patients and correlation with disease. J Infect Dis. 1995;171:857–63.
56. Hatipoglu HG, Sakman B, Yuksel E. Magnetic resonance and diffusion-weighted imaging findings of herpes simplex encephalitis. Herpes. 2008;15:13–7.
57. Kusuhara T, Nakajima M, Inoue H, et al. Parainfectious encephalomyeloradiculitis associated with herpes simplex virus 1 DNA in cerebrospinal fluid. Clin Infect Dis. 2002;34:1199–205.
58. Anderson MS, Abzug MJ. Hydrops fetalis: an unusual presentation of intrauterine herpes simplex virus infection. Pediatr Infect Dis J. 1999;18:837–9.
59. Corey L, Wald A. Maternal and neonatal herpes simplex virus infections. N Engl J Med. 2009;361:1376–85.
60. Kimberlin DW, Lin CY, Jacobs RF, et al. Natural history of neonatal herpes simplex virus infections in the acyclovir era. Pediatrics. 2001;108:223–9.
61. Kimberlin DW, Gutierrez KM. Herpes simplex virus infection. In: Wilson CB, Nizet V, Maldonado YA, et al., editors. Remington and Klein's infectious diseases of the fetus and newborn infant. 8th ed. Philadelphia: Elsevier Saunders; 2016. p. 843–65.
62. Curfman AL, Glissmeyer EW, Ahmad FA, et al. Initial presentation of neonatal herpes simplex virus infection. J Pediatr. 2016;172:121–6.
63. Wasserman R, August CS, Plotkin SA. Viral infections in pediatric bone marrow transplant patients. Pediatr Infect Dis J. 1988;7:109–15.
64. Naraqi S, Jackson GG, Jonasson O, et al. Prospective study of prevalence, incidence, and source of herpesvirus infections in patients with renal allografts. J Infect Dis. 1977;136:531–40.
65. Whitley RJ, Levin M, Barton N, et al. Infections caused by herpes simplex virus in the immunocompromised host: natural history and topical acyclovir therapy. J Infect Dis. 1984;150:323–9.
66. Crane LR, Gutterman PA, Chapel T, et al. Incubation of swab materials with herpes simplex virus. J Infect Dis. 1980;141:531.
67. Wald A, Huang ML, Carrell D, Selke S, Corey L. Polymerase chain reaction for detection of herpes simplex virus (HSV) DNA on mucosal surfaces: comparison with HSV isolation in cell culture. J Infect Dis. 2003;188:1345–51.
68. Pouletty P, Chomel JJ, Thouvenot D, et al. Detection of herpes simplex virus in direct specimens by immunofluorescence assay using a monoclonal antibody. J Clin Microbiol. 1987;25:958–9.
69. Melvin AJ, Mohan KM, Schiffer JT, et al. Plasma and CSF herpes simplex virus levels at diagnosis and outcome of neonatal infection. J Pediatr. 2015;166:827–33.

70. Sudesh S, Laibson PR. The impact of the herpetic eye disease studies on the management of herpes simplex virus ocular infections. Curr Opin Ophthalmol. 1999;10:230–3.
71. James SH, Whitley RJ. Treatment of herpes simplex virus infections in pediatric patients: current status and future needs. Clin Pharmacol Ther. 2010;88:720–4.
72. Stanberry LR, Spruance SL, Cunningham AL, et al. Glycoprotein-D-adjuvant vaccine to prevent genital herpes. N Engl J Med. 2002;347:1652–61.
73. Stanberry LR, Cunningham AL, Mindel A, et al. Prospects for control of herpes simplex virus disease through immunization. Clin Infect Dis. 2000;30:549–66.

COVID: Upper Respiratory Involvement 72

Rezarta Taga Senirli and Erdem Atalay Çetinkaya

72.1 Introduction

Coronaviruses are a group of enveloped, positive-stranded RNA viruses. Their electron microscope view is crown-like due to the spike glycoproteins in their envelopes [1]. They are known as zoonotic viruses, usually infecting mammals and birds. Anyway, there are human-infecting viruses within the coronaviridae family. The most popular ones are SARS CoV, Middle East Respiratory Syndrome (MERS) CoV, and one of recent date, SARS CoV-2 or better known as COVID-19 [2–4].

It was alluded that SARS CoV-2 is genetically similar to a strain found in bats and probably evolved from it. But the exact source needs to be understood anyway [5].

COVID-19 made a swift and noisy entry into our lives, causing numerous cases and pathologies within a few months. After nearly 2 years of pandemic, as of March 2022, over 460 million people had been infected and more than six million died [6].

SARS-CoV-2 showed significant mutations since the time it was first identified. The major mutations seen during the pandemic are Alpha, Beta, Gamma, Delta, and Omicron. The lately seen variant, Omicron, seemed to have increased transmissibility [7]. Additionally, it was hypothesized that Omicron had a greater predilection for the upper airways compared to earlier variants. As support for this hypothesis, when Omicron was more dominant, publications from different countries [8, 9] pointed to an increased and more severe COVID-19 association.

Fortunately, lower respiratory tract infections were reported to be less common in children and mortality was lower (0.1%) compared to adults (5–15%) [10].

Studies pointed out that children infected with COVID-19 usually showed a mild presentation of the disease, with cough and fever being the typical symptoms [8,

R. T. Senirli · E. A. Çetinkaya (✉)
Department of Otorhinolaryngology, Antalya Training and Research Hospital, University of Health Sciences, Antalya, Turkey

H. Yüksel et al. (eds.), *Pediatric Airway Diseases*, Comprehensive ENT, https://doi.org/10.1007/978-3-031-74853-0_72

11]. Preliminary studies in Wuhan Children's Hospital showed that up to 15% of COVID-19-infected patients were asymptomatic [12]. Later, extensive systematic reviews of the literature revealed that about 13.7% of the children presented with upper respiratory symptoms such as rhinorrhea, sneezing, or nasal congestion. Similarly, throat pain or pharyngitis symptoms were observed in about 28.9% of them [11, 13]. Nevertheless, pneumonia remains one of the most feared outcomes of COVID-19 in pediatric patients.

In this chapter, we discuss COVID-19 from an otolaryngological point of view, debating the relationship & upper respiratory tract involvement.

72.2 Upper Respiratory Tract Infection

Upper respiratory tract infections refer to a group of infections that primarily affect the nose, throat, and other parts of the upper airway. These infections are common and usually caused by viruses. They can be categorized into several subgroups based on the specific area of the upper respiratory tract they affect:

72.2.1 Nasal Infections

72.2.1.1 Rhinitis

Rhinitis is the inflammation of the nasal mucosa, causing symptoms like a runny or congested nose, sneezing, and itching. Acute rhinitis is usually divided into allergic and respiratory viral infections. Allergic rhinitis is the subject of another study, but we would like to remind you that acute viral rhinitis is one of the most common infections in humans [14]. Acute viral rhinitis is well-known as a self-limiting pathology unless any bacterial infection superimposes.

Human rhinoviruses (HRV) are responsible for up to half of the cases of upper respiratory infections [15]. Other known agents for this pathology are coronaviruses, adenoviruses, respiratory syncytial virus (RSV), influenza, and parainfluenza viruses.

Articles from various countries published before COVID-19 report that seroprevalence of Human Coronaviruses rate about 5% among children with upper respiratory tract infection [16–19]. Although an apparent ratio related to the post-COVID-19 period is not found in the literature, it is reported that SARS-CoV-2 upper respiratory tract infections in pediatric patients tend to be mild and that almost 15% of these patients are asymptomatic [12].

72.2.1.2 Sinusitis

Sinusitis refers to the inflammation of the sinuses, often leading to headache, facial pain, and nasal congestion. Often showing a polymicrobial pattern, this pathology is one of children's most common health problems [20]. We find it essential to mention a study conducted in the previous years. In this prospective study, Revai et al. investigated children between 6 and 35 months of age [21]. They pointed out that these young children had an incidence of six episodes of viral upper respiratory tract infections per year and that 8% (that means 0.5 episodes per patient-year) of these attacks were complicated by acute rhinosinusitis.

Regarding the COVID-19 period, perhaps we did not see this percentage of complications, but serious concerns for invasive fungal rhinosinusitis have been raised. Post-COVID-19 fungal rhinosinusitis has been described primarily in adult patients [22, 23], but sporadic pediatric cases have also been reported from India. It is crucial to note that all seven reported pediatric fungal sinusitis cases were immunosuppressed.

72.2.2 Pharyngeal Infections

72.2.2.1 Pharyngitis

Pharyngitis is the inflammation of the membranes and underlying structures of the throat. Acute pediatric pharyngitis is mainly caused by viruses and usually during the cold time of the year. Primary viral agents are the ones we know as respiratory viruses: rhinovirus, coronavirus, influenza virus, and adenovirus. The typical examinational findings are tonsillopharyngeal erythema and anterior lymphadenopathy, which are usually expected to self-limit.

Pharyngitis was also one of the presenting clinical findings during COVID-19. Limited studies on pediatric patients report pharyngitis among initial clinical findings at rates ranging from 8.3% to 46.2% [11].

72.2.2.2 Tonsillitis

Tonsillitis refers to the inflammatory process of the palatine tonsils. Although it is usually seen in school-aged children, almost all are affected at least once in their lifetime. Numerous microorganisms can cause acute tonsillitis, but it is generally known to be a bacterial infection. Viral pathogens usually contributing to acute tonsillitis are Epstein Barr Virus, rhinovirus, enterovirus, influenza, and adenovirus [24].

Different studies published during the COVID-19 pandemic reported a decreased frequency of acute tonsillitis [8, 11, 25]. But this is thought to be a result of less interaction due to the massive lockdown.

72.2.3 Laryngeal Infections

72.2.3.1 Laryngitis

Laryngitis is the inflammation of the laryngeal mucosal layer resulting in voice changes, hoarseness, inspiratory wheezing, or cough. Hoarseness is a well-known voice problem, especially among children between 8 and 14 [26], but laryngitis is mainly seen in children between 6 months and 3 years old. It is also important to remind us of croup, which involves the upper airway by explicitly affecting the subglottic region. Occasionally, this pathology can become a life-threatening condition.

During the COVID-19 pandemic, especially during Omicron variant dominance, many articles [8, 27] highlighted increased croup cases and the more severe course of these patients.

72.3 Management

From now on, December 2019 marks the time of the generation of a new coronavirus, which was later named SARS CoV-2. Soon after the beginning of the pandemic, it was understood that the primary spreading way is infected patients & aerosols they produce [5, 28]. It is important to note that placental seeding or, in some way, vertical transmission was not documented [29]. After an incubation time of an average of 7 days (max. 12.5 days), the actual devastating infection appears [30]. Even though severe infection was seen in adults, pediatric patients were primarily affected. According to a study conducted in Italy [5], 1.6% of COVID-19 patients were aged 0–18. Almost always, a household source was present in pediatric cases.

Children themselves were accused of being significant spreaders [31].

Considering all the essential items mentioned so far, let us have a look at the treatment of COVID-19 (+) pediatric ENT patients. Treatment of these patients can be classified in some groups:

1. **Symptomatic Treatment**

   The supportive care meant for patients with mild infections & who do not need hospitalization is similar to the common cold or any other viral infection; it should contain sufficient calories, water intake, and other supportive treatments [32]. Another critical issue is isolating the patient from the outer environment or household.
2. **Antibiotics**

   Normally, there is no need for antibiotherapy in pediatric COVID-19 patients. In case of any secondary bacterial infections, in correlation with laboratory & radiologic findings, antibiotics can be given.
3. **Glucocorticoids**

   WHO does not recommend glucocorticoid treatment unless it is strictly indicated. This indication often implies lower respiratory tract infections or acute attacks of obstructive pulmonary diseases [32].
4. **Antiviral Therapy**

   There exists no approved antiviral therapy for pediatric COVID-19 patients.
5. **SARS CoV-2 Vaccines**

   It was previously mentioned that young children and adolescents tend to show mild COVID-19. Anyway, immunization is essential for them, too. According to the WHO reports, among 175 vaccine candidates authorized for a clinical trial, 13 vaccines received Emergency Use Authorization [33]. Some of these got authorization for use in children, too. For some vaccines, authorization was given for children up to 6 months.

72.4 Conclusion

The last 3 years have been quite difficult times for mankind. Fortunately, children were a bit luckier than adults. Different studies revealed that pediatric patients show mild infections.

References

1. Zhu N, Zhang D, Wang W, et al. A novel coronavirus from patients with pneumonia in China, 2019. N Engl J Med. 2020;382(8):727–33.
2. Wu F, Zhao S, Yu B, et al. A new coronavirus associated with human respiratory disease in China. Nature. 2020;579(7798):265–9.
3. Hu B, Guo H, Zhou P, Shi ZL. Characteristics of SARS-CoV-2 and COVID-19. Nat Rev Microbiol. 2021;19(3):141–54.
4. Chan JF, Yuan S, Kok KH, et al. A familial cluster of pneumonia associated with the 2019 novel coronavirus indicating person-to-person transmission: a study of a family cluster. Lancet. 2020;395:514–23. https://doi.org/10.1093/infdis/jiaa077.
5. Cascella M, Rajnik M, Cuomo A, Dulebohn SC, Napoli RD. Features, evaluation, and treatment coronavirus (COVID-19). Treasure Island (FL): StatPearls Publishing; 2020 Jan. Last update: 2020 Mar 20.
6. World Health Organization. Weekly epidemiological update on COVID-19. 2022 Mar 16.
7. World Health Organisation. Statement on Omicron sublineage BA.2 [Internet]. 2022 [cited 2022 Apr 3]. Available from: https://www.who.int/news/item/22-02-2022-statement-on-omicron-sublineage-ba.2#:~:text=Studies%20have%20shown%20that%20BA,most%%20 20common%20Omicron%20sublineage%20reported
8. Cheng AT, Watson AL, Picardo N. Lessons learnt from the COVID-19 pandemic in pediatric otolaryngology. Curr Otorhinolaryngol Rep. 2022;10:456–63. https://doi.org/10.1007/s40136-022-00422-5.
9. Brewster RCL, Parsons C, Laird-Gion J, et al. COVID-19-associated croup in children. Pediatrics. 2022;149(6):e2022056492. https://doi.org/10.1542/peds.2022-056492.
10. Kabeerdoss J, Pilania RK, Karkhele R, et al. Severe COVID-19, multisystem inflammatory syndrome in children, and Kawasaki disease: immunological mechanisms, clinical manifestations and management. Rheumatol Int. 2021;41:19–32. https://doi.org/10.1007/s00296-020-04749-4.
11. Patel NA. Pediatric COVID-19: systematic review of the literature. Am J Otolaryngol. 2020;41:102573. https://doi.org/10.1016/j.amjoto.2020.102573.
12. Guan W, Ni Z, Hu Y, et al. Clinical characteristics of coronavirus disease 2019 in China. New Engl J Med Mass Med Soc. 2020;382:1708–20. https://doi.org/10.1101/2022.02.17.22271030 .
13. Tezer H, Demirdağ TB. Novel coronavirus disease (COVID-19) in children. Turk J Med Sci. 2020;50(SI-1):592–603. https://doi.org/10.3906/sag-2004-174.
14. Slavin RG, Spector SL, Bernstein IL, et al. The diagnosis and management of sinusitis: a practice parameter update. J Allergy Clin Immunol. 2005;116:S13–47.
15. Winther B, Gwaltney JM Jr, Mygind N, et al. Viral-induced rhinitis. Am J Rhinol. 1998;12(1):17–20.
16. Zhang SF, Tuo JL, Huang XB, et al. Epidemiology characteristics of human coronaviruses in patients with respiratory infection symptoms and phylogenetic analysis of HCoV-OC43 during 2010–2015 in Guangzhou. PLoS One. 2018;13(1):e0191789.
17. Lau SKP, Woo PCY, Yip CCY, et al. Coronavirus HKU1 and other coronavirus infections in Hong Kong. J Clin Microbiol. 2006;44(6):2063–71.

18. Chiu SS, Hung Chan K, Wing Chu K, et al. Human coronavirus NL63 infection and other coronavirus infections in children hospitalized with acute respiratory disease in Hong Kong. China Clin Infect Dis. 2005;40(12):1721–9.
19. Papa A, Papadimitriou E, de Souza Luna LK, et al. Coronaviruses in children, Greece. Emerg Infect Dis. 2007;13(6):947–9.
20. Brook I. Acute sinusitis in children. Pediatr Clin N Am. 2013;60(2):409–24. https://doi.org/10.1016/j.pcl.2012.12.002.
21. Revai K, Dobbs LA, Nair S, et al. Incidence of acute otitis media and sinusitis complicating upper respiratory tract infection: the effect of age. Pediatrics. 2007;119:e1408–12.
22. El-Kholy NA, El-Fattah AMA, Khafagy YW. Invasive fungal sinusitis in post-COVID-19 patients: a new clinical entity. Laryngoscope. 2021;131:2652–8. https://doi.org/10.1002/lary.29632.
23. Gur ÖE, Sonbay Yılmaz ND, Yavuz S, et al. Rhino-orbital mucor mycosis in the elderly population after COVID-19. Turk J Geriatr. 2022;25(4):592–9. https://doi.org/10.31086/tjgeri.2022.318.
24. Brodsky L, Poje C. Tonsillitis, tonsillectomy and adenoidectomy. In: Bailey BJ, editor. Head and neck surgery – otolaryngology. 4th ed. Philadelphia: Lippincott Williams and Wilkins; 2006. p. 1184–99.
25. Stansfield J, Dobbs S, Harrison R, et al. Management of ENT emergencies during the coronavirus disease 2019 pandemic. J Laryngol Otol. 2021;135:117–24. https://doi.org/10.1017/S0022215121000530.
26. Angelillo N, Di Costanzo B, Angelillo M, et al. Epidemiological study on vocal disorders in paediatric age. J Prev Med Hyg. 2008;49:1–5.
27. Pitstick CE, Rodriguez KM, Smith AC, et al. A curious case of croup: laryngotracheitis caused by COVID-19. Pediatrics. 2021;147(1):e2020012179.
28. Stoecklin BS, Rolland P, Silue Y, et al. First cases of coronavirus disease 2019 (COVID-19) in France: surveillance, investigations, and control measures, January 2020. Euro Surveill. 2020;25(6):2000094.
29. Schwartz DA. An analysis of 38 pregnant women with COVID-19, their newborn infants, and maternal-fetal transmission of SARS-CoV-2: maternal coronavirus infections and pregnancy outcomes. Arch Pathol Lab Med. 2020;144(7):799–805. https://doi.org/10.5858/arpa.2020-0901-SA.
30. Huang C, Wang Y, Li X, et al. Clinical features of patients infected with 2019 novel coronavirus in Wuhan, China. Lancet. 2020;395(10223):497–506. https://doi.org/10.1016/S01406736(20)30183-5.
31. Cao O, Chen Y, Chen C. Chiu C.SARS-CoV-2 infection in children: transmission dynamics and clinical characteristics. J Formos Med Assoc. 2020;119(3):670–3. https://doi.org/10.1016/j.jfma.2020.02.009.
32. Chen Z, Fu J, Shu Q, et al. Diagnosis and treatment recommendations for pediatric respiratory infection caused by the 2019 novel coronavirus. World J Pediatr. 2020;16(3):240–6. https://doi.org/10.1007/s12519-020-00345-5.
33. COVID-19 vaccines with WHO emergency use listing. Available from: https://extranet.who.int/pqweb/vaccines/vaccinescovid-19-vaccine-eul-issued

MIX
Papier aus verantwortungsvollen Quellen
Paper from responsible sources
FSC® C105338

If you have any concerns about our products,
you can contact us on
ProductSafety@springernature.com

In case Publisher is established outside the EU,
the EU authorized representative is:
Springer Nature Customer Service Center GmbH
Europaplatz 3, 69115 Heidelberg, Germany

Printed by Libri Plureos GmbH
in Hamburg, Germany